STRATEGIC APPROACHES
IN
CORONARY INTERVENTION

STRATEGIC
APPROACHES
IN
CORONARY
INTERVENTION

EDITORS

STEPHEN G. ELLIS, MD

DIRECTOR, SONES CARDIAC CATHETERIZATION LABORATORIES
DEPARTMENT OF CARDIOLOGY
THE CLEVELAND CLINIC FOUNDATION
CLEVELAND, OHIO

PROFESSOR OF MEDICINE
OHIO STATE UNIVERSITY
COLUMBUS, OHIO

DAVID R. HOLMES, JR., MD

CONSULTANT, DIVISION OF CARDIOVASCULAR DISEASES
AND INTERNAL MEDICINE
MAYO CLINIC AND MAYO FOUNDATION

PROFESSOR OF MEDICINE
MAYO MEDICAL SCHOOL
ROCHESTER, MINNESOTA

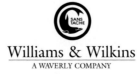

Williams & Wilkins
A WAVERLY COMPANY

BALTIMORE • PHILADELPHIA • LONDON • PARIS • BANGKOK
BUENOS AIRES • HONG KONG • MUNICH • SYDNEY • TOKYO • WROCLAW

Editor: Jonathan W. Pine, Jr.
Managing Editor: Molly L. Mullen
Production Coordinator: Raymond E. Reter
Copy Editor: Elizabeth Mahoney
Designer: Dan Pfisterer
Illustration Planner: Wayne Hubbel
Cover Designer: Dan Pfisterer
Typesetter: Graphic World, Inc., St. Louis, Mo.
Printer: Maple Press Co., York, Pa.
Binder: Maple Press Co., York, Pa.

351 West Camden Street
Baltimore, Maryland 21201-2436 USA

Rose Tree Corporate Center
1400 North Providence Road
Building II, Suite 5025
Media, Pennsylvania 19063-2043 USA

Accurate indications, adverse reactions and dosage schedules for drugs are provided in this book, but it is possible that they may change. The reader is urged to review the package information data of the manufacturers of the medications mentioned.

Printed in the United States of America

Library of Congress Cataloging-in-Publication Data

Strategic approaches in coronary intervention / [edited by] Stephen G. Ellis, David R.
  Holmes, Jr.
    p. cm
  Includes bibliographical references and index.
  ISBN 0-683-02797-2
  1.Coronary heart disease—Treatment.   2. Endarterectomy.   3. Coronary heart
disease—Surgery—Complications.   I. Ellis, Stephen G. (Stephen Geoffrey), 1951- .
II. Holmes, David R.,1945- .
    [DNLM: 1. Coronary Disease—therapy. WG 300 S8977 1996]
  RD598.M95S77 1996
  617.4'12—dc20
  DNLM/DLC
  for Library of Congress   94-23645
                                                             CIP

*The publishers have made every effort to trace the copyright holders for borrowed material.
If they have inadvertently overlooked any, they will be pleased to make the necessary
arrangements at the first opportunity.*

95 96 97 98 99
1 2 3 4 5 6 7 8 9 10

To my family (Sandy, Jessica, and Gary) and my mentors (the late Andreas Gruentzig, Spencer King III, and John Douglas), without whose help and understanding this book would not have been possible.
Stephen G. Ellis

To my family and wife, who, because of their support and tolerance, have given me the opportunity to work on this and the myriad of other fascinating activities.
David R. Holmes, Jr.

Preface

Since its inception in 1977 percutaneous coronary intervention has undergone dramatic evolution. Early therapy was appropriately limited in scope to "simple" lesions since equipment was primitive by today's standards. As equipment and operator experience improved, by the mid to late 1980s interventionalists had begun to extend their reach and even encroach on the prior domain of cardiac surgeons—patients with multivessel disease and/or impaired ventricular function, but efforts and success were somewhat limited because of the remaining problems of abrupt vessel closure, restenosis, and difficulty in traversing totally occluded vessels.

Now in the 1990s, when many new devices have become widely available, the options for treatment have become increasingly numerous and complex, but the limitations of balloon angioplasty have not been completely circumvented. In fact, new treatments have brought with them new complications. At the same time, economic constraints have begun to focus on these procedures as those with high cost and, in some instances, with unproven or untested benefit relative to other forms of therapy.

For these reasons it has become increasingly important to have a rational basis for choosing between treatment options. We believe that there is now ample evidence that the results of various percutaneous interventions are to a certain extent predictable. The acute results depend on lesion morphology, and the long-term results depend on the inital results achieved. Angiography remains the "gold standard" by which both morphology and results are assessed, but intravascular ultrasound and perhaps angioscopy are likely to become increasingly important. As a predictor of outcome, ventricular function is also, of course, important. These predictors differ dramatically from those of the results of bypass surgery, which depend not on the lesions bypassed, but rather primarily on the nature of the distal "target" vessel, ventricular function, and other concomitant problems such as the presence of mitral regurgitation.

Thus a strategic approach to possible percutaneous treatment of a patient with coronary disease should involve an assessment of the location, severity, and morphology of important stenoses, as well as an assessment of ventricular function, other illnesses, and the needs and desires of the patient. Obviously, the options of medical and surgical therapy should also be entertained. The pivotal importance of lesion morphology in determining results has led us to develop this textbook, *Strategic Approaches in Coronary Intervention,* focusing on the choices faced by the practicing cardiologist who must deal with individual patients and their unique coronary lesions.

The first section of the text (Chapters 1 through 11) reviews the use of each of the major percutaneous devices, with an emphasis on technique and optimizing results. Chapters 9 and 10 deal with the emerging role of ultrasound and angioscopy in supplementing angiography to predict outcome and evaluate results. The next important chapter 12A, B, C discuss the varied means of comparing treatment results—randomized trials, case-control studies, registries and empirical observation. Chapters 13 and 14 delve further into the key issues of assessing the severity of a given lesion and whether the asymptomatic patient with coronary disease should be revascularized.

The emphasis of the text (Chapters 15–37), in contradistinction to most other major texts of interventional cardiology, is on the problem-oriented approach to treatment—serially discussing the varied types of lesions and other problems faced by the interventionalist. The opinions of many experienced practitioners in the field were sought, each chosen for their expertise in dealing with the problem at hand. In some instances consensus is seen and in others a marked disparity of thought. Knowledge of both is critical for the practicing physician.

Finally, the appropriate use of adjunctive medications to optimize the balance between freedom from coronary thrombosis and excessive systemic bleeding, as well as to possibly limit subsequent restenosis, are addressed in Chapters 38–40.

This textbook is directed at the practicing interventionalist, hopefully providing guidance in dealing with difficult day-to-day problems. Noninterventional cardiologists, internists, and surgeons may also find it useful in understanding the promise and the limitations of percutaneous treatment as they consider the appropriate referral of their patients. It will have achieved its purpose if more patients receive appropriate treatment and have extended and high-quality lives.

Coordination and publication of this text has only been possible by virtue of the tremendous effort of many talented people. Over 90 authors with special expertise contributed. We are particularly indebted to these contributors and to the staff of Williams & Wilkins for processing their work. The experience-based insights and overall coordination of this effort provided by Jonathan Pine and Molly Mullen, respectively, were invaluable. Finally, we would never have been able to accomplish this task without the patience and the diligent and innovative assistance of our secretaries, Patti Durnwald and Shari Gardner, and without the understanding of our families. For all this support we are tremendously grateful.

STEPHEN G. ELLIS
DAVID R. HOLMES, JR.

Contributors

Alaa E. Abdelmeguid, M.D., Ph.D.
Division of Cardiovascular Medicine
Henry Ford Hospital
Detroit, Michigan

Eric R. Bates, M.D.
Associate Professor
Department of Internal Medicine
University of Michigan
Ann Arbor, Michigan

C. Bauters, M.D.
Université de Lille
Hopital Cardiologique
Service de Cardiologie et Hemodyamique
Lille, France

Malcolm R. Bell, M.B.B.S., F.R.A.C.P.
Assistant Professor of Medicine
Mayo Medical School
Senior Associate Consultant
Division of Cardiovascular Diseases and Internal
  Medicine
Mayo Clinic and Mayo Foundation
Rochester, Minnesota

Michel Bertrand, M.D.
Professor of Medicine (Cardiology)
Chief, Division of Cardiology
Universite de Lille
Hopital Cardiologique
Lille, France

John A. Bittl, M.D.
Assistant Professor of Medicine
Harvard Medical School
Director of Interventional Cardiology
Brigham and Women's Hospital
Boston, Massachusetts

James D. Boehrer, M.D.
Texas Cardiology Consultants
Dallas, Texas

Martial G. Bourassa, M.D.
Professor of Clinical Medicine
Department of Medicine
Medical Director
Department of Medicine
Montreal Heart Institute
University of Montreal
Montreal, Quebec, Canada

John A. Bresnahan, M.D.
Associate Professor of Medicine
Mayo Medical School
Consultant, Division of Cardiovascular Diseases
Mayo Clinic
Rochester, Minnesota

Maurice Buchbinder, M.D.
Associate Professor of Clinical Medicine
Department of Medicine/Cardiology
University of California at San Diego Medical Center
San Diego, California

Bernard Burnad, M.D., M.P.H.
Associate Professor
Clinical Epidemiology Unit
Institute of Social and Preventive Medicine
Lausanne, Switzerland

Douglas M. Burtt, M.D.
Assistant Professor of Medicine
Brown University School of Medicine
Interventional Cardiologist
The Miriam Hospital
Director, Cardiac Catheterization Laboratory
Roger Williams Medical Center
Providence, Rhode Island

Robert M. Califf, M.D.
Associate Professor of Medicine
Director of Cardiac Care Unit
Director, Clinical Epidemiology and Biostatistics
Department of Medicine
Duke University
Durham, North Carolina

Peter F. Cohn, M.D.
Professor of Medicine & Chief of Cardiology
Department of Medicine
State University of New York at Stony Brook
 Health Sciences Center
Stony Brook, New York

Keith E. Davis, M.D.
Interventional Cardiology Fellow
University of California at San Diego Medical
 Center, Naval Medical Center
San Diego, California

Anthony C. De Franco, M.D.
Secton of Interventional Cardiology
The Cleveland Clinic Foundation
Cleveland, Ohio

Nadia Debbas, M.D., Ph.D.
Department of Cardiology
Centre Hospitalier Universitaire Vaudois
Lausanne, Switzerland

Ezra Deutsch, M.D.
Associate Professor of Medicine
Director, Cardiac Catheterization Laboratory
Department of Medicine
Temple University School of Medicine
Philadelphia, Pennsylvania

Paul W. Diggs, M.D.
Department of Cardiology
State University of New York at Stony Brook
Stony Brook, New York

Thomas J. Donohue, M.D.
Assistant Professor of Medicine
Department of Medicine
St. Louis University Medical Center
St. Louis, Missouri

John S. Douglas, Jr., M.D.
Associate Professor of Medicine
Emory University School of Medicine
Co-Director, Cardiovascular Laboratory
Emory University Hospital
Atlanta, Georgia

Eric Eeckhout, M.D.
Cardiologist
Department of Cardiology
University Hospital
Lausanne, Switzerland

Neal L. Eigler, M.D.
Associate Professor
Department of Medicine
University of California, Los Angeles School of
 Medicine
Co-Director
Cardiovascular Intervention Center
Cedars-Sinai Medical Center
Los Angeles, California

Stephen G. Ellis, M.D.
Professor of Medicine
The Ohio State University
Director, Sones Cardiac Catheterization Laboratories
Department of Cardiology
The Cleveland Clinic Foundation
Cleveland, Ohio
Columbus, Ohio

Raimund Erbel, M.D., F.A.C.C., F.E.S.C.
Director of the Department of Cardiology
Universitatsklinkum Essen
Zentrum Fur Innere Medizin
Essen, Germany

David P. Faxon, M.D.
Professor of Medicine
Chief, Division of Cardiology
University of Southern California School of Medicine
Los Angeles, California

Robert Federici, M.D.
Duke University Medical Center
Durham, North Carolina

Tim A. Fischell, M.D.
Associate Professor of Medicine
Director, Cardiac Catheterization Laboratory
Division of Cardiology
Vanderbilt University
Nashville, Tennessee

David L. Fischman, M.D.
Division of Cardiology
Thomas Jefferson University
Philadelphia, Pennsylvania

Peter J. Fitzgerald, M.D., Ph.D.
Assistant Professor of Medicine (Cardiology)
Department of Interventional Cardiology
Stanford University
Stanford, California

Riley D. Foreman, D.O.
Interventional Cardiology Fellow
University of California San Diego Medical Center
Naval Medical Center
San Diego, California

Kirk N. Garratt, M.D.
Assistant Professor of Medicine
Mayo Medical School
Consultant
Division Of Cardiovascular Diseases
Mayo Clinic
Rochester, Minnesota

Junbo Ge, M.B., M.Sc., M.D.
Department of Cardiology
University of Essen
Essen, Germany

Harry H. Gibbs, M.B., B.S.
Vascular Medicine Unit
Princess Alexandra Hospital
Brisbane, Queensland
Australia

Sheldon Goldberg, M.D.
Professor of Medicine
Director, Division of Cardiology
Thomas Jefferson University
Philadelphia, Pennsylvania

Jean-Jacques Goy, M.D.
Associate Professor
Department of Cardiology
University Hospital
Lausanne, Switzerland

Paul A. Gurbel, M.D.
Assistant Professor
Director of Interventional Cardiology
University of Maryland School of Medicine
Baltimore, Maryland

Robert A. Harrington, M.D.
Assistant Professor of Medicine
Division of Cardiology
Duke University Medical Center
Durham, North Carolina

Andreas Hartmann, M.D. Ph.D.
Department of Cardiology
J.W. Goethl University Medical Center
Frankfurt, Germany

Geoffrey O. Hartzler, M.D.
Mid-America Heart Institute
Kansas City, Missouri

Michael Haude, M.D.
Internist, Kardiologie
Oberarzt der Abt. fur Kardiologie
Zentrum fur Innere Medizin
Essen, Germany

William Hillegass, M.D.
Duke University Medical Center
Durham, North Carolina

Tomoaki Hinohara, M.D.
Director, Cardiac Catheterization Laboratory
Sequoia Hospital
Redwood City, California

David R. Holmes, Jr., M.D.
Professor of Medicine
Mayo Medical School
Consultant, Division of Cardiovascular Diseases
    and Internal Medicine
Mayo Clinic and Mayo Foundation
Rochester, Minnesota

Michel Hurni, M.D.
Cardiovascular Surgery
Centre Hospitalier Universitaire Vaudois
Lausanne, Switzerland

Jeffrey M. Isner, M.D.
Professor of Medicine
Tufts University School of Medicine
Chief, Cardiovascular Research
St. Elizabeth's Hospital
Boston, Massachusetts

Alice K. Jacobs, M.D.
Associate Professor of Medicine
Boston University School of Medicine
Director, Cardiac Catheterization Laboratory
Boston University Medical Center
Boston, Massachusetts

James G. Jollis, M.D.
Assistant Professor of Medicine
Duke University Medical Center
Durham, North Carolina

Joel K. Kahn, M.D.
Attending Cardiovascular Interventionalist
Department of Internal Medicine
William Beaumont Hospital
Royal Oak, Michigan

Martin Kaltenbach, M.D., Ph.D.
Professor of Medicine
Department of Cardiology
J.W. Goethe University Medical Center
Frankfurt, Germany

Lukas Kappenberger, M.D., F.G.S.C., F.A.C.C.
Professor
Department of Medicine
Centre Hospitalier Universitaire Vaudois
Lausanne, Switzerland

Urs. P. Kaufmann, M.D.
Director of Interventional Cardiology
Department of Cardiology
University Hospital
Bern, Switzerland

Laurence R. Kelley, M.D.
Division of Cardiovascular Diseases
Scripps Clinic and Research Foundation
La Jolla, California

Morton J. Kern, M.D.
Professor of Medicine
Director, J.G. Mudd Cardiac Catheterization
  Laboratory
St. Louis University Hospital
St. Louis, Missouri

Takeshi Kimura, M.D.
Department of Cardiology
Kokura Memorial Hospital
Kitakyushu, Japan

Spencer B. King III, M.D.
Professor of Medicine (Cardiology)
Director of Interventional Cardiology
Emory University Hospital
Atlanta, Georgia

Kevin R. Kruse, M.D.
Duke University Medical Center
Durham, North Carolina

J.M. Lablanche, M.D.
Professor of Cardiology
Université of Lille
Lille, France

Christopher J.W.B. Leggett, M.D.
Duluth, Georgia

Frank Litvack, M.D.
Co-Director, Cardiovascular Intervention Center
Cedars-Sinai Medical Center
Associate Professor of Medicine
UCLA School of Medicine
Los Angeles, California

Fengqi Liu, M.D.
Department of Cardiology
Division of Internal Medicine
University of Essen
Essen, Germany

Daniel B. Mark, M.D., M.P.H.
Associate Professor of Medicine
Cardiovascular Division
Duke University Medical Center
Durham, North Carolina

Eugene McFadden, M.D.
Université de Lille
Hopital Cardiologique
Service de Cardiologie et Hemodynamique
Lille, France

Bernhard Meier, M.D., F.A.C.C., F.E.S.C.
Professor and Head of Cardiology
University Hospital
Bern, Switzerland

Michael B. Mock, M.D.
Professor of Medicine
Mayo Medical School
Consultant
Department of Cardiovascular Division
Mayo Clinic
Rochester, Minnesota

David J. Moliterno, M.D.
Department of Cardiology
The Cleveland Clinic Foundation
Cleveland, Ohio
Assistant Professor of Medicine
The Ohio State University
Columbus, Ohio·

William L. Mullen, M.D.
Senior Research Fellow
Department of Cardiology
University of California San Francisco
San Francisco, California

David W.M. Muller, M.B.B.S.
Assistant Professor
Department of Internal Medicine
University of Michigan
Ann Arbor, Michigan

Steven E. Nissen, M.D.
Vice Chairman
Department of Cardiology
The Cleveland Clinic Foundation
Cleveland, Ohio

Masakiyo Nobuyoshi, M.D.
Department of Cardiology
Kokura Memorial Hospital
Kitakyushu, Japan

William W. O'Neill, M.D.
Director, Cardiology Division
Department of Internal Medicine
William Beaumont Hospital
Royal Oak, Michigan

E. Magnus Ohman, M.D.
Assistant Professor of Medicine
Coordinator of Clinical Trials in Interventional
*   Cardiology*
Duke University Medical Center
Durham, North Carolina

Nowamagbe Omoigui, M.D.
Associate Professor of Medicine
Director, Division of Cardiology
Department of Medicine
University of South Carolina
Richland Medical Park
Columbia, South Carolina

Alfred F. Parisi, M.D.
Professor of Medicine, Brown University School of
*   Medicine*
Chief of Cardiology, Brown University School of
*   Medicine*
Chief of Cardiology, The Miriam Hospital
Providence, Rhode Island

Harry R. Phillips III, M.D.
Associate Professor of Medicine
Co-Director, Interventional Cardiovascular
*   Program*
Duke University Medical Center
Durham, North Carolina

Joseph F. Pietrolungo, D.O., M.S.
The Heart Group, Inc.
Ravenna, Ohio

P. Quandalle, M.D.
Université de Lille
Hopital Cardiologique
Service de Cardiologie et Hemodynamique
Lille, France

Stephen R. Ramee, M.D.
Director, International Cardiology
Section of Cardiology
Ochsner Clinic
New Orleans, Louisiana

Guy S. Reeder, M.D.
Professor of Medicine
Mayo Graduate School
Director, Coronary Care Unit
Mayo Affiliated Hospitals
Rochester, Minnesota

Reimer Riessen, M.D.
Research Associate
Department of Cardiovascular Research
St. Elizabeth's Hospital
Boston, Massachusetts

Keith A. Robinson, Ph.D.
Assistant Professor
Department of Medicine (Cardiology)
Emory University School of Medicine
Atlanta, Georgia

Uri Rosenschein, M.D.
Attending Physician
Cardiac Catheterization Laboratory
Tel Aviv Medical Center
Tel Aviv University
Tel Aviv, Israel

Gary S. Roubin, M.D.
Professor of Medicine
Director of Interventional Cardiology and
*   Radiology*
Adult Cardiac Catheterization Laboratory
University of Alabama at Birmingham
Birmingham, Alabama

Patrick Ruchat, M.D.
Service de Chirurgie Cardio-Vasculaire
Centre Hospitalier Universitaire Vaudois
Lausanne, Switzerland

Hossein Sadeghi, M.D.
Professor
Service de Chirurgie Cardio-Vasculaire
Centre Hospitalier Universitaire Vaudois
Lausanne, Switzerland

Robert D. Safian, M.D.
Director, Interventional Cardiology
Division of Cardiology
William Beaumont Hospital
Royal Oak, Michigan

Timothy A. Sanborn, M.D.
Professor of Medicine
Department of Medicine
Cornell University Medical College
Director, Cardiac Catheterization Laboratory
The New York Hospital
New York, New York

Michael P. Savage, M.D.
Associate Professor of Medicine
Division of Cardiology
Department of Medicine
Thomas Jefferson University
Philadelphia, Pennsylvania

Vicky Savas, M.D.
Interventional Cardiologist
William Beaumont Hospital
Royal Oak, Michigan

Richard A. Schatz, M.D.
Cardiovascular Interventions
Heart, Lung and Vascular Center
Scripps Clinic and Research Foundation
La Jolla, California

Robert S. Schwartz, M.D.
Mayo Clinic
Rochester, Minnesota

Patrick W. Serruys, M.D., Ph.D.
Professor of Interventional Cardiology
Erasmus University Rotterdam and
  Interuniversity Cardiology Institute of the
  Netherlands
Catheterisation Laboratory, Thoraxcenter
Erasmus University Rotterdam
Rotterdam, The Netherlands

Joel A. Shapiro, M.D., Ph.D.
Cardiovascular Intervention Center
Cedars-Sinai Medical Center
Los Angeles, California

Fayaz A. Shawl, M.D., F.A.C.C.
Clinical Associate Professor of Medicine
  (Cardiology)
George Washington University School of Medicine
Washington, D.C.
Director, Interventional Cardiology
Washington Adventist Hospital
Takoma Park, Maryland

Conrad Simpfendorfer, M.D., F.A.C.C.
Department of Cardiology
Section of Interventional Cardiology
The Cleveland Clinic Foundation
Cleveland, Ohio

Michael H. Sketch, Jr., M.D.
Director, Interventional Cardiac Catherization
  Laboratory
Duke University Medical Center
Durham, North Carolina

Artur M. Spokojny, M.D.
The New York Hospital-Cornell Medical Center
New York, New York

Kumar Sridhar, M.D.
Thomas Jefferson University Hospital
Philadelphia, Pennsylvania

Richard S. Stack, M.D.
Associate Professor of Medicine
Department of Medicine
Director, Interventional Cardiovascular Program
Duke University Medical Center
Durham, North Carolina

Jean-Christophe Stauffer, M.D.
Me'decin Associe'
Department of Cardiology
Centre Hospitalier Universitaire Vaudois
Lausanne, Switzerland

Simon H. Stertzer, M.D., F.A.C.C.
Clinical Professor of Medicine
Division of Cardiovascular Medicine
Stanford University Medical Center
Stanford, California

Frank Stumpe, M.D.
Medecin Associe
Chirurgie Cardio-Vasculaire
Centre Hospitalier Universitaire Vaudois
Lausanne, Switzerland
Chir. Cardiague
Hopital De Sion
Sion, Switzerland

James E. Tcheng, M.D., F.A.C.C.
Assistant Professor of Medicine
Duke University Medical Center
Durham, North Carolina

Paul S. Teirstein, M.D.
Director, Interventional Cardiology
Scripps Clinic and Research Foundation
La Jolla, California

Alan Tenaglia, M.D.
Duke University Medical Center
Durham, North Carolina

On Topaz, M.D., F.A.C.C.
Associate Professor of Medicine
Director, Interventional Cardiac Catheterization
    Laboratory
Department of Cardiology
Medical College of Virginia
Richmond, Virginia

Eric J. Topol, M.D.
Professor of Medicine
The Ohio State University
Chairman, Department of Cardiology
The Cleveland Clinic Foundation
Cleveland, Ohio

E. Murat Tuzcu, M.D.
Staff Physician
Department of Cardiology
The Cleveland Clinic Foundation
Assistant Professor of Medicine
The Ohio State University
Columbus, Ohio

Andonis G. Violaris, M.B., M.R.C.P.
Wellcome International Research Fellow
Catheterisation Laboratory
Thoraxcenter
Erasmus University Rotterdam
Rotterdam, The Netherlands

Pierre Vogt, M.D.
Medecin Adjoint
Division de Cardiologie
Centre Hospitalier Universitaire Vaudois
Lausanne, Switzerland

Paul Walinsky, M.D.
Division of Cardiology
Thomas Jefferson University
Philadelphia, Pennsylvania

Steven W. Werns, M.D.
Assistant Professor
Department of Internal Medicine
University of Michigan
Ann Arbor, Michigan

Christopher J. White, M.D.
Health Care International
Clydebank, Scotland

Patrick L. Whitlow, M.D.
Department of Cardiology
The Cleveland Clinic Foundation
Cleveland, Ohio

John S. Wilson, M.D.
Interventional Cardiologist
Allegheny General Hospital
Pittsburgh, Pennsylvania

Paul G. Yock, M.D.
Director, Center for Research in Cardiovascular
    Interventions
Stanford University School of Medicine
Stanford, California

Contents

SECTION V.
SUMMARY AND FUTURE DIRECTIONS

NEW TECHNIQUES OF CORONARY REVASCULARIZATION AND IMAGING

1. Directional Coronary Atherectomy: Current Prospects

TOMOAKI HINOHARA

The directional coronary atherectomy (DCA) catheter was the first non-balloon interventional device approved by the Food and Drug Administration (FDA) for the treatment of coronary artery disease. Since approval of this device in 1990, DCA has been widely performed. It was estimated that approximately 50,000 cases were performed in 1993 worldwide. The concept of atherectomy (removal of atheroma) was introduced by J.B. Simpson to overcome some of the limitations of percutaneous transluminal coronary angioplasty that are associated with uncontrolled damage to the arterial wall caused by balloon dilatation (Fig. 1.1) (1–3).

The unique feature of DCA is the combination of "directional" control and "debulking" (Fig. 1.2). Operators should maximize this feature to obtain optimal results. Controlled debulking of obstructive tissue creates a large, smooth lumen. In addition, partial removal of tissue changes the compliance of the vessel wall and allows even stretching of the vessel wall (facilitated angioplasty) without creating significant dissections. The directional nature of this procedure is unique compared with other interventional techniques. Debulking obstructive tissue by orientation of the window toward the plaque enables the operator to create an effective lumen with low risk of complication. In addition, adjustment of the supportive balloon pressure gives some control over the depth of tissue excised. All these aspects of DCA help the operator perform a more precise and controlled intervention.

To perform DCA safely and effectively, the operator needs to understand the concept and procedure of DCA because of differences in technique compared with percutaneous transluminal coronary angioplasty (PTCA). Without a clear understanding of the DCA procedure, the outcome of DCA may be suboptimal and more hazardous.

DCA OUTCOME

Outcome of Procedure

Since the introduction of this procedure in 1988, many studies have demonstrated the safety and efficacy of DCA (Table 1.1) (4–8). Studies by the Multicenter Registry, company sponsor (DVI), and new approaches of coronary intervention (NACI) sponsored by NIH during the relatively early stages of the DCA experience demonstrated a high success rate and a low major complication rate. In the CAVEAT (coronary angioplasty versus excisional atherectomy trial) study done in 1990, though the primary end point of the study was to compare restenosis against PTCA, the initial angiographic success rate determined quantitatively was significantly higher with DCA compared with PTCA (89% versus 80%) (7). Major complication rates were similar: death—DCA 0% versus PTCA 0.4%; CABG—DCA 3% versus PTCA 2%; and Q-wave myocardial infarction—DCA 2% versus PTCA 2%. The incidence of non-Q-wave myocardial infarction (CK MB elevation greater than twice normal) was significantly higher following DCA (DCA 19%

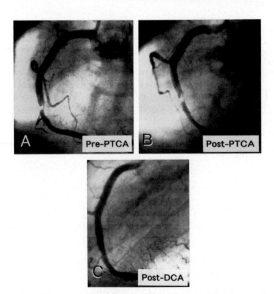

Figure 1.1. Example of successful DCA following initial failed attempt at PTCA. This case demonstrates the different mechanisms between PTCA and DCA. **A.** *Pre-PTCA:* Extremely eccentric lesion in the middle segment of the right coronary artery. **B.** *Post-PTCA:* Despite full expansion of 3.5-mm balloon, there is significant eccentric stenosis. Lesion morphology following PTCA suggests significant elastic recoil. **C.** *Post-DCA:* Excellent result with DCA, with excision of obstructive tissue.

DIRECTIONAL CORONARY ATHERECTOMY

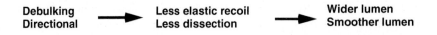

| Debulking Directional | → | Less elastic recoil Less dissection | → | Wider lumen Smoother lumen |

Figure 1.2. Features of DCA.

Table 1.1
DCA: Overall Results

	Number of Lesions	DCA Success (%)	Procedure Success (%)	Death (%)	Q-Wave MI (%)	CABG (%)
DVI registry (4)	1015	85	92	0.5	0.9	4.0
NACI registry	986	82	97	0.6	1.3	1.3
Sequoia Hosp (5) (1986–88)	447	90	94	0.3	0.8	3.1
Beth Israel Hosp (6)	225	91	98	0	0	0.5
CAVEAT (7)	512		88[a] (96)[b]	0	2.0	4.0
CCAT (8)	138	81	96	0	0.7	1.5

[a]Defined by the Angiographic Core Lab.
[b]Defined by each center.

Table 1.2
DCA: Sequoia Experience

Period: April 1988 to December 1993
Outcome
Number of procedures	1732
Number of lesions	2061
Successful catheter placement	95%
Tissue excised	16.4 mg
Residual stenosis	17.7%
Post-DCA diameter	2.6 mm
DCA success rate	91.9%
DCA/PTCA success rate	95.5%

Complications
Major complications (%)	3.2
Death	0.4
CABG[a]	3.0
Q-wave MI	0.4

Other complications (%)
CK MB elevation	12.4
Distal embolization	1.8
Groin repair	1.0
Stroke	0.4
In-hospital occlusion	1.0
Perforation (no CABG)	0.4

[a]CABG for perforation 0.4%.

versus PTCA 8%). In contrast, the CCAT (Canadian coronary atherectomy trial) showed no difference in the complication rate, including incidence of myocardial infarction (8).

The experience at Sequoia Hospital since 1988 is summarized in Table 1.2. The DCA success rate was 92%. An additional 4% of lesions were successfully treated with PTCA following an initial failed DCA, bringing the overall procedural success rate to 96%. Over the last several years, with improvement of equipment and operator skills, the DCA success rate has improved significantly, particularly in primary lesions (Fig. 1.3). Currently, the DCA success rate, similar for both primary and restenosis lesions, exceeds 95%. In the past the success rate for primary lesions was significantly lower than for restenosis lesions. Major complications occurred in 3.2% (death 0.4%, Q-wave MI 0.4%, and CABG 3.0%) (see Complications in detail). The reasons for DCA failures are multifactorial; one of the major causes is failure to reach or to cross the lesion with the device. Once the device is placed across the lesion, DCA failure is rather infrequent. DCA success rates and major complication rates for vessels are summarized in Figure 1.4.

The outcome of DCA is influenced by patient condition, vessel condition, and lesion characteristics (Table 1.3) (5, 9). The success rate is lower among older patients or patients with extremely unstable angina. Many of AHA/ACC type B lesions are effectively treated with DCA; however, the outcome of DCA for lesions in calcified vessels, calcified lesions, lesions in tortuous vessels, lengthy lesions, lesions at an angle, or lesions in a diffusely diseased vessel is somewhat suboptimal.

Complications

Some complications of the DCA procedure are similar to PTCA, while others are rather

CHANGES IN DCA SUCCESS RATE

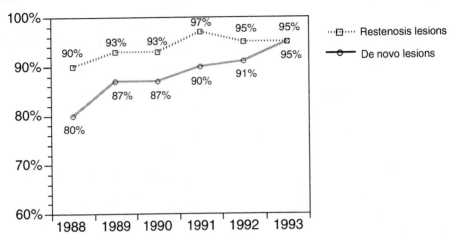

Figure 1.3. Changes in DCA success rate over 6 years at Sequoia Hospital. Significant improvement of the DCA success rate was observed, particularly in primary lesions.

specific to DCA (Table 1.4) (11). A summary of complications of Sequoia Hospital is found in Table 1.2. One of the clinically significant complications, though rather infrequent (2 to 5%), is acute occlusion (5, 10). The location of the occlusion and potential causes of acute occlusion are summarized in Table 1.5. Acute occlusion at the lesion tends to occur either when the device fails to cross the lesion or when inadequate atheroma was removed because of calcification or a technical problem. The causes of these acute occlusions are likely dissection, flap, or thrombus formation. When adequate tissue is removed from a lesion and an optimal lumen size is achieved, acute or subacute occlusion is extremely rare. Acute occlusions proximal to the lesion are often related to aggressive manipulation of the device; this complication can be avoided with appropriate case selection and gentle handling of the device.

The most serious and somewhat unique complication associated with DCA is perforation. The incidence of perforation is low (0.8%: Sequoia experience) compared with PTCA, and perforation causing tamponade is very rare (0.1%). Despite the low incidence of perforation, it is important to avoid this potentially lethal complication (Table 1.6). Most perforations can be avoided with adequate case selection and appropriate technique, and DCA should be considered contraindicated for significantly angulated lesions, lesions with extensive dissection, and lesions in small arteries. Use of an inappropriately oversized device or use of high balloon inflation pressures during the initial cuts may cause perforation. Appropriate positioning of the device at the lesion and orientation of the window toward the plaque borders are key factors in preventing perforation. The risk of perforation is higher if cuts are made in the normal vessel wall. Most perforations have occurred in the normal segment of the vessel

Vessels and DCA Success Rate

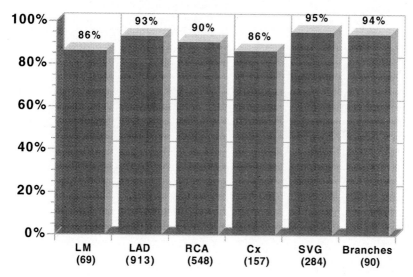

A   p < 0.001

Vessels and DCA Complication Rate

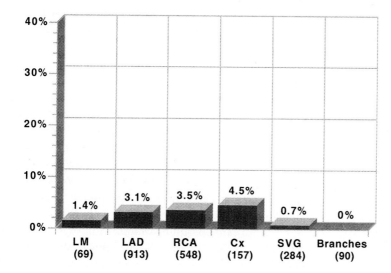

B

Figure 1.4.   A. Target vessel and DCA success rate. **B.** Target vessel
and major complication rate (death, Q-wave MI, or CABG).

Table 1.3
Clinical and Angiographic Risk Factors in DCA Outcome

Clinical factors
    Old age (>70)
    Unstable angina (extreme)
    Recent thrombolytic therapy
    Multivessel disease
Angiographic factors
    Calcification
    Lengthy lesion (≥20 mm)
    Proximal tortuosity
    Bend stenosis
    Diffusely calcified vessel
    Diffuse disease

Table 1.4
DCA-Specific Complications

DCA-Specific Complications (Unusual for PTCA)
  Perforation
  Nose-cone trauma distal to lesion
    Dissection
    Worsening of lesion
  Guidewire fracture
Complications More Frequent Than With PTCA
  Distal embolization (vein graft)
  Guide catheter-induced dissection (right coronary artery)
  Side branch loss
  Groin complication
  Mild creatine kinase elevation without clinical sequelae

Table 1.5
Acute Occlusion

Occlusion proximal to lesion
  Guide-induced dissection (RCA)
  Aggressive device manipulation (existing mild disease)
Occlusion at lesion
  Failure to cross
  Salvage PTCA for failure to cross—dissection
  Device-induced dissection
  Thrombus
  Inadequate tissue removal
  Spasm
Distal to lesion
  Nose cone trauma—dissection, thrombus
  Spasm

Table 1.6
Perforation: Potential Causes

Case selection
  Severe angulation
  Extensive or spiral dissection
  Small vessel (<2.0 mm)

Procedure
  Oversize device
  High balloon inflation pressure
  Inappropriate device positioning
  Inappropriate window orientation (extremely eccentric
    lesion)
  Spasm

when the device had been placed proximal or distal to the lesion. A small perforation (minimal dye staining or localized leaking of contrast) can be effectively sealed by a prolonged balloon inflation for 10 to 15 minutes. For significant perforations or patients with hemopericardium or tamponade, however, CABG should be considered as the primary approach.

Angiographic distal embolization caused by excised tissue or thrombus is a rather rare complication in native coronary arteries; however, a small elevation of the CPK more frequently observed following DCA compared with PTCA may be associated with microembolism. In contrast, distal embolization in diffusely diseased vein grafts is much more frequent (11%: Sequoia experience). Case selection in vein grafts is important to avoid embolism; DCA should be performed

only for focal lesions in otherwise nondiseased vein grafts, and diffusely diseased vein grafts should be avoided.

Restenosis

One of the goals of DCA is to reduce restenosis. DCA prevents elastic recoil by debulking obstructive tissue; thus it may prevent mechanical causes of restenosis. Furthermore, obtaining a large postinterventional lumen may prevent clinically significant restenosis (large lumen concept proposed by Dr. Don Baim et al) (1, 2). With a large postinterventional lumen a larger space is available for tissue growth (smooth muscle cell proliferation and matrix formation) during the healing process. Thus this process may cause only partial renarrowing of the lesion without clinically significant restenosis when a large postinterventional lumen is obtained. In contrast, if only a small postin-terventional lumen is obtained, a small amount of the mass growth will obliterate the lumen, causing significant restenosis. In the CAVEAT study the most significant predictor for follow-up lumen size was postinterven-tional minimal lesion diameter (MLD) (7). Kuntz et al. demonstrated that late loss (post-MLD minus follow-up MLD) is usually simi-lar among the devices and is not device-dependent, with approximately 1 mm of loss (13). When the results of DCA and stent (Schatz coronary stent) were compared, in their experience, the restenosis rate was 30% for DCA and 26% for stents. A larger post-MLD was obtained with stents compared with DCA and this difference reflected a larger fol-low-up MLD for stents (14).

The restenosis experience at Sequoia Hos-pital is summarized in Figure 1.5. The inci-dence of restenosis was lowest among primary lesions in native coronary arteries and highest among restenosis lesions in saphenous vein grafts. Analysis of restenosis based on the "large lumen concept" among primary lesions in native coronary arteries is summarized in Figure 1.6. Restenosis in vessels greater than 3 mm was 24%, in lesions treated with the 7 Fr device was 18%, and post-MLD >3 mm was 22%. Based on these data, DCA is effec-tive long-term therapy when the procedure is done in a relatively large vessel (>3 mm) using a 7 Fr device, obtaining a large post-MLD.

CAVEAT was a randomized trial compar-ing the restenosis rates for DCA and PTCA in 1012 lesions (7). This study demonstrated a slightly lower restenosis rate defined by quan-titative angiograms among 862 lesions (50% for DCA and 57% for PTCA, $P = .06$); how-ever, there was no clinical benefit between the two devices with similar incidence of subse-quent revascularization. The results from the CCAT (Canadian coronary atherectomy trial)

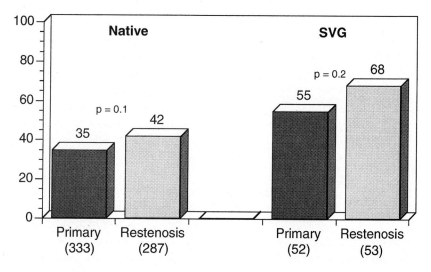

Figure 1.5.   Restenosis rate following DCA in native coronary artery and saphenous vein graft. The lesion was categorized as primary (de novo) lesions and restenosis lesions from previous PTCA. Restenosis was defined as greater than 50% steno-sis by quantitative measurement at follow-up angiography. The follow-up compliance rate was approximately 78%.

RESTENOSIS (Primary Lesions)

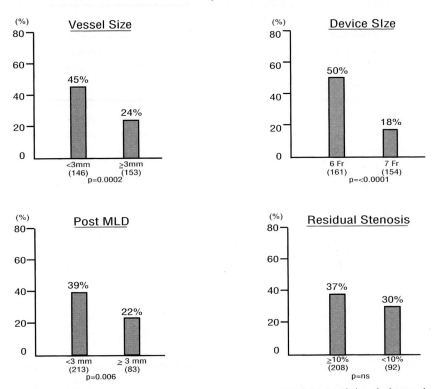

Figure 1.6.   Restenosis rate in primary native coronary artery based on vessel size, device used, post-MLD, and residual stenosis.

Table 1.7
Restenosis Following DCA

Study	Vessel size (mm)	Post-MLD (mm)	Residual stenosis (%)	Restenosis rate (%)
Beth Israel Hosp (6)	3.2	3.0	7	32
Sequoia Hosp	3.3	2.9	13	31
CAVEAT (7)	2.9	2.0	29	50
CCAT (8)	2.9	2.3	26	46

study were similar to CAVEAT (8). The potential explanations of the relatively high incidence of restenosis without obvious benefit of clinical outcome following DCA compared with PTCA in these studies are as follows: (a) some case-selection bias with possible exclusion of extremely eccentric lesions or ostial left anterior descending artery (LAD) lesions; (b) use of first-generation SCA-1 device rather than the current EX device; (c) no standardized technique among the operators, with significant variation in technique; and (d) relatively high residual stenosis following DCA compared with other previously published studies.

It has been shown previously that DCA creates a large postinterventional lumen compared with PTCA with less incidence of dissection (15); however, the residual stenosis following DCA was much higher in both the CAVEAT and CCAT studies compared with previous observational studies (Table 1.7). This high residual stenosis may be one of the potential reasons for relatively high restenosis rates. To reduce the restenosis rates, the postinterventional residual stenosis needs to

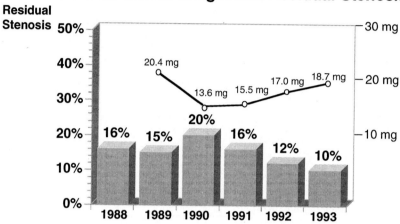

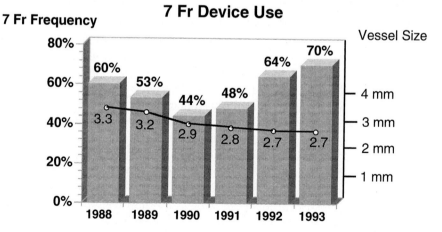

Figure 1.7. Changes in procedure method and outcome over the last 4 years at Sequoia Hospital. **A.** Amount of tissue excised and residual stenosis. **B.** Vessel size and use of 7 Fr device.

be minimal (<10% residual stenosis), not accepting a "successful result" with a moderate degree of residual stenosis. With adequate case selection and appropriate technique, unlike PTCA, DCA is a procedure capable of achieving optimal lumen size with minimal residual stenosis.

OPTIMAL DCA

Over the last several years, in addition to equipment improvements, the procedure has evolved. Because it was a new technique, there was no standardization of the procedure, with significant variations among the operators in the past. Our technique at Sequoia Hospital has evolved significantly over the last 4 years, as shown in Figure 1.7. More recently, despite vessels being somewhat smaller, use of the 7 Fr device has increased. Using optimally sized devices with low balloon inflation pressures, the amount of excised tissue has increased, associated with lower residual stenosis. Currently, the residual stenosis at the end of the procedure is approximately 10%.

Based on analysis of restenosis information, it is essential to minimize residual stenosis, obtaining the largest postinterventional lumen possible without complications. The goal of DCA is to excise an appropriate amount of tissue (15 to 20 mg) and obtain a large diameter with minimal residual stenosis (<10 to 15%) by quantitative analysis. To achieve these results, the operators should retrain their eyes to evaluate post-DCA results. The usual "PTCA success" is not acceptable for DCA. When one compares the visual estimation to quantitative analysis, the visual estimation underestimates residual stenosis; minimal residual stenosis by visual estimation usually reflects 20 to 30% stenosis by quantitation and no residual stenosis by visual estimation is approximately 10% by quantitative analysis. Therefore, if on-line quantitative analysis is not used, the operator should aim for no residual stenosis by visual estimation to minimize residual stenosis.

Table 1.8
Optimal DCA

1. Selection of appropriate sized device
     Vessel 2.5 mm to 3 mm   6 Fr EX
     Vessel ≥3 mm   7 Fr EX
     Vessel ≥4 mm   7 Fr EX or 7 Fr G
2. Precise device position at lesion
     Check position frequently with contract injection
3. Precise device orientation
     45 degree rotation if possible
     More cuts toward eccentric plaque
4. Balloon pressure
     Start with low pressure, 5 to 10 psi
     Gradually increase pressure
5. Multiple cuts
     At least 10 to 20 cuts
     In many cases >20 cuts
6. Post-DCA assessment
     Contrast flow around the device in place
     Angiogram <10%
     Adequate tissue removal (15 to 20 mg; nose cone full)
7. For residual stenosis
     Step-up device size if adequate
     Use higher balloon pressure
     Post–balloon dilatation (encourage in more cases unless
        no residual stenosis)

The recommended DCA procedure for optimal DCA is summarized in Table 1.8. Carelessly aggressive DCA attempting to excise as much tissue as possible may increase the risk of perforation. To avoid perforation, the selection of an appropriately sized device, the precise location of the device, and the use of low initial balloon pressure are important. Generally, post-DCA balloon dilatation is a safe method to increase the postinterventional lumen size without significant risk of dissection or perforation. At the present time the data for post–balloon dilatation are limited; however, many operators currently elect to postdilate routinely in most cases after initial debulking of the lesion by DCA. Following debulking, low balloon inflations will stretch the vessel evenly without causing dissection. Post-DCA balloon dilatation should be done if >10% residual stenosis remains and also may be considered or encouraged for <10% residual stenosis. Use of a slightly larger balloon (balloon vessel ratio 1.2:1) with relatively low pressure (2 to 3 atm) is recommended. Further analysis of the balloon effect following DCA should be available in the near future through currently ongoing randomized trials: OARS (optimal atherectomy restenosis study) and BOAT (balloon angioplasty versus optimal atherectomy trial).

Use of IVUS (intravascular ultrasound) is often helpful to perform optimal atherectomy. IVUS supplies information regarding morphology and characteristics of the lesion that are not available from an angiogram. Examining the eccentricity of the plaque and the nature of the calcification (superficial calcium versus deep wall calcium) will assist in determining case selection, as well as the approach of DCA. The ring of calcium in the lumen indicates that excision of the calcification with DCA will be extremely difficult. Following the initial atherectomy procedure, reviewing the results with IVUS often provides further information for residual plaque

burden. In addition, IVUS gives more precise measurement of the artery for selection of the device, as well as the balloon selection for postdilatation.

CASE SELECTION AND APPLICATION

The DCA procedure is more difficult to perform than PTCA; thus the application of DCA may differ significantly based on the operator's skill and experience. For the operator with no previous experience or only minimal experience (less than 10 cases) the ideal lesion (a noncalcified, focal lesion in a proximal segment of a large vessel) should be selected for DCA. With more experience with this procedure, a more complex lesion can be approached safely and effectively. Case selection should be based on patient condition, left ventricular dysfunction, accessibility to the lesion, and lesion morphology (Table 1.9).

Table 1.9
DCA Case Selection

Levels of Difficulty: Scoring System (Sequoia Guideline)							
Vessel		Location		Vessel Size		Type	
LM	3	Ao-Ost	6	≥ 3 mm	0	Primary	2
LAD	0	Non Ao-Ost	4	≤ 3 mm	1	Restenosis	0
RCA	2	Prox	0	≤ 2.5 mm	2		
LCX	4	Mid	2	< 1.5 mm	C		
Diagonal	2	Distal	4				
SVG-RCA	0						
SVG-Left	3						

Diffuse Disease		Lesion Length		Tortuosity		Angulation		Calcification	
None	0	< 5 mm	0	None	0	None	0	None	0
Mild	2	5–10 mm	1	Mild	2	Mild	2	Mild	4
Moderate	6	10–15 mm	3	Moderate	4	Moderate	4	Moderate	8
Severe	C	15–20 mm	6	Severe	C	Severe	C	Severe	C
Degenerative		20–30 mm	8						
Vein-Graft	C	≥ 30 mm	C						

C, Contraindication. (In addition, spiral or extensive dissections are also contraindicated.)

Using a combined score from the above sections, determine the Level of Difficulty in approaching a particular lesion with DCA on the scale below.

DCA Procedure: Levels of Difficulty								
Easy		Moderate		Difficult		Very Difficult		
2	4	6	8	10	12	14	16	18

Accessibility

Because of the profile and stiffness of the device, approaching a lesion with this device is more limited than with PTCA. Accessibility of the device to the lesion is determined by various factors: (a) guiding catheter position; (b) ostial location; (c) vessel size; (d) location of the lesion; (e) vessel compliance and stiffness; (f) curvature, tortuosity of the vessel; and (g) hardness of the lesion. The lesion in the circumflex artery is less approachable because of difficulty inserting the device into the circumflex artery. Approachable circumflex lesions are characterized by (a) the short left main; (b) the large left main; and (c) the short take-off of the circumflex artery. Most saphenous vein grafts are approachable; however, a steep take-off of the saphenous vein graft from the aorta (mostly saphenous vein graft to the left coronary artery) may be a difficult site. DCA should be considered contraindicated if the vessel is markedly tortuous. Aggressive manipulation to pass through a tortuous vessel should be avoided because of the risk of injury to the vessel wall. Lesions with moderate tortuosity in noncalcified, nondiffusely diseased, relatively large-sized vessels can be approached with this procedure by an experienced operator. Calcified vessels usually indicate lack of compliance. Vessel compliance is needed for the device to pass through the proximal segment of the vessel. A noncompliant vessel does not accommodate passage of the device, and minimal curvature of a noncompliant vessel inhibits advancement of the device.

Lesions Suitable for DCA

The application of the DCA procedure is summarized in Table 1.10. Ideal lesions for PTCA (AHA classification: type A lesion) are generally good for DCA. The type A lesion in a proximal segment and in a relatively large vessel is ideal for DCA because of its high success rate and relatively low restenosis rate. When using a 7 Fr device in a vessel >3

Table 1.10
Applications of DCA (Sequoia Recommendation)[a]

- Type A lesion in large vessel ≥3 mm), easy access
- Severely eccentric lesion
- Abnormal contour
  - Ulceration
  - Flap
  - Limited dissection
- Ostial lesion
  - Nonaorta: LAD, (CX), (diagonal)
  - Aorta: LM, SVG, RCA
- Moderately lengthy lesion (10–20 mm) in large vessel
- Large bifurcation lesion
- Salvage for failed PTCA

[a]These applications are based on experience at Sequoia Hospital. *CX*, Circumflex coronary artery; *LAD*, left anterior descending coronary artery; *LM*, left main coronary artery; *RCA*, right coronary artery; *SVG*, saphenous vein graft.

mm, the restenosis rate should be approximately 20%.

Eccentric lesions are effectively treated by DCA because of the directional nature of this procedure. Removing obstructive tissue selectively from the eccentric location results in a wide postlesion diameter with less recoil or dissection. Debulking obstructive tissue from a lesion with ulceration or limited dissection also effectively creates a large lumen. A lesion in the coronary ostium is not usually treated effectively with PTCA because of the significant elastic recoil following balloon dilatation. Debulking from this location prevents elastic recoil and creates an effective lumen with a low incidence of dissection. Left anterior descending ostial lesions are ideal for DCA with a predictable outcome in this important location. In addition, diagonal ostial lesions are often treated effectively with a short-window device, with excellent results. Right coronary artery ostial lesions are effectively treated with DCA; however, the treatment of this particular location is technically more difficult and requires operator expertise. Debulking obstructive tissue from tubular lesions prevents dissections or intimal flaps and helps to create a large postlumen diameter. PTCA for bifurcation lesions in large vessels is often ineffective because of elastic recoil of the ostium and shifting of the plaque from one side to the other during balloon dilatation. Debulking by DCA prevents plaque shifting and the result of this procedure is more satisfactory than PTCA. The short-window device is the device of choice for a somewhat angulated take-off of the branch lesion. Many lesions following a failed PTCA attempt are effectively treated with DCA. The accessibility of the device to the lesion and causes of PTCA failure should be carefully evaluated. DCA is most effective when PTCA has failed as a result of elastic recoil or a limited localized dissection in the plaque itself. Spiral dissection should be avoided because of the risk of perforation. One of the potential advantages of salvage DCA compared with a stent following failed PTCA is the ease of patient care following the procedure: the patient does not require anticoagulation following DCA, and subacute occlusion without anticoagulation remains low following DCA.

Lesions Unsuitable for DCA

The presence of calcification in either the vessel wall or the lesion is the most influential factor for the outcome of DCA. It is difficult to advance the catheter through a noncompliant calcified vessel in a proximal segment and to cross a calcified lesion with this high-profile device. Furthermore, despite successful placement of the device, tissue is often difficult to excise from a calcified lesion with the current cutter design. In addition, severely tortuous vessels or diffusely diseased arteries are generally not suitable for DCA because of the potential risk of complications. Operator experience will help to approach some of the selected lesions in this setting. Severely angulated lesions should be considered contraindicated for DCA because of difficulty crossing the lesion and the increased risk of perforation with deep cuts in the angulated segment. Lesions greater than 20 mm, particularly primary lesions, contain significant plaque burden and are not suitable for DCA because of the risk of complications such as dissection and acute occlusion. Extensive dissections (spontaneous or post-PTCA) are contraindicated because of the increased risk of perforation when attempting removal of a spiral dissection with compromised vessel wall integrity. Diffusely diseased saphenous vein grafts, particularly in patients with left ventricular dysfunction, should be avoided because of increased risk of embolism by debris from the graft.

CURRENT PROBLEMS AND THE FUTURE OF DCA

Although many improvements have been made over the last several years, it is important to consider that DCA is still an evolving procedure. Further improvements of the guiding catheter and atherectomy catheter are required to make this procedure more user-friendly and effective. Compared with PTCA, DCA is technically more difficult and the operator needs to be trained properly for this procedure. The result of DCA depends on the operator's skills and experience. Further improvements of the atherectomy device and guiding catheter will assist the inexperienced operator in performing the DCA procedure much more easily and safely. A new catheter (GTO—"greater torque output") with improved torque has been introduced for clinical use. This catheter will allow the operator to orient the window more precisely and easily. Presently, many calcified lesions cannot be excised because of the limitations of the cutter. An enhanced cutter, which will be introduced in the near future, will enable the operator to cut calcified plaque more effectively. This may improve the performance of the device, as well as expand some of the DCA indications. Furthermore, a flexible housing to accommodate some of the curvature encountered during advancement of the device is under development. Some of the limitations of the current procedure include how to precisely excise tissue and when to stop the procedure. To reduce the restenosis rate following DCA, it is important to perform effective debulking and obtain an excellent postinterventional lumen. This requires more aggressive atherectomy and thus may increase the risks of perforation. Use of intravascular ultrasound (IVUS) has helped in performing more aggressive atherectomy, in selecting the appropriately sized device, and in achieving a more precise orientation of the window to excise eccentric plaque. However, it is rather complex and time-consuming to use the IVUS device for routine atherectomy. In addition, often the orientation of the window of the DCA device is still based on the feeling of the operator using fluoroscopy. On-line information by ultrasound will obviously give more feedback to the operator during the atherectomy procedure. The combined DCA and IVUS catheter (guided atherectomy catheter) will overcome many of the current limitations of using the DCA and IVUS catheters in a sequential way. Development of a guided atherectomy catheter is currently under way, and in the future atherectomy can be performed more effectively and safely with this new device.

REFERENCES

1. Simpson JB. Future interventional techniques. In: Califf RM, Mark DB, Wagner GS, eds. Acute coronary care in the thrombolytic era. Chicago: Year Book Medical, 1988.
2. Simpson JB, Selmon MR, Robertson GC, Cipriano PR, Hayden WG, Johnson DE, Fogarty TJ. Transluminal atherectomy for occlusive peripheral atherectomy disease. Am J Cardiol 1988;61:96G–101G.
3. Hinohara T, Selmon MR, Robertson GC, Braden L, Simpson JB. Directional atherectomy: new approaches for treatment of obstructive coronary and peripheral vascular disease. Circulation 1990;81:IV 79–91.
4. Baim DS, Hinohara T, Holmes D, Topol E, Pinkerton C, King SB III, Whitlow P, et al for the US Directional Coronary Atherectomy Investigator Group. Results of directional coronary atherectomy during multicenter preapproval testing. Am J Cardiol 1993;72:6E–11E.
5. Hinohara T, Robertson GC, Simpson JB. Directional coronary atherectomy. In: Topol EJ, ed. Textbook of interventional cardiology. Philadelphia: WB Saunders, 1994.
6. Safian RD, Gelbfish JS, Erny RE et al. Coronary atherectomy: clinical, angiographic, and histologic findings and observations regarding potential mechanisms. Circulation 1990;82:69.
7. Topol EJ, Leya F, Pinkerton CA et al. A comparison of directional atherectomy with coronary angioplasty in patients with coronary artery disease. N Engl J Med 1993; 329:221–227.
8. Adelman AG, Cohen EA, Kimball BP et al. A comparison of directional atherectomy with balloon angioplasty for lesions of the left anterior descending coronary artery. N Engl J Med 1993;329:228–233.
9. Ellis SG, De Cesare NB, Pinkerton CA, Whitlow P, King SB III, Ghazzal ZM, Kereiakes DJ et al. Relation of stenosis morphology and clinical presentation to the procedural results of directional coronary atherectomy. Circulation 1991;84:644–653.
10. Popma JJ, Topol EJ, Hinohara T, Pinkerton CA, Baim DS, King SB III, Holmes DR Jr et al for the Directional Atherectomy Investigator Group. Abrupt vessel closure after directional coronary atherectomy. J Am Coll Cardiol 1992; 19:1372–1379.
11. Hinohara T, Robertson GC, Selmon MR, Vetter JW, McAuley BJ, Sheehan DJ, Simpson JB. Directional coronary atherectomy complications and management. Cathet and Cardiovasc Diagn 1993;1:61–71.
12. Baim DS, Kuntz RE. Directional coronary atherectomy: How much lumen enlargement is optimal? Am J Cardiol 1993;72:65E–70E.
13. Kuntz RE, Safian RD, Levine MJ et al. Novel approach to the analysis of restenosis after the use of three new coronary devices. J Am Coll Cardiol 1992;19:1493.
14. Kuntz RE, Hinohara T, Robertson GC, Safian RD, Simpson JB, Baim DS. Influence of vessel selection on the observed restenosis rate after endoluminal stenting or directional atherectomy. Am J Cardiol 1992;70:1101–1108.
15. Rowe MH, Hinohara T, White NW, Robertson GC, Selmon MR, Simpson JB. Comparison of dissection rates and angiographic results following directional coronary atherectomy and coronary angioplasty. Am J Cardiol 1990; 66:49–53.

2. Rotational Atheroablation/Atherectomy

KEITH E. DAVIS, RILEY D. FOREMAN, and MAURICE BUCHBINDER

In the early 1980s Dr. David Auth, working at the time as director of the Laser Surgery Laboratory at the University of Washington, began investigating the possibility of using a rotational device as an alternative, mechanical means of debulking atheromatous plaque. In an effort to improve the results of percutaneous revascularization and perhaps reduce the restenosis rates seen with conventional balloon angioplasty, he began to develop several designs that ultimately evolved into the Rotablator (Heart Technology, Inc., Bellevue, WA). The Rotablator is a high-speed, rotating, abrasive burr–tipped catheter that selectively ablates inelastic, atheromatous plaque creating a smooth channel through diseased peripheral and coronary arteries (Fig. 2.1). This device has proven to be especially effective where complex lesion characteristics such as calcification, tortuosity, small caliber, ostial location, and diffuse disease typically increase the risk of intervention with conventional balloon catheters.

THE DEVICE

The cutting element of this particular device consists of a "football" shaped, elliptical, metal burr attached to a flexible, stainless steel, helical driveshaft. The front half of the abrasive burr is impregnated with diamond microchips measuring 20 to 30 microns in diameter. The burr is available for coronary use in 0.25-mm increments from 1.25 mm to 2.5 mm in diameter. (There is also a 2.15-mm burr.) The driveshaft is covered by a thin, Teflon™ sheath throughout its length allowing for saline infusion during activation of the burr, thereby minimizing frictional heat. The

shaft and burr are connected to an advancer housing unit, which has a lockable, sliding control knob that allows the advancement and retraction of the burr in relation to the distal end of the sheath during ablation. Compressed-air drive tubing, an infusion port, and fiberoptic tachometer cables are attached to the advancer housing along with a guidewire brake release button. The compressed air tubing and tachometer cables are in turn connected to a control box, which allows adjustment and display of the rotational speed of the burr.

The Rotablator is typically advanced over a special, 310-cm-long, 0.009-inch-diameter guidewire. The Rotablator guidewire has a radiopaque, distal tip, which enlarges to 0.017 inches in diameter to prevent embolization of the burr in the unlikely event that the burr separates from the shaft during ablation.

MECHANISM OF ABLATION

During the ablation procedure, the burr spins at approximately 160,000 to 190,000 rpm allowing the diamond microchips to pulverize atherosclerotic plaque into fine microparticles. The device is a low-torque system, thereby minimizing the likelihood of producing dissection flaps. Unlike any other device for vascular intervention, the Rotablator selectively removes harder, atherosclerotic plaque while deflecting more elastic, nondiseased segments of the vessel wall (Fig. 2.2). This application of "differential cutting" is analogous to the effect of a fingernail file on the flesh of a finger compared to its effect on a fingernail. Initial studies in canine coronaries showed that damage to normal arterial wall was largely confined to the intima with removal of only 10 to 30% of the internal elastic lamina without evidence of medial dissection typically seen with balloon angioplasty (1). The result of rotational ablation is usually a smooth, cylindrical, polished-appearing surface without dissection (Fig. 2.3) or thrombus (2–4).

Since its inception, a variety of aspiration designs have been evaluated early in the Rotablator development, but these were eventually discarded because of technical difficulty in producing aspiration conduits that were flexible, durable, and able to rotate

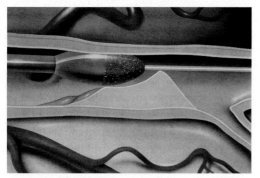

Figure 2.1. Illustration of Rotablator burr in section of a diseased artery. (Courtesy of Heart Technology, Bellevue, WA.)

at the necessary speeds. Furthermore, since 88% of the particulate debris produced during rotablation in human cadavers appears to be less than 12 microns with 77% being less than 5 microns, most of the debris passes readily through the microcirculation and is subsequently cleared by the reticuloendothelial system (5, 6). In a separate study evaluating particulate debris, 98% of the particles from atherosclerotic rabbit iliac arteries were found to be less than 10 microns in diameter (7). The physiologic effect of Rotablator debris was investigated in a study in which particles produced by rotablation were injected into canine coronary arteries. Bolus injection of 32 mm^3 of debris produced no measurable change in mean blood flow. However, very large boluses of heavily calcified debris, 42 mm^3 and 96 mm^3, respectively, did result in a decrease in mean blood flow and produced hemodynamic compromise (5). Echocardiographic monitoring of left ventricular function during rotablation has yielded the finding of transient echo contrast enhancement in the distribution of the treated lesion without associated wall motion abnormalities. Because the contrast enhancement occurred prior to the advancement of the burr and cleared rapidly, and because injection of atherosclerotic Rotablator debris in an exper-

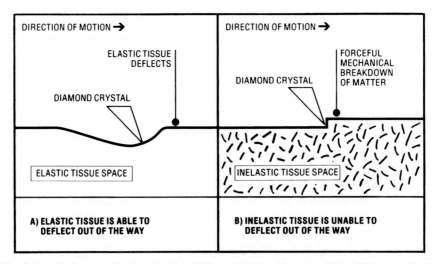

Figure 2.2. Schematic demonstrating the principle of differential cutting. (Courtesy of Heart Technology, Bellevue, WA.)

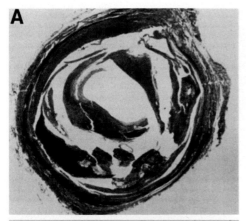

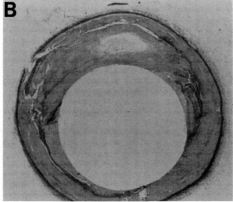

Figure 2.3. Photomicrograph of arterial cross sections. **A.** After balloon angioplasty with resultant plaque fracturing, as well as multiple medial and intimal dissections. **B.** After rotational atherectomy with resultant near complete removal of atheromatous plaque and a smooth lumen without apparent dissections.

imental model failed to produce the same degree of enhancement, this enhancement has been attributed to the formation of microcavitation bubbles produced by the spinning burr. These bubbles have been reproduced under experimental conditions using the Rotablator (8).

RESULTS IN COMPLEX LESIONS

To date clinical trials of rotational ablation have confirmed its efficacy in a wide variety of coronary lesions with a 95% overall success rate in 3424 lesions. This includes a 95% success rate in patients with type B lesions and a 91% success rate in type C lesions. Suc-

cess, defined as less than 50% residual stenosis and the absence of major complications, was 85% with rotablation alone, increasing to well over 90% when low-pressure, adjunctive balloon dilatation was done (9).

Calcified, noncompliant lesions constitute a significant obstacle to conventional balloon angioplasty. However, unlike standard angioplasty, analysis of the Rotablator multicenter registry data has shown that the success with rotablation combined with balloon angioplasty was unaffected by the degree of calcification (Fig. 2.4) and that previously *undilatable* lesions could be treated successfully in 97% of patients using such a combined approach (10, 11). Generally, it is believed that rotational ablation may facilitate subsequent balloon angioplasty by improving the vessel's compliance, thereby increasing the efficacy of balloon dilatation while decreasing the risk of significant dissection. In a comparative analysis of primary balloon angioplasty with rotational ablation, intravascular ultrasound demonstrated medial dissection in 43% of those treated with balloon angioplasty alone, while none of the patients treated with rotational ablation alone or combined with complementary balloon angioplasty demonstrated medial dissection, supporting the concept of improved vessel compliance following mechanical debulking (12).

Despite the advent of long balloons, longer lesions remain a difficult challenge for interventional cardiologists. Excellent success rates may be achieved in the majority of patients with long lesions treated with rotablation combined with balloon percutaneous transluminal coronary angioplasty (PTCA). In the Rotablator multicenter registry, procedural success was achieved in 92% of patients with lesions 1.5 to 2.5 cm in length. These longer lesions were associated with a slightly higher non-Q-wave MI rate of 6.2% and a Q-wave MI rate of 2.8%. This compares to rates of 4.0% and 0.7%, respectively, for lesions less than 1 cm in length (13). In an early study of 42 patients with diffuse coro-

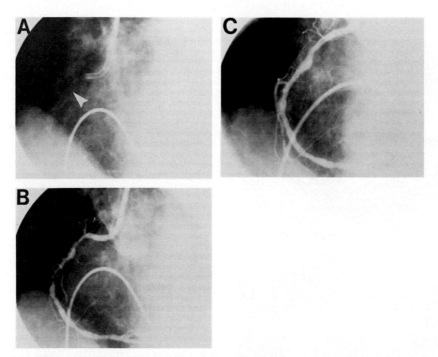

Figure 2.4. Successful rotational atheroablation of a highly calcified diffusely diseased right coronary artery (RCA). **A.** Demonstration of highly calcified RCA. **B.** Diffusely diseased mid RCA with 90% stenosis in the left anterior oblique (LAO) projection. **C.** After rotational atherectomy with complimentary percutaneous transluminal coronary angioplasty (PTCA) with no significant residual stenosis.

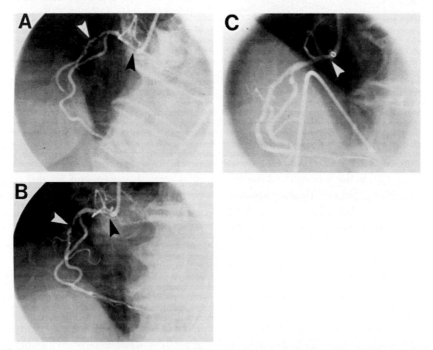

Figure 2.5. Successful rotational atherectomy of sequential RCA lesions. **A.** Right anterior oblique (RAO) projection of right coronary artery (RCA) with black arrow demonstrating ostial 70 to 90% lesion. **B.** RCA on left anterior oblique (LAO) projection with black arrow demonstrating ostial stenosis and white marker demonstrating focal mid 90% stenosis. **C.** After rotational atherectomy. RCA in LAO projection with excellent result at both lesion sites.

nary artery disease who were generally poor candidates for balloon PTCA or CABG, *stand-alone* rotablation was successful in 92% of those patients with lesions less than 1 cm in length and in 70% of those with lesions greater than 1 cm. However, success was limited by failure to cross the lesion with a guidewire in four patients, by eight non-Q-wave myocardial infarctions, and by one abrupt closure. Of those patients with non-Q-wave infarction, the four patients who developed regional wall motion abnormalities on the postprocedural left ventriculograms demonstrated recovery of function on follow-up ventriculography (14).

The high success rates achieved in complex lesions have been confirmed in several single-center reports such as the series reported by Stertzer and colleagues. They obtained a 95.4% overall success rate in 346 lesions, an impressive result given that nearly half of these patients had undergone previous angioplasty with only 13% success. In their series, complications included Q-wave infarctions in 2.5% and non-Q-wave infarctions (defined as isolated CPK isoenzyme elevations) in 11%, rates similar to those experienced in their contemporaneous balloon angioplasty series (15).

In addition to noncompliant, calcified, and long lesions, encouraging results have been reported in ostial (Fig. 2.5), protected left main, bifurcating, and angulated lesions (16) (Fig. 2.6). Goudreau and Cowley et al. reported success in 30 of 31 ostial lesions attempted with minimal complications, including one patient with non-Q-wave infarction, one occlusion, and two intimal dissections (17). Lesions involving bifurcation points (Fig. 2.7) were likewise associated with a high, 95% procedural success rate. Although the incidence of branch vessel occlusion was low at 1.5%, there was a small but significant increase in the inci-

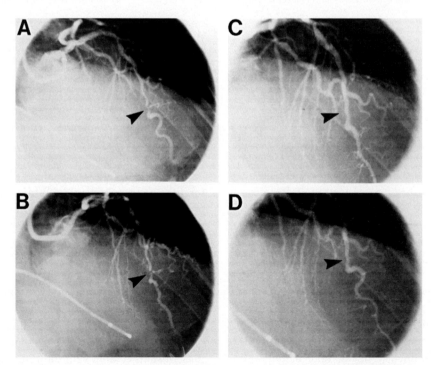

Figure 2.6. Rotational atheroablation of calcified, angulated, tortuous, mid left anterior descending (LAD) lesion. **A.** Right anterior oblique (RAO) with cranial projection of mid vessel stenosis. **B.** After passage of type C guidewire with straightening of distal artery. **C.** After procedure with no significant residual stenosis. Type C guidewire remains in place. **D.** After procedure and after removal of type C guidewire.

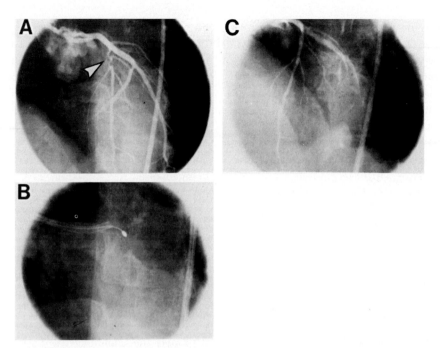

Figure 2.7. Successful rotational atherectomy of tortuous mid-proximal left anterior descending (LAD). **A.** Tortuous diffuse lesion narrowing to 70% immediately after bifurcation of LAD. First diagonal branch in left anterior oblique (LAO) cranial projection. **B.** A 1.75-mm Rotablator burr in proximal LAD. **C.** No residual stenosis after rotational atherectomy with complimentary percutaneous transluminal coronary angioplasty (PTCA), and the first diagonal branch was left undisturbed.

dence of complications in this particular subset with Q-wave infarctions occurring in 2.2% compared to 0.6% in nonbifurcation lesions (18, 19).

RESTENOSIS

Although acute outcome appears improved by rotational ablation, the long-term effect remains uncertain. The actual restenosis rates are difficult to assess accurately because of incomplete angiographic follow-up. Using the most liberal definition of restenosis, namely greater than 50% luminal narrowing at the treatment site, the angiographic restenosis rate was 39% in 78% of 874 possible lesions in patients available for repeat angiography (20). In Stertzer's series of 242 patients, angiographic follow-up was available in 87 patients and clinical follow-up in 182. The combined clinical and angiographic restenosis rate was estimated to be 37% (15).

In a European multicenter series, follow-up angiography was performed in 60% of 129 patients. Restenosis was found in 46% of those who underwent rotablation alone compared with 30% in those patients who had rotational ablation combined with adjunctive balloon angioplasty (21). Angiographic follow-up was available for 91% of a series of 42 patients undergoing stand-alone rotablation for *diffuse* coronary disease. While this select group of patients with narrowings greater than 1 cm in length demonstrated angiographic restenosis in 75%, those with lesions less than 1 cm experienced a low, 22% restenosis rate despite having diffuse disease and stand-alone rotablation (15). These rates compare favorably with restenosis rates in similar lesions treated with balloon angioplasty, especially considering that many of these lesions treated with the Rotablator had failed or were felt to be suboptimal for balloon angioplasty. Direct comparison of restenosis rates following rotablation with other interventions must await the results of randomized trials.

TECHNIQUE

Preprocedural pharmacotherapy is similar to that administered before standard balloon PTCA. All patients are given aspirin and a calcium channel blocker prior to the procedure. All patients receive heparin during the procedure to maintain an activated clotting time (ACT) greater than 350 seconds. It has been our practice to avoid beta-blockers when possible because of concerns of potentially aggravating coronary spasm seen commonly during rotational ablation (22). Intravenous and intracoronary nitroglycerin are routinely administered during the procedure. Venous access is routinely obtained to facilitate placement of a temporary transvenous pacemaker, which is inserted prophylactically for RCA, dominant circumflex, and diffusely diseased, long LAD lesions. Rotablation of lesions in these vessels is commonly associated with transient AV block. This phenomenon is most likely secondary to passage of microparticulate debris or microcavitation bubbles through the vessels perfusing the AV node, SA node, or infranodal conduction tissue.

Guiding catheter selection is identical to balloon PTCA except that the internal diameter must be large enough to accommodate the largest anticipated burr. The routine use of large lumen, 9 Fr guides with sideholes allows passage of burrs up to 2.15 mm. For larger burrs, namely the 2.25 mm and 2.50 mm burrs, 10 Fr guides are needed. Following proper engagement of the guiding catheter, an exchange length, 0.009-inch Rotablator guidewire is usually advanced across the lesion and positioned distally in the artery. Initially, the "bare or free" wire technique can be used. The small-diameter guidewire can be more difficult to manipulate and has less torque than standard angioplasty wires. At times it may be necessary to cross the lesion with a regular PTCA wire and subsequently exchange for the Rotablator wire using a low-profile transfer catheter with a lumen large enough to accommodate the 0.017-inch wire tip.

Once the wire is in place, one can select the initial burr. In general, we recommend using the step technique, which involves starting with a smaller, 1.25 mm to 1.75 mm burr with the intention of sizing up on subsequent passes. We believe that with the step approach, the amount of debris produced per pass and the potential for dissection is drastically reduced. This is especially true in diffusely diseased vessels with limited distal runoff. As far as optimal sizing is concerned, studies utilizing intravascular ultrasound have suggested that the luminal diameter following rotablation exceeds the largest burr diameter by 1.19-fold ($\pm$ 0.19-fold); therefore we have recommended a 0.7 to 0.8 burr-to-artery ratio for optimal and safe debulking (3). Stertzer et al. reported a trend toward higher complications if too large a burr was used initially or if too large a step was used during the progression toward final burr sizes. Several pseudoaneurysms were encountered when attempting to achieve a burr-to-artery ratio of 0.9 to 1.0 (15).

Once a Rotablator catheter is selected, it is loaded onto the guidewire and the burr is advanced manually to the Y-adapter where it is briefly tested and the rotational speed adjusted to approximately 190,000 to 200,000 rpm. With a wire clip placed on the end of the wire, the burr is advanced to the lesion under fluoroscopic observation. Considerable resistance may be met as the burr nears the end of the guiding catheter. Significant negative tension must be applied to the guidewire to advance the burr into the artery. At times it may be necessary to briefly activate the burr in the proximal artery to negotiate tortuosity en route to more distal lesions. Activation of the burr relieves the friction between the burr and wire through the principle of orthogonal displacement of friction facilitating advancement or withdrawal of the burr while maintaining wire position. With the burr positioned slightly proximal to the lesion, rotablation is initiated by advancing the burr in a very slow, pecking motion, very gently withdrawing and readvancing if necessary to prevent the buildup of torque with a subsequent drop in rpms, which could potentially lead to dissections. The burr is gradually advanced across the stenosis several times, each pass lasting 30 to 45 seconds, until the burr passes easily across the lesion site. During withdrawal of the device the air break, which automatically catches the wire, is deactivated while the wire is held externally using a wire clip. Progressively larger burrs are used to achieve the desired burr-to-artery ratio. If deemed necessary, adjunctive balloon dilatation can be performed. It is currently our practice to employ low-pressure balloon inflations (2 to 4 atms) if the residual stenosis is in excess of 20 to 30%. Following completion of the procedure, the patient usually remains on intravenous nitrates, along with oral calcium channel blockers, aspirin, and systemic anticoagulation with heparin for 24 to 36 hours.

Immediately following rotablation, coronary spasm may be present. It occurred in 27% in one report, usually at or distal to the lesion and may be related to vibratory action releasing local, vasoactive mediators (20). This spasm usually recedes following liberal use of intracoronary and intravenous nitroglycerin, but at times may be refractory to pharmacologic intervention. In such cases, we have found that short, low-pressure balloon inflations combined with intracoronary nitrates will usually abate the spasm.

Occasionally, diminished coronary flow associated with symptoms and EKG evidence of ischemia can be seen. This syndrome has been referred to as the "slow-reflow phenomenon." It is most commonly seen following rotablation of longer lesions, particularly in heavily calcified, diffusely diseased arteries with compromised distal vascular beds. One study reported "slow flow" in 9.5% of 286 patients with non-Q-wave MI and Q-wave MI subsequently developing in 33% and 9% of these patients, respectively (23). This has been attributed to delayed capillary clearance of atherosclerotic debris, or perhaps short-lived, microcavitation bubbles. Most of these episodes resolve spontaneously over several minutes; occasionally intensive hemodynamic support with vasopressors and intraaortic balloon pump (IABP) may be required. In our experience, most of these instances of "slow-flow" resolve within 45 minutes to an hour with complete restoration of the baseline hemodynamic status.

Recent experience indicates that patients with high-risk lesions (type B2 or C) or those with decreased left ventricular function may have lower periprocedural complications when elective IABP counterpulsation is used. In our experience with 159 consecutive patients, who on clinical or angiographic criteria were considered to be at high risk for an adverse outcome, those who received elective IABP placement prior to rotational ablation demonstrated a clear decrease in procedural complications. A cohort of 28 patients of these 159 high-risk patients received elective IABP counterpulsation. While slow flow was observed in 18% and 17% of IABP and non-IABP recipients, respectively, periprocedural non–Q-wave myocardial infarction did not occur in any of the IABP patients. In contrast, nine (7%) of the non-IABP recipients suffered a periprocedural non–Q-wave myocardial infarction (O'Murchu B, Foreman R, Peterson K, Buchbinder M, unpublished data, 1995).

CURRENT STATUS

The device was temporarily recalled voluntarily in June 1992 following reports of mechanical malfunction related to the drive-shaft malfunction. The recall was subsequently lifted and clinical investigational use resumed without further incident. The device received FDA approval in June 1993.

At present we are primarily utilizing the Rotablator in any lesion that appears to have morphologic predictors for suboptimal results with balloon PTCA. These predictors include but are not limited to calcification, tortuosity, and ostial location, as well as lesions that are undilatable, are unable to be crossed with a balloon catheter, or result from restenosis from prior intervention. It is recommended that the rotablator not be used in the presence of visible thrombus or in saphenous vein graft lesions.

SUMMARY

High-speed coronary rotational ablation with the Rotablator provides a safe, effective method of revascularization of complex lesions deemed to be suboptimal for standard balloon angioplasty. Restenosis rates in these complex lesions appear to be similar to those seen in less complex lesions treated with balloon angioplasty. Long-term patency with the Rotablator must be considered in the context that many of the lesions being treated are not amenable to balloon angioplasty. The role of rotational ablation in less complex lesions must await randomized trials comparing success, complications, and restenosis with other percutaneous revascularization techniques. As it becomes more evident that mechanical solutions alone are not likely to solve the restenosis problem, the Rotablator will certainly continue to play a useful role in recanalization of difficult lesions, often refractory to balloon dilatation.

REFERENCES

1. Hansen D, Auth D, Hall M, Ritchie J. Rotational Endarterectomy in normal canine coronary arteries: preliminary report. J Am Coll Cardiol 1988;11:1073–1077.

2. Fourrier J, Stonkowiak C, Lablance J, Prat A, Brunetaund J, Bertrand M. Histopathology after rotational angioplasty of peripheral arteries in human beings. J Am Coll Cardiol 1988;11:109.

3. Mintz G, Potkin B, Keren G, Satler L, Pichard A, Kent K, Popma J et al. Intravascular ultrasound evaluation of the effect of rotational atherectomy in obstructive atherosclerotic coronary artery disease. Circulation 1992;86: 1383–1393.

4. Bass T, Gilmore P, White C, Chami Y, Kircher B, Jain S, Conetta D. Surface luminal characteristics following coronary rotational atherectomy vs balloon angioplasty: angioscopic, ultrasound, and angiographic evaluation. J Am Coll Cardiol 1993;21:444A.

5. Prevosti L, Cook J, Unger E, Sheffield C, Almagor Y, Bartorelli A, Leon M. Particulate debris from rotational coronary atherectomy: size, distribution, and physiologic effect. Circulation 1988;78:II-83.

6. Ahn S, Auth D, Marcus D. Removal of focal atheromatous lesions by angiographically guided high-speed rotary atherectomy. J Vasc Surg 1988;7:292.

7. Hansen DD, Auth DC, Vracko R, Ritchie JL. Rotational atherectomy in rabbit iliac arteries. Am Heart J 1988; 115:160–165.

8. Zotz R, Erbel R, Philipp A, Judt A, Wagner H, Lauterborn W, Meyer J. High-speed rotational angioplasty-induced echo contrast in vivo and in vitro optical analysis. Cathet Cardiovasc Diag 1992;26:98–109.

9. Rotablator multicenter registry data through April 1993.

10. Altman D, Popma J, Kent K, Satler L, Pichard A, Mintz G, Keller M, et al. Rotational atherectomy effectively treats calcified lesions. J Am Coll Cardiol 1993;21:443A.

11. Reisman M, Leon M, Rivera I, Pichard A, Satler L, Buchbinder M. Use of the Rotablator in patients with "undilatable" coronary lesions. Circulation 1991;84:II-82.

12. Koschyk D, Terres W, Weber P, Chen C, Hamm C. Less vascular injury after coronary rotablation combined with lo-pressure angioplasty? Investigation with intravascular ultrasound. J Am Coll Cardiol 1993;21:444A.

13. Reisman M, Cohen B, Warth D, Fenner J, Gocka I, Buchbinder M. Outcome of long lesions treated with high-speed rotational ablation. J Am Coll Cardiol 1993;21:443A.

14. Tierstein P, Warth D, Haq N, Jenkins N, McCowan L, Aubanel-Reidel P, Morris N et al. High-speed rotational coronary atherectomy for patients with diffuse coronary artery disease. J Am Coll Cardiol 1991;18:1694–1701.

15. Stertzer S, Rosenblum J, Shaw R, Sugeng I, Hidalgo B, Ryan C, Hansell H et al. Coronary rotational ablation: initial experience in 302 procedures. J Am Coll Cardiol 1992;21:287–295.

16. Rosenblum J, O'Donnell M, Stertzer S, Schechtmann N, Baciewicz P, Hidalgo B, Myler R. Rotational ablation of a severely angulated stenosis previously not amenable to balloon angioplasty. Am Heart J 1991;122:1766–1768.

17. Goudreau E, Cowley M, DiSciascio G, DeBottis D, Vetrovec G, Sabri N. Rotational atherectomy for aorto-ostial and branch ostial lesions. J Am Coll Cardiol 1993;21:31A.

18. Cowley M, Warth D, Whitlow P, Kipperman D, Buchbinder M. Factors influencing outcome with coronary rotational ablation: multicenter results. J Am Coll Cardiol 1993; 21:31A.

19. Whitlow P, Cowley M, Bass T, Warth D. Risk of high-speed rotational atherectomy in bifurcation lesions. J Am Coll Cardiol 1993;21:445A.

20. Buchbinder M, Leon M, Warth D, Marco J, Dorros G, Zacca N, Erbel R. Multicenter registry of percutaneous coronary rotational ablation using the Rotablator. J Am Coll Cardiol 1992;19:333A.

21. Bertrand M, Lablanche J, Leroy F, Bauters C, Jaegere P, Serruys P, Meyer J et al. Percutaneous transluminal coronary rotary ablation with Rotablator (European experience). Am J Cardiol 1992;69:470–474.

22. Nanas J, Sutton R, Alazraki N, Tsagaris T. Acute myocardial infarction in post infarct patient possible through beta blocker–induced coronary artery spasm. Am Heart J 1987;113:388–391.

23. Ellis S, Franco I, Satler L, Whitlow P. Slow reflow and coronary perforation after Rotablator therapy—incidence: clinical, angiographic and procedural predictors. Circulation 1992;86:I-652.

3. Extraction Atherectomy

KEVIN R. KRUSE, MICHAEL H. SKETCH, JR., and RICHARD S. STACK

Since percutaneous transluminal coronary angioplasty (PTCA) was first clinically performed in 1977 by Andreas R. Gruentzig (1), there has been an explosion of new technologic devices to treat atherosclerotic coronary disease (2). Although balloon angioplasty remains the standard treatment strategy for percutaneous revascularization (3), several patient and lesion morphology characteristics have been identified that increase procedural risk, including acute coronary syndromes, ostial location, calcification, thrombus, angulation, eccentric plaque, presence of major side branches, length >20 mm, total occlusions, and degenerated saphenous vein grafts (4–6). The new interventional devices were developed to address these specific limitations of balloon angioplasty. Identifying the potential niches and applying this new technology with the limited clinical data remain the ongoing challenges to all interventional cardiologists.

The transluminal extraction-endarterectomy catheter (TEC) was developed in conjunction with Duke University Medical Center and manufactured by Interventional Technologies Inc. (San Diego, CA). This chapter will focus on the use of the TEC in a practical, problem-solving approach to high-risk lesions often unapproachable by conventional angioplasty.

DESCRIPTION OF THE TEC DEVICE

The TEC device is a percutaneous, over-the-wire, motor-driven cutting and aspiration system (Fig. 3.1). The distal cutting tip has a conical configuration consisting of two stainless steel blades with adjacent windows. Advancement of the TEC cutter requires a unique 0.014-inch TEC guidewire with a radiopaque floppy tip and a 0.021-inch terminal ball. The guidewire is stiff with extra support allowing straightening of the artery and coaxial cutting to avoid vessel perforation. The terminal 0.021-inch distal ball was specifically designed to avoid wire entrapment by the cutting blades. The cutting head is attached to a hollow flexible torque tube that is connected to a handheld catheter drive unit. The drive unit contains the motor and has sites for attachment of a remote battery power source and a detachable vacuum bottle. A trigger on the drive unit simultaneously activates the distal cutting head and vacuum allowing continuous excision and extraction of atherosclerotic plaque and thrombus.

TEC PROCEDURE

Preprocedural treatment follows the same guidelines as routine balloon angioplasty. All patients receive 325 mg of aspirin starting 24 to 48 hours prior to the scheduled procedure. Percutaneous femoral arterial access is obtained using a 10.5 Fr arterial sheath. Once access is obtained, 10,000 units of heparin are administered with additional boluses as required to maintain an activated clotting time (ACT) of 350 to 400 seconds. Routinely following and maintaining an elevated ACT is particularly important when treating lesions in degenerated bypass grafts containing intraluminal thrombus.

The 10.5 Fr arterial sheath allows insertion of a 10 Fr guide catheter, which is required to enable passage of all TEC cutter sizes and to provide adequate opacification of the distal

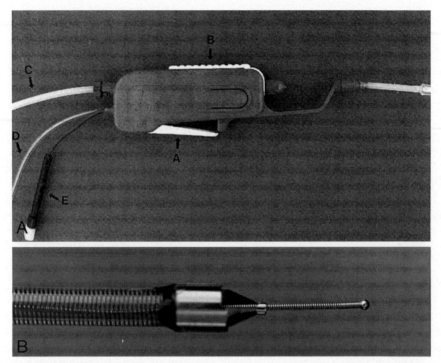

Figure 3.1. **A** The transluminal extraction-endarterectomy catheter (TEC) drive unit. *A,* Trigger; *B,* advancement control level; *C,* rear extension tubing; *D,* suction tubing; *E,* power connector. **B** A close-up of the cutter head and torque tube of the transluminal extraction-endarterectomy catheter over a 0.014-inch TEC guidewire. (From Sketch MH, Phillips HP, Lee M, Stack RS. Coronary transluminal extraction-endarterectomy. J Invest Cardiol 1991;3:23–28 with permission.)

artery. To avoid arterial wall trauma during passage of this large guide catheter to the aortic root, the guide catheter should be advanced over a 0.063-inch J-tip guidewire or a 7 Fr tapered tip multipurpose introducer catheter with a 0.035-inch J-tip guidewire. In patients with peripheral vascular disease a giant-lumen, 9 Fr guide catheter can be used in conjunction with the 5.5 or 6 Fr device.

Once the coronary ostium is engaged, intracoronary nitroglycerin (100 to 200 μg) is administered and preintervention scout injections are obtained. After the lesion is visualized, the TEC guidewire is advanced across the lesion and positioned as far distally as possible to ensure cutting on the stiff radiolucent portion.

The TEC device is assembled, flushed with saline, and tested prior to intracoronary use. Next, the cutter size is selected. Cutter sizes available for coronary use include 5.5 to 7.5 Fr (1.8 to 2.5 mm), and sizes up to 15 Fr are available for peripheral application. In general the cutter is undersized by 1 mm in relationship to the reference vessel diameter. Smaller sizes are initially used for severely stenotic vessels, while larger sizes are used to facilitate primary thrombus extraction.

The selected cutting head is advanced over the wire and positioned several millimeters proximal to the lesion. Intracoronary nitroglycerin is administered prior to cutter activation to minimize coronary vasospasm. To facilitate aspiration of excised material, a pressurized lactated Ringer's solution is infused through the guide catheter. The trigger on the bottom of the housing unit that controls the cutting blade rotation and the vacuum suction is then activated. The cutter rotates at 750 rpm and is manually advanced using a lever at the top of the housing unit. A continuous flow of blood should be seen collecting in the vacuum bottle throughout the procedure and during cutter advancement. After one to three passes across the lesion lasting 10 to 15 seconds each, the lesion is again angiographically visualized. If necessary, progressively larger cutters can be utilized. The material can thus be collected for analysis or histologic examination. If the angiographic results remain unsatisfactory, adjunctive balloon angioplasty can be performed. Sheaths are removed 4 to 6 hours after the procedure unless additional heparin is required.

PRACTICAL APPLICATION

As new technology evolves and clinical experience accumulates, the patient and lesion specific inclusion and exclusion criteria must be reassessed. Initially, the TEC device was used in proximal, discrete, concentric coronary lesions in native vessels. With refinements in the device and enhanced operator experience, these inclusion criteria were successfully expanded to include ostial lesions, degenerated vein grafts, and lesions containing intraluminal thrombus. Balloon angioplasty of these lesions has been associated with high risk and low procedural success. Therefore these lesion characteristics are considered potential niches for TEC application (Table 3.1).

The specific exclusion criteria are listed in Table 3.2. Severe proximal vessel tortuosity can inhibit advancement, especially when larger cutter sizes are required. Moderately to heavily calcified lesions are resistant to debulking and can also restrict advancement of the cutting head. Lesions that are associated with an increase risk of vessel perfora-

Table 3.1
Potential Niches

- Ostial lesions
- Presence of intraluminal thrombus
- Degenerated saphenous vein grafts
- Acute myocardial infarction with large thrombus burden

Table 3.2
TEC Exclusion Criteria

- Tortuous anatomy proximal to the target lesion
- Moderately to heavily calcified lesion
- Severe eccentricity or angulation of the target lesion
- Major dissection
- Bifurcation lesions
- Lesions in vessels less than 2.5 mm in diameter
- Total occlusion unable to be successfully recanalized with a guidewire
- Severe peripheral vascular disease

tion include severely eccentric plaque, angulation >45 degrees, and prior spontaneous dissection. Each individual case must be assessed for the risk of vessel perforation, and extreme care must be maintained to avoid this complication. Bifurcation lesions are not approachable since the side branch cannot be protected with a guidewire during cutting. The other exclusion criteria listed apply to all percutaneous interventional procedures and include inability to cross the stenosis with a guidewire and severe peripheral vascular disease.

RESULTS

U.S. TEC Multicenter Registry

The U.S. TEC Multicenter Registry contains the largest reported experience and consists of 1318 lesions in 1147 patients performed at 29 sites in the United States from July 1988 to January 1992 (24–30). The baseline patient and lesion demographics are outlined in Tables 3.3 and 3.4. This group is unique in that nearly 50% of the patient population was treated for saphenous vein graft stenosis and 28% of these grafts contained thrombus. The mean bypass-graft age was 8.3 years. In native coronary arteries, lesion length was >10 mm in 55% and 14% contained thrombus. Therefore the U.S. TEC Multicenter Registry included high-risk patients in which PTCA has a reduced procedural success rate.

The overall success rates are shown in Table 3.5. Lesion success was defined as reduction in luminal stenosis by at least 20%

Table 3.3
Baseline Demographics

	U.S. TEC Multicenter Registry		NACI Registry
Characteristic	Native Vessels n = 609	Saphenous Vein Grafts n = 538	Native Vessel and SVG n = 211
Age (mean years)	60	65	64
Male	76%	82%	71%
Multivessel disease	44%	89%	81%
Prior MI	32%	50%	62%
Acute MI[a]	18%	14%	NR
Prior CHF	7%	13%	NR
Ejection fraction	NR	NR	49.6%
Graft age (mean years)	N/A	8.3	NR

[a]Percentage of patients who presented with an acute myocardial infarction and subsequently underwent TEC atherectomy for a residual postinfarct stenosis.

TEC, transluminal extraction-endarterectomy catheter; NACI, new approaches to coronary intervention; SVG, saphenous vein grafts; MI, myocardial infarction; CHF, congestive heart failure; NR, not reported; N/A, not applicable.

Table 3.4
Lesion Morphology

	U.S. TEC Multicenter Registry		NACI Registry
Characteristic	Native Vessels n = 668	Saphenous Vein Grafts n = 650	Native Vessel and SVG n = 240
Length > 10 mm	55%	43%	34%
Thrombus	14%	28%	41%
Ostial	9%	9%	NR
Calcification	24%	8%	13%
Total occlusion	5%	10%	9%
SVG age > 3 years	N/A	87%	NR

TEC, Transluminal extraction-endarterectomy catheter; NACI, new approaches to coronary intervention; SVG, saphenous vein grafts; NR, not reported; N/A, not applicable.

Table 3.5
Success Rate

	U.S. TEC Multicenter Registry		NACI Registry
Characteristic	Native Vessels n = 668	Saphenous Vein Grafts n = 650	Native Vessel and SVG n = 240
Lesion success[a]	93%	93%	80%
TEC alone	88%	86%	
TEC + PTCA	95%	96%	
Characteristic	Native Vessels n = 609	Saphenous Vein Grafts n = 538	Native Vessel and SVG n = 211
Patient success[b]	89%	89%	78%
TEC alone	82%	81%	
TEC + PTCA	91%	91%	

[a]Lesion success defined as a reduction in the stenosis by at least 20%, with a residual stenosis ≤50%.

[b]Patient success defined as lesion success for all lesions treated without occurrence of major complication.

TEC, Transluminal extraction-endarterectomy catheter; NACI, new approaches to coronary intervention; SVG, saphenous vein grafts; PTCA, percutaneous transluminal coronary angioplasty.

with a residual narrowing of ≤50%. Patient success was defined as lesion success for all treated lesions without occurrence of major complications. The success rates did not differ between native vessels and saphenous vein grafts with 93% lesion success and 89% patient success. Adjunctive PTCA was required in 76% of native coronary vessels and was associated with an improvement in lesion success to 95% with a patient success of 91%. Treatment of bypass grafts required the use of adjunctive PTCA in 74% of cases and was associated with an increase in lesion success to 96% with a patient success of 91%. Therefore adjunctive PTCA is often utilized and can improve the angiographic result without the occurrence of major complications.

Analysis of major complications is extremely important since it reflects not only patient morbidity and mortality but also increased medical costs. The major complications and overall complication rate are depicted in Figure 3.2. For native coronary

arteries, there was a 5.9% overall complication rate with a 1.2% occurrence of Q-wave myocardial infarction, a 3.6% need for coronary artery bypass grafting, and a 1.6% in-hospital mortality. Compared to native coronary arteries, treatment of saphenous vein bypass grafts had a lower overall complication rate of 4.3%, which was statistically insignificant. The development of Q-wave myocardial infarction was 0.7%, the need for coronary artery bypass grafting was statistically less at 0.4% ($P = .01$), and the associated mortality rate was higher at 3.2% ($P = .09$). Additional complications associated with treatment of bypass grafts included distal embolus 3.7%, perforation 1.0%, transient no-reflow 1.8%, and acute closure 2.9%.

Restenosis remains a significant limitation of balloon angioplasty and has not been shown to be reduced by the application of transluminal extraction atherectomy. The U.S. TEC Multicenter Registry collected information on restenosis, which is summa-

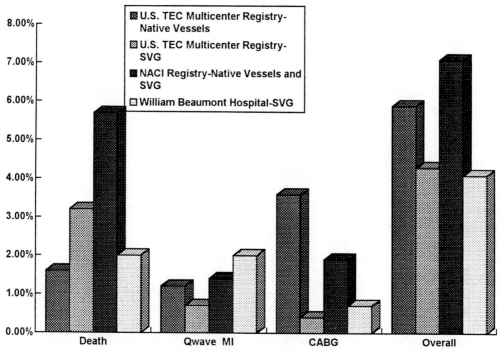

Figure 3.2. Major complications.

Table 3.6
U.S. TEC Multicenter Registry: Restenosis rate

	Native Vessel	Saphenous Vein Grafts
Angiographic follow-up	73%	65%
Angiographic restenosis[a]	51%	60%
TEC alone	54%	66%
TEC + PTCA	49%	59%

[a]Angiographic restenosis defined as lumen diameter narrowing >50% and an increase of at least 30% from the immediate postprocedure stenosis.

TEC, Transluminal extraction-endarterectomy catheter; *PTCA*, percutaneous transluminal coronary angioplasty.

rized in Table 3.6. The angiographic restenosis rate was defined as an increase of at least 30% from the immediate postprocedure stenosis and greater than 50% luminal narrowing at 6-month follow-up. For native vessels there was a 73% angiographic follow-up of eligible patients with a reported restenosis rate of 51%. The angiographic follow-up was 65% for saphenous vein grafts with a restenosis rate of 60%.

Additional information on restenosis is provided by the Duke Multicenter Coronary TEC Registry. Patients were enrolled at five centers between July 1988 and April 1991. A total of 351 lesions in 313 patients were treated with a 6-month angiographic follow-up rate of 84% in 256 eligible patients. Restenosis defined as 50% or greater diameter stenosis occurred in 48% of patients (103 of 215). Overall lesion restenosis rate was 45% (native artery: 45%; vein graft: 46%). Although the total numbers are small, subgroup analysis revealed that a <25% residual stenosis in native arteries led to a 34% restenosis rate. When TEC alone produced a <25% residual stenosis, an 18% restenosis rate was observed (31).

Other studies have supported the concept that restenosis appears to be directly related to acute procedural gain, which is known as the "bigger is better" theory (32). A specific study to address this theory examined 146 cineangiograms using TEC atherectomy from 20 centers (33). The overall restenosis rate

(≥50% diameter stenosis) was 55%. For lesions with a final diameter stenosis of <30%, the restenosis rate was 46%. If a less than 20% diameter stenosis was obtained, the restenosis rate was 35%. When aggressively attempting to minimize the residual diameter stenosis, caution must always be maintained to avoid an increase in acute procedural complications.

NACI Registry

Additional nonrandomized data are now available from the new approaches to coronary intervention (NACI) registry (34). From November 1990 to November 1992, fourteen participating centers collected data on transluminal extraction atherectomy involving 240 lesions in 211 patients. Although both native vessel and saphenous vein graft lesions were included, saphenous vein graft lesions comprised 64% of the total population. The baseline patient demographics and lesion morphologies are summarized in Tables 3.3 and 3.4. In this cohort of patients, 24% were considered inoperable/high risk, 81% had two- to three-vessel coronary artery disease, and 62% had a prior myocardial infarction. The lesion morphology was also high risk since 34% of lesions were >10 mm in length and 41% contained thrombus. Success was defined as either device success (stenosis improvement by ≥20% and residual stenosis <50% after device alone), lesion success (stenosis improvement by ≥20% with a final residual stenosis <50%), or procedural success (lesion success without major complications). There was a 48% device success with requirement of adjunctive PTCA in 89% of cases to achieve an 80% lesion success rate. The overall procedural success rate was 78% (Table 3.5). Although the success rates were comparable to other studies, the complication rates were higher than previously reported (Fig. 3.2). The overall complication rate was 7.1% with 1.4% Q-wave myocardial infarction, 1.9% CABG, and 5.7% in-hospital mortality rate. Since this is a nonrandomized observational study, the preferential treatment of a higher-risk patient population with high-risk lesion morphology, including degenerative saphenous vein grafts, may contribute to this observed complication rate.

POTENTIAL NICHE APPLICATIONS

With the rapid introduction of new interventional technologies comes the need to define potential niches for each revascularization device. A major limitation in determining potential niches for the TEC device is the absence of a randomized trial. Since randomized trial results are not available, application is currently based on clinical experience and observational data. Potential niches for the TEC device are ostial lesions, degenerative saphenous vein grafts, and lesions with intraluminal thrombus; however, further rigorous testing is warranted to confirm these niche applications (35–40). Patients with these lesion characteristics have previously been defined as a high-risk group with poor success when treated with standard PTCA. Of all the potential niche applications, the TEC device appears to be most suitable for treatment of degenerative saphenous vein-graft lesions and thrombus. The treatment of degenerated saphenous vein grafts, especially those associated with thrombus, presents a difficult treatment dilemma and warrants further discussion.

Understanding the mechanisms of saphenous vein-graft atherosclerosis is essential in managing patients who present with graft closure and stenosis. The mechanisms of graft closure include thrombus, intimal hyperplasia, and atherosclerosis. These processes can occur simultaneously within a saphenous vein-graft conduit, but often operate at different times following graft implantation.

In the early postoperative period, platelets and the coagulation system interact predisposing to early graft closure. Predisposing factors to early thrombosis include injury to venous endothelium during harvesting, implantation anastomosis trauma, graft tension, and sudden exposure to high arterial pressure. Poor distal runoff and graft-to-distal vessel mismatch with resultant slow vein-graft blood flow can predispose to thrombosis. Previous studies have demonstrated that antiplatelet therapy with aspirin and dipyridamole will reduce the risk of acute graft closure (41), and that this therapy appears particularly important during the first year (42).

If grafts remain patent without acute thrombosis, they develop intimal hyperplasia, which produces additional graft narrowing and contributes to the graft attrition rate by the first postoperative year. These lesions are typically focal and are particularly amenable to percutaneous revascularization. Arteriosclerosis appears to predominate in late graft stenoses and leads to the development of degenerative vein grafts. Microscopically, this lesion appears similar to native atherosclerotic lesions with lipid-laden macrophages, smooth muscle cells, cholesterol clefts, organized thrombus, fibrocollagenous tissue, and calcified deposits. However, an observed increased quantity of foam cells can predispose to plaque fissure and rupture with the development of superimposed thrombosis (43–49). It is the presence of this friable tissue that has previously defied percutaneous attempts at revascularizing degenerative saphenous vein grafts.

Because of these mechanisms, the graft attrition rate has been reported to be 15 to 22% during the first year, 1 to 2% per year between the first and sixth years, and 4 to 5% per year between the sixth and tenth years for saphenous vein bypass grafts (50–52). The process of graft occlusion and stenosis contributes to the recurrence of angina and reduced survival after 7 to 10 years. The treatment of patients who require revascularization is particularly challenging. The morbidity and mortality of reoperation are greater than the initial surgery and vary according to operative experience and institution. Recent studies have noted a 2.5 to 7.5% thirty-day operative mortality and a 4.0 to 9.2% perioperative myocardial infarction rate. Patients have less early relief of angina associated with reoperation during the first postoperative year; however, 5- to 10-year follow-up shows similar mortality rates (53).

As the number of coronary artery bypass procedures increases (now more than 350,000 per year) and the patient population ages, there has been an increasing pool of post-bypass patients who present for management of recurrent ischemia. In the initial 1979 report on nonoperative dilatation of coronary artery stenosis by Gruentzig and colleagues (1), saphenous vein angioplasty was shown to be feasible with an angiographic success rate of 71% (five out of seven attempted procedures). Unfortunately, restenosis was noted to occur in three of five grafts during follow-up. In 1983 Douglas and associates reported on a larger series to examine this attractive alternative to reoperation (54). A total of 62 patients were treated for saphenous vein graft lesions, and the success rate (defined as >30% reduction in stenosis) was 94%. The restenosis rate was reported on 41 patients and was 34%. Although this initial report was promising, the study represented a low-risk group of patients in that 62% of grafts were less than 1 year old and 55% of lesions occurred at the anastomosis site.

A more recent review by De Feyter and associates summarized the results of previous trials totaling 1571 patients treated for saphenous vein-graft lesions (55). The overall clinical success was 88%, and the 6-month restenosis rate was 42% (restenosis rate by site was 58% proximal, 52% body, and 28% anastomosis). Procedural complications were low with a <4% occurrence of myocardial infarction, a <2% need for urgent CABG, and a <1% mortality. Risk factors, which were identified to predict unfavorable outcome, included diffuse disease, graft age >4 to 6 years, presence of thrombus, proximal or body stenosis, and chronically occluded saphenous vein grafts. It is likely that the more difficult high-risk-lesion morphologies

were excluded from these observational reports. In fact, a study by Platko and associates identified graft age as an independent predictor of poor outcome (56). Between 1981 and 1987, 101 patients were treated for saphenous vein-graft stenosis. A total of 107 bypass grafts were dilated at 117 sites. The angiographic follow-up was 56.3% and the clinical follow-up was 96.7%. Of the 53 patients with graft age <36 months, there were no complications, the angiographic restenosis rate was 42%, and the continued clinical success (survival without myocardial infarction, repeat angioplasty, bypass surgery, or symptom recurrence) was 67% at 54-month follow-up. The 48 patients with graft age >36 months suffered an overall complication rate of 14.9% with a 12.5% incidence of myocardial infarction, a 4% need for coronary bypass surgery, and a 4% mortality. In addition, these patients had an 83% angiographic restenosis rate with continued clinical success in only 36%. Since these initial series, interventional cardiologists continue to struggle with revascularizing the higher-risk saphenous vein-graft lesions.

To help clarify the role of TEC atherectomy, a recent study reported on a consecutive institutional patient experience in treating saphenous vein grafts (57). Between December 1988 and June 1992 TEC atherectomy was performed on 158 lesions in 146 patients. The mean graft age was 8.3 years, and lesion morphology was complex, including lesion length of >10 mm (54%), aorto-ostial location (21%), eccentricity (64%), and associated thrombus (28%). Although acute myocardial infarctions were excluded, total occlusions represented 6% of the lesions treated. In this high-risk group, transluminal extraction atherectomy produced a 39.2% device success rate and required adjunctive PTCA in 91.2% to achieve a procedural success rate of 84%. The complication rates were similar to the U.S. TEC Multicenter Registry data and included a 4.1% overall complication rate with a 2% incidence of

Q-wave myocardial infarction, a .7% need for CABG, and a 2% mortality rate (Fig. 3.2). Unfortunately, application of TEC atherectomy to saphenous vein grafts may be limited by distal embolization (11.9%), no-reflow (8.8%), abrupt closure (5.0%), and a restenosis rate of 69%.

As mentioned previously, the U.S. TEC Multicenter Registry provides information on the treatment of a larger series of saphenous vein-graft lesions (30). A total of 650 lesions (mean graft age was 8.3 years) were treated with TEC atherectomy with an overall lesion success rate of 93%. For saphenous vein grafts >3 years, the success rate was 94%, and, for those grafts containing intraluminal thrombus, the success rate was 90%. Although TEC atherectomy had a high procedural success rate, it was associated with in-hospital morbidity, a mortality rate of 3.2% (2.4% in patients not treated during acute MI) and a late restenosis rate of 50 to 60%. It is uncertain whether these complications are intrinsic to the TEC catheter or related to the high-risk lesions and patient population. Although the TEC atherectomy should be used cautiously, it can be recommended as a potential niche device to treat diffusely diseased degenerative saphenous vein grafts.

Case Reports and Technical Considerations

The following case reports are included to illustrate the technical aspects and practical application of transluminal extraction atherectomy.

CASE 1

A 58-year-old man initially presented 6 years ago with an inferior myocardial infarction. Subsequent cardiac catheterization revealed an ejection fraction of 52% with moderate inferior hypokinesis and severe, three-vessel coronary artery disease. A four-vessel coronary artery bypass grafting procedure was performed with placement of a right internal mammary artery (RIMA) to the right coronary artery, a left internal mammary artery (LIMA) to the left anterior descending artery, and saphenous vein grafts to the ramus intermedius and the second obtuse marginal.

He presented with a 2-month history of progressive refractory angina despite maximum medical therapy. Therefore he underwent a cardiac catheterization, which showed an ejection fraction of 66% with mild mitral regurgitation. The native coronary arteries were remarkable for a 95% left anterior descending artery, 50% left circumflex, and 75% obtuse diagonal stenosis with occlusion of the second obtuse marginal and the right coronary artery. The right and left internal mammary arteries were patent without stenosis. The saphenous vein graft to the obtuse diagonal was occluded and the saphenous vein graft to the second obtuse marginal had a 95% diffuse proximal stenosis (Fig. 3.3 A).

This case illustrates an interesting treatment dilemma. Although the saphenous vein graft is only 6 years old, the lesion is diffuse with the appearance of thrombus and friable tissue consistent with a degenerated saphenous vein graft. In addition, the abrupt angulated origin places this stenosis at high risk for percutaneous revascularization. Primary balloon angioplasty without debulking would likely be associated with a lower procedural success and a higher restenosis rate. Stenting would be technically difficult because of the acute angulated origin, which could impede stent advancement. Successful treatment would also require multiple overlapping stents. Since the lesion is diffuse, it is not particularly amenable to debulking with directional atherectomy. Laser application is limited in the treatment of diffuse degenerated saphenous vein grafts containing thrombus. Therefore the transluminal extraction atherectomy catheter was selected as the initial device to facilitate thrombus extraction and plaque debulking.

A 10 Fr hockey stick catheter was used and provided exceptional backup support. After initial heparin bolus, an activated clotting time (ACT) of 426 seconds was achieved. A 0.014-inch TEC guidewire was advanced across the lesion and positioned as far distally as possible. Two passes were made with a 7 Fr cutter, and the excised material was collected in the vacuum bottle. A post-TEC angiogram showed marked angiographic improvement (Fig. 3.3 B). After tissue debulking, a 40 mm 4.0 balloon catheter was positioned across the residual stenosis and inflated to 8 atm for three minutes. This produced a successful final angiographic result of 25% with minor dissection (Fig. 3.3 C). There were no procedural or in-hospital complications.

This case report illustrates the application of the TEC device to diffusely diseased, degenerative saphenous vein-graft lesions. The initial plaque debulking achieved by tissue and thrombus extraction allowed for successful balloon angioplasty. Although proximal vessel tortuosity and lesion angulation are contraindica-

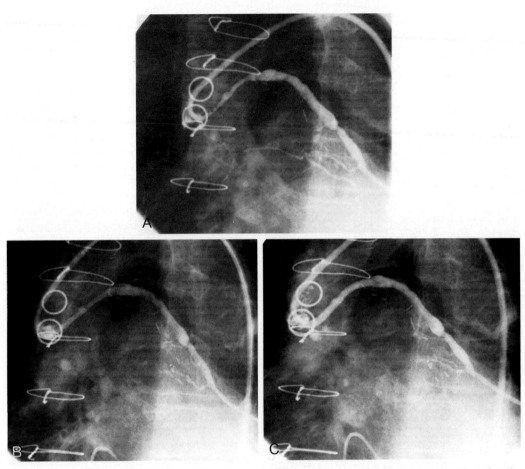

Figure 3.3. **A** Angiogram demonstrating a 95% diffuse stenosis in the proximal body of the saphenous vein graft to the second obtuse marginal. **B** Repeat angiogram in the right anterior oblique projection after two passes with a 7 Fr TEC cutter. **C** Final result obtained after adjunctive balloon angioplasty.

tions to transluminal extraction atherectomy, the cutter and torque tube system is flexible and in this case allowed passage across the angulated saphenous vein-graft origin. To avoid vessel perforation, caution must be maintained to ensure advancement over the stiff portion of the guidewire and adequate blood flow into the vacuum bottle.

CASE 2

A 74-year-old woman underwent coronary artery bypass grafting 12 years ago for unstable angina with placement of saphenous vein grafts to the right coronary artery and left anterior descending artery. She developed recurrent angina 5 years later, which was successfully treated medically. A 2-month history of unstable angina culminated in her current admission for a non-Q-wave myocardial infarction. The hospital course was complicated by transient atrial fibrillation, mild congestive heart failure, and recurrent angina. A diagnostic cardiac catheterization revealed an ejection fraction of 35% with anterior hypokinesis. The native coronary anatomy was remarkable for total occlusion of the left anterior descending and right coronary arteries with a 50% obstruction of the first obtuse marginal. The saphenous vein graft to the right coronary artery was patent. The infarct-related artery was the saphenous vein graft to the left anterior descending, which had a 95% mid-body stenosis with a filling defect. She was transferred on intravenous heparin for further management. Although relook preintervention injections revealed a decrease in the size of the filling defect, there was a persistent haziness in a focal lattice-type configuration (Fig. 3.4 *A*).

There were multiple treatment options available, including directional atherectomy, intracoronary stenting, balloon angioplasty, intracoronary thrombolytic therapy, or continued medical management. Because of the history of postinfarction angina and the concern over persistent thrombus following angiography, transluminal extraction atherectomy was chosen as the initial therapeutic intervention to facilitate evacuation of persistent clot and/or friable saphenous vein-graft material.

A 10 Fr JR-4 guide catheter and a 0.014-inch TEC guidewire were used. The lesion underwent two passes with a 7 Fr TEC cutter reducing the stenosis to 25% with a minor dissection and evidence of a reduced but persistent angiographic intraluminal filling defect. Next, a 20 mm 3.5 balloon catheter was inflated to 10 atm for 5 minutes resulting in an improved angiographic appearance. The final residual stenosis was <25% without persistent dissection (Fig. 3.4 B). There were no procedural complications, and the patient denied any recurrent angina during her hospital course.

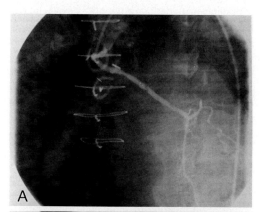

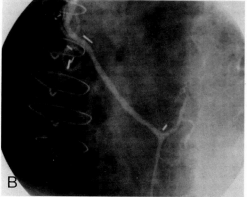

Figure 3.4.   **A** Saphenous vein graft to the left anterior descending artery with a 75% stenosis and an intraluminal filling defect suggestive of thrombus. **B** Final result following TEC atherectomy and adjunctive balloon angioplasty.

It is often technically difficult to distinguish thrombus from friable plaque tissue by angiography. Angioscopy has shown promise in differentiating clot from dissection flaps in saphenous vein grafts. Transluminal extraction atherectomy has the advantage in this setting to treat lesions with a high clinical suspicion for associated thrombus. If a significant filling defect had persisted after the initial cuts and if the vessel size had permitted, consecutively larger cutters could be used to facilitate further clot extraction.

CASE 3

A 39-year-old man presented 6 years ago with a myocardial infarction and subsequently underwent coronary artery bypass grafting. He was successfully revascularized with placement of a left internal mammary artery to the left anterior descending artery and saphenous vein grafts to the first diagonal and the first obtuse marginal. Over the ensuing years he required multiple hospital admissions for recurrent angina but was treated medically. Six months ago he underwent cardiac catheterization that revealed an ejection fraction of 60%, patent bypass grafts, and tandem 95% lesions in the native right coronary artery. The balloon angioplasty procedure of the right coronary artery was complicated by a myocardial infarction. Repeat cardiac catheterization 2 months later revealed an occluded right coronary artery that was managed medically. Despite medical therapy, he developed recurrent chest pain and presented with a non-Q-wave myocardial infarction. The culprit lesion was the saphenous vein graft to the first diagonal, which showed a 75% ulcerated body stenosis with a large intraluminal filling defect by angiography (Fig. 3.5 A). Coumadin anticoagulation therapy was initiated. Five days after discharge he required readmission for recurrent angina and was referred for further management.

Given the patient's young age, obtaining an adequate result and reducing the rate of restenosis are imperative. Although extensive research on medical therapies involving antiplatelet agents, antithrombotic agents, calcium channel blockers, antiproliferative agents, lipid-lowering agents, angiotension-converting enzyme inhibitors, and growth factor inhibitors has shown conflicting results, no overall benefit has been demonstrated (3, 22). The EPIC trial demonstrated a reduction in clinical restenosis for a specific class of antiplatelet drugs that block the platelet glycoprotein IIb/IIIa receptor (58–59). In the BENESTENT and STRESS trials, angiographic restenosis was reduced by 25 to 30% in de novo coronary lesions treated with the Palmaz-Schatz stent. Although the degree of intimal proliferation is not diminished, the Palmaz-Schatz stent

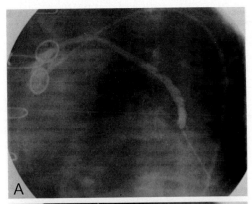

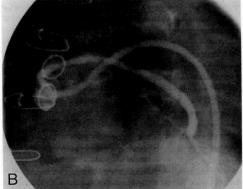

Figure 3.5. **A** Angiogram demonstrating a 75% stenosis in the body of the saphenous vein graft to the first diagonal. Associated intraluminal thrombus was confirmed by angioscopy. **B** Final result obtained after TEC atherectomy and placement of a Palmaz-Schatz stent.

creates a larger initial lumen (60, 61). This is consistent with the "bigger is better" theory of coronary restenosis. In this case, multiple device technologies were applied to achieve the best angiographic result with the largest luminal dimension.

Initial preintervention injections revealed a 75% body stenosis of the saphenous vein graft to the first diagonal. A 10 Fr hockey stick guiding catheter and a 0.014-inch TEC guidewire were used. Angioscopy was performed and revealed red thrombus material occupying 80% of the cross-sectional area. Because of the persistent intraluminal thrombus, a 7.5 Fr TEC cutter was selected, and three passes were performed without complications. A post-TEC angiographic filling defect was documented by angioscope to represent a large intraluminal dissection flap. Without evidence of persistent intraluminal thrombus, a Palmaz-Schatz stent was deployed. To obtain the largest luminal diameter, the stent was expanded with a 5.0 balloon catheter. Angioscopy documented complete deployment, and the final angiogram showed no residual stenosis (Fig. 3.5 *B*). This case demonstrates the adjunctive use of new interventional technologies to successfully treat high-risk-lesion morphology.

SUMMARY

The transluminal extraction-endarterectomy catheter is a unique interventional device that utilizes distal rotating and cutting blades to both excise and aspirate atheromatous plaque. The U.S. Food and Drug Administration has approved the TEC device for use in peripheral arteries, coronary arteries, and saphenous vein bypass grafts. Because of its unique design, the TEC catheter has potential niche application in the treatment of ostial lesions, degenerated saphenous vein grafts, and intraluminal thrombus. Of these niches, degenerated bypass grafts appear particularly suitable for revascularization with the transluminal extraction atherectomy catheter. Although no comparative experience with balloon angioplasty exists for this cohort of patients, previous studies have documented the high risk involved in treating old (<36 month) bypass grafts, especially in the presence of intraluminal thrombus. Determining the optimal revascularization strategy is currently based on observational series and will require confirmation by well-designed randomized trials.

As clinical experience accumulates and technology advances, the strategies for percutaneous revascularization will continue to evolve. An area of future development for the TEC device includes an expandable cutting head. This design has potential application in saphenous vein grafts to facilitate use as a stand-alone device, to extract thrombus, and to minimize the residual luminal diameter.

REFERENCES

1. Gruentzig AR, Senning A, Siegenthaler WE. Nonoperative dilation of coronary-artery stenosis: percutaneous transluminal coronary angioplasty. N Engl J Med 1979; 301:61–68.
2. Stack RS, Califf RM, Phillips HR, Pryor DB, Quigley PJ, Bauman RP, Tcheng JE et al. Interventional cardiac catheterization at Duke Medical Center. Am J Cardiol 1988;62:3F–24F.
3. Landau C, Lange RA, Hillis LD. Percutaneous transluminal coronary angioplasty. N Engl J Med 1994;330:981–993.
4. Myler RK, Shaw RE, Stertzer SH, Hecht HS, Ryan C, Rosenblum J, Cumberland DC et al. Lesion morphology and coronary angioplasty: current experience and analysis. J Am Coll Cardiol 1992;19:1641–1652.

5. Weintraub WS, Kosinski AS, Brown CL, King SB. Can restenosis after coronary angioplasty be predicted from clinical variables? J Am Coll Cardiol 1993;21:6–14.

6. Killip T. Twenty years of coronary bypass surgery. N Engl J Med 1988;319:366–368.

7. Topol EJ, Ellis SG, Cosgrove DM, Bates ER, Muller DW, Schork NJ, Schork MA et al. Analysis of coronary angioplasty practice in the United States with an insurance-claims data base. Circulation 1993;87:1489–1497.

8. Detre K, Holubkov R, Kelsey S, Cowley M, Kent K, Williams D, Myler R et al. Percutaneous transluminal coronary angioplasty in 1985–1986 and 1977–1981. The NHLBI registry. N Engl J Med 1988;318:265–270.

9. Waller BF. "Crackers, Breakers, Stretchers, Drillers, Scrapers, Shavers, Burners, Welders and Melters"—the future treatment of atherosclerotic coronary artery disease? A clinical-morphologic assessment. J Am Coll Cardiol 1989; 13:969–987.

10. Block PC, Myler RK, Stertzer S, Fallon JT. Morphology after transluminal angioplasty in human beings. N Engl J Med 1981;305:382–385.

11. Simpfendorfer C, Belardi J, Bellamy G, Galan K, Franco I, Hollman J. Frequency, management and follow-up of patients with acute coronary occlusions after percutaneous transluminal coronary angioplasty. Am J Cardiol 1987; 59:267–269.

12. Ellis SG, Roubin GS, King SB, Douglas J, Weintaub WS, Thomas RG, Cox WR. Angiographic and clinical predictors of acute closure after native vessel coronary angioplasty. Circulation 1988;77:372–379.

13. Detre KM, Holmes DR, Holubkov R, Cowley MJ, Bourassa MG, Faxon DP, Dorros GR et al. Incidence and consequences of periprocedural occlusion: The 1985–1986 NHLBI percutaneous transluminal coronary angioplasty registry. Circulation 1990;82:739–750.

14. Lincoff AM, Popma JJ, Ellis SG, Hacker JA, Topol EJ. Abrupt vessel closure complicating coronary angioplasty: clinical, angiographic and therapeutic profile. J Am Coll Cardiol 1992;19:926–935.

15. Serruys PW, Foley DP, Kirkeeide RL, King SB. Restenosis revisited: insights provided by quantitative coronary angiography. Am Heart J 1993;126:1243–1267.

16. Nobuyoshi M, Kimura T, Ohishi H, Horiuchi H, Nosaka H, Hamasaki N, Yokoi H et al. Restenosis after percutaneous transluminal coronary angioplasty: pathologic observations in 20 patients. J Am Coll Cardiol 1991;17:433–439.

17. Liu MW, Roubin GS, King SB. Restenosis after coronary angioplasty: potential biologic determinants and role of intimal hyperplasia. Circulation 1989;79:1374–1387.

18. Dzau VJ, Gibbons GH, Cooke JP, Omoigui N. Vascular biology and medicine in the 1990s: scope, concepts, potentials, and perspectives. Circulation 1993;87:705–718.

19. Gibbons GH, Dzau VJ. The emerging concept of vascular remodeling. N Engl J Med 1994;330:1431–1438.

20. Mcbride W, Lange RA, Hillis LD. Restenosis after successful coronary angioplasty: pathophysiology and prevention. N Engl J Med 1988;318:1734–1737.

21. Califf RM, Fortin DF, Frid DJ, Harlan WR, Ohman EM, Bengtson JR, Nelson CL et al. Restenosis after coronary angioplasty: an overview. J Am Coll Cardiol 1991;17: 2B–13B.

22. Hermans WR, Rensing BJ, Strauss BH, Serruys PW. Prevention of restenosis after percutaneous transluminal coronary angioplasty: the search for a "magic bullet." Am Heart J 1991;122:171–187.

23. Waller BF, Pinkerton CA, Orr CM, Slack JD, VanTassel JW, Peters T. Restenosis 1 to 24 months after clinically successful coronary balloon angioplasty: a necropsy study of 20 patients. J Am Coll Cardiol 1991;17:58B–70B.

24. O'Neill WW, Kramer BL, Sketch MH, Meany TB, Pichard AD, Knopf WD, Grines CL et al. Mechanical extraction atherectomy: report of the U.S. transluminal extraction catheter investigation. Circulation 1992;86:I-779 (abstract).

25. Meany T, Kramer B, Knopf W, Pichard A, Sketch M, Juran N, Stack R et al. Multicenter experience of atherectomy of saphenous vein grafts: immediate results and follow-up. J Am Coll Cardiol 1992;19:262A (abstract).

26. Sketch MH, O'Neill WW, Galichia JP, Feldman RC, Walker CM, Sawchak SR, Tcheng JE et al. The Duke multicenter coronary transluminal extraction-endarterectomy registry: acute and chronic results. J Am Coll Cardiol 1991;17:31A (abstract).

27. Sketch MH, O'Neill WW, Tcheng JE, Walker C, Galichia JP, Sawchak S, Cress S et al. Early and late outcome following coronary transluminal extraction-endarterectomy: a multicenter experience. Circulation 1990;82:III-310 (abstract).

28. Sutton JM, Gitlin JB, Casale PN. Major complications after TEC atherectomy: preliminary analysis derived from the multicenter registry experience. Circulation 1992;86:I-456 (abstract).

29. Sketch MH, Phillips HP, Lee MM, Stack RS. Coronary transluminal extraction-endarterectomy. J Invasive Cardiol 1991;3:13–18.

30. Labinaz M, Sketch MH, O'Neill WW, Stack RS. Transluminal extraction-endarterectomy. In: Roubin GS, Califf RM, O'Neal WW, Phillips HR, Stack RS, eds. Interventional cardiovascular medicine: principles and practice. New York: Churchill Livingstone, 1994.

31. Sketch MH, O'Neill WW, Galichia JP, Feldman RC, Walker CM, Sawchak SR, Meany TB et al. Restenosis following coronary transluminal extraction-endarterectomy: the final analysis of a multicenter registry. J Am Coll Cardiol 1992;19:277A (abstract).

32. Kuntz RE, Baim DS. Defining coronary restenosis: newer clinical and angiographic paradigms. Circulation 1993; 88:1310–1323.

33. Popma JJ, O'Neill WW, Kramer B, Moses J, Sketch MH, Whitlow PL, Knopf W et al. A quantitative analysis of late angiographic outcome after transluminal extraction-endarterectomy (TEC). Circulation 1992;86:I-457.

34. Baim DS, Kent KM, King SB, Safian RD, Cowley MJ, Holmes DR, Roubin GS et al. Evaluating new devices: acute (in-hospital) results from the new approaches to coronary intervention registry. Circulation 1994; 89:471–481.

35. Guzman LA, Villa AE, Whitlow P. New atherectomy devices in the treatment of old saphenous vein grafts: are the initial results encouraging? Circulation 1992;86:I-780 (abstract).

36. Lincoff AM, Guzman LA, Casale PN, Ellis SG, Whitlow PL. Impact of atherectomy devices on the management of saphenous vein graft lesions with associated thrombus. Circulation 1992;86:I-779 (abstract).

37. Kramer B, Larkin T, Niemyski P, Parker M. Coronary atherectomy in acute ischemic syndromes: implications of thrombus on treatment outcome. J Am Coll Cardiol 1991;17:385A (abstract).

38. O'Neill WW, Meany TB, Kramer B, Knopf WD, Pichard AD, Sketch MH, Stack RS. The role of atherectomy in the management of saphenous vein grafts disease. J Am Coll Cardiol 1991;17:384A (abstract).

39. Popma JJ, Leon MB, Mintz GS, Kent KM, Satler LF, Garrand TJ, Pichard AD. Results of coronary angioplasty using the transluminal extraction catheter. Am J Cardiol 1992; 70:1526–1532.

40. Leon MB, Pichard AD, Kramer BL, Knopf W, O'Neill W, Stack R. Efficacious and safe transluminal extraction atherectomy in patients with unfavorable coronary lesions. J Am Coll Cardiol 1991;17:219A (abstract).

41. Chesebro JH, Clements IP, Fuster J, Elueback LR, Smith HC, Bardsley WT, Frye RL et al. A platelet-inhibitor-drug trial in coronary-artery bypass operations: benefit of perioperative dipridamole and aspirin therapy on early postoperative vein-graft patency. N Engl J Med 1982; 307:73–78.

42. Goldman S, Copeland J, Moritz T, Henderson W, Zadina K, Ovitt T, Kern K et al. Long-term graft patency (3 years) after coronary artery surgery: effects of aspirin. Results of a VA cooperative study. Circulation 1994;89:1138–1143.

43. Walts AE, Fishbein MC, Matloff JM. Thrombosed, ruptured atheromatous plaques in saphenous vein coronary artery bypass grafts: ten years' experience. Am Heart J 1987; 114:718–723.

44. Vlodaver Z, Edwards JE. Pathologic changes in aortic-coronary arterial saphenous vein grafts. Circulation 1971; 44:719–728.

45. Bulkley BH, Hutchins GM. Accelerated "atherosclerosis": a morphologic study of 97 saphenous vein coronary artery bypass grafts. Circulation 1977;55:163–169.

46. Kalan JM, Roberts WC. Morphologic findings in saphenous veins used as coronary arterial bypass conduits for longer than 1 year: necropsy analysis of 53 patients, 123 saphenous veins, and 1865 five-millimeter segments of veins. Am Heart J 1990;119:1164–1184.

47. Waller BF, Rothbaum DA, Gorfinkel HJ, Ulbright TM, Linnemeier TJ, Berger SM. Morphologic observations after percutaneous transluminal balloon angioplasty of early and late aortocoronary saphenous vein bypass grafts. J Am Coll Cardiol 1984;4:784–792.

48. Shelton ME, Forman MB, Virmani R, Bajaj A, Stoney WS, Atkinson JB. A comparison of morphologic and angiographic findings in long-term internal mammary artery and saphenous vein bypass grafts. J Am Coll Cardiol 1988; 11:297–307.

49. Lawrie GM, Lie JT, Morris GC, Beazley HL. Vein graft patency and intimal proliferation after aortocoronary bypass: early and long-term angiopathologic correlations. Am J Cardiol 1976;38:856–862.

50. Lytle BW, Loop FD, Cosgrove DM, Ratliff NB, Easley K, Taylor PC. Long-term (5 to 12 years) serial studies of internal mammary artery and saphenous vein coronary bypass grafts. J Thorac Cardiovasc Surg 1985;89:248–258.

51. Frey RR, Bruschke AV, Vermeulen FE. Serial angiographic evaluation 1 year and 9 years after aorto-coronary bypass. J Thorac Cardiovasc Surg 1984;87:167–174.

52. Fitzgibbon GM, Burton JR, Leach AJ. Coronary bypass graft fate: angiographic grading of 1400 consecutive grafts early after operation and of 1132 after one year. Circulation 1978;57:1070–1074.

53. Cameron A, Kemp HG, Green GE. Reoperation for coronary artery disease: 10 years of clinical follow-up. Circulation 1988;78(Suppl):I-158–162.

54. Douglas JS, Gruentzig AR, King SB, Hollman J, Ischinger T, Meier B, Craver JM et al. Percutaneous transluminal coronary in patients with prior coronary bypass surgery. J Am Coll Cardiol 1983;2:745–754.

55. De Feyter PJ, Van Suylen RJ, De Jaegere PT, Topol EJ, Serruys PW. Balloon angioplasty for the treatment of lesions in saphenous vein bypass grafts. J Am Coll Cardiol 1993;21:1539–1549.

56. Platko WP, Hollman J, Whitlow PL, Franco I. Percutaneous transluminal angioplasty of saphenous vein graft stenosis: long-term follow-up. J Am Coll Cardiol 1989; 14:1645–1650.

57. Safian RD, Grines CL, May MA, Lichtenberg A, Juran N, Schreiber TL, Pavlides G et al. Clinical and angiographic results of transluminal extraction coronary atherectomy in saphenous vein bypass grafts. Circulation 1994; 189:302–312.

58. Califf RM and the EPIC investigators. Use of a monoclonal antibody directed against the platelet glycoprotein IIb/IIIa receptor in high-risk coronary angioplasty. N Engl J Med 1994;330:956–961.

59. Topol EJ, Califf RM, Weisman HF, Ellis SG, Tcheng JE, Worley S, Ivanhoe R et al. Randomised trial of coronary intervention with antibody against platelet IIb/IIIa integrin for reduction of clinical restenosis: results at six months. Lancet 1994;343:881–886.

60. Fischman DL, Leon MB, Baim DS, Schatz RA, Savage MP, Penn I, Detre K et al. A randomized comparison of coronary-stent placement and balloon angioplasty in the treatment of coronary artery disease. N Engl J Med 1994; 331:496–501.

61. Serruys PW, DeJaegere P, Kiemeneij F, Magaya C, Rutsch W, Heyndrickx G, Emanuelsson H et al. A comparison of balloon-expandable-stent implantation with balloon angioplasty in patients with coronary artery disease. N Engl J Med 1994;331:489–495.

4. Excimer Laser Coronary Angioplasty

FRANK LITVACK, and NEAL L. EIGLER

In the early 1980s the concept of applying laser energy transmitted via fiberoptics for removing atherosclerotic vascular obstructions emerged as a promising research technique. Early investigations were simplistic and utilized little more than off-the-shelf laser technologies. Expectations were overblown probably by the same trait that Alexis de Tockueville in the 19th century observed as Americans' ever-optimistic belief, bordering on faith, in the inevitability of progress. Early clinical investigation was focused on the continuous-wave, thermally acting lasers, and results were unsatisfactory secondary to excessive thermal injury and vascular damage. Excimer lasers produce nanosecond pulses of short wavelength, ultraviolet energy (1). These lasers were first studied in inorganic systems where it was observed that they were capable of etching material with minimal thermal injury. Excimer energy was first applied to vascular tissue in 1983. Since that time significant effort was expended developing, refining, and studying clinical excimer laser angioplasty systems—a process that remains ongoing. This chapter will provide an overview of the clinical experience to date with the technology and a personal approach to its appropriate clinical application.

BACKGROUND

The term "excimer" is an acronym for excited dymer. Excimer lasers emit directly in the ultraviolet portion of the spectrum from 193 to 351 nanometers. The wavelength of emission of the laser is dependent on the nature of the gas mixture. For a more extensive review of the physical chemistry of excimer lasers, the reader is referred elsewhere (2, 3). For the purposes of cardiovascular application, the xenon chloride 308 nanometer laser is most appropriate.

Continuous-wave lasers ablate by inducing intense localized heating of the tissue. Such lasers would include the argon ion, the carbon dioxide, and the Nd:YAG, all of which were investigated for vascular application in the early 1980s (4, 5). Histologic examination of atherosclerotic plaque ablated by any of these continuous-wave lasers demonstrates typical thermal injury characterized by concentric zones of carbonized material, eosinophilic coagulum, and vacuolization. Excimer lasers typically produce relatively few of these thermal effects, and ablated specimens range from craters etched with scalpel-like precision to relatively small zones of thermal and blast injury (1). The precise histopathologic results depend on the excimer wavelength use, the mode of transmission (air versus fiberoptic), and the medium in which the tissue ablation has occurred. Recently, experimental data have been presented that has challenged the notion that excimer lasers remove tissue with minimal collateral damage. Van Leeuwen et al. (6) have carefully studied excimer laser ablation in animal models and in vitro under a variety of conditions. These investigators contend that the vaporization of blood that occurs during in vivo excimer laser angioplasty results in important acoustic transients that cause tissue dissection and disruption. They further state that the clean craters seen during in vitro irradiation in the air are not reproduced during in vivo excimer laser angioplasty. These findings are in contrast of those Isner et al. who have reported on their examination of atherectomized specimens of atherosclerotic plaque following excimer laser angioplasty in peripheral arteries. In these specimens relatively limited thermal or acoustic damage was seen, and the authors concluded that in vivo ablation has similar histopathologic findings to those demonstrated during experimental in vitro study under ideal conditions (7). The findings of Van Leeuwen et al. would, however, help to explain the angiographic dissection not infrequently seen following coronary excimer laser angioplasty and discussed later in this chapter.

Low peak power laser energy is relatively easy to transmit through fiberoptics. A 308 nanometer excimer laser, however, because of its nanosecond pulse duration (peak power = energy/pulse ÷ pulse duration), produces an enormous peak power. Such peak powers are capable of destroying the transmitting fiberoptic bundle. The development of clinical excimer laser angioplasty systems has therefore required a great deal of engineering with respect to the laser unit and the fiberoptic transmission systems (catheters). Lasers specifically designed for medical application and with all the safety features incumbent on this use needed to be engineered and constructed. An entire new discipline—the transmission of high peak power pulses through fiberoptics—was developed. In the early days of laser angioplasty, the focus was the laser source. As with coronary angioplasty, the functional characteristics of the catheter are of critical importance to the efficacy of procedure. From the cardiologist's perspective, the ideal excimer laser source would be (a) inexpensive, (b) low maintenance, and (c) user-friendly. The functionally effective laser catheter needs to be (a) sufficiently flexible to navigate through tortuous coronary artery systems, (b) efficient in the ablation of even calcified tissue, (c) compatible with conventional angioplasty technique,

(d) associated with a low incidence of complications, and (e) directable so that the laser energy ablates obstructive plaque with minimal ablation of normal vascular tissue.

CLINICAL DATA

Excimer laser coronary angioplasty (ELCA) as performed today utilizes over-the-wire catheter technique. All excimer catheters are constructed of multiple individual fiberoptics arranged either concentrically or eccentrically around a guidewire lumen. The concentric catheter design includes catheters ranging in diameter from 1.3 mm to 2.2 mm. The eccentric design is 1.8 mm in diameter. Catheters are constructed of individual fibers of approximately 50 microns fused into bundles. The eccentric catheter is torqueable and has a protective tip through which the guidewire runs. The concept is to torque the catheter placing the ablative fiberoptic surface in contact with the atherosclerotic plaque. The protective tip opposes the normal arterial wall, shielding it from laser irradiation (Fig. 4.1).

In the United States most of the clinical excimer laser angioplasty experience has been obtained using devices from two manufacturers. Our group has been involved with the development and clinical application of the Advanced Interventional Systems device. We have reported our registry experience with

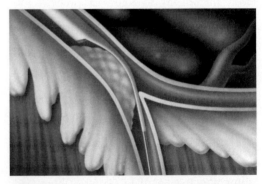

Figure 4.1. Schematic of 1.8-mm directional laser catheter. The eccentric fiber bundle may be "torqued" to oppose the lesion, giving the operator "directional" control.

the first of 3000 patients treated at 33 medical centers (8). Seventy-five percent of patients were male, and the mean age was 62 ± 10 years. Sixty-eight percent of patients were CCSFC class III or IV. Approximately one-third of patients have undergone prior balloon angioplasty or other interventional therapy. The cohort consisted of 3592 lesions of which 90% were stenoses. Approximately 8% were aorto-ostial in location, and 20% lesions were longer than 20 mm in length. Laser success, defined as $\geq 20\%$ reduction in lumen diameter and the achievement of a lumen near the diameter of the largest catheter used, was 84%. Procedure success, defined as a final stenosis less than 90% without major ischemic complication, was 90%. Of note, there was no difference in the procedure success rates between the first 2000 patients treated and the last 1000 patients. Seventy-nine percent of the entire cohort underwent adjunctive balloon angioplasty; however, there was a significant change in this pattern in the last 1000 patients in whom 95% underwent adjunctive balloon angioplasty.

The baseline mean diameter stenosis by visual observation was $86 \pm 12\%$, and this decreased to $50 \pm 22\%$ after excimer angioplasty. The mean final diameter stenosis was $27 \pm 19\%$. Of significance, there was no difference in laser or procedure success rates when stratified by lesion length. Data on comprehensive lesion morphology collected prospectively in 775 patients and 919 lesions from the latter portion of the study revealed that 77% of patients had ACC/AHA type B2 or C lesions. There were no significant differences in success rates between complex lesions (types B2 and C) and simple lesions (types A and B).

Table 4.1 shows success and major complication rates by lesion length. It demonstrates that 49% of lesions were longer than 10 mm in length. The laser success and procedure success did not vary from the short through the intermediate and long lesions. Similarly, the rate of major ischemic compli-

Table 4.1
Success and Major Complication Rates by Lesion Length and Type

Lesion Length (mm)	Procedure Success (%)	Major Ischemic Complications (%)
<10	91	6.0
10–19	92	4.6
20–29	89	6.6
≥30	87	7.3
Lesion type		
Aorto-ostial	89	6.9
Vein graft	92	3.9
Total occlusion[a]	89	2.4
Other	90	6.4

[a]Crossed by guidewire.

cations, including in-hospital death, Q-wave MI, and bypass surgery, did not vary between groups. Table 4.1 also shows success in major complication rates for select complex lesions. Laser success but not procedure success varied depending on lesion morphology. Of note, the lowest laser success rate was achieved in the "other" lesion category, which includes all lesions not fitting into one of the other three groups, such as short and nonostial, subtotal but nonocclusive, and highly eccentric lesions. Similarly, there was some variation in major ischemic complication rates, the lowest being seen for total occlusions and vein grafts and the highest for ostial lesions and the "other" category.

In-hospital death occurred in 0.5% of patients and Q-wave myocardial infarction in 2.1% of patients. In-hospital bypass surgery occurred in 3.8% of patients. Laser perforation occurred in 1.2% of patients, but decreased from 1.6% in the first 2000 treated to 0.4% in the last 1000 patients. This diminution in perforation rate resulted from better case selection as operators became more aware of relative contraindications. Sixty-two percent of patients with overt perforation had no major complications and were treated conservatively. However, 35% required bypass surgery, 2.7% developed Q-wave myocardial infarction, and in-hospital death occurred in 5.4% of patients.

A major and persistent limitation of excimer laser angioplasty has been coronary dissection. In the registry experience, coronary dissection was reported on the case report forms in 13% of lesions. Sustained occlusion was seen in 3.1% and transient occlusions in 3.4% of lesions. Coronary dissection will be discussed more completely elsewhere in this chapter. When dissection did occur, it was associated with a major ischemic complication more frequently than when it was not seen. Fifteen percent of patients who suffered dissection had a major ischemic complication opposed to 4.1% in patients who did not have coronary dissection.

Eigler et al. have reported the results of excimer laser coronary angioplasty in aorto-ostial lesions (9). Between December 1989 and May 1992, 260 aorto-ostial excimer laser coronary angioplasty procedures were performed on 209 stenoses in 200 patients. Canadian Cardiovascular Society class III or IV angina was present in 76%. Fifty-nine percent of lesions were in the right coronary artery, 28% in vein grafts, and 12% in the left main coronary artery. Adjunctive balloon-angioplasty (PTCA) was performed in 72% of patients, and the procedure success rate was 90%. This included a procedure success rate of 92% in the left main lesions, 89% in right coronary lesions, and 90% in saphenous vein grafts. Quantitative angiographic analysis showed a baseline minimum luminal diameter (MLD) of 0.8 ± 0.5 mm and a baseline stenosis of $76 \pm 14\%$. At the completion of the procedure, MLD averaged 2.1 ± 0.6 mm and percent diameter stenosis was $36 \pm 15\%$ ($P < .01$). A major complication during hospitalization occurred in 3.9% of patients (death 0%, Q-wave myocardial infarction 0.5%, and bypass surgery 3.4%). Six-month angiographic follow-up available in just over half the patients revealed an angiographic restenosis rate ($>50\%$ diameter stenosis) of 39%. Of note, the restenosis rate in the left main lesion was 64% but in the right coronary

lesions was 35%. From these data the authors concluded that excimer laser coronary angioplasty was an effective and safe therapy in patients with aorto-ostial stenoses. Six-month restenosis and adverse event rates were at an acceptable level though significantly increased in the left main lesions.

Recent data from the multicenter New Approaches to Coronary Intervention (NACI) registry have further substantiated the notion that excimer angioplasty can be safely performed even in selected complex lesion types (10). Multiple logistic regression models were used to analyze the influence of clinical and lesion characteristics on success rates and major complications in 400 consecutive patients. Mean age was 64 years, 68% of patients were male, 36% had prior PTCA, 36% had prior CABG, 18% had severe concomitant disease, and 19% were inoperable or high risk. Fifty-three percent had multivessel disease. Lesion morphology included 34% tubular or diffuse, 26% moderate or severe tortuosity, 60% eccentric, 14% total occlusion, and 35% calcified. Procedure success rate was 89%. MLD increased from 0.57 mm to 2.09 mm ($P < .001$); percent stenosis decreased from 80 to 26% ($P < .001$). Major complications were death 1.3%, emergency CABG 2%, and Q-wave MI 0.8%. Of all clinical characteristics only "severe concomitant diseases" correlated with major complications (relative risk = 3.21; 95% CI = 1.001, 10.44). No significant risk factor was found in analysis of major complications versus lesion characteristics. Analysis of procedure success in lesion characteristics revealed only larger vessel size to be inversely correlated with procedure success (relative risk = 0.034 for 1 mm increment of vessel size; 95% CI = 0.01, 0.10). These data demonstrated that in the NACI registry ELCA was performed in patients with predominantly complex lesion characteristics. Further, regression models showed that the usual angiographic features associated with lower success and higher complication rates following PTCA are not operative with ELCA. Patients with severe concomitant medical illness are at higher risk for major ischemic complications, as is the case with other interventional therapies.

In recent months, data on three other potentially important studies have been presented in abstract form. The ERBAC study was a three-way randomized trial comparing conventional balloon angioplasty with excimer laser angioplasty and rotational atherectomy. In the view of these authors the study was methodologically flawed. The three-way randomization excluded chronic total occlusions and extremely long lesions—the two lesion subsets that probably do best with excimer angioplasty. Nonetheless, the data are potentially important. The study demonstrated that rotational atherectomy did better in acute procedural outcome as compared with excimer angioplasty. It did, however, note disturbingly high angiographic restenosis rates in all three groups. The 6-month restenosis rates were 54% for PTCA, 60% for excimer angioplasty, and 62% for rotational atherectomy. These numbers did not achieve statistical significance; nonetheless, they are higher than any that have been previously reported with excimer angioplasty. Of note, the acute complication rate for the excimer patient was significantly higher than that reported in the American NACI Registry (11).

Pieak et al. have presented results of the AMRO trial. This was a Dutch trial comparing balloon angioplasty with excimer laser angioplasty for lesions longer than 10 mm. This study showed no difference in the long-term angiographic results or in the follow-up adverse events between the two cohorts. This study was performed early in the experience of excimer angioplasty and did not use the saline technique, the optimal laser technique with aggressive debulking and balloon dilation. Nonetheless, the results place the onus to produce substantiating data on those individuals who believe that excimer angioplasty

provides an advantage (12).

Deckelbaum et al. have presented data on the effect of intracoronary saline infusion on dissection during excimer laser coronary angioplasty in a randomized trial. Following laser catheter passage through the lesion, the presence and extent of dissection was assessed angiographically and graded on a scale of 0 (none) to 5 (total occlusion) based on a modified NHLBI classification. Analysis of dissections in the 59 lesions revealed a mean dissection grade of 0.73 ± 1.38 for the blood medium versus 0.19 ± 0.42 for the saline medium. Moderately severe or worse dissections (greater than or equal to grade II) occurred in seven of 33 lesions (21%) for blood medium and one of 26 lesions (4%) for saline medium. Acute occlusion caused by laser-induced dissection occurred in one case in the blood medium. These authors concluded that intracoronary saline infusion decreased the incidence and severity of arterial dissection during excimer laser angioplasty and should be incorporated in all procedures to improve acute outcome (13).

CASE SELECTION

Based on available data from the multicenter registry, the NACI database, and our personal experience, it appears that excimer laser coronary angioplasty is best suited for select complex lesions that are suboptimal for conventional balloon angioplasty. These lesion types include (a) long lesions, (b) diffuse, tight lesions, (c) aorto-ostial lesions, (d) chronic total occlusions (even long occlusions) crossable by a guidewire, (e) eccentric and bifurcation lesions (treated with the directional catheter only), and (f) some saphenous vein grafts, especially those that are relatively small in diameter with long lesions. In these lesion categories, excimer laser angioplasty as an adjunct to balloon angioplasty can, in most cases, achieve satisfactory acute results. Another lesion type in which the excimer laser may be applicable would be densely calcified lesions or lesions that are difficult or impossible to dilate using conventional balloon technology. Though not universally effective in these settings, excimer angioplasty, even with a small diameter, 1.3-mm catheter, can often pass through an undilatable lesion. The resultant lumen is not sufficient, but there appears to be some photoacoustic or other mechanical effect on the atherosclerotic plaque that then renders a lesion pliable and amenable to conventional balloon dilatation at low to moderate pressure.

Excimer angioplasty is perhaps the most simple of the new interventional technologies to perform. The technique uses conventional guide catheters and wires, and passage of the laser catheter is similar to that with conventional balloon angioplasty. This notwithstanding, the procedure can be frustrating and ineffective when inappropriately applied. Proper case selection is paramount to optimizing clinical results. A thorough understanding of the limitations of existing catheter technology, as well as limitations and effects of intravascular laser irradiation, is required. Clinical experience has demonstrated that using the concentric catheters in lesions that are highly eccentric, on angulated segments, or at bifurcations is associated with undue risk of failure and/or complication. The directional catheter, though early in its clinical application, appears to circumvent the limitation of applying excimer angioplasty to eccentric and bifurcation lesions.

LESION ELIGIBILITY (CONCENTRIC CATHETERS)

As with all devices, case selection is the key to satisfactory results. Analysis of ELCA registry data and of report experience of our investigators has allowed us to identify lesion types most appropriate for ELCA, as well as lesion types contraindicated for the procedure. We categorize lesions as (a) desirable, (b) acceptable, and (c) contraindicated.

   A. Desirable Lesions
     1. Diffuse

     2. Long
     3. Total occlusion
     4. Aorto-ostial
     5. Saphenous vein grafts
     6. Nondilatable or noncrossable lesions by PTCA
   B. Acceptable Lesions
     1. Ostial lesions of LAD if only the LAD is a "straight shot" from the left main. An angulated or highly superior LAD take-off has been associated with perforation in at least one case.
     2. Restenotic lesions.
     3. Highly degenerative or thrombotic vein grafts.
     4. Lesions involving a side branch.
   C. Relatively Contraindicated Lesions
     1. Bifurcation lesions as differentiated from a lesion that gives off a branch. (In a true bifurcation lesion the trajectory of the catheter actually changes. In a branch point lesion the trajectory of the catheter is unchanged because of the branch.)
     2. Highly eccentric lesions.
     3. Lesions involving tight radius bends.
     4. Mid-LAD lesions that terminate in a tight-radius intramyocardial or intraventricular groove "dip."
     5. Any evidence of prior dissection either laser or balloon induced.

LESION ELIGIBILITY (1.8-MM-DIAMETER DIRECTIONAL CATHETER)

Native vessel diameter should be 2.5 to 3.5 mm in diameter.

DESIRABLE LESION MORPHOLOGY

     1. Eccentric lesions (mild to moderate calcification).
     2. Bifurcation lesions: (a) the plaque is immediately distal to the bifurcation and (b) the plaque is immediately proximal to the bifurcation.
     3. Lesions on a bend, especially in the lesser curvature.

TECHNICAL APPROACH (ALL CATHETERS)

     1. Always use a well-supported guide catheter so that it remains engaged during laser firing to avoid unintentional back-and-forth motion of the laser catheter, which may induce trauma (dissection or perforation).
     2. Cross the lesion with a conventional or "extra tracking" guidewire. We recommend initiating the procedure with a 300-cm wire or extending the wire following crossing the lesion. We recommend "free wiring" all lesions.
     3. For chronic total occlusions, the use of the 0.018-inch or 0.025-inch Terumo wire has improved crossability.
     4. Always keep guidewire tip as far distal as possible to allow for tracking over stiff body wire.
     5. Use energy densities between 45 and 60 mJ/mm^2 at frequencies of 10 to 30 Hertz.

6. Always position laser catheter in direct proximity to the lesion at the beginning of laser ablation. That is, the catheter should be in contact with the lesion so as to minimize ablation of blood and the normal arterial wall. Ablation of blood can be associated with acoustic shock and dissection.

7. Flush 20 cc of saline through the guide catheter via a control syringe. One should initiate flushing just prior to initiating lasing and terminate the flushing after laser energy has been stopped.

8. Laser energy should be applied for 1 to 3 seconds and then stopped with a "waiting" of 1 to 3 seconds. Never apply laser energy for more than 3 seconds, and it is in fact desirable to limit laser energy to 1 to 2 seconds. Always ensure that the guidewire is taut while advancing.

9. Perform only one pass and then withdraw the laser catheter and assess luminal patency. If a lumen diameter equal to the size of the laser catheter has been achieved, no further laser pass should be performed. If a sufficient lumen diameter is not achieved and if the operator is sure that there is no luminal dissection, another laser pass may be performed.

TROUBLESHOOTING

1. Guidewire motion is "freezing" in catheter: Remove catheter and vigorously flush wire lumen and wet wire again.

2. No flow in distal artery following laser pass: Unless there is obvious dissection or guide catheter obstruction, attempt use of intracoronary nitroglycerin if clinically appropriate. If no response, then attempt adjunctive PTCA.

3. Laser catheter does not fully cross lesions around a bend: The problem here may be inability of the catheter tip to make the bend. Forcing a laser catheter may result in perforation.

4. Dissection has occurred following laser pass: Either observe or treat with balloon or appropriate mechanical device, depending on severity, flow, etc. *Never* apply further laser energy.

PERFORATION

As mentioned above, excimer angioplasty is a procedure that requires careful attention to case selection and technical detail. Complications occur not infrequently when the technology is applied outside the defined therapeutic parameters. Perforation, a serious but not universally catastrophic complication of excimer angioplasty, should occur in well under 0.5% of cases. Using the concentric catheter, perforation has been noted in the fol-

lowing instances: (a) applying laser energy to a highly eccentric lesion, especially when that lesion is on a tight radius bend; (b) applying laser energy at the site of a bifurcation, wherein perforation at the "carina" may occur; (c) applying a laser catheter that is near equal to or greater than the diameter of the native vessel; (d) applying laser energy in a previously dissected vascular segment, whether this dissection was laser-induced or induced by balloon or a rather interventional technique; and (e) failure to "back off" when the laser catheter is not successfully crossing the lesion.

The most successful laser results occur when the laser catheter crosses the lesion with minimum force and resistance. The operator must be able to react when the laser catheter does not easily cross the lesion. If a 1.3-mm diameter catheter is being used, applying further force for a period of 1 to 2 seconds only and/or increasing the laser repetition rate to 30 Hertz is sometimes effective. If these maneuvers do not result in successful passage across the lesion, the laser component of the procedure should be terminated. Applying excessive laser energy (greater than 2 to 3 seconds) in one location to a catheter that is not crossing the lesion is often associated with dissection and/or acute occlusion.

The incidence of vascular perforation should be below 0.5%. Anatomic factors predisposing to perforation have been discussed above. Avoidance of this situation should result in marked reduction of the incidence of perforation. Perforation may result in hemodynamic compromise in approximately one-third of the cases, depending on flow rate, underlying heart disease, and status of the pericardium. When it does occur, hemodynamic compromise can develop in less than 1 minute. Tamponade is best treated by inflating a balloon at the perforation site plus appropriate medical therapy and pericardiocentesis, if necessary. Bypass surgery is usually required.

If dye extravasation is noted in the patient,

make sure to maintain guidewire position and rapidly inflate a conventional or perfusion balloon. Bypass surgery should be considered in these patients, even if stabilized and no further extravasation is noted. Although not uniform, delayed hemodynamic compromise (48 hours) has been reported following apparent stabilization. The patients that may be "safest" from this complication are those with previously opened pericardium and those with intramuscular dye extravasation. Those that may be at highest risk for delayed compromise are those with pericardial extravasation and intact pericardium.

Minimizing Dissection

As described above, dissection can occur in an unpredictable fashion. It appears likely that dissection is the result of vaporization of blood and consequent acoustic transients with mechanical trauma to the vessel wall. This may explain the fact that dissection is more frequent in type A than in tubular or diffuse lesions. The tubular, diffuse lesion or the calcified lesion may be less pliable and therefore less likely to dissect. Further, the type A lesion is more likely to have normal wall adjacent to it with a wide luminal diameter. Consequently, the blood in the normal area is vaporized and tears the normal intima. We believe that lasing in a saline medium will reduce photoacoustic effects and dissection. As such, we recommend saline infusion via the guide catheter as described above. Of note, there is significant ongoing research on developing a laser-catheter firing system that releases energy from only a portion of the fiberoptics at any given time. For example, if the active tip of the laser catheter is divided into 4 equal quadrants, then each section could be fired in sequence very rapidly. In vitro research, including high-speed filming and histologic analysis, has shown that this markedly reduces the photoacoustic effect on tissue. We believe it is probable that this "multiplexing" will rapidly be applied to clinical excimer laser angioplasty systems in conjunction with saline infusion and that the dissections seen in approximately 15% of cases will be significantly reduced.

SUMMARY

In summary, excimer laser angioplasty is a useful technique for treating select complex lesions that either are not amenable to or are poor candidates for balloon angioplasty. Using concentric catheters, the lesions to be treated would include diffuse, long, ostial, calcified, undilatable, vein graft, and total occlusions. Using the newer directional catheter, it may also be possible to treat highly eccentric or bifurcation lesions. As with all new interventional technologies, case selection is paramount, and if cases are selected poorly or if technique is not careful, serious complications may ensue. Coronary dissection, the most unpredictable of the excimer laser complications, may potentially be reduced in frequency by the use of saline flush and/or "multiplexing" systems.

REFERENCES

1. Grundfest WS, Litvack F, Forrester JS, Goldenberg T, Swan HJC, Morgenstern L, Fishbein M et al. Laser ablation of human atherosclerotic plaque without adjacent tissue injury. J Am Coll Cardiol 1985;5:929–933.

2. Laudenslager JB. Ion-molecule processes in lasers. In: Ausloos P, ed. Kinetics of ion-molecule reactions. New York. Plenum, 1978.

3. Boulnais JL. Photophysical processes in recent medical laser developments: a review. Lasers Med Sci 1986; 1:47–66.

4. Sanborn TA, Faxon DP, Haudenschild CC, Ryan TJ. Experimental angioplasty: circumferential distribution of laser thermal injury with a laser probe. J Am Coll Cardiol 1985;5:934–938.

5. Welch AJ. The thermal response of laser irradiated tissue. IEEE J Quantum Electron 1984;QE-20:1471–1481.

6. van Leeuwen TG, van Ervin L, Meertens JH, Motamedi M. Post MJ, Borst C. Origin of arterial wall dissections induced by pulsed excimer and mid-infrared laser ablation in the pig. J Am Coll Cardiol 1992;19:1610–1618.

7. Isner JM, Rosenfeldt K, White CJ, Ramme S, Kearney M, Pieczek A, Langevin RE et al. In vivo assessment of vascular pathology resulting from laser radiation. Analysis of 23 patients studied by directional atherectomy and immediately after laser angioplasty. Circulation 1992; 85(6):2185–2196.

8. Litvack F, Eigler N, Margolis J et al. Percutaneous excimer laser angioplasty: results of the first consecutive 3000 patients. J Am Coll Cardiol 1994;23:323–329.

9. Eigler N, Weinstock B, Douglas JS, Goldenberg T, Hartzler G, Holmes D, Leon M et al. Excimer laser coronary angioplasty of aorto-ostial stenoses: results of the excimer laser coronary angioplasty (ELCA) registry in the first 200 patients. Circulation 1993;88:2049–2057.

10. Litvack F, Lai SM, Margolis J, Mehta S, Detre K, Eigler N. Excimer laser coronary angioplasty: influence of clinical and angiographic characteristics on outcome—an NACI registry report. Circulation 1993;88:I-23 (abstract).

11. Vandormael M, Reifart N, Preusler W, Schwarz F, Storger H, Hofmann M, Klopper J et al. Six-month follow-up results following excimer laser angioplasty, rotational atherectomy and balloon angioplasty for complex lesions: ERBAC study. Circulation 1994;90(4):1143 (abstract).

12. Piek JJ, Appelman YE, Strikwerda S, Koolen JJ, David GK, de Feyter PJ, Serruys PW et al. Excimer laser coronary angioplasty versus balloon angioplasty used in long coronary lesions: the in-hospital results of the AMRO trial. Circulation 1994;90(4):1778 (abstract).

13. Deckelbaum LI, Strauss BH, Bittl JA, Rohlfs K, Scott J, and the PELCA investigators. Effect of intracoronary saline infusion on dissection during excimer laser coronary angioplasty: a randomized trial. Circulation 1994;90:(4)1774 (abstract).

5. Solid-State Laser: The Holmium:YAG System

ON TOPAZ

LASER TECHNOLOGY

A realization of the limitations of traditional percutaneous transluminal coronary angioplasty stimulated the development of several new mechanical and photo-optical technologies, including laser devices, which themselves have created considerable expectation (1). Cardiovascular laser angioplasty is intended to ablate atherosclerotic plaque material, in contrast to balloon angioplasty where the target stenosis is compressed or displaced (2). At first *continuous-wave* lasers, whose activity is based on photothermal mechanisms (3), were utilized. As a distinct limitation, these lasers required a certain amount of water to be present for the photothermal ablation to occur. Thus ablation of heavily calcified atherosclerotic plaques is not possible. In addition, these lasers created significant damage to adjacent arterial wall as a result of peak tissue temperatures higher than 160°C (4). With further development *pulsed-wave* lasers were introduced as a strategy for vaporizing atherosclerotic plaques with significantly less thermal damage to the arterial wall than with continuous-wave lasers and for efficient ablation of calcified plaques.

The mechanism of plaque removal by pulsed-wave lasers involves rapid delivery of short, high-peak, energy pulses using a combination of a brief pulse duration with an adequately long pulse interval, ensuring that the thermal relaxation time of the irradiated plaque is not exceeded, therefore minimizing thermal injury. In pulsed-wave, *solid-state* lasers the active laser material is a collection of ions, molecules or atoms in the form of a solid material. Energy from an external source is transferred into the lasing medium to raise the energy level above the ground state, a process called *excitation mechanism.* This process is conducted by a brilliant flash lamp (5). Once there are more atoms in an excited energy state than in a lower energy state, a single photon emitted by some other atom triggers a process of *stimulated emission* in which excited atoms are stimulated to emit their energy coherently with the trigger photon. At the back end of the active-medium chamber a mirror, which is totally reflective, returns photons of light back into the active medium where additional excited atoms undergo further amplification. On the other side of the chamber containing the active medium a partially reflective mirror releases a predetermined fraction of the light through, and that light beam is the operative laser beam. *Solid-state* lasers that operate in the *mid-infrared* zone include erbium, holmium, thulium, neodymium, and ruby. A number of solid-state, mid-infrared lasers have been investigated for application in laser angioplasty, including the Nd:YAG laser, operating at 1.94 microns; the cobalt magnesium fluoride laser (Co:MgF), which has output at 1.94 microns; the thulium:YAG laser, which operates at 2.01 microns and 1.96 microns; and the holmium:YAG laser, tunable to 2.09 microns. All of these lasers, operating close to the 1.93-micron water-absorption peak, should provide excellent tissue removal capability with little or no thermal damage to the adjacent arterial wall. Although excimer laser reportedly performs well in clinical studies (6), the above-mentioned solid-state lasers have potential advantages over excimer lasers, as they are much smaller, easier to maintain, more cost-effective, and provide higher reliability (7). Probably the most exciting mid-infrared, pulsed-wave, solid-state laser source recently introduced for coronary interventions in the holmium:YAG (yttrium; aluminum; garnet) laser, which emits pulses of light at the 2.09-micron wavelength. This chapter delineates basic mechanisms involved and the clinical experience gained with this laser and provides strategic approaches to its application in coronary interventions.

The Device

There are several manufacturers of holmium: YAG laser devices. We have gained a large clinical experience with the solid-state, pulsed-wave Eclipse 2100 model (Eclipse Surgical Technologies, Palo Alto, CA). Laser output from the generator is activated with a foot pedal, delivering pulses of 250 microseconds, pulse width of 250 to 600 mJ/pulse, at a frequency of 5 Hz. The device requires 220-volt, 20-ampere, single-phase power. Its weight is 250 kg (495 lbs). Laser light with a 2.09-micron wavelength is transmitted through multiple, optical low-OH silica fibers. The fibers are constructed in a close-packed circular array surrounding a central lumen that accepts 0.014-inch or 0.018-inch guidewires. A soft tip provides easy maintenance of coaxial alignment, and an atraumatic wrap protects the vessel wall from the fibers' edges. As the laser light is emitted from the distal tip of the catheter in front-firing mode, ablation is obtained in either close or direct contact with the target plaque along the coaxial length of the guidewire within the coronary artery. Currently, six sizes of multi-fiber catheters are utilized: 1.2 mm (27 optical fibers, 75 microns each), 1.3 mm (20 optical fibers, 100 microns each), 1.4 mm (40 optical fibers, 50 microns each), 1.5 mm (26 optical fibers, 100 microns each), 1.7 mm (49 optical fibers, 50 microns each), and 2.0 mm (12 optical fibers, 100 microns each). The tissue absorption depth for this laser is approximately 400 microns (8), which is ten-fold deeper than that of the excimer laser. This device, which is an investigational coronary laser system, is currently applied to patients with a protocol approved by the Food and Drug Administration in an observational, nonrandomized, multicenter study involving medical centers in the United States and abroad.

The Biologic Interaction

The interactions between laser light and biologic material include (a) *reflection* of the light from the surface without any effect on the material, (b) *transmittance* of laser light through the material without producing any effect, (c) *scattering* of light from the material's surface or from inside as the light passes through it, and (d) *absorption* of the laser light, a process that produces heat within the material. Only the latter interaction leads to laser-based treatment. In the coronary arteries the interaction between the laser and the atherosclerotic tissue includes removal of the atherosclerotic plaque and its accompanied thrombus through evaporation.

Preliminary experimental studies with the holmium:YAG laser in wet-field ablation of diseased, soft, and calcified atheromas typically showed tissue histology with little thermal damage but severe acoustic damage caused by shock waves, resulting in the formation of fissures and surface irregularities. It was postulated that shock-wave effects arise from the short pulse (~200 microseconds) and high peak powers (~5000 watts) of the holmium laser. A concern was raised about the application of the holmium laser to calcified atheromas creating large shock waves that could fragment calcified atheroma, creating irregular surfaces and large fragments that might diminish acute and long-term patency of recanalized vessels (8). Other issues of concern were the capability of the holmium laser to effectively ablate calcified tissues with acceptable threshold fluences and the in vitro demonstration of high incidence of thrombotic occlusions (9).

Once clinical experience was gained, it soon became clear that the reported in vitro phenomenon of acoustic damage related to shock waves is rarely clinically manifested. The holmium laser was found to be remarkably efficient in evaporization of atherosclerotic plaques, calcified lesions, and thrombi alike. Analysis of the unfavorable results from the above-mentioned in vitro experiments disclosed that in most of these experiments lasing was conducted by stiff fibers with markedly different lasing parameters and technique than with those utilized in human application. Subsequently, a large body of in vitro studies was established corroborating the clinical impression of favorable laser-tissue interaction. McKay et al. (10) showed that the holmium laser can selectively ablate atheromatous plaques with only minimum thermal damage. Isner demonstrated no thermal injury when ablation was carried out at a low fluency, as applied clinically, while thermal injury was produced once high fluencies, not used in clinical application, were delivered (11). Aretz examined human cadaver aorta after holmium laser application and found charring at a high fluency at 600 mJ and severe thermal damage at 900 mJ. At 1 week after holmium lasing of canine arteries, Aretz found mild intimal hyperplasia, very little fibrosis, maintenance of elastin structure, and no inflammatory response (12). Hirota and his colleagues at Tokyo Women's Medical College, Tokyo, Japan, analyzed the effect of the holmium: YAG on rabbit's heart muscle and on rabbit's atherosclerotic aorta. These investigators found that the lasing-site margins were smooth and that adequate plaque evaporation was achieved without vacuolization or charring (13). Thus significant acoustic damage and shock waves may occur, but only if high fluencies of irradiation, contraindicated in clinical practice, are applied.

The Multicenter Clinical Experience

Since May 1990 there has been an ongoing multicenter observational study assessing the feasibility and safety of a holmium:YAG laser system (the Eclipse) in treatment of atherosclerotic lesions in native coronary arteries and vein grafts (14). Patients with ischemia related to lesions amenable to balloon angioplasty or bypass surgery are considered for this study. Morphologically, the target lesions include sequential or diffuse occlusions, calcific lesions, total or subtotal stenoses that fail to be crossed by a conventional balloon catheter, restenosis at the site of previous angioplasty,

Table 5.1
Holmium Laser Multicenter Registry—1994

No. of patients	1340
No. of lesions	1457
Patient age	61.3 ± 11.1
Males	73.4%
Pts. Hx (%)	
MI	43.8
CHF	9.1
Diabetes	20.6
Hypertension	52.6
Smoking	45.4
Hypercholesterolemia	55.2
Prior angioplasty	29.2
Prior CABGs	16.2
Indication for procedure (%)	
Positive exercise test	5.4
Stable angina	23.6
Unstable angina	66.0
Acute MI	5.0
ACC/AHA lesion classification (%)	
A	14.4
B1	22.5
B2	37.2
C	25.9
Lesion location (%)	
LAD	42
RCA	32
CX	16
SVG	10
Lesion length (mm)	12 ± 10
% stenosis	
Prelaser	89 ± 10
Postlaser	62 ± 21
Final	22 ± 19
Mean pulses	115 ± 96
Laser success	86%
Overall success	93%

Table 5.2
Analysis of Four Groups of Patients Treated by the Holmium:YAG Laser

	SVG Lesions	Total Occlusion	Calcified Lesions	Diffuse Lesions
No. of patients	130	155	365	159
No. of lesions	146	156	392	163
% Prelaser stenosis	90.2 ± 10.7	100%	88.8 ± 10.1	91.4 ± 10.1
%Postlaser stenosis	59.7 ± 21.2	71.9 ± 21.5	64.6 ± 21.0	67.3 ± 20.1
% Final stenosis	21.6 ± 18.7	20.9 ± 22.5	25.4 ± 21.9	23.1 ± 21.9
Procedure success	91.8%	93.6%	89.5%	92.0%
Death	2.3%	0.6%	1.3%	1.2%
Emergency CABGS	3.4%	0.6%	3.1%	2.5%
MI: Q-wave	1.4%	0%	1.8%	1.2%
Non–Q-wave	8.2%	3.2%	1.8%	3.7%
Dissection: Major	0%	2.9%	5.1%	6.6%
Minor	3.4%	2.9%	6.6%	3.8%
Abrupt closure	1.4%	1.9%	1.8%	1.0%
Perforation: Local	1.4%	0.6%	1.5%	2.5%
Nonlocal	0%	0.6%	0.5%	0%
Thrombus	3.4%	1.9%	1.8%	1.2%
Distal embolism	7.5%	3.2%	0.5%	1.8%
Spasm	4.8%	7.7%	8.7%	11.0%

and ostial coronary or saphenous vein graft stenoses. Procedural success is defined as a reduction of stenosis ≤50% after adjunctive balloon angioplasty and the absence of a major clinical complication (in-hospital death, emergency coronary artery bypass surgery, and Q-wave myocardial infarction). By the time of this writing, 1340 patients with a mean age of 61.3 ± 11.1 years were studied. Patient clinical characteristics are depicted in Table 5.1. A total of 1457 lesions have been treated. Sixty-six percent of the patients had unstable angina, 23.6% had stable angina, 5.4% had positive exercise tests, and 5% were treated for acute myocardial infarction. Forty-two percent of the lesions were located in the LAD, 32% in the RCA, 16% in the circumflex artery, and 10% in saphenous vein grafts. By the ACC/AHA classification (15) 14.4% were type A lesions, 22.5% were type B1, 37.2% type B2, and 25.9% type C. The mean lesion length was 12 ± 10 mm; 115 ± 96 laser pulses were emitted per patient. The laser decreased the stenosis from 89% ± 10% to 62 ± 21%, and adjunct balloon angioplasty achieved a final mean residual stenosis of 22 ± 19%. Laser

success was achieved in 87% of the patients (defined as complete crossing of the target lesion by the laser and reduction of ≥20% in stenosis), and final procedural success (defined as ≤50% residual stenosis and no major complication) was 93%. At 6 months repeat angiography was performed in 29% of the lesions and showed restenosis in 47% of these. When analyzing the effect of lesion length on the procedural success and related major complications, we found no difference between lesions longer than 20 mm and lesions of either 10 to 20 mm or those shorter than 10 mm. In comparing procedural success in restenosis lesions (post–balloon angioplasty) to that of de novo lesions, it was found that the laser achieved similar success rates (86.7% and 86.5%) and low major complication rates in both types of lesions.

Table 5.2 depicts subgroup analysis of the multicenter registry. Four categories of lesions considered not ideal for balloon angioplasty are presented. In three out of the four—saphenous vein grafts, chronic total occlusions, and diffuse long lesions—procedural success exceeded 91% and in the fourth, calcified stenoses, it reached 89.5%. As expected, major complications most frequently occurred in patients with old, degenerated saphenous vein grafts.

COMPLICATIONS IN THE MULTICENTER STUDY

Table 5.3 depicts the occurrence of major and minor complications in the multicenter experience. The incidence of major complications was as follows: death 0.7%, emergency bypass surgery 2.9%, acute Q-wave myocardial infarction 1.1%, and acute non–Q-wave myocardial infarction 3.2%. This incidence is considered acceptable for percutaneous revascularization. Other complications included major dissections 4.1%, nonsignificant dissections 5.5%, acute closure 2.7%, perforation 1.9%, thrombus formation 2.5%, distal embolus 1.3%, and arterial spasm 11.7%. Of note, the majority of the dissections were not flow limiting. Spasm appears to be readily treated by short balloon inflations. Centers that adopted the *"pulse and retreat"* lasing technique report a significantly lower complication rate than that of the multicenter registry.

INDICATIONS AND CONTRAINDICATIONS

Table 5.4 depicts indications for holmium coronary laser angioplasty based on the multicenter experience. This laser can be safely and effectively applied to certain lesions that are known to respond poorly to balloon angioplasty. These include long, diffuse lesions (lesion length >10 mm), lesions in old saphenous vein grafts (Fig. 5.1), aorto-ostial coronary and saphenous vein stenoses (Fig. 5.2), complex lesions, moderately and heavily calcified lesions, total occlusions that can be crossed with a guidewire, and balloon dilatation failures. The target lesions can either be de novo or restenotic. Complex-type and thrombotic lesions are considered best treated by holmium angioplasty. This niche for application is unique to holmium:YAG laser (16). The patients selected for holmium laser treatment can have a solitary lesion (Fig. 5.3) or multiple lesions and single- or multiple-vessel disease, if treating the latter does not pose unacceptable risk to the patient. Contraindications for application of holmium laser include unprotected left main coronary artery, lesions located at a bend of >60°, lesions in arteries with a diameter smaller than the laser catheter size, lesions not traversable by a guidewire, and inability of the guidewire to be advanced to a safe distal position in the target artery. Decreased left ventricular ejection fraction per se is not considered a contraindication.

Table 5.3
Complications in the Holmium Multicenter Registry (n = 1340 pts)

Complication	Percent
Death	0.7
Emergency CABGS	2.9
Myocardial infarction	
Q-wave	1.1
Non–Q-wave	3.2
Dissection (total)	9.6
Significant	4.1
Nonsignificant	5.5
Acute closure	2.7
Perforation	1.9
Thrombosis	2.5
Distal embolus	1.3
Arterial spasm	11.7

Table 5.4
Indications and Contraindications for Holmium Coronary Laser Angioplasty

Indications
  Lesions that cannot be dilated or crossed with a balloon
  Total occlusions—provided that they can be crossed with a guidewire
  Long lesions (>20 mm long)
  Aorto-ostial lesions
  Calcified lesions
  Complex lesions; de novo or restenotic; thrombotic
Contraindications
  Unprotected left main artery
  Bend lesions >60°
  Lesions in arteries with a caliber smaller than the laser catheter size
  Lesions not traversable by a guidewire
  Inability to advance guidewire to a safe distal position

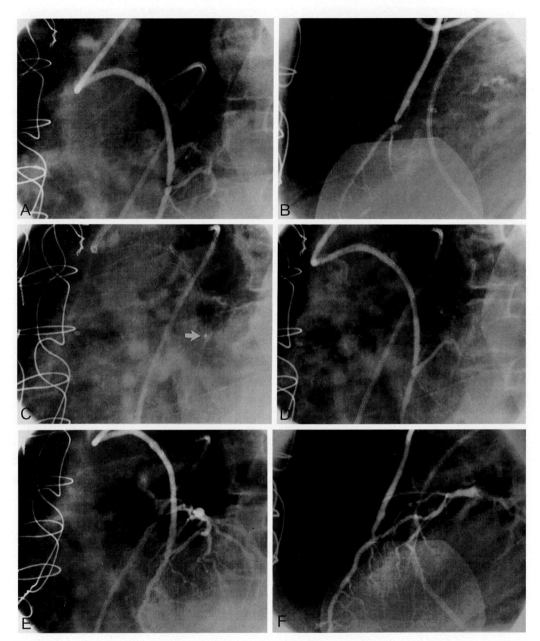

Figure 5.1. A high-risk laser angioplasty. A 63-year-old man with severe unstable angina and anterior wall ischemia, 6 months after CABG. Cardiac catheterization demonstrated total occlusion of the three native coronary arteries and total occlusion of two out of three saphenous vein grafts. Echocardiogram revealed left ventricular ejection fraction (LVEF) = 40%. The patient was not considered a candidate for repeat CABG. As the saphenous vein graft to the left anterior descending artery is a "sole supplier" to the myocardium, an intraaortic balloon pump (IABP) was placed prior to lasing. **A.** Angiogram is cranial left anterior oblique projection demonstrating a critical stenosis at the anastomosis of the saphenous vein graft to the left anterior descending artery. **B.** The lesion in left lateral projection. **C.** LaserPrime (Eclipse) 1.4-mm and 1.5-mm catheters (tip marked by an arrow) were utilized over a 0.014-inch Nitinol (Microvena/Medtronic) guidewire delivering a total of 46 pulses. **D.** Postlasing angiogram showing reduction of the stenosis, with a recanalization corresponding to the size of the 1.5-mm laser catheter. **E.** Final angiogram in left anterior oblique projection demonstrating results after adjunct PTCA. **F.** Final results in left lateral projection.

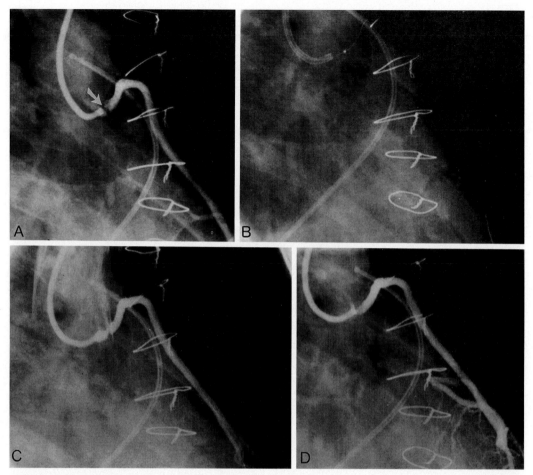

Figure 5.2. Angiograms from a patient with severe peripheral vascular disease, COPD, who was considered to be a poor candidate for repeat CABG. The patient experienced severe unstable angina and anterolateral ischemia. **A.** Critical ostial stenosis *(arrow)* of a saphenous vein graft to the left anterior descending artery. **B.** Via the left brachial approach an 8 Fr LCB (Medtronic) guiding catheter and a 0.014-inch guidewire (ACS) were introduced. LaserPrime (Eclipse) catheters (1.2, 1.4, and 1.5 mm) delivered a total of 104 pulses to the target lesion. **C.** Immediate postlasing angiogram revealing reduction of the stenosis. **D.** Final angiogram following balloon angioplasty demonstrating adequate patency.

LASING EQUIPMENT

As with balloon angioplasty, the Judkins femoral approach is most commonly used. However, in patients with severe peripheral vascular disease at the McGuire VA Medical Center of the Medical College of Virginia, the percutaneous brachial approach has been utilized successfully from either the left or the right arm. For patients whose procedure is considered high risk, such as those with very low ejection fraction or with a target vessel that is the "sole remaining supplier" to the

coronary circulation, it is preferable to place an intraaortic counterpulsation balloon pump prior to actual lasing. Selecting the appropriate guiding catheter is important. A Judkins-shaped catheter is selected for lesions located in the LAD, proximal, nontortuous circumflex, and RCA. An Amplatz-shaped guiding catheter can be used for lesions that require significant guiding catheter support. Use of the Cordis giant lumen 8 Fr or 9 Fr (Cordis, Miami, FL) is recommended for its easy handling, adequate opacification, and stable sup-

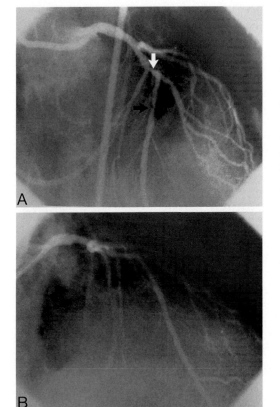

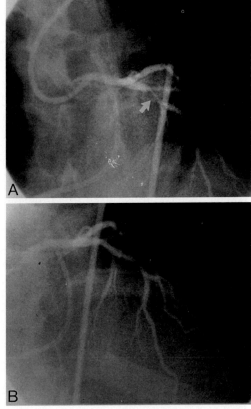

Figure 5.3. A patient with unstable angina associated with ischemia in the anterior wall. **A.** Two lesions (marked by arrows) in the left anterior descending artery. **B.** Final angiogram following lasing with a 1.7-mm LaserPrime (Eclipse) catheter and adjunct balloon angioplasty. The patient is asymptomatic 1 year after the procedure with a negative exercise thallium test.

Figure 5.4. Combined laser atherectomy for a patient with unstable angina. **A.** Severe eccentric lesion *(arrow)* in the left anterior descending artery. **B.** Results after laser followed by adjunct atherectomy.

port. The Medtronic Sherpa (Medtronic, Minneapolis, MN) guide catheter is another good choice for adequate delivery of the laser catheters. In cases in which directional atherectomy will follow laser irradiation, a 10 Fr DVI (DVI, Redwood City, Cal) directional atherectomy guiding catheter provides excellent support and opacification capability (Fig. 5.4).

The ACS Extra Strength 0.018-inch or 0.014-inch guidewire (ACS, Santa Clara, California) provides adequate support in most cases. However, in difficult lesions that require significant, stable guidewire support the Nitinol (Medtronic/Microvena, Min-

neapolis, MN) 0.014-inch or 0.016-inch guidewire is an excellent choice. Another advantage with these wires is protecting side branches during lasing. If a transluminal extraction catheter (TEC) procedure is planned to follow lasing, a 0.014-inch TEC (Interventional Technologies Inc., San Diego, CA) wire, with its excellent support capability, is suitable for delivery of laser catheters. In patients who need laser-assisted recanalization for total occlusions, we successfully applied the ACS 0.010-inch (ACS, Santa Clara, California) guidewire. In such cases this wire can provide adequate support, and lasing appears to be safe. However, we do not recommend using this guidewire in vessels that are not totally occluded, as the dead space between the catheter and the wire may adversely affect the results.

The present holmium laser catheters generate lumens similar to the diameter of the catheter itself. It should be remembered that laser catheters are nonexpandable devices. Thus the traditional approach of matching the balloon size to the healthier, adjacent segment of the dilated artery should herein not be applied. The laser operator should concentrate on the target lesion itself. As a general rule, the more severe the stenosis, the smaller the catheter size should be. Our experience suggests that for lesions of 90% stenosis or greater, lasing should begin with the smallest catheter available—1.2 mm. Then, after successful recanalization, the size of the catheter can be increased. This approach is essential to avoid unnecessary dissections caused by a too-large catheter's "shoulders," which push and disrupt the plaque's edges and its adjacent luminal wall. For lesions of 80 to 90% stenosis, a catheter no larger than 1.4 mm should be applied first.

LASING TECHNIQUE STRATEGY

There is an agreement between experienced laser operators that the most important part of the laser procedure, other than case selection, is delivery and activation of the laser to the target site. Debulking techniques such as lasing require a great deal of patience and accurate judgment from the operator. It is dangerous to treat lasing sessions as if they were balloon inflations. Operators who utilize solid-state, pulsed-wave lasers should take into account unique physical phenomena associated with lasing. During plaque ablation the atherosclerotic tissue is vaporized and gas is formed. VanLeewen and colleagues demonstrated that dissections are caused during holmium and excimer lasing by forceful expansion of the vapor gas bubble within the laser treatment site (17). Abela studied the mechanism of acute closure during coro-

nary lasing and demonstrated that it is attributed to the "Mille-Feuilles" effect. This phenomenon occurs when high-energy pulses create a cavitation bubble that produces shock waves following the collapse of the bubble. The shock waves create multiple layers of dissections that "puff" up the arterial wall like the many layers seen in the French pastry "mille feuilles" (thousand leafs). As a result, acute vessel closure occurs. The effect cannot be relieved by nitrates and requires balloon dilations for remodeling of the dissected arterial layers (18). Other related phenomena are coronary spasm and the obstruction to forward flow in the treated artery. While the latter is caused by the presence of the laser catheter, the former is caused by the heat generated during lasing (19).

To reduce heat formation and allow forward coronary flow to cool the lasing site and to eliminate the formation of forcefully expanded gas bubbles, we have introduced a lasing technique called the "pulse and retreat" technique (20). The operator places the catheter 1 to 3 mm away from the proximal end of the target lesion, as the holmium laser with its deep penetration depth can initially be used as a noncontact catheter, and then the catheter is slowly advanced toward the lesion, delivering 8 to 12 pulses only. The laser catheter is then retracted into the guiding catheter or into a proximal, large portion of the target artery. A pause of 45 seconds is taken prior to the next lasing session and 50 to 100 mcg of intracoronary nitroglycerin is injected. This maneuver permits restoration of forward blood flow with its coolant effect on the plaque and ensures adequate coronary vasodilation. Combining tactile feedback and contrast injections, the catheter is readvanced to the target plaque for another session of 8 to 12 pulses, and the process is repeated until the laser catheter passes smoothly across the lesion. It is also recommended to consider injections of cold saline after each lasing session, as Lee et al. (21) have demonstrated lower peak temperatures, faster tissue cooling, and subsequently, less tissue injury with perfusion of cold saline during lasing. It is of paramount importance that lasing not be performed immediately following contrast injections because dye can cause explosion of the artery by a potentiating effect on the peak pressure waves (22). With an experience exceeding 120 procedures since the introduction of the new lasing technique, no perforation or acute vessel closures were encountered by this author; only dissection occurred and spasm was eliminated as well.

Energy delivery parameters are provided by the manufacturer. If a laser catheter does not ablate at the initial level of energy, the fluence can be increased provided it remains within the recommended range for a given size of a catheter. If after one adjustment of delivered energy the catheter is still unable to be adequately advanced, the lasing option should be reconsidered. Ginsburg (23) described a useful method of how to advance the laser catheter; it involves a slight tug on the guidewire during lasing to permit the necessary, very slow, forward movement of the catheter tip through the lesion. There is no doubt that attempts to advance the catheter too quickly through a lesion results in complications such as dissections and acute vessel closure. The laser catheter needs to perform the ablation and be advanced mainly by self-propagation along its created channel, while the operator combines tactile feedback, fluoroscopy, and repeat contrast injections.

Complications unique to laser usage include acute vessel closure, perforation, and spasm. In addition, dissections merit special attention. The recognition, identification, and adequate management of complications are mandatory to ensure a safe laser program.

ROLE IN ACUTE MYOCARDIAL INFARCTION

The holmium laser, whose wavelength coincides with strong water-absorption peaks, seems appropriate for acute thrombolysis; a fresh thrombus is known to have a high water content that results in a large thermal sink and, consequently, dissipation of laser thermal energy (24). The utilization of this laser in acute myocardial infarction for both thrombolysis and plaque ablation (16, 25) may be warranted as many acute infarction patients fail to qualify to receive thrombolytic drugs (26), and significant numbers of patients fail to benefit from these agents. Furthermore, considering the need to open an infarct-related artery for improved prognosis (27), mechanical revascularization is warranted for patients with contraindications for thrombolytic agents or who clinically failed to respond to thrombolysis. Application of direct balloon angioplasty as the first line of therapy in acute myocardial infarction is still controversial, especially if the infarct-related artery contains a complex lesion and/or large thrombus (28). The immediate and short-term follow-up results include up to a 15% acute closure rate and a restenosis rate up to 60% within 6 months (29–31). Investigators from the University of Miami were the first to utilize the holmium laser in acute myocardial infarction (32). To date, we have gained experience with 24 patients with complicated acute myocardial infarction, 10 of whom were in cardiogenic shock at the time of emergency catheterization (Fig. 5.5). By quantitative coronary angiography, laser reduced the mean percent stenosis from $84 \pm 17\%$ to $55 \pm 22\%$ ($P < .001$), and adjunct PTCA achieved $37 \pm 15\%$ ($P < .001$) residual narrowing. Minimal luminal diameter (mm) was increased from 0.6 ± 0.6 to 1.6 ± 0.9 ($P < .002$) by laser and to 2.1 ± 0.5 by adjunct PTCA ($P = .003$). Mean flow increased from TIMI 0.7 to 2.8 ($P < .001$). Clinical success (elimination of ischemia and chest pain; <50% residual stenosis; adequate thrombolysis; no death, CABG, perforation, major dissection, or extension of myocardial infarction) was achieved in 23 of 24 patients. The finding that 23 out of these 24 patients survived the complicated acute infarction further attests to the potential of this technol-

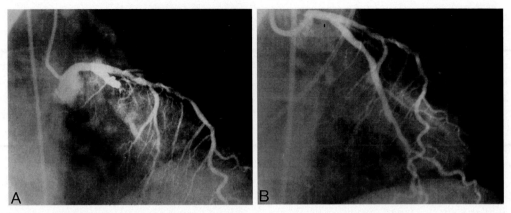

Figure 5.5. A patient with severe chest pain, marked ischemia, and hypotension 10 hours after the onset of acute myocardial infarction. **A.** Total occlusion of the Cx artery, the infarct-related vessel. **B.** Final results after lasing and adjunct balloon angioplasty. Patency was achieved within 15 minutes. No thrombolytics were needed.

Table 5.5
Excimer[a] Versus Holmium[b] Laser-Assisted Coronary Angioplasty for Lesions Containing Thrombus

	Thrombus		No Thrombus		P Value	
Complication	Excimer (n = 12)	Holmium (n = 66)	Excimer (n = 130)	Holmium (n = 46)	Excimer	Holmium
Embolization	3 (25%)	2 (3%)	1 (1%)	0 (0%)	<0.001	NS
MI	4 (33%)	2 (3%)	2 (2%)	0 (0%)	<0.001	NS
Abrupt closure	2 (17%)	3 (4.5%)	5 (4%)	0 (0%)	0.049	NS
Spasm	0 (0%)	3 (4.5%)	1 (1%)	3 (6.5%)	NS	NS
Emergency CABGS	0 (0%)	1 (1.5%)	2 (2%)	0 (0%)	NS	NS
Major dissection	0 (0%)	1 (1.5%)	6 (5%)	0 (0%)	NS	NS
Minor dissection	1 (8%)	6 (9%)	10 (8%)	2 (4.5%)	NS	NS
Perforation	0 (0%)	0 (0%)	3 (2%)	0 (0%)	NS	NS

[a]From Estella P et al. J Am Coll Cardiol 1993;21:1550.
[b]From Topaz O et al. Am Heart J 1995 (submitted for publication).

ogy. Thus our initial clinical experience suggests that this technology can be safely and successfully applied in selected patients with acute myocardial infarction complicated by ongoing ischemia and angina (33). Some authorities predict that utilization of the holmium laser will open the door to a new approach in treatment of this critical clinical condition (34).

THROMBOTIC LESIONS

The presence of intracoronary thrombus in unstable, ischemic coronary syndromes has been associated with an increased risk of complications during coronary balloon angioplasty (35). Estella and coworkers (36) have

demonstrated that success of the excimer laser is significantly compromised when thrombus is angiographically detected. In contrast, in our experience with the holmium laser, the presence of angiographically detected thrombus did not significantly increase the risk of poor clinical outcome and did not compromise the safety and efficacy of the holmium laser-assisted coronary angioplasty (37). This observation is substantiated by data presented in Table 5.5, which delineates a comparison between holmium and excimer treated thrombotic and nonthrombotic lesions. These data support the hypothesis that the holmium:YAG laser may have an important effect on thrombotic tissue in humans.

CONCLUSIONS

The holmium:YAG laser is reliable, compact, nontoxic, easy to maintain and less expensive than other coronary laser systems. Accumulated clinical experience with this device indicates that it is a feasible and safe technology for revascularization in selected patients with symptomatic coronary artery disease. The device has a special niche in treatment of complex and calcified stenoses, as well as thrombotic lesions, complete occlusions, and acute myocardial infarction. Presently, laser-created neolumen is usually inadequate and requires adjunctive balloon angioplasty or directional atherectomy to achieve an optimal result. Newer, directional or eccentric, multifiber laser catheters may be able to achieve larger, adequate neolumens. Similar to other debulking devices such as excimer laser and directional atherectomy, the likelihood of the holmium laser alone yielding a high percentage of long-term patent vessels is still remote.

ACKNOWLEDGMENT

Many thanks to Laurie Topaz, Shirley McCray, Anne-Marie de Merlier, and Michelle Martin whose skills and patience were essential in preparation of this chapter.

REFERENCES

1. Litvack F, Grundfest WS, Segalowitz J et al. Interventional cardiovascular therapy by laser and thermal angioplasty. Circulation 1990;81(Suppl IV). IV-109–116.
2. Deckelbaum LI. Coronary laser angioplasty. Lasers Surg Med 1994;14:101–110.
3. Bouinais JL. Photophysical processes in recent medical laser developments: a review. Lasers Med Sci 1986; 1:47–66.
4. Litvack F, Grundfest WS, Papaioannou T, Mohr FW, Jakubowski AT, Forrester JS. Role of laser and thermal ablation devices in the treatment of vascular diseases. Am J Cardiol 1988;61:81G–86G.
5. Johnson J. Laser physics and its relevance to applications in medicine. In: Abela GS, ed. Lasers in cardiovascular medicine and surgery: fundamentals and techniques. Boston: Kluwer Academic, 1990.
6. Litvack F, Eigler N, Margolis J et al. Percutaneous excimer laser coronary angioplasty: results in the first consecutive 3000 patients. J Am Coll Cardiol 1994;23:323–329.
7. Fry SM. Laser Angioplasty—a physician's guide. 1st ed. Hanalei: SBDI, 1990.
8. Bonner RF, Smith PD, Prevosti LG, Bartorelli A, Almagor Y, Leon MB. Laser sources for angioplasty. In: Abela GS, ed. Lasers in cardiovascular medicine and surgery: fundamentals and techniques. Boston: Kluwer Academic, 1990.
9. Hassenstein S, Hanke H, Hanke S et al. Incidence of thrombotic occlusions in experimental holmium laser angioplasty compared to excimer laser angioplasty. Circulation 1991;84(Suppl II):124 (abstract).
10. McKay CR, Landas S, Robertson D et al. Histologic and angiographic effects of a new pulsed holmium:YAG laser in normal and atherosclerotic human coronary arteries. J Am Coll Cardiol 1991;17:207A.
11. Isner JM. Pathology. In: Isner JM, Clarke RH, eds. Cardiovascular laser therapy. 1st ed. New York: Raven, 1989.
12. Aretz HT, Butterly JR, Jewell ER et al. Effects of holmium-YSGG laser irradiation on arterial tissues: preliminary results. Soc Photo-Optical Instrument Engin 1989; 177:1067.
13. Hirota J, Shiikawa A, Nakano H et al. Early results of operative transluminal laser coronary angioplasty. Proceedings of the fifth annual meeting of the Japanese Society of Cardioangioscopy and Laser Cardioangioplasty, Tokyo, Japan, 1991.
14. Topaz O. Holmium:YAG laser angioplasty: the multicenter experience. In: Topol EJ, ed. Textbook of interventional cardiology. 2nd ed. Philadelphia: WB Saunders, 1993.
15. Ryan TJ, Faxon DP, Gunnar RU et al. Guidelines for percutaneous transluminal coronary angioplasty. A report of the American College of Cardiology/American Heart Association Task Force on Assessment of Diagnostic and Therapeutic Cardiovascular Procedures (Subcommittee on Percutaneous Transluminal Coronary Angioplasty). Circulation 1988;78:486.
16. Topaz O. Holmium laser coronary thrombolysis—a new treatment modality for revascularization in acute myocardial infarction: review. J Clin Laser Med Surg 1992; 10:427–431.
17. VanLeewen TG, Motamedi M, Meerteus JH et al. Origin of aortic wall dissections induced by ultraviolet and infrared pulsed laser ablation. Circulation 1991;84(Suppl II):361 (abstract).
18. Abela GS. Abrupt closure after pulsed laser angioplasty: spasm or a "Mille-Feuilles" effect? J Intervent Cardiol 1992;5:259–262.
19. Deckelbaum LI, Isner JM, Donaldson RF et al. Reduction of laser-induced pathologic tissue injury using pulsed energy delivery. Am J Cardiol 1985;56:662–667.
20. Topaz O. A new, safer lasing technique for laser-facilitated coronary angioplasty. J Intervent Cardiol 1993;6:297–306.
21. Lee BI, Rodriguez ER, Notargiocomo A et al. Thermal effects of laser and electrical discharge on cardiovascular tissues. Implications for coronary artery recanalization and endocardial ablation. J Am Coll Cardiol 1986;8:193–200.
22. Baumbach A, Hasse KK, Rose C, Oberhoff M, Hanke H, Harsch KR. Formation of pressure waves during in vitro excimer laser irradiation in whole blood and the effect of dilution with contrast media and saline. Lasers Surg Med 1994;14:3–6.

23. Ginsburg R. Laser angioplasty technique. In: Ginsburg R, Geschwind HJ, eds. Primer on laser angioplasty. 2nd ed. Mount Kisco: Futura, 1992.

24. Abela GS, Barbeau GR. Laser angioplasty: potential effects and current limitations. In: Topol EJ, ed. Textbook of interventional cardiology. 1st ed. Philadelphia: WB Saunders, 1990.

25. Topaz O, Rozenbaum EA, Battista S, Peterson C, Wysham DG. Laser-facilitated angioplasty and thrombolysis in acute myocardial infarction complicated by prolonged or recurrent chest pain. Cathet Cardiovasc Diagn 1993;28:7–16.

26. Murray N, Lyons J, Layton C, Balcom R. What proportion of patients with myocardial infarction are suitable for thrombolysis? Br Heart J 1987;57:144–147.

27. Cigarroa RG, Lange RA, Hillis LD. Prognosis after acute myocardial infarction in patients with and without residual anterograde coronary blood flow. Am J Cardiol 1989; 64:155–160.

28. Simoons ML, Arnold AER, Betri UA et al. Thrombolysis with tissue plasminogen activator in acute myocardial infarction: no additional benefit from immediate percutaneous coronary angioplasty. Lancet 1988;1:197–203.

29. Rothbaum DA, Linnemeir TJ, Landin RJ et al. Emergency PTCA in acute myocardial infarction: a three-year experience. J Am Coll Cardiol 1987;10:264–272.

30. Hopkins J, Savage M, Zanlunski A. Recurrent ischemia in the zone of prior myocardial infarction: results of coronary angioplasty of the infarct-related vessel. Am Heart J 1988;115:14–19.

31. Ellis SG, Roubin GS, King SB III, Douglas JS Jr, Weintraub WS, Thomas RG, Cox WR. Angiographic and clinical predictors of acute closure after native vessel coronary angioplasty. Circulation 1988;77:372–379.

32. deMarchena E, Mallon S, Posada JD, Garvey-Patsias K, Joshi B, Correa L, Sequeira R et al. Direct holmium laser-assisted balloon angioplasty in acute myocardial infarction. Am J Cardiol 1993;71:1223–1225.

33. Topaz O, Minisi AJ, Luxenberg M, Rozenbaum E. Laser angioplasty for lesions unsuitable for PTCA in acute myocardial infarction: quantitative coronary angiography and clinical results. Circulation 1994;90(Suppl I):I-434.

34. Heuser R. Editorial commentary. Cathet Cardiovasc Diagn 1993;28:17.

35. Vetrovec GW, Cowley MJ, Overton H, Richardson DW. Intracoronary thrombus in syndromes of unstable myocardial ischemia. Am Heart J 1981;102:1202–1208.

36. Estella P, Ryan TJ, Landzberg JS et al. Excimer laser-associated coronary angioplasty for lesions containing thrombus. J Am Coll Cardiol 1993;21:1550–1556.

37. Topaz O, Rozenbaum EA, Luxenberg MG, Wysham DG, Schumacher A. Holmium:YAG laser-facilitated coronary angioplasty for treatment of thrombotic and nonthrombotic lesions: clinical and quantitative coronary angiographic results in 112 patients. Am Heart J 1995 (submitted for publication).

6. Coiled Metallic Stents

CHRISTOPHER J.W.B. LEGGETT, and GARY S. ROUBIN

Despite new technologic improvements in equipment for percutaneous transluminal coronary angioplasty (PTCA) and the advent of newer devices for debriding atherosclerotic plaque from stenotic coronary arteries, the incidence of acute or threatened closure remains significant, between 2 and 10% depending on the complexity of the lesion treated (1–4). An additional 30 to 50% of patients go on to have late restenosis of the treated lesion. The reasons for acute closure and late restenosis are multifactorial, but arterial dissection of plaque and vessel wall recoil represent the most powerful contributors. Intracoronary stenting therefore emerged out of a need by interventional cardiologists to provide patients with an alternative to emergent coronary artery bypass grafting (CABG) and immediate or delayed myocardial infarction in the setting of acute vessel closure complicating PTCA. Despite the subsequent development of perfusion balloon technology facilitating prolonged inflations, coronary stenting has evolved as a more reliable technique for treating arterial dissection and impending vessel closure. It has been recently appreciated that vessel wall plaque recoil and remodeling can be favorably influenced by coronary stenting. In addition, it has been demonstrated that the stents have a beneficial effect on late restenosis.

HISTORICAL BACKGROUND

Initial work on the expandable coil version of the intracoronary stent by Cesare Gianturco began in the early 1980s. In 1985, through collaboration with Gary S. Roubin, M.D., stent deployment experimentation expanded into the coronary arteries of dogs and swine and the atherosclerotic iliac arteries in rabbits. In 1987 the Food and Drug Administration (FDA) authorized a phase I study in humans under Roubin's investigation. In this study the stent was used as a bridge to surgery in the setting of acute closure complicating PTCA. Initially all patients underwent coronary artery bypass grafting (CABG); none experienced transluminal myocardial infarction, and all were discharged from the hospital within 8 days (5). On the basis of this favorable data with regard to myocardial salvage, the FDA gave approval for a phase II study, which permitted the use of the intracoronary stent for treatment of acute and threatened vessel closure following PTCA. The device was subsequently approved by the FDA on June 1, 1993, for coronary use in the setting of acute or threatened closure.

Since the initiation of the phase II study and its subsequent approval by the FDA for clinical application, the largest experience in the treatment of acute or impending closure complicating coronary interventional procedures has been gained with the Gianturco-Roubin Flexible metallic coil stent (FlexStent, Cook Inc., Bloomington, IN). Both single-center and multicenter experiences have confirmed the efficacy of coronary artery stenting in reducing the incidence of myocardial infarction, emergency CABG, and overall mortality associated with acute closure (6, 7). A recent prospective randomized trial has also suggested the efficacy of this device for reducing late restenosis (8). Larger multicenter studies are under way to further confirm these findings.

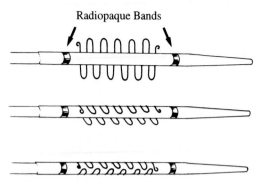

Radiopaque Bands

Figure 6.1. Schematic representation of the Gianturco-Roubin (Cook, Inc.) coiled metallic stent. The diagrams show the "clamshell"-like function. If stents are undersized, and then overexpanded, plaque may prolapse within the stent.

STENT DESIGN

This device is made of a monofilamentous, surgical stainless steel wire, 0.006 inch in diameter, wrapped in a serpentine manner around a compliant polyethylene (PE) balloon catheter so that every 360° the wire makes a 180° turn (Fig. 6.1). This design results in a series of interdigitating U- and inverted U-shaped loops and allows the coil to expand in a clamshell manner as the balloon is inflated. Currently, stents increasing in diameter by 0.5-mm increments are available from 2.0 to 4.0 mm. The stent is available in 20-mm and 12-mm lengths, measured from complete coil to complete coil. There are two markers delineating the proximal and distal portions of the stent. The first complete loop of the stent is 2 to 3 mm inside each radiopaque marker. The balloon used to deliver the 12-mm device is 20 mm in length; the balloon used to deliver the 20-mm stent is 30 mm in length.

The balloon catheter has a 4.3 Fr shaft. The maximum guidewire size compatible with the balloon catheter is 0.018 inch. The amount of metal involved is relatively small, covering approximately 12% of the surface area of the artery. With proper deployment the wires are embedded into the intimal layer of the vessel wall, further reducing the area of exposed metal.

Unique properties of this flexible coil stent include (a) flexibility to allow deployment to most segments of the coronary tree, including vessels with acute takeoff and moderate tortuosity, saphenous vein bypass grafts, and internal mammary artery grafts; (b) the relatively small metal surface allows positioning at branch-points with minimal compromise in flow; and (c) the length of the stent does not shorten with deployment.

Limitations of this device include the following: First, the irregular surface of the stent as it is mounted on the balloon can make deployment through calcified and tortuous vessels relatively difficult even for experienced operators. Second, the open nature of the coil construction fails to restrain small flaps and prolapsing plaque in some situations. Solutions to these and other technical problems will be discussed in the following pages.

PATIENT SELECTION

All patients undergoing PTCA in whom the target vessel is between 2.5 and 4.0 mm should be considered as possible candidates for intracoronary stenting should the appropriate clinical situation develop. Although the final decision to utilize intracoronary stenting is made in the catheterization laboratory at the time of angiography, the consideration for potential stenting should be estimated and seriously discussed well in advance of the patient arriving at the catheterization laboratory (generally the night before). The use of the stent in angioplasty salvage may require intensive postprocedural anticoagulation with heparin, aspirin, ticlopidine, and warfarin; thus patients need to be screened before angioplasty for risk factors that may preclude anticoagulation. The majority of patients, however, can be managed on aspirin and ticlopidine therapy only.

CONTRAINDICATIONS

Possible contraindicators to stenting include recent cerebral or gastrointestinal hemorrhage, vessel diameter <2.0 to 2.5 mm, significant vessel tortuosity or proximal atherosclerosis prohibiting adequate guide catheter support, large amount of untreated thrombus at lesion site, and bleeding diatheses that limit the use of antiplatelet agents and anticoagulant therapy. Other relative contraindications include history of carcinomatosis, laser-treated diabetic retinopathy, chronic pulmonary or gastrointestinal inflammatory disease, active peptic ulcer disease, active menstruation, and anemia of unknown origin. Nonetheless, the risk of bleeding needs to be balanced against the risk of acute closure and the likely outcome of emergency CABG. At any rate, if long-term anticoagulation is not possible, the stent can still be useful as a bridge to bypass surgery. It is important to note, however, that in many patients intensive anticoagulation is not required to maintain stent patency and that patients can be managed on antiplatelet therapy only.

It is extremely important for the operator to understand those factors that contribute to stent thrombosis and, in turn, the need for intensive anticoagulation. Indications for stenting will depend on the risk benefit ratio for any individual patient. Stent thrombosis is rare, <1.0% in large vessels (≥3.0 mm) stented with large stents (≥3.5 mm), especially if used in an elective or semielective setting (8). Optimal angiographic results (see later technical discussion) are critical in lowering stent thrombosis.

Optimal initial results include good distal runoff, minimal residual narrowing, no residual dissection (particularly distal to stent), and no intraluminal filling defects. In such cases intense anticoagulation is not necessary and good antiplatelet therapy alone will be sufficient. Accordingly, a recent history of retinal hemorrhage in such a patient would not be a contraindication to stenting.

Alternatively, vessels with poor distal runoff (particularly infarct-related vessels within 14 days of a myocardial infarction), small vessels, long dissections, a lesion requiring multiple stents, and a lesion with large thrombus burden are at higher risk of thrombosis. These patients require intense anticoagulation, including the combination of antiplatelet, coumadin, and heparin therapy. Accordingly, these vessels should only be stented if the risk of bleeding is considered to be less than the risk associated with the alternative management option.

PRETREATMENT

As closure is unpredictable, patients who meet the criteria for stenting are routinely given soluble aspirin (325 mg twice a day) and ticlopidine 250 mg b.i.d. on the evening before PTCA. Even in patients in whom intensive anticoagulation is not being considered, high-dose antiplatelet therapy is critically important. Once the patient arrives in the cardiac catheterization laboratory, 10,000 units of heparin are routinely given at the beginning of angioplasty. Activated clotting time (ACT) is measured and supplemental boluses of heparin are administered to maintain an ACT between 250 secs and 300 secs.

To ensure adequate anticoagulation, an ACT should be checked every 30 minutes throughout the case. Once the decision to stent is made, and often at the outset of cases with lesions that are high risk for stenting, a 10% solution of dextran-40 may be administered to the patient. A rapid infusion of 200 cc is given, and a drip is maintained at 25 cc per hour. To prevent allergic reactions, 250 mg methylprednisolone and 20 cc (150 mg/cc) Promit is routinely administered intravenously. Current opinion is that dextran is not an essential element of the stent drug regimen.

It is strongly advisable to begin the PTCA procedure with equipment that will facilitate stenting should it become necessary. There are six primary objectives that must be met to consistently practice stenting techniques that will ensure stent placement success.

1. Know what ancillary equipment is required for successful stenting.
2. Know how and when to initiate the anticoagulation protocol.
3. Know how to select a stent of the appropriate diameter.
4. Know how to prepare the vessel for stenting.
5. Review the present checklist.
6. Know the fundamentals of stent deployment to ensure a successful stent implantation.

ANCILLARY EQUIPMENT (SEE TABLE 6.1)

Guiding Catheters

Advanced planning is critical. It is easier and safer to select guide catheter equipment at the outset of a case that will permit vessel stenting should stenting become necessary. Stents ranging in size from 2.0 mm to 3.0 mm in diameter pass easily through 8 Fr large-lumen guiding catheters with an interior diameter of ≥0.077 inch (e.g., Marathon, Inc.; Baxter Inc.). Alternatively, 3.5-mm and 4.0-mm stents require 8 Fr guiding catheters with ≥0.086-inch internal diameter (i.e., Cook, Schneider, Cordis, Mansfield) or large-lumen 9 Fr guiding catheters. It is best to utilize a guiding catheter that will remain firm and supportive during the angioplasty procedure. If you chose a guiding catheter that softens during the procedure, you will quickly find that it is unsuitable for the stenting procedure. For left coronary lesions we recommend beginning the case with a short-tipped left Judkins guide. This device provides excellent support and allows for maneuver-

ability, including "Amplatzing" if necessary for tracking of a difficult stent. The left Amplatz guiding catheter is suitable for left circumflex, left vein grafts and right coronary arteries (particularly right coronary arteries with upgoing or shepherd's crook configuration). The Judkins right is ideal for right coronary lesion and the multipurpose guiding catheter for right vein graft lesions.

Large-lumen Tuohey-Borst adapters (USCI, Billerica, MA; ACS, Santa Clara, CA; Medtronic, Inc., Minneapolis, MN; Cook, Inc., Bloomington, IN; Microvena Corp., St. Paul, MN) are needed to allow passage of the stent. It is advisable to routinely utilize these large Tuohey-Borst adapters for all PTCA procedures.

Guidewires

Our standard choice are 0.018-inch extra-support guidewires (Cook Inc., Microvena). Satisfactory deployment of the flexible coil stent is greatly enhanced by the use of these wires. They optimize guide catheter support, provide maximal coaxial alignment, straighten out curves in the vessel, and facilitate tracking of the stent around angular segments in the vessel. Use of these wires is facilitated by use of a 0.018-inch compatible balloon catheter, which permits easy exchange of the standard, flexible, steerable coronary wire for an extra-support wire should stenting become necessary. Stent placement is achieved by placing the balloon tip catheter distal to the dissection and then exchanging the wire. The extra-support wire reduces vessel tortuosity, straightens the proximal vessel, and provides a firm rail over which to track the stent. To this end, the tip of the wire should be placed as distally as possible to ensure the stiff shaft of the wire is across the lesion. In simple anatomic straight vessels usage of standard 0.016-inch and 0.018-inch wires may be adequate, but for the interventionalist less experienced with stenting, maximum guidewire support with extra-support wires is strongly recommended.

Table 6.1
Catheterization Laboratory Equipment

- ACT analyzer
- Intraaortic balloon pump
- Large-bore Tuohey-Borst adaptors
- Large-lumen 8 Fr (0.086 inch) guide catheter
- 2.0, 2.5, 3.0, 3.5, and 4.0 mm Cook stents will easily pass through new 8 Fr Lumax Cook guide catheter with 0.086-inch lumen. (Recommended because of unusual "stiffness" and support)
- Extra-support guidewire—0.018-inch (Cook Roadrunner), 0.018-inch extra-support (ACS), 0.018-inch stabilizer (Cordis)
- 0.018-inch compatible PTCA balloon catheter
- Medications (aspirin, dipyridamole, dextran, methylprednisolone, promit).

Angioplasty Balloon Catheters

Use of the above-mentioned guidewires requires routine use of 0.018-inch compatible angioplasty balloon catheters. A number of manufacturers produce suitable over-the-wire, as well as monorail, balloons with ideal crossing profiles. Before the release of the Synergy catheter (Mansfield/Boston Scientific Corp, Watertown, MA), use of the monorail system had a major drawback because of the inability to exchange guidewires for an extra-support wire when needed for stent placement. If a 0.014-inch system is used, inexpensive exchange catheters (e.g., Cook, Inc.) are available for changing to a 0.018-inch extra-support wire.

INDICATIONS FOR STENTING

Indications for use of the flexible coil stent are evolving. The stent can be used successfully in the following situations: acute and threatened closure, including extensive (>6 cm) arterial dissections; prevention of restenosis in lesions showing suboptimal results from initial balloon dilation; treatment of resistant focal coronary spasm; and focal systolic compression by myocardial bridges. The device has been placed in all segments of the coronary arteries, including ostial locations and distal branches such as the posterior descending, obtuse marginal, and diagonal arteries. The device can be safely placed across major side branches, including the left main bifurcation. Clearly, this last maneuver requires special circumstances and patient management. The device has also been successfully used in saphenous vein grafts (≤4.0 mm in diameter) and left and right internal mammary conduits. It can be used across distal anastomosis sites, tapering vessels, and extremely tortuous segments. It is not suitable for small vessels <2.0 to 2.5 mm and, given the present design constraints, vessels ≥4.0 mm. The device is difficult to deploy in tortuous, noncompliant, calcified arteries. When there exists documented acute vessel closure with TIMI 0 or TIMI I flow and persistent ischemia after angioplasty and the patient has no contraindications, the decision to stent is straightforward. (It is usually prudent to undertake stenting before acute closure occurs.) Impending or threatened closure, however, is difficult to define. A residual stenosis ≥50% and significant dissection characterized by lumen compromise, a length ≥10 mm with extraluminal contrast staining, and an observed angiographic deterioration over the minutes after the last inflation are harbingers of impending closure. For example, when dilating a critical last remaining vessel, it is often more advisable to stent any visible dissection flap than to run the risk of acute closure and immediate hemodynamic collapse.

Sizing/Balloon Stent Relationships

To achieve the best possible immediate and late clinical results, accurate sizing of the coronary stent is critical. Undersizing the stent results in significant residual stenosis with increased risk of early thrombosis and likelihood of restenosis. The stent is mounted on a compliant angioplasty balloon of standard construction with a covering sheath. A 3.0-mm stent is delivered on a compliant balloon that may reach a nominal size of 3.5 mm when expanded at 6 atm unconstrained on the bench top. However, stents are typically deployed at low pressures, approximately 4 to 5 atm, and the compliant balloon and stent are constrained at these pressures by the vessel wall. At high inflation pressures of 6 to 8 atm the balloon may continue to expand compliance, and there exists the potential for arterial damage and distal dissection. It has been recently shown at the University of Alabama at Birmingham that the diameters achieved at low pressures are substantially less than the nominal diameter (9). For example, when deployed at low pressures a 4.0-mm stent has a 3.6-mm diameter, a 3.5-mm stent has a 3.2-mm diameter, and a 3.0-mm stent has a 2.8-mm diameter. Accordingly, one should choose a stent with nominal size approximately 0.5 mm larger than the reference diameter of the target vessel.

Current recommendations are as follows: vessels 2.0 to 2.4 mm in diameter should be supported with a 2.5-mm stent; those 2.5 to 2.9 mm in diameter with a 3.0-mm stent; those 3.0 to 3.4 mm in diameter with a 3.5-mm stent; and those 3.5 to 4.0 mm in diameter with a 4.0-mm stent. All stents should be initially deployed at low pressure between 4 and 5 atmospheres. Follow-up inflation with a noncompliant balloon at high pressures (14–16) is now routinely recommended to optimize stent placement and expansion. Sizing of the noncompliant follow-up balloon should be based on diameter of adjacent normal segments.

STENTING TECHNIQUE

Step One

Once the decision to stent has been made, the first step is to place an extra-support guidewire into the coronary artery. This can be achieved by placing a 0.018-inch guidewire compatible balloon as far distally as possible in the vessel to be stented. The existing guidewire is removed and the extra-support guidewire is advanced, via the lumen of the balloon catheter, and placed as distal as possible. Either an extension-length wire or an extended wire should be used. At 300 cm the Roadrunner extra-support wire by Cook is of sufficient length such that an extension is not necessary (Fig. 6.2).

Step Two

It is critical that the target lesion be adequately dilated prior to placement of the stent. This includes predilating moderate stenosis proximal to the lesion to allow smooth passage of the stent. Occasionally, even lesions distal to the dissection must be carefully dilated to facilitate stent positioning. Before starting the procedure be certain the distal limits of the dissection have been well defined.

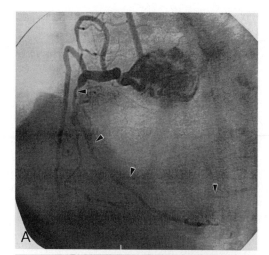

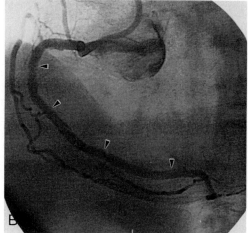

Figure 6.2. Stenting of acute closure caused by a long, spiral dissection. **A** shows occlusion of the vessel beginning from a proximal bend point and extending to the distal posterior descending artery. The dissection was first wired using a standard flexible coronary guidewire. A balloon was then advanced into the posterior descending artery (PDA) to confirm that a true lumen had been reestablished. Multiple inflations were performed to establish brisk antegrade flow and to precisely determine the distal limits of the dissection. This balloon was then readvanced into the PDA, and the flexible wire was replaced with an 0.018-inch Cook Roadrunner guidewire. Beginning at the PDA, a series of 3.0-, 3.5-, and 4.0-mm stents were placed distally from the PDA to the proximal right coronary artery to reconstruct the vessel. The final result is shown in **B.**

Step Three

The stent balloon is prepared in the standard negative-pressure fashion. The operator should make certain that the stent is intact on the balloon. Using the stent on the current balloon design, the rather stiff balloon tip can be softened by "working" the tip of the balloon. Operator gloves should be clean and free of debris or thrombus. Do not attempt to place a stent if any of the tightly wrapped stent coils have been loosened (or disrupted) during preparation of the device.

Step Four

The extended guidewire is held straight, and the stent is easily tracked over the wire and advanced to the Tuohey-Borst Y adapter. The Y adapter is then opened widely to allow for passage of the stent without any resistance. This is critical because hasty passage through the Y adapter can cause the stent to be "accordioned" and damaged. It is critical that the operator feel no resistance to the passage of the stent through the Tuohey-Borst adapter. Inexperienced operators are encouraged to use a pull-away sheath provided with the stent. The pull-away sheath is first placed through the Y adaptor; this ensures that the stent will not be damaged. Use of the pull-away sheath requires the use of very large bore & adaptors, that is, Cook (provided with stent), DVI, Microvena, or Angion. The stent is advanced over the wire to the tip of the coronary guiding catheter. This is achieved with the operator's assistant providing constant back pressure on the wire as stent is advanced forward. This should be performed under fluoroscopy to prevent inadvertent pulling back of wire across the lesion.

Before advancing the stent into the coronary artery, it is important to ensure maximum guide catheter support. Again, for the left coronary system this can be achieved with deep intubation of the left main with a soft, short-tipped, left Judkins catheter. Counterclockwise rotation is best for access into the left anterior descending artery, (LAD) while clockwise rotation facilitates entrance into the left circumflex ostium (left Amplatz guides are also helpful with left circumflex stenting). The native right coronary artery is best intubated with right Judkins or left Amplatz guides. Maximum coaxial support can be best visualized in right anterior oblique projection with gentle clockwise torque. Right bypass grafts are best cannulated with a multipurpose guide, while Amplatz-shaped guides perform well for left bypass grafts. It is of critical importance to ensure that the guiding catheter is well intubated into the artery and well supported before advancing the stent.

Step Five

When the operator's assistant applying gentle backward tension on the guidewire, the stent is advanced out of the guide into the coronary artery. The operator should advance the stent in the following fashion: the fingers of the left hand should steady and maintain the position of the guide catheter to the vascular sheath, and the Tuohey-Borst adapter should rest between the middle and ring fingers of the right hand while the stent balloon catheter is advanced between the index finger and the thumb with a constant steady forward pressure (never pull the stent back into the guide once it has exited). Again, it is important for the assistant to pull back on the guidewire to allow forward movement of the stent balloon. This is referred to as the "push-pull" technique. The operator must coordinate this maneuver by instructing the assistant exactly when to pull back on the extra-support wire. In right coronary and left circumflex arteries a well-coordinated deep breath from the patient will also assist passage of the stent. Repeated small injections of contrast are necessary to ensure proper positioning of the stent. While the stent wires cannot be visualized, the proximal and distal markers serve as landmarks for proper positioning of the stent. Complete stent coils begin approximately 2 to 3 mm inside the markers of the stent. One should always err on the side of distal placement of the stent to ensure that the distal dissection has been covered.

Step Six

Once the stent has been delivered to the desired location, the balloon is rapidly inflated to 4 to 5 atm under fluoroscopy. Allow adequate time for the balloon to fully expand the stent; this can usually be achieved in 30 to 60 seconds. Occasionally, pressures of 5 atm for 60 to 90 seconds may be required. If necessary, the stent can be very rapidly dilated by rapidly inflating to 6 to 7 atm. If this is done, deflate the balloon immediately after the coils are fully expanded. Caution: the stent balloon is extremely compliant and pressure exceeding 5 atm may result in unwanted dissection distal to the stent. After stent deployment the balloon is deflated and removed with the operator removing the balloon and the assistant advancing the guidewire. To avoid damage to the proximal vessel and even the stent in proximal locations, it is necessary for the operator to hold back on the guiding catheter as it tends to be "pulled" deeply into the artery as the "bulky" balloon is withdrawn. Subsequently, the first postdeployment angiogram is acquired.

Step Seven

One should consider the stent balloon simply as a vehicle for reliable delivery of the stent to the lesion and for initial deployment of the stent at low pressures. Following stent deployment the following situations may be encountered: (a) a smooth result with full coverage of the dissection and good distal runoff; (b) residual proximal dissection requiring an additional stent; (c) an uncovered distal dissection; or (d) no evidence of residual dissection, but rather evidence of either filling defects or a hazy appearance within the stented segment. Each of these scenarios requires a different solution, but high-pressure inflations with a noncompliant balloon are mandatory in all situations.

SMOOTH RESULTS

In this situation we recommend follow-up inflation with a high-pressure, low-profile, noncompliant balloon sized to the vessel.

Balloon should be inflated to 14 to 16 atm. To avoid dissection high-pressure inflations should be restricted to within the stent coils. Slight oversizing of the balloon (i.e., a 3.5 balloon in a 3.2 vessel) will produce good results. To ensure smooth transition from stent to distal vessel, first place the distal tip of the balloon just distal to the stent and expand to 2 to 3 atm of pressure. Slowly withdraw the balloon into the stent, only going to high pressures once the balloon is fully restrained by the stented segment (Fig. 6.3).

RESIDUAL PROXIMAL DISSECTIONS

This simply requires placement of a second stent proximal to the first with some overlap. This overlap is essential to prevent any potential prolapse of atherosclerotic material between the two stents. One must keep in mind when positioning the stent that the first complete stent loop is 2 to 3 mm inside the stent markers (see Fig. 6.2).

UNCOVERED DISTAL DISSECTION

This can be a difficult problem to overcome for it has a few inherent potential hazards. Occasionally, a small residual distal dissection may respond to a prolonged balloon inflation. If this is unsuccessful, an attempt to deploy a second stent distal to and via the first stent can be made. If available a 12-mm stent is preferable as it usually passes somewhat more easily through an existing 20-mm stent. The obvious danger is coil overlap with potential clutching and subsequent contortion or "accordioning" of one or both stents, and this can obviously result in vessel thrombosis and occlusion. To avoid this problem first dilate the proximal stent with a larger, high-pressure balloon and use 0.018-inch extra-support wire and good guide support. In every case it is best to avoid this problem by (a) carefully identifying the dissection extent prior to stenting, (b) if in doubt placing the first stent more distally, and (c) deploying the stent at the lowest pressure that will expand the stent.

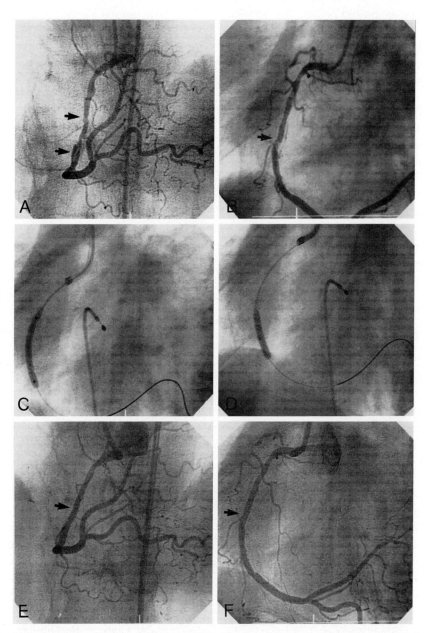

Figure 6.3. Dissection in the mid right coronary artery RAO views **(A)** and LAO views **(B)**. Having carefully identified the limits of the dissection, a single stent sized larger than the artery is placed over an 0.018-inch extra-support wire **(C)**. A high-pressure (16A) inflation is then performed within the stent **(D)**, and final results with 0% residual narrowing is achieved RAO **(E)** and LAO **(F)**.

FILLING DEFECTS/HAZY-VESSEL APPEARANCE

In this situation a noncompliant, high-pressure balloon is placed within the stented segment and inflated to 14 to 16 atm for several minutes. If haziness persists, one must make a judgment call concerning the relative contribution of plaque prolapsing between the stent wires or thrombus. The former problem is more likely to be observed in badly dissected fibrotic lesions associated with chronic anginal syndromes. Management involves placing a second stent with the first stent (see previous section). If thrombus is suspected or there is soft plaque, unstable anginal syndromes, or PTCA for acute MI, then a side-hole infusion catheter should be placed within the stent (Cook, Inc.; Target Therapeutics) and urokinase infused at 80,000 units/hour IV for 6 to 12 hours.

COMPLEX STENTING TECHNIQUES

Side Branch Stenting

Because of the construction of the Cook Stent with interdigiting loops (gaps between the loops), flow down major side branches is rarely compromised. It is acceptable to place a stent in a main vessel at a branch point and then pass a wire via the stent down the side branch or use a fixed wire balloon to treat lesions in the side branch (Fig. 6.4). Any resistance to passage of the balloon should elicit caution from the operator. Potential problems include passage of the wire underneath a stent strut with subsequent abutting of the balloon against the coil of the stent and side-to-side resistance of passage of the balloon through the stent because of the balloon profile or vessel tortuosity. When recrossing stents for any reason, but particularly in tortuous segments, unused, low-profile balloons are preferable.

If branch point dissection occurs and main vessel with side branch stenting is necessary, double wiring of the side branch and main vessel should be performed to protect both vessels simultaneously. Once both vessels have been safely wired, stenting of the side branch should be performed first with all coils strategically placed within the side branch (ostium, distally). Operator experience is important in these situations because if one stents the main vessel first with the wire in place down the side branch, the operator would have created a difficult problem by trapping the side branch wire underneath the coil and between the coil and the wall of the vessel. Ideally, stenting of the side branch is undertaken first; subsequently, the side branch wire is removed followed by stenting of the main vessel. Most often it is prudent to stent the main vessel first and simply place a balloon through the side of the stent to dilate the side branch. Often there exists some residual narrowing at the ostium of the side branch, but anticoagulation usually ensures patency. When stenting the side branch first, be careful not to leave the side branch stent coils protruding into the main lumen and thus prohibiting adequate placement of the stent into the main vessel (Fig. 6.5). Clinical situations may arise where the operator will not have time to stent both vessels because of ischemia or acute closure, for example; the decision must then be made regarding which vessel is clinically most important. Although it is generally easy to wire the side branch through the side of stent, it is extremely difficult and usually impossible to pass a stent through an existing stent and then out the side of the stent. If this is attempted, it usually first requires placing the balloon partially in the main vessel and partially in the side branch to stretch the coils as far apart as possible to allow passage of the second stent. Obviously, the main limitations are metal-to-metal contortion and the stent becoming accordioned. Occasionally, it is necessary to perform "kissing balloon techniques" within the stented bifurcation to optimize the result (Figs. 6.5 and 6.6).

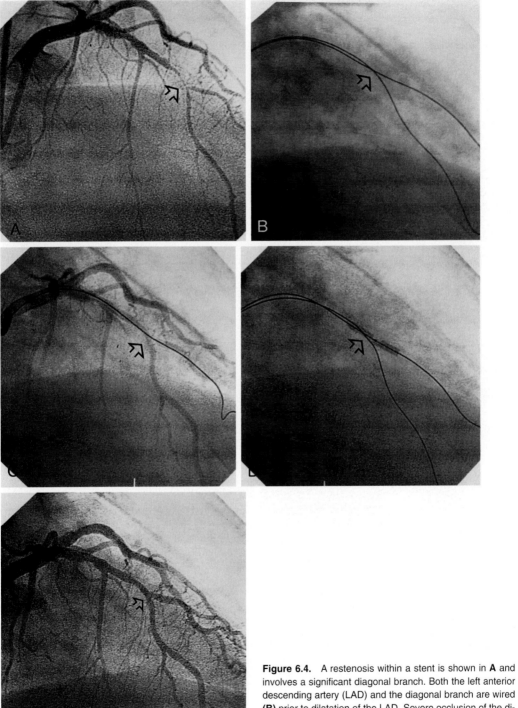

Figure 6.4. A restenosis within a stent is shown in **A** and involves a significant diagonal branch. Both the left anterior descending artery (LAD) and the diagonal branch are wired **(B)** prior to dilatation of the LAD. Severe occlusion of the diagonal results. A balloon is passed through the stent wires **(D)**, and the lesion is dilated. The final result is shown in **E.**

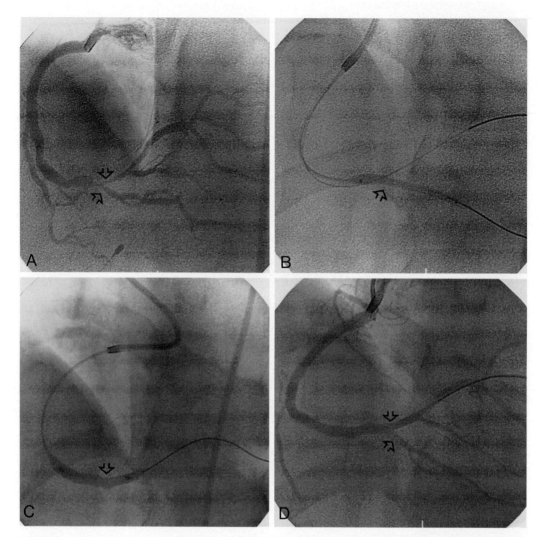

Figure 6.5. Dual stenting of side branches. **A.** A complex lesion involving the bifurcation of the right coronary artery into a large posterolateral branch and a large posterior descending artery. Ultrasound examination of the vessel prior to stenting revealed that at the bifurcation the diameter from media to media was 3.8 mm. The vessel tapered rapidly after the bifurcation. **B.** Each branch was wired and predilated with 0.018-inch compatible balloon systems. The flexible wires were then replaced with 0.018-inch Cook Roadrunner wires, and a 3.0-mm stent was advanced into the posterior descending artery. At least one coil of the stent was left in the main right coronary artery. The wire in the posterior descending artery was then removed, and a low-profile balloon was advanced across the lesion in the posterolateral branch. Inflation of this balloon ensured that the remaining coil was well compressed against the ostium of the posterior descending artery. **C.** A 4.0-mm stent was then advanced into the posterolateral segment artery (PLSA) branch. **D.** After deployment of this stent, there was once again some compromise of the previously placed 3.0-mm stent. **E.** A 4.0-mm balloon was then placed through the "barrel" of the 4.0-mm stent in the posterolateral branch, and a 3.0-mm fixed wire device was placed through the 4.0-mm stent and down the barrel of the 3.0-mm stent. Simultaneous inflations produced an excellent angiographic result with no residual stenosis apparent in either of these major branches **(F)**.

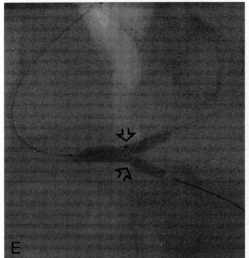

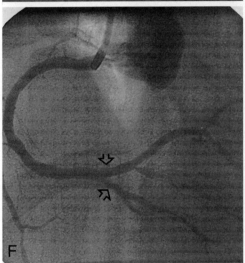

Figure 6.5E, F

Tapering Vessels

The Cook stent can be fashioned to accommodate tapering vessels (Figs. 6.7 and 6.8). First, deploy the stent at lowest pressures in the tapered vessel to allow for coil expansion. Then partially withdraw the balloon into the proximal, larger vessel and inflate at higher pressures to increase the diameter of the stent and mold it to fit the more proximal vessel. (Remember the stent balloon is very compliant at higher pressures.)

Multivessel Stenting

There is no contraindication to multivessel stenting once the decision has been made to stent. In patients with several stenotic sites in different vessels one can generally safely proceed to angioplasty of the second vessel when the first vessel is stented. The operator's threshold for placing additional stents in different vessels or in the same vessel at a different site should be low once the patient is committed to anticoagulation. The use of multiple stents during a single procedure has not been associated with an increased incidence of stent thrombosis or restenosis. Coil stents can be used effectively in vein grafts up to 4 mm in diameter (Fig. 6.9).

Stenting Ostial Sites

A clear view of the ostial lesion is critical. One must obtain a view that permits maximal visualization throughout stent placement. Initially, the stent is advanced into the vessel partially beyond the ostial site. After disengaging the guide from the ostium, the stent is carefully pulled back until the proximal marker is approximately 4 mm outside the vessel to ensure coverage of the ostial lesion (Fig. 6.10). Since the first coil is 2 mm inside the marker, only approximately 2 mm of stent coil is exposed in the aorta (in RCA lesions) or the distal left main in left circumflex lesions. There does not appear to be a problem with leaving part of the stent in the aorta or distal left main. With other stent designs, subsequent catheterization can fishmouth the opening of the stent, preventing further access. This has not been a problem with the coil stent. It is, however, very important to cover the ostial lesion while leaving as little unprotected coil exposed as possible.

Stenting in Acute Myocardial Infarction

Prolonged intracoronary urokinase infusion at 80,000 to 100,000 units per hour is mandatory if one elects to stent an acutely infarcted

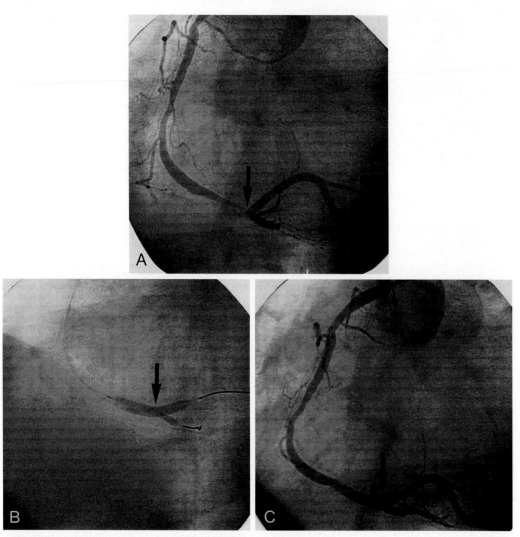

Figure 6.6. Stenting of a bifurcation lesion utilizing the "kissing-balloon" technique within the stent. **A** shows a high-grade lesion at the origin of the posterior descending and posterolateral segments of the right coronary artery. A 3.5-mm stent was placed within the lesion and extended into the posterolateral branch. After placement of the stent, the origin of the posterior descending artery was compromised. **B.** A 3.5-mm balloon was placed through the "barrel" of the stent, and a 3.0-mm fixed wire balloon system was placed through the stent and into the posterior descending artery. **C.** Simultaneous inflations were performed, and the final angiographic result was excellent.

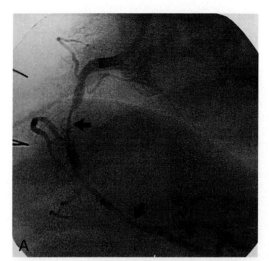

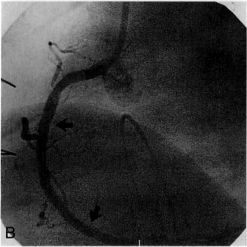

Figure 6.7.   Elective stenting to prevent restenosis in severe, diffuse disease. **A.** This diabetic female patient had undergone seven previous angioplasties to this right coronary artery and one previous bypass surgery. The vein graft to this vessel was occluded. There was a high-grade proximal lesion and a long, diffuse distal segment. Although the lumen appeared to be no more than 2.5 mm in diameter, ultrasound examination revealed the vessel was 3.5 mm distally and 4.0 mm proximally. **B.** A series of 3.5- and 4.0-mm stents were placed in the vessel producing the angiographic result.

vessel. Depending on logistics, 6 to 18 hours of infusion in the coronary care units is necessary. Poststent lucency and high thrombogenic potential in this setting make intracoronary urokinase a necessity.

Retrieving Stents

In situations where the stent cannot be adequately deployed or when the stent has accordioned during passage, the stent balloon unit should be slowly withdrawn to the mouth of the guiding catheter. Similar to deployment of the stent, never pull the stent back into mouth of the guide as "degloving" of the stent off the balloon can occur. Once the stent is at the mouth of guide, the guide catheter and stent are withdrawn as one unit through the arterial sheath (see Fig. 6.2). The 0.18-inch extra-support coronary guidewire certainly facilitates this maneuver. If the stent becomes "hung up" on the valve of the sheath, one should remove the sheath along with the guide catheter and stent balloon over the guidewire. Obviously, this above process should be carefully performed under fluoroscopy. As a safeguard the wire is not removed with the stent balloon or guide catheter. This allows the stent to remain on the wire in the unfortunate circumstance of degloving of the stent off the balloon during the retrieval process. If the stent does come off onto the wire, endomyocardial bioptones or the special Cook retrieval device can be used to clamp the stent and remove it. Finally, another more technically difficult option is to attempt to thread the balloon through the stent once the wire has crossed and to inflate to low pressure within or distal to the stent and then to withdraw.

Intraaortic Balloon Pump (IABP) Support

It is crucial to consider stenting as part of an overall strategy for managing acute closure and, simultaneously, optimizing the patient's hemodynamic status. Use of IABP has proven invaluable in circulatory support, augmentation of coronary blood flow, and even helping to "stent open" the dissection by raising the intracoronary perfusion pressure after PTCA. Furthermore, stent placement can take a long time in cases of complex anatomy requiring

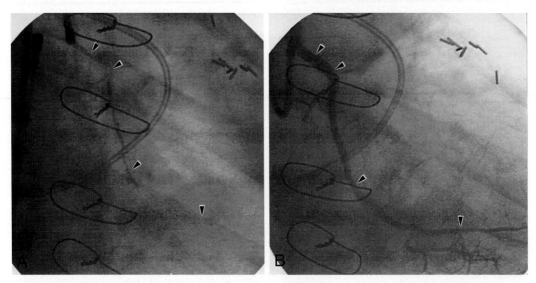

Figure 6.8. Endoluminal reconstruction of chronically occluded vessels. **A.** A chronically occluded left main and large obtuse marginal branch were accessed with a 0.018-inch guidewire (Terumo) and a 0.016-inch standard wire prior to dilatation and stenting. **B.** After the distal lumen was established and brisk antegrade flow was observed, a series of 3.0-, 3.5-, and 4.0-mm Cook stents were placed from the distal obtuse marginal vessel to the left main stem.

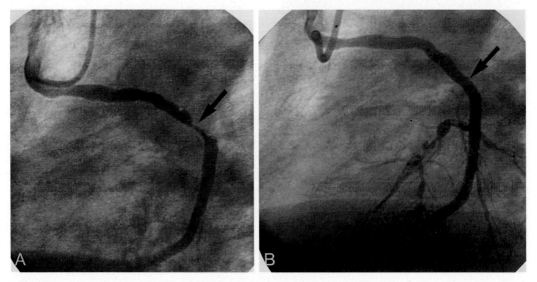

Figure 6.9. Stenting saphenous vein bypass grafts. **A.** A complex lesion is seen in a diffusely diseased saphenous vein bypass graft to a left anterior descending artery. **B.** After balloon dilatation, a suboptimal result remained, and a 4.0-mm stent was advanced into the graft over a 0.018-inch Roadrunner guidewire producing a good angiographic result.

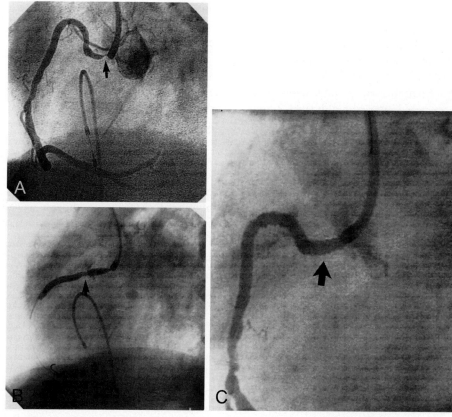

Figure 6.10. An ostial RCA lesion **(A)** is dilated with a high-pressure balloon prior to stent placement **(B)**. In stenting ostial lesions we prefer to leave at least one coil of the stent outside the artery. The stent is then postdilated with a high-pressure, noncompliant balloon with the final results shown **(C)**. No untoward sequelae have been observed.

prolonged deep guiding catheter intubation. The intraaortic balloon pump has been critical in permitting these aggressive maneuvers.

Intravascular Ultrasound Imaging

Intravascular ultrasound assessment prior to stenting facilitates correct stent sizing (see Fig. 6.7). The emergence of this technique has permitted interventionalists to reliably compare what is often angiographically called zero percent residual stenosis following stent deployment to an accurate intravascular lumen diameter. We have found that despite the angiographic appearance of 0% residual stenosis that the initial minimal lumen diameter visualized by intravascular ultrasound can be appreciably increased with a subsequent high-pressure balloon inflation.

It is the achievement of this maximal lumen diameter that we believe gives our patients the best opportunity to maintain a patent artery, decreasing the risk of both stent thrombosis and late restenosis. Because of our intracoronary ultrasound observations we strongly advocate high-pressure noncompliant, appropriately sized, follow-up balloon inflation after every stent is placed.

POSTSTENT MANAGEMENT

Following the procedure the patient is transferred back to the floor with sheaths in place. If used, dextran is continued at 25 cc/hour (less in patients with impaired left ventricular function). If sheaths are to be pulled the same day, heparin is stopped and an ACT is checked every hour until it is <170 seconds.

At that time sheaths are removed and compressive pressure is applied with a mechanical C clamp (Clamp Ease, Pressure Products, Inc., Malibu, CA) for 60 minutes or until hemostasis is adequately achieved. In the majority of patients who require heparin, the drug is resumed approximately 1 to 2 hours after adequate hemostasis, without bolus usually at 1000 units/hour. PTT (partial thromboplastin time) is checked in 4 hours and then rechecked every 6 hours, keeping the patient between 55 to 75 seconds. After two successful therapeutic PTTs Dextran is discontinued. It is important to avoid large boluses with heparin or at any time overanticoagulating the patient. All patients receive soluble aspirin, ticlopidine, calcium channel blocker, stool softener, and an H_2 receptor antagonist to prevent gastrointestinal upset.

The anticoagulation options are in evolution. The "standard" stent anticoagulation protocol recommends continuation of heparin until full anticoagulation with coumadin is established. In this now outdated protocol we aimed for an international normalized ratio (INR) of 3 to 4 or a prothrombin time (PT) of 17 to 20 for the reagents used in our laboratory. This process typically requires 3 to 5 hospital days. After achieving the desired anticoagulation level, heparin is gradually tapered over 12 hours. Abrupt cessation of heparin has been reportedly associated with rebound thrombosis.

In patients at low risk of thrombosis we are currently recommending an alternative anticoagulation protocol. The selection of which anticoagulation protocol to utilize is based on a number of factors, including number of stents deployed, size of stent deployed, vessel appearance after stenting, vessel type (native versus vein graft), and setting of stent deployment (e.g., myocardial infarction). A useful approach to selecting an appropriate anticoagulation regimen is shown in Tables 6.2 and 6.3. In Table 6.2 we show a scheme that classifies patients into having a high (++++) risk of thrombosis and those with a negligible (+) risk, depending on the presence or absence of risk factors present. Moderate- (+++) and low-risk patients (++) lie somewhere between these two extremes. In Table 6.3 we show examples of four different anticoagulation regimens (super, standard, expedited, and no anticoagulation) that can be applied to these four groups. This logical approach to anticoagulation has worked well in our practice. Subcutaneous heparin can be administered three times a day doses of 5000 to 15,000 IU, depending on PTT measurements done 6

Table 6.2
Thrombosis Risk After Stenting

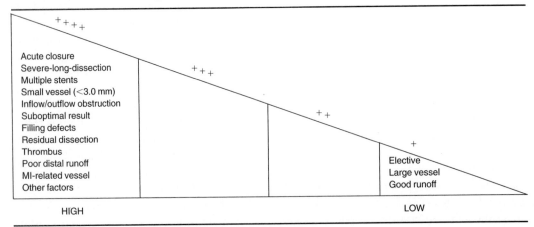

Table 6.3
Anticoagulation Regimens

	++++	+++	++	+
	Super Anticoagulation	Standard Anticoagulation	Expedited Anticoagulation	No Anticoagulation
Sol. ASA	✔	✔	✔	✔
Ticlopidine	✔	✔	✔	✔
IV Dextran	✔	✔	✔	✔
±IC Urokinase				
IV Heparin	✔	✔	✔	✔
S/Q Heparin	✔		✔	
Coumadin				
Discharge				
Coumadin	✔	✔		
S/Q Heparin	✔ (3 wks)		✔ (3 wks)	
Antiplatelet Rx	✔	✔	✔	✔

hours after dosing. Low–molecular-weight heparin (Lovenox) is preferable and can be used in weight-adjusted doses between 30 mg and 60 mg twice a day as shown in Table 6.3. Ticlopidine and aspirin in combination should be used in all patients.

If aggressive anticoagulation protocols are chosen, the poststent patient mobilization protocol is critical to the entire stenting process. To minimize bleeding complication at the puncture site, a 4-day gradual mobilization program has been recommended. The protocol is more critical with the standard and enhanced regimens. Day #1 the patient is flat in bed with head elevation <20°. Day #2 the patient can sit up in bed and after 36 hours can dangle legs over the side of bed and use a bedside commode. Day #3 the patient can sit up out of bed and walk to the bathroom. Day #4 the patient is freely mobile and may be discharged if PT >17 seconds.

With the newer anticoagulation protocols hospital stay can be appropriately shortened.

COIL STENTING WITHOUT ANTICOAGULATION

Coil stenting without anticoagulation has been investigated over the last 18 months in a number of centers in Europe and North America. Patients are managed with aspirin 325 mg twice a day and Ticlopidine 250 mg twice a day. No heparin is administered after the procedure, and the patients can be ambulated and discharged the day after stenting. No coumadin is used in this protocol. Ticlopidine is administered for 4 weeks. Because of the occasional (0.4%) episode of leukocytopenia associated with the use of ticlopidine, a white cell count is done at 2 to 3 weeks. After 4 weeks, aspirin can be continued once daily in an enteric-coated preparation.

In patients selected for this regimen, thrombosis rates have been less than 1% and bleeding problems have been rare and similar to standard PTCA. Most importantly, hospital stay and charges have been markedly reduced. The no-anticoagulation approach to coil stenting has been used in a variety of clinical situations, including threatened closure, severe dissection, total occlusions prior to PTCA, multiple stent use, and multivessel stenting.

Success with this technique is predicated on using properly sized stents and adjunctive high-pressure inflations with noncompliant balloons to optimize the angiographic results. Routine intravascular ultrasound assessment of the stent results has been advocated by some investigators, but the majority of centers using no anticoagulation have had excellent results without the routine use of intracoronary ultrasound.

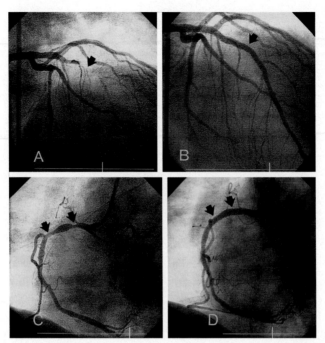

Figure 6.11. Multivessel stenting without anticoagulation. **A.** A totally occluded left anterior descending artery is opened and stented with tandem 3.5-mm and 4.0-mm stents. **B.** A tapered 4.0- to 3.5-mm noncompliant balloon was used to post-dilate the stent to 16 atm. **C.** A 4.0-mm stent was placed in the proximal right coronary artery and similarly dilated with the same high-pressure balloon. **D.** Sheaths were removed the same day. No heparin or coumadin was administered, and the patient was discharged within 48 hours on aspirin and ticlopidine.

The largest experience with this approach in North America has come from the University of Alabama at Birmingham. As of February 1995, 54 patients receiving 71 coil stents had been managed without anticoagulation with no episodes of stent thrombosis, patient hemorrhage, need for vascular repair, or blood transfusion. An illustrative example of multistent, multivessel stenting without anticoagulation is shown in Figure 6.11. Coil stenting without anticoagulation is now recommended by the authors in all patients who have optimal stent deployment.

COMPLICATIONS AFTER STENTING

Bleeding Complications

In the multicenter stent registry the incidence of bleeding complications has fallen from 25% in the early experience to approximately 5% in the latter part of the study. In centers not using anticoagulation bleeding complications no longer represent a problem. The most common site of bleeding remains the femoral puncture site, while gastrointestinal, genitourinary, pulmonary, and intracranial bleeding have all been reported. Greater experience, more individual and careful observance of heparin use, and gradual mobilization programs have been the primary factors responsible for reduction of bleeding complications. Most puncture-site bleeding occurs within the first 2 to 3 days postprocedure. Usually, bleeding can be controlled with temporary cessation of heparin and direct compression to the arterial bleeding site. If at any time significant bleeding occurs, all anticoagulation should be stopped while keeping the patient only on antiplatelet therapy. If there is a life-threatening bleed from any site (i.e., GI hemorrhage, respiratory hemorrhage), all anticoagulation and antiplatelet therapy should be stopped and careful patient observation undertaken. Most importantly, bleeding complications can be abolished by not using anticoagulation regimens.

Stent Thrombosis

Stent thrombosis usually occurs within the first few days after stent placement. Stent thrombosis is a function of poor patient selection and suboptimal stent deployment technique. Although the multicenter registry data only reports an incidence of 7.8% stent thrombosis, this event accounts for one-third to one-half of the myocardial damage with stenting (6). The major predictors of stent thrombosis appear to be (a) residual arterial dissection not covered by the stent and (b) use of stents ≤2.5 mm. Of 300 vessels (288 patients) stented at our institution from October 1989 to February 1992, stent thrombosis developed in 22 patients (22 vessels, 7%) at 6 ± 3 days (range 0 to 11 days) after stenting. Poststent residual dissection was associated with a thrombosis rate of 29% compared with 5% when dissection was absent. Use of stents ≤2.5 mm was associated with a thrombosis rate of 13% compared with 2% when stents ≥3.0 mm were used. Vessels with a residual filling defect were associated with a thrombosis rate of 12% compared with 7% when a residual filling defect was absent. Twenty-one of the 22 patients (95%) with stent thrombosis had either stents ≤2.5 mm, residual dissection, or a residual filling defect. When both a residual dissection or luminal filling defect and a small stent were present, the incidence of thrombosis was 9 out of 30 (30%). When none of these characteristics were present and stents ≥3.0 mm were utilized, the incidence of thrombosis was only 1 out of 125 (1%, $P < .001$). The learning curve appears to play a part. As the operators became more experienced, stents were sized more generously, greater care was taken to adequately cover all dissection, and anticoagulation was managed more meticulously. In that series

of patients stented with severe dissection, threatened closure, or established closure, the incidence of stent thrombosis was 12% for the first 50 vessels stented, 8% for the next 50 vessels, and 6% for the last 200 vessels stented. A parallel fall has also been observed in the multicenter registry. In our most recent series of 100 patients stent thrombosis has been less than 2% despite not using anticoagulation in more than 80% of patients.

MANAGEMENT OF STENT THROMBOSIS

Fortunately, stent thrombosis usually occurs while the patient is in a hospital. In all cases, except a patient with bleeding complications, a bolus of 10,000 units of heparin is given while preparations are made for urgent recatheterization. The options usually include (a) redilatation with or without bolus thrombolytic therapy or (b) redilatation with or without overnight intracoronary urokinase infusion. In patients who are not candidates for redilatation or thrombolysis or in cases of repeat stent thrombosis, emergent bypass surgery should be considered.

SUMMARY

The flexible coiled metallic stent has clearly demonstrated significant benefits in the setting of acute and threatened closure. It has decreased overall patient mortality and morbidity and the need for urgent bypass surgery in angioplasty settings. The accumulating information suggests that these stents will also reduce restenosis rates in patients with suboptimal results after PTCA. With greater attention to the technical aspects of stent placement and sizing and with subsequent high-pressure inflations to ensure adequate deployment of stents into the vessel wall, the incidence of stent thrombosis and restenosis will continue to decline. In addition, the employment of less aggressive anticoagulation protocols will reduce bleeding complications and shorten the hospital stay poststenting. The coupling and refining of these strategies will allow interventional cardiologists the opportunity to offer their patients safer therapies in the management of coronary artery disease.

REFERENCES

1. Ellis SG, Vandormael MG, Cowley MJ et al. and the Multi-vessel Angioplasty Prognosis Study Group. Coronary morphologic and clinical determinants of procedural outcome with angioplasty for multivessel coronary disease. Implications for patient selection. Circulation 1990;82:1193–1202.

2. Detre KM, Holmes DR Jr., Holubkov R et al. and the coinvestigators of the National Heart, Lung and Blood Institute's Percutaneous Transluminal Coronary Angioplasty Registry. Incidence and consequence of periprocedural occlusion. The 1985–1986 NHLBI PTCA registry. Circulation 1990; 82:739–750.

3. Ellis SG, Roubin GS, King SB III et al. In-hospital cardiac mortality after acute closure after coronary angioplasty. Analysis of risk factors from 8207 procedures. J Am Coll Cardiol 1988;11:211–216.

4. Simpfendorfer C, Belardi J, Bellamy G et al. Frequency, management and follow-up of patients with acute coronary occlusions after percutaneous transluminal coronary angioplasty. Am J Cardiol 1987;59:267–269.

5. Roubin GS, Douglas JS Jr, Lembo NJ et al. Intracoronary stenting for acute closure following percutaneous transluminal coronary angioplasty. Circulation 1988;78(Suppl I):407 (abstract).

6. Roubin GS, Cannon AD, Agrawal S et al. Intracoronary stenting for acute and threatened closure complicating PTCA. Circulation 1992;85:916–927.

7. George BS, Voorhees WE III, Roubin GS et al. Multicenter investigation of coronary stenting to treat acute or threatened closure after percutaneous transluminal coronary angioplasty: clinical and angiographic outcomes. J Am Coll Cardiol 1993; 22:135–143.

8. Rodriguez AE, Santaera O, Larribau M, Fernandez M, Sarmiento R, Nestor PB, Roubin GS et al. Coronary stenting decreases restenosis in lesions with early loss (24 hours after) in minimal luminal diameter after successful PTCA. Circulation 1995 (in press).

9. Ho DSW, Liu MW, Iyer SS et al. Sizing the Gianturco-Roubin coronary flexible coil stent. Cathet Cardiovasc Diagn 1994;32:242–248.

7. Slotted-Tube Metallic Stents

LAURENCE R. KELLEY, PAUL TEIRSTEIN, and RICHARD A. SCHATZ

The Palmaz-Schatz coronary stent (Fig. 7.1) has been demonstrated to be both safe and effective in the treatment of selected patients with coronary artery disease. Enthusiastic response to the initial experience with the Palmaz-Schatz stent has generally reflected dissatisfaction with suboptimal results from balloon angioplasty. It appears that a definite niche for stenting is evolving for large vessels, de novo lesions, and dissected segments with impending vessel closure. A lesion-specific approach to coronary intervention with multiple-device availability, both singly and sequentially, supports a trend in coronary revascularization toward anatomic stratification of patient subsets. While such a lesion-specific approach will most likely continue to direct interventional choices, more recent data suggest that indications for stenting with the Palmaz-Schatz stent may broaden remarkably to include primary treatment of de novo lesions, ostial lesions, type C lesions, and saphenous vein grafts, as well as restenotic and acutely dissected lesions. Early results from two recently completed multicenter, international, randomized trials (BENESTENT and STRESS), designed to compare percutaneous transluminal coronary angioplasty to stenting with the Palmaz-Schatz stent (Johnson and Johnson Interventional Systems, Warren, NJ), are encouraging. These early data appear to support the thesis that in de novo lesions initial complications and restenosis may be significantly less with stenting than with percutaneous transluminal coronary angioplasty.

This chapter is designed to present an approach to the clinical utilization of the Palmaz-Schatz stent. This technique reflects a knowledge acquired in response to practical, as well as intellectual, developments in coronary revascularization since 1987. We will highlight the safety and efficacy of this device. Moreover, we suggest that with meticulous attention to a series of sequentially related, simple details the Palmaz-Schatz stent may be a useful adjunct to coronary intervention. Nevertheless, this chapter should optimally serve as a primer for the safe treatment of patients with the Palmaz-Schatz stent.

PATIENT SELECTION

Candidates for percutaneous coronary revascularization are selected on the basis of established clinical and angiographic criteria. The eligible population for stenting with the Palmaz-Schatz stent encompasses most of this established group of stable patients without regard for age (1) or sex, with few important exceptions.

The intensive anticoagulation regimen that may be required following stenting to prevent thrombosis may exclude certain patients. From the moment of stent implantation until endothelialization of the stainless steel stent occurs (estimated about 28 days), there is a decreasing risk of stent thrombosis with an abrupt decline after the first week. Stent thrombosis is potentially the most catastrophic event following implantation, resulting in subacute vessel closure, possible myocardial infarction, or even death. The incidence of thrombotic occlusion has decreased with increased operator and institutional experience (2). In the STRESS (3)

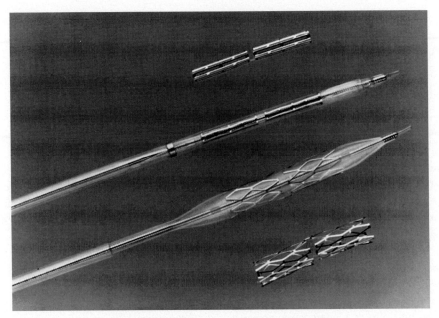

Figure 7.1.   The Palmaz-Schatz coronary stent.

trial, the incidence of subacute thrombosis with stenting was 3.5%. A low incidence of stent thrombosis is achieved by proper stent deployment and scrupulous maintenance of the anticoagulation schedule. Therefore prior to stent implantation patients should be carefully screened for potential hemorrhagic complications of anticoagulation. Recent upper or lower gastrointestinal bleeding, severe epistaxis, recent hemorrhagic cerebrovascular event, and bleeding diathesis are examples of contraindications to stenting. Prior to stenting, we liberally examine patients with esophagogastroduodenoscopy and have proceeded safely where active bleeding has not been identified. Menorrhagia, particularly severe, diabetic retinopathy with neovascularization but without hemorrhage, and bronchiectasis might be considered examples of relative contraindications to stenting. Menses may be temporarily suppressed prophylactically with Megace. A history of allergy, idiosyncratic reaction, untoward response, or intolerance to any aspect of the anticoagulation regimen should also be considered a contraindication to stenting.

Ultimately, each patient should be viewed in the context of their own predicament and disease. Judgment rests with the clinician to estimate in the balance the risk of ongoing ischemia and suboptimal revascularization versus the risk of bleeding and stent thrombosis. The physician must also assess the psychosocial context of their patient's ability to tolerate a possibly prolonged hospital course, a rigorous anticoagulation regimen, and undeviating follow-up. The clinician may regard a physically or mentally disabled patient or an unreliable patient as ineligible for elective stenting, but may reverse that decision in an emergent situation where no reasonable alternative is available.

Patients with unstable angina may also be treated safely with the Palmaz-Schatz stent with a restenosis rate comparable to that achieved for stable patients (4). Ideally, however, these patients are not treated with stenting acutely because of the instability of the lesion itself. If thrombus is angiographically apparent, stenting with the Palmaz-Schatz stent should be postponed or avoided because of the unacceptable risk of subacute thrombosis in this situation (5). Moreover, it is likely that in many of these situations angiographically inapparent but clinically significant thrombus may be present. Angiographically inapparent thrombus or a prothrombotic milieu may also be present in the lesion acutely dissected at balloon angioplasty or other percutaneous revascularization. Angioscopy may be useful in clarifying this issue, but may be impractical in an unstable situation. Ideally, these unstable lesions are "stabilized" medically with 5 days of continuous heparin. A more expedient alternative might be a 6- to 24-hour infusion of intracoronary urokinase prior to stent implantation. These measures may stabilize the precipitant plaque adequately to limit subacute thrombosis. Finally, these patients who constitute a group at relatively high risk for subacute thrombosis require a more aggressive approach to anticoagulation in the first 7 days following stent placement. A high therapeutic partial thromboplastin time in the range of 90 to 100 seconds in the period from day 2 to day 7 may provide adequate protection from this untoward event.

PATIENT PREPARATION

Eligible patients for coronary revascularization with the Palmaz-Schatz stent should be cognizant of the possible ardors of the procedure itself, the 18 to 24 hours of bed rest following sheath removal, a 3- to 5-day (7 days in "high-risk" patients) hospitalization, and the careful and frequent follow-up. All patients are treated with a noncoated aspirin at 325 mg orally daily and more recently we and others have used ticlopidine 250 to 500 mg daily as the only other anticoagulant. Dextran and persantine are no longer utilized, and warfarin is used only in the nonelective setting or when an optimal result cannot be achieved when the stent is deployed electively. Other pharmacologic intervention is directed toward patient comfort and prevention of complications. Those with a history of peptic ulcer disease without re-

cent activity may benefit from empiric treatment with an H-2 receptor antagonist or sucralfate.

VESSEL AND LESION SELECTION

The mechanism of benefit of stenting provides insight into the limitations of the Palmaz-Schatz stent. Long-term success following stenting is derived from the attainment of a maximal luminal diameter (7). The metallic stent prevents recoil and allows full expansion of the lesion with minimal dissection. The apparent mechanism of stenting and improved restenosis is clearly not in the prevention or minimization of intimal proliferation but in the achievement of full expansion of the vessel.

This benefit is limited mechanically in vessels of <3.0 mm diameter where the amount of steel present per area of exposed vessel may exceed a threshold beyond which the risk of thrombosis is high and restenosis is not diminished. It is helpful to note that a properly deployed stent merely provides a thin albeit strong lattice framework that supports the disarrayed architecture of a diseased vessel. This trusslike concept allows minimal surface area to provide maximal structural support. It follows therefore that the larger the vessel the more ideally suited it may be for stenting with less metal exposed per surface area of the vessel and intuitively less risk of thrombosis and restenosis. Success with stenting in large peripheral vessels without intensive anticoagulation supports this concept (8). Thus appropriate vessels for stenting are >3.0 mm and <5.0 mm in cross-sectional diameter. This upper limit may reflect only a limitation of supporting equipment with current prototypes.

Vessels of adequate size and significance should be considered potential candidates. Insignificant distribution of the involved vessel supplying a small amount of myocardium or poor distal runoff places the stent at risk for thrombosis, and such a vessel should be avoided. An unprotected left main coronary artery lesion should also be avoided except under the most unusual circumstances.

Vessels in which stenting is being contemplated should be carefully screened for two potentially problematic characteristics: tortuosity and other obstructive disease. Proximal vessel tortuosity may be sufficient to prevent safe passage of the stent delivery system. The currently available 4.9 Fr stent delivery system is still relatively bulky when compared to a balloon catheter. A well-seated guiding catheter in a "power position" is required to advance the device into the coronary vessel. Vessel tortuosity must be assessed in anticipation of difficulty in safe passage of the stent delivery system.

The presence of other significantly obstructive disease in the involved vessel or in a significant branch conjures up further potential for complications that require thoughtful provision. Mindful that the stent once deployed is irretrievable, the clinician must anticipate future pathologic developments in the vessel and its branches. Stenting of a segment that involves the origin of a significant branch will effectively lock that branch in "stent jail" and preclude further catheter-based intervention in that branch. One can anticipate, nevertheless, that side branches without obstructive lesions that are placed in stent jail will maintain normal flow acutely and in follow-up (9). However, side branches with obstructive lesions of significant size or distribution to merit bypassing should not be isolated by stenting.

Stenting in the presence of significant distal disease is hazardous. The implied slow flow and poor runoff of distal obstruction exposes the stent to an increased risk of thrombosis. Conversely, the subsequent percutaneous treatment of obstructive disease in the distal vessel may be limited by the presence of a stent in the proximal vessel, which may inhibit balloon delivery or retrievability. Ironically, if the distal vessel is >3.0 mm, the most cautious approach may be to stent both lesions in the same seating beginning

distally. If the distal vessel is <3.0 mm, then it is not advised to attempt percutaneous transluminal coronary angioplasty of the distal vessel in the same session as proximal stenting.

A strategy for multiple lesions in the target vessel may be a staged approach with initial balloon angioplasty of the distal or branch disease. If the lesion remains stable and the results satisfactory after a period of observation of not less than 12 hours, then the proximal lesion may be stented with reasonable assurance of no significantly increased risk. Regardless of the location of the secondary lesion, it appears reasonable to treat a vessel segment with stenting after all other lesions have been addressed and their outcome is assured. This approach should minimize the exposure of the stent to the prothrombotic milieu of an acute closure at percutaneous transluminal coronary angioplasty, poor distal runoff, and low-flow states.

The maximum lesion length for elective stenting is currently <15 mm. This too is a function of the prototypical stent and delivery system designs and may be modified as further developments occur. Commensurate with the previous discussion of matching metal exposed to surface area of vessel, we look to the future when shorter stents may be applied to shorter lesions, thus minimizing unnecessary blood-metal interface. As we become more precise at customizing stent length to lesion length, we must also remember that a slight reduction in stent length occurs with stent expansion, which may occasionally become clinically significant. Lesions longer than 15 mm currently would require at least two stents overlapping, which is both technically challenging and may be associated with a higher risk of thrombosis and restenosis (10) if there is excessive overlap. For these reasons, lesions longer than 15 mm should not be electively stented. However, in a non-elective setting the situation may require multiple stents, the operator accepting the increased risk of restenosis rather than ongoing ischemia or bypass surgery. A caveat, however, is that one should always leave room in the length of the vessel for placement of a bypass graft, should the need arise.

Lesion characteristics that have been found to predict complications with balloon angioplasty do not portend unfavorably with stenting (2). Singh et al. (11) reported a core angiographic laboratory evaluation of lesion severity in 658 target lesions treated with stenting and found no significant difference in subacute thrombosis, myocardial infarction, coronary bypass graft surgery, or death within 30 days between type A, B, and C lesions. A second center angiographically evaluated 88% of 222 patients 6 months following stenting with the Palmaz-Schatz stent and found a low restenosis rate in spite of the fact that 97% of the lesions had one or more risk factors for restenosis and angioplasty (12). Leon et al., in a multicenter retrospective review of stent implantation in saphenous vein grafts and native coronaries, found similar acute and long-term results in both conduits (10).

The most important lesion characteristic that is predictive of a poor outcome with stents is the intralesional presence of thrombus. Lesion complexity, ostial location, prior restenosis, total occlusion, and saphenous vein bypass graft location should not be regarded as adverse predictors of acute or long-term complications with stenting.

GUIDING CATHETER SELECTION

Guiding catheters should be of adequate internal luminal diameter to accommodate the stent delivery system. The minimal acceptable internal diameter is 0.082 inches, although 0.084 inches will provide somewhat easier stent delivery, as well as improved flow for coronary injections during "fine tuning" and localization at time of deployment. Usually, this can be accomplished with an 8 Fr guiding catheter.

When compared to the low-profile, sleek balloons currently available, the newer interventional devices, including the Palmaz-Schatz stent delivery system, are more bulky with higher profiles and inflexible segments. Thus they are more difficult to deliver. This has resulted in a resurgence in the importance of guiding catheter curve selection. Selection of a guiding catheter is a pivotal decision made early in the procedure of stent placement that becomes crucial in the setting of proximal vessel tortuosity, sharp-angled vessel origin such as a shepherd's crook right coronary artery, and unstable lesions. A simple maneuver referred to as the "push test" may be used to anticipate how well a selected guiding catheter will transmit force applied to the proximal end. Ideally, with forward advancement of the catheter, fluoroscopy will demonstrate a tendency of the guiding catheter to intubate further into the target vessel rather than prolapse toward the aortic root. We have found this "push test" to be very helpful in predicting the success or failure of the guiding catheter to provide adequate power for stent delivery in individual situations. The operator should be extremely careful in performing the "push test" to avoid vessel trauma. Failure to pass the "push test" should result in rejection of the guiding catheter in favor of one that can be anticipated to perform adequately at the critical moment of stent delivery. The catheter exchange at this time, prior to the crossing of the lesion with a wire, is performed easily and without concern for compromising the goal of successful angioplasty.

ARTERIAL ACCESS

Early reports of stenting described a high incidence of groin complications. This initial problem has not been borne out with subsequent operator experience and familiarity. In the STRESS (3) trial the incidence of either surgical vascular repair or bleeding requiring transfusion was 8.8% with stenting versus 4.5% with angioplasty, or roughly twice that seen with angioplasty. Groin complications may be minimized by scrupulous attention to the details of arterial access, sheath removal, and anticoagulation. Thus femoral arterial access should be obtained by the primary operator with a "clean" anterior wall puncture of a compressible segment of the common femoral artery. We favor the use of fluoroscopy to identify the location of the femoral head in all but the most straightforward femoral approaches.

Following the successful deployment of the Palmaz-Schatz stent, heparin is withheld and the activated clotting time (ACT) is measured every half hour until the ACT is <150 seconds. When the ACT is <150 seconds, the femoral sheath is removed in the usual manner, with direct compression manually or mechanically applied until hemostasis is achieved. After hemostasis is obtained, mechanical compression is resumed at a nonocclusive intensity to be gradually withdrawn over 2 hours. Heparin, if deemed necessary, is resumed 6 hours following sheath removal with a 2500-unit bolus followed by a constant infusion. The partial thromboplastin time is monitored with a goal of 50 to 70 seconds while in the hospital. In the patient considered at high risk for subacute thrombosis, we modify our PTT goal to 90 to 100 seconds after 48 hours of treatment at the lower dose. The patient is maintained on strict bed rest for 18 to 24 hours following sheath removal.

STENT SIZING

Recent explanations for the mechanism of stent restenosis attribute success with stenting to the acute gain derived from the maximum luminal diameter (7, 13). Thus physician selection of stent size directly influences optimal long-term results for each patient. True vessel size is best estimated with digital enhancement of orthogonal angiographic views or intravascular ultrasound both proximal and distal to the lesion. Stent delivery system size is chosen such that the stent, once deployed, is slightly larger than the estimated vessel diameter in a ratio of approximately 1.1:1.0. This should ultimately leave an an-

giographic appearance of a slight "step up" to the proximal edge and a "step down" at the distal edge of the stent. In actuality, stents within the various sizes of delivery systems are identical. While the stents themselves are of uniform size, delivery-system balloons are sized according to package labeling. The balloons in the system are compliant, polyethylene balloons that are nominally inflated at 4 to 6 atm. The compliant aspect of the balloons may result in angiographically obvious asymmetric expansion along the long axis of the stent, usually resulting in a dumbbell appearance. We have also discovered at intravascular ultrasound more angiographically subtle, or even visually inapparent, oval asymmetry of the circular axis, representing incomplete stent expansion within the stented vessel. Final stent expansion should be optimized by the use of a noncompliant, balloon-dilating catheter in all situations. We now follow virtually every stent deployment with a high-pressure inflation using a noncompliant balloon to achieve optimum implantation and expansion with or without ultrasound guidance (Fig. 7.2).

TECHNIQUE

Having considered indications, possible complications, and necessary equipment and thoughtfully provided for the limitation of misadventure, the clinician must initiate the procedure itself. The pharmacologic treatment should be reviewed, as well as the patient's clinical status. The prior administration of aspirin and ticlopidine should be verified. After arterial sheaths are in place, heparin is administered in bolus format with an ACT goal of 300 seconds at the time of stent implantation. The guiding catheter must be of sufficient internal diameter to allow smooth passage of the stent delivery system. The catheter will have demonstrated coaxial alignment with the proximal portion of the target vessel and vessel intubation with the "push test."

Angiographic "mapping" views of coro-

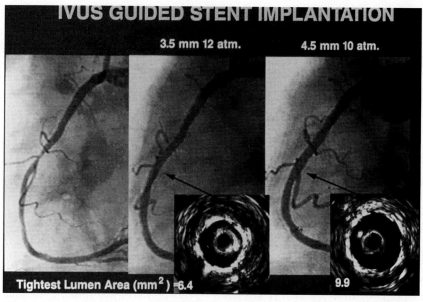

Figure 7.2. Improved luminal geometry after final stent dilatation with a noncompliant balloon.

nary injections are obtained. These best high-light not only the lesion and distal vessel but also demonstrate markers in the fluoroscopic field that can be used to localize the lesion at the time of deployment when the stent delivery system may obstruct the flow of coronary injections. Such markers may be anatomic such as vessel calcification, bends, side branches, and bone or nonanatomic landmarks such as surgical clips and sternotomy wires. The "mapping" views are thoroughly studied for any evidence of thrombus and any clues that may aid in the irrevocable process of stent implantation.

The internal diameter of the delivery balloon will accommodate a guidewire of no greater diameter than 0.014 inches. In anticipation of at least one balloon exchange, an exchange-length wire is always selected.

Delivery of the stent system to the lesion is facilitated by predilation of the target lesion. Every effort is made toward the endpoint of smooth stent delivery. Dottering maneuvers or excessive pressure against resistance must be avoided as these may dislodge the stent. Stent dislodgement or even

partial migration may be undetected because of the radiolucency of the Palmaz-Schatz stent, even with optimal fluoroscopic imaging equipment. Thus ideal guiding-catheter size and support and now predilation must be employed to ease the smooth advancement of the stent delivery system across the lesion. A 2.5-mm balloon-dilating catheter is always utilized for predilation, even for larger vessels.

Two purposes are served by predilation. The first is the facilitation of the passage of the stent delivery system. The goal, of course, is *not* a perfect balloon angioplasty result, thereby eliminating the angiographic features of the lesion itself, which are landmarks for ultimate stent deployment. The second purpose is achieved by careful observation of the inflation of the angioplasty balloon. A lesion that resists balloon inflation may resist full stent expansion. Such a lesion may be anticipated to have limited acute gain and be predisposed to thrombosis and restenosis. A truly nondistensible lesion might be better treated with a device other than the Palmaz-Schatz stent.

PREPARATION OF THE STENT DELIVERY SYSTEM

The stent delivery system is a factory-assembled unit that includes the stent premounted on a delivery balloon and delivery sheath.

The Palmaz-Schatz stent is a 15-mm, stainless steel, slotted tube that is comprised of two 7-mm segments connected by a 1-mm articulation. The stent is constructed such that the metal struts assume a rectangular configuration when the stent is crimped down onto the delivery balloon. When the balloon is inflated, the configuration of the struts is expanded and transformed into a series of open diamonds. This diamond-shaped or truss configuration confers the structural strength to the device.

The stent arrives from the factory already crimped down upon the delivery balloon. The balloon itself is a fairly compliant angioplasty balloon 20 mm in length with two radiodense markers spaced centrally 17 mm apart. Proximally, there is a Y adapter with a side port for balloon inflation and a central port for wire passage. The balloon catheter arrives from the factory within a delivery sheath, which is 4.9 Fr diameter and has a single distal radiodense marker. The proximal end of the delivery sheath has a Y adapter. The central port is a Tuohy-Borst adapter and accommodates the delivery balloon and wire. The side port is a flush port that is rarely utilized.

There is a clamshell device attached to the sheath and balloon proximally when the system is removed from the package. This should be removed immediately as it inhibits adjustments in the device. After the clamshell device is removed, the side port of the balloon catheter is always capped. This will prevent flushing of this port by an overzealous assistant with inadvertent balloon dilatation and stent dislodgement. The balloon itself is never preinflated nor is negative pressure applied prior to intended deployment. The central port of the balloon catheter and the central and side ports of the delivery sheath should, however, be flushed with sterile saline.

Next, attention should be directed toward adjustments in the relationship of the components of the catheter. First, the position of the stent and the delivery balloon and its relationship to the two bracketing radiodense markers should be carefully noted. As the stent itself is radiolucent, these markers may be the only gauge to estimate stent location during delivery. The locations of the radiodense marker on the delivery sheath should also be noted, as well as its relationship to the other markers. The position of the stent may be adjusted and manually crimped by loosening the Tuohy-Borst valve of the delivery sheath and advancing the balloon catheter sufficiently to manipulate the stent. Finally, the balloon catheter with stent is incompletely withdrawn into the sheath such that the distal portion of the balloon with about 1 mm of the stent remains exposed outside of the sheath. This arrangement best approximates a graded transition from guidewire to balloon to stent to sheath. This may minimize the risk of snagging of the stent delivery system when advanced into the vessel. After careful adjustment and inspection, the tightened Tuohy-Borst valve of the delivery sheath should secure the components of the system.

A final assessment for "pistoning" is designed to mimic resistance to catheter advancement. The tip of the balloon catheter may be gently gripped between two fingers and pushed into the delivery sheath. Ideally, the balloon catheter will not "piston" back into the sheath more than minimal retraction. Excessive "pistoning" may result in snagging. Minute manipulation of the balloon catheter and sheath relationship may be needed to achieve an acceptable transition with minimal "pistoning."

DELIVERY

At the time of delivery, the stent delivery system is introduced into a satisfactorily seated guiding catheter over an exchange-length guidewire. Once the stent delivery system has crossed the aortic arch, the system is carefully advanced under fluoroscopic guidance into the vessel. The left hand is placed on the guiding catheter at the femoral sheath, and firm pressure is applied simultaneously while the right hand advances the delivery system. An assistant should constantly maintain negative tension on the guidewire. It is essential that sudden jerking movements or force against resistance be avoided. One must remember that such movements may move or even embolize the stent. Because of its radiolucency, however, this may not be apparent to the operator until after balloon inflation. Thus dottering should never be used to advance the delivery system. If significant resistance is found, then the system may safely be removed prior to sheath retraction and stent exposure and a second predilatation may be required. Usually, however, persistent gentle pressure on both the guiding catheter and the system with effective guidewire tension will result in successful stent delivery.

Sheath retraction and stent exposure should be considered a "point of no return" in stenting with the Palmaz-Schatz stent. Once the sheath has been retracted, there is no safe way to make more than minor adjustments in positioning of the balloon with confidence that the stent has not become dislodged. One should never attempt to resheath an exposed stent as this will surely embolize an unexpanded stent.

Therefore prior to sheath retraction the operator should confirm ideal localization of the stent within a diseased portion of the vessel by careful angiographic inspection of the vessel, anatomic landmarks, other landmarks, and their relationship to the radiodense markers of the stent delivery balloon. The stent itself occasionally may be visualized, but usually its location within the vessel is only estimated by observation of the catheter markers and their spatial relationship prior to catheter insertion. Several angiographic views may be required to ensure exact matching of the stent to the lesion.

It is sometimes advisable to place the stent slightly off-center to avoid the central articulation coinciding with a focal lesion.

The stent is exposed by loosening the Tuohy-Borst valve of the delivery sheath and retracting the delivery sheath completely to the hub of the Y connector of the balloon catheter. This maneuver should be performed carefully under fluoroscopic observation and without any sudden movements. Final adjustments may be made but must be small and carefully performed without the protection of the sheath to prevent stent migration. The moment of stent exposure should be considered irrevocable and represents a commitment to stent deployment. At this point, the balloon port is uncapped and the balloon prepared with a single negative aspiration. A final angiographic assessment may be performed and minimal adjustments made.

Actual deployment occurs with a rapid inflation of the delivery balloon to a nominal pressure of 6 atm. The balloon need only be inflated for 10 to 15 seconds. Following a single inflation, the balloon catheter may be withdrawn from the guiding catheter and discarded as it will not be used again.

Initial angiographic assessment of the result is performed immediately. Again, the stent may not be visible on fluoroscopy. The stented segment should demonstrate a "step up" from normal vessel proximally and a "step down" to normal vessel distally. It is important to confirm stent deployment and the degree of expansion within the diseased segment. Subacute thrombosis, possibly caused by local turbulence and restenosis, are dependent on ideal localization and full expansion of the stent within the area of stenosis.

The entire involved vessel should be inspected for patency, flow, distal runoff, side branch occlusion, and thrombus. If distal flow or runoff is poor, distal embolization should be suspected. Treatment of distal embolization with intracoronary verapamil at a dose of 100 to 200 μg may result in improvement in flow. If thrombus is present or suspected, then a bolus of intracoronary urokinase in a dose of 250,000 units infused over 3 to 5 minutes is indicated.

Stent deployment is then optimized by the use of a noncompliant balloon appropriately sized to embed the end struts of the stent into the vessel wall and fully expand the stent with no residual stenosis. Even if the angiographic appearance is excellent, a final full inflation with a noncompliant balloon 16 to 20 atm is recommended. At the completion of the procedure, the final angiographic appearance should include a "step up" and "step down" before and after the area of stenting with no residual stenosis within the lesion.

At the completion of the stenting procedure, the patient is transferred to an intermediate care unit with the femoral artery sheath sewn in place. Heparin is not continued immediately following the procedure. The ACT should be monitored every 30 minutes until the results have decreased to 150 seconds, at which time the femoral sheath is removed and hemostasis obtained with direct compression for a minimum of 20 minutes. Following direct compression, we also place a mechanical compressive device over the arterial puncture site to be gradually released over 2 hours. We enforce bed rest following sheath removal for 18 to 24 hours.

Six hours following sheath removal and when necessary, heparin is resumed with a bolus of 2500 units followed by a constant infusion with a PTT goal of 50 to 70 seconds.

The postprocedural oral pharmacologic regimen includes a nonenteric-coated aspirin at 325 mg daily and ticlopidone 250 mg twice daily, dipyridamole 75 mg three times a day. Warfarin is begun the evening of a complicated procedure, usually with an initial dose of 10 mg, and adjusted on subsequent days. With the intention of inhibiting coronary vasospasm, a calcium channel blocker or nitroglycerin is almost always used following stenting with the Palmaz-Schatz stent.

If warfarin is to be used, the patient is maintained on the above regimen for 3 to 5 days while warfarin is being "loaded." The goal of the prothrombin time is 16 to 18 seconds (1.5 to 2.0 international normalized ratio (INR). Once this desired level is achieved, we continue heparin for an overlap of at least 24 hours. Heparin is discontinued the morning of discharge and a final prothrombin time off heparin is confirmed in the therapeutic range. Warfarin is generally continued for one month.

The exact need for ticlopidone remains to be determined. When it is used patients should be cautionated to report signs of infection immediately to physician as neutropenia is reported in about 2% of patients. This is generally reversible by withdrawal of the drug. We suggest continuing ticlopidone for only 4 weeks and checking the white blood cell count every other week.

THE FINAL RESULTS OF THE STRESS TRIAL

The STRESS trial (STent REStenosis Study) is a large randomized trial designed to compare elective coronary stenting with the Palmaz-Schatz coronary stent (PSS) to PTCA in patients with de novo lesions of native coronary arteries. Between January 1991 and February 1993, 407 patients were randomly assigned to PSS (N = 205) or PTCA (N = 203). When reviewing the results of this trial, it is important to bear in mind that low-pressure stent delivery and warfarin, rather than contemporary stent delivery techniques, were used.

Primary success by quantitative coronary analysis (QCA) was 96% in the stent group compared to 83% in the PTCA group. Crossover from stent to PTCA occurred in eight of the 205 patients (3.9%), but these were all *nonischemic* driven events compared with the 20 of 202 (9.9%) *ischemic* crossover events from PTCA to stent bailout.

Late thrombosis occurred in 3.5% of the patients randomized to PSS and 1.5% in those randomized to PTCA (all bailout stent patients). There was a significant decrease in in-hospital major complications in the PSS group when crossovers were included as "events." There was less recoil (13% versus 27%, $P \leq .0001$) and fewer dissections (7% versus 34%, $P \leq .0001$) in the stent group as well. There was no significant difference in *major* bleeding complications (6.8% versus 5.0% = NS).

Six-month angiographic follow-up was achieved in 88% of the patients and showed a significant improvement in MLD in the stent patients (1.77 mm versus 1.53 mm, $P = .0005$). QCA analysis revealed that this improved MLD was the result of a greater increase in acute gain (1.71 mm versus 1.17 mm, $P = .0001$) and persisted despite greater late loss (0.74 mm versus 0.44 mm, $P = .0001$).

When analyzed as a continuous variable, event-free survival was significantly improved in stent patients (80% versus 73%, $P = .023$) and target vessel revascularization was less in stent patients (10% versus 16%, $P = .035$).

In conclusion, the study showed the following:

1. The primary success rate is greater following PSS.
2. Ischemic in-lab events are eliminated with PSS.
3. Subacute thrombosis is a rare but late complication in PSS.
4. Both elastic recoil and dissections are significantly decreased with PSS.
5. In-hospital complications are significantly decreased with PSS.
6. There is a 34% reduction in angiographic restenosis at 6 months with PSS.
7. There is a trend toward increased event-free survival and decreased target-vessel revascularization with PSS.

The improved clinical outcomes in patients randomized to the Palmaz-Schatz coronary stent was offset by a longer hospital stay and a trend toward an increase in *total* bleeding complications. Nonetheless, the evidence for greater short- and long-term

success following PSS is compelling, and therefore coronary stenting should be considered in *all* patients with focal lesions of large native coronaries greater than 3 mm in diameter.

CONCLUSION

The Palmaz-Schatz coronary stent is firmly established as a safe tool in the armamentarium of the interventional cardiologist. As further developments in both stent and ancillary equipment design occur, we anticipate that the role and relative safety of the Palmaz-Schatz stent will expand. Effective utilization of this device, however, is predicated on prudent patient and lesion selection and meticulous attention to the details of the procedure itself and patient management thereafter.

REFERENCES

1. Saenz CB, Killinger JF, Baim DS, Curry RC. Palmaz-Schatz intracoronary stent in the elderly: NACI experience. J Am Coll Cardiol 1992;19:109A (abstract).
2. Carrozza JP Jr, Kuntz RE, Levine MJ et al. Angiographic and clinical outcome of intracoronary stenting: immediate and long-term results from a large single-center experience. J Am Coll Cardiol 1992;20:328–337.
3. Fischman DL, Leon MB, Baim D et al. A randomized comparison of coronary stent placement and balloon angioplasty in the treatment of coronary artery disease. N Engl J Med 1994;331:496–501.
4. Heuser RR, Strumpf RK, Walker CM, Cleman MW, Schatz RA. Coronary stenting in unstable angina: no greater risk than in stable angina. J Am Coll Cardiol 1992;19:178A (abstract).
5. Herrmann HC, Buchbinder M, Clemen MW et al. Emergent use of balloon-expandable coronary artery stenting for failed percutaneous transluminal coronary angioplasty. Circulation 1992;86:812–819.
6. Kaplan AI, Sabin S. Dextran-40: another cause of drug-induced noncardiogenic pulmonary edema. Chest 1975;68:376–377.
7. Kumura T, Nosaka H, Yokoi H, Iwabuchi M, Nobuyoshi M. Serial angiographic follow-up after Palmaz-Schatz stent implantation: comparison with conventional balloon angioplasty. J Am Coll Cardiol 1993;21:1557–1563.
8. O'Laughlin MP, Slack MC, Grifka RG, Perry SB, Lock JE, Mullins CE. Implantation and intermediate-term follow-up of stents in congenital heart disease. Circulation 1993;88:605–614.
9. Fischman D, Savage M, Cleman M et al. Fate of lesion-related side branches following coronary artery stenting. J Am Coll Cardiol 1991;17:208A (abstract).

10. Leon MB, Kent KM, Baim DS et al. Comparison of stent implanation in native coronaries and saphenous vein grafts. J Am Coll Cardiol 1992;19:263A (abstract).

11. Rocha-Singh KJ, Fischman DL, Savage MP, Goldberg S, Teirstein PS, Schatz RA. Influence of angiographic lesion characteristics on early complication rates after Palmaz-Schatz stenting. J Am Coll Cardiol 1993;21:292A (abstract).

12. Carrozza J, Kuntz R, Pomerantz R et al. Encouraging acute and long-term angiographic and clinical outcome of coronary stenting: a large single-center experience. J Am Coll Cardiol 1992;19:48A (abstract).

13. Kuntz RE, Gibson CM, Nobuyoshi M, Baim DS. Generalized model of restenosis after conventional balloon angioplasty, stenting and directional atherectomy. J Am Coll Cardiol 1993;21:15–25.

8. Bioabsorbable Stents

ROBERT S. SCHWARTZ

Despite the widespread application of coronary balloon angioplasty, several limitations remain in the application of this useful procedure. These problems center on both mechanical and biochemical causes. The issues (Table 8.1) are not limited to balloon angioplasty, but also affect most new devices for revascularization.

Pharmacologic therapy for percutaneous revascularization requires treatment of the entire body for a problem limited to only a few centimeters in the coronary artery. In consideration of therapies for these problems, it is clear that a properly designed intracoronary stent capable of local drug elution could potentially eliminate most of the problems. The desirable properties of an ideal stent are listed in Table 8.2.

METALLIC STENTS: THE FIRST GENERATION

The first generation of metallic intracoronary stents has shown great promise in clinical trials to date (1–11). The foundations of stenting originated with Dotter's early work in 1969. Many early concepts have not changed in over 20 years (12). The current metallic stent design implementations include balloon-expandable (Palmaz-Schatz, Medtronic Wiktor, Cordis, Strecker, Gianturco-Roubin) and self-expending (Medinvent) varieties. The metals used in these devices include spring-tempered stainless steel and elemental tantalum. The physical and mechanical properties of these metals make them easily deployable using the standard operator skills of balloon angioplasty. Adequate radial strength results from both balloon- and self-expanding designs after deployment. Metal stents are well tolerated from a histopathologic standpoint (Fig. 8.1).

Ease of deployment and excellent tissue biocompatibility have demonstrated that the metal stent will clearly become a major part of the interventionalist's armamentarium. These stents have functioned well, generally permitting alternatives to emergency coronary bypass surgery by reestablishing patency of an acutely occluded coronary artery through mechanical support of dissections and prevention of recoil. The long-term angiographic and clinical results with metallic stents are also acceptable, especially in view of the acute setting in which they are implanted (13, 14). These stents should remain in the coronary arteries without chemical or physical degradation for the life of the patients in whom they are implanted.

At least one metal stent design appears to show significant impact on restenosis as well. To have preliminary restenosis data directly comparing balloon angioplasty with the Palmaz-Schatz slotted tubular stent was a purpose of the BENESTENT trial (15). This European trial was coordinated through the Thoraxcenter in Rotterdam and enrolled 260 patients. Patients were randomized for suitable lesions and received either the Palmaz-Schatz slotted tubular stent or balloon angioplasty only. Angiographic endpoints in this trial were 6-month minimal luminal diameter (MLD) determined by quantitative coronary arteriography. Clinical endpoints were also studied in this trial and included the need for repeat procedures, recurrent angina, or evidence of ischemia, stroke, myocardial infarc-

Table 8.1
Problems With Percutaneous Interventions for Revasularization

Acute/chronic elastic recoil
Thrombus at the angioplasty site
Intimal dissection
Restenosis
Chronic total occlusion

Table 8.2
Properties of the Ideal Stent

Property	Application
Radial strength	Support intimal dissections, limit recoil
Antithrombotic	Eliminate need for systemic anticoagulation
Antirestenotic	Eliminate neointimal hyperplasia

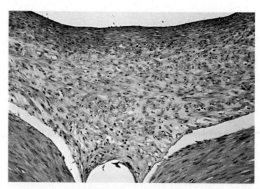

Figure 8.1. Neointima and media at the site of stent placement in a porcine coronary artery 28 days following stent implant. The stent wire was tantalum and was well tolerated on a cellular basis, as evidenced by lack of inflammatory cells in both arterial layers. Neointima in the porcine coronary artery formed as a result of the arterial *injury* from the stent wire, rather than from the wire itself, as in reference 44. Hematoxylin/Eosin Stain, magnification × 50.

Table 8.3
Reported Overall Restenosis Rates of Various Metal Stents

Device	Design	Restenosis Rate (%)	Reference
Palmaz-Schatz Stent	Stainless steel; slotted tubular	17–45	(4, 45, 46)
Wiktor Stent	Tantalum; wire/ balloon expandable	37	(3, 47, 48)
Gianturco-Roubin Stent	Stainless steel; wire/balloon expandable	20–61	(49, 50)
Wallstent	Stainless steel; self-expanding		(51, 52)

tion, or death. Clinically, there were ten subacute occlusions, six in the PTCA group and four in the stent group.

Using an intention-to-treat analysis, the restenosis rates were 20% for the stent versus 31% for angioplasty. Repeat intervention was required in 13% of stent patients and 29% of angioplasty patients. The postprocedural MLD for stents was significantly higher, possibly explaining the difference in restenosis rates (follow-up median MLD: 1.64 mm in balloon-treated patients versus 1.90 mm in the stent group, $P < .05$). This trial is unique in that it is among the earliest of either drugs or devices to definitively show impact on restenosis.

Other metallic stent designs may be associated with higher restenosis rates (Table 8.3), comparable to those of balloon angioplasty. This conclusion cannot be proven until randomized trials of stenting and balloon angioplasty are performed.

PROBLEMS WITH METAL STENTS

While clear structural and delivery advantages of metallic stents exist, there are limitations as well. These limitations relate primarily to two problems: (a) acute and subacute *thrombosis* and (b) *restenosis*. While metal stent technology provides excellent mechanical support, it will not solve either of these problems.

Stents placed for acute closure are at high risk of thrombosis because of the presence of preformed thrombus. The vessel-scaffolding effect may further increase this thrombogenic potential, since circumferential expansion of a freshly dilated artery may expose *more* thrombogenic subintimal surface to flowing blood. This thrombogenic environment requires strong countermeasures such as dextran infusion, in addition to heparin during stent implant. Oral anticoagulation typically prolongs hospitalization for 3 to 4 days after implant and must be continued for a few months. The anticoagulation requirement is a direct consequence of stent-blood incompatibility.

Metallic stents also result in more rigid arterial segments than the nearby native artery. This mechanical mismatch may partly cause higher long-term restenosis and occlusion rates, particularly at the ends or articulation points. Prosthetic vascular grafts suffer similar problems since they are also stiffer than native vessels. Neointimal hyperplasia similarly develops at the anastomotic points of prosthetic grafts (16).

The long-term effects of metal implants in patients have been considered another disadvantage. However, substantial precedent exists for chronic metallic implants, showing outstanding tissue tolerance (wire sutures, pacemakers and leads, staples, etc.). This issue has not been a problem with stents in over 7 years of follow-up to date. Whether it becomes a problem in the very long-term remains to be seen.

Finally, clinical results show that purely mechanical solutions are not likely to have substantial impact on restenosis alone. Newer revascularization methods such as atherectomy (17–19), rotary abrasion (20, 21), laser angioplasty (22–24), and various heating methods (25, 26) all show restenosis rates similar to conventional dilation. It is thus likely that adjunctive pharmacologic methods will be necessary to solve the restenosis problem. While metallic stents alone cannot deliver drugs, coatings may allow local, high-concentration drug delivery.

POTENTIAL SOLUTIONS: FUTURE STENTS

Possible solutions to thrombosis and restenosis include a totally absorbable stent or a hybrid stent that is partially absorbable and partly permanent. In either case pharmaco-logic intervention by the stent itself will be a requirement. Recent biomaterial advances permit consideration of alternative, non-metallic intracoronary stents. Improvements would result in devices being easily deployed with good fluoroscopic visibility. Nonthrombogenicity (or possibly "antithrombogenicity") could allow short-term systemic anticoagulation, as in current balloon angioplasty practice. The stent might be temporary, remaining in place only as needed to allow adequate arterial healing. Besides beneficial effects on thrombosis, it should abolish restenosis. This would entail formation of a thin endothelialized layer of neointimal hyperplasia. The large diameter, natural tissue conduit left by the stent would allow good blood flow and should remain unchanged for the remainder of the patient's life.

SYNTHETIC BIOCOMPATIBLE POLYMERS

Synthetic biocompatible polymers may be an alternative to purely metallic devices, since good results occur with vascular prostheses made from these polymers. Biocompatible polymers contain many repeating molecular structural subunits. Most polymers used in biologic application today were developed for industrial purposes and later found to have biomedical applications.

The biologic behavior of a polymer depends both on its repeating subunit configurations and on conformations of the polymerized molecule. In most macroscopic polymers the polymerized chains have many different lengths. The polymers' gross and biologic properties can be strongly influenced by the range and shape of the molecular weight distribution.

Polymeric blood compatibility is dominated by the molecular layers in contact with blood, making the polymer surface critical for blood contact applications (27, 28). Surface polymer characteristics may vary substantially from the bulk polymer to only a few molecular layers deep to that surface. Agents used to synthesize the polymer or to give it

Table 8.4
Chemical Structure of Common Polymers With Cardiac Application

Polymer Name	Structure	Cardiac Use
Polyethylene		Catheters, PTCA balloons
Polytetrafluoroethylene (PTFE), Teflon, Goretex		Synthetic grafts, catheters
Polypropylene, Prolene		Vascular suture
Polyethylene terephthalate, Dacron, Mylar		PTCA balloons
Polyurethane		Pacing leads

desirable physical features such as flexibility (plasticizing agents) frequently migrate to the polymer surface, potentially altering biocompatibility. Polymer surface properties and modifications are thus critical to understanding blood and biocompatibility.

A polymeric intracoronary stent will need good bulk properties for practical intracoronary delivery. It will also require surface properties that prevent thrombosis and avoid stimulating neointimal hyperplasia. Surface-modifying technology may help to satisfy both needs.

Typical polymers used for biomedical devices today exhibit good tissue compatibility (Table 8.4), although they vary in their ability to deliver drugs. While most of these are "biocompatible," they still are thrombogenic.

STENT THROMBOGENICITY

Studies of foreign surface and blood interfaces showed the importance of surface electric charge, thermodynamic surface energy, surface chemistry,[a] and texture (29). However, these studies may have oversimplified the interactions. For example, materials with net negative surface charge (negative electrochemical potentials) were thought highly blood compatible; this hypothesis is now known to be an erroneous simplification. No simple rules govern the interactions of blood and foreign materials (30, 31). These

[a]One measure of the surface energy in a polymer is to measure the angle formed between the surface and a bead of water placed on that surface. The more hydrophobic, the larger the surface free energy and, some believe, the more blood compatible.

interactions begin by the attachment of plasma proteins (the "conditioning film"), usually albumin, fibrinogen, or fibrin. This film initiates a second phase of biologic interaction, platelet adhesion and aggregation. Complement activation by C3 and C5 occurs early in foreign material-blood interactions. Following platelet adhesion and aggregation, activation of the extrinsic clotting system completes the clotting process. Currently, many problems remain with biopolymers; there is no blood compatible foreign material. This recently was called "the blood compatibility catastrophe" by Ratner in an editorial (32).

An important distinction must thus be made between materials that are *blood compatible* and those that are *biocompatible* (soft tissue compatible). Materials that are blood compatible are biocompatible, but the converse is not generally true. Blood compatibility requirements appear substantially more stringent. Little is known about blood compatibility of many polymers, and no universally accepted evaluation standards exist.

BIODEGRADABLE POLYMERS: USES IN STENTS

Many polymers are gradually absorbed in tissue. Some biocompatible polymers currently in use for intramuscular, intraperitoneal, and subcutaneous drug delivery applications are listed in Table 8.5. These polymers disintegrate by chemical hydrolysis of the backbone chain. Polymer degradation occurs either by

**Table 8.5
Bioabsorbable Polymers With Possible Stent Applications**

Polylactic acid/polyglycolic acid
Polyanhydrides
Polyorthoesters
Polyphosphate esters
Polyiminocarbonates
Polyurethanes (absorbable)
Polyhydroxy butyrates
Polycaprolactones
Polytrimethylene carbonates

homogeneous or heterogeneous means. Heterogeneous degradation occurs at the polymer surface only, while gross structural integrity of the polymer remains, much like ice melting in a glass of warm water. Homogeneous degradation occurs evenly throughout the structure. This causes fragmentation and structural integrity loss soon after implantation, much like the piecemeal breakup of an iceberg. Most bioabsorbable polymers degrade via both mechanisms. Hydrophobic polymers undergo heterogeneous degradation, while hydrophilic polymers degrade by homogeneous dissolution through hydration. Degradation times can range from a few hours to many years, even for the same polymer. Degradation times depend on bulk polymer configuration, additives, and fabrication methods.

Biodegradability provides a means for controlled release of incorporated drugs. This scheme allows continuous, concentrated, local elution of desired bioactive agents. High local concentrations translate into better-tolerated, low, systemic doses.

BIODEGRADABLE STENTS

Fabrication and animal testing of biodegradable stents have recently begun; little prior testing of polymers in the coronary arteries has been reported. Experience from three collaborating centers showed disappointing results for many polymers, both biostable and biodegradable (33, 34).

Polymers were tested in these studies using a standard tantalum Wiktor stent, an arc (roughly 90°) of which contained a thin polymer stripe (Fig. 8.2). This configuration allowed the polymer to be firmly placed against the coronary artery. The opposite side of the stent had no polymer, making for a control close to the polymer-artery contact site. The studies were done to establish the compatibility of the polymers themselves, although these polymers could elute drugs.

The biodegradable polymers tested included polyorthoester, polyglycolic/polylactic acid, polyhydroxybutyrate, polycaprolactone, and polyethylene oxide/polybutylene terephthalate in the stripe configuration. All were implanted in porcine coronary arteries for 28 days. The polymers were carefully cleaned with saline, but were not sterilized out of concern that the sterilizing agent might be taken up by the polymer and yield artifactual results. Residual solvent elution from the polymers was tested and was non-existent.

Unfortunately, all biodegradable polymers resulted in a substantial amount of neointimal thickening as shown in Figure 8.3 and Table 8.6. Similarly, the biostable polymers tested (polyethylene terephthalate, medical-grade silicone, and polyurethane) as well caused neointimal thickening (Table 8.6).

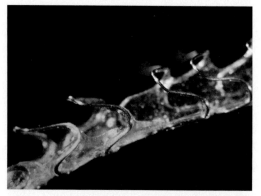

Figure 8.2. Polymer stripe configuration on tantalum stent for testing in porcine coronary arteries. The polymer subtends an arc of about 90 degrees and is pressed against the vessel wall for evaluation of the polymer response. The absence of polymer on the opposite wall permits a control site in close proximity.

Table 8.6

Neointimal Thickening With Bioabsorbable and Biostable Polymers Porcine Coronary Arteries, 28 days

Bioabsorbable Polymers	Number of Arteries	Mean Neointimal Thickness (mm)
Polycaprolactone	6	.79
Poly-hydroxy butyrate-valerate	4	.68
Poly-glycolic/poly-lactic acid	8	.50
Poly-orthoester	8	1.62
Polyethylene oxide- polybutylene terephthalate	10	.63
Biostable Polymers		
Polyurethane (medical grade)	8	1.12
Silicone (medical grade)	6	1.59
Polyethylene terephthalate	8	.42

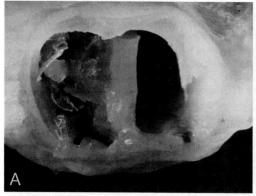
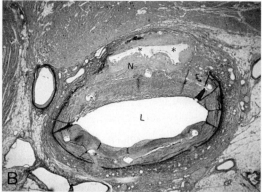

Figure 8.3. **A.** Gross photograph of polymer coronary artery implant shown in Figure 8.2. There was a severe response to the polymer as shown, while on the opposite side there was a lesser response to the bare stent wire. The lumen was substantially compromised by the reaction to the polymer. **B.** Low-power photomicrograph of a different porcine coronary artery 28 days following stripe stent implant. Note the polymer has been responsible for neointimal formation around the sites of vessel contact. This is substantially more than from the tantalum stent wires themselves along the lower portion of the figure. L, Lumen; *, location of polymer (removed for histologic processing); N, neointima at site of polymer location. Elastic van Gieson stain, magnification × 7.5.

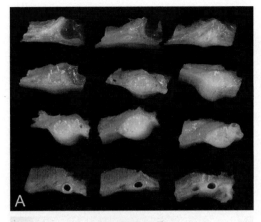

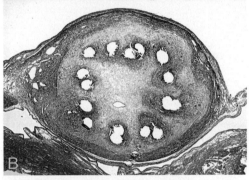

Figure 8.4. **A.** Configuration of self-expanding polyethylene terephthalate (PET) stent for intracoronary implant. **B.** Representative serial sections (2 mm thick) showing the results of PET stent implant 28 days after implant. Severe neointimal hyperplasia has totally occluded this vessel. **C.** Low-power photomicrograph of an occluded arterial section from PET stent implant. Total occlusion is evident. Holes are from the PET strands. Darker areas indicate inflammation and foreign-body reaction by the artery.

In a prior study of the polymer, polyethylene terephthalate (PET) strands (0.006-inch) were woven into a self-expanding, dual, counterhelical stent design. Much neointima was found to result from this design as well, although PET is biostable with an estimated biologic survival of more than 30 years. All hearts showed myocardial infarction in the distribution of the stent-implanted coronary artery (35). Coronary artery examination revealed total occlusion in all animals (Fig. 8.4). Microscopic examination showed areas of severe neointimal hyperplasia associated with organizing thrombus. Besides the neointimal hyperplasia, giant cells and eosinophils were noted near the PET stent struts, consistent with a mild foreign-body response. It is likely that thrombus deposition occurred on this biostable polymeric stent, associated with the severe neointimal thickening. Although the reasons for this reaction are unclear, it is likely that the reaction resulted from two causes: chronic thrombus formation on the polymer and an inflammatory response induced by the polymer. Both mechanisms have been previously described as part of the neointimal thickening process in the pig coronary artery following angioplasty injury.

These results are in stark contrast to those of Zidar and colleagues who studied the short- and long-term response to a stent fabricated from poly-L-lactide (PLLA) (36). These studies were performed in canine coronary arteries and were from 2 hours to 18 months in duration. Results showed that this material was bioabsorbable, biocompatible, and noninflammatory over all time periods. Additional in vitro studies of thrombogenicity showed low thrombogenic potential (37).

Reasons for the discrepancies in these studies remain unclear. Differences in the polymers themselves might be for one reason. PLLA is a polyester and has been studied the most comprehensively of all degradable and drug-eluting polymers. The first use of polyester was in absorbable sutures, which documented that the PLLA erodes relatively homogeneously to lactic acid, water, and carbon dioxide. These degradation products have little toxicity, but have been reported to cause an inflammatory response in nonarterial applications (38). Rods of poly-lactide-glycolide copolymer for internal-bond fixation have been studied in human orthopedic applications. In 516 patients a foreign-body reaction occurred in 7.9%, consisting of fluctuant swellings, sterile abscesses, and sinus formation frequently re-

Figure 8.5. Demonstration of neointimal formation around stent wires in a porcine coronary artery. **A.** A small amount of fibrin has deposited at the stent wire site. This stent was placed 4 days before sacrifice. The fibrin has covered the stent wire and extended laterally to cover part of the vessel media. Monocytes and lymphocytes *(arrows)* have begun infiltrating the fibrin mass from the luminal side. *L,* Lumen; *, stent wire hole; *M,* media; *F,* mural fibrin. Hematoxylin and eosin stain, magnification × 100. **B.** Early neointimal hyperplasa forming over fibrin stent wire deposition. A "cap" of smooth muscle cells has formed along the luminal surface of the fibrin 13 days after injury. This cap will progressively increase in thickness, downward toward media, as thrombus is resorbed, leaving a healed neointima. The primary component of this tissue is smooth muscle cells. Monocytes and lymphocytes are seen deeper in the fibrin layer, presumably resorbing this fibrin. The results will be total fibrin resorption and replacement by neointima. *L,* Lumen; *S,* smooth muscle cell "cap" over mural fibrin; *, stent wire hole; *M,* media; *F,* mural fibrin. Hematoxylin and eosin stain, magnification × 50.

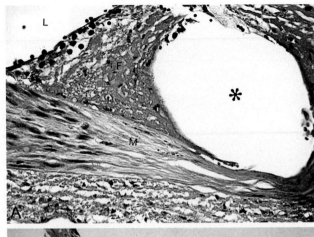

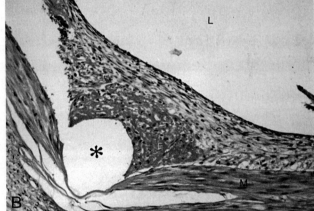

quiring surgical drainage (39). It is possible that higher-molecular-weight polymers of PLLA may be better tolerated, since the degradation time is prolonged.

A second possible difference is test species. Dogs are known to have an attenuated neointimal arterial response to coronary artery injury. They also have very active thrombolytic potential and have lower whole blood platelet concentration than do pigs (40). This question of species differences may be resolved when the Duke bioabsorbable stent is implanted in pigs or in other species such as the nonhuman primate.

An explanation for the differences will likely yield useful information regarding the restenosis process. Neointimal hyperplasia is a polymer-related problem for synthetic vascular grafts also. Synthetic grafts cannot be implanted smaller than 6 mm without developing severely occlusive neointima, eventually causing prosthetic thrombosis. A polymeric solution to the stent problem would thus have important ramifications elsewhere in vascular medicine. No material with suitable blood interface properties for small prosthetic grafts has been found despite much research. The problem of the polymeric intracoronary stent thus shares many similarities with that of the small-diameter graft; solutions in one area should yield insight into the other.

HYPERPLASIA FOLLOWING POLYMER IMPLANTATION: A RESPONSE TO "INJURY"?

The synthetic polymers tested in porcine arteries stimulate neointimal hyperplasia. It is possible that the proper polymer was not found. Another possibility is that neointimal hyperplasia forms universally with *any* synthetic implant. The hyperplastic polymer response may be viewed from the perspective of the injured artery, entailing thrombosis, inflammation, and final healing with smooth muscle cell infiltration (41–43). Figure 8.5 illustrates the normal stages of neointimal formation with early fibrin deposition. A pronounced inflammatory response of lymphocytes and monocytes follows, with eventual infiltration by smooth muscle cells to form a neointimal layer.

The pessimistic view that *all* polymers cause neointimal hyperplasia by similar mechanisms allows that some polymers may incite more neointimal hyperplasia than others. Hypothetical mechanisms include different degrees of fibrin deposition and inflammatory response. The species differences between dogs and pigs may, as noted, represent less thrombus and/or less inflammation from the implanted polymer.

The polymer-hyperplasia paradigm allows for the apparent "biocompatibility" of the some polymers over others. The requirements for arterial implants are more stringent than subcutaneous or other nonarterial applications. The polymer must be *both* tissue and blood compatible since both thrombus and

inflammation result in neointimal hyperplasia.

Geometric constraints also complicate the problem. A 3-mm coronary artery will develop a 50% stenotic lesion from a neointimal layer only 0.75 mm thick.[a] Traditional medical applications of polymers such as subcutaneous implants, sutures, and orthopedic applications do not suffer from neointimal formation of as little as 0.75 mm. This example shows that commonly used polymers may all be unsuitable for small-caliber arterial applications, including stent use. This serious concern has recently been reflected in the biomaterial literature as noted.

THE FIBRIN-FILM STENT

Concern about failure of synthetic polymers in the porcine coronary studies led to considerable reflection about other solutions. Exogenous fibrin-film sleeves may represent such a solution. Fibrin forms naturally from the blood at sites of arterial injury. It is both "biocompatible" and biodegradable.

---

[a]A diameter reduction of 50% in a 3.0-mm coronary artery corresponds to a diameter of 1.5 mm. Neointima need be only 1.5 mm/2 = 0.75 mm thick to create this reduction since its thickness appears as a reduction in radius.

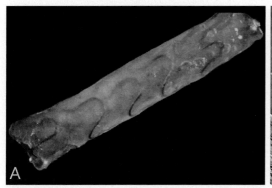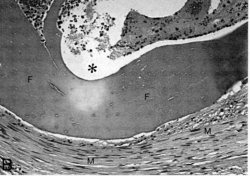

Figure 8.6. **A.** Fibrin-film stent with the film completely covering the tantalum wire. The viscoelastic properties of the fibrin film make it easily crimped on an angioplasty balloon and easily expanded in place at the desired arterial site. **B.** Photomicrograph of the fibrin film placed acutely in a porcine coronary artery. The fibrin is held against the media of the vessel. *F,* Fibrin film from stent; *L,* lumen; *,* stent wire location; *M,* media. Hematoxylin and eosin stain, magnification × 75.

Fibrinogen is easily isolated from whole blood and can be processed into fibrin film through polymerization with thrombin. Fibrin has many properties making it practical as a material for interventional cardiology: its viscoelastic characteristics make it formable into a stent configuration and deliverable by standard methods. It can be sterilized, dehydrated, and rehydrated for later use. It is capable of drug incorporation for chronic elution.

The applications of fibrin technology in coronary stents have been under study in our laboratory. A very thin (0.1-mm) fibrin film is formed on a standard, tantalum, balloon-expandable stent, completely encasing the metal wires (Fig. 8.6). Early results have shown the feasibility of a relatively nonthrombogenic device that heals into a vessel wall with small amounts of neointima. Studies using fibrin films in porcine coronary arteries are in the early stages.

The principle of fibrin in the coronary arteries may extend to other biomaterials: processed proteins, collagens, or glycosaminoglycans may represent a new era in biomaterials technology. Hybrid devices such as the fibrin-film tantalum stent can capitalize on the advantages of both types of material to create new solutions for many clinical problems.

CONCLUSION

Advances in the technology of interventional cardiology have literally made the entire coronary tree and most atherosclerotic lesions accessible to dilation. The major limitations of percutaneous revascularization include thrombus formation, uncontrolled dissection and acute closure, restenosis, and successful approaches to chronic total occlusions. It is easy to conceive of new stent technology that would simultaneously solve these problems: mechanical support of the dilated vessel with local drug elution to limit thrombosis and neointimal hyperplasia. Such a device could render angioplasty an outpatient procedure.

Continued development with collaboration among clinicians, bioengineers, and basic scientists will be required to develop this device.

ACKNOWLEDGMENT
The authors would like to express thanks to the J Holden DeHaan foundation for financial support, and to Rod Wolff, Mike Dror, and Ron Tuch of Medtronic, Inc. for collaboration in much of the work described in this manuscript.

REFERENCES

1. Baim DS, Levine MJ, Leon MB, Levine S, Ellis SG, Schatz RA. Management of restenosis within the Palmaz-Schatz coronary stent: the U.S. multicenter experience. The U.S. Palmaz-Schatz Stent Investigators. Am J Cardiol 1993; 71:364–366.
2. Bonan R, Bhat K, Lefevre T et al: Coronary artery stenting after angioplasty with self-expanding parallel wire metallic stents. Am Heart J 1991;121:1522–1530.
3. Burger W, Krieken T, de-Jaegere P et al. Mid-term follow-up after Wiktor stent implantation for prevention of restenosis. J Am Coll Cardiol 1993;21:30A (abstract).
4. Colombo A, Maiello L, Almagor Y et al. Coronary stenting: single institution experience with the initial 100 cases using the Palmaz-Schatz stent. Cathet Cardiovasc Diagn 1992; 26:171–176.
5. Haude M, Erbel R, Straub U, Dietz U, Schatz R, Meyer J. Coronary stent implantation in acute vessel closure 48 hours after an unsatisfactory coronary angioplasty. Cathet Cardiovasc Diagn 1990;21:263–265.
6. Haude M, Erbel R, Straub U, Dietz U, Schatz R, Meyer J. Results of intracoronary stents for management of coronary dissection after balloon angioplasty. Am J Cardiol 1991;67:691–696.
7. Popma JJ, Ellis SG. Intracoronary stents: clinical and angiographic results. Herz 1990;15:307–318.
8. Roubin GS, Robinson KA, King SB, III et al. Early and late results of intracoronary arterial stenting after coronary angioplasty in dogs. Circulation 1987;76:891–897.
9. Roubin GS, King SB, III, Douglas JS Jr, Lembo NJ, Robinson KA. Intracoronary stenting during percutaneous transluminal coronary angioplasty. Circulation 1990;81(Suppl IV):92–100.
10. Schatz RA. Introduction to intravascular stents. Cardiol Clin 1988;6:357–372.
11. Schartz RA, Goldberg S, Leon M et al. Clinical experience with the Palmaz-Schatz coronary stent. J Am Coll Cardiol 1991;:155B–159B.
12. Dotter C. Transluminally placed coilspring endoarterial tube grafts. Long-term patency in canine popliteal artery. Invest Radiol 1969;4:327–332.
13. Mehl JK, Schieman G, Dittrich H, Buchbinder M. Emergent saphenous vein graft stenting for acute occlusion during percutaneous transluminal coronary angioplasty. Cathet Cardiovasc Diagn 1990;21:266–270.

14. Sigwart U, Urban P, Golf S et al. Emergency stenting for acute occlusion after coronary balloon angioplasty. Circulation 1988;78:1121–1127.

15. de-Jaegere P, Serruys P, Kiemeneij F et al. Clinical and angiographic results of the pilot phase of the BENESTENT study. J Am Coll Cardiol 1993;21:30A (abstract).

16. Leborgne O, Samson M, Suryapranata H et al. Implantation of endoprostheses in aortocoronary bypass. Preliminary experience at the Thoraxcenter of Rotterdam. Arch Mal Coeur 1989;82:1595–1599.

17. Fishman RF, Kuntz PE, Carrozza JPJ et al. Long-term results of directional coronary atherectomy: predictors of restenosis. J Am Coll Cardiol 1992;20:1101–1110.

18. Foley D, Hermans W, de Jaegere P et al. Is "bigger" really "better"? A quantitative angiographic study of immediate and long-term outcome following balloon angioplasty, directional atherectomy and stent implantation. Circulation 1992;86:I–530.

19. Garratt KN, Holmes DR Jr, Bell MR et al. Restenosis after directional coronary atherectomy: differences between primary atheromatous and restenosis lesions and influence of subintimal tissue resection. J Am Coll Cardiol 1990;16:1665–1671.

20. Bertrand ME, Lablanche JM, Leroy F et al. Percutaneous transluminal coronary rotary ablation with Rotablator (European experience). Am J Cardiol 1992;69:470–474.

21. Niazi K, Brodsky M, Friedman H, Gangaharan V, Choksi N, O'Neill W. Restenosis after successful mechanical rotary atherectomy with the Auth Rotablator. J Am Coll Cardiol 1990;15:57A.

22. Litvack F, Margolis J, Cummins F et al. Excimer laser coronary angioplasty (ELCA) registry: report of the first consecutive 2080 patients. J Am Col Cardiol 1992;19:276A (abstract).

23. Margolis JR, Litvack F, Krauthamer D, Trautwein R, Goldenberg T, Grundfest W. Excimer laser coronary angioplasty: American multicenter experience. Herz 1990;15:223–232.

24. Buchwald AB, Werner GS, Unterberg C, Voth E, Kreuzer H, Wiegand V. Restenosis after excimer laser angioplasty of coronary stenoses and chronic total occlusions. Am Heart J 1992;123:878–885.

25. Reis GJ, Pomerantz RM, Jenkins RD et al. Laser balloon angioplasty: clinical, angiographic and histologic results. J Am Coll Cardiol 1991;18:193–202.

26. Spears JR, Reyes VP, Wynne J et al. Percutaneous coronary laser balloon angioplasty: initial results of a multicenter experience. J Am Coll Cardiol 1990;16:293–303.

27. Baier R. Role of surface energy in thrombogenesis. Bull NY Acad Sci 1972;48:235.

28. De Palma V, Baier R, Ford J, Gott V, Furusse A. Investigation of three surface properties of several metals and their relation to blood compatibility. J Biomed Mat Res Sym 1972;3:137–145.

29. Sawyer P, Srinivasan S. Role of electrochemical surface properties in thrombosis at vascular interfaces. Bull NY Acad Sci 1972;48:235.

30. Andrade J, Hlady V. Plasma protein adsorption: the big twelve. In: Leonard E, Turitto V, Vroman L, eds. Blood in contact with natural and artificial surfaces.

31. Greisler H. Interactions at the blood/material interface. Ann Vasc Surg 1990;4:98–103.

32. Ratner B. The blood compatibility catastrophe. J Biomed Mat Res 1993;27:283–287.

33. Lincoff A, Schwartz R, van der Giessen W et al. Biodegradable polymers can evoke a unique inflammatory response when implanted in the coronary artery. Circulation 1992;86:I–801.

34. Lincoff A, van der Giessen W, Schwartz R et al. Biodegradable and biostable polymers may both cause vigorous inflammatory responses when implanted in the porcine coronary artery. J Am Coll Cardiol 1993;21:179A.

35. Murphy JG, Schwartz RS, Edwards WD, Camrud AR, Vlietstra RE, Holmes DR Jr. Percutaneous polymeric stents in porcine coronary arteries. Initial experience with polyethylene terephthalate stents. Circulation 1992;86:1596–1604.

36. Zidar J, Mohammad S, Culp S, Culp S, Brott B, Phillips H, Stack R. In vitro thrombogenicity analysis of a new bioabsorbable, balloon-expandable, endovascular stent. J Am Coll Cardiol 1993;21:483A.

37. Zidar J, Gammon R, Chapman G et al. Short- and long-term tissue response to the Duke bioabsorbable stent. J Am Coll Cardiol 1993;21:439A.

38. Suganuma J. Biological response of intramedullary bone to poly-L-lactic acid. J Appl Biomat 1993;4:13–27.

39. Bostman O, Hirvensalo E, Makinen J. Foreign-body reactions to fracture fixation implants of biodegradable synthetic polymers. J Bone Joint Surg 1991;72-B:592–596.

40. Mason R, Read M. Some species differences in fibrinolysis and blood coagulation. J Biomed Mater Res 1971;5:121–128.

41. Schwartz R, Edwards W, Camrud A, Holmes DJ. Developmental stages of restenotic neointimal hyperplasia following porcine coronary artery injury: a morphologic review. J Vasc Med Biol 1993;

42. Schwartz R, Holmes D Jr, Topol E. The restenosis paradigm revisited: an alternative proposal for cellular mechanisms. J Am Coll Cardiol 1992;20:1284–1293.

43. Schwartz RS, Edwards WD, Huber KC et al. Coronary restenosis: prospects for solution and new perspectives from a porcine model. Mayo Clin Proc 1993;68:54–62.

44. Schwartz R, Huber K, Murphy J et al. Restenosis and the proportional neointimal response to coronary artery injury: results in a porcine model. J Am Coll Card 1992;19:267–274.

45. Ellis SG, Savage M, Fischman D et al. Restenosis after placement of Palmaz-Schatz stents in native coronary arteries. Initial results of a multicenter experience. Circulation 1992;86:1836–1844.

46. Haude M, Erbel R, Straub U, Dietz U, Meyer J. Short- and long-term results after intracoronary stenting in human coronary arteries: monocentre experience with the balloon-expandable Palmaz-Schatz stent. Br Heart J 1991;66:337–345.

47. Buchwald A, Unterberg C, Werner GS, Voth E, Kreuzer H,

Wiegand V. Short- and long-term results following implantation of the new Wiktor stent in acute coronary occlusion following PTCA. Z Kardiol 1990;79:837–842.

48. de Jaegere PP, Serruys PW, Bertrand M et al. Wiktor stent implantation in patients with restenosis following balloon angioplasty of a native coronary artery. Am J Cardiol 1992;69:598–602.

49. Raizner A, Minor S, Pinkerton C, George B, Fearnot N, Voorhees W. Quantitative assessment of the six-month restenosis rates of the Gianturco-Roubin stent. Circulation 1991;84:II–589 (abstract).

50. Ellis S, Verlee P, Muller D. Comparison of outcome after coil vs. slotted tube stainless steel coronary stent implantation to prevent restenosis—lessons from a single group experience. J Am Coll Cardiol 1993;21:293A (abstract).

51. Lau KW, Gunnes P, Williams M, Rickards A, Sigwart U. Angiographic restenosis after successful Wallstent stent implantation: an analysis of risk predictors. Am Heart J 1992;124:1473–1477.

52. Strauss BH, Serruys PW, Bertrand ME et al. Quantitative angiographic follow-up of the coronary Wallstent in native vessels and bypass grafts (European experience—March 1986 to March 1990). Am J Cardiol 1992;69:475–481.

9. Percutaneous Coronary Angioscopy

CHRISTOPHER J. WHITE and STEPHEN R. RAMEE

The broad application of percutaneous coronary revascularization, first performed in 1977 by Dr. Gruentzig (1), has completely changed the clinical approach to coronary artery disease. Advances in catheter technology and design have allowed us to maintain a high procedural success rate and minimize complication rates as more complex and difficult lesions are accepted for percutaneous treatment.

These improvements in catheter technology have included both therapeutic and diagnostic devices. One of these new diagnostic devices is the angioscope (2–30). The angioscope is a percutaneous, catheter-based system designed to allow direct visual inspection of the endoluminal surface of the coronary arteries. The promise of the angioscope is that direct visual examination of the surface morphology of a coronary artery will provide more specific, more sensitive, and more accurate information than angiography, "the gold standard" for identifying subtle differences in atherosclerotic plaque morphology. Our hypothesis is that this enhanced ability to detect subtle details of plaque morphology will yield improved clinical outcomes for patients with complex lesions.

THE ANGIOSCOPE

The imaging system is made up of components, including illumination fibers, imaging fibers, a charge coupled device (CCD) television camera and monitor, and a videotape recorder. The illumination source provides a high-intensity "cold" light to avoid thermal damage to the vessel being imaged. The imaging bundle consists of at least 2000 optical fibers for adequate resolution. The video recorder provides an archival storage medium for review of the images.

The angioscope (Fig. 9.1) (Imagecath, Baxter Edwards, Irvine, CA) is a catheter within a catheter. The inner member of the catheter contains 3000 image fibers and is guided within the coronary artery over a 0.014-inch angioplasty guidewire. The outer catheter measures 4.5 Fr in diameter and has a lumen for inflating and deflating the occlusion balloon at its distal tip. Both the inner and outer catheters are guided by the same angioplasty guidewire in a "monorail" fashion. The occlusion balloon is a compliant balloon that achieves a variable final diameter depending on the volume of liquid introduced by hand-injection up to a maximum diameter of 5.0 mm. In the space between the inner catheter and outer catheter, there is room for a flush solution to be infused to clear the field of view during inflation of the occlusion balloon. The inner catheter may be advanced or withdrawn independently of the outer catheter a distance of 6 cm so that many segments of the vessel lumen can be examined.

IMAGING PROCEDURE

To perform angioscopy, an 8 Fr conventional angioplasty guiding catheter is advanced to the coronary ostium of interest, and 10,000 units of heparin are administered. A 0.014-inch angioplasty guidewire is placed into the distal portion of the coronary artery. The angioscope is then connected to the light source, the television camera, and the flush line. It is necessary to adjust the focus and to white-balance the scope. The angioscope, which is a

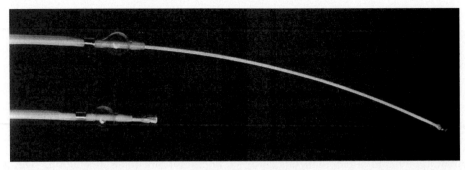

Figure 9.1   Photograph of the angioscope with the occlusion balloon inflated and inner image bundle extended *(top)* and retracted *(bottom)*.

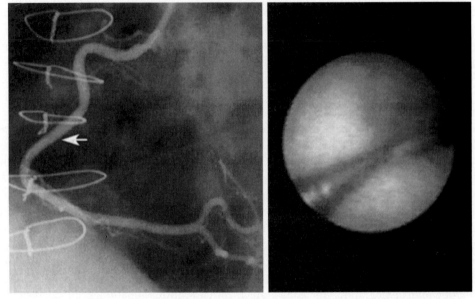

Figure 9.2   Angiography and angioscopy of a normal right coronary artery 1 year posttransplantation.

"monorail" design, is advanced over a guide-wire and into the coronary artery proximal to the segment of the vessel to be imaged. The flush lumen of the angioscope is connected to a power injector for infusion of warmed, lactated Ringer's at a rate of 0.5 to 1.0 cc per second. The occlusion balloon is hand-inflated with a 1-cc syringe filled with a 50:50 mixture of saline and radiographic contrast. Special care is taken not to overinflate the balloon. The inner catheter (imaging bundle) is then advanced over the guidewire to view the intraluminal surface of the vessel. Each imaging sequence lasts approximately 30 to 45 sec-

onds after which the balloon is deflated and the flush discontinued. These steps can be repeated several times until the region of interest has been adequately investigated.

When angioscopy is performed with angioplasty, imaging may be performed before and/or after treatment. When imaged before angioplasty, the lesion is generally not crossed because of the size of the angioscope catheter. Complete imaging of the vessel can be performed after dilation to examine the distal segments of the vessel not accessible prior to angioplasty. The entire sequence from introducing the angioscope to obtaining images can usually be accomplished in less than 5 minutes.

There may be occasions when the angioscope image is suboptimal. In this case, the first step is to refocus the scope and repeat the white-balancing procedure. Repeat white-balancing will often correct color distortions. The most common reason for a suboptimal image is that the scope will always face the outside wall in a sharply curving segment of a tortuous artery. By using a more rigid guidewire, the scope can be directed more toward the lumen of the vessel; however, we commonly choose not to attempt angioscopy in tortuous coronary segments for this reason. Another cause of suboptimal imaging is failure to clear the lumen of opaque blood either because the occlusion balloon is not adequately tamponading antegrade flow or because collateral blood flow is overcoming the distal flush of clear crystalloid solution. By increasing the flush rate through the distal scope lumen (up to a maximum of 1 cc/second) and ensuring that the compliant occlusion balloon is inflated properly, this problem can almost always be overcome.

CORONARY MORPHOLOGY

Atherosclerotic Plaque

The coronary angioscope provides a unique opportunity to observe the surface morphology of the coronary arteries during cardiac catheterization or intervention. One of the most distinctive features of a diseased coronary artery is the contrast between atherosclerotic plaque and normal arterial endothelium. The normal coronary artery intima has a smooth, glistening, white surface (Fig. 9.2). In contrast, atherosclerotic plaque is frequently pigmented ranging from yellow to yellow-brown in color (Fig. 9.3). White plaque, probably representing a fibrotic lesion, is more commonly seen in patients with restenosis following balloon angioplasty (Fig. 9.4).

Surface features of plaque include textures that may appear corrugated or smooth. Complex plaque morphologies such as ulcerations and dissections are seen more commonly in patients with unstable angina. In saphenous vein bypass grafts, plaque may appear as friable material loosely attached to the vessel wall.

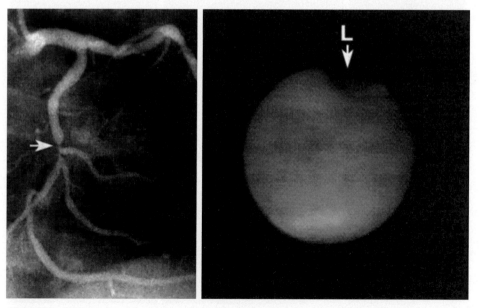

Figure 9.3 Angiography and angioscopy of an atherosclerotic plaque in the left circumflex coronary artery.

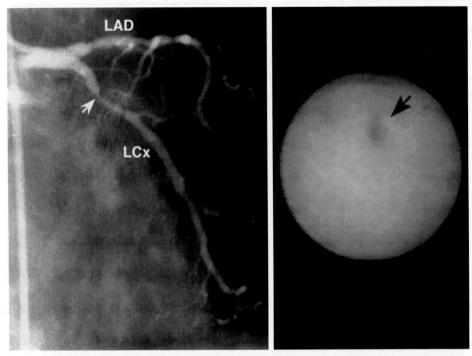

Figure 9.4   Angiography and angioscopy of a restenosic lesion in the left circumflex artery.

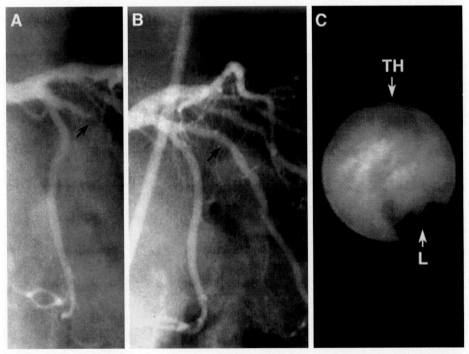

Figure 9.5   A. Angiography demonstrating total occlusion of an obtuse marginal branch of the circumflex artery in a patient with unstable angina pectoris. **B.** Angiography following PTCA. **C.** Angioscopy following PTCA of the dilated lesion showing a large mural thrombus *(TH). L,* Lumen.

Intracoronary Thrombi

Intracoronary thrombus is characterized by its red color against the white or yellow background of atherosclerotic plaque. It is our impression that the relative age of thrombi can be assessed, with more recent clots having a brighter red color and older thrombi having a duller, darker red–brown color. Intraluminal occlusive thrombi have the appearance of globular masses, are attached to the vessel wall, and protrude into the lumen. Mural thrombi, patches of red color that lie flat against the vessel wall (Fig. 9.5), are commonly associated with ulcerated lesions seen in patients with unstable angina.

Dissection

Superficial dissections are visualized as flimsy disruptions of the intimal surface. They may appear as white fronds of tissue seeming to dangle into the lumen, analogous to bedsheets hanging on a clothesline. Deep dissections appear as crevices or cracks in atherosclerotic plaque that extend into the media of the arterial wall. These deep dissections may expose the subsurface of the plaque as aggregates of yellow lipid or pink smooth muscle fibers of the media. Such intimal disruptions are more commonly seen in patients with acute ischemic syndromes, most often following balloon angioplasty.

CLINICAL STUDIES

Stable Angina Pectoris

Intracoronary angioscopy was performed before (n = 11) and/or after (n = 14) coronary angioplasty in patients with stable angina (Table 9.1). Atherosclerotic plaque was visualized in all patients. Intracoronary thrombus was identified in one (9%) patient by angioscopy. Intimal disruption or dissection was detected in two (18%) patients by angioscopy prior to angioplasty. Following balloon angioplasty, plaque fracture and dissection were seen in 12 (86%) stable angina patients.

Unstable Angina Pectoris

INTRACORONARY THROMBI

In patients with unstable angina, angioscopy was performed before (n = 40) and/or after (n = 54) angioplasty in patients with unstable angina. All of these patients had atherosclerotic plaque associated with their coronary lesions, which most commonly were yellow to yellow-brown in color. Before angioplasty, intracoronary thrombi were visualized angioscopically in 23 of 40 (57%) patients. Following angioplasty, intracoronary thrombi were seen in 36 of 54 (66%) patients (Table 9.1). These results confirmed the intraoperative angioscopy study by Sherman et al. (12) in which a surprisingly high incidence of intracoronary thrombi in patients with unstable angina, as well as the insensitivity of angiography for detecting these thrombi, was first documented. These *in vivo* findings are consistent with postmortem studies suggesting that the pathophysiology responsible for the occurrence of unstable angina is plaque rupture and thrombus formation.

Preliminary data from 122 patients who underwent angioscopy and angioplasty suggest that the presence of intracoronary thrombus is related to adverse in-hospital outcomes. Intracoronary thrombus was identified in 74 of 122 (61%) patients by angioscopy versus only 24 of 122 (20%) patients by angiography ($P < .001$). In the 24 vessels with

Table 9.1
Angioscopy Versus Angiography for Detecting Thrombi and Dissection

	Thrombus n (%)	Dissection n (%)
Pre-PTCA		
Stable angina (n = 11)	1 (9)	2 (18)
Unstable angina (n = 40)	23 (57)[a]	26 (65)[b]
Post-PTCA		
Stable angina (n = 14)	3 (21)	12 (86)
Unstable angina (n = 54)	36 (66)[a]	47 (87)

[a]$P \le .01$ vs stable angina.

[b]$P = .02$ vs stable angina. *PTCA*, Percutaneous transluminal coronary angioplasty.

angiographic evidence of thrombi, angioscopy confirmed the presence of intracoronary thrombus in only 20 (83%) vessels.

A major in-hospital complication (death, MI, emergency bypass surgery) occurred following successful PTCA in 10 of 74 (14%) patients with angioscopic thrombus versus 1 of 48 (2%) patients without thrombus ($P = .03$). An in-hospital ischemic event (recurrent angina, repeat PTCA, or abrupt occlusion) occurred in 19 of 74 (26%) patients with thrombi versus only 5 of 48 (10%) patients without angioscopic thrombi ($P = .03$). Relative-risk analysis demonstrated that angioscopic thrombus was strongly associated with adverse outcomes (either a major complication or a recurrent ischemic event) following PTCA (relative risk 3.11; 95% CI 1.28, 7.60; $P = .01$) and that angiographic evidence of thrombi was not associated with these complications (relative risk 0.85; 95% CI 0.36, 2.00; $P = .91$).

The presence of angioscopic intracoronary thrombus is strongly linked to in-hospital adverse outcomes following angioplasty. To determine whether angioscopic thrombus is merely an *innocent bystander* or the actual culprit in lesions more likely to fail angioplasty will require a prospective randomized trial to see if removal of the thrombus with thrombolytic agents can reduce the incidence of complications in this high-risk subgroup.

DISSECTIONS

Dissections were classified either as superficial, delicate white fronds of tissue that appeared to be shallow intimal dissections, or as deep plaque fractures that extended into the arterial wall. Prior to angioplasty, angioscopy revealed that 26 of 40 (65%) patients had dissections and ruptured plaques. Following angioplasty, dissections were seen angioscopically in 47 of 54 (87%) unstable angina patients (Table 9.1). This superior ability of the angioscope to detect intimal disruptions is because of the high-resolution optics that enable the operator to image subtle details of the artery's surface morphology. The majority of the arterial dessections seen were superficial tears that may not have been large enough for angiography to detect.

Restenosis After Angioplasty

We performed angioscopy in five patients presenting with clinical and angiographic evidence of restenosis following coronary balloon angioplasty (31). Atherosclerotic plaque in this group of patients was distinctive in that, in four of the five patients, the lesions were white and appeared fibrotic. The white fibrotic appearance of the restenosic lesions supported speculation that restenosis is secondary to fibrointimal proliferation. The single lesion that contained yellow pigmentation was from a patient who had early restenosis 6 weeks after successful balloon angioplasty. Angioscopically, there was evidence of a very large dissection that had healed in such a manner that the lumen of the coronary artery was significantly narrowed.

Saphenous Vein Grafts

The results of percutaneous angioscopy and angiography for detecting critical elements of surface lesion morphology were compared in 21 patients undergoing balloon angioplasty of saphenous vein coronary bypass grafts (29). Angioscopy and angiography were performed before and after angioplasty of "culprit lesions" in bypass grafts. All but one of the patients had unstable angina. The mean age of the saphenous vein coronary bypass grafts was 10.1 ± 2.4 years (range 5 to 15 years). Restenosis at a prior angioplasty site was present in seven patients. Intravascular thrombi were seen in 15 of 21 (71%) grafts by angioscopy and in four of 21 (19%) grafts by angiography ($P < 0.001$). Dissection was identified in 14 of 21 (66%) grafts by angioscopy and in 2 of 21 (10%) grafts by angiography ($P < 0.01$). The presence of friable plaque lining the luminal surface of the vein graft was detected in 11 of 21 (52%) grafts by

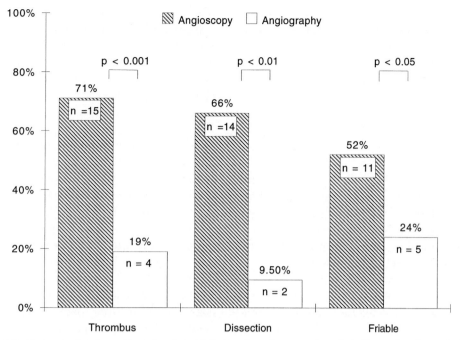

Figure 9.6   Bar graph of angiographic and angioscopic findings in saphenous vein grafts before and/or after angioplasty.

angioscopy and in 5 of 21 (24%) grafts by angiography ($P <.05$). There was no correlation between age of the bypass graft and presence of friable plaque. We concluded that angioscopy is superior to angiography for detecting complex lesion morphology in bypass grafts and for detecting the presence of friable plaque, which does not preclude an uncomplicated angioplasty result (Fig. 9.6).

To determine whether angioscopy can predict the incidence of embolic complications in bypass grafts will require a larger number of patients to be studied. Certainly, the risk for distal embolization is increased in a graft with friable plaque compared with graft with smooth fibrous plaque; but the magnitude of that risk is not yet known.

Abrupt Occlusion After Angioplasty

Percutaneous coronary angioscopy was performed in 10 patients following abrupt occlusion after balloon angioplasty. All of the patients had failed to respond to the administration of intracoronary nitroglycerin and therefore were undergoing single-vessel

angioplasty of a culprit lesion causing unstable angina. Although the angiographic characteristics of patients with high risk for abrupt occlusion have been described, no data exist regarding angioscopic findings in this population.

Intravascular thrombi were observed at the site of the abrupt occlusion in nine of 10 (90%) patients and were occlusive in two (20%) patients. Fragmented plaque and tissue flaps secondary to dissection of the artery wall were seen in all 10 patients and were occlusive in eight patients. The primary cause of the abrupt occlusion was thrombus in two patients and occlusive dissection in eight patients. Seven of the occlusive dissections were associated with nonocclusive mural thrombi, and the two occlusive thrombi were associated with superficial (nonocclusive) dissections. One patient had evidence of an occlusive dissection without thrombus present.

Angioscopy revealed the cause of abrupt occlusion in each case by allowing direct visual inspection at the site of occlusion (Fig. 9.7). It is of interest that although the primary cause of abrupt occlusion was most often an occlusive dissection, incidental, nonocclusive intracoronary thrombi were associated with these dissections in all but one case. Angioscopy may be useful in selecting the specific therapy for abrupt occlusion (thrombolysis for thrombus; long balloon inflations, atherectomy, or stents for dissection).

Angioscopically Guided Interventions

To improve the immediate and long-term results of percutaneous coronary intervention, a number of new methods of angioplasty have been developed and tested in clinical trials. Ultimately, angioscopy will not be a clinically relevant tool unless it can be used to influence the short-term and long-term outcomes of these percutaneous interventions. We have performed angioscopy in small numbers of patients after a variety of new interventions, including directional atherectomy, intracoronary stenting, and laser angioplasty, and have obtained interesting results.

Following directional atherectomy (Devices for Vascular Intervention, Temecula, CA) a smooth, widely patent lumen is commonly seen angiographically. Angioscopy, however, typically reveals a roughened endovascular neolumen with large amounts of residual plaque present. Dissections and semicircular troughs in the vessel wall, caused by incomplete plaque removal, are also commonly seen angioscopically (Fig. 9.8).

Intracoronary stenting has been utilized in clinical trials as a method of treating abrupt reocclusion and restenosis after balloon angioplasty. Unfortunately, both abrupt reocclusion and restenosis can occur even within stented vessels. In one such patient with restenosis after stenting, nonpigmented neointimal proliferation could be seen overlying the struts of a rigid, balloon-expandable stent by angioscopy. After angioplasty the bare stent struts were apparent. Coronary angioscopy has also been performed following Holmium:YAG coronary laser angioplasty. Although there was no gross evidence of charring, angioscopy did demonstrate superficial intimal tears and a brown discoloration that were not previously seen in native atherosclerosis and may have been caused by thermal energy dissipation.

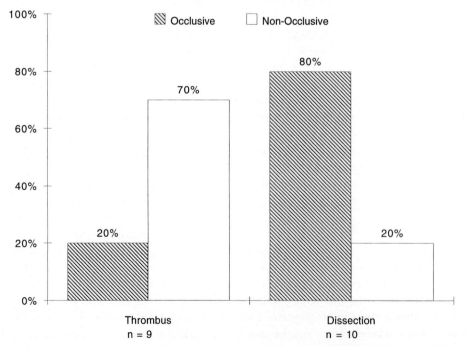

Figure 9.7 Bar graph of angioscopic findings in arteries with abrupt occlusion following attempted angioplasty.

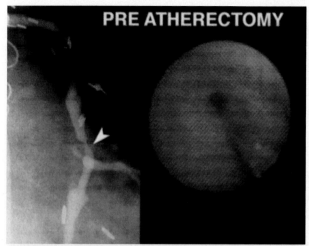

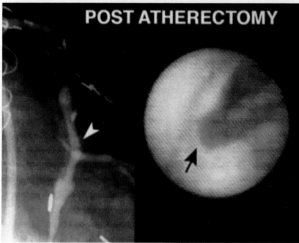

Figure 9.8 Angioscopy of a lesion before *(above)* and after *(below)* directional atherectomy. Note the eccentric lumen created as we attempted to make circumferential cuts.

POTENTIAL CLINICAL UTILITY
Natural History Studies

The correlation of atherosclerotic lesion morphology with clinical outcomes has been the cornerstone of our understanding of this disease and has guided our treatment of these patients. The landmark study by DeWood et al. (32) made clear the role of intracoronary thrombosis in the pathogenesis of myocardial infarction and dramatically changed the standard therapy of this disease from supportive care to interventional therapy with thrombolytic agents. Angiographic morphology studies of coronary arteries in patients with stable and unstable angina have allowed us to stratify patients with high-risk lesions (33–35). These studies have been limited by the documented insensitivity of angiography for detecting subtle changes in coronary artery surface morphology such as plaque fractures, dissections, and intracoronary thrombi and for assessing residual stenosis following angioplasty (36–50).

When compared with angiography, angioscopy offers a superior sensitivity and specificity for identifying subtle changes in atherosclerotic plaque morphology. Like angiography, this is a percutaneous technique that can be used during diagnostic angiography to more closely examine suspicious regions or lesions and, hopefully, provide more precise data concerning the progression of coronary disease. Angioscopy allows the in vivo examination of the surface pathology present in the coronary artery. Our early studies suggest that angioscopy has the potential to improve our understanding of coronary artery lesion morphology in patients with acute ischemic syndromes, restenosis following angioplasty, atherosclerotic allograft coronary disease, and saphenous vein graft disease.

Guiding Interventional Therapy

Percutaneous coronary angioscopy may play a role in guiding interventional coronary therapy. Angioscopy, in comparison with angiography, is better able to detect small amounts of intracoronary thrombus, which may have a negative impact on the outcome of angioplasty in patients with acute ischemic syndromes. Preliminary studies suggest that angioscopic detection of intracoronary thrombus in patients undergoing balloon angioplasty can identify those at higher risk for complications of the procedure. Perhaps the administration of adjunctive thrombolytic therapy, either before or after balloon dilation, will be guided by angioscopic findings.

Other seemingly useful roles for angioscopy require further investigation. The angioscope could possibly play a role in reducing the risk of reocclusion in infarct arteries by more completely visualizing the intracoronary thrombus after intravenous thrombolytic therapy. The angioscope may have clinical utility in stratifying the risk of complications after angioplasty in arteries that have a "hazy" appearance by angiography. In patients with abrupt occlusion following angioplasty, the angioscope should be able to reliably differentiate thrombotic occlusion from intimal dissection. This distinction would lead to more specific therapy for the occluded artery and possibly increase the success of salvage angioplasty, thereby reducing the need for emergency coronary bypass surgery. As alternative angioplasty techniques such as atherectomy, laser angioplasty, and stent implantation are more com-

monly used, perhaps the surface morphology of coronary lesions will become an important factor in determining indications for these procedures.

Our early experience with angioscopy in patients with stenotic saphenous vein coronary bypass grafts has demonstrated the ability to differentiate shaggy atheroma from smooth fibrotic-appearing lesions that has not been possible with angiography alone. This suggests that the risk of distal embolism in older vein grafts following balloon dilation may be better assessed by angioscopy and that the choice of revascularization procedure in patients with stenotic bypass grafts could be guided by angioscopic findings.

Conclusion

The future of coronary angioscopy as an everyday tool for the interventional cardiologist is uncertain at present. Clearly, angioscopy has superior sensitivity for intracoronary pathology when compared with angiography. The question is whether the information provided by angioscopy will have a significant impact on improving the current results of coronary angioplasty.

Coronary angioscopy will not replace diagnostic angiography as the "gold standard" for imaging stenotic lesions in coronary arteries. Angiography provides a rapid method for identifying critical lesions and for mapping the coronary artery tree. However, there may well be a clinical niche for a technology that gives accurate information regarding a specific lesion if the information can be used to improve the acute or chronic outcome of the interventional procedure.

Angioscopy appears to offer such technology. Angioscopy allows us to examine the surface morphology of coronary arteries during cardiac catheterization. With angioscopes we now have clinical access to information regarding arterial wall pathology that heretofore has only been available at necropsy. Whereas angiography provides us with a two-dimensional, black and white image of the coronary vessels, angioscopy complements this with a full-color, three-dimensional perspective of the intracoronary surface morphology.

REFERENCES

1. Gruentzig AR, Senning A, Siegenthaler WE. Nonoperative dilatation of coronary-artery stenosis. Percutaneous transluminal coronary angioplasty. N Engl J Med 1979; 301:61–68.

2. Mizuno K, Kurita A, Imazeki N. Pathological findings after percutaneous transluminal coronary angioplasty. Br Heart J 1984;52:588–590.

3. Cutler EC, Levine, Beck CS. The surgical treatment of mitral stenosis: experimental and clinical studies. Arch Surg 1924;9:689–821.

4. Harken DE, Glidden EM. Experiments in intracardiac surgery. II. Intracardiac visualization. J Thorac Surg 1943;12:566–572.

5. Bolton HE, Bailey CP, Costas-Durieux J, Gemeinhardt W. Cardioscopy—simple and practical. J Thorac Surg 1954; 27:323–329.

6. Sakakibara S, Ikawa T, Hattori J, Inomata K. Direct visual operation for aortic stenosis: cardioscopic studies. J Int Coll Surg 1958;29:548–562.

7. Litvack F, Grundfest WS, Lee ME et al. Angioscopic visualization of blood vessel interior in animals and humans. Clin Cardiol 1985;8:65–70.

8. Grundfest WS, Litvack F, Sherman T et al. Delineation of peripheral and coronary detail by intraoperative angioscopy. Ann Surg 1985;202:394–400.

9. Sanborn TA, Rygaard JA, Westbrook BM, Lazar HL, McCormick JR, Roberts AJ. Intraoperative angioscopy of saphenous vein and coronary arteries. J Thorac Cardiovasc Surg 1986;91:339–343.

10. Lee G, Garcia JM, Corso PJ et al. Correlation of coronary angioscopic to angiographic findings in coronary artery disease. Am J Cardiol 1986;58:238–241.

11. Grundfest WS, Litvack F, Glick D et al. Intraoperative decisions based on angioscopy in peripheral vascular surgery. Circulation 1988;78(Suppl I):I-13–I-17.

12. Sherman CT, Litvack F, Grundfest W et al. Coronary angioscopy in patients with unstable angina pectoris. N Engl J Med 1986;315:913–919.

13. Spears JR, Spokojny AM, Marais HJ. Coronary angioscopy during cardiac catheterization. J Am Coll Cardiol 1985; 6:93–97.

14. Susawa T, Yui Y, Hattori R et al. Direct observation of coronary thrombus using a newly developed ultrathin (1.2 mm) flexible angioscope. J Am Coll Cardiol 1987;9(Suppl A): 197A (abstract).

15. Takahashi M, Yui Y, Susawa T et al. Evaluation of coronary thrombus by a newly developed ultra-thin (0.75 mm) flexible quartz microfiber angioscope. Circulation 1987; 76(Suppl IV):IV-282 (abstract).

16. Uchida Y, Furuse A, Hasegawa K. Percutaneous coronary angioscopy using a novel balloon guiding catheter in patients with ischemic heart diseases. Circulation 1987; 76(Suppl IV):IV-185 (abstract).

17. Uchida Y, Tomaru T, Nakamura F, Furuse A, Fugimori Y, Hasegawa K. Percutaneous coronary angioscopy in patients with ischemic heart disease. Am Heart J 1987; 114:1216–1222.

18. Inoue K, Kuwaki K, Ueda K, Shirai T. Angioscopy guided coronary thrombolysis. J Am Coll Cardiol 1987;9(Suppl A): 62A (abstract).

19. Morice M-C, Marco J, Fajadet J, Castillo-Fenoy A. Percutaneous coronary angioscopy before and after angioplasty in acute myocardial infarction: preliminary results. Circulation 1987;76(Suppl IV):IV-282 (abstract).

20. Inoue K, Kuwaki K, Ueda K, Takano E: Angioscopic macropathology of coronary atherosclerosis in unstable angina and acute myocardial infarction. J Am Coll Cardiol 1988;11(Suppl A):65A (abstract).

21. Kuwaki K, Inoue K, Ueda K, Shirai T, Ochiai H. Percutaneous transluminal coronary angioscopy during cardiac catheterization: the results of experiences in the first 30 patients. Circulation 1987;76(Suppl IV):IV-186 (abstract).

22. Uchida Y, Hasegawa K, Kawamura K, Shibuya I. Angioscopic observation of the coronary luminal changes induced by percutaneous transluminal angioplasty. Am Heart J 1989;117:769–776.

23. Uchida Y. Percutaneous coronary angioscopy by means of a fiberscope with a steerable guidewire. Am Heart J 1989;117:1153–1155.

24. Ramee SR, White CJ, Collins TJ, Mesa JE, Murgo JP. Percutaneous angioscopy during coronary angioplasty using a steerable microangioscope. J Am Coll Cardiol 1991; 17:100–105.

25. White CJ, Ramee SR. Percutaneous coronary angioscopy: Methods, findings, and therapeutic implications. Echocardiography 1990;7:485–494.

26. Mizuno K, Arai T, Satomura K et al. New percutaneous transluminal coronary angioscope. J Am Coll Cardiol 1989;13:363–368.

27. Ventura HO, White CJ, Ramee SR et al. Percutaneous coronary angioscopy findings in patients with cardiac transplantation. J Am Coll Cardiol 1991;17:273A (abstract).

28. Ventura HO, White CJ, Ramee SR, Collins TJ, Mesa JE, Jain A. Coronary angioscopy in the diagnosis of graft coronary artery disease in heart transplant recipients. J Heart Lung Transplant 1991;10:488 (letter).

29. White CJ, Ramee SR, Collins TJ, Mesa JE, Jain A. Percutaneous angioscopy of saphenous vein coronary bypass grafts. J Am Coll Cardiol 1993;21:1181–1185.

30. White CJ, Ramee SR, Collins RJ, Jain A, Mesa JE, Ventura HO. Percutaneous coronary angioscopy: applications in interventional cardiology. J Interv Cardiol 1993;6:61–67.

31. White CJ, Ramee SR, Mesa J, Collins TJ. Percutaneous coronary angioscopy in patients with restenosis after coronary angioplasty. J Am Coll Cardiol 1991;17(Suppl B): 46B–49B.

32. DeWood MA, Spores J, Notske R et al. Prevalence of total coronary occlusion during the early hours of transmural myocardial infarction. N Engl J Med 1980;303:897–902.

33. Ambrose JA, Winters SL, Stern A. Angiographic morphology and the pathogenesis of unstable angina pectoris. J Am Coll Cardiol 1985;5:609–616.

34. Rehr R, Disciascio G, Vetrovec G, Cowley M. Angiographic morphology of coronary artery stenoses in prolonged rest angina: evidence of intracoronary thrombosis. J Am Coll Cardiol 1989;14:1429–1437.

35. Levin DC, Fallon JT. Significance of the angiographic morphology of localized coronary stenoses: histopathologic correlations. Circulation 1982;66:316–320.

36. Vlodaver Z, Frech R, Van Tassel RA, Edwards JE. Correlations of the antemortem coronary arteriogram and the postmortem specimen. Circulation 1973;47:162–169.

37. Grondin CM, Dyrda I, Pasternac A, Campeau L, Bourassa MG, Lesperance J. Discrepancies between cineangiographic and postmortem findings in patients with coronary artery disease and recent myocardial revascularization. Circulation 1974;49:703–708.

38. Pepine CJ, Feldman RL, Nichols WW, Conti CR. Coronary arteriography: potentially serious sources of error in interpretation. Cardiovasc Med 1977;2:747–752.

39. Arnett EN, Isner JM, Redwood DR et al. Coronary artery narrowing in coronary heart disease: comparison of cineangiographic and necropsy findings. Ann Intern Med 1979;91:350–356.

40. Isner JM, Kishel J, Kent KM, Ronan JA, Ross AM, Roberts WC. Accuracy of angiographic determination of left main coronary arterial narrowing: angiographic-histologic correlative analysis in 28 patients. Circulation 1981; 63:1056–1064.

41. Spears JR, Sandor T, Baim DS, Paulin S. The minimum error in estimating coronary luminal cross-sectional area from cineangiographic diameter measurements. Cathet Cardiovasc Diagn 1983;9:119–128.

42. White CW, Wright CB, Doty DB et al. Does visual interpretation of the coronary arteriogram predict the physiologic importance of a coronary stenosis? N Engl J Med 1984; 310:819–824.

43. Isner JM, Donaldson RF. Coronary angiographic and morphologic correlation. Cardiol Clin 1984;2:571–592.

44. Gould KL. Quantification of coronary artery stenosis in vivo. Circ Res 1985;57:341–353.

45. Zijlstra F, van Ommeren J, Reiber HC, Surruys PW. Does the quantitative assessment of coronary artery dimensions predict the physiologic significance of a coronary stenosis? Circulation 1987;75:1154–1161.

46. Marcus ML, Skorton DJ, Johnson MR, Collins SM, Harrison DG, Kerber RE. Visual estimates of percent diameter coronary stenosis: "A battered gold standard." J Am Coll Cardiol 1988;11:882–885 (editorial).

47. Katritsis D, Webb-Peploe M. Limitations of coronary angiography: an underestimated problem? Clin Cardiol 1991;14:20–24.

48. Block PC, Myler RK, Stertzer S, Fallon JT. Morphology after transluminal angioplasty in human beings. N Engl J Med 1981;305:382–385.

49. Duber C, Jungbluth A, Rumpelt HJ, Erbel R, Meyer J, Thoenes W. Morphology of the coronary arteries after combined thrombolysis and percutaneous transluminal coronary angioplasty for acute myocardial infarction. Am J Cardiol 1986;58:698–703.

50. Essed CE, Van Den Brand M, Becker AE. Transluminal coronary angioplasty and early restenosis: fibrocellular occlusion after wall laceration. Br Heart J 1983;49:393–396.

10. Intravascular Ultrasound

PAUL G. YOCK, PETER J. FITZGERALD, and WILLIAM L. MULLEN

Over 5 years have now passed since the first clinical use of an intravascular ultrasound catheter. There has been considerable technical refinement during this time and a building of enthusiasm among interventionalists for the clinical utility of ultrasound imaging. A number of centers are integrating ultrasound routinely into their approach to various interventions, helping to clarify our understanding of applications for the technology. This chapter will summarize the results of this early experience with imaging, with the overall goal of outlining a practical strategy for applying ultrasound imaging in the context of a multidevice interventional practice.

CATHETER AND EQUIPMENT SETUP

Stand-alone ultrasound imaging catheters are of two basic designs: multielement (solid-state) and single element (mechanical). There is currently one commercially available solid-state catheter, which has 64 imaging elements located in a cylindrical array at the tip (1). The catheter has a profile of 3.5 Fr and is configured in a standard over-the-wire design with 0.014-inch guidewire compatibility. The imaging catheter is connected to a pole-mounted relay unit, a monitor/recording station close to the patient table, and a larger image processing computer (which need not reside in the room). Advantages of the solid-state approach include absence of any moving parts and coaxial catheter design.

The other major design—single element with mechanical rotation—has been adopted by several companies (2). In this design a flexible cable traveling the length of the catheter is used to rotate a transducer configuration at the tip of the catheter. Some of these catheters incorporate a special mirror or reflector, which allows higher quality images to be generated immediately at the catheter surface. The currently available mechanical catheters range in size from 2.9 to 3.9 Fr and are delivered in some version of a "rapid exchange" or "rail" configuration. The major advantage of the mechanical catheters is superior image quality in terms of penetration of the signal, dynamic range (gray-scale capability), and effective resolution. These catheters are connected to a motor drive unit, which, in turn, is attached to an integrated image processing unit and display console.

Catheter setup varies somewhat with the type of catheter used in the laboratory. For the multielement, solid-state catheter there is no special flushing or preparation before insertion in the guide. One extra step is necessary before entering the target vessel, however, to remove a halo (ring-down) artifact that is seen around the catheter. With the catheter free in the aorta or within a large segment of vessel, a mask of the artifact is made and digitally subtracted from subsequent images. The mechanical catheters require careful flushing with fluid (water or saline) before insertion into the guide to clear air from the transducer housing. Even small bubbles trapped within this housing can substantially degrade the images. Once the flushing is performed, the catheters can be delivered directly into the segment of interest and imaging can be begun immediately.

System settings are also somewhat variable among the different manufacturers, but in general are quite similar to the parameters available to control noninvasive echo scanners. Adjustments can typically be made in "zoom," overall gain, time-gain compensation (gain as a function of depth from the catheter), compression (the gray-scale "map" of the image), and reject (a control for removing noise from the image, which suppresses all signals with an amplitude below the level selected by the operator). The greatest potential for operator error is in these last two adjustments of image presentation, compression and reject. It is important to develop an image with the widest possible display of tissue gray levels—rather than a very black and white, or "bistable" image. In practice this means adjusting the settings so that low-level imaging of blood within the lumen is noted; this will appear as a finely speckled, fairly homogeneous pattern that changes between systole and diastole. There is a tendency at first to adjust the system settings so that the blood disappears entirely, leaving a very distinct black appearance to the lumen. The danger in this strategy is that soft plaque or thrombus, which can have levels of ultrasound backscatter just slightly higher than blood, may be erased from the image as well.

Once the catheter is delivered into an artery, the imaging protocol is fairly straightforward. The most difficult task is coordinating the position of the ultrasound image with the angiographic location of the catheter tip in the vessel. Largely, this is a function of experience, but there are a few practical guidelines that may be of use. First, it is helpful to connect the system electronics so that one of the catheterization laboratory monitors is dedicated to the ultrasound image. This allows the operator to make fine adjustments in catheter position while studying the fluoroscopic and ultrasound images side-by-side. Some of the ultrasound scanners provide an alternative approach with a "picture-in-picture" capability on the scanner screen. In our experience it is most useful for orientation purposes to place the ultrasound image in the smaller, inset window and the fluoroscopic

image in the full-screen window. It is also helpful to record fluoroscopic images on the ultrasound videotape for subsequent review. In our laboratory we have configured the system so that when fluoro is on, this image is laid down on tape; when fluoro is off, the ultrasound image is recorded.

Orientation is also greatly facilitated by use of a controlled pullback technique. The catheter is delivered well distal to the target lesion, and then is pulled back in a slow and steady fashion to systematically cover the region of interest. A very slow rate of pullback is important to capture fine detail: a rate of 1 mm/second is reasonable (so that a pullback through a 4-cm region of interest takes 40 seconds). Once this imaging sequence is completed, the catheter can be withdrawn from the vessel and the images reviewed on videotape. This gives the operator time to review the images free of any ischemia for the patient and provides an organized method for understanding the relative positions of the ultrasound images. Several companies provide motorized pullback assist devices that ensure a slow and steady scanning of the vessel. Perhaps more important is a new generation of mechanical catheters in which the rotating imaging element is able to move longitudinally within the catheter body. The catheter is introduced beyond the region of interest, and the imaging element is slowly retracted in a spiral fashion. This provides a smooth accumulation of the image without the discontinuities that can be encountered when attempting to move the entire catheter within a tortuous and/or irregular lumen.

BASICS OF IMAGE INTERPRETATION

The utility of intravascular ultrasound hinges on a "quirk" of nature—that the layers of the arterial wall have sufficiently different acoustic behavior to be distinguishable at high frequencies of ultrasound. The media of muscular arteries such as the coronaries is particularly distinct ultrasonically, since it contains relatively low amounts of elastin and collagen compared with plaque/intima or adventitia. As a result the media tends to stand out as a thin, dark band on the ultrasound image (Fig. 10.1), providing a very useful marker defining the outer boundary of a plaque. With severe athereosclerotic disease the media may be so thin that it is not visible as a separate layer; in these cases the outer border of plaque is still fairly easy to identity, since the appearance of the plaque is quite different from the normal vessel wall (Fig. 10.2). It is generally not possible to differen-

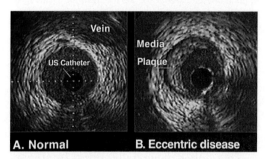

Figure 10.1. Examples of intravascular ultrasound scans from normal and atherosclerotic (eccentric) vessel segments. **A.** In the truly normal segment, no three-layered appearance is seen. An adjacent vein is imaged through the wall of the artery. Calibration marks are 0.5 mm per tick. **B.** An eccentric plaque is seen between 7 and 2 o'clock. The media is identified as a thin, dark stripe underlying the plaque.

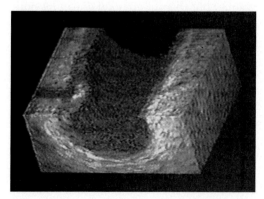

Figure 10.2. A three-dimensional reconstruction of a "hemisection" of a coronary artery. The plaque is the relatively thin carpet of soft gray material lining the vessel wall. An area of localized calcium deposit is seen on the left. Note the shadowing caused by this small accumulation of calcium.

tiate the adventitia from the periadventitial tissues because of the similar levels of acoustic reflectance. Imaging of the intimal layer depends on sufficient intimal thickening being present to provide a definable target on the ultrasound scan. In a truly normal vessel in a young person (thickness of intima less than 150 microns) the intima will not appear as a separate layer in the ultrasound scan (Fig. 10.1) (3). Since the average intimal thickness for a 40-year-old male is over 200 microns, however, most patients coming to the catheterization laboratory for an intervention will have a distinctly visualized intima and the so-called three-layered appearance [(i) plaque-plus-intima, (ii) media, (iii) adventitia-plus-periadventitia] evident throughout the coronary tree.

Identification of the lumen contour is generally straightforward, particularly when the lumen is large enough that there is significant standoff distance between the catheter and the vessel wall. Occasionally, when the catheter size is close to the lumen caliber, it may be more difficult to define the edge of the lumen. Compounding this problem is the fact that the reflectivity of blood increases markedly at low velocities, so that if the catheter is partially occlusive, the ultrasound signal within the lumen can approach the level of the vessel wall. In this situation it may be useful to inject radiographic contrast or saline through the guiding catheter. There is generally enough cavitation during an injection to create microbubbles, which provide a contrast effect that helps to outline the area of flowing blood.

Differentiation of plaque components is generally possible based on their appearance on the ultrasound scan. The most important of these components from the standpoint of performance of a therapeutic device—and, coincidentally, the easiest to identify—is calcium. Just as in noninvasive echo, calcium is identified by its bright reflectance and the fact that the ultrasound beam is not able to penetrate beyond it to deeper tissues (the "shad-

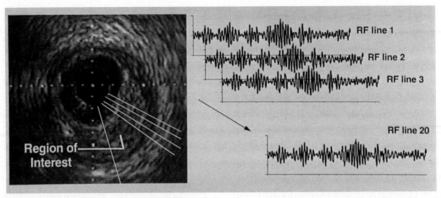

Figure 10.3. Raw radiofrequency (RF) data *(right)* are shown, corresponding to the vectors in the image on the left. The RF data contain more specific information about tissue type than the processed image and are the basis for "tissue characterization" techniques.

owing" phenomenon) (see Fig. 10.2) (4). Very dense deposits of fibrous tissue may give a similar appearance to calcium (with shadowing), but will also have a similar impact on the biomechanics of plaque response (see below). The distinction between soft fibrous tissue and fibrofatty tissue can be subtle. Fatty components have a lower echogenicity than fibrous tissue, and so appear darker on the ultrasound scan. It is often possible to see dark areas within a plaque that may represent lipid "pools"; however, the operator needs to be alert for several possible confounding factors. If the dynamic range (gray scale capability) of the catheter is poor, even fibrous plaque will tend to have dropout of echoes within the plaque substance ("sonolucent" zones), giving the false appearance of a lipid-rich core. Even with a catheter having good imaging characteristics, zones deep within a large plaque accumulation may appear relatively echo-poor because of inadequate time-gain compensation settings (not enough adjustment for signal loss because of the long signal path through deep plaque). False lumens within the plaque can give a similar appearance, a phenomenon which is encountered more commonly in peripheral than in coronary imaging. More accurate assessment of the lipid content of plaques may await so-called tissue characterization methods, where

computer-based analysis of features of the signal, in addition to amplitude, is used to extract more information about tissue type (Fig. 10.3). The clinical importance of being able to define the lipid content of plaques remains unclear at this point.

One other potentially difficult area of image interpretation is the discrimination between soft plaque and thrombus. These tissues can have comparable amplitudes of backscatter, leading to a generally similar appearance on the ultrasound scan. Thrombus tends to have a more homogeneous and "scintillating" tissue appearance than soft plaque, but this differentiation can be quite subtle. Again, this may be an area where tissue characterization methods are ultimately brought into service. The identification of thrombus is an area where angioscopy has considerable advantage over intravascular ultrasound.

PREINTERVENTION IMAGING FOR DEVICE SELECTION

The current size and delivery characteristics of stand-alone ultrasound imaging catheters allow preprocedure imaging to be accomplished in a significant majority—perhaps 70 to 80%—of cases (5). Because all available catheters have a "side-looking" transducer configuration, it is necessary to cross a lesion to image it. Undoubtedly, some degree of mechanical expansion (Dottering) of lesions occurs with passage of the catheters when they are the first catheter delivered into the vessel. Whether this is perceived to be a problem by the operator will obviously depend on the lesion and the therapeutic device ultimately selected. With directional atherectomy, for example, the ease with which the imaging catheter passes provides a good indication of how difficult it will be to deliver the atherectomy device—and the imaging catheter may also "predilate" the lesion to some extent.

The single most useful piece of information to gather from preinterventional scanning is the presence and location of any calcium deposits within the plaque. Ultrasound is considerably more sensitive than angiography in detecting calcium deposits. In the studies that have addressed this issue, calcium is detected by fluoroscopy in 20 to 40% of lesions, compared to a 60 to 70% detection rate by ultrasound (4–7). As a rough rule, two quadrants or more of calcification (an arc greater than 180 degrees) must be present on the ultrasound scan before there is sufficient mass of calcium to register on fluoroscopy.

Besides indicating the presence of calcification within a lesion, ultrasound is able to identify where the calcium deposits occur within a plaque—deep at the medial border, at the luminal surface, within the plaque substance, or a mixture of these (Fig. 10.4). The position of the calcium deposits has a critical influence on the performance of the various therapeutic catheters. This effect is perhaps most pronounced with the directional atherectomy device. When calcium is located superficially in the plaque at the luminal surface, cutting by the current atherectomy device is significantly impaired. In a recent study tissue retrieval was reduced by half in this situation compared to lesions where calcium was located deep at the medial border, or was absent altogether (7). In a so-called "napkin-ring" lesion, where superficial calcium encircles the lumen for an arc of greater than two quadrants, tissue retrieval drops to one-third. Final lumen areas show the same magnitude of dependence on the pattern of calcification as does tissue weight—lesions with superficial calcium result in a much lower postprocedure lumen area.

Experience with imaging guidance of rotational atheroablation has confirmed the claims that, unlike the directional atherectomy catheter, this device is capable of removing calcified portions of plaque (8). In the setting of superficial calcification or dense fibrotic plaque, the postprocedure lumen appears round and regular by ultrasound, with a final lumen diameter approximately equal to the definitive burr size (Fig. 10.5). With soft plaque, on the other hand, the final lumen tends to be significantly smaller in caliber than the largest burr, averaging approximately 50% in our experience. This may reflect a combination of postprocedural spasm (which may be more prominent in soft plaque) and a tendency for the Rotablator to push aside rather than cut soft plaque.

Figure 10.4. Two examples of calcification within lesions. **A.** An arc of calcium is deposited deep at the media border between the 9- and 11-o'clock positions. **B.** Superficial calcium is layered at the luminal surface in two segments between the 3- and 12-o'clock positions.

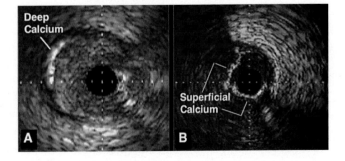

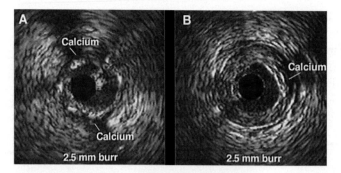

Figure 10.5. Examples of Rotablator cases. In both cases there is calcification present, with the characteristic shadowing. The lumens are relatively round and regular, which is a typical result for this device in hard plaque.

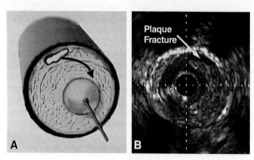

Figure 10.6. Tearing of plaque in association with localized calcium. **A.** This schematic shows the tearing forces that originate adjacent to a calcium deposit and extend out into the lumen. **B.** A typical plaque fracture occurring immediately next to a rim of calcium.

Combining these findings for the two atherectomy devices suggests that a plausible triage strategy can be based on the presence or absence of significant (one quadrant or greater) calcification at the luminal border. In the presence of this type of calcification, initial treatment with the Rotablator is more likely to be effective. On the other hand, in a lesion with deep calcification, tissue retrieval will probably be more extensive with directional atherectomy. The fairly frequent finding of a rim of calcium at the medial border (Fig. 10.4*A*) is ideal for directional atherectomy, since the soft overlying plaque can be removed by the device, but the calcium will effectively protect against deep cuts into media or adventitia.

Lesion response to balloon angioplasty is also strongly influenced by the presence of localized calcium deposits. When calcium is present within a softer plaque matrix, the high shear forces that occur between the calcium

and soft plaque cause plaque tears to originate at this point (Fig. 10.6) (9). These tears may not necessarily be deleterious, however: a recent study suggests that greater acute lumen gain is seen in lesions that tear (and hence, in lesions with localized calcium deposits) (10). In addition, the calcium-associated tears tend to be confined within the plaque substance and do not extend to media or adventitia, a situation that may trigger higher rates of intimal proliferation. We do not yet understand enough about the long-term implications of these findings, however, to know whether finding localized calcium within a lesion might rationally influence the decision to perform balloon angioplasty.

Even less is understood at this point about the impact of local calcification on the behavior of stents. Anecdotal reports of incomplete or irregular stent expansion in areas of calcification are circulating, but a consistent picture has not yet emerged.

Besides the pattern of calcification, a second category of potentially relevant information that ultrasound can provide with respect to device selection is the amount and distribution of plaque present within a vessel and target lesion. The decision to perform directional atherectomy, at least on the part of some operators, is influenced positively by the perception from the angiogram that the plaque is eccentric. Comparative studies between angiography and intravascular ultrasound have demonstrated that the accuracy of judging eccentricity by angiography is at best moderate, with one-third or more lesions being incorrectly categorized (10). Whether the amount of plaque present in a lesion has any significant influence on which device or approach is optimal for treatment is unknown at this point.

MONITORING AND ENDPOINT ASSESSMENT

Once an approach is selected for a given lesion, ultrasound imaging may provide useful information in monitoring the procedure. In the case of balloon angioplasty, ultrasound provides a more accurate assessment of the response of the vessel segment to dilatation than the angiogram. Plaque tears and dissections are detected in 50 to 70% of coronary angioplasties by ultrasound, compared to 20 to 40% by angiography (10). One early study has suggested that tearing is a significant predictor of restenosis (11); this finding remains to be verified by larger trials. Other studies have shown that acute gain is greater in lesions that tear compared with those that do not tear, a factor that by itself would predict a better long-term outcome for the lesions that tear (12). Whether there are types of tears that are associated with greater amounts of late loss (and resulting restenosis) is not yet known.

Besides the ability to detect tears, ultrasound provides a more accurate measure of true lumen dimensions following angioplasty than is possible with angiography alone (12). Ultrasound has shown that the "hazy" angiographic appearance following PTCA covers a wide spectrum of actual morphologic findings, ranging from thrombus to the presence of an "arm" of dissected plaque tissue projecting into the lumen. When these irregular lumens following angioplasty are quantitated by ultrasound, it is not surprising that the areas do not match the measurements by quantitative angiography. Whether a more accurate determination of lumen area post-procedure by ultrasound will in fact increase the power of lumen area as a predictor of outcome remains to be seen. Preliminary reports

from ongoing studies (13, 14) suggest that lumen cross-sectional area and percent cross-sectional narrowing (ratio of lumen to lumen plus plaque) are highly significant predictors of long-term outcome. Larger numbers and prospective trials will be necessary to confirm this association. At this point in our understanding of ultrasound-determined morphology and PTCA, the main practical application of imaging appears to be in lesions with a "surprising" appearance by ultrasound—that is, lesions that appear to be well dilated by angiography, but on ultrasound have a very small cross-sectional area.

The use of ultrasound as a monitoring tool is more straightforward in the case of directional atherectomy. Here the ability to identify the areas of deepest plaque accumulation by ultrasound provides useful information for the positioning and rotational orientation of the cuts. Correlating the location of plaque seen on ultrasound with angiographic markers that can be used to orient the atherectomy housing requires some experience. The strategy here depends on finding a reference branch close to or within the lesion that can be used to cross-correlate the ultrasound and angiographic information. For example, in working in the left anterior descending artery, a diagonal branch close to the lesion is selected. The ultrasound catheter is placed at the ostium of the diagonal, and the position of the ostium (referenced to the hours of the clock) is noted. The catheter is then advanced into the lesion and the orientation of the plaque is noted. By this method the rotational orientation of the deepest area of plaque accumulation relative to the ostium of the diagonal can be determined (Fig. 10.7). The imaging catheter is then withdrawn and the atherectomy device inserted and rotated into the position known to have the greatest depth of plaque. If the plaque is truly eccentric, with normal vessel on other sides of the wall, the cuts are made only in this area. Repeat imaging can be performed as the housing of the atherectomy device is being

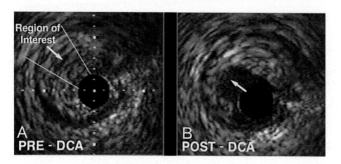

Figure 10.7. Example of directed atherectomy using ultrasound. In **A** the "region of interest" for cutting plaque was identified on the ultrasound scan and correlated with the rotational position judged from the angiogram. Panel **B** shows the results of several cuts with the atherectomy device in this area.

emptied of tissue samples. The images of the remaining plaque afford a guide to help decide whether to perform further cuts, cuts at higher pressures, or cuts with a larger device. One potential limitation of this orienting method arises from an occasional problem with the mechanical imaging catheters that has been dubbed "NURD" (nonuniform rotational distortion). This refers to an angular distortion of the image caused by uneven drag on the drive cable. If this occurs during an image orientation sequence for directional atherectomy, there may be some inaccuracy in registering the precise position of the plaque. This is only a problem if the NURD occurs between the target lesion and the reference branch.

Ultrasound imaging studies of atherectomy in which angiography alone was used for guidance (and ultrasound performed after angiographic completion) have suggested that, on average, greater than 60% of the vessel cross-sectional area is filled by plaque even after angiographically successful atherectomy. This occurs despite the relatively frequent occurrence of subintimal sampling— that is, retrieval of media or adventitia by the device. Our unpublished experience with imaging-guided atherectomy suggests that plaque residuals can be reduced to 20 to 40% using ultrasound, with a concomitant reduction in subintimal sampling to 10 to 20%. In many cases lower plaque residuals cannot be achieved because the "reach" of the device itself becomes a limitation. Whether more aggressive and targeted plaque removal has a

significant impact on long-term recurrence rates with directional atherectomy is unknown at this point. A combined imaging/directional atherectomy device developed by our group is currently undergoing early clinical evaluation. This catheter has the ultrasound transducer mounted immediately behind the cutter, providing "on-line" imaging guidance for atherectomy.

Monitoring of rotational atherectomy or concentric laser ablation by imaging follows a different strategy, since these are intrinsically symmetrical plaque removal devices. With either technology, the knowledge that there is extensive calcification in the lesion may modify the operator's "attack rate" on the plaque. The major utility of ultrasound, however, is in helping to make a decision about upsizing to a larger device. In our early experience with the Rotablator,[a] the ultrasound images motivated increasing the definitive burr size in over half of the cases treated. The images were also useful in helping to determine what proportion of lumen compromise in a particular segment was caused by spasm versus residual plaque. There are ongoing ultrasound studies to assess the efficacy of postablation angioplasty to achieve further expansion of the lumen. With the eccentric laser catheter, the strategy for orienting the fiber with respect to the plaque accumulation using ultrasound is similar to the protocol for directional atherectomy.

---

[a]In collaboration with Simon Stertzer, MD, of the San Francisco Heart Institute.

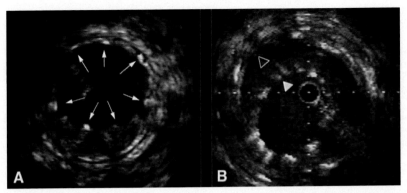

Figure 10.8. Complete **(A)** and incomplete **(B)** apposition of a Palmaz-Schatz stent. **A.** The struts of the stent appear as bright points *(small arrows)*. Note in **B** that the stent *(solid arrow)* fails to reach the vessel wall *(open arrow)*.

Experience with monitoring of stent placement by ultrasound is accumulating rapidly. Several of the centers with extensive experience in both ultrasound imaging and stenting have reported a significant incidence—perhaps in the range of 10 to 30%—of incomplete apposition of the stents detected by intravascular ultrasound postdeployment when balloon inflation pressures are 12 to 16 atm. (Fig. 10.8). The images reveal that at some segment along the length of the stent there is failure for the metallic struts to reach the vessel wall. Given the issue of thrombogenicity, incomplete apposition of a stent with the resultant flow disturbance and increased exposure of metal may be undesirable. There is further, yet unpublished experience to suggest that angiographically undetected, incomplete *expansion* of stents occurs in a much larger percent of cases—perhaps 80% or higher. It is not yet clear whether certain types of lesions—for example, those with an extensive matrix of calcification—are more susceptible to this problem.

RESEARCH DIRECTIONS

A large number of the clinically relevant questions concerning the role of imaging guidance in coronary interventions remain unanswered at present. The technology has just recently reached the point where reasonably high quality images can be obtained on a routine basis, with a significant proportion of cases capable of being imaged prior to intervention. The highest priority for clinical research at this point is to establish whether there are any morphologic predictors of outcome that can be determined by ultrasound—for example, the presence and depth of tears, the degree of calcification, the true cross-sectional area of the lumen, or the volume and type of plaque. A clear understanding of the relative importance of these and other factors will help in the design of randomized trials to definitively test the clinical utility and cost-effectiveness of ultrasound imaging.

REFERENCES

1. Nissen SE, Grines CL, Gurley JC et al. Application of a new phased-array ultrasound imaging catheter in the assessment of vascular dimensions. Circulation 1990; 81:660–666.

2. Yock PG, Fitzgerald PJ, Linker DT, Angelsen BAJ, Tech DR. Intravascular ultrasound guidance for catheter-based coronary interventions. J Am Coll Cardiol 1991;17:39B–45B.

3. Fitzgerald PJ, St. Goar FG, Connolly AJ, Pinto FJ, Billingham ME, Popp RL, Yock PG. Intravascular ultrasound imaging of coronary arteries: Is three layers the norm? Circulation 1992;86:154–158.

4. Mintz GS, Douek P, Pichard AD et al. Target lesion calcification in coronary artery disease: an intravascular ultrasound study. J. Am Coll Cardiol 1992;20:1149–1155.

5. Pichard AD, Mintz GS, Satler LF, Kent KM, Popma JJ, Kovach JA, Leon MA. The influence of pre-intervention intravascular ultrasound imaging on subsequent transcatheter treatment strategies. J Am Coll Cardiol 1993; 21:133A (abstract).

6. Honye J, Mahon DJ, Jain A et al. Morphologic effects of

coronary balloon angioplasty in vivo assessed by intravascular ultrasound imaging. Circulation 1992;856:1012–1025.

7. Fitzgerald PJ, Muhlberger VA, Moes NY et al. Calcium location within plaque as a predictor of atherectomy tissue retrieval: an intravascular ultrasound study. Circulation 1992;86(Suppl I):I-516 (abstract).

8. Mintz GS, Potkin BN, Keren G et al. Intravascular ultrasound evaluation of the effect of rotational atherectomy in obstructive atherosclerotic coronary artery disease. Circulation 1992;86:1383–1393.

9. Fitzgerald PJ, Ports TA, Yock PG. Contribution of localized calcium deposits to dissection after angioplasty. Circulation 1992;86:64–70.

10. Fitzgerald PJ, Mullen WL, Yock PG, and the GUIDE Trial investigators. Discrepancies between angiographic and intravascular ultrasound appearance of coronary lesions undergoing intervention. A report of phase I of the GUIDE Trial. J Am Coll Cardiol 1993;21:118A (abstract).

11. Tenaglia AN, Buller CE, Kissle KB, Phillips HR, Stack RS, Davidson CJ. Intracoronary ultrasound predictors of adverse outcomes after coronary artery interventions. J Am Coll Cardiol 1992;20:1385–1390.

12. Hodgson JM, Reddy KG, Suneja R, Nair R, Lesnefsky EJ, Sheehan HM. Intracoronary ultrasound imaging: correlation of plaque morphology with angiography, clinical syndrome and procedural results in patients undergoing coronary angioplasty. J Am Coll Cardiol 1993;21:35–44.

13. Tobis JM, Colombo A, Gaglioni A et al. Intravascular ultrasound guidance of interventional procedures: a randomized trial. Circulation 1993;88(Suppl):I-660.

14. Mintz GS, Pichard AD, Ditrano CJ, Harvey M, Leon MB. Intravascular ultrasound predictors of angiographic and restenosis. Circulation 1993;88(Suppl):I-598.

11. New Techniques

A. Pullback Atherectomy

TIM A. FISCHELL

Despite advances in both balloon dilatation equipment and technique, percutaneous transluminal coronary angioplasty (PTCA) continues to be limited by abrupt vessel closure, restenosis, and limitations in safely treating complex coronary lesions. The pullback atherectomy catheter (PAC, Arrow International, Inc., Reading, PA) is one of the most recently developed devices for mechanical atherectomy, with the goal of improving on the results achievable with balloon angioplasty. The PAC was designed to allow relatively safe and efficient debulking of plaque, while minimizing the risks of distal embolization and of vessel perforation. The retrograde cutting mechanism is designed to obtain better coaxial cutting than antegrade cutting atherectomy because of the mechanics of pulling, rather than pushing, a sharp cutting blade over a flexible guidewire. Initial clinical experience in peripheral vessels has also suggested that this design is well suited for the treatment of bifurcation lesions and, theoretically, should perform well when cutting across ostial stenoses. The device is currently undergoing phase 2 of investigation for both the treatment of peripheral vascular disease and obstructed dialysis fistulas. The phase 1 trial of the coronary device is expected to begin in the spring or summer of 1995. Thus far this device has shown potential for overcoming some of the limitations of balloon angioplasty, and may ultimately prove useful for treating lesions that might be poorly treated by balloon angioplasty.

RETROGRADE ATHERECTOMY: TECHNICAL ASPECTS

The PAC is an over-the-wire device that consists of an inner, movable "cut-collect" catheter contained within a flexible, outer "closing" catheter (Figs. 11A.1 and 11A.2). The tapered distal ("Dottering") tip, which is attached to the cut-collect catheter, contains a hollow collecting chamber and a cylindrical stainless-steel cutting blade that rotates at approximately 2000 rpm driven by a handheld, disposable, motor drive unit (Rotator). Once the device has crossed a target lesion, the closing catheter is pulled back through the lesion creating a gap between the distal tip (with the cutting blade) and the closing catheter (Figs. 11A.1 and 11A.2). The plaque then recoils around a "nonspinning cannula" connected to the distal cutting blade/chamber. With the handheld Rotator activated, the cut-collect catheter is then pulled back through the lesion with the excised atheroma collected in the distal tip's collection chamber. The cut-collect catheter is then secured in a closed position by tightening an Tuohy-Borst fitting at the proximal end of the device. One of the key safety features of the PAC is the finite distance between the cutting blade and the nonspinning cannula (see Fig. 11A.1), which limits the maximal cut thickness to 0.5 to 0.7 mm per pass depending on the device used. Thus it is not possible, under most circumstances, to make a deep cut with any single cutting pass. In addition, the nonspinning cannula is relatively stiff, preventing displacement of the blade during cutting and maintaining a cut aligned nearly coaxially with the arterial segment's true lumen.

The peripheral device is available in 9 Fr and 7.5 Fr outer diameter versions. More re-

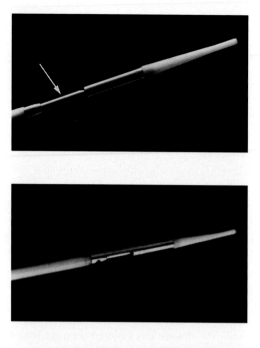

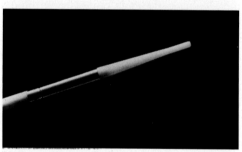

Figure 11A.1. Photographs of pullback atherectomy catheter (PAC). In the top panel the distal end of a 9.0 Fr peripheral device is shown in its open configuration. Arrow points to the "nonspinning cannula" connected to the distal tip of the cut-collect catheter. In the middle panel a 9.0 Fr, peripheral, "shielded" PAC with a 120° cutting surface is shown in its open configuration. In the lower panel the PAC is shown in its closed configuration (e.g., for crossing lesions or after completing a cutting pass).

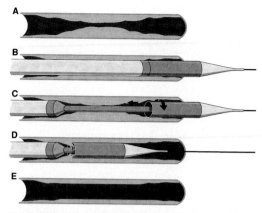

Figure 11A.2. Schematic showing the steps in treating an atherosclerotic lesion with the pullback atherectomy catheter (PAC). **A.** Untreated lesion. **B.** Device is passed through lesion in closed configuration. **C.** Closing catheter is pulled back. **D.** Cut-collection catheter is "pulled back" through lesion shaving and collecting plaque. **E.** Final result. (Reproduced with permission from Miller Freeman, Inc., *Cardio Interventions*.)

cently clinical trials have begun using a 6 Fr peripheral device intended for the treatment of infrapopliteal disease. In addition, a new "shielded" device has also been approved for clinical use in the treatment of peripheral vascular disease. This device has a shield covering up to 240° of the cylindrical cutter, allowing one to direct a cut with a 120° arc toward an eccentric plaque (see

Fig. 11A.1, *middle panel*). Active development efforts are under way to produce a standard and a shielded PAC with the capability to also perform intravascular ultrasonic imaging. It is hoped that this technology may improve the ability to debulk plaque while limiting the cutting to the intima in a large majority of cases. The peripheral device tracks readily over 0.018-inch, or smaller, guidewires. The coronary device is now being tested using 6.0 Fr and 7.2 Fr sizes. The coronary device tracks over a 0.014-inch coronary guidewire.

PRELIMINARY EVALUATION

Preclinical testing of PAC was performed initially in 13 severely diseased cadaveric superficial femoral arteries. After one to three passes with a 7.5 Fr device, followed by 9 Fr and/or 10.5 Fr devices, there was a reduction in mean diameter stenosis from 95% to 21% without adjunctive balloon angioplasty (1, 2). The device was effective in cutting calcified plaques. Histologic examination demonstrated a generally smooth, cylindrical residual lumen (Fig. 11A.3) with the cut limited to the intima in all but one case.

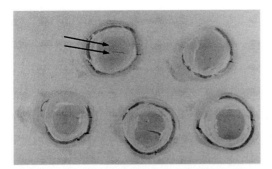

Figure 11A.3. Histopathologic cross sections (1-mm intervals) after pullback atherectomy of a totally occluded cadaveric superficial femoral artery. The grey staining material *(arrows)* is barium gelatin mixture used to pressure fix the specimen after cutting and outlines the round neolumen created by PAC.

PAC TREATMENT OF PERIPHERAL ARTERY DISEASE

A trial of pullback atherectomy for the treatment of symptomatic peripheral vascular disease was begun as a pilot study in 1990. In 1991 the trial was expanded to a multicenter trial. Since then 179 patients with 225 lesions have been treated with pullback atherectomy. The trial has recently been expanded to include a total of 20 clinical sites in the United States and Great Britain (see Acknowledgements). Early clinical results in the treatment of superficial femoral and popliteal artery lesions have been encouraging with a high primary success rate and a relatively low complication rate. To create a lumen larger than the outer diameter of the PAC, a novel technique using external leg compression during the atherectomy has been employed in most of the cases in phase 2 of the peripheral vessel trial. Using this technique of "compressional" pullback atherectomy, a blood pressure cuff is placed around the patient's leg prior to starting the procedure. After the PAC has crossed the lesion and the closing catheter is pulled back, exposing the cutting blade, the cuff is inflated to a pressure of 10 to 100 mm Hg greater than systolic blood pressure. This effectively compresses the plaque into the path of the cutting blade, allowing one to debulk the plaque.

Once the compressional pass is completed, the cuff is deflated. Multiple passes with compression may be used to further debulk the lesion and to create neoluminal dimensions larger than the outer diameter of the PAC device.

The inclusion criteria for the peripheral trial includes patients with lifestyle-limiting claudication or resting limb ischemia, who have angiographically important (>50% diameter stenosis) lesion(s), ≤7 cm in length. Detailed data from the first 99 patients and 135 lesions, treated within the investigational protocol, are summarized below.

A guidewire was passed successfully across all 135 lesions, and the PAC was advanced successfully across the stenosis or occlusion in 134 of 135 (99%) lesions. In one case a 9 Fr PAC could not be advanced across the lesion, and it was successfully treated with balloon angioplasty. Obstructive tissue was removed successfully in 100% of the cases treated with pullback atherectomy. Stand-alone pullback atherectomy was performed in 75 of 134 cases (56%), with adjunctive balloon angioplasty (PTA) performed in the other cases.

Thirteen percent of the lesions treated were total occlusions (17 of 134). The remaining 117 lesions had a mean diameter stenosis of 74%. Of the lesions treated 72% were focal and 28% diffuse; 57% were eccentric with 43% concentric. Nearly half (43%) had calcification evident in the lesion during fluoroscopy. The average lesion length was 2.2 cm with a range of 0.4 to 7.0 cm. Four of the treated lesions occurred in arterial grafts.

Acute procedural success, defined as a less than 50% diameter stenosis with an improvement of at least 20% without major complications, was achieved in 94 of 99 cases (95%). For the 130 native vessel lesions treated in which study inclusion criteria were met, the average initial diameter stenosis by caliper methods was 82%. The average postatherectomy stenosis was 30% and the average post-procedural stenosis was 22%

Table 11A.1
SCIVR Clinical Categories of Limb Ischemia

Category	Grade	Clinical Description	Objective Criteria
0		*Asymptomatic,* no hemodynamically significant occlusive disease	Normal results of treadmill test (5 min at 2 mph on a 12° incline)
1	I	*Mild claudication*	Treadmill exercise completed, postexercise AP is greater than 50 mm Hg but more than 25 mm Hg less than normal
2		*Moderate claudication*	Symptoms between those of categories 1 and 3
3		*Severe claudication*	Treadmill exercise cannot be completed, postexercise AP is less than 50 mm Hg
4	II	*Ischemic rest pain*	Resting AP of 60 mm Hg or less, flat or barely pusatile ankle or metatarsal plethysmographic tracing, tow pressures less than 40 mm Hg
5	III	*Minor tissue loss,* nonhealing ulcer, focal gangrene with diffuse pedal ischemia	Resting AP of 40 mm Hg or less, ankle or metatarsal plethysmographic tracing flat or barely pulsatile, toe pressure less than 30 mm Hg
6		*Major tissue loss,* extending above metatarsal level, functional foot no longer salvageable	Same as category 5

AP, Ankle pressure.

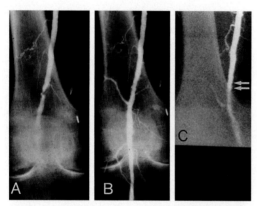

Figure 11A.4. Angiographic result following pullback atherectomy of a heavily calcified and eccentric lesion in the superficial femoral artery. **A.** Initial lesion appearance with evidence of calcification. The middle panel **(B)** shows acute result and right panel **(C)** shows a 5-month follow-up angiogram without evidence of restenosis. The heavily calcified (bonelike) plaque removed in this case is shown in Figure 11A.5.

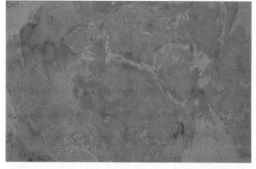

Figure 11A.5. Light microscopic section (hematoxylin and eosin) from intimal plaque removed from the lesion shown in Figure 11A.4. Section shows dense calcification with osteoid formation (i.e., actual bone formation within the intimal plaque).

(after adjunctive PTA). For the four graft lesions the average initial stenosis was 77% with a postatherectomy stenosis of 25%.

The ankle-brachial index (ABI) was measured before and after PAC treatment in all 99 patients. The mean ABI prior to the procedure was 0.62, with an average ABI of 0.88 24 hours following the procedure. SCVIR change in limb status (Table 11A.1) demonstrated an improvement of +3 in 58% of cases, +2 in 33%, +1 in 6%, and no change in 5%.

Intravascular ultrasonic imaging after PAC has demonstrated a generally cylindrical neolumen without subintimal dissection or "scalloping" in the majority of cases studied. The device has worked very well in calcified and eccentric lesions (Figs. 11A.4 and 11A.5). The device has also shown some promise in the treatment of bifurcation lesions such as at the tibial artery. These lesions typically respond poorly to PTA, but have been well treated by PAC (Fig. 11A.6).

Histopathologic analysis is available in 95 of the 99 cases. The average plaque weight removed was 232 mg per lesion, with a mean of 101 mg/cm of lesion length treated. Intimal tissue was removed in 94 of 95 cases (99%). There are no comparable published data available to allow the comparison of the amount of plaque removed with PAC as compared with the devices for vascular intervention (DVI) device in peripheral vessels. However, by comparison, in one published coronary trial using primarily a 7 Fr Atherocath, the mean plaque weight removed was 16.5 mg with a range of 4 to 45 mg (4). Medial tissue was observed in 64 of 95 cases (67%), and adventitial tissue was seen in 15 of 95 cases (15%). These data, with regard to depth of cutting, are similar to that reported with the use of directional atherectomy in both the peripheral (medial cutting in 55%) (3) and coronary circulations (4, 5). Plaque calcification was present in 33 of 95 cases (35%) with organized (old) thrombus in 29%. It appears that this relatively high incidence of medial and adventitial tissue retrieval is the result of compression with the 360° cutter, which may preferentially compress more normal wall constituents into the cutting path. It is likely that the deeper cutting seen with this compressional technique can be reduced using the shielded PAC with compression, particularly in large vessels (>5.0 mm) with eccentric lesions, or by using the 360° cutter without compression in smaller (<4.0 mm) vessels.

A summary of the adverse events related to PAC is outlined in Table 11A.2. Data are available from the first 110 patients and 150 lesions treated. Despite the early (learning curve) nature of these data, there were surprisingly few major complications, defined as those resulting in limb loss or necessitating surgical intervention. There were no cases of limb loss attributable to the PAC procedure in these first 110 cases. There was only one small and self-limited perforation (0.7%), despite the use of compression. The only complications requiring surgical intervention were three cases (2.7%) of vascular repair related to injury at the sheath entry site (one dissection and two pseudoaneurysms). All three of these were treated successfully by surgery. None of these groin complications were the direct result of the use of the PAC device.

Figure 11A.6. Angiographic *(upper panels)* and angioscopic *(lower panels)* appearance before and after pullback atherectomy of a high-grade stenosis at tibial bifurcation. In the lower left-hand panel there is virtually no apparent lumen by angioscopy before atherectomy (arrow points to luminal opening). After treatment with PAC a smooth and cylindrical luminal opening is apparent *(lower right panel).*

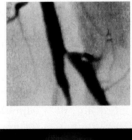
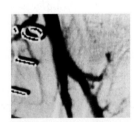
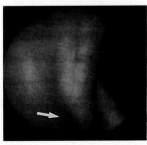
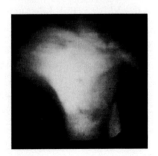

Table 11A.2
Complications: Pullback Atherectomy in Peripheral Vessels

Total number of patients	110
Total number of sites treated	150
Major complications	
Death	0/110 (0%)
PAC-related vascular complications → surgery	0/150 (0%)
Vascular entry site complications → surgery	3/110 (2.7%)
Limb Loss	0/110 (0%)
Minor complications	
Distal emboli resolved without surgery	2/150 (1.3%)
Thrombus formation (resolved without surgery)	8/150 (5.3%)
Perforation (minor, self-limiting)	1/150 (0.7%)
Intimal dissection (minor, non–flow limiting)	2/150 (1.3%)
Minor groin complications	14/110 (12.7%)

Of the 41 successfully treated cases with 6-month clinical follow-up who have had SCVIR ischemia category data (see Table 11A.1) collected, 20 of 41 (49%) were asymptomatic, 6 of 41 (15%) were minimally symptomatic (SCVIR category of 1), and 15 of 41 (36%) had SCVIR ischemia categories of 2 or greater. The ABI data is available in 35 patients at 6 months and shows a mean reduction from 0.88 post-PAC to 0.74 at follow-up. In 19 patients the mean ABI at 1 year was 0.83 versus 0.89 post-PAC.

There is relatively limited long-term angiographic follow-up data available. Using the definition of a greater than 50% residual diameter stenosis as the criteria for angiographic restenosis, there was an overall restenosis rate of 44% (18 of 41 lesions; 38 superficial femoral artery and 3 popliteal lesions) at 6-month angiographic follow-up. It should be noted, however, that 10 additional patients who were asymptomatic refused 6-month follow-up angiography, thus potentially biasing these angiographic follow-up data. If these patients, who are assumed to have a patent treatment site, were included in the 6-month analysis, the calculated restenosis rate would be 35% (18 of 51). Only one of seven patients (14%) who have

had 1-year angiographic follow-up have met the above criteria for angiographic restenosis (one patient with a 51% diameter stenosis). Clinical restenosis, as judged by a return of symptoms to as severe or more severe than the presenting symptoms, based on SCVIR ischemia category was observed in approximately 30% of patients at 6 months. These rates of restenosis are similar to previously published data from a similar group of patients with femoral or popliteal arterial lesions treated with either directional atherectomy (restenosis rate 39%) (3) or balloon angioplasty (6- to 12-month restenosis rates = 25 to 67%) (6–8).

Using the compressional pullback atherectomy technique, there appears to be a significant effect on the adequacy of plaque debulking and on the incidence of restenosis. If the lesion was debulked to a residual diameter stenosis of less than 30%, at the end of the procedure the angiographic restenosis was observed in 5 of 16 cases (31%) versus approximately 60% in cases with residual stenosis of greater than 40%. Interestingly, preliminary and limited data suggest a very low risk of restenosis (one of nine cases, 11%) if there is adequate debulking (residual stenosis <30%), cutting is limited to the intimal layers, and no adjunctive balloon angioplasty is performed. This restenosis rate is similar to that reported with directional atherectomy when substantial debulking is performed with that device (i.e., restenosis rate 18% when <30% residual stenosis is achieved [9]). It is hoped that this type of result may be more easily obtainable with the shielded device in peripheral vessels (with compression) and in the coronary arteries with a closer match between vessel and cutter diameters (no compression). It remains to be determined whether plaque debulking, with a cylindrical neolumen and without deep injury from cutting, stretching, or thermal injury, can yield improved long-term results with this device as compared with balloon angioplasty or directional atherectomy.

CORONARY DEVICE

The coronary device has been evaluated in preclinical testing for approximately two years. The device has been used to successfully debulk atheromatous plaque in a cholesterol-fed rabbit iliac model and has been tested in normal pig coronary arteries. The device was very "trackable" in the preclinical testing, using 9 and 10 Fr guiding catheters for support in the pig coronary tests. In this porcine coronary testing the coronary PAC was advanced without difficulty around 45 to 60° bends in both the left anterior decending and circumflex coronary arteries and to the apex of the heart in the left anterior descend-

ing coronary artery. It was the impression of the operators that the PAC device was more trackable than the DVI Atherocath having comparable outer diameters. The total length of the "stiff" inflexible cutter and collection apparatus in the 6 Fr PAC is 15 mm versus 17 mm for the 6 Fr DVI Atherocath.

The first successful human coronary pullback atherectomy case was performed in December 1994 with Dr. Helmut Drexler in Frieburg, Germany. In this case a high-grade eccentric left anterior descending coronary lesion was treated with two cutting passes with the 2.0-mm (6 Fr) device. A fibrous piece of plaque was removed, improving the mini-

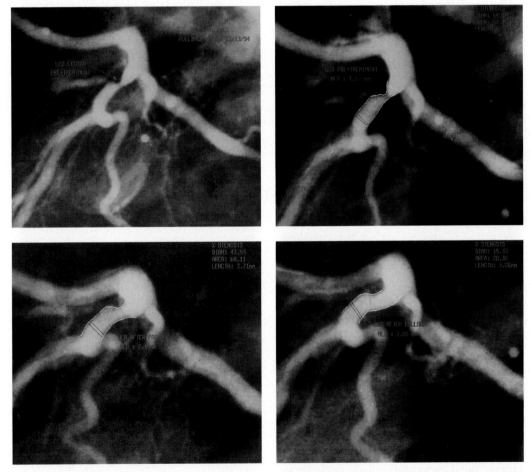

Figure 11A.7. Angiographic result in first successful human coronary pullback atherectomy case. Pretreatment, high-grade LAD lesion (*upper panels;* left without quantitative measurements, right with quantitative angiography). Lower left shows result after cutting pass with 2.0-mm PAC. Final result after single balloon inflation is shown in lower right panel.

mum luminal diameter from 1.1 mm to 2.1 mm. Given the large size of the vessel, adjunctive balloon angioplasty was performed yielding a final minimum luminal diameter of 3.1 mm and a 7 to 15% diameter stenosis (quantitative angiography) with a smooth luminal contour (Fig. 11A.7). There were no complications.

At the time of this writing plans are under way for expansion of a European and Canadian clinical trial. Phase I FDA approval for the coronary application of pullback atherectomy is expected by the summer of 1995.

CONCLUSIONS

Although further clinical trials are required to better define the safety and efficacy of pullback atherectomy, the PAC seems to have several potentially desirable characteristics. For example, like rotational atherectomy, PAC appears to leave a smooth cylindrical lumen (10) but with the advantage of collecting the atheromatous debris for examination, thereby avoiding distal embolization of the Rotablator and the potential for significant blood loss with the aspiration technique of the transluminal extraction catheter (TEC). Theoretically, the PAC should maintain better coaxial alignment during cutting than antegrade atherectomy because of the mechanics of pulling rather than pushing over a flexible guidewire. The coronary device may have the advantage of being relatively user-friendly compared with the Atherocath, and should be able to debulk with one or two cutting passes requiring not more than 30 to 40 seconds per pass. In addition, the device appears capable of debulking even relatively heavily calcified plaque. For the coronary applications the PAC does still have the disadvantage, compared with balloons, of being relatively stiff and of large profile. Although this device has some potential, relatively little can be said about its exact clinical niche, particularly in the treatment of coronary artery disease, at this early stage.

ACKNOWLEDGMENTS

We would like to thank Steven Stiles and *Cardio Intervention,* for the permission to reproduce a figure used in a prior publication of *Cardio Intervention.*

We would also like to acknowledge the assistance of Dr. David Fischell for assisting in the data collection, and the PAC principal investigators who have contributed to the ongoing clinical trial in peripheral vascular disease. These include Dr. Arina van Breda (Alexandria Hospital, Alexandria, VA), Dr. Stephen Kaufman (Emory University, Atlanta, GA), Dr. Andrew H. Cragg (Fairview Riverside Medical Center, Minneapolis, MN), Dr. Edward B. Diethrich (Humana Hospital, Phoenix, AR), Dr. Floyd Osterman (Johns Hopkins Hospital, Baltimore, MD), Dr. Michael Rees (Killingbeck Hospital, Leeds, England), Dr. Barry Katzen (Miami Vascular Institute, Miami, FL), Dr. Jay Hollman (Oschner Clinic, Baton Rouge, LA), Dr. Robert Sanchez (Presbyterian Hospital, Albuquerque, NM), Dr. Anna Belli (Saint Georges Hospital, London, England), Dr. Jonathan Levy (Scottsdale Memorial Hospital, Scottsdale, AR), Dr. Christopher Cates (SJA, Atlanta, GA), Dr. Barry Toombs (St. Lukes Episcopal Hospital, Houston, TX), Dr. Peter C. Block (St. Vincent's Hospital, Portland, OR), Dr. Lewis Wexler (Stanford University, Stanford, CA), Dr. Constantin Cope (U. Pennsylvania, Philadelphia, PA), Dr. E. Bruce McIff (Utah Valley Regional Medical Center, Provo, UT), Dr. Richard Gray (Washington Hospital Center, Washington, DC), and Dr. Robert White Jr. (Yale Univ. Medical Center, New Haven, CT).

REFERENCES

1. Fischell TA, Fischell RE, White RI, Chapolini R. Ex-vivo results using a new pullback atherectomy catheter (PAC). Cathet Cardiovasc Diagn 1990;21:287–291.
2. Fischell TA, Fischell RE, White RI, Chapellini R. Ex-vivo and preliminary clinical results using a new pullback atherectomy catheter (PAC). J Am Coll Cardiol 1991; 17(2):204A (abstract).
3. Von Polnitz A, Nerlich A, Berger H, Hofling B. Percutaneous peripheral atherectomy: angiographic and clinical follow-up of 60 patients. J Am Coll Cardiol 1990;15:682–688.
4. Penny WF, Schmidt DA, Safian RD, Erny RE, Baim DS. Insights into the mechanism of luminal improvement after directional coronary atherectomy. Am J Cardiol 1991; 67:435–437.
5. Garratt KN, Kaufman UP, Edwards WD, Vliestra RE,

Holmes DR Jr. Safety of percutaneous coronary atherectomy with deep arterial resection. Am J Cardiol 1989; 64:538–540.

6. Greenfield A. Femoral popliteal and tibial arteries: percutaneous transluminal angioplasty. Am J Roentgenol 1980; 135:927–935.

7. Probst P, Cerny P, Owens A, Mahler F. Patency after femoral angioplasty: correlation of angiographic appearance with clinical findings. Am J Roentgenol 1983; 140:1227–1232.

8. Johnston KW, Rae M, Hogg-Johnston SA et al. Five-year results of a prospective study of percutaneous transluminal angioplasty. Ann Surg 1987;206(4):403–413.

9. Simpson JB, Selmon MR, Robertson GC et al. Transluminal atherectomy for occlusive peripheral vascular disease. Am J Cardiol 1988;61:96G–101G.

10. Fourrier JL, Stankowiak C, Lablanche CM, Prat A, Brunetaaud JM, Bertrand ME. Histopathology after rotational angioplasty of peripheral arteries in human beings. J Am Coll Cardiol 1988;11:109A (abstract).

B. Physiologic Low Stress Angioplasty

EZRA DEUTSCH

Percutaneous transluminal coronary angioplasty (PTCA) is confronted with a number of problems that both impact on the initial success and limit the long-term effectiveness of the procedure. Remodeling of coronary artery stenoses by PTCA in man is achieved through the application of radial compressive forces to the atherosclerotic arterial wall. There is mechanical compression of atheroma and concurrent splitting or fracture of noncompliant, calcified aspects of obstructive plaque. The more compliant components of the arterial wall are stretched (1). There is exposure of subendothelial surfaces and thrombus formation at the dilation site, which may evolve to threaten or even cause acute closure of the dilated vessel. Histologic analysis of atherosclerotic arteries immediately following balloon dilation in both animal and necropsy specimens reveals endothelial denudation, linear and spiral tears in the intimal surface that often extend into the media, and subintimal hemorrhage and thrombus formation

at the angioplasty site (2, 3). Dissection is observed angiographically in up to 30% of cases (4). The presence of intimal flaps and thrombus formation postangioplasty in man have been confirmed by angioscopy (5). Restenosis after successful PTCA occurs with an observed incidence ranging from 30 to 50% (6) and is the primary limitation of the procedure. Certain angiographic and morphologic predictors of restenosis after PTCA have been described, implying that the cost of arterial remodeling in eccentric, severe stenoses (minimum luminal diameter <0.5 mm) is reflected in an increased incidence of restenosis (7, 8). Thus the localized barotrauma that occurs during arterial recanalization in balloon angioplasty gives rise to the conditions that predispose to these acute and long-term complications.

Platelet activation and loss of local vasodilatory responses contribute greatly to the process of restenosis (9–15). Histologic examination of angioplasty sites in experimental models and in human necropsy studies consistently reveals intimal hyperplasia or thickening, irrespective of whether there is angiographic evidence of restenosis (16, 17). The extent to which neointimal hyperplasia occurs may thus be dependant on the degree of arterial damage that occurs as a result of the remodeling process during PTCA. Restenosis lesions are typically concentric, suggesting that the process of renarrowing caused by neointimal hyperplasia involves the entire dilated segment in a circumferential fashion (8).

RATIONALE OF THERMAL ANGIOPLASTY

The concept of applying thermal energy during angioplasty evolved from observations that the principal complications of PTCA—acute closure, caused by significant dissection and/or thrombus formation, and restenosis, the result of neointimal hyperplasia—could be effectively treated by the simultaneous application of heat (at 85° to 120°C) and pressure during angioplasty laser balloon angioplasty (LBA) (18). The geometry of the disrupted tissue planes at the luminal surface post-PTCA produces zones of separated flow that serve as the substrate for ongoing platelet aggregation and microthrombus formation (18). Welding of these dissected tissue planes should provide a smooth, non-thrombogenic lumen with restoration of laminar flow. Elastic recoil following balloon dilatation has been well described (18, 19). Thus the residual lumen post-PTCA is typically less than the desired endpoint, in part related to the viscoelastic properties of the arterial wall. Thermal angioplasty abolishes elastic recoil after PTCA (20), likely the result of straightening of elastic fibers (21–23) and medial smooth muscle cell damage (21). Inhibition of smooth muscle cell proliferation by direct damage to the cells during the initial thermal angioplasty might also impede the restenosis process.

PLOSA

Physiologically controlled low-stress angioplasty (PLOSA) is a technique based on the premise that the application of heat at 60°C and a minimal balloon distending pressure during angioplasty would permit arterial remodeling with less intimal disruption than is observed with conventional angioplasty. Phase change of the cholesteryl ester components of atherosclerotic plaque might occur utilizing thermal energy at these temperatures in vivo. The "softened" plaque could subsequently be dilated at lower inflation pressures. Thus, in PLOSA, the angioplasty component of arterial remodeling would be achieved with "low-stress" inflation pressures. A reduction in the extent of arterial barotrauma that occurs during conventional PTCA would theoretically minimize the extent of intimal damage and dissection, paralleled by a diminished likelihood of acute thrombotic closure and subsequent neointimal hyperplasia.

The hypothesis of PLOSA is based on the observation that the lipid component of human atheroma comprises as much as 30 to 65% of the total dry weight (24) and is thus the major constituent of the atherosclerotic plaque. Fatty streaks (often forming in childhood) are seen in the intimal surface of the arterial wall and are the result of cellular cholesterol uptake in excess of excretion. Over time there is nucleation of cholesterol to form inert crystals, paralleled by cell necrosis and plaque formation. Atherosclerotic plaques are thus stratified. The most rigid cholesterol crystals comprise the base of the plaque, and the softer, more recently deposited cholesterol esters (cholesteryl oleate, linoleate, and palmitate) are found on the luminal aspect of the intima (24).

The distribution of lipids in the arterial wall is divided between three major populations: phospholipid, free cholesterol, and cholesterol esters. The lipid content of normal intima is approximately 5% of cell constituents. In contrast to normal intima, atherosclerotic intima may be composed of as much as 30 to 65% lipid (24). As the plaque develops, there is a shift from a phospholipid-rich to a cholesterol ester–rich state. This is demonstrated clinically by the age-related increase in LDL-like lipids.

These three classes of lipid have marked differences in their thermal properties in vitro. Both phospholipid and cholesterol monohydrate have melting points of 85°C. In contrast, cholesterol esters exhibit a complex thermal behavior. Cholesteryl oleate melts from a crystal to a liquid at 51°C. On cooling, first a cholesteric state forms at 47.5°C, followed by a stable smectic state below 42°C. Cholesteryl linoleate melts from crystal to liquid at 42°C. Cholesteryl palmitate does not melt to a liquid state until 83.5°C (24). Further, it is likely that the higher melting point cholesterols soften before melting, perhaps at temperatures under 85°C. These physiochemical properties may thus permit thermal remodeling of atherosclerotic plaque in the temperature range of 50 to 60°C.

THE PLOSA SYSTEM

The PLOSA system (Boston Scientific Corporation, Natick, MA) consists of a modified conventional angioplasty balloon catheter and a control unit. Two platinum electrodes are mounted on the catheter shaft inside the balloon and are attached to the control unit by wires. A radiofrequency potential is applied at 650 kHz across these resistive elements. As current flows between the electrodes, heat is generated by resistive power loss in the fluid inside the balloon (typically a 50/50 mixture of 0.9 M NaCl and ionic contrast). This heat is in turn transmitted to the arterial wall by conduction. No radiofrequency energy passes through tissue; it is confined to the balloon. The temperature of the fluid is selectable by the operator and is accurate to within ±2°C. A temperature sensor mounted on the catheter shaft inside the balloon is in direct contact with the balloon fluid and is connected to a feedback system in the control unit. This thermistor provides continuous temperature monitoring to the control unit, which instantaneously regulates radiofrequency input, thus preventing temperature overshoot. Uniform heating of the balloon to 60°C, as confirmed by thermal map profiles, is achieved within seconds. Cooling of the saline/contrast mixture inside the balloon to 37°C occurs after cessation of radiofrequency energy input. Data from our laboratory have demonstrated that only those areas of the arterial wall in direct contact with the PLOSA balloon will be heated. The PLOSA balloon is depicted in Figure 11B.1.

One striking difference between PLOSA and other devices that utilize thermal energy to treat obstructive coronary stenoses is the relatively low temperature of 60°C employed during PLOSA. Thermal ablation of atherosclerotic plaque, initially thought to be a beneficial effect of laser therapy (temperature range 100 to 400°C), produces a charred endothelial surface that may result in vascular spasm and resultant thrombosis (25, 26). The incidence of restenosis has not been dimin-

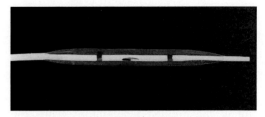

Figure 11B.1. The PLOSA balloon is a modified conventional angioplasty balloon catheter. Two platinum radiofrequency electrodes are mounted on the catheter shaft, inside the balloon. A thermistor is also located on the catheter shaft, centered inside the balloon. Both electrodes and the thermistor are connected to a control unit (not shown) by wires inside the catheter shaft.

ished by laser therapy, either as independent therapy or in conjunction with balloon angioplasty (1, 25–27). Laser balloon angioplasty (applied temperature estimated at 85 to 120°C, inflation pressures of 6 to 10 atm) also has a high restenosis rate when applied as either primary or adjunctive therapy (28). One explanation for the significant incidence of restenosis with these devices is that thermal injury, with attendant cell necrosis, occurs at these temperatures. In contrast, only minimal medial cell injury was observed following PLOSA at 60°C in an in vivo porcine coronary artery angioplasty model (21). It is interesting to note that the extent of cell damage in this model was significantly increased when PLOSA was performed at 70°C.

One distinct advantage of the PLOSA system is the use of radiofrequency energy as the source of thermal output. The magnitude of energy output can be closely regulated, permitting tight control of the applied temperature. Early studies using prototype bipolar radiofrequency balloon angioplasty catheters with electrodes on the balloon surface demonstrated that thermal "molding" of postmortem human atherosclerotic arterial segments could be successfully performed, and that larger luminal diameters were achieved, with no evidence of subsequent elastic recoil (29). These authors demonstrated that thermal energy was applied only to that segment of artery in contact with the balloon system. However, there was histologic evidence of medial myocyte damage with this system. A major concern in the design of the initial radiofrequency system with surface electrodes was the inability to have precise control of the applied temperature. Thus the PLOSA system was modified such that two radiofrequency electrodes were mounted on the catheter shaft inside the balloon. Radiofrequency energy applied between these electrodes is confined to the balloon and results in heating of the contrast/saline mixture inside the balloon. Thermal energy reaches the arterial wall by thermal conduction. A thermistor is also mounted on the catheter shaft inside the balloon. The balloon temperature in the present system can be regulated by a control unit to within 1°C.

EXPERIMENTAL STUDIES

Proof of Principle—In Vitro Cadaver Atherosclerotic Iliac Artery Studies

The initial evaluation of the PLOSA system was performed in freshly-excised cadaver atherosclerotic human iliac arteries. Range-finding experiments with this experimental system demonstrated that 60°C and 2 atm were optimal temperature and pressure settings necessary to achieve stenosis reduction utilizing a single 60-second treatment. Lower temperatures (40 to 50°C) required inflation pressures of 6 atm to reduce the initial stenoses and were associated with an equivalent incidence of dissection to PTCA. There was no additional improvement in angiographic or angioscopic outcomes at temperatures above 60°C when compared with the 60°C treatments at 2 atm.

In this model PLOSA resulted in improved stenosis reduction, a lower incidence of dissection, and a significant reduction in the extent of intimal disruption compared with conventional angioplasty (30). On morphometric analysis of histologic arterial cross sections, only 4.6% ± 2.6% of the intimal surface was damaged following PLOSA,

which contrasts sharply with the 29.3% ± 10.4% observed after conventional angioplasty. These effects are not the result of balloon inflation at a lower pressure, as the incidence of dissection and the extent of intimal disruption in a cohort of segments dilated at low pressure and 37°C was significantly higher than that observed in the PLOSA group.

EFFECTS OF PLOSA ON ARTERIAL ELASTIC PROPERTIES

Further insight into the mechanism of PLOSA comes from studies examining the effect of simultaneous application of heat at 60°C and a minimal distending pressure on the elastic properties of intact porcine iliac vessels (31). Progressive inflation of a conventional angioplasty balloon in an appropriately sized, freshly excised, porcine common iliac artery generates a pressure-volume curve that describes the compliance of the arterial segment. Inflation of a PLOSA balloon at 60°C in the contralateral, paired arterial segment resulted in a rightward shift of this pressure-volume curve, even at a minimal balloon volume. Thus the compliance of the artery is increased when subjected to heating at 60°C and progressive inflation of the PLOSA balloon. Histologic straightening of elastic fibers was observed in PLOSA-treated segments, in parallel with this alteration in arterial compliance. These alterations in arterial compliance, likely the result of combined thermal-pressure effects on elastic fibers, may have important effects on arterial remodeling in man.

TIME COURSE OF TRANSMURAL ARTERIAL HEATING

To gain further insight into the mechanism of PLOSA, we examined the time course of transmural heating and the relationship between arterial wall thickness and temperature gradients in normal and atherosclerotic rabbits (32) in vivo. The heating profiles of normal and atherosclerotic aorta are quite different. Heat transfer during PLOSA is rapid in atherosclerotic arteries and is amplified in areas of larger plaque thickness. Thermal energy may thus be focused to the area of greatest plaque burden in PLOSA. This observation suggests that plaque and the surrounding media and adventitia are a rapid conductor of heat in this model. The eccentric nature of atherosclerotic plaque may also account for the rapid heat transfer, as more surface area of the plaque is in direct contact with the balloon surface and thus receives augmented thermal input.

PRESERVATION OF ARTERIAL VASOREACTIVITY

The effects of balloon angioplasty on coronary arterial vasoreactivity in man are well known (19). There is persistent vasoconstriction, which may in part be caused by the uniform endothelial denudation in those areas of the coronary artery in direct contact with the balloon surface. This results in the loss of synthesis of endogenous vasodilators such as endothelium-dependent relaxing factor and prostacyclin. In addition, stretching and tearing of medial smooth muscle fibers results in progressive coronary vasoconstriction after angioplasty, both at the site of the dilatation and in the distal vessel. This phenomenon can be reversed with intracoronary nitroglycerin and is thought to occur because of direct balloon injury to medial smooth muscle. As PLOSA is performed at significantly lower inflation pressures, the attendant reduction in arterial barotrauma might result in preservation of endothelium and smooth muscle architecture and thus in preserved vascular responsiveness.

To assess the effect of PLOSA on arterial vasoreactivity, the vasomotor responses of arterial rings of atherosclerotic rabbit abdominal aorta subjected to either PLOSA, conventional balloon angioplasty, or no intervention were evaluated (33). Contraction and relaxation responses to norepinephrine and nitroglycerin were similar in the three groups and paralleled the responses of normal (nonatherosclerotic) aortic rings. However, methacholine-induced vasorelaxation was observed only in normal rings and in atherosclerotic rings treated with PLOSA. The vasodilator response to methacholine in this model requires intact endothelium and implies that endothelial function is preserved after PLOSA but not after conventional angioplasty.

In Vivo Atherosclerotic Rabbit Studies

The acute and long-term effects of PLOSA were directly compared with conventional angioplasty in the atherosclerotic rabbit. In both the acute and long-term animals, angiographic and histologic outcomes after arterial remodeling using the PLOSA system were significantly better than after conventional balloon angioplasty. A mean of 82.2% of the intimal surface was damaged after balloon angioplasty, as compared with only 35.5% damage of the intimal circumference following PLOSA. The minimal extent of arterial barotrauma after PLOSA contrasts the difference in mechanisms of plaque reduction between PLOSA and balloon angioplasty (34).

The long-term outcomes in this atherosclerotic model reflect the observations made in those animals studied acutely (35). Using a measure of neointimal hyperplasia defined as the region of arterial wall from the endothelial surface at the lumen to the luminal margin of the media (36), the cross-sectional area of neointima (in mm^2) was significantly less in PLOSA treated segments than in paired arteries treated with conventional angioplasty. This finding was consistent in the animals studied either at 30 days or at 60 days. Quantitative analysis of follow-up angiograms at 30 and 60 days demonstrated a significant increase in the minimum luminal diameter in the PLOSA group at 30 days compared with the angioplasty cohort, with a trend to significance at 60 days. These data show that the less traumatic mechanism of arterial remodeling in PLOSA impacts favorably on the incidence of restenosis in this model and suggests that PLOSA may offer similar benefits in man.

CLINICAL EXPERIENCE

Phase I Human Coronary Trial

STUDY DESIGN

The initial human coronary cases were performed in Europe and Canada prior to the onset of the United States phase I clinical trial. The inflation protocol was designed in such a fashion as to derive a maximal benefit from the application of thermal energy at 60°C to "soften" the atherosclerotic plaque such that only a minimum distensile force (applied by the balloon) would be required to remodel the coronary stenosis. The PLOSA balloon is made of a unique blend of polyethylene tetraphalate and exhibits minimal compliance, achieving nominal size at 1 atm, with less than a 2% increase in size at 5 atm. This design minimizes the potential for any isolated angioplasty effect. Exact sizing of the balloon to the arterial diameter of the stenosed segment is thus necessary to achieve optimal stenosis reduction. These first cases demonstrated that PLOSA was a safe and effective percutaneous technique of remodeling atherosclerotic coronary stenoses. One critical observation was that a significant period (approximately 1 second of cooling for each second of heating) was required for the saline/contrast mixture inside the balloon to cool from 60 to 42°C prior to deflation after each PLOSA treatment.

The inflation sequence for the United States phase I protocol is outlined in Table 11B.1. The first inflation is limited to a peak pressure of 2 atm. A peak pressure of 5 atm can be employed during the second inflation, in an effort to provide additional dilating force without overexpansion of those aspects of the balloon unopposed by obstructive plaque. After two inflations the operator may elect to upsize the balloon by 0.25 mm in diameter. Indeed, if straightening of elastic fibers occurs after the initial inflations, a larger balloon may be required to achieve complete

Table 11B.1
PLOSA Human Coronary Protocol

Inflation #	Balloon:Artery Ratio	Peak Pressure	Maximum Inflation Time
1	1:1	2 atm	90 sec
2	1:1	5 atm	90 sec
3	>1:1	2 atm	90 sec
4	>1:1	5 atm	90 sec

Inflations 2 and 4 may be repeated multiple times at the investigator's discretion.

An angiographic endpoint of <20% residual stenosis is desired.

remodeling of the stenosed coronary segment. A residual stenosis of less than 20% is the desired endpoint.

The phase I protocol permits treatment of a single lesion with PLOSA. Patients with de novo lesions or lesions that have restenosed after previous treatment with conventional angioplasty are considered eligible for participation in this protocol. Angiographic inclusion criteria require greater than 70% stenosis in a vessel 2.5 to 3.5 mm in diameter, and lesions must be less than 20 mm in length. Patients suffering an acute myocardial infarction or who have received thrombolytic therapy less than 1 week prior to intervention are excluded from this study, as are patients with severe left ventricular dysfunction (LVEF <35%). Patients who are pacemaker-dependent (permanent or temporary) are also ineligible for this protocol. Other angiographic criteria that preclude consideration for this study are an unprotected left main stenosis >50%, 100% occluded lesions, and the presence of either intracoronary thrombus or a severely calcified lesion.

Seventy-two patients comprised the human coronary experience (37). Forty-six patients had an isolated coronary stenosis, twenty-two had two vessel disease, and five had three vessel disease. Mean left ventricular ejection fraction was 63%. Anginal symptoms were present in 90%, and 30% of patients with angina were unstable (Canadian Cardiovascular Society class IV) at the time of the procedure. Risk factors for coronary artery disease include a family history of premature coronary artery disease in 52%, tobacco abuse in 72%, hyperlipidemia in 59%, hypertension in 36%, and diabetes in 14%.

Seventy-three stenoses (52 de novo, 20 restenotic) were treated with PLOSA. Fifty lesions were type B, 20 were type A, and two were type C morphology (American College of Cardiology/American Heart Association typology). All patients received 325 mg of aspirin the morning of the procedure. All oral and intravenous cardiac medications were continued for each patient. Anticoagulation with intravenous heparin was achieved after insertion of arterial and venous femoral cannulas. Additional heparin was administered as needed throughout the case to maintain an activated clotting time of >350 sec. All patients described typical anginal chest discomfort during PLOSA inflations; in addition, a number of patients described a sensation of "heat" in parallel with temperatures over 55°C.

An angiographic success was achieved in 93% of patients. A mean initial stenosis of 80.6 ± 1.5% (mean ± sem) was reduced to 30.8 ± 1.7%. Mean MLD increased from 0.57 ± 0.04 mm preprocedure to 2.06 ± 0.06 mm 5 minutes after PLOSA, with no evidence of elastic recoil at 15 minutes (MLD 2.01 ± 0.06 mm). Localized dissection at the PLOSA site occurred in 11 patients (15%). Adjunctive PTCA was performed in six patients. In two cases PTCA was utilized in an effort to further improve the arterial lumen at the site of the stenosis. In two patients a perfusion balloon catheter was employed to treat a dissection after PLOSA. In one case a low-pressure inflation was performed with a conventional PTCA balloon to break up arterial thrombus at the PLOSA site. There was one instance of abrupt closure of the treated vessel that occurred following premature deflation of the PLOSA balloon at 60°C. This patient required emergent CABG surgery (37).

In each case arterial remodeling was achieved at a significantly lower inflation pressure than would be expected with conventional balloon angioplasty (mean 3.85 ± 0.12 atm). Longer inflation times were required, accounted for in part by 30- to 90-second periods as the device cooled to 42°C prior to deflation, after individual heating inflations of 55 to 90 seconds. Total heating time ranged from 55 to 480 seconds (mean 190 seconds). A mean of 3.5 ± 1.5 inflations were performed. A mean of 1.3 ± 0.4 balloons were employed per case (37). The typical angiographic appearance of an arterial segment after treatment with PLOSA is a smooth, tubular lumen that resembles the shape of the fully inflated balloon. Intracoronary ultrasound reveals a minimum of intimal disruption and a smooth, circular lumen. A representative case is shown in Figure 11B.2.

To directly compare the procedural variables and angiographic outcomes of PLOSA with PTCA, we performed a retrospective, case-matched, control study of 20 human coronary lesions treated with PLOSA as sole therapy with 35 randomly selected lesions, matched for lesion location and arterial location, that were treated with PTCA (38). Angiograms were analyzed at a core laboratory using a computer-based, edge-detection system (39). Stenosis reduction was achieved with significantly lower inflation pressures after PLOSA than with conventional angioplasty. Although longer inflation periods were required during PLOSA, the number of inflations per case was similar in the two groups. Initial lesion severity, as measured both by percent stenosis and minimum luminal diameter, was similar in the PLOSA and PTCA cohorts. However, the residual stenosis postprocedure was significantly less after PLOSA, paralleled by a significantly greater minimum luminal diameter in the PLOSA group. These procedural variables and angiographic outcomes are outlined in Table 11B.2.

Arterial recoil is a commonly observed phenomenon after PTCA. Utilizing the PLOSA and case-matched control PTCA cohort described above, quantitative analysis

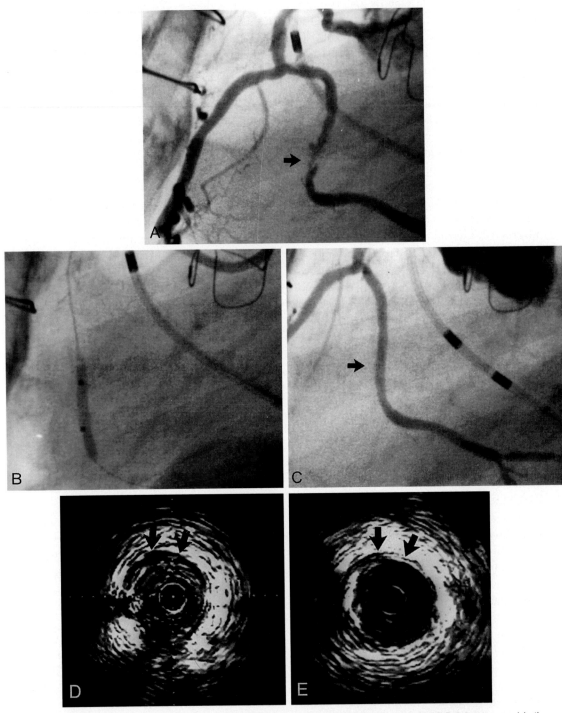

Figure 11B.2. PLOSA of a distal right coronary artery stenosis. **A.** An initial 90% stenosis (MLD 0.3 mm, *arrow*) in the distal right coronary artery is depicted. The angiographic appearance is that of an ulcerated, ruptured plaque. **B.** The PLOSA balloon is fully inflated at 2 atm in the lesion. **C.** This lesion was reduced to a 7% narrowing after 2 inflations with a 3.25-mm PLOSA balloon (MLD 2.82 mm, *arrow*). **D.** Intracoronary ultrasound of the lesion pre-PLOSA. There is a large plaque burden and a spontaneous dissection superiorly *(arrows)*. **E.** Intracoronary ultrasound of the same lesion after PLOSA. There is a smooth, circular lumen. The dissection plane has been sealed *(arrows)*.

Table 11B.2
PLOSA Versus Conventional Angioplasty: Procedural Variables and Angiographic Outcomes

	PTCA	PLOSA	P value
Peak pressure (atm)	8.2 ± .32	3.7 ± .22	.0001
# of inflations	3.5 ± .25	2.8 ± .25	ns
Total inflation time (sec)	224 ± 24	402 ± 44	.0003
% Diameter stenosis (pre)	80 ± 1.8	85 ± 1.5	.04
% Diameter stenosis (post)	31 ± 2.0	24 ± 1.9	.03
Minimum luminal diameter (pre)	0.62 ± .06	0.49 ± .05	ns
Minimum luminal diameter (5 min post)	2.04 ± .07	2.41 ± .11	.005
Minimum luminal diameter (15 min post)	1.79 ± .07	2.37 ± .11	.0001

of angiograms performed 5 and 15 minutes after the final inflation in each case revealed no change in the minimum luminal diameter in the PLOSA group. However, minimum luminal diameter declined 0.25 mm 15 minutes after PTCA, representing an 18% loss of the acute gain. Thus a greater initial improvement in minimum luminal diameter and the absence of elastic recoil are observed after PLOSA in comparison with PTCA (37).

One further insight into the mechanism of PLOSA comes from analysis of changes in lesion eccentricity. To compare the coronary arterial remodeling that occurs with PLOSA and conventional PTCA, the eccentricity of the vessel wall at the site of stenosis was assessed from preintervention and postintervention angiograms using a computer-based, edge-detection system. Changes in the morphology of each side of the vessel wall were separately assessed based on changes in the standard deviation of the radius of curvature (SDC) averaged across the stenotic zone. An eccentricity index was generated from a ratio of the SDCs of the opposing vessel walls. This technique permits evaluation of lesion eccentricity independent of the course of the arterial segment in space. Lesion eccentricity was similar in the PLOSA and case-matched groups before intervention. However, lesions were significantly less eccentric after PLOSA. The more diseased side of the arterial wall (evidenced by the greatest SDC preintervention) was significantly more parallel to the midline with PLOSA than with PTCA.

These data suggest that the mechanism of stenosis reduction is different in PLOSA than in PTCA. PLOSA thus results in more concentric dilatation with facilitated remodeling of regions with greater plaque burden (40).

TREATMENT OF SUBOPTIMAL PTCA CAUSED BY ACUTE ARTERIAL RECOIL

Suboptimal dilatation complicating PTCA may occur as the result of elastic recoil. Based on the observations that PLOSA results in straightening of elastic fibers in experimental models and that there is no acute recoil of dilated segments after PLOSA in man, the inclusion criteria for PLOSA were expanded to permit acute PLOSA treatment of patients who have a suboptimal result after conventional angioplasty because of recoil at the dilatation site. Eight patients have been treated with PLOSA for this indication. Five lesions were de novo and three were restenotic. Three lesions were in the LAD, four were in the left circumflex, and there was one RCA stenosis. During conventional PTCA a mean of 4.9 ± 0.4 inflations were performed to a peak of 11.5 ± 1.1 atm with at least 1:1 balloon:artery sizing. In each case at least two inflations were performed where the PTCA balloon was fully expanded. PLOSA was then performed using a balloon of comparable size to the largest PTCA balloon. An average of 3.6 PLOSA inflations were performed, with a mean total heating time of 281 ± 69 seconds at a peak of 4.0 ± 0.4 atm. MLD increased from 0.76 ± 0.13 mm pre-

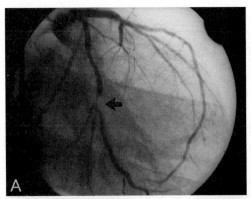

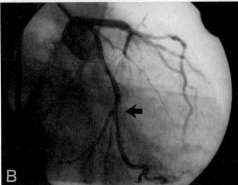

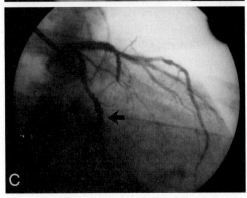

Figure 11B.3.   Suboptimal PTCA caused by elastic recoil successfully treated with PLOSA. **A.** A restenosis lesion in a large, obtuse marginal branch of the left circumflex artery *(arrow)*. **B.** A 54% residual narrowing is present after multiple inflations above the nominal inflation pressure with an appropriately sized angioplasty balloon (peak 10 atm) *(arrow)*. **C.** A minimum residual narrowing (23%) is seen *(arrow)* after 2 inflations with a PLOSA balloon of identical size (peak inflation pressure 3 atm).

SUMMARY

The application of heat at 60°C and a minimal distending pressure distinguishes PLOSA from other percutaneous forms of coronary remodeling. The magnitude of the initial gain achieved after PLOSA is significantly greater than that observed after PTCA. It has recently been proposed that greater acute gains in coronary minimum luminal diameter are associated with a reduced incidence of subsequent restenosis (41). In PLOSA the large increase in minimum luminal diameter is achieved at lower inflation pressures than are typically required with either conventional angioplasty or other balloon-facilitated coronary remodeling techniques. Experimental studies with PLOSA demonstrate that the application of heat and only minimal inflation pressure minimizes the extent of barotrauma and permits a significant degree of functional preservation of vascular endothelium. The effects of PLOSA on arterial recoil are likely the direct result of thermal energy on the elastic elements of the arterial wall. Ongoing examination of long-term outcomes after PLOSA will broaden our understanding of the thermal behavior and subsequent responses of atherosclerotic coronary vasculature. Future studies, including concurrent intraluminal imaging and thermal-mediated drug delivery, may further optimize this technique for better acute and long-term outcomes.

PTCA to $1.1 \pm .10$ mm post-PTCA, with a further increase to $1.67 \pm .11$ mm post-PLOSA ($P = .01$). This corresponded to a reduction in residual percent stenosis from $59.0 \pm 4.1\%$ post-PTCA to $35.6 \pm 5.6\%$ after PLOSA treatment. Thus the application of thermal energy appears to have beneficial effects on the elastic properties of coronary vasculature in this setting. One such patient treated in our laboratory is illustrated in Figure 11B.3.

REFERENCES

1. Waller BF. "Crackers, breakers, stretchers, drillers, scrapers, shavers, burners, welders and melters"—the future treatment of atherosclerotic coronary disease? A clinical-morphologic assessment. J Am Coll Cardiol 1989; 13:969–987.
2. Faxon DP, Weber VJ, Haudenschild C, Gottsman SB, McGovern WA, Ryan TJ. Acute effects of transluminal angioplasty in three experimental models of atherosclerosis. Arteriosclerosis 1982;2:125–133.
3. Block PC, Baughman KL, Pasternak RC, Fallon JT. Transluminal angioplasty: correlation of morphologic and angio-

graphic findings in an experimental model. Circulation 1980;61:778–785.

4. Matthews BJ, Ewels CJ, Kent KM. Coronary dissection: a predictor of restenosis? Am Heart J 1988;115:547–554.

5. Ramee SR, White CJ, Collins TJ, Mesa JE, Murgo JP. Percutaneous angioscopy during coronary angioplasty using a steerable microangioscope. J Am Coll Cardiol 1991; 17:100–105.

6. Hirshfeld JW Jr, Schwartz JS, Jugo RS et al. Restenosis after coronary angioplasty: a multivariate model to relate lesion and procedure variables to restenosis. J AM Coll Cardiol 1991;18:647–656.

7. Deutsch E, Hirshfeld JW Jr, Pepine CJ, Bove AA. Analysis of initial lesion characteristics and arterial remodelling six months after angioplasty in a stable population. J Am Coll Cardiol 1992;19:258A.

8. Deutsch E, Gerber RS, Martin JL, Burke JA, Combs WG, Bove AA. Initial lesion eccentricity predicts restenosis after successful coronary angioplasty. J Am Coll Cardiol 1993;21:89A.

9. Chesebro JH, Lam YHT, Badimon L, Fuster V. Restenosis after arterial angioplasty: a hemorrheologic response to injury. Am J Cardiol 1987;60:10B–16B.

10. Lucas MA, Deutsch E, Hirshfeld JW, Barnathan ES, Laskey WK. Influence of heparin therapy on PTCA outcome in patients with coronary thrombus. Am J Cardiol 1990; 65:179–182.

11. Fuster V, Badimon L, Cohen M, Ambrose J, Badimon JJ, Chesebro JH. Insights into the pathogenesis of acute ischemic syndromes. Circulation 1988;77:1213–1220.

12. Wilcox JN. Thrombin and other potential mechanisms underlying restenosis. Circulation 1991;84:432–434.

13. Ross R. The pathogenesis of atherosclerosis: an update. N Engl J Med 1986;314:488–500.

14. McNamara CA, Sarembock IJ, Gimple LW, Fenton JW III, Coughlin SR, Owens GK. Thrombin stimulates proliferation of cultured rat aortic smooth muscle cells by a proteolytically activated receptor. J Clin Invest 1993;91:94–98.

15. Liu MW, Roubin GS, King SB. Restenosis after coronary angioplasty: potential biologic determinants and role of intimal hyperplasia. Circulation 1989;79:1374–1387.

16. Austen GE, Ratliff NH, Hollman J, Tabei S, Phillips DF. Intimal proliferation of smooth muscle cells as an explanation for recurrent coronary artery stenosis after percutaneous transluminal coronary angioplasty. J Am Coll Cardiol 1985;6:369–375.

17. Giraldo AA, Esposo OM, Meis JM. Intimal hyperplasia as a cause of restenosis after percutaneous transluminal coronary angioplasty. Arch Pathol Lab Med 1985;109:173–175.

18. Spears JR. Percutaneous transluminal coronary angioplasty restenosis: potential prevention with laser balloon angioplasty. Am J Cardiol 1987;60:61B–64B.

19. Fischell TA, Derby G, Tse TM, Stadius ML. Coronary artery vasoconstriction routinely occurs after percutaneous transluminal coronary angioplasty. Circulation 1988;78:1323–1334.

20. O'Neill BJ, Title LM, Makowski S, Martin JL, Bove AA, Fram DB, McKay RG et al. Absence of early recoil after

successful physiologic low-stress angioplasty. Circulation 1993;88:1–150.

21. Fram DB, Aretz TA, Fisher JP, Mikan JS, Reisner A, Mitchel JF, Gillam LD et al. In vivo radiofrequency balloon angioplasty of porcine coronary arteries: histologic effects and safety. J Am Coll Cardiol 1992;19:217A.

22. Jenkins RD, Sinclair IN, Leonard BM, Sandor T, Schoen FJ, Spears RJ. Laser balloon angioplasty vs balloon angioplasty in normal rabbit iliac arteries. Lasers Surg Med 1989;9:237–247.

23. Sinclair IN, Jenkins RD, James LM, Sinofsky EL, Wagner MS, Sandor T, Schoen FJ et al. Effect of laser balloon angioplasty on normal dog coronary arteries in vivo. J Am Coll Cardiol 1988;11(Suppl):108A.

24. Small DM. Progression and regression of atherosclerotic lesions: insights from lipid physical biochemistry. Arteriosclerosis 1988;8:103–129.

25. Forrester JS, Litvak F, Grundfest W. Vaporization of atheroma in man: the role of lasers in the era of balloon angioplasty. Int J Cardiol 1988;20:1–7.

26. Sanborn TA. Laser angioplasty. What has been learned from experimental and clinical trials? Circulation 1988; 78:769–774.

27. Spears JR, Reyes VP, Wynne J et al. Percutaneous coronary laser balloon angioplasty: initial results of a multicenter experience. J Am Coll Cardiol 1990;16:293–303.

28. Reis GJ, Pomerantz RM, Jenkins RD, Kuntz RE, Bainm DS, Diver DJ, Schnitt SJ et al. Laser balloon angioplasty: clinical, angiographic and histologic results. J AM Coll Cardiol 1991;18:193–202.

29. Lee BI, Becker GJ, Waller BF, Barry KJ, Connolly RJ, Kaplan J, Shapiro AR et al. Thermal compression and molding of atherosclerotic vascular tissue with use of radiofrequency energy: implications for radiofrequency balloon angioplasty. J Am Coll Cardiol 1989;13:1167–1175.

30. Deutsch E, Martin JL, Budjak R, Goldman BI, Heilbrunn SM, Abele JE, Bove AA. Low-stress angioplasty at 60°C: attenuated arterial barotrauma. Circulation 1990;82:III-72.

31. Mitchel JF, Fram DB, Fisher JP, Sanzobrino BW, Maffucci LM, Dyckman WP, Gillam LD et al. Low-grade (60°C) heating increases vascular compliance during balloon angioplasty. Circulation 1991;84:II-300.

32. Deutsch E, Martin JL, Budjak R, Bove AA. Time course of transmural heating during low-stress at 60°C in the atherosclerotic rabbit: preferential heating of plaque. Cathet Cardiovasc Diagn 1992;22:75.

33. Morley D, Zhang XY, Budjak R, Martin JL, Bove AA, Deutsch E. Preservation of arterial vasoreactivity following low-stress angioplasty at 60°C in the atherosclerotic rabbit. Circulation 1991;84:II-299.

34. Deutsch E, Morley D, Martin JL, Budjak R, Bove AA. Conventional angioplasty vs low-stress angioplasty at 60°C in the atherosclerotic rabbit iliac artery: angiographic and histologic outcomes and platelet deposition. Circulation 1991;84:II-299.

35. Deutsch E, Martin JL, Budjak R, Goldman BI, Bove AA. Low-stress angioplasty at 60°C in the atherosclerotic rabbit results in reduced neointimal hyperplasia. Circulation 1992;86:I-185.

36. Stary HC, Blankenhorn DH, Chandler AB, Glagov S, Insull W Jr, Richardson M, Rosenfeld ME et al. A definition of the intima of human arteries and of its atherosclerosis-prone regions. Circulation 1992;85:391–405.

37. Deutsch E, Martin JL, Makowski S, O'Neill BJ, McKay RG. Acute and chronic outcomes after physiologic low stress angioplasty (PLOSA) of de novo coronary stenoses: results of the phase I trial. Circulation 1993;88:I-646.

38. O'Neill BJ, McKay RG, Martin JL, Makowski S, Fram DB, Bove AA, Title LM et al. Physiologic low stress angioplasty at 60°C: comparison to matched controls undergoing conventional coronary angioplasty. Circulation 1992;86:I-457.

39. Bove AA, Holmes DR, Owen RM et al. Estimation of the effects of angioplasty on coronary stenosis using quantitative video angiography. Cathet Cardiovasc Diagn 1985; 11:5–9.

40. Martin JL, Deutsch E, McKay RG, Fram DB, O'Neill BJ, Makowski S, Bove AA. Coronary remodelling with low-stress angioplasty at 60°C vs conventional angioplasty in man: analysis of changes in plaque eccentricity. J Am Coll Cardiol 1993.

41. Kuntz RE, Baim DS. Defining coronary restenosis: newer clinical and angiographic paradigms. Circulation 1993; 88:1310–1323.

C. Ultrasound Angioplasty

URI ROSENSCHEIN

The priests blew their horns . . . and the wall fell down flat.—Joshua 6:20

Sound waves are a class of mechanical waves that consist of vibrations of the atomic or molecular particles of a substance about the equilibrium position of those particles. These waves propagate ideally through solids and, to a lesser extent, through liquids and gases. The range of sound audible to the human ear is from 20 to 18,000 Hz. Sound waves above the audible range lie in the ultrasound range. There are roughly two classes of ultrasound applications, those of low power and those of high power. The low-power class includes instruments that perform diagnostic tests and measurements, while the high-power class includes devices that change the physical and/or chemical state of the material on which they operate. Classically, ultrasound was employed in cardiology in diagnostic echocardiography—a low-power class device. Recently high-power ultrasound has

been harnessed in transcatheter technology for ablation of arterial stenoses (Fig. 11C.1).

High-power ultrasound devices were used in medicine mainly for the fragmentation of calculi (1), in surgery with the ultrasound "scalpel" (2), and for decalcification of aortic valves (3). Tissues containing a heavy matrix of collagen and elastin such as arterial wall, bladder, or heart valves are resistant to ultrasound. Tissues without elastic support such as thrombus, atherosclerotic plaque, or calcific deposits are easily disrupted by high-power ultrasound. This inherent selective ablation of high-power ultrasound led us to the hypothesis that high-power ultrasound can induce the selective injury required for successful transluminal intervention. Ultrasound had potential for ablating the occlusion without damaging the ultrasound-resistant arterial wall.

PERIPHERAL VESSEL EXPERIENCE

In 1986 we developed a prototype of an ultrasound angioplasty device for the recanalization of peripheral arteries. The device consists of a solid metal, flexible ultrasound catheter coupled at its proximal end to an ultrasound transducer in the handpiece. The transducer consists of piezoelectric crystals that convert electrical energy, supplied by a small portable power generator, to high-power, 20 kHz, ultrasonic energy (Fig. 11C.2). The ultrasound is transmitted by the ultrasound catheter to the target lesion in the arterial system. This design is the classic design of all current ultrasound angioplasty devices, whether for peripheral or coronary applications. This design differs from the design of intravascular ultrasound imaging devices. In the latter the piezoelectric crystals generate low-power high-frequency ultrasound and are mounted at the tip of the catheter that carries only the electrical signal.

In vitro we have studied the effects of ultrasound on thrombi, atherosclerotic plaques, and arterial wall. Ultrasound efficiently ablated thrombi. Following sonication for

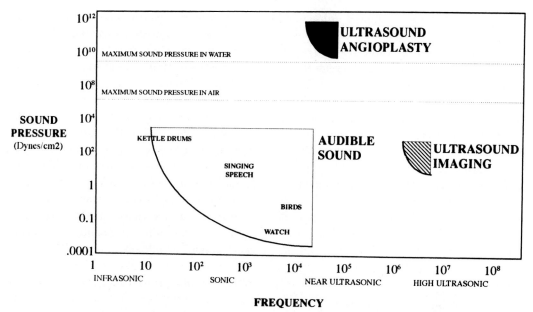

Figure 11C.1.   Graphic presentation of the spectrum of sound. The intensity and frequency of several sonic phenomena are roughly delineated. Ultrasound imaging devices operate in the low-power, high-frequency (3 to 10 MHz) range. Ultrasound angioplasty employs high-power ultrasound at the lower end of the ultrasound range (20 to 45 kHz).

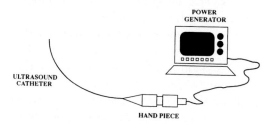

Figure 11C.2.   Schematic drawing of the generic design of ultrasound angioplasty devices.

20 seconds, the weight of the solid thrombi was reduced from a mean of 1.6 g to a mean of 0.4 g. The solid thrombus was liquified and did not recoagulate after 60 minutes. Following sonication the liquified thrombus tested very positive for fibrin degradation products and revealed an abundance of fibrin fragments on blood films. Mechanical penetration of the thrombus did not induce any significant change in its weight, excluding a "Dotter" effect.

Plaque ablation was studied using atherosclerotic aortic segments. Fatty plaques were found to be more susceptible to ultrasound ablation than complicated plaques—less than 30 seconds were required to ablate an area of 1 cm² of fatty plaque, while the clinically relevant complicated plaques required up to 180 seconds to ablate a similar area. Following sonication there was no damage to the media or adventitia. In normal aortic segments exposed to 4 minutes of high-power ultrasound, only a zone of endothelial injury was noted at the site of sonication (4). Ernst et al. have defined the "therapeutic index" of ultrasound angioplasty by measuring the time required to penetrate the aorta and atherosclerotic plaques. When the device was operated within therapeutic levels (tip displacement of 90 μ), the time taken to penetrate the aorta was approximately three times longer than that taken to penetrate an atherosclerotic plaque. This wide "therapeutic index" almost disappeared when higher intensities of ultrasound were used (5).

In vivo we have attempted ultrasound recanalization in thrombus-rich occlusions in peripheral arteries in a canine model. Thrombotic occlusion was induced by crush injury followed by temporary segmental ligation of the artery and injection of thrombin into the ligated segments. In each dog the left femoral artery was sonicated and the right femoral artery was mechanically penetrated ("Dottered") with the ultrasound device. Application of ultrasound for 2 minutes reduced the obstruction from a mean of 93% stenosis to wide-open arteries, with a mean residual stenosis of 18% and a TIMI grade 3 flow. Dottering thrombi in the control group did not achieve significant changes in the degree of obstruction, excluding a "Dotter" effect (4). Ultrasound angioplasty was performed in vivo on explanted human atherosclerotic arteries by Siegel et al. In these experiments 80% of the sonicated arteries did not achieve 50% or less residual stenosis (mean residual stenosis 62%) with ultrasound as a stand-alone modality; for acceptable results the procedure had to be completed with balloon angioplasty (mean final residual stenosis 29%) (6). This far-from-ideal result of ultrasound recanalization of occlusive atherosclerotic plaques contrasts sharply with the dramatic levels of recanalization attained with ultrasound angioplasty of thrombotic occlusions.

We scored the damage to arterial walls following ultrasound angioplasty in the thrombus-rich lesion canine model. The level of damage was similar both in the ultrasound and the "Dottered" control groups. The baseline level of damage was probably associated with the experimental protocol that included crush injury to the artery.

We have studied ultrasound angioplasty in totally occluded femoral arteries during femoral-popliteal bypass surgery. The design of the protocol enabled us to obtain angiograms, as well as tissue, after the procedure. In the control group, totally occluded arteries were "Dottered" with the device. The excised arteries were pressure-fixed and underwent morphometric analysis to calculate the cross-sectional area of the recanalized lumen. The sonicated arteries had significantly larger cross-sectional areas of recanalization than the "Dottered" control arteries (mean of 5.9 versus 1.7 mm^2, $P < .05$). The control arteries had a lumen similar in area to that of the ultrasound device (2.0 mm^2, $P =$ ns). It was noted that differences in the responses of the occlusive lesions to ultrasound were associated with their composition. Fibrous plaques were ablated just enough to permit adequate recanalization (19% cross-sectional area), while thrombotic occlusions were almost completely ablated (91% cross-sectional area). Histology did not reveal damage to the arterial wall (7). In a clinical study in peripheral arterial disease, conducted by Siegel et al., the stenosis decreased from $94 \pm 10\%$ to $55 \pm 23\%$ after ultrasound angioplasty. The procedure was supplemented with balloon angioplasty to achieve a final result of $12 \pm 8\%$ stenosis (8). These investigators had 16% mechanical arterial dissections and perforations. These mechanical complications were related more to the stiff catheter design and to its manipulation at unfavorable angles than to ultrasound application. In both studies angiography did not reveal any evidence of embolization, spasm, or thrombosis. Siegel and coworkers have described and documented the vasodilatory effects of catheter-delivered, low-frequency, high-power ultrasound. In two patients vasospasm was relieved by short exposure (mean 60 seconds) of the artery to energized ultrasound catheter (9). A study conducted by Fischell et al. has documented in vitro that catheter-delivered, high-power, low-frequency ultrasound induces a dose-dependent, endothelium-independent, smooth muscle relaxation. The ultrasound's relaxation effect was capable of reversing both receptor-mediated and voltage-dependent vasoconstriction independent of damage to smooth muscle cells and thermal effect (10).

To date the experience with ultrasound angioplasty in peripheral arteries suggests that thrombus-rich lesions might be the ideal lesion type to be treated with ultrasound. Arterial walls are resistant to high-power ultrasound at power levels found to be clinically effective. The inherent selectivity of ultrasound ablation makes the technique potentially effective and safe for percutaneous recanalization of thrombus-rich lesions.

CORONARY ARTERY EXPERIENCE

In the development of a coronary device, several technologic challenges have to be addressed:

1. To attain acceptable levels of miniaturization, the diameter of the transmission wire needs to be reduced to optimal dimensions. This will invariably increase compressional and tensile forces, which may lead to catheter fatigue problems.

2. Ultrasound is transmitted best in a solid metal wire, in proportion to the cross-sectional area of the wire. Thus the issue of the flexibility of the wire versus the quantity of usable energy has to be dealt with in the development of a coronary device.

3. Acoustic energy is attenuated at curves (i.e., aortic arch). This theoretically may result in loss of acoustic energy and unacceptable heat generation.

Recently the development of new coronary ultrasound angioplasty devices was reported (11–13). The device we have been using to investigate coronary ultrasound angioplasty consists of an ultrasound catheter (140 cm long) with a distal flexible multiwire segment connected to a 1.6-mm tip designed specially to optimize the cavitation effect (Angiosonics, Wayne, NJ) (Fig. 11C.3). The multiwire flexible segment uses solid metal wire for effective ultrasound transmission, but is still able to maintain the desired flexibility. The multiwire flexible segment behaves acoustically in a manner similar to that of fiberoptics, which effectively transmits light waves through glass and yet maintains its flexibility. The device fits into a standard 9 Fr angioplasty guide catheter and accepts, in a "monorail" fashion, a 0.014-inch angioplasty guidewire. The ultrasound transducer is in a small tubular handpiece (102-mm length, 25-mm diameter) and consists of a piezoelectric element controlled by a portable integrated computer (216 mm $\times$ 406 mm $\times$ 420 mm, 20.5 kg). The system is designed to ensure resonance and constant power output under the variable loading conditions encountered during the procedure. The frequency used by this system is 45 kHz. The range of power output, measured as longitudinal displacement at the tip, is 40 to 50 μ.

Hartnell et al. evaluated, in vitro, fresh thrombus ablation by this coronary ultrasound angioplasty device (12). The experiments were conducted in a custom-made test apparatus simulating closely the distance, curves, orientation, and physical environment the device will encounter during coro-

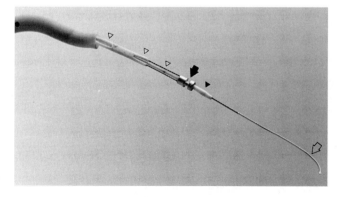

Figure 11C.3. Coronary ultrasound angioplasty device inserted in a 9 Fr guide catheter coaxially mounted in a "monorail" fashion over a 0.014-inch high-torque floppy guidewire *(open arrow)*. The multiwire flexible element *(open arrowhead)* allows the use of a solid metal wire for effective ultrasound transmission while maintaining the designed level of flexibility needed for coronary use. The tip *(solid arrow)* is designed especially to optimize the cavitation effect. A nose cone with a distal marker *(solid arrowhead)* extends from the tip. The system is controlled by integrated computer design to ensure constant resonance and power output.

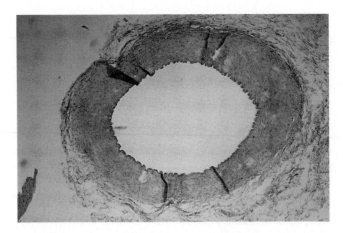

Figure 11C.4. A representative, histopathologic specimen of left circumflex artery following sonication at energy levels sufficient to induce effective thrombolysis (18 W, 80% duty cycle). The overall integrity of the arterial wall and its elastic structures are intact. There is no cellular damage.

nary ultrasound thrombolysis in the proximal left anterior descending artery (LAD). Fresh human thrombi, 2 to 3 cm in length and 3 mm in diameter, were placed in the phantom LAD. The ultrasound catheter was introduced into the test apparatus inside a 10 Fr guiding catheter and was positioned near the thrombi. Ultrasound was then applied until the thrombi were completely ablated, the affluent was collected for analysis and intraluminal temperature was measured. The investigators found that the device is quite efficient in ablating thrombi. Ultrasound-generated acoustic streaming "pulled" the thrombi (140 to 270 mg in weight) toward the tip where they were ablated in less than 2 minutes. There were no visible particles in the affluent. Subcapillary size filters (5 and 0.4 μ) collected most of the material, which consisted of aggregates of platelets and of red blood cells trapped in the fibrin meshwork. The intraluminal temperature was always below 46°C. The device has acceptable flexibility and is compatible with the standard interventional hardware used during the experiments. These results are consistent with those of a study by Phillipe et al., where high-power ultrasound applied by a 130-cm-long probe ablated thrombi efficiently with 96% of the debris being <10 μ in size (11).

In vivo studies of coronary ultrasound thrombolysis are currently in progress. In a study conducted by our group the acute effects of high-power ultrasound in intact canine coronary arteries are being investigated and compared with PTCA. Ultrasound angioplasty was found not to be accompanied by adverse effects. During sonication the animals were hemodynamically stable and without changes in the heart rate or rhythm. None of the experiments showed any angiographic evidence of adverse effects: there were no dissections, perforations, thrombi, changes in the TIMI grade flow or in the diameter of the sonicated artery. Histopathology revealed no injury after sonication of intact canine arteries (Fig. 11C.4). The myocardium revealed no ischemic changes, necrosis, or hemorrhage. Following sonication there was no evidence of significant hemolysis, change in the coagulation millieu, or release of CK-MB (14).

A study designed to determine the efficacy of coronary ultrasound angioplasty, by the Angiosonics' device, to induce ultrasound thrombolysis in vivo is currently under way. Occlusive thrombotic occlusions are induced in the LAD in a closed-chest canine model employing combined mechanical and electrical injury. Preliminary data showed that sonication resulted in full angiographic recanalization of the arterial lumen (personal communication, A. Michael Lincoff, M.D.,

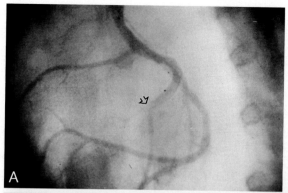

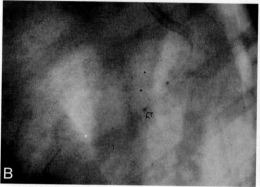

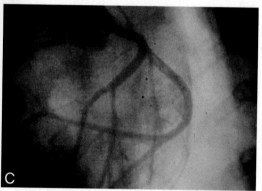

Figure 11C.5. Representative coronary angiography of ultrasound angioplasty in a canine model. **A.** Following combined mechanical and electrical injury, an occlusive thrombotic occlusion is induced in the mid LAD *(arrow)*. **B.** The ultrasound thrombolysis device during sonication in the mid LAD. The marker *(arrow)* is at the distal nose cone. **C.** Sonication of the thrombotic occlusion resulted in full angiographic recanalization of the arterial lumen without angiographic evidence of adverse effects. (Courtesy of A. Michael Lincoff, M.D.)

Cleveland Clinic Foundation, Cleveland, OH) (Fig. 11C.5). Histopathology revealed no damage to the sonicated arterial segment. There were variable degrees of residual nonocclusive thrombus.

Our experience suggests that the ultrasound angioplasty device is compatible with the cardiac catheterization laboratory environment. The skills required for operating the percutaneous coronary system are similar to those required for coronary balloon angioplasty. The catheter was easily delivered to the distal coronary arterial segment without guiding catheter "backup" problems. During ablation with ultrasound, neither the catheter being precisely coaxial in the artery nor the power application time were crucial. Slight operator errors did not damage the ultrasound-resistant arterial wall. However, it seems to be important that the ultrasound device be in close contact with the thrombotic occlusion during the procedure.

Steffen et al. have studied ultrasound angioplasty in a similar animal model using a single-wire design device (Baxter-Edwards LIS, Irvine, CA). In this study, ultrasound (19.5 kHz; 25 watts at acoustic horn) recanalized five out of seven thrombotically occluded arteries. Following recanalization angiography revealed no evidence of residual thrombi. Histopathology revealed nonocclusive residual thrombus and mild mechanical injury. The damage to the artery found by Steffen et al. may be the result of the perhaps less flexible, single-wire design of the ultrasound probe rather than ultrasound related (13).

The accumulated data suggest that coronary ultrasound thrombolysis may be a safe and effective clinical method for mechanical recanalization of thrombus-rich lesions. Acute myocardial infarction (AMI) is the prototype clinical condition caused by a thrombus-rich lesion in the coronary tree.

An occlusive thrombus superimposed on a "nonsignificant," ruptured plaque is the hallmark of AMI (15). More than a decade of clinical experience with pharmacologic thrombolytic therapy established the beneficial effects of clot lysis and reperfusion of the arterial lumen in the setting of AMI. Early, effective, and sustained patency of the infarct-related artery has been associated with improved survival and preserved left ventricular function. Pharmacologic thrombolytic therapy for AMI still suffers considerable shortcomings. Meta-analysis of eight trials showed that only about 20% of AMI patients had thrombolytic therapy (16). The situation outside the clinical trials is similar: in 1992 only about 162,000 patients in the United States were treated with thrombolytic agents out of about 675,000 patients admitted yearly with AMI (17). Recent studies suggest that in up to 45% of the patients treated with thrombolytic therapy the drugs fail to achieve a meaningful degree of reperfusion—that is a TIMI grade 3 flow (18, 19). Even in the face of successful reperfusion, the very potent thrombogenic stimulus of the residual thrombus (20) results in reocclusion of the infarct-related artery in up to 29% of patients (21). Thus, out of 100 patients admitted with AMI, only about 12 patients will be treated with thrombolytic therapy and will have successful and sustained reperfusion. These data and the recent success of primary PTCA in achieving reperfusion in AMI in rigorous randomized trials (22, 23) suggest that "the door has been opened" for a device solution for occlusive thromboses in the coronaries. Thus in our first clinical trial the safety and efficacy of ultrasound angioplasty will be studied in AMI patients. This will be a mechanistic study in which the ability of ultrasound angioplasty to induce successful and sustained reperfusion will be studied.

NONINVASIVE ULTRASOUND ABLATION

A beam of ultrasound has many properties similar to those of a beam of light. Both obey general wave equations, and each travels at a characteristic velocity that depends on the properties of the medium in which it travels. Ultrasonic beams, like light beams, can be focused, and very high levels of energy can be concentrated at a focal point at a specific distance from the source of energy (24).

We have hypothesized that high-power, focused, acoustic energy from an external acoustic generator can travel easily through tissue, deep into the body, similar to lithotripsy. This focused acoustic energy will induce a noninvasive and selective ablation of a target thrombus. The feasibility of noninvasive acoustic thrombus ablation was studied in vitro in a thrombotic artery model. Fresh thrombus was prepared in vitro, weighed, and inserted into human arterial segments. A shock-wave lithotripter was used as a source for focused, high-power acoustic energy. In this device 90% of energy is focused at a point approximately 2 cm in diameter. The thrombotic arterial segments were immersed in a water bath at the focal point. An x-ray location system, employing two image-conversion systems, verified the 3-D positioning of the thrombotic segment at the focal point. The test arteries were exposed to focused shock waves, while the control group underwent identical treatment but without exposure to shock waves. The residual solid thrombus was reweighed. The extent of thrombus ablation was evaluated from the change in solid thrombus weight. To elucidate the mechanism of shock-wave thrombus ablation, a 5-MHz ultrasound transducer imaged the arterial segment in the water bath before, during, and after each experiment. Application of shock waves reduced the weight of a solid thrombus by 91% as compared with a 42% decrease in the control group ($P = .0001$). The change in thrombus weight in the control group was attributed mostly to physiologic clot retraction. Following application of shock waves there were no gross or microscopic signs of damage to the arterial segments. Ultrasound images obtained during the experiment showed, immediately after the application of shock waves, the formation of a localized field of transient cavitation in the zone of the focal point, encompassing the thrombotic arterial segment (25). Other investigators have observed that externally applied ultrasound can accelerate thrombolysis by r-tPA in vitro (26, 27). It should be noted that all these studies were conducted with high-frequency, low-power ultrasound, without focusing the energy field. Harpaz et al. have shown that when ultrasound and r-tPA are applied simultaneously, a better and early thrombolysis is achieved, as compared with the r-tPA-only control group. In the ultrasound-only group, thrombolysis was not observed. These data suggest that the cavitation effect is not involved in the acceleration of pharmacologic thrombolysis by low-power, high-frequency ultrasound (26).

Lauer et al. have studied in vivo the effect of low-power, 1-MHz ultrasound on thrombolysis in a rabbit jugular vein thrombosis model. They documented a trend toward better thrombolysis when ultrasound was applied together with r-tPA. However, the results were not statistically significant, probably because of the small sample size (27).

The current embryonic stage of this technology and the lack of more in vivo and clinical data leave many important issues open. These open issues include the ability to focus ultrasound deeper into the tissue, patient discomfort, and the potential effects of ultrasound on the heart's electrical activity (28).

MECHANISM OF ULTRASOUND ABLATION

Transient acoustic cavitations are produced in liquid media subjected to high-power acoustic irradiation when the negative acoustic pressure during the rarefaction phase of the cycle becomes so great that the tensile strength of the water is not sufficient to maintain continuity. The liquid is then disrupted and vapor-filled microbubbles form. When the positive pressure phase begins, the cavitation collapses violently. During the final stage of collapse, transient cavitations generate local high pressures (29) and temperatures (30) in the liquid medium. One bubble was calculated to deposit about 300×10^6 eV of energy on collapse (31). These forces are sufficient to induce depolymerization in a variety of polymers (32). Transient acoustic cavitations were previously observed to be generated by the ultrasound angioplasty device at the power levels employed during ultrasound angioplasty (7).

We have studied in vitro the relationships between ultrasound ablation, cavitation, and tissue elasticity. These investigators found that ultrasound thrombus ablation is evident only when the cavitation threshold has been exceeded, suggesting that the cavitation effect is involved in the mechanism of ultrasound thrombus ablation. Above the cavitation threshold there was a good correlation between the speed at which a thrombus is ablated and ultrasound power (33). These investigators also found a negative correlation between ultrasound ablation and tissue elasticity. The high elasticity of the arterial wall makes it resistant to the disruptive effects of ultrasound, while the low elasticity of the thrombus makes it sensitive to ultrasound ablation. The data suggest that the differences in elasticity between arterial wall and thrombi delineate the wide margins of safety of ultrasound angioplasty.

SUMMARY

Ultrasound angioplasty has the potential to be a safe and effective catheter-based therapeutic modality, mainly for the treatment of thrombus-rich lesions. Results from clinical trials are needed to define the clinical niche for ultrasound angioplasty. Noninvasive ultrasound thrombolysis is an in vitro phenomenon. More work is needed to study its in vivo and clinical feasibility. Ultrasound has the potential to be an important energy with therapeutic, as well as diagnostic, application.

REFERENCES

1. Marberger M. Disintegration of renal and urethral calculi with ultrasound. Urol Clin North Am 1983;10:729–741.

2. Weitz J, Hodgson WJB, Loscalzo LJ, McElhinney. A bloodless technique for tongue surgery. Head Neck Surg 1981;3:244–246.

3. Brown AH, Davies PG. Ultrasonic decalcification of calcified cardiac valves and annuli. Br Med J 1972; 143:1088–1089.

4. Rosenschein U, Bernstein JJ, DiSegni E, Kaplinsky E, Bernheim J, Rozenszajn L. Experimental ultrasonic angioplasty: disruption of atherosclerotic plaques and thrombi in vitro and arterial recanalization in vivo. J Am Coll Cardiol 1990;15:711–717.

5. Ernst A, Schenk EA, Gracewski S et al. Ability of high-intensity ultrasound to ablate human atherosclerotic plaques and minimize debris size. Am J Cardiol 1991;68:242–246.

6. Siegel RJ, DonMichael TA, Fishbein MC et al. In vivo ultrasound arterial recanalization of atherosclerotic total occlusions. J Am Coll Cardiol 1990;15:345–351.

7. Rosenschein U, Rozenszajn LA, Kraus L et al. Ultrasonic angioplasty in totally occluded peripheral arteries: initial clinical, histological and angiographic results. Circulation 1991;83:1976–1986.

8. Siegel RJ, Gaines P, Crew JR, Cumberland DC. Clinical trial of percutaneous peripheral ultrasound angioplasty. J Am Coll Cardiol 1993;22:480–488.

9. Siegel RJ, Gaines P, Procter A, Fischell TA, Cumberland DC. Clinical demonstration that catheter-delivered ultrasound energy reverses arterial vasoconstriction. J Am Coll Cardiol 1992;20:732–735.

10. Fischell TA, Abbas MA, Grant GW, Siegel RJ. Ultrasonic energy: effects on vascular function and integrity. Circulation 1991;84:1783–1795.

11. Philippe F, Drobinski G, Bucherer C et al. Effects of ultrasound energy on thrombi in vitro. Cathet Cardiovasc Diagn 1993;28:173–178.

12. Hartnell GG, Saxton JM, Friedl SE, Abela GS, Rosenschein U. Ultrasonic thrombus ablation: in vitro assessment of a novel device for intracoronary use. J Interven Cardiol 1993;6:69–76.

13. Steffen W, Fishbein MC, Luo H, Lee DY, Nita H, Cumberland DC, Tabak SW et al. High-intensity, low-frequency catheter-delivered ultrasound dissolution of occlusive coronary artery thrombi: an in vitro and in vivo study. J Am Coll Cardiol 1994;24:1571–1579.

14. Rosenschein U, Rozenszajn LA, Bernheim J, Keren G, Alter A, Frimerman A, Laniado S et al. Safety of coronary ultrasound angioplasty: effects of sonication in intact canine coronary arteries. Cathet Cardiovasc Diagn (in press).

15. Fuster V, Badimon L, Badimon J, Chesebro JH. The pathogenesis of coronary artery disease and the acute coronary syndromes. N Engl J Med 1992;326:242–250.

16. Muller DWM, Topol EJ. Selection of patients with acute myocardial infarction for thrombolytic therapy. Ann Intern Med 1990;113:949–960.

17. Topol EJ, Califf RM. Thrombolytic therapy for elderly patients. N Engl J Med 1992;327:45–47.

18. Karagounis L, Sorensen SG, Menlove RL, Moreno F, Anderson JL. Does thrombolysis in myocardial infarction (TIMI) perfusion grade 2 represent a mostly patient artery or a mostly occluded artery? Enzymatic and electrocardiographic evidence from the TEAM-2 study. J Am Coll Cardiol 1992;19:1–9.

19. Lincoff AM, Topol EJ, Califf RM, Sigmon KN, Lee KL, Ohman EM, Rosenschein U et al for the Thrombolysis and Angioplasty in Myocardial Infarction Study Group. Significance of coronary artery with TIMI grade 2 flow "patency." Am J Cardiol (in press).

20. Gulba DC, Westhoff-Bleck M, Claus G, Piper J, Lichtlen PR. Residual coronary thrombus—a major risk factor for early reocclusion after thrombolysis in acute myocardial infarction. Circulation 1991;84(Suppl II):2271 (abstract).

21. Meijer A, Verheugt FWA, Werter CJPJ, van der Poll JMJ, Lie KJ, de Swart H. Aspirin versus Coumadin in prevention of reocclusion and recurrent ischemia after successful thrombolysis. A prospective placebo-controlled angiographic study: results of the APRICOT study. Circulation 1993;87:1524–1530.

22. Grines CL, Browne KF, Marco J et al. A comparison of immediate angioplasty with thrombolytic therapy for acute myocardial infarction. N Engl J Med 1993;328:673–679.

23. Gibbons RJ, Holmes DR, Reeder GS, Bailey KR, Hopfenspirger MR, Gersh BJ. Immediate angioplasty compared with the administration of a thrombolytic agent followed by conservative treatment for myocardial infarction. N Engl J Med 1993;328:685–691.

24. Lynn JG, Zwemer RL, Chick AJ, Miller AE. A new method for the generation and use of focused ultrasound in experimental biology. J Gen Phys 1942;26:179–193.

25. Rosenschein U, Yakubov SJ, Guberinich D et al. Shockwave thrombus ablation, a new method for noninvasive mechanical thrombolysis. Am J Cardiol 1992;70:1358–1361.

26. Harpaz D, Xucai C, Francis CW, Marder VJ, Meltzer RS. Ultrasound enhancement of thrombolysis and reperfusion. J Am Coll Cardiol 1993;21:1507–1511.

27. Lauer CG, Burge R, Tang DB, Bass BG, Gomez ER, Alving BM. Effect of ultrasound on tissue-type plasminogen activator–induced thrombolysis. Circulation 1992; 86:1257–1264.

28. Smailys A, Dulevicius Z, Muckus K, Dauksa K. Investigation of the possibilities of cardiac defibrillation by ultrasound. Resuscitation 1981;9:233–242.

29. Henry GE. Ultrasonics. Sci Am May 1954, p. 55–63.

30. Flint EB, Suslick KS. The temperature of cavitation. Science 1991;253:1397–1399.

31. Apfel R. Acoustic cavitation. In: Methods of experimental physics: ultrasonics. New York: Academic Press, 1981.

32. Kost J, Leong K, Langer R. Ultrasound-enhanced polymer degradation and release of incorporated substances. Proc Natl Acad Sci 1989;86:7663–7666.

33. Rosenschein U, Frimerman A, Laniado S, Miller HI. Study of the mechanism of ultrasound angioplasty from human thrombi and bovine aorta. Am J Cardiol 1994;74:1263–1266.

D. Stenosis Severity Assessment with Intracoronary Doppler

MORTON J. KERN AND THOMAS J. DONOHUE

Angiography is known to be an imperfect method to determine the physiologic significance of a coronary stenosis (1, 2). Although quantitative angiography has been employed to improve the correlations between anatomy and physiology, it too has its limitations (3). Decisions regarding intervention are often based on noninvasive, indirect testing of lesion significance with radionuclide perfusion imaging or pharmacologic stress studies, which are not available to the patient in the catheterization laboratory.

Coronary vasodilatory reserve measured with Doppler catheters in the 1980s has not been a reliable indicator of the physiologic impact of stenoses (4). The weaknesses of intracoronary Doppler catheter methods are related to limitations of catheter size and restriction to measurements made only in regions proximal to the coronary stenosis in question. Proximal coronary flow reserve measurements are diagnostically limited because they concurrently assess regions of varying vasodilatory reserve and must therefore reflect a weighted average of these disparate zones. Further correlations between quantitative angiography, myocardial perfusion scintigraphy, and translesional pressure gradients have been poor (5). A technical advance in Doppler methodology involves the satisfactory manufacture of a Doppler-tipped angioplasty guidewire, 0.014 to 0.018 inch in diameter (Flowire, Cardiometrics, Inc., Mountain View, CA) (Fig. 11D.1), which now permits measurement of flow velocity both proximal and distal to a lesion, supplying information on lesion resistance and distal myocardial hyperemic capacity (6). Directly measured basal and hyperemic blood flow distal to coronary stenoses can now pro-

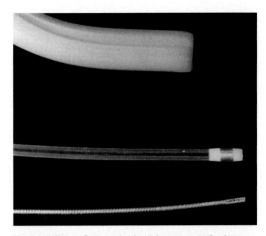

Figure 11D.1. Catheterization laboratory methods to assess coronary flow. 8 Fr angiographic (Doppler) catheter *(top)*. 2.2 Fr pressure gradient catheter *(middle)* (Target Therapeutics). Doppler Flowire 0.014-inch diameter *(bottom)* (Cardiometrics, Inc., Mountain View, CA).

vide more accurate means of assessing the physiologic impact of angiographic coronary narrowings (6).

FLOW VELOCITY, VOLUMETRIC FLOW, AND BRANCHING ARTERIES

The use of distal flow velocity for assessment of lesion significance is predicated on two major principles. First, flow velocity accurately reflects coronary blood flow volume when the cross-sectional area of a vessel remains constant. Based on the first principles of Doppler ultrasound physiology, volumetric coronary blood flow is the product of the velocity of the red cells moving through a conduit of a known cross-sectional area. The velocity (cm/sec) and cross-sectional area (cm^2) product yields flow values in cm^3/sec, the volumetric translation of velocity. The second major concept involves the human coronary circulation, which is a system of branching conduits diminishing in size into the distal myocardium (Fig. 11D.2). Because of branching, both volumetric flow and cross-sectional vessel area diminish from the proximal to distal myocardial regions, and therefore a velocity value is maintained from the proximal to the distal locations. Thus a ratio

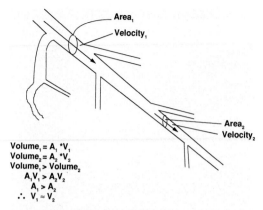

$$Volume_1 = A_1 * V_1$$
$$Volume_2 = A_2 * V_2$$
$$Volume_1 > Volume_2$$
$$A_1 V_1 > A_2 V_2$$
$$A_1 > A_2$$
$$\therefore V_1 \approx V_2$$

Figure 11D.2. Diagram of coronary branching arteries with diminishing proximal to distal volume flow rate and cross-sectional area resulting in velocity normalization.

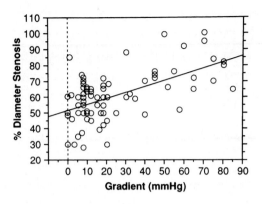

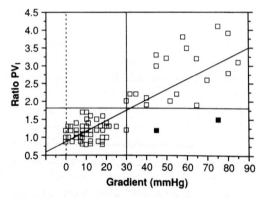

Figure 11D.3. Correlation between angiography (% diameter stenosis) and translesional pressure gradients (mm Hg) *(top).* Correlation between the ratio of proximal to distal total velocity integral (ratio PV$_i$) and translesional pressure gradients (mm Hg) *(bottom).* The two black boxes represent the proximal right coronary artery stenoses occurring prior to any branch points (see text for discussion). (With permission from Wilson RF et al. Circulation 1990;82:1595–1606.)

of proximal to distal velocity can be used to assess the severity of lesions. In arteries with non–flow-limiting lesions, this ratio should approach 1.

Significant lesions produce increased resistance diverting blood flow to other proximal branches in front of the lesion, reducing flow distal to significant lesions. Initial studies in our laboratory (7, 8) have demonstrated that flow velocity is maintained from the proximal to distal region in normal arteries and that loss of distal velocity relative to proximal velocity (proximal:distal velocity integral ratios >1.7) can be directly related to translesional pressure gradients >30 mm Hg (8) (Fig. 11D.3). Translesional pressure gradients >30 mm Hg have been associated with myocardial ischemia on stress testing (9). Translesional pressure gradients <20 mm Hg have been considered suitable endpoints after angioplasty (10). Whether translesional pressure gradients of ≤20 mm Hg require angioplasty is under investigation. However, lesions that are not flow limiting generally should not require mechanical intervention.

THE DOPPLER GUIDEWIRE

The 0.018-inch floppy angioplasty-style guidewire is 175 cm long and equipped with a 12-

MHz Doppler crystal at the tip. The Doppler signal is processed by on-line, fast Fourier transformation to yield a spectral flow velocity displayed on a bedside video recorder with a hard-copy thermal page printer. The spectral velocity envelope is outlined with computer-assisted edge detection. Automatic analysis provides phasic, mean and peak velocities, as well as the total, diastolic, and systolic flow velocity integrals (time-area of flow). These data are easily acquired and automatically processed without operator-dependent adjustments (11, 12).

METHOD OF CORONARY FLOW VELOCITY MEASUREMENTS

Using a standard femoral angioplasty approach, 6 Fr or larger sheaths and guiding catheters are inserted followed by administration of 5000 to 10,000 units of IV heparin. The 0.018-inch Flowire (Cardiometrics, Inc., Mountain View, CA) is advanced into the guide catheter through a standard Y-connector and positioned across the lesion. For translesional gradient measurements, a 2.2 Fr tracking catheter (Target Therapeutics) can be used over the Flowire. For assessment during diagnostic angiography, the Flowire can be passed through 5 and 6 Fr diagnostic catheters with similar technique.

Figure 11D.4. **A.** Frames from a coronary cineangiogram in the left anterior oblique projection (LAO) and right anterior oblique projection (RAO) of the left anterior descending artery demonstrating a 60% diameter narrowing (84% area) of the proximal segment by QCA in the "worst" projection. **B.** Coronary blood flow velocity proximal and distal to the left anterior descending stenosis at baseline and during maximal hyperemia with 12 mcg of intracoronary adenosine (flow velocity scale = 0 to 200 cm/sec). Proximal flow is normal (mean velocity 32 cm/sec) with normal phasic pattern (DSVR 1.9). Proximal but not distal hyperemia is normal. The ratio of proximal to distal flow velocity is 1.9. Distal hyperemia was impaired with a flow reserve ratio of approximately 1.42. **C.** The distal flow velocity after angioplasty demonstrated an increase of the distal velocity equivalent to proximal velocity with restoration of the phasic flow signal and hyperemia of 2.1 times basal flow *(top)*. Translesional gradient before and after angioplasty at baseline and during maximal hyperemia *(bottom)*. Hemodynamic tracings show electrocardiogram, aortic pressure and distal coronary pressure, both phasic and mean (from the top down, 0-200 mm Hg scale). Mean resting gradient is 40 mm Hg, which widens to approximately 50 mm Hg at maximal hyperemia. Following angioplasty, mean baseline gradient is 8 mm Hg, which widens to approximately 20 mm Hg during maximal hyperemia. (With permission from Segal J et al. J Am Coll Cardiol 1992;20:276–286.)

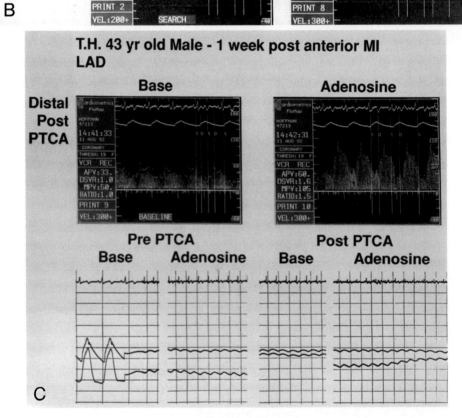

Figure 11D.4.B and C.

ASSESSMENT OF THREE CORONARY STENOSES

With this background the assessment of left anterior descending stenoses of nearly equal angiographic characteristics and severity in three patients will be discussed. Each lesion has unique flow findings that cannot be differentiated from angiography alone.

Patient #1

A 43-year-old man had an acute anterior myocardial infarction (13). Coronary angiography revealed a 60% diameter narrowing in the proximal left anterior descending coronary artery (Fig. 11D.4A). A thallium-201 low-level exercise test had been performed, which showed reversible anterior and apical effects. Before angioplasty, translesional flow velocity assessment of the stenosis was performed.

Basal and hyperemic flow velocity data was obtained proximal (3 to 4 artery diameters) to the stenosis. Maximal intracoronary hyperemia was then produced by 12 to 18 mcg of adenosine administered through the guiding catheter (14). The stenosis was then traversed with the Doppler guidewire and distal (at least 10 artery diameters, ≈2 cm) basal and hyperemic flow responses were again recorded (Fig. 11D.4B).

Assessment of the left anterior descending coronary lesion showed that proximal flow velocity was normal in magnitude, phasic pattern, and coronary hyperemic capacity (Fig. 11D.4B). Flow velocity distal to the left anterior descending coronary stenosis was abnormal. The proximal average peak velocity was 32 cm/sec, distal was 17 cm/sec with a proximal:distal ratio of 32:17 = 1.9. In addition, the phasic nature of the diastolic:systolic velocity ratios was abnormally low (1.3; normal left coronary diastolic:systolic velocity ratio >1.5) (8). Distal hyperemia was also impaired (distal flow [hyperemic:basal] reserve = 1.42). The translesional gradient measured with the tracking catheter was 40 mm Hg, corresponding to the abnormal proximal:distal ratio (Fig. 11D.4C). This gradient increased to 48 mm Hg during maximal hyperemia (Fig. 11D.4C, bottom). Coronary angioplasty was successfully performed, reducing the stenosis to <30% diameter narrowing with restoration of the normal distal phasic flow velocity patterns (diastolic:systolic ratio = 1.6), improvement of basal flow (mean velocity = 33 cm/sec) and distal hyperemia (distal flow reserve = 1.96) (Fig. 11D.4C, top panels). The final gradient was 8 mm Hg at rest, which increased to 20 mm Hg during maximal hyperemia.

Patient #2

A 59-year-old man with typical and atypical chest pain had cardiac catheterization (15). A thallium scintigraphy exercise study showed a minimal anterior-apical defect. Angiography showed an eccentric severe lesion in the left anterior descending coronary artery. In the left anterior oblique (LAO) view (Fig. 11D.5A), the lesion is severe (>70%). In the right anterior oblique (RAO) view, the lesion is moderate (<50%).

Translesional flow velocity was measured before angioplasty. Translesional flow velocity spectra (Fig. 11D.5B, top panels) and pressure gradients (Fig. 11D.5B, lower panels) were obtained at rest and during maximal hyperemia with adenosine (12 mcg intracoronary). Proximal and distal flow velocity are nearly identical with a proximal:distal velocity ratio of 1.05. The resting gradient is zero. With adenosine, distal flow increases ≥2.5 × baseline. The hyperemic gradient is 10 mm Hg. No angioplasty was performed. The patient's symptoms abated, and he was well at 14-month follow-up.

Patient #3

A 43-year-old man who had chest pain and an abnormal stress test with reversible scintigraphic defects in the anterior and anteroapical regions was scheduled for angioplasty. Coronary arteriography in the left anterior oblique projection revealed a 58% diameter stenosis of the left anterior descending (Fig. 11D.6A). Flow velocity and translesional pressure gradients were obtained during the study. Proximal mean flow velocity was approximately 30 cm/sec, distal velocity was 25 cm/sec with a proximal to distal velocity ratio of 1.2 (Fig. 11D.6B). The translesional pressure gradient was approximately 20 mm Hg. Distal coronary flow velocity after 18 mcg of intracoronary adenosine increased to 2.9 × basal flow with distal mean velocity reaching 87 cm/sec. Of note, during hyperemia the resting gradient increased to approximately 46 mm Hg (Fig. 11D.6B, bottom right). Although flow velocity was normal, the resting translesional gradient was marginal. Coronary angioplasty was successfully performed (Fig. 11D.6A, bottom). The residual stenosis was 33% diameter by quantitative angiography. Distal flow velocity following the angioplasty was recorded at 5 and 15 minutes after the procedure to assess immediate physiologic results, as well as alterations in coronary vasodilator reserve after a successful dilation (Fig. 11D.6C). Five minutes after angioplasty, distal basal mean velocity was 27 cm/sec, unchanged from before the procedure. Distal hyperemia at 5 minutes was 53 cm/sec for a coronary vasodilatory reserve of 2.1. After 15 minutes, baseline flow velocity had fallen slightly to a mean value of 18 cm/sec and hyperemia remained unchanged at 52 cm/sec for a coronary reserve value of 2.7, nearly identical to that observed before angioplasty. The pressure gradient following the procedure was 3 mm Hg with maximal hyperemic flow velocity increasing the gradient to 25 mm Hg. Basal and hyperemic flow were unchanged by this angiographically successful procedure. The thallium scan, however, remained abnormal. Clinically, the patient has done well.

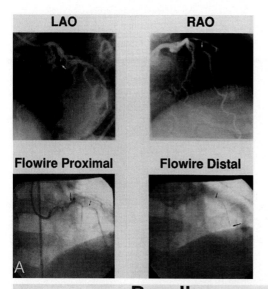

Figure 11D.5. A. Angiographic views of eccentric lesion in the left anterior descending coronary artery in a 59-year-old man with atypical chest pain. In the left anterior oblique (LAO) view, the lesion is severe (>70%). In the right anterior oblique (RAO) view, the lesion is moderate (<50%). The lower panels show the sites at which flow velocity and gradient data was obtained. Small arrow is lesion; larger arrow is guidewire position, proximally *(left)* and distally *(right)*. **B.** Flow velocity spectra *(top panels)* and translesional gradients *(lower panels)* at rest and during maximal hyperemia with adenosine (12 mcg intracoronary). Proximal and distal flow velocity are nearly identical with a ratio of 1.05. The mean resting gradient is zero. With adenosine, distal flow increases 2.5 × baseline and the mean hyperemic gradient is 10 mm Hg. A thallium scintigraphy exercise study showed a minimal apical defect, and no angioplasty was performed. The patient's symptoms abated spontaneously, and he was well at 8-month follow-up. (With permission from Wilson RF, et al. Circulation 1990;82:1595–1606).

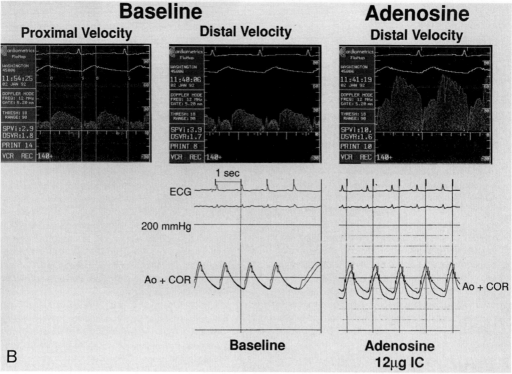

43 yr old Male, LAD, Pre PTCA

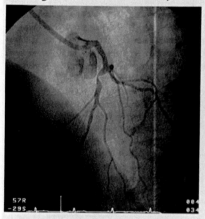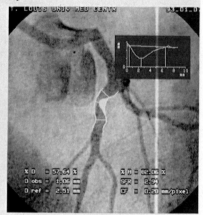

43 yr old Male, LAD, Post PTCA

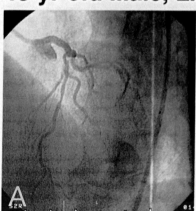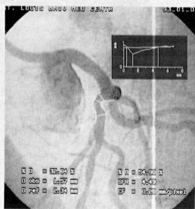

Figure 11D.6. A. Angiographic frames of a left anterior descending lesion (58% diameter narrowed) with an abnormal stress test. Before *(top)* and after *(bottom)* angioplasty. **B.** Translesional flow velocity and pressure gradient before angioplasty. Proximal and distal flows are nearly equivalent with proximal:distal ratio 1.2. Distal hyperemia is 2.9 × basal flow. The mean resting gradient of 20 mm Hg increases to 46 mm Hg during hyperemia. **C.** After angioplasty, distal flow is similar both at rest and during hyperemia. The resting gradient of 2 mm Hg increases to 20 mm Hg with 2.7 × basal flow increase. The thallium scan remained positive. Did angioplasty improve blood flow? (See text.)

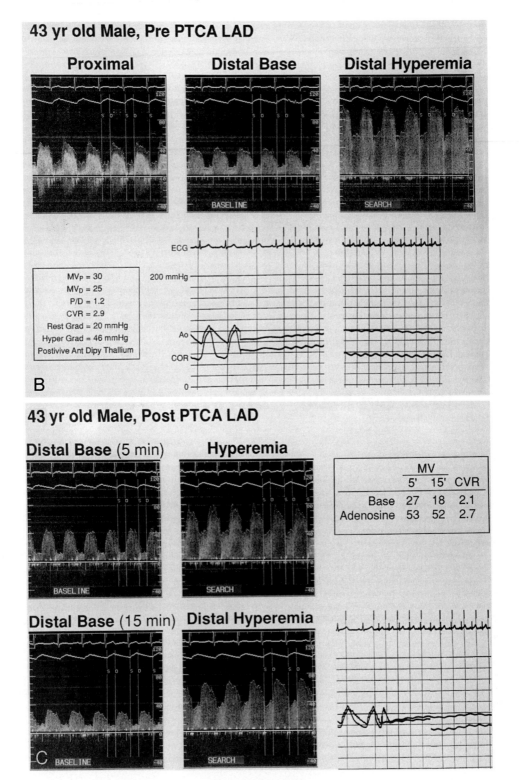

Figure 11D.6.B and C.

DISCUSSION

Case #3, more than the first two, highlights the clinically important question of which of the major physiologic indicators should be accepted in determining the need for angioplasty and the success after a mechanical intervention. The thallium scan remained positive following the angioplasty, despite the fact that the gradient was relieved. Normal distal flow before angioplasty was unchanged after angioplasty. The marginal pressure gradient of 20 mm Hg was reduced to 3 mm Hg without any alteration in distal flow. The thallium scan likely represented a false-positive finding. Without improvement in distal flow or distal hyperemia, it is difficult to say that reduction of the translesional gradient was significant. Also, a hyperemic gradient of 45 mm Hg, in view of a distal flow velocity that can increase three times basal values, likely had little physiologic significance in this particular patient. Since augmentation of distal flow is the objective of antiischemic interventions, this parameter may be the most significant indicator of lesion significance.

The use of flow velocity in the assessment of a coronary stenosis prior to the decision for angioplasty has important clinical impact on patients now undergoing coronary interventions. Many interventions are performed with no objective evidence of ischemia (16). Further, it is well known that noninvasive risk stratification tests carry a relatively high incidence of false positives in some patient groups. In some centers, positive stress testing may be as high as 30% in patients with normal coronary angiography (17, 18). As shown in the three case examples, significant lesions often cannot be differentiated by angiography, but may be separated by flow velocity. Flow velocity data obtained in hemodynamically significant lesions demonstrate three findings: (a) increased proximal to distal flow velocity ratio, (b) loss of the normal phasic diastolic to systolic flow velocity ratio, and (c) impaired distal (but not necessarily proximal) hyperemic responses to vasodilators

Table 11D.1

Translesional Flow Velocity Criteria for Hemodynamically Significant Lesions

1. Proximal to distal flow velocity integral ratio >1.7 = translesional pressure gradient >30 mm Hg. (Applies only in branching arteries. See below.)[a]
2. Distal coronary vasodilatory reserve >2.0.
3. Distal diastolic:systolic mean velocity ratio:

	Normal
Left anterior descending	>1.7
Circumflex	>1.5
Right coronary artery	>1.2 (proximal)
Right coronary artery	>1.4 (posterior descending, posterolateral branch)

[a]Proximal:distal ratio not applicable in diffuse distal disease, serial or tandem lesions, and ostial lesions (no proximal location).

(Table 11D.1). In patients with multiple coronary artery narrowings, direct translesional flow dynamics can indicate one lesion as significant (13, 15). Angioplasty of flow-normal stenoses may be unnecessary, thus reducing risks, costs, and complications associated with coronary angioplasty. Lesions of angiographically intermediate severity may not be hemodynamically significant despite abnormal ischemic stress testing (19). The selection of an appropriate intervention based on translesional hemodynamics offers the patient and physician the opportunity to defer an unnecessary intervention.

PROXIMAL:DISTAL FLOW VELOCITY RATIO

The physiologic rationale for using a proximal to distal flow velocity ratio is based on classical hydrodynamic theory and confirmed with directly measured translesional gradient data (8). In branching arteries, where the continuity equation cannot be employed, proximal arterial flow input can be diverted to the areas of lower vascular resistance caused by a moderate stenosis producing resistance to flow. Diversion of flow through more proximal branch points diminishes distal flow (velocity). The proximal to distal ratio cannot be used in single conduits, ostial lesions, diffuse distal disease, or tandem or serial lesions where distal velocity may be accelerated. In addition, attainment of an accurate proximal

Figure 11D.7.   Relation of proximal to distal flow velocity ratio to caliper—measured percent diameter stenosis in 119 coronary stenoses. A ratio greater than 1.7 is rarely seen with a stenosis >50%, but many apparently more severe stenoses (by calipers) have velocity ratios ≤1.7.

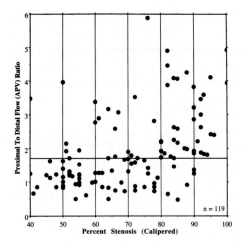

	Percent Stenosis					
	40 - 50%	51 - 60%	61 - 70%	71 - 80%	81 - 90%	91 - 100%
Total Number	16	22	19	21	26	15
Number > 1.7	2	5	7	9	20	15
Percent > 1.7	13%	23%	37%	43%	77%	100%

flow velocity value requires sampling far enough away from the lesion and zone of flow convergence. In data from our laboratory (8), proximal to distal flow velocity ratios (using the total flow velocity integral) of >1.7 are nearly always (98%) associated with translesional gradients of >30 mm Hg in branching arteries. Figure 11D.7 illustrates the relation of proximal:distal velocity ratio to measured percent coronary stenosis.

TRANSLESIONAL GRADIENTS AND DISTAL FLOW VELOCITY

Translesional pressure gradients are currently not used in isolation for several reasons. The technique is cumbersome and subject to signal artifact from catheter kinking and vessel tortuosity. The earlier studies used larger-diameter, 4 Fr, first-generation angioplasty catheters to measure gradients. Pressure gradients, at times, conflicted with angiography and thus were considered unreliable. More important is the fact that a translesional pressure gradient reflects only half of the information needed to judge a lesion as significant. Pressure gradients are directly related to the flow. As shown in case examples during hyperemia, when flow increases, the gradient increases in a curvilinear relationship reflecting lesion resistance. A gradient of 25 mm Hg may be trivial if distal flow can increase >3 × basal values. The ability to assess both relative pressure and flow with the distal flow velocity is a distinct advantage of the velocity guidewire method over the pressure gradient technique.

What constitutes a clinically significant, translesional flow velocity-pressure gradient is under investigation. From a historical review of coronary hemodynamics obtained at the time of angioplasty, translesional pressure gradients of <20 mm Hg and residual coronary artery diameter narrowings of <30% were accepted as satisfactory final results associated with reduced late restenosis rates and a lower incidence of postprocedural abrupt closure. Unlike experimental animal studies relating coronary hemodynamics to ischemia, however, there is little data in patients to identify a level of resting translesional flow-pressure gradient that provides a reliable predictor of provokable myocardial ischemia. Although it is desirable to have a zero translesional gradient within the coronary tree, some lesions in patients may have pressure gradients without demonstrable evidence of exercise- or drug-induced myocardial ischemia.

The hemodynamic criteria correlating with inducible ischemia further depend on the size of the perfusion bed, coronary artery, aortic and left ventricular pressures, myocardial oxygen demand, and coronary vasomotor tone. The pressure-flow (velocity) relationship of any lesion should correlate to clinical findings and postprocedural outcome. Translesional pressure-velocity relationships, previously difficult to obtain clinically, are currently entering the clinical arena for more accurate lesion assessment with miniaturization of sensor-tipped guidewires. Since restoration of blood flow is the endpoint of an intervention, dilating lesions with normal translesional blood flow is unlikely to be helpful.

LIMITATIONS

The limitations of translesional velocity assessment should be noted. Occasionally, it may be difficult to find the maximal distal flow velocity signals and one could falsely conclude that a significant flow reduction is present because of a significant lesion. Therefore the Doppler guidewire tip in the distal region should be rotated in several different orientations in all patients to identify the maximal and most intense spectral flow velocity signals that have a complete Doppler envelope. In tortuous segments, stable distal signals can usually be obtained. However, more guidewire manipulation is often needed to achieve satisfactory signals. In some patients guidewire manipulation may not be suitable because of tortuosity or lesion complexity. In these instances the Doppler Flowire can be exchanged for a finer, smaller, and softer guidewire. After the guidewire traverses the lesion, a tracking catheter is placed distally. The Flowire can then be exchanged for the softer guidewire. Both pressure and flow velocity across the lesion can now be mea-

sured. An elevated distal flow velocity and falsely normalized proximal to distal flow velocity ratio, suggesting an insignificant lesion, might be seen if the distal measurements are made in a region with distal disease where there is flow acceleration secondary to distal luminal narrowing. In patients with serial lesions or diffuse distal disease, the proximal to distal flow ratio should not be used. In these cases confirmation of lesion significance with coronary vasodilatory reserve and translesional pressure gradients may be needed.

Guide catheter obstruction to inflow at the ostium of the coronary artery may interfere with interpretation of both proximal and distal velocity signals. For this reason intermediate lesions can be assessed at the time of diagnostic catheterization with 6 Fr diagnostic or guiding catheters with outside diameters of <0.05 inch.

Finally, the translesional resting hemodynamics may not reflect ischemia-producing conditions that could occur during coronary vasoconstriction nor exacerbation of lesions as a result of increased myocardial demand during exercise or emotional stimulation (20). Translesional pressure gradients will be increased to various degrees corresponding to the increase in flow and lesion resistance. Whether clinical benefit would be conferred by dilating a lesion with a marginal resting pressure gradient and normal flow compared with medical therapy remains under investigation.

SAFETY OF GUIDEWIRE INSTRUMENTATION

Angioplasty guidewire instrumentation of severe lesions is rarely associated with lesion disruption. The incidence of lesion injury with moderately narrowed lesions should be equal or less. In a nationwide survey of users, <5 out of 4000 patients have had any type of coronary dissection or closure reported with the Flowire manipulation. The safety of guidewire instrumentation in normal and mildly diseased arteries is high. In a preliminary examination of the first 200 patients undergoing guidewire instrumentation who did not have angioplasty with moderate lesions, no patient was noted to have a complication of wire insertion either early or on late follow-up at 6 months (21).

SUMMARY

Using translesional flow velocity as a marker of the physiologic significance of a lesion, a more accurate and objective determination for the necessity of intervention can be obtained. This approach is especially important for angiographically intermediately severe lesions. Given the limitations of noninvasive testing for coronary stenoses, patients with clinical requirements for coronary interventions may be spared unnecessary procedures by having lesions assessed with direct intracoronary flow measurements.

ACKNOWLEDGMENT

The authors wish to thank the J.G. Mudd Cardiac Catheterization Team and Donna Sander for manuscript preparation.

REFERENCES

1. Roberts WC, Jones AA. Quantitation of coronary arterial narrowing at necropsy in sudden coronary death. Am J Cardiol 1979;44:39–44.
2. White CW, Wright CB, Doty DB, Hiratza LF, Eastham CL, Harrison DG, Marcus ML. Does visual interpretation of the coronary arteriogram predict the physiologic importance of a coronary stenosis? N Engl J Med 1984;310:819–824.
3. Deleted in proof.
4. Wilson RF, Laughlin DE, Ackell PH et al. Transluminal subselective measurement of coronary artery blood flow velocity and vasodilator reserve in man. Circulation 1985;72:82–92.
5. Marcus ML, Armstrong ML, Heistad DD et al. A comparison of three methods of evaluating coronary obstructive lesions: postmortem arteriography, pathological examination and measurement of regional myocardial perfusion during maximal vasodilation. Am J Cardiol 1982;49:1699–1706.
6. Kern MJ, Anderson HV, eds. A symposium: the clinical applications of the intracoronary Doppler guidewire flow velocity in patients: understanding blood flow beyond the coronary stenosis. Am J Cardiol 1993;71:1D–86D.
7. Ofili EO, Kern MJ, Labovitz AJ, St Vrain JA, Segal J, Aguirre F, Castello R. Analysis of coronary blood flow velocity dynamics in angiographically normal and stenosed arteries before and after endoluminal enlargement by angioplasty. J Am Coll Cardiol 1993;21:308–316.
8. Donohue TJ, Kern MJ, Aguirre FV, Bach RG, Wolford T, Bell CA, Segal J. Assessing the hemodynamic significance of coronary artery stenoses: analysis of translesional pressure-flow velocity relationships in patients. J Am Coll Cardiol 1993;22:449–458.
9. Wijns W, Serruys PW, Reiber JHC, van den Brand M, Simoons ML, Kooijman CJ, Balakumaran K et al. Quantitative angiography of the left anterior descending coronary artery: correlations with pressure gradient and results of exercise thallium scintigraphy. Circulation 1985;71:273–279.
10. Hodgson JM, Reinert S, Most AS, Williams DO. Prediction of long-term clinical outcome with final translesional pressure gradient during coronary angioplasty. Circulation 1986;74:563–566.
11. Doucette JW, Corl PD, Payne HM et al. Validation of a Doppler guidewire for intravascular measurement of coronary artery flow velocity. Circulation 1992;85:1899–1911.
12. Segal J, Kern MJ, Scott NA, King SB III, Doucette JW, Heuser RR, Ofili E et al. Alterations of phasic coronary artery flow velocity in humans during percutaneous coronary angioplasty. J Am Coll Cardiol 1992;20:276–286.
13. Kern MJ, Flynn MS, Caracciolo EA, Bach RG, Donohue TJ, Aguirre FV. Use of translesional coronary flow velocity for interventional decisions in a patient with multiple intermediately severe coronary stenoses. Cathet Cardiovasc Diagn 1993;29:148–153.
14. Wilson RF, Wyche K, Christensen BV, Zimmer S, Laxson DD. Effects of adenosine on human coronary arterial circulation. Circulation 1990;82:1595–1606.
15. Kern MJ, Donohue TJ, Aguirre FV, Bach RG, Caracciolo EA, Ofili E, Labovitz AJ. Assessment of angiographically intermediate coronary artery stenosis using the Doppler Flowire. Am J Cardiol 1993;71:26D–33D.
16. Topol EJ, Ellis SG, Cosgrove DM, Bates ER, Muller DWM, Schork NJ, Schork MA et al. Analysis of coronary angioplasty practice in the United States with an insurance-claims data base. Circulation 1993;87:1489–1497.
17. American College of Physicians. Efficacy of exercise thallium-201 scintigraphy in the diagnosis and prognosis of coronary artery disease. Ann Intern Med 1990;113:703–704.
18. Ritchie JL, Trobaugh GB, Hamilton GW, Gould KL, Narahara KA, Murray JA, Williams DL. Myocardial imaging with thallium-201 at rest and during exercise: comparison with coronary arteriography and resting and stress electrocardiography. Circulation 1977;56:66.
19. Bodenheimer MM, Banka VS, Helfant RH. Nuclear cardiology. II. The role of myocardial perfusion imaging using thallium-201 in diagnosis of coronary artery disease. Am J Cardiol 1980;45:674–684.
20. Ganz P, Abben RP, Barry WH. Dynamic variations in resistance of coronary arterial narrowings in angina pectoris at rest. Am J Cardiol 1987;59:66–70.
21. Mechem CJ, Kern MJ, Aguirre F, Cauley M, Stonner T. Safety and outcome of angioplasty guidewire Doppler instrumentation in patients with normal or mildly diseased coronary arteries. Circulation 1992;86(4):I-323 (abstract).

DECISION MAKING IN INTERVENTIONAL CARDIOLOGY

12. The Role of Randomized Trials, Registries, and Experience-Based Common Sense

A. The Duke Perspective

ROBERT M. CALIFF

The practice of invasive cardiology has undergone a revolution as it has moved from a purely diagnostic subspecialty to one with well-documented potential for both improving patient health and creating iatrogenic complications. Beginning with the innovative development of the angioplasty technique by Andreas Grüntzig, the field has developed to a point where practitioners now have a variety of tools from which to choose in the management of each patient. This revolution has been more than technologic, however. Over the same period the biology of atherosclerosis has come to be understood at a basic level as never before, the economics of procedure-based medicine have been through a "golden era," enhanced approaches to defining the natural history of coronary artery disease have been developed, and methods of risk stratification have evolved. Finally, the evolution of computer systems has been so rapid that access to summary data about patients and medical outcomes is no longer the small, peculiar interest of clinical epidemiologists, but rather is available both to administrators and to those who pay for medical care. One outgrowth of these changes has been an emerging sense of concern that the selection of patients for particular procedures by individual practitioners may not be a consequence of a scientific evaluation of the risks and benefits of the procedure for that patient, but may instead represent a biased choice with undue influence of the physician's beliefs and financial incentives.

The point of view expressed in this chapter has developed from a decade of clinical practice coupled with intense involvement in both observational studies and randomized clinical trials in several areas of cardiology. It represents a synthesis of concepts arising from the collaborative efforts of investigators from several disciplines in the Duke Databank for Cardiovascular Disease (1, 2). This organization was initiated in the late 1960s in an effort to understand the long-term implications of treatment selection in patients with ischemic heart disease (3). At a practical clinical level the goal of the organization is to provide each patient with the best possible estimate of the expected outcome for different treatment options. For the past $2\frac{1}{2}$ decades this group has been developing approaches to the evaluation of outcome data to understand clinical decision making and the consequences of treatment selection. In this effort opinions have been formed about the strengths and weaknesses of each approach, providing information to support therapeutic decision making and the role of practicing clinicians in the acquisition of new information about the outcomes related to procedures. This chapter attempts to articulate an approach to clinical care, including the current role of the practitioner in the acquisition and interpretation of objective information, what is likely to happen in the future, and how the practitioner must become part of the process of rapid assimilation of objective information about medical practice.

Table 12A.1.
Clinical Research Designs in Increasing Order of Rigor

No controls (case reports, case series)
Literature controls
Historical controls
Concurrent controls
Concurrent controls with multivariate analysis
Randomized controlled trial

HIERARCHY OF EVIDENCE

When attempting to make a decision about the best treatment for a patient, a variety of information can be used, ranging from the memory of the individual practitioner to the multicenter, randomized clinical trial (Table 12A.1). The goal when using these information sources is to provide the practitioner and the patient with an estimate of the most likely outcomes with different treatment choices. The basic information needed for rational, clinical decision making is fundamental knowledge about the disease and its therapy, an understanding of the wishes of the patient, and the humility that derives from knowing that for almost every therapy currently available the outcome of the application of that therapy cannot be predicted with absolute certainty. One is always left with a series of probabilities that must be weighed using the best evidence possible. Interventional cardiology provides an almost ideal paradigm for the study of this issue because of the discrete nature of the treatment (compared with multiple doses of a medication or years of risk factor modifications), the readily measurable clinical outcomes, and the large amount of health care resources used by the practitioner.

RANDOMIZED CLINICAL TRIALS

The randomized clinical trial is considered the paramount scientific method for evaluating therapy. Its primary advantage is that it controls for differences in baseline characteristics, thus eliminating the influence of confounding factors. The straightforward analysis afforded by randomized trial data assumes that potential differences in baseline characteristics have been equalized by the process of random allocation of treatment. Many have argued that the inferences drawn from statistical comparisons in randomized trials are in fact dependent on the random allocation of treatment (4). No matter how much effort is expended attempting to adjust for differences in baseline characteristics in observational studies, one is still left with uncertainty about whether unmeasured factors could have accounted for these differences.

Randomized trials may have substantial problems that often are overlooked by advocates for clinical trials. When applying the results of randomized trials to clinical practice, the clinician should always ask two fundamental questions: are the results valid and are the results generalizable? Particularly in trials involving operator-dependent technology, a number of difficult issues arise. Were patients who were put into the trial representative of practice? Was the technology as applied similar to the current application in practice? Were the relevant endpoints appropriate for clinical decision making, and were they measured completely and accurately? Just as the observational study is vulnerable to questions about unmeasured confounding factors, the randomized trial can always be accused of inadequacy on these measures. The best defenses against such criticism, of course, are developing consensus within the scientific and clinical community about the relevance of the proposed trial before it is begun and maintaining documentation of trial procedures, including some accounting for patients not randomized, as the trial proceeds. In the case of intracranial/extracranial bypass, for instance, review of the registry associated with the trial seemed to indicate that the best surgical candidates were not randomized, leaving the generalizability of the results open to question (5). Despite these potential criticisms, the brief history of randomized trials has proven their relevance and dominant position in the hierarchy of clinical evidence. When the application of a procedure is clearly different from previous approaches to a clinical problem and it is thought to represent a clinical advance, the ideal goal would be to subject that procedure to a randomized clinical trial before it is placed into widescale clinical use. Otherwise, those who develop new technology will be exposed to the criticism that could arise when, months to years later, the new technique may be shown to be equivalent or perhaps even detrimental compared with the old therapy.

The argument is often made that randomized trials are too expensive and that a trial cannot be performed to evaluate every issue (3). As the information age advances, the incremental cost of randomizing, given a pre-existing database, will continue to diminish. The existing information infrastructure will increasingly absorb the majority of the cost of data collection and analysis. Nevertheless, because in the current era the cost of setting up a randomized trial infrastructure is significant, trials should be reserved for significant changes in technology or medical therapy. The judgment about this issue in the case of a specific technology is subjective and debatable.

OBSERVATIONAL DATABASES

Contemporaneous Controls

A comparison of treated patients and contemporary controls can provide an excellent estimate of treatment effect (6). In our own experience a carefully constructed, observational treatment comparison of surgery and medical therapy for coronary artery disease has reproduced the results observed in the major clinical trials in this area. Such comparisons are not simple, however, and in our estimation require a structure with certain critical elements, as outlined by Hlatky (7) and Pryor (2). First, the cohort of patients to be evaluated must be prospectively defined. Second, the critical baseline characteristics known to affect prognosis in the disease state of interest must be defined and measured. Third, prospective data collection on well-defined forms must be part of the process; retrospective chart review is too often inadequate to provide the kind of accuracy needed to adjust for baseline characteristic differences, and small differences in interpretation of baseline characteristics can lead to improper statistical adjustment. Fourth, endpoints to be studied should also be defined prospectively and measured without bias. For mortality measurement this requirement is not difficult, but for measurement of nonfatal endpoints, a system of prospective follow-up, preferably blinded to initial treatment, should be the standard. Fifth, a satisfactory computer system avoiding the common problems of clinical databases such as failure to distinguish between missing data and negative data should be in place. Sixth, ideally, there should be a mechanism to identify missing or incorrect data in real time to prevent the bias inherent in selective chart recall. Finally, an interdisciplinary team of clinicians, biostatisticians, and computer scientists should work together to define the best possible analysis strategy and interpretation of the data. Such an analysis group should include invasive practitioners to allow for inclusion of appropriate expertise into interpretation of the results, but both noninvasive physicians and invasive physicians not involved in the care of the patients should be included in the primary analysis to avoid bias (8). The subtle bias that occurs when the professional reputation or referral practice of the investigator depends on the clinical result can be counterbalanced by a multidisciplinary team without losing the expertise necessary for the best research in interventional cardiology.

The statistical analysis of observational treatment comparisons is not simple and requires careful consideration with the same concerns as a randomized trial. For example, many recent comparisons evaluating therapies or health care systems have failed to take into account the sample sizes needed to detect significant differences. This approach is particularly troublesome in health policy, where a type II statistical error (assuming no difference when a difference actually exists) can be made easily as part of the continuous quality improvement process. When an inadequately sized study is conducted, a high likelihood exists that new advances in therapy will be judged to be ineffective.

In addition to the general concerns of statistical analysis of outcome data, the methods of adjusting for differences in baseline characteristics are difficult and require considerable expertise. One particularly common and egregious error is to tabulate baseline characteristics in the two treatment groups and to report "no significant differences" in them. Unfortunately, many small "insignificant" differences in baseline characteristics can add up to substantial differences in expected outcomes in one group compared with another if the sample sizes are appropriate (9).

A second common trap in the comparative analyses of randomized trials and observational data is the assumption that when a P value is larger than .05 one can assume that there is no difference in outcomes between the two therapies. This issue of assuming "equivalence" without properly assessing the likelihood of a type II error has been reviewed extensively (10). In general, the sample size to prove "equivalence" is larger than the sample size required to prove whether that difference is present. For example, if a current device has an abrupt closure rate of 3 to 5% in a group of patients with a particular set of anatomic characteristics and a new device designed to prevent restenosis has an unknown risk of creating abrupt closure, Table 12A.2 gives the sample size for each group in a comparative randomized trial required to "rule out" various increases in the rate of abrupt closure.

Thirdly, the goal of an observational treatment comparison is to develop a statistical

Table 12A.2.
Sample Sizes to Rule Out Increase in Risk of Abrupt Vessel Closure

Rate in Control Group (%)	Rate Desired to Rule Out With New Therapy (%)	Sample Size Needed
5	6	11,119
	7	3061
	8	1483
	9	903
	10	621
3	4	7295
	5	2114
	6	1067

$\alpha = .05$; $\beta = .90$; two-sided testing.

Table 12A.3.
Improper Conclusions Due to Lack of Consideration of Differences in Baseline Characteristics

Baseline Morphology	Treatment A (n = 2000) (%)	Treatment B (n = 2000) (%)
Stenosis severity	80	80
Eccentric	56	75
Thrombus	12	12
Lesion length >10 mm	20	40
Angulated	20	20
Bifurcation	10	10
Abrupt closure rate	5.2	7.0[a]

[a]$P = .029$

model that will accurately predict the likely outcome for an individual patient if given each of the treatments being evaluated. Accordingly, a properly performed treatment comparison will include substantial prior work on statistical modeling of outcomes. The predictive models should have been assessed for reliability, or the concordance between predicted and observed outcomes, and for discrimination, or the ability to separate patients with and without the outcome of interest. These components of predictive accuracy must be developed in one population and tested in another, or must be developed in a large enough sample that the predictive ability can be validated independently. Without such validation of the ability to predict outcome in multiple populations with the disease process under study, adjustments for differences in baseline characteristics cannot be made with any degree of certainty in an observational treatment comparison.

An example of the difficulty that could arise in an observational comparison of devices with regard to abrupt closure is seen in Table 12A.3. Using the point estimates from a study of the relationship between lesion morphology characteristics and likelihood of abrupt closure from a study done at Duke, two populations are shown with slightly different lesion morphology characteristics, none of which by themselves are significantly different between the two groups. In an observational treatment comparison, the naive investigator who did not prospectively measure these characteristics would conclude that device A significantly $(P = .03)$ reduced the abrupt closure rate. In reality the device had no effect: the observed difference in abrupt closure rate is the result of the differences in underlying lesion morphology in the two populations.

In summary, contemporaneous observational databases can be used for treatment comparisons, but the level of certainty is a step below the randomized trial. The generalizability may be greater, since every patient treated can be included in the analysis. The statistical issues are much more complex than randomized trials, so that observational treatment comparisons should not be accepted unless they have been subjected to the scrutiny of careful and fundamental involvement by a multidisciplinary team of researchers using the same principles of data collection and management as the controlled clinical trial.

HISTORICAL CONTROLS FROM DATABASES

The history of medicine is replete with new therapies that were thought to be major advances based on a comparison with historical controls, but too often these therapies have failed the scrutiny of properly controlled trials. Classic examples included gastric freezing and suppression of asymptomatic ventricular arrhythmias by encainide, fle-

cainide, and ethmoczin. In many cases, by retrospectively applied current standards these comparisons were clearly fatally flawed. However, more subtle difficulties can mar even the most well-intended comparison with historical controls, and there is ample reason to believe that these problems are substantial in the evaluation of interventional therapies. The milieu of interventional therapy has continued to change, predominantly because of better antithrombotic therapy during the procedures but also because of better equipment and improved understanding of the goals and techniques of therapy. Definitions of baseline characteristics and methods of acquisition of measured factors that could affect outcome usually are not replicated. A particularly important issue because of its effect on both acute complications and restenosis is the characterization of unstable angina, which unfortunately has been defined differently by almost every study. Thus any study using historical controls should be placed at a much lower level of importance than studies with contemporary controls and rigorous analysis, even when the historical data were collected in a computerized database. The advantage of the database, even for historical controls, is that efforts can be made to control for baseline characteristics differences in individual patient data, which allows for a much more powerful adjustment than attempting to compare group means.

HISTORICAL CONTROLS FROM THE LITERATURE

Using historical controls from the medical literature is treacherous. Expected complication rates and restenosis rates from interventional procedures can vary up to twofold, depending on the composition of baseline characteristics. These are often not reported completely for the group, and without individual patient data proper adjustment for baseline differences cannot be made. In the absence of any other data, the historical control group from the literature can be used to place the findings of an observational study in perspective to determine whether a prospective study should be recommended, but only in extreme circumstances should further extrapolation to routine practice be made.

CASE SERIES

Even a notch below historical controls is the observational case series without controls. Such series have led to fundamental miscalculations of event rates in the new population being evaluated because of a failure to recognize the lack of generalizability of the observation. This mistake has led to erroneous impressions about the new therapy because of assumptions about what the event rate would have been with the old therapy. Case series, however, provide the impetus to develop new concepts, and only when a positive case series is reported should a prospective study be designed and carried out.

PERSONAL EXPERIENCE

Day-to-day decision making must be based on a synthesis of information from the above sources and the personal experience and skills of the cardiologist (11). In our clinical practice, however, we have been humbled by learning that our "personal experience" was misleading in the use of antiarrhythmics to suppress harbinger rhythm disturbances, calcium channel blockers in the treatment of patients with depressed left ventricular function, and directional atherectomy to produce a more "predictable" result. Three fundamental aspects of personal-experience recall must be considered to place this issue in perspective.

First, studies of human cognition have verified the well-known "last case phenomenon (12)." Because memory becomes more blurred with time, we tend to remember our last case most vividly. Knowing that the outcome of the individual patient is a complex result of multiple factors, including the patient's disease state in terms of pathophysiology that we do or do not understand, as well

as our treatment of it, the irrational nature of the "last case phenomenon" is readily apparent. Secondly, we tend to operate via heuristics, or rules of thumb (13). Such heuristics tend to be based on simplifications of complex probability functions such as "if a patient has left main disease, surgery is indicated," but heuristic thinking makes it difficult to integrate multiple factors impinging on the same patient. Finally, we tend to be distracted by irrelevant information. The physician evaluating a patient must process large amounts of data while attempting to focus on the critical patient characteristics that are most likely to affect outcome. A number of studies have now shown that relatively simple statistical models can do as well as expert clinicians in predicting the likelihood of medical outcomes in a variety of illnesses (14–16).

To have a realistic perspective concerning therapies in ischemic heart disease, one must have a healthy respect for the play of chance and the relatively minor role of therapy in determination of the overall outcome. The outcomes of patients with ischemic heart disease are based on many factors, only a modest part of which is the procedure they are undergoing at the time. Our therapies are not curative and carry new risks to which the patient would not have been exposed without the intervention. Even the highest risk form of coronary disease, left main stenosis, is associated with a 50% chance of survival 5 years later with medical therapy. Thus the common feeling among clinicians that a good patient outcome is truly attributable to the treatment and a bad outcome is a reasonable price to pay for the effort because the patient would have done badly without intervention may be unfounded. Analyses of the relative importance of surgery and of thrombolytic therapy in predicting survival in a patient with coronary disease reinforce the concept that the major determinants of outcome are not the treatment but the age of the patient and the degree of impairment of left ventricular function at the time of the evaluation.

Clinicians must become more aware that the sample sizes needed to make personal inferences are no different from the sample sizes needed for clinical trials. Essentially, this means that an individual physician would never see enough patients in his or her personal career to determine which thrombolytic agent is associated with the lowest mortality or whether one approach or another lowers restenosis rates by 10 to 20% in the practice of angioplasty.

One particularly troublesome aspect of interventional cardiology is that the interventionist is intensely involved with the patient for a short period, and yet the time course of ischemic heart disease must be measured in years. The intuitive instinct to act within an acute zone of comfort could be counterproductive in some cases for the procedure-oriented specialist when the long-term interest of the patient is considered. Most patients do not return frequently to the interventional cardiologist for follow-up, and even if they did return more frequently, the ability of the cardiologist to integrate outcomes of hundreds of patients over time outstrips human capacity.

APPROACH TO THE PROBLEM

Based on the above discussion, therapeutic decision making must integrate these different types of information to make the best decision for the individual patient. A current approach to the problem is to place therapeutic decisions into categories. When a therapy has been shown to be superior in randomized clinical trials, it should be used unless a specific reason can be found not to do so. When a well-designed observational study with contemporary controls is available, it should be used for decision making in preference to other data when a randomized trial is not available. In the absence of the above, personal experience based on pathophysiologic reasoning is our next best guide. A review of recent misadventures in medical therapeutics should lead to a humble attitude on the part of the clinician, however. Many clini-

cians felt they were helping patients by suppressing premature ventricular beats with antiarrhythmic drugs or by "unloading" the ventricle with calcium channel blockers. Yet both therapies were found to be detrimental when subjected to the scrutiny of properly designed trials (17, 18).

Since published literature is subject to being outdated by new technology or other aspects of the therapeutic environment, we consider maintenance of an observational database to be critical to sound practice. The database serves several purposes. By continually observing patient outcomes, one can develop an enhanced understanding of the impact of therapy on long-term outcome. Practice patterns can be observed to determine whether they fit with expected behavior. (For example, is surgery being done on patients with left main disease and what is the current overall complication rate?) In a more controversial vein, the quality of care as measured by medical outcomes can be assessed to determine whether individual and group results are in the range to justify current choice of therapy.

The general area of choice among medical therapy, percutaneous intervention, and coronary surgery provides an example of how randomized trials, databases, and personal experience must be melded. With a background of surgery prolonging survival in patients with multivessel disease and impaired left ventricular function, a concept that has been greatly reinforced by a better understanding of the sample size issue (19), we face the difficult issue of recommending percutaneous intervention in the absence of definitive, randomized trial data to support such a recommendation. The clinician is tempted to make decisions about treatment recommendations based on published studies or personal experience, evaluating anatomic subsets for acute success rates. Although this information is valuable, and more of it should be available, the therapeutic choice is actually much more complex. Ideally, the clinician would like to

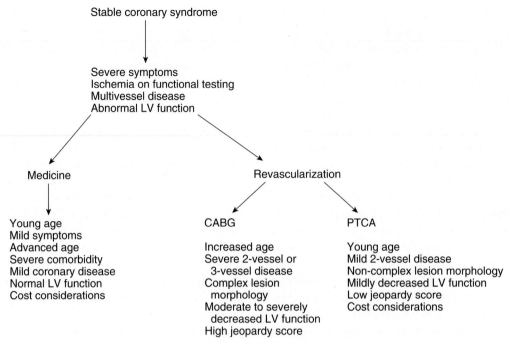

Figure 12A.1.   Treatment algorithm for patients with stable ischemic syndromes.

know both the short-term and the long-term expected outcome with all three approaches: continued medical therapy, surgery, or percutaneous intervention. We have used a combination of data from randomized trials and our own experience to construct a set of principles on which we make therapeutic decisions (Fig. 12A.1) (20, 21). Within this set of principles the individual clinician must make decisions considering special medical characteristics and preferences of the patient. When these guidelines are violated, for example, failing to revascularize a patient with severe multivessel disease and left ventricular dysfunction, additional justification is needed.

DEVELOPMENT OF NEW THERAPIES

When a new approach to therapy is introduced, the performance of the procedure is tracked from the beginning. If the procedure is considered experimental or developmental, institutional review-board approval should be required. The results of the procedure should be continuously compared with expected results from technology and with procedures already in general use. When investigators reach a certain level of confidence that the procedure is beneficial, randomized trials are strongly encouraged (22–24). When a randomized trial is not feasible, efforts are made to perform observational studies with careful contemporary adjustment for baseline differences using individual patient variables (25).

In the development of new devices, we advocate a staged strategy. When a new device or significant enhancement of an old device is conceived, the target patient population should be carefully delineated and a series of patients should undergo the procedure with informed consent. Generally, the technology and the patient population need considerable refinement during the early stages of device development. As the device matures, the clinical outcome of interest should be compared with outcomes of patients in a well-defined database with the same characteristics using multivariate modeling techniques to attempt to adjust for baseline differences. Using confidence limits for clinical outcomes, the developers can gauge their degree of confidence with the advantage of the new technology. This potential clinical advantage must be weighed against the cost of development and the cost of implementation to the medical care system. A device that will increase the cost of care must be clearly superior to current technology if it is to be introduced into wide-scale clinical practice. Alternatively, a device that will likely reduce the cost of medical care need only be equally effective. If the device or approach is a substantial departure from current approaches, a randomized clinical trial is the only way to ensure that it is truly an advance. Such a trial should be initiated as soon as the device has reached a point at which the clinicians and scientists involved are confident *based on empiric data* that the approach is beneficial and worthy of proliferation in practice. When a minor enhancement is made in the design of a device, we believe that it should be evaluated by careful observational studies, preferably employing the level of rigor outlined under the section on observational studies with contemporary controls.

ADMINISTRATIVE USES OF DATABASES

The advent of sophisticated computerized information systems has now made baseline clinical and outcome data available to a variety of observers, including physicians, administrators, and payors. Access to these data has allowed government and private sources to construct "scorecards" relating the relative outcomes of hospitals, physicians, and health care systems (26). Resisting the increasing use of databases to assess quality of care is a strategy doomed to failure. Rather, physicians should strive to ensure that proper data are collected and that the best possible methods of adjusting for differences in baseline characteristics are used when scorecards are developed. Sophisticated regression algorithms can be used to calculate actuarial and expected-event rates so that physicians are not punished for agreeing to perform high-

risk procedures. These algorithms are only as good as the data collected to go into them, however, and developing valid and generalizable equations requires the same sort of multidisciplinary approach described for observational treatment comparisons.

THE FUTURE

In the future we hope that administrative databases, clinical databases, and randomized trials will emanate from a series of networks of hospitals and physicians dedicated to the use of high-quality information in the everyday practice of medicine. Because an observational database will be required to justify quality and price in the new, more competitive health care system, maintenance of networks will become routine. When a randomized trial needs to be performed, the questions related to the randomization can simply be overlaid on the existing information structure. In the absence of physician leadership in this area, the process will move forward under the control of administrators and business.

REFERENCES

1. Rosati RA, Lee KL, Califf RM, Pryor DB, Harrell FE Jr. Problems and advantages of an observational data base approach to evaluating the effect of therapy on outcome. Circulation 1982;65:27–32.
2. Pryor DB, Califf RM, Harrell FE Jr, Hlatky MA, Lee KL, Mark DB, Rosati RA. Clinical data bases. Accomplishments and unrealized potential. Med Care 1985;23:623–647.
3. Califf RM, Pryor DB, Greenfield JC Jr. Beyond randomized clinical trials: applying clinical experience in the treatment of patients with coronary artery disease. Circulation 1986; 74:1191–1194.
4. Temple R. Problems in the use of large data sets to assess effectiveness. Int J Technol Assess Health Care 1990; 6:211–219.
5. Fields WS, Maslenikov V, Meyer JS et al. Joint study of extracranial arterial occlusion. V. Progress report of prognosis following surgical or nonsurgical tests for transient ischemic attacks and cervical carotid artery lesions. JAMA 1970;211:1993.
6. Hlatky MA, Califf RM, Harrell FE Jr, Lee KL, Mark DB, Pryor DB. Comparison of predictions based on observational data with the results of randomized controlled clinical trials of coronary artery bypass surgery. J Am Coll Cardiol 1988;11:237–245.
7. Hlatky MA, Califf RM, Harrell FE Jr, Lee KL, Mark DB,

Muhlbaier LH, Pryor DB. Clinical judgment and therapeutic decision making. J Am Coll Cardiol 1990;15:1–14.

8. Thompson DF. Understanding financial conflicts of interest. N Engl J Med 1993;329:573–576.

9. Lee KL, McNeer JR, Starmer CF, Harris PJ, Rosati RA. Clinical judgment and statistics: lessons from a simulated randomized trial in coronary artery disease. Circulation 1980;61:508–515.

10. Frieman JA, Chalmers TC, Smith H Jr, Kuebler RR. The importance of beta, the type II error, and sample size in the design and interpretation of the randomized controlled trial. N Engl J Med 1978;299:690–694.

11. Antman EM, Lau J, Kupernick B, Mosteller R, Chalmers TC. A comparison of results of meta-analyses of randomized control trials and recommendations of clinical experts: treatments for myocardial infarction. JAMA 1992; 268:240–248.

12. Detsky AS, Redelmeier D, Abrams HB. What's wrong with decision analysis? Can the left brain influence the right?. J Chronic Dis 1987;40:831–836.

13. Eraker SA, Politser P. How decisions are reached: physician and patient. Ann Intern Med 1982;97:262–268.

14. Jackman JD Jr, Zidar JP, Tcheng JE, Overman AB, Phillips HR, Stack RS. Outcome after prolonged balloon inflations of greater than 20 minutes for initially unsuccessful percutaneous transluminal coronary angioplasty. Am J Cardiol 1992;69:1417–1421.

15. Lee KL, Pryor DB, Harrell FE Jr, Califf RM, Behar VS, Floyd WL, Morris JJ et al. Predicting outcome in coronary disease. Statistical models versus expert clinicians. Am J Med 1986;80:553–560.

16. Kong DF, Lee KL, Harrell FE Jr, Boswick JM, Mark DB, Hlatky MA, Califf RM et al. Clinical experience and predicting survival in coronary disease. Arch Intern Med 1989; 149:1177–1181.

17. The Cardiac Arrhythmia Suppression Trial (CAST) Investigators. Preliminary report: effect of encainide and flecainide on mortality in a randomized trial of arrhythmia suppression after myocardial infarction. N Engl J Med 1989; 321:406–412.

18. Packer M. Calcium channel blockers in chronic heart failure: the risks of "physiologically rational" therapy. Circulation 1990;82:2254–2257.

19. Yusuf S, Zucker D, Peduzzi P, Fisher LD, Takaro T, Detre K, Kennedy JW et al. Effect of coronary artery bypass graft surgery on survival: overview of ten-year results from randomised trials by the coronary artery bypass surgery trialists collaboration. Lancet 1994;344:563–570.

20. Califf RM, Harrell FE Jr, Lee KL, Rankin JS, Hlatky MA, Mark DB, Jones RH et al. The evolution of medical and surgical therapy for coronary artery disease. A 15-year perspective. JAMA 1989;261:2077–2086.

21. Mark DB, Nelson CL, Califf RM, Harrell FE Jr, Lee KL, Jones RH, Fortin DF et al. The continuing evolution of therapy for coronary artery disease: initial results from the era of coronary angioplasty. Circulation 1994;89:2015–2025.

22. Topol EJ, Leya F, Pinkerton CA, Whitlow PL, Hofling B, Simonton CA, Masden RR et al. for the CAVEAT Study Group. A comparison of directional atherectomy with coronary angioplasty in patients with coronary artery disease. N Engl J Med 1993;329:221–227.

23. Ohman EM, George BS, White CJ, Kern MJ, Gurbel PA, Freedman RJ, Lundergan C et al. for the Randomized IABP Study Group. The use of aortic counterpulsation to improve sustained coronary artery patency during acute myocardial infarction: results of a randomized trial. J Am Coll Cardiol 1993;21:397A (abstract).

24. Ohman EM, Marquis J, Ricci DR, Brown RIG, Knudtson ML, Kereiakes DJ, Samaha JK et al. for the Perfusion Balloon Catheter Study Group. A randomized comparison of gradual prolonged versus standard primary balloon inflation on early and late outcome: results of a multicenter clinical trial. Circulation 1994;89:1118–1125.

25. Tenaglia AN, Zidar JP, Jackman JDJ, Fortin DF, Krucoff MW, Tcheng JE, Phillips HR et al. Treatment of long coronary artery narrowings with long angioplasty balloon catheters. Am J Cardiol 1993;71:1274–1277.

26. Topol EJ, Califf RM. Scorecard cardiovascular medicine: its impact and future directions. Ann Intern Med 1994; 120:65–70.

B. The Mayo Clinic Perspective

MICHAEL B. MOCK

The first possibly effective myocardial revascularization procedure was introduced in 1950 by Vineberg who blindly implanted an internal mammary artery into the ventricular myocardium (1). However, it was not until the 1960s when Sones and Judkins developed safe and effective angiographic techniques for radiographically analyzing the human coronary artery circulation that the modern era of myocardial revascularization became feasible (2, 3). Utilizing coronary angiography to define the underlying obstructive coronary disease and to strategically define the placement of bypass vein grafts, Favaloro vastly expanded the effectiveness of myocardial revascularization (4). Soon after the introduction of the coronary bypass surgery, conflict arose about which patients would benefit from the procedure. Ischemic heart disease presents a broad clinical spectrum that for some, unfortunately, can mean a sudden premature death, while, on the other hand, others more fortunate can live for many years in spite of significant angina and recurrent myocardial infarctions. The recognition that prognosticating survival in patients with coronary artery disease is difficult with multiple factors that can influence both longevity and quality of life has made selection criteria for new methods of myocardial revascularization controversial (5). The debate about the real role of coronary bypass in treating coronary artery disease led to the development of three major multicenter randomized trials comparing coronary bypass with medical treatment: The Veterans Administration Cooperative Study of Treatment of Angina (6), The European Coronary Surgery Study (7), and the NHLBI Coronary Artery Surgery Study (CASS) (8). These three major studies were widely debated. Most cardiologists and cardiovascular surgeons agreed that overall coronary bypass has a small impact on survival. There is proven survival benefit only for the subset of patients presenting with significant left main coronary disease and patients with three-vessel disease and impaired left ventricular function. On the other hand, the majority of patients receiving coronary bypass were found to have improvement over medical treatment in the relief of angina resulting in a better quality of life. Just about the time that the controversy of determining who should be revascularized by coronary bypass was resolved, Dr. Andreas Grüntzig in 1977 introduced per cutaneous transluminal coronary angioplasty (PTCA) (9).

At a time when there was great emphasis on the technique of randomized clinical trials for evaluating new therapies, it is not surprising that early in the development of his new nonoperative approach to myocardial revascularization Dr. Grüntzig called for a randomized trial to compare this new procedure with the more established coronary bypass (10).

To track the use of this new technique of myocardial revascularization from its inception, the NHLBI Cardiac Diseases Branch established a voluntary PTCA registry, which included the initial cases of the founder of the technique along with those of other pioneers, including Drs. Myler, Stertzer, Dorros, Kent, and Block and investigators from 29 other centers. Data on cases treated at these centers through August 1980 were included in this interim or initial PTCA registry. Of the 631 patients enrolled in this interim registry, 80% had single-vessel disease. The success rate was 59%, the periprocedure myocardial infarction rate was 4%, emergency CABG rate was 6%, and in-hospital mortality was 1%. When a workshop on PTCA was convened in Bethesda, Maryland, in June 1979, a major recommendation for an expanded registry was made rather than the initiation of a randomized trial that was argued by some participants (11).

The second phase of the NHLBI PTCA registry began in August 1980 with the Data Coordinating Center at the University of Pittsburgh. There was great enthusiasm for the registry with 105 centers entering data from 3079 patients by the close of the registry in September 1981. The general results were similar to the initial data with 81% of the patients having single-vessel disease and without change in the hospital mortality or periprocedure myocardial infarction rate, which remained respectively at 29% and 5%.

The NHLBI PTCA registry, which enrolled early and late data on patients receiving PTCA from 1977 through 1981 at a large number of medical centers, helped establish the risks and benefits of this less-invasive method of myocardial revascularization. It also permitted the establishment of a learning curve by demonstrating that with more experience there are fewer complications (12). Although the registry was important for selecting the patients for which PTCA was feasible and for identifying the immediate risks of the procedure, I think the most important accomplishment of this early registry was that it helped create a "community of investigators" who became friends and colleagues, voluntarily sharing not only their data but their ideas and enthusiasm for this new technique and the process of clinical investigation. This spirit was made possible in large part by the cooperation and enthusiasm of Dr. Andreas Grüntzig.

From its inception the NHLBI registry was understood to be a useful tool for providing preliminary data for planning randomized trials. When we compare two different therapies for a disease, a randomized clinical trial is the most effective method for providing definitive answers on the relative efficacy of the two therapies, since the randomization procedure ensures that the patients assigned to the two treatment groups are similar in both known and unknown variables. Also, with a randomized trial, we minimize selection bias for the two therapies being tested. Still another benefit for the randomized trial is the ability to assess the probability that a given set of findings could have occurred by chance if there were no differences in the outcomes for the two treatments. In the NHLBI workshop on PTCA held in 1983, the design of potential clinical randomized trials using estimates from the data from the Coronary Artery Surgery Study (CASS) was presented (13). It was considered that randomized studies could be carried out in patients with proximal subtotal occlusion in one or more coronary arteries. Medical therapy could be considered as a control for patients with one-vessel coronary artery disease, medical or surgical therapy for two-vessel coronary disease, and surgical therapy for patients with three-vessel disease. In response to using mortality as an endpoint, it was concluded that the required sample size would be in the thousands even for multivessel disease. Trials evaluating myocardial infarction and angina would require 500 patients in each treatment group.

In conducting a trial in patients presenting with angina, functional testing improves the objectivity of evaluating for recurrence of ischemia by combining patient symptoms with electrocardiographic or imaging data.

The establishment of controlled laboratories to independently evaluate certain endpoint data without knowledge of treatment assignment improved the objectivity of the assessment.

From the initial experience with PTCA to the present, the high frequency of restenosis of successfully dilated lesions has been the Achilles' heel of PTCA. Therefore patients undergoing PTCA often require multiple retreatments with PTCA or crossover to coronary bypass. Therefore, in designing comparative randomized studies for PTCA and coronary bypass surgery, it is important to consider that the patients are randomized to either a treatment strategy of initial PTCA or initial coronary bypass and to recognize that a repeat PTCA or a subsequent coronary bypass will be required in a significant minority of patients assigned to the initial PTCA treatment strategy and to a lesser degree in those patients assigned to the initial surgical strategy.

Angiographic endpoints are important in determining the comparability of the extent of disease and the assessment of myocardial jeopardy. There is added advantage of a subsequent independent assessment, ideally by a central angiographic laboratory. By studying large angiographic databases, an attempt can be made at better predicting lesion outcome. By assessing later angiographic endpoints, it can be determined if there is any relationship between the baseline morphologic features and late angiographic findings, including patency of grafts and dilated lesions. This would also permit evaluation of any relationship between early and late angiographic features and revascularization status and adverse clinical outcomes such as recurrence of angina, interval myocardial infarctions, and poor exercise capacity. The most important test of comparability between PTCA and coronary bypass is in patients with symptomatic multivessel disease, particularly if there is impairment of the left ventricular function. If PTCA can be shown to be as effective as coronary bypass in these patients in relieving angina and improving functional capacity without increasing the risk of death or myocardial infarction, its clinical usefulness will be considerably enhanced.

An important issue to be resolved in randomized trials comparing multivessel PTCA versus coronary bypass surgery is the completeness of revascularization. In studies of both PTCA and coronary bypass there has been good correlation between the relief of angina in the subsequent clinical course and the completeness of revascularization (14, 15). On the other hand, in studying the survival of the nonoperated patients in the Coronary Artery Surgery Study registry, patients with stenosis in two vessels but with only one proximal obstruction have the same survival as those without a proximal stenosis, and patients with two proximal obstructions have a significantly poorer survival, similar to patients with three-vessel disease with two proximal stenoses (16).

Randomized trials comparing PTCA with coronary bypass in patients with multivessel disease will provide important data to help resolve the issue of the value of "completeness of revascularization" if there are adequate patients in each treatment group.

The issue of health reform has placed great current emphasis on cost reduction. Since ischemic heart disease accounts for a large portion of our health care costs and since myocardial revascularization procedures are high-ticket items in providing ischemic heart disease care, cost must be included as an endpoint in randomized trials comparing these procedures. PTCA has attraction as an alternative for coronary bypass because of its allegedly shorter periods of hospitalization and disability and lower costs. There have been short-term comparisons showing some lower costs for PTCA in mostly single-vessel disease (17).

Randomized trials of adequate sample size and with long-term, follow-up cost studies are required to resolve the cost issue since restenosis with PTCA often results in the recurrence of symptoms and this triggers repeat hospitalization, arteriography, and revascularization procedures. The need for these additional procedures can quickly eradicate the earlier reduced costs and disability in patients receiving initial PTCA.

The view of the 1983 National Heart, Lung and Blood Institute Workshop on the Outcome of Percutaneous Transluminal Coronary Angioplasty in regard to randomized clinical trials was summarized by the chairman, Dr. Valler Willman, as follows: "Many investigators fully endorse a prospective clinical randomized trial and believe that in the absence of such information, clinical practice will be on uncertain footing. Although this proposal was not fully endorsed, there was no categorical substantiative counterargument. It appears likely that trials will be proposed and evaluated on their individual merits." Perhaps in retrospect, it was the great success of the National Heart, Lung and Blood Institute Registry for PTCA that, by providing high-quality multicenter data on PTCA, including long-term follow-up, helped delay randomized trials. Another reason given for delaying randomized clinical trials comparing PTCA and coronary bypass was the rapidly progressing technical progress of the equipment used in coronary angioplasty. However, when a similar argument was made by cardiac surgeons at a time in the late '60s and early '70s when cardiologists were calling for randomized trials comparing coronary bypass with medical treatment, Chalmers wrote that not only was early randomization ethical (to determine that the new treatment was not worse than the old) but to postpone randomization would be unethical because patients might be "sacrificed" (18). Perhaps it took longer to mount comparative trials because to the cardiologist PTCA was seen as a way of replacing a major surgical procedure requiring anesthesia with a less invasive catheter procedure performed in an arena in which they were more comfortable. There is no question that randomized trials to compare PTCA with coronary bypass took much longer to initiate than did trials comparing medical treatment with coronary bypass for whatever the reason (19). Nearly 15 years after the initiation of PTCA by Grüntzig and after the NHLBI Workshop on PTCA calling for randomized trials to compare PTCA with more established treatments, data from randomized trials are beginning to appear. The only randomized trial comparing medical treatment with PTCA is the Angioplasty Compared to Medicine (ACME) trial from the Veterans Administration (20). In this trial 107 patients were randomized to stepped-care medical treatment, which included nitrates, beta blockers, and calcium antagonists either alone or in various combinations, and 105 patients were assigned to PTCA.

Three years of follow-up have now been reported from this important trial, which notably showed prolonged exercise capacity and reduced angina for the patients assigned to PTCA. This was shown at 6 months and has persisted for 36 months. No difference in survival or the occurrence of myocardial infarction was noted between the medically assigned or PTCA-assigned patients. With such a low sample size we would not expect the ACME trial to show any difference in survival or the occurrence of myocardial infarction. A study of the long-term follow-up of patients suitable for PTCA with single-vessel disease from the Coronary Artery Surgery Study would indicate the need for thousands of patients to have been enrolled in the ACME trial to prove improved survival with PTCA over medical therapy (21).

In clinical practice there is often concern about the patient with isolated, severe, proximal disease in the left anterior descending artery. This concern is heightened if the patient is shown to have a large area of ischemia involving the anterior wall and septum with functional testing. Such patients trigger the question of whether these lesions truly are "widow makers." During the planning phase for the National Heart, Lung, and Blood Institutes Bypass Angioplasty Revascularization Investigation (BARI) study, an attempt was made to include patients with proximal, isolated, left anterior descending disease for randomization to either PTCA or surgical grafting with a left internal mammary artery graft. There was not support within the study group to include these patients. Recently, Goy and colleagues reported the results of a small-scale randomized trial of PTCA compared with surgical grafting in this population (see Chapter 29B). One hundred thirty-four patients were randomized. At 2-year follow-up, patients randomized to PTCA had a slightly higher incidence of death or infarction (12% versus 5%, $P = .21$). When repeat revascularization was also considered, the benefit of surgery became more marked (55% versus 13%, $P < .01$).

The Emory Angioplasty Versus Surgery Trial (EAST) was originated by Dr. Andreas Grüntzig after he relocated to Atlanta. The EAST trial screened approximately 5000 patients to randomize 392 patients with an average age of 62 years. Most patients presented with class III or IV angina. All patients had multivessel coronary disease, and 60% had two-vessel disease. Dr. King has reported 3 years of follow-up (22). The survival is similar at 93% for the PTCA versus 94% for the surgical patients. The occurrence of nonfatal myocardial infarction did not statistically differ in the two treatment groups nor did the occurrence of a large defect on thallium functioning testing. However, at 3 years there was more recurrent class III or IV angina in the patients assigned to PTCA (20% versus 12%) (22). The greater recurrence of angina in the patients assigned to PTCA accounts for a much larger number of the patients assigned to PTCA requiring additional revascularization procedures during 3 years of follow-up compared with the surgically assigned patients (66% versus 12%). At 3 years, left ventricular function was equal in the two treatment groups (69%). We shall await with interest the 5-year follow-up results planned for the EAST trial.

The German Angioplasty versus Bypass Investigation (GABI) randomized 359 patients with classes III and IV angina and multi-vessel disease. This is similar to the EAST trial. The GABI trial has reported preliminary 1-year follow-up data. At 1 year the percentage of patients free of death and/or non-fatal myocardial infarction was similar in the groups assigned to PTCA and coronary bypass (88% versus 94%). The GABI trial reported that both treatment groups showed similar levels of angina and exercise tolerance at 1 year. However, as in the EAST trial, a significantly larger number of the patients assigned to PTCA required an additional revascularization procedure than those assigned to coronary bypass (44% versus 6%). The GABI trial has reported a 6-month angiogram for 61% of the randomized patients. This follow-up angiogram showed that by 6 months following PTCA 35% of the patients had lesions ≥50%, but only 10% of this group with angiographic evidence of restenosis reported angina, which was similar to the surgical group (23).

The Randomized Intervention Treatment of Angina (RITA) organized in the United Kingdom randomized 1011 patients with a ≥70% lesion in one vessel and ≥50% lesions in two vessels (24). Approximately one-half of the randomized patients had single-vessel disease. This study has reported endpoints for 2½ years with the combined mortality and nonfatal infarction similar in the PTCA and coronary bypass groups (9.8% versus 8.6%). As in the other trials reported to date, there was a significantly higher utilization of repeat revascularization procedures in those patients assigned to PTCA compared with the surgical patients at 2½ years of follow-up (31.2% versus 7.8%).

The largest and most comprehensive randomized clinical trial comparing PTCA with coronary bypass is the National Heart, Lung and Blood Institutes Bypass Angioplasty Revascularization Investigation (BARI) study (25). This multicenter trial enrolled patients at 14 primary clinical sites and five coinvestigational sites in the United States and Canada between August 1988 and July 1, 1991. The patients are being followed at the clinical sites with a 10-year follow-up planned. Although the baseline data of the 1829 randomized patients (PTCA 915, CABG 914), 2013 eligible but not randomized patients, and 422 patients excluded from randomization because of angiographic findings unsuitable for PTCA have been reported, no endpoint data has been released from the BARI study. Current plans call for submitting the 5-year follow-up data from the BARI study for presentation at the Scientific Sessions of the American College of Cardiology in March 1996. The BARI study is the only randomized study that has sufficient numbers of randomized patients to permit a statistically sound comparison of survival between PTCA and coronary bypass.

The BARI study's large registry of eligible but not randomized patients and a prospectively enrolled subset of patients excluded from randomization because of angiographic findings making the patient unsuitable for randomization will provide very important information to put in perspective the findings of the randomized trial. When the extracranial-intracranial arterial bypass study was reported in 1985, there was great criticism that the results were not of clinical importance because so many eligible patients were not randomized and no data were available in the eligible but not randomized group (26). In a strong editorial in the *British Medical Journal*, Dudley makes an important statement regarding the importance of a registry of eligible but not randomized patients who should be followed such as is being done in the BARI trial. "The clinical trial is a powerful tool for uncovering therapeutic truth, and it can continue to be used provided . . . the reality of the equality of follow-up for those excluded is recognized" (27).

The scientific importance of the BARI study will also be enhanced by the Central Angiographic Laboratory, which analyzes all baseline and follow-up angiograms (28). A subset of BARI randomized patients have agreed to have 1-year and 5-year prescheduled follow-up angiograms regardless of subsequent clinical symptoms. The BARI study Central Electrocardiographic Laboratory interprets all baseline and follow-up electrocardiograms and the follow-up exercise ECG at 3 months, 1 year, 3 years, and 5 years. Since no endpoint data have yet been reported from the largest clinical trial comparing PTCA and coronary bypass, it is important that we do not make premature definitive conclusions based on the preliminary data that have been released from the smaller trials.

At this point, however, we can say that the current available data have demonstrated the early safety and effectiveness of PTCA in selected patients with multivessel disease. This is important data for those treating patients with symptomatic multivessel coronary disease. Before we had randomized clinical trial data, there were many who questioned the use of PTCA in revascularizing patients with multivessel disease. The early data from the randomized trials would indicate that it is reasonable to consider PTCA and coronary bypass as equally appropriate initial revascularization options in those patients with lesions suitable for angioplasty. There is a clear consensus from all of the trials reporting preliminary data that those patients assigned to initial angioplasty are much more likely in the early follow-up interval to require an additional revascularization procedure. On the other hand, because of the use of the incremental revascularization procedures, the success of both procedures in relieving angina at 1 year is

approximately 90%, and there is no excess death or nonfatal myocardial infarction in either treatment group in accomplishing this laudable goal. It is important to reflect that, based on follow-up angiography in GABI at 6 months and in EAST at 1 and 3 years, there is less complete revascularization in those patients assigned to PTCA. However, in spite of this, the relief of angina is not significantly different since reinterventions have been selectively directed toward those patients with recurrent or persistent symptoms and the repeat procedures are more common in the patients assigned to PTCA in this early phase of follow-up.

The current data allow for the individualization of choice by patients and their physicians. For the patient who, because of lifestyle or personality, wants *one* procedure and a low risk of early repeat hospitalization and who can accept the early disability and discomfort of a major surgical procedure the choice is coronary bypass.

For the patient who is terrified by the thought of anesthesia and a major surgical procedure and who can accept the possible early recurrence of symptoms and repeat coronary angiography and the greater chance of continuing on more medication, the current data would indicate they can have an 80% chance of avoiding surgery by having initial PTCA (assuming they had anatomy that would have qualified them for inclusion in these trials). In the meantime we must look to the long-term follow-up data from the larger BARI study for additional information that may modify the current options. The study of Economics and Quality of Life (SEQOL) ancillary study under way at seven of the BARI clinical sites will also provide important data on which to base the most economic choice for myocardial revascularization.

While follow-up is continuing, there will be additional advances in PTCA such as the use of stents and new drug therapy, which already show promise for reducing by up to one-third the restenosis rate after PTCA.

Increasingly, cardiac surgeons are applying the use of the internal mammary artery for bypass grafting. Therefore we can expect continuing improvement in both revascularization procedures being evaluated. These advances in technology will only enhance the long-term results of trials evaluating the study of either *initial PTCA* or *initial coronary bypass* in treating patients presenting with symptomatic obstructive coronary artery disease.

REFERENCES

1. Vineberg AM, Niloff PH. The value of surgical treatment of coronary artery occlusion by implantation of the internal mammary artery into the ventricular myocardium: an experimental study. Surg Gynecol Obstet 1950;91:551–561.
2. Sones FM Jr, Shirey EK. Cine coronary arteriography. Mod Concepts Cardiovasc Dis 1962;31:735–738.
3. Judkins MP. Selective coronary arteriography: a percutaneous transfemoral technic. Radiology 1967;89:815–824.
4. Favalaro RG. Saphenous vein graft in the surgical treatment of coronary artery disease. J Thorac Cardiovasc Surg 1969;58:178.
5. Emond M, Mock MB, Davis KB et al. Long-term survival of medically treated patients in the Coronary Artery Surgery Study (CASS) Registry. Circulation 1994;90:2645.
6. Murphy ML, Hultgren HN, Detre K, Thomsen J, Takaro T, participants of the Veterans Administration Cooperative Study. Treatment of chronic stable angina: a preliminary report of survival data of the Randomized Veterans Administration Cooperative Study. N Engl J Med 1977; 297:621–627.
7. European Coronary Surgery Study Group. Long-term results of prospective randomised study of coronary artery surgery in stable angina pectoris. Lancet 1982;2:1173–1180.
8. CASS principal investigators and their associates. Coronary Artery Surgery Study (CASS): a randomized trial of coronary artery bypass surgery: survival data. Circulation 1983;68:939–950.
9. Grüntzig AR, Meyler RK, Hanna ES, Turina MI. Coronary transluminal angioplasty. Circulation 1977;55(3):84 (abstract).
10. Grüntzig AR, Senning A, Siegenthaler WE. Nonoperative dilatation of coronary artery stenosis: percutaneous transluminal coronary angioplasty. N Engl J Med 1979; 301:61–68.
11. Proceedings of the Workshop on Percutaneous Transluminal Coronary Angioplasty. US Department of Health, Education and Welfare Publ. No. (NIH) 80-2030.
12. Kelsey S, Mullin S, Detre K, Mitchell H, Cowley MJ, Gruentzig AR, Kent KM. Effect of investigator experience on percutaneous transluminal coronary angioplasty. Am J Cardiol 1984;53:56C–64C.
13. Fisher LD, Holmes DR Jr, Mock MB et al. Design of comparative clinical studies of percutaneous transluminal coronary angioplasty using estimates from the Coronary Artery Surgery Study. Am J Cardiol 1984;53:138C–145C.
14. Bell MR, Gersh BJ, Schaff HV et al. Effect of the completeness of revascularization on the long-term outcome of patients with three-vessel disease undergoing coronary bypass surgery: a report from the Coronary Artery Surgery Study Registry. Circulation 1992;86:446–457.
15. Reeder GS, Holmes DR Jr, Detre K, Costigan T, Kelsey SF. Degree of revascularization in patients with multivessel coronary disease: a report from the National Heart, Lung, and Blood Institute Percutaneous Transluminal Coronary Angioplasty Registry. Circulation 1988;77:638–644.
16. Ringquist I, Fisher LD, Mock MB et al. Prognostic value of angiographic indices of coronary artery disease from the Coronary Artery Surgery Study (CASS). J Clin Invest 1983;711:1854–1866.
17. Reeder GS, Krishan I, Nobrega FT et al. Is percutaneous angioplasty less expensive than bypass surgery? N Engl J Med 1984;311:1157–1162.
18. Chalmers TC. Randomization and coronary artery surgery. Ann Thorac Surg 1971;14:323–327.
19. Mock MB, Reeder GS, Schaff HV et al. Percutaneous transluminal coronary angioplasty versus coronary artery bypass: isn't it time for a randomized trial? N Engl J Med 1985;312:916–918.
20. Parisi AF, Folland ED, Hartigan P on behalf of the Veterans Affairs ACME Investigators. A comparison of angioplasty with medical therapy in the treatment of single-vessel coronary artery disease. N Engl J Med 1992;326:10–16.
21. Holmes DR Jr, Vlietstra RE, Fisher LD et al. Follow-up of patients from the Coronary Artery Surgery Study (CASS) potentially suitable for percutaneous transluminal coronary angioplasty. Am Heart J 1983;106:981–988.
22. Zhao X-Q, Grown BG, Stewart DK, Hillger LA, King SB III, EAST Angiographic Coordinating Center. Arteriographic Endpoints from Emory Angioplasty vs. Surgery Trial (EAST). Circulation 1993;88:I-506 (abstract).
23. Rupprecht HJ, Hamm CW, Reimers J, Trautmann S, Meyer J for the GABI-Study-Group. Angiographic follow-up of the German Angioplasty vs. Bypass Investigation (GABI-Trial). Circulation 1993;88:I-506 (abstract).
24. RITA trial participants. Coronary angioplasty versus coronary artery bypass surgery: the Randomized Intervention Treatment of Angina (RITA) trial. Lancet 1993; 341:573–580.
25. Protocol for the Bypass Angioplasty Revascularization Investigation. Circulation 1991;84(Suppl V):V1–V27.
26. The EC/IC Bypass Study Group. Failure of extracranial bypass to reduce the risks of ischemic stroke: results of the international randomized study. N Engl J Med 1985; 313:1191–1200.
27. Dudley HA. Extracranial-intracranial bypass. I. Clinical trials. Br Med J 1987;294:1501–1502 (editorial).
28. Alderman EL, Stadius M. The angiographic definition of the Bypass Angioplasty Revascularization Investigation. Coronary Artery Disease 1992;3:1189–1207.

C. The Thoraxcenter Perspective

ANDONIS G. VIOLARIS and PATRICK W. SERRUYS

Percutaneous transluminal coronary angioplasty (PTCA), introduced by Grüntzig in the late 1970s, has been a major breakthrough in the treatment of obstructive coronary artery disease. Increasing operator experience and improvements in balloon catheter technology have resulted in a high immediate success rate and a low incidence of complications, which in turn has resulted in an increasing number of patients with more advanced coronary artery disease now being considered candidates for balloon angioplasty. Substantial limitations still remain, however, which include technical factors relating to the coronary anatomy that limit the intervention to particular subgroups of patients with coronary artery disease, acute occlusion resulting in increased morbidity and mortality, and longer-term restenosis in 30 to 40% of patients. Because of these limitations inherent in balloon angioplasty, pharmacologic agents to reduce restenosis and a plethora of new devices designed to improve the short- and long-term results of catheter-based revascularization have been introduced.

Considerable difficulties exist, however, in assessing long-term restenosis and making valid comparisons between the different treatment modalities available. We therefore need a means of rapidly and effectively assessing not only the acute efficacy and safety of new devices but also of comparing their long-term results with those of balloon angioplasty. Randomized trials, registries, and personal experience all go some way toward answering these questions. In this monograph we review the use of these three methods and propose a compromise approach, based on matching patient and lesion characteristics, that may result in the more rapid and efficient assessment of new devices and pharmacologic agents.

RANDOMIZED STUDIES

The best way to compare the short- and long-term clinical and angiographic results of different coronary interventions or pharmacologic agents is with a randomized study. The proper design of a randomized study to compare different interventional techniques requires the selection of the appropriate angiographic variables reflecting the restenosis process. In a recent study we examined which angiographic parameter best described functional status 6 months after successful single-vessel coronary angioplasty (1). Sensitivity and specificity curves for the prediction of anginal status and exercise electrocardiography of four quantitative angiographic variables were constructed, and the point of highest diagnostic accuracy for the variables was determined at the intersection of the sensitivity and specificity curves. The points of highest diagnostic accuracy using minimal luminal diameter were similar for both anginal status and exercise electrocardiography at 1.45 and 1.46 mm, respectively. This suggests that the minimal luminal diameter at follow-up may be useful for predicting clinical events such as recurrence of angina. In addition, the use of a central angiographic core lab, using a well-validated system of quantitative coronary angiography, with the expertise required to ensure the accuracy of all collated data and to minimize the possibility of introducing methodologic errors and bias is required. Also required are a sufficient number of patients undergoing repeat angiography at a predetermined time. This number depends on the variability in outcome among the patients, the magnitude of the difference in outcome, and the alpha and beta errors. Changing the power of the study in one way or another will affect the number of patients needed. Accepting a larger chance of missing an effective treatment (large beta error and thus a reduction in power) means substantially less patients are needed.

A randomized study has several theoretical advantages. It guarantees population homogeneity in terms of clinical and angiographic variables and thus allows the direct comparison of different therapeutic treatment modalities with no bias regarding selection of treatment. Furthermore a well-designed randomized study may ensure that if a device is used, the device has a fair trial by requiring adequate expertise of all participating investigators. For example, with most devices there is often a steep learning curve, and therefore to ensure the fair evaluation of a device a minimum requirement would be that participating personnel have performed a set number of procedures using the device, with acceptable success and complication rates.

Problems Related to All Studies

Despite the above advantages randomized studies also have some inherent, logistic limitations. These include patient exclusions by virtue of the inclusion/exclusion criteria and inconsistencies in the timing of randomization, follow-up duration, and definitions of clinical and angiographic primary endpoints. We would like to expand on these using as an example four, recently completed, multicenter, restenosis trials: MERCATOR (randomized, double-blind, placebo-controlled, restenosis prevention trial of cilazapril 5 mg) (2), MARCATOR (randomized, double-blind, placebo-controlled, restenosis prevention trial of cilazapril 1, 5, or 10 mg) (3), CARPORT (randomized, double-blind, placebo-controlled, restenosis prevention trial of a thromboxane A_2 receptor antagonist) (4), and PARK (randomized, double-blind, placebo-controlled trial of ketanserin 40 mg) (5).

Patient Selection Bias—Inclusion/Exclusion Criteria

The inclusion/exclusion criteria for a study may have a substantial influence on both the power of a study and the applicability of the results to the general angioplasty population. The main inclusion/exclusion criteria in most studies relate to the coronary anatomy (single-vessel versus multivessel disease)/lesion morphology, the pattern of angina (stable versus unstable), a previous history of myocardial infarction, and concomitant drug therapy or device use.

SINGLE-VESSEL VERSUS MULTIVESSEL DISEASE

Large centers likely to participate in randomized studies often report that a large proportion of their patients have multivessel disease requiring multilesion angioplasty. If you therefore confine your study to single-vessel disease, you will limit the number of eligible patients. If you decide to include multivessel angioplasty, however, the problem then arises of how to handle restenosis. Do you perform a lesion- or a patient-related analysis. If you choose a patient-related analysis, how do you handle three dilated lesions in the same patient? It is much easier in statistics to work with single numbers than a collection of numbers. Because restenosis is likely to be a lesion-related rather than a patient-related problem (even the so-called patient-related factors such as unstable angina or recent angina actually reflect lesion instability) (6), we tend to reconcile lesion with patient analysis by using the average MLD (minimal luminal diameter) of multiple lesions obtained from multiple views so that statistically you deal with one MLD per patient. It is interesting, however, that despite the onus in the planning stage to include multivessel dilation, over 80% of patients randomized in the large multicentre trials have single-vessel disease with 16% two-vessel disease and 4% three-vessel disease.

STABLE VERSUS UNSTABLE ANGINA PECTORIS

One reason for including unstable patients is that in multivariate analysis the greatest loss in MLD occurs in the unstable patients.

For example, in the CARPORT study the change in MLD at follow-up was -0.37 ± 0.59 mm in patients with duration of angina <2.3 months (n = 210), while it was only -0.26 ± 0.53 mm in patients with duration of angina >8.5 months (n = 229). A similar pattern was seen in the MERCATOR study where the change in MLD at follow-up was -0.33 ± 0.55 mm in patients with duration of angina <86 days (n = 252), while it was only -0.19 ± 0.48 mm in patients with duration of angina >305 days (n = 256). The importance of this is in the power calculation. If unstable patients are excluded, then the calculation of the power of the trial becomes extremely difficult and large numbers of patients are required. In the ongoing FLARE study looking at fluvastatin for restenosis, the drug has to be started 3 weeks prior to PTCA which means unstable patients are excluded from the study, increasing the number of patients required.

If you do decide to include patients with unstable angina, the problem then arises that there is no accepted definition of this term. A practical definition, used in the CARPORT study, was pain at rest controlled by intravenous nitrates. Even within this group, however, there is a marked heterogeneity of patients, and a better definition and subdivision of unstable angina is needed. In the ongoing HELVETICA study (randomized, double-blind, placebo-controlled, restenosis prevention trial of recombinant hirudin) patients are entered using the Braunwald classification, which will hopefully provide better information on the long-term restenosis rate in the various subgroups of unstable angina.

PREVIOUS MYOCARDIAL INFARCTION

Most studies have systematically excluded patients with recent myocardial infarction from trial entry. In the MERCATOR study, for example, patients with a myocardial infarct within 3 weeks were excluded (Table 12C.1). In the MARCATOR study an amendment was passed 3 months into the trial allowing patients within 5 days of myocardial infarction to be entered into the study. This high rate of recent myocardial infarction may be responsible for the increased loss in MLD in the MARCATOR compared with the MERCATOR study (0.37 versus 0.28 mm).

Table 12C.1.
Screening Results of 17 Log-Keeping Clinics Participating in the MERCATOR Multicenter Randomized Study of Cilazapril[a]

Reason for Exclusion	Number[b]	%
History of sustained essential hypertension	271	21.2
Previous and/or failed PTCA at the same site	268	21.0
Q-wave MI less than 4 weeks prior to study entry	174	13.6
Follow-up coronary angiography unlikely	109	8.5
Logistic reasons	67	5.2
Significant concomitant disease	50	3.9
Older than 75 years	43	3.4
Dilatation of bypass graft	40	3.1
Primary perfusion therapy	39	3.1
No informed consent given	39	3.1
Current evidence of prior history of heart failure	28	2.2
Participation in other trial	14	1.1
Atherectomy/stent	13	1.0
Other reasons[c] (less than 1% each)	122	9.6

[a]From MERCATOR study group. Circulation 1992; 86–100–101 with permission.

[b]Screening results of 17 clinics which recruited 65% of the patients.

[c]Left main disease, history of type II hypercholesterolemia, previous cerebro-vascular accident, previous participation in MERCATOR, hypotension, contraindication to ACE inhibition/aspirin, women of childbearing potential, insulin-dependent diabetes, miscellaneous.

EXCLUSION CRITERIA BASED ON TRIAL MEDICATION

The trial medication may also play a significant role in selection bias by excluding patients with contraindications to the medication or those on concomitant therapy that may interact with the trial medication. For example, in the MERCATOR and MARCATOR studies hypertension was a major exclusion criterion because of the associated hypotensive effect of cilazapril (Table 12C.1). In the MERCATOR study 15% of all patients screened were excluded because of sustained essential hypertension. In the CARPORT and PARK studies the use of platelet-inhibiting or nonsteroidal antiinflammatory drugs within 7 days preceding the study was responsible for the exclusion of 28% of patients. The use of oral anticoagulants at the time of the procedure excluded a further 9% of patients.

EXCLUSION CRITERIA BASED ON TECHNOLOGY

Most randomized pharmacologic studies on restenosis have specifically excluded the use of new devices. This means that when the results are published, a possible criticism will be that they do not reflect and therefore do not apply to the real world. Statistically, as long as the use of new devices occurs in less than 10% of randomized patients, dealing with them is not a problem. Once they reach 50%, however, stratification of patients according to treatment modality would be required. Future trials are thus likely to include all new technologies, apart from stents. It is of interest, however, that in the ongoing HELVETICA study, where the use of new technology is allowed, these only occur in 4% of the patients entered, so there is no need for posthoc stratification.

Stringent entry criteria designed to minimize the randomization of high-risk patients mean that only a minority of eligible patients may be recruited for a particular study. In the MERCATOR study, for example, 1755 patients were screened but only 478 (27.2%)

were actually recruited into the study. The reasons for exclusion included a history of sustained essential hypertension (271 patients, 15.4%) and previous and/or failed PTCA at the same site (268 patients, 15.3%), as well as a variety of other less frequent factors (Table 12C.1). In the PARK study even fewer screened patients were enrolled into the study (704/5636, 12.5%).

The exclusion of high-risk patients may have a significant influence, however, on the power of a trial. Historically, the loss in MLD during follow-up has been around 0.4 mm (7). For the trial power calculations, for a 30% reduction in the treatment group the expected loss would be 0.25 mm. For all the recent trials, however, the MLD loss has been much lower (CARPORT 0.31 mm, MERCATOR 0.30 mm, PARK 0.26 mm), resulting in a reduction in the power of the trials and making it more difficult to demonstrate significant benefit. This is because they have taken the minimalist approach toward patient recruitment—only enrolling patients with single-vessel disease and stable angina pectoris and specifically excluding high-risk patients such as those with recent myocardial infarction and unstable angina.

Inclusion of such patients should increase the loss in MLD during follow-up and hence increase the power of a trial. Thus future trials are likely to take a "maximalist" approach by including patients with multivessel disease, unstable angina, recent myocardial infarction, and previous PTCA and restenosis. In the ongoing HELVETICA trial, for example, only difficult unstable patients are included, which will hopefully increase the power of the study.

In addition, often little indication is given of the proportion of eligible patients entered into the study and the likely outcome of patients excluded from the study. Therefore the results of a study may not apply to the large proportion of patients seen in clinical practice.

Timing of Randomization

The optimal timing of randomization is also unclear. Do you randomize the patients before the procedure as in the PARK, HELVETICA, and CARPORT studies, or do you only randomize them once the procedure has been successfully performed as in the MERCATOR and MARCATOR studies? In the PARK and CARPORT studies, since the mechanism of drug action implied that it would prevent both acute occlusion caused by platelet aggregation–induced thrombus formation and late restenosis caused by platelet aggregation–induced hyperplasia, trial medication was started before the procedure, that is, before wall injury occurred. This had major consequences for the definition of the clinical endpoint. On the one hand, all failure between first balloon inflation and the end of the procedure could have been influenced by the trial medication and were therefore counted as clinical endpoints. On the other hand, as the aim of this trial was to study the effect of ketanserin on the inhibition of neointimal hyperplasia following balloon wall injury, it seemed reasonable to exclude from the analysis of the main clinical endpoints those patients in whom no balloon inflation had occurred.

In the MERCATOR and MARCATOR studies, concern was voiced over the possible hypotensive effect of the medication if it was given prior to the procedure. The debate centered around whether the medication should be given prior to the procedure and any perioperative hypotension treated with volume expansion or whether it would be safer to administer the study medication after the procedure. Since preliminary animal experiments had shown no major difference in inhibition of neointimal proliferation whether the drug was given 1 hour before or within 2 days after wall injury, we were able to screen patients before the procedure but only enroll those who had undergone a successful coronary angioplasty into the study. This approach eliminated problems relating to the influence

of the drug on the success of the procedure but may also have introduced selection bias. For example, if the investigator noted the presence of thrombus postangioplasty, this may have influenced the likelihood of a patient being subsequently entered into the study. This may explain why in a multivariate analysis of the CARPORT study the presence of thrombus was associated with the relative loss, whereas this was not the case in the MERCATOR study.

Timing of Follow-Up Duration

One of the consequences of having systematic, follow-up angiography at 6 months is that it distorts the natural occurrence of clinical endpoints (reinterventions). As a consequence, all indications for a revascularization procedure that have been triggered by the 6-month repeat angiogram are counted as endpoints, provided that the indication is also substantiated by anginal symptoms or positive findings at exercise testing. In the CARPORT study clinical events were counted up to the 6-month angiogram minus 2 weeks. This meant that the therapeutic implications of the diagnostic angiogram were circumvented, resulting in a lower rate of events compared with similar studies. This led to two problems. Firstly, it reduced the power of the study to detect a difference in restenosis, and secondly, it may have tempted investigators to await recatheterisation before further therapy. To overcome these problems, in the MERCATOR study we increased the cutoff point to 7 months. This, however, tended to overestimate the clinical event rate by including cosmetic dilatations following the 6-month angiograms and thus introduced a different problem into the analysis. For the PARK study we again extended the study to 7 months, but excluded cosmetic dilatation by insisting that for a repeat PTCA to be a clinical event the clinician had to justify his decision on the basis of objective evidence of ischemia. Furthermore, the decision to redo the PTCA was counted as a clinical event

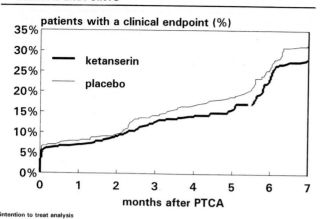

PARK
CUMULATIVE DISTRIBUTION of
CLINICAL ENDPOINTS

intention to treat analysis

Figure 12C.1. Cumulative distribution curve of clinical endpoints for the Post Angioplasty Restenosis Ketanserin (PARK) trial. Note the distribution of endpoints and how the timing of recatheterization may influence the results. (Reprinted by permission from Serruys PW et al. Circulation 1993;88:1588–1601.)

even if it did not physically occur during the follow-up period. This did not completely solve the problem, however, as certain patients were marked down for repeat interventions that never occurred for a variety of reasons. Thus the optimal time for restudy may play a role in the clinical endpoints as shown graphically in Figure 12C.1.

It may be best in the future therefore to have a primary endpoint at 7 months and a secondary endpoint at 12 months.

Definition of Primary Endpoints

The primary goal in restenosis trials is an improvement in the short- and long-term clinical outcome in patients undergoing PTCA. It is assumed that the improvement in clinical outcome relates directly to the prevention of the stenosis recurrence. This may not be completely true, however.

CLINICAL ENDPOINTS

For the MERCATOR study as our primary clinical endpoints we chose a combination of the major untoward clinical events, namely, death, myocardial infarction, referral for coronary artery bypass surgery, or an indication for repeat angioplasty. The advantages are obvious in that if the endpoint is based on these so-called "hard" criteria, the endpoint

is evaluable in all randomized patients and leads to simple effect estimates with corresponding 95% confidence intervals. Because hard endpoints only occur, however, in approximately 20% of cases, our ability to detect even a 50% difference in restenosis rate between intervention and control requires a very large sample size with all the associated logistic problems. Surrogate, soft endpoints such as recurrence of angina or noninvasive evidence of myocardial ischemia may also be introduced to increase the event rate to 50% and hence to reduce the sample size required (Table 12C.2). Because of the subjective nature of these, however, bias is introduced into the study.

For example, in trials testing pharmacologic compounds with possible antiischemic or antianginal effects unrelated to postinjury hyperplasia, subjective, soft endpoints may be misleading and obscure the reasons for observed improvement. In the MERCATOR study fewer patients in the cilazapril-treated group experienced anginal pain during exercise testing compared with the control group, despite similar workloads, double product, and ST-segment changes (Table 12C.3). This was regardless of angiographically similar restenosis rates suggesting that cilazapril had no effect on intimal hyperplasia but perhaps

Table 12C.2.
Total Number of Events and Ranking Scale in the CARPORT Study[a]

	Total No. of Events During 6-Month Follow-Up				Ranking of Clinical Status 6 Months After PTCA			
	Control N = 346		GR32191B N = 351		Control N = 346		GR32191B N = 351	
Death								
-Late	6		4					
-All	6	(2%)	4	(1%)	6	(2%)	4	(1%)
Myocardial infarction								
-Procedural	5		5					
-Early	11		7					
-Late	6		6					
-All	22	(6%)	18	(5%)	22	(6%)	18	(5%)
CABG								
-Procedural	3		7					
-Early	5		2					
-Late	18		18					
-All	26	(8%)	27	(8%)	19	(6%)	22	(6%)
Repeat angioplasty								
-Early	9		6					
-Late	59		54					
-All	68	(20%)	60	(17%)	52	(15%)	49	(14%)
*@CCS IV	5	(2%)	1	(0.3%)	5	(2%)	1	(0.3%)
*@CCS III	19	(6%)	18	(5%)	11	(3%)	11	(3%)
*@CCS II	36	(11%)	47	(14%)	23	(7%)	30	(9%)
*@CCS I	26	(8%)	32	(9%)	14	(4%)	19	(5%)
None	254	(75%)	249	(72%)	194	(56%)	197	(56%)

[a]From Serruys PW et al. Circulation 1991; 84:1568–1580 with permission.

*, For 687 patients alive at 6-month follow-up; @, secondary endpoint; *CCS,* Canadian Cardiovascular Society angina classification.

Table 12C.3.
Exercise Test Results of 564 Patients Randomized in the MERCATOR Study[a]

	Control N = 291 Pts		Cilazapril N = 273 Pts		P Value
Maximum workload (Watts)	146 ± 39		151 ± 44		NS
Exercise time (sec)	446 ± 124		454 ± 127		NS
Systolic blood pressure at peak exercise (mm Hg)	196 ± 27		192 ± 28		NS
Heart rate at peak exercise (bpm)	142 ± 22		142 ± 21		NS
Double product (mm Hg 100/bpm)	279 ± 65		275 ± 66		NS
ST deviation >1 mm	102	(36%)	99	(37%)	NS
Anginal symptoms during test	74	(25%)	42	(15%)	0.03
Combination of ST >1 mm and symptoms	39	(13%)	25	(9%)	NS

[a]From MERCATOR study group. Circulation 1992; 86:100–101 with permission.

Pts, Patients.

may have affected endothelial function. A similar effect was seen in the PARK study where patients receiving ketanserin demonstrated a trend toward a lower incidence of revascularization procedures (77 versus 95 in the control group). This may have been secondary to the arteriolar dilating effect of ketanserin, resulting in left ventricular unloading, or perhaps to its effect on rheologic parameters, resulting in increased coronary blood flow.

A further confounding variable is the fact that not all variables are of equal importance. For example, death is of a different order of magnitude from myocardial infarction, which in turn is of a different order of magnitude from repeat angioplasty. Furthermore, the total count of events only gives a general impression of complications as events are not mutually exclusive and may overlap. A patient may, for example, sustain an acute occlusion resulting in myocardial infarction and subsequent death despite emergency coronary artery bypass grafting; in terms of total count of events this patient might be counted four times.

Ranking endpoints in terms of relative descending importance (Table 12C.2) may overcome some of these problems, but the problem of quantifying each complication and its relative importance then arises. For example, how many myocardial infarctions are equivalent to death? Such methods are standard in the field of decision analysis, however, and a similar composite endpoint has been recently proposed for late follow-up after coronary angioplasty (8, 9). Although such an approach requires prospective valuation, it clearly provides the ability to combine both clinical and angiographic endpoints and may thus be useful in early, phase 2 clinical trials to improve statistical power.

In attempting to address these questions other models have also been proposed. Friedrich and colleagues showed that the constant-hazard model cannot be applied to coronary interventional techniques as the risk is not constant but varies over time (10). Furthermore, this rate combines two underlying hazards: an early time-dependent hazard caused by restenosis of the target vessel and a more constant hazard caused by the progression of coronary atherosclerosis or comorbid disease. This temporal sequence of events is highest at the time of the initial procedure and at the follow-up catheterization, where there is an artificial increase in the rate of events (Fig. 12C.1).

An alternative means of overcoming some of these problems is also with the use of event-free survival curves. These provide in a graphic form information on the time course, as well as on the incidence of endpoints.

NONINVASIVE EVALUATION OF RESTENOSIS

As far as detection of restenosis by noninvasive diagnostic tests is concerned, it can generally be said that an abnormal exercise ECG response or myocardial perfusion defect on a thallium-201 scintigram is usually associated with either an angiographically demonstrable restenosis of the dilated segment, a functionally inadequate original dilation, or the presence of additional disease. The sensitivity and specificity of the test may therefore be increased by performing the test prior to the procedure to document a baseline result, immediately after angioplasty to filter out the presence of additional disease or inadequate functional dilation, and subsequently at 6 months to document restenosis.

Logistic problems arise, however, in trying to perform the exercise test. Firstly, most of the centers participating in large multicenter studies are regional referral centers draining large areas, whose first contact with the referred patient is at the time of the procedure. It is logistically difficult for them therefore to ensure that all patients have an exercise test prior to the procedure. Secondly, problems arise in performing the exercise test immediately after the procedure with doubts raised as to the safety of this policy. Thus insurmountable difficulties arise in trying to arrange the exercise test prior to and immediately after angioplasty. The concept is advanced, however, that perhaps we do not need to do this and, since all we are doing is comparing two groups—an active and a placebo group, perhaps we should just exercise test all patients at 6 months. For the reasons outlined above, however, the positive predictive value of late treadmill testing varies from 39 to 64% (Table 12C.4), making it difficult to make valid intergroup observations. The only useful role we have found for the exercise test is to substantiate the need for a repeat therapeutic PTCA at follow-up.

Similar arguments can also be used against the role radioisotopes. The need for pre-, immediate, post-, and follow-up scans also raises two additional issues. Firstly, objections are raised regarding the repeated use of radioisotopes and the long-term result of doing so. Secondly, problems arise in the objective assessment of the results as there is still no agreed standardized procedure for image acquisition and interpretation.

For all the above reasons exercise testing or thallium scintigraphy are of little value in the assessment of long-term restenosis. Their only role may be to substantiate the therapeutic procedure if repeat angiography is suggestive of a significant restenosis.

ANGIOGRAPHIC ENDPOINTS

The most accurate way to quantify the proliferative response as part of restenosis would be with the direct measurement of neointimal thickening following coronary intervention. This is not, however, currently possible in man, although the advent of new imaging modalities such as angioscopy and, more especially, intravascular ultrasound may one day make it possible. For debulking devices that may alter both acute dimensional gain and the later proliferative response, currently quantitative coronary angiography is the most objective and reproducible method available to describe the changes in stenosis geometry following intervention. Although it only measures the process indirectly without defining its nature (recoil, organized mural thrombus, neointimal hyperplasia), it has nonetheless become the accepted gold standard in documenting restenosis.

There is still, however, no agreed on angiographic definition of restenosis (11, 12). To date there have been a total of 13 different definitions used in the literature, but none have become widely accepted. Although the clinician is best served by the "present/not present" assessment of restenosis, the biologic process of restenosis itself may be best analyzed by measuring the ab-

Table 12C.4.
Detection of Restenosis by Exercise Treadmill Testing[a]

Author	Angiographic Follow-Up %	Restenosis %	PPV %	NPV %	Timing of Test
O'Keefe	100	13	29	73	<1 month
Scholl	83	12	40	27	1 month
Wijns[b]	74	35	50	65	3–7 weeks
Wijns[b]	89	40	60	52	3–8 weeks
Bengston	96	51	39	84	6 months
Rosing	100	34	47	76	8 months
Ernst	100	4	50	95	4–8 months
Honan	88	58	57	64	6 months
Scholl	83	12	64	50	6 months

[a]Modified from Califf et al. Restenosis: the clinical issues. In: Topol EJ, ed. Textbook of interventional cardiology. Philadelphia: WB Saunders, 1990.

[b]Thoraxcenter

PPV, Positive predictive value; *NPV*, negative predictive value.

solute angiographic dimensions on a continuous scale. This is for two main reasons. Firstly, as we have previously demonstrated, all lesions undergo restenosis to some extent during follow-up in a Gaussian distribution. Secondly, if we treat restenosis as a continuous variable, more information can be gleaned from the available data regarding the underlying process. Furthermore, the use of a continuous variable in statistical analysis allows us to reduce the number of patients required to demonstrate benefit in a specific study by two-thirds. For example, if treatment reduces the loss of luminal diameter from 0.40 mm under placebo to 0.25 mm under active medication (SD = 0.5 mm), 233 patients per group would be required to have a power of 90%. The above reduction corresponds to restenosis rates (defined as a loss of minimal luminal diameter of 0.72 mm) of 25% and 17.5%, respectively. This difference, however, can be statistically detected with a power of 90% with 620 patients per treatment group. Thus the quantitative outcome determined from direct measurements of continuous variables can be evaluated statistically with only one-third the number of patients required for the categorical outcome.

The minimal luminal diameter provides more reliable and meaningful information than percentage diameter stenosis with regard to the hemodynamic significance of a coronary artery lesion and has been shown to correlate at follow-up with the recurrence of angina or exercise-induced myocardial ischemia (1). The minimal luminal diameter at follow-up thus best describes the lesion severity at this point in time, while the process of restenosis can best be addressed by measuring the changes in luminal diameter from postintervention to follow-up in pharmacologic studies looking at restenosis. In studies examining devices, however, because of differences in the initial gain/loss, it is impossible to use the change in luminal diameter at follow-up and is best to look at a static parameter such as the MLD at follow-up to assess restenosis.

Are Quantitative Angiographic Parameters a Good Surrogate for Clinical Events?

One of our convictions is that the difference in minimal luminal diameter at follow-up between two populations will be translated into clinical terms. This has been generally true, as illustrated recently by the results of the BENESTENT and STRESS trials. A discordance, however, was noted in the CAVEAT I trial wherein a modest improvement in luminal dimensions at follow-up after directional atherectomy compared with PTCA did not "translate" into clinical benefit.

A more detailed analysis is available for the CARPORT study. In that study the mean difference in coronary diameter between postangioplasty and follow-up angiogram was similar in the control and GR32191B groups (-0.31 ± 0.54 mm and -0.31 ± 0.55 mm, respectively), and this was reflected in similar rates of clinical events. If you separate the population into two, however, on the basis of symptoms or positive ergometry, the cumulative distribution curves for change in minimal luminal diameter clearly separate (Fig. 12C.2), suggesting that the change in MLD may indeed reflect clinical events. Furthermore, in the MERCATOR study when the patient population was stratified according to the minimal lumen diameter at follow-up (Table 12C.5), the percentage of patients reaching one of the predefined clinical endpoints was as high as 65% in the worst category (MLD at follow-up <1.15), whereas the percentage of event-free patients ranged from 63 to 78% in the other categories. Additionally, 41% of the patients in the worst versus only 6% in the best anatomic category had reintervention irrespective of the initial dilatation site. Besides the prognostic value, the anatomic results also had a clear functional impact because only 2% of the patients in the best anatomic category had a positive exercise test versus 26% in the worst.

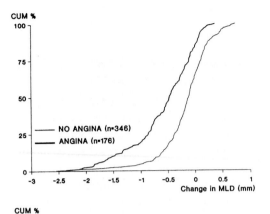

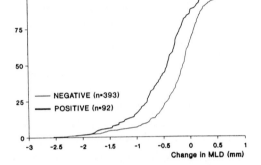

Figure 12C.2. Top panel. Cumulative distribution (CUM %) curve for change in minimal luminal diameter (MLD) for symptomatic and asymptomatic patients at follow-up angiography. **Bottom panel.** Cumulative distribution (CUM %) curve for change in minimal luminal diameter (MLD) for patients with positive and negative ergometry at follow-up angiography. (Reprinted by permission from Serruys PW et al. Circulation 1991; 84:1568–1580.)

Limitations of Differences in MLD Between Various Trials

Over the last few years it has become apparent that the loss in MLD in different trials could vary considerably, and in the placebo groups the loss in MLD ranged from 0.24 to 0.36 mm. The reasons for this are unclear, although one possibility is that these differences in mean luminal diameter at follow-up reflect differences in baseline demographic data. Factors such as the percentage of recruited patients in angina class 4, patients with recent onset of angina, unstable patients, and diabetic patients and the frequency of total occlusion have a major impact on the loss in MLD at follow-up. Popma and colleagues suggest that in future trials high-risk patients not be excluded to therefore avoid a misrepresentation of the population of typical patients undergoing angioplasty (9). Furthermore, they suggest that by selecting elective patients the expected late loss in MLD may be reduced, resulting in a requirement for a larger study population.

Limitations of Quantitative Angiography

Quantitative coronary angiography (QCA) provides an outline of the vessel lumen and not the vessel wall, which is where the un-

Table 12C.5.
Prognostic Value of Minimal Luminal Diameter at Follow-Up in the Preprotocol MERCATOR Population Divided Into Five Equal Segments[a]

MLD Follow-Up (mm)	Exercise Test		Clinical Outcome							
	<1 mm STT Changes and No Chest Pain	≥1 mm STT Changes and Chest Pain	MI		Reintervention		Angina		None	
<1.10	70 (75%)	24 (26%)	5	(4%)	49	(41%)	24	(20%)	41	(35%)
1.10 to 1.39	88 (88%)	12 (12%)	1	(1%)	18	(15%)	25	(21%)	74	(63%)
1.39 to 1.63	103 (90%)	11 (10%)	2	(2%)	10	(8%)	31	(26%)	77	(64%)
1.63 to 1.91	99 (93%)	8 (7%)	1	(1%)	7	(6%)	21	(15%)	89	(75%)
1.91 or more	111 (98%)	2 (2%)	1	(1%)	7	(6%)	18	(15%)	94	(78%)
	471 Pts	57 Pts	10 Pts		91 Pts		119 Pts		375 Pts	

[a]From MERCATOR study group. Circulation 1992; 86:100–101 with permission.

MLD, Minimal luminal diameter; *mm*, millimeter; *MI*, myocardial infarction; *Pts*, patients.

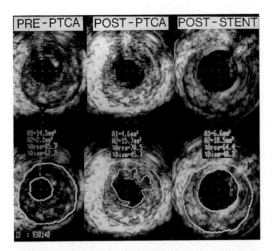

Figure 12C.3. Ultrasound imaging prior to balloon angio-plasty and following angiographically successful balloon dilatation. It can be clearly seen post-PTCA that the angio-graphic success is as a result of eccentric tears in the vessel wall with only a small increase in the residual luminal area (pseudosuccess). Following successful stent implantation there is a good residual luminal area. (Images courtesy of Dr. C. diMario, Thoraxcenter, Erasmus University, Rotterdam, The Netherlands.)

derlying pathologic process is occurring. Thus much of what may be an angiographic success may turn out to be a pseudosuccess, perhaps because of cracks and dissection planes in the vessel wall giving the impression of a successful result whereas in reality there may be little increase in the actual luminal area (Fig. 12C.3). Thus a split in the vessel wall may provide an angiographically successful result (a pseudosuccess), but subsequent apposition of the split-wall layers may result in an angiographic restenosis (a pseudorestenosis), a lesion being classified as restenosis whereas in fact it was never an actual success.

Thus we may have to separate the clinical outcome, which may be measured by QCA, from the pathologic process occurring in the vessel wall. Whether new concepts in the visualisation of the vessel wall such as angioscopy or, perhaps more importantly, intravascular ultrasound can refine our understanding of the underlying pathologic

process is still unclear but holds a great deal of promise.

Ideal Trial

As outlined above, although randomized studies are the best means we have of comparing the acute and long-term results of different interventional devices and the impact of pharmacologic therapies, they remain limited by inherent logistic problems. Our ideal randomized trial would be based purely on clinical follow-up of hard endpoints at 1 year. This would assess the effect of the intervention, whether it is drug therapy or a device compared with stand-alone angioplasty without the interference from the recatheterization procedure.

MATCHING STUDIES

In view of the large number of pharmacologic and mechanical interventions available to us and the time, energy, and financial burdens involved in conducting a large randomized trial, we have developed the concept of matching to use as a surrogate for a randomized study. Matching may offer insight into the effects of different interventional techniques, screen devices, and yield statistically helpful information such as a required sample size for the proper design of a randomized trial.

The principles of matching by quantitative angiography are threefold. Firstly, the angiographic dimensions of matched lesions are assumed to be identical. Secondly, the observed differences between the two identical lesions must be within the range of system-analysis reproducibility (0.1 mm; 1 SD). Finally, the reference diameter of the lesions to be matched must be selected to be within a range of ±0.3 mm (3 SD; confidence limits 99%). Matching can also be extended to include lesion location and clinical parameters such as male sex, stable/unstable angina, diabetes, total occlusions, and other risk factors that may confound the incidence of restenosis.

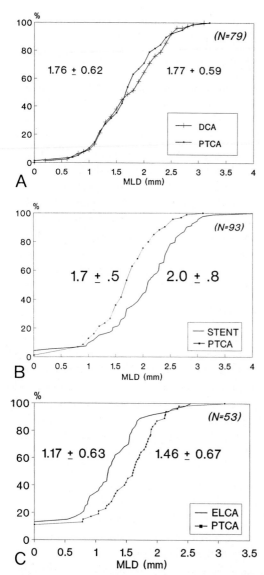

Figure 12C.4. Cumulative distribution curves of MLD at follow-up for matched populations. **A.** Atherectomy versus PTCA. **B.** Stent implantation versus PTCA. **C.** Excimer laser versus PTCA.

Matching in Action

We have used the principles outlined above to assess late luminal renarrowing in atherectomy, stent implantation, and excimer laser versus balloon angioplasty (Fig. 12C.4).

In atherectomy versus balloon angioplasty we demonstrated that matching for clinical and angiographic variables resulted in two comparable groups with identical baseline stenosis characteristics (13). Atherectomy resulted in a more pronounced increase in minimal luminal diameter than did balloon angioplasty (1.17 ± 0.29 to 2.44 ± 0.42 mm versus 1.21 ± 0.38 to 2.00 ± 0.36 mm), but this favorable immediate result was subsequently lost during late angiographic follow-up, as the minimal luminal diameter at follow-up did not differ between the two groups (1.76 ± 0.62 versus 1.77 ± 0.59 mm, atherectomy versus balloon angioplasty) (Fig. 12C.4A). This suggests that in matched populations, atherectomy induces a greater initial gain in minimal luminal diameter than balloon angioplasty but that the greater vascular wall injury induced by this device is associated with a more pronounced late loss. The results of this study were subsequently reflected in the CCAT and CAVEAT studies.

Using coronary stenting we demonstrated that Wallstent implantation results in a superior immediate increase in minimal luminal diameter (from 1.22 ± 0.34 to 2.49 ± 0.40 mm) compared with balloon angioplasty (from 1.21 ± 0.29 to 1.92 ± 0.35 mm) (14). Despite a greater decrease in minimal luminal diameter after Wallstent implantation compared with balloon angioplasty (0.48 ± 0.74 versus 0.20 ± 0.46 mm), the minimal luminal diameter at follow-up was significantly greater after stent implantation (2.01 ± 0.75 versus 1.72 ± 0.54 mm) (Fig. 12C.4B). Although different stents were evaluated, our results paralleled those of the recently reported BENESTENT and STRESS trials.

Using excimer laser we demonstrated that despite similar acute increases in minimal luminal diameter (from 0.73 ± 0.47 to 1.77 ± 0.41 mm, excimer laser, versus 0.74 ± 0.46 to 1.78 ± 0.34 mm, coronary angioplasty), the minimal luminal diameter after excimer laser was significantly lower at follow-up (1.17 ± 0.63 versus 1.46 ± 0.63 mm) (Fig. 12C.4C), suggesting that in successfully treated matched coronary lesions there is reduced long-term efficacy after excimer laser compared with balloon angioplasty. Whether these preliminary results will be reflected in clinical outcome will be answered in the ongoing AMRO randomized study of excimer laser versus balloon angioplasty.

Limitations of Matching

The major limitation of a matching study is its retrospective design and the inevitable presence of selection bias. It controls for bias only in those variables taken into account. It is not possible to match for all variables because of practical difficulties in finding patients who meet all the matching criteria. Moreover, if categories of matching are relatively crude, there may be room for substantial differences between matched groups. For example, if clinical variables such as unstable angina or perhaps diabetes, which are known to predispose to a higher restenosis rate, are not included in the matching, substantial differences will occur between the two groups that may influence the validity of statistical comparisons.

Role in Clinical Decision Making

The use of matching studies as a surrogate for randomized studies offers the potential to rapidly screen a number of devices and to assess which are most likely to represent advances in balloon angioplasty. These can then be examined in larger randomized studies. Furthermore, matching yields statistically helpful information regarding the proper design of subsequent randomized trials such as required sample size.

REGISTRIES

The advantage of a registry is that data are collated in a coordinating center that allows information to be gleaned regarding the success and acute complications in a self-selected group of patients from a variety of centers with varying expertise. It therefore gives an impression of the acute results at the ground level and may, if adequate follow-up is encouraged, give an indication of the long-term restenosis rate. Information is obtained at little expense in terms of time or money as it is normally freely available at each institution.

There are a number of major limitations to extrapolating the results from registries to the general population, however. Firstly, the patients are entered on an ad hoc basis by the operator and may not be representative of the totality of patients on whom the device was used. This may explain, for example, why the *reported complication rates from registries are consistently lower than the complication rates observed in clinical practice.* Secondly, there are usually no central angiographic core lab and no independent verification or audit of the data supplied by the investigator to ensure accuracy and reproducibility. Furthermore, the angiographic analysis is normally performed by the operator with visual assessment of the coronary angiogram, a technique introducing bias and inaccuracies. Finally, the analysis is usually performed on a post hoc basis with multiple statistical comparisons being made on a small number of selected patient subgroups.

Because of the inherent limitations outlined above it is difficult to interpret the data from the various registries and to draw meaningful conclusions (15). The only useful information that may be gleaned from registries may be some idea about trends in various patient subgroups; for example, that calcification may not be good for atherectomy.

EXPERIENCE-BASED COMMON SENSE

Whatever the results of large randomized studies, it is ultimately the skill and judgment of the individual doctor in assessing and treating a particular lesion in an individual patient that will determine the safety and efficacy of the procedure. The main advantage of experience-based common sense is that it will limit cardiologists to the use of specific devices that are safe in their hands on specific lesions in their particular circumstances. Experience-based common sense, however, will tell them little regarding long-term restenosis.

Furthermore, there are a large number of other potential limitations to experience-based common sense. Virtually all new devices have a steep learning curve so that an individual doctor may never do enough cases to get past this learning curve. Thus an operator who has never attained a sufficient level of skill in using the device will be prejudiced against it and perhaps only use it in specific patient subgroups. This combination of individual expertise and selection bias means that the safety and efficacy of particular devices can never be adequately quantified and that any differences between devices would be extremely difficult to prove.

SUMMARY

Adverse coronary anatomy, acute occlusion, and long-term restenosis remain major limitations of coronary angioplasty. Over the last 5 years atherectomy, stenting, and laser techniques have been introduced as potentially safer alternatives to balloon angioplasty with improved short- and long-term results. Considerable difficulty exists, however, in making valid comparisons between the different modalities with regard to the above outcome measures. Device registries may be useful for the initial assessment of the initial safety and success of the device. Matching studies may help to screen devices for subsequent randomized studies to delineate the precise role of each new device. We must never forget, however, that irrespective of the results of registries and matching and randomized studies, the final arbiter of the success or failure of the procedure will be the cardiologist and the team treating the individual patient.

REFERENCES

1. Rensing BJ, Hermans WRM, Deckers JW, de Feyter PJ, Serruys PJ. Which angiographic parameter best describes functional status 6 months after successful single-vessel coronary angioplasty? J Am Coll Cardiol 1993;21:317–324.
2. MERCATOR study group. Does the new angiotensin converting enzyme inhibitor Cilazapril prevent restenosis after percutaneous transluminal coronary angioplasty? Results of the MERCATOR study: a multicenter, randomized, double-blind placebo-controlled trial. Circulation 1992; 86:100–110.
3. The MARCATOR study group. Angiotension converting enzyme inhibition and restenosis: the final analysis of the MARCATOR trial. Circulation 1992;86(Suppl):I-53 (abstract).
4. Serruys PW, Rutsch W, Heyndrickx GR et al. Prevention of restenosis after percutaneous transluminal coronary angioplasty with thromboxane A$_2$-receptor blockade. A randomized double-blind, placebo-controlled trial. Circulation 1991;84:1568–1580.
5. Serruys PW, Klein W, Tijssen JPG et al. Evaluation of ketanserin in the prevention of restenosis after percutaneous transluminal coronary angioplasty: a multicenter randomized double-blind placebo-controlled trial. The Post-Angioplasty Restenosis Ketanserin (PARK) trial. Circulation 1993;88:1588–1601.
6. Gibson CM, Kuntz RE, Nobuyoshi M, Rosner B, Baim DS. Lesion-to-lesion independence of restenosis after treatment by conventional angioplasty, stenting or directional atherectomy. Circulation 1993;87:1123–1129.
7. Serruys PW, Luijten HE, Beatt KJ et al. Incidence of restenosis after successful coronary angioplasty: a time-related phenomenon. A quantitative angiographic study in 342 consecutive patients at 1, 2, 3, and 4 months. Circulation 1988;77:361–371.
8. Califf RM, Topol EJ, Stack RS et al. An evaluation of combination thrombolytic therapy and timing of cardiac catheterization in acute myocardial infarction: the TAMI-5 randomized trial. Circulation 1991;83:1543–1556.
9. Popma JM, Califf RM, Topol EJ. Clinical trials of restenosis after coronary angioplasty. Circulation 1991;84:1426-36.
10. Friedrich SP, Gordon PC, Leidig GA et al. Clinical events following new interventional devices are determined by time-dependent hazards. Circulation 1993;86:I-785 (abstract).
11. Beatt KJ, Serruys PW, Hugenholtz PG. Restenosis after coronary angioplasty: new standards for clinical studies. J Am Coll Cardiol 1990;15:491–498.
12. Serruys PW, Foley DP, de Feyter PJ. Restenosis after coronary angioplasty: a proposal of new comparative approaches based on quantitative angiography. Br Heart J 1992;68:417–424.
13. Umans VA, Hermans WRM, Foley DP, Strikwerda S, van der Brand M, de Jaegere PP, de Feyter PJ et al. Restenosis after directional coronary atherectomy and balloon angioplasty: a comparative analysis based on matched lesions. J Am Coll Cardiol 1993;21:1382–1390.
14. de Jaegere PP, Hermans WR, Rensing BJ, Strauss BH, de Feyter PJ, Serruys PW. Matching based on quantitative coronary angiography as a surrogate for randomized studies: comparison between stent implantation and balloon angioplasty of native coronary artery lesions. Am Heart J 1993;125:310–319.
15. Topol EJ. Promises and pitfalls of new devices for coronary artery disease. Circulation 1992;83:689–694.

CLINICAL PROBLEMS

13. Evaluating Stenosis Severity: Quantitative Angiography, Coronary Flow Reserve, and Intravascular Ultrasound

STEVEN E. NISSEN, E. MURAT TUZCU, ANTHONY C. De FRANCO, and DAVID J. MOLITERNO

Accurate quantitative and qualitative assessment of potential target lesions plays a central and critical role in interventional decision making. Traditionally, evaluation has consisted of simple visual inspection of the angiogram to estimate the percentage reduction in luminal diameter or cross-sectional area. This approach relies on visual comparison of the lumen size in the culprit lesion and an adjacent "normal" reference segment. After defining the target lesions, most operators also employ subjective visual criteria to estimate absolute vessel caliber, the degree of curvature, and the extent of involvement of side branches.

More recently, practitioners have employed qualitative evaluation of culprit lesion morphology to assist selection of the preferred revascularization technique. The most important morphologic criteria include identification of intraluminal filling defects suggestive of thrombus and visual assessment of the presence or absence of fluoroscopic calcification. However, nearly all morphologic criteria rely on subjective visual methods for lesions classification. Thus visual inspection of the angiogram determines whether revascularization is warranted and guides selection of the optimal type and size of interventional device.

During the intervention, the traditional approach to percutaneous revascularization also employs visual assessment by fluoroscopy or digital angiography to guide the procedure and evaluate its success. Accordingly, the decision to employ a larger balloon, perform additional atherectomy cuts, upsize to a larger Rotablator burr, or place a coronary stent has typically depended on visual analysis of angiographic images. Recognition of potentially catastrophic complications such as extensive dissection or intraluminal thrombus has also relied on subjective visual criteria.

Despite the nearly universal acceptance of "eyeball angiography," disquieting reports have appeared over several decades demonstrating important limitations for simple visual assessment of coronary lesions (1–7). A series of reports have questioned the accuracy of visual evaluation of angiograms as means to quantify lesion severity, classify vessel morphology, assess calcification, and evaluate procedural success.

Recent technical advances in imaging and computer technology have enabled development of more objective techniques for lesion assessment. Two approaches, quantitative coronary angiography and intravascular ultrasound, are now widely applied in research and clinical practice. Although not routinely used in most interventional laboratories, these newer modalities offer important advantages in quantitative and qualitative evaluation of coronary stenoses. A third approach, calculation of coronary flow reserve from digital angiography, is not now commonly used, but offers valuable insights into stenosis evaluation methods. Accordingly, a working knowledge of these techniques is a fundamental requirement of the advanced interventional laboratory.

LIMITATIONS OF VISUAL ASSESSMENT

Despite the universal application of visual analysis of angiograms, careful examination has revealed major deficiencies in this approach to quantitative assessment of coronary lesions. Studies have established that subjective visual interpretation of angiograms exhibits large and clinically significant intraobserver and interobserver variability (6). Other investigations have compared lesion severity by angiography with quantitative histologic examination of necropsy specimens (2, 4, 5). These reports have demonstrated major differences between the apparent angiographic severity of luminal narrowings and postmortem assessment. Importantly, investigators have also documented significant discrepancies between visual assessment of lesion severity and independent measurements of the physiologic effects of the stenoses (7).

The well-documented limitations of visual methods for stenosis quantification originate from several predictable inadequacies. Angiography portrays the complex cross-sectional anatomy of the coronary lesion as a planar silhouette of the contrast-filled vessel lumen. However, both necropsy studies and intravascular ultrasound demonstrate that coronary obstructions are often complex with a markedly distorted or eccentric luminal shape. Mechanical coronary interventions further complicate this intrinsic problem by fracturing or dissecting the atheroma within the lesion, thereby exaggerating the magnitude of luminal eccentricity (8). Thus the angiographic appearance of a complex post-intervention vessel often consists of an enlarged, although frequently "hazy" lumen. With extensive plaque fracture and increased luminal eccentricity, the hazy, broadened angiographic silhouette of a lu-

men may overestimate the actual vessel diameter and misrepresent the true gain in lumen size.

Limitations of Percent Stenosis

Traditional methods for characterizing lesion severity by angiography depend on visual determination of the percentage reduction in luminal diameter or area at the stenosis site. This process requires estimation of minimum luminal dimensions both within the coronary lesion and at an adjacent, seemingly uninvolved "normal" reference segment. However, necropsy studies often reveal a diffuse, rather than focal, pattern of plaque distribution in atherosclerotic coronary disease (4). A diffusely diseased vessel may contain no truly normal segment from which to precisely calculate the percent stenosis. In such cases visual assessment of the percentage of luminal reduction will underestimate lesion severity.

However, coronary disease may produce vessel ectasia, a phenomenon in which atherosclerosis produces destruction of the media, resulting in pathologic dilation of the involved segment. Segmental ectasia can represent an important confounding variable precluding accurate determination of the percent stenosis. In the presence of an abnormally dilated reference vessel, simple visual inspection will always overestimate the severity of the obstruction. Accordingly, a lesion with an adequate minimum lumen diameter will appear severely stenotic if compared to an adjacent segment with abnormal ectasia. Thus the traditional approach to lesion quantification, which defines the stenosis relative to another vessel segment, can both overestimate and underestimate the luminal narrowing.

QUANTITATIVE CORONARY ANGIOGRAPHY
Historical Background

First described by Brown and Dodge in the late 1970s, quantitative coronary angiography (QCA) was introduced as a more objective measure of lesion severity to supplement subjective visual methods (9). In its original and simplest form, QCA employs computer measurements of manually traced vessel borders to determine the relative lumen size within the lesion and at an adjacent reference segment. Although this calculation yields only a percent stenosis, correction for radiographic magnification permits the method to generate absolute values for lumen diameter. Because quantitative angiography antedates modern digital angiography, QCA was initially applied only to 35-mm cineangiographic film. The original method required projection of a single, selected 35-mm frame on a reflective screen with careful manual tracing of the vessel borders by a trained operator. The traced vessel outlines are subsequently digitized using a hand-operated electronic cursor to enable computer measurement of the arterial diameter and percent diameter reduction.

Initial scientific studies demonstrated several potential benefits of quantitative computer assessment of coronary cineangiography. Proponents demonstrated that the technique significantly reduces intraobserver and interobserver variability in determination of percent stenosis (10). Early investigators also demonstrated excellent short-term reproducibility for serial measurements of arterial dimensions at the same site (11). However, the accuracy of repeated measurements demands a high degree of precision in operator technique, including meticulous attention to angiographic projections and the digitization procedure. Potential sources of error include differences in film type or processing, miscalculation of radiographic magnification, and interobserver differences in tracing vessel borders (12). Serial measurements of the same vessel or lesion also require careful recording of the radiographic projection at the time of initial study with return to these precise angles for subsequent examinations.

Refinements to QCA

Proponents of QCA introduced many improvements to quantitative angiography technique during the decade of the 1980s. Important advances included direct digitization of film using a video camera mounted on the cineangiographic projector. Initially, this refinement did not obviate the requirement for a trained operator to manually trace the arterial contour. However, subsequent development of automated computer methods for edge detection eventually reduced or eliminated the necessity to employ subjective visual methods for identifying vessel borders. The initial applications of automated border determination were notoriously slow and cumbersome, often inaccurate, and frequently required the operator to manually correct the computer interpretation of the arterial borders. More recently, development of increasingly powerful computers and improved algorithms have greatly improved the performance of automated border detection methods (Fig. 13.1). Nevertheless, no currently available computer algorithm can precisely draw the contour of every vessel encountered in interventional practice.

Most early implementations of quantitative angiography relied on a single, carefully chosen angiographic projection to determine lesion diameter and percent stenosis. However, advocates of the QCA technique quickly recognized the eccentric nature of many coronary stenoses and introduced biplane approaches to quantitation of lesion severity. Strictly applied, biplane methods require two mutually orthogonal angiographic projections with border determination and individual correction for radiographic magnification. Biplane algorithms can calculate lesion diameter and percent stenosis as an average of the two views or apply more complex geometric shape models. Although biplane quantitative angiography represents a more rational approach, the difficulty in obtaining optimal radiographic projections limits application to a distinct subset of vessels.

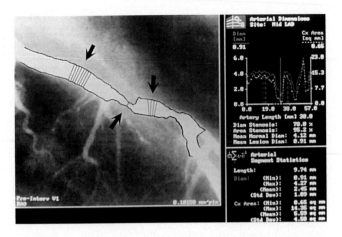

Figure 13.1. Example of quantitative angiography using automated border detection. In the left panel the arrows indicate the proximal reference segment, the minimal luminal diameter in the stenosis, and the distal reference segment. Note that the proximal and distal reference segments are measured at multiple locations and the results averaged. The right panel shows the graphic and numeric display of the results of quantitative measurements.

Absolute Lesion Dimensions

Percent stenosis, as previously stated, represents only a relative measure of the severity of a coronary obstruction. Accordingly, percent stenosis will poorly reflect the severity of the lesion whenever the "normal" reference segment is either diffusely diseased or ectatic. Recognizing this potentially important flaw, many proponents of quantitative angiography have proposed absolute coronary dimensions as a more precise measure of stenosis severity. This value is typically reported as the minimum luminal diameter (MLD), which can be expressed as a linear measurement or converted by simple geometry to a cross-sectional area (Fig. 13.1). Clinical studies have supported this approach, demonstrating that symptomatic patients with positive exercise studies generally exhibit lesional cross-sectional areas of 0.8 mm^2 or less.

Although measurement of MLD is now widely applied, there are several important potential sources of error underlying this approach. For any single lesion, uncertainty exists regarding the amount of myocardium supplied by the vessel. Intuitively, a 0.8-mm^2 stenosis will have greater physiologic impact in a first-order vessel with a large perfusion bed than in a smaller second- or third-order coronary. Further uncertainty arises from complex lesional features, variability in stenosis length, and the presence of serial or branch lesions within a single perfusion bed. Accurate assessment of true MLD generally requires high-quality angiograms obtained using at least two orthogonal coronary projections. Unfortunately, the presence of overlapping vessels and inability to image at extremely oblique angles often complicates attempts to acquire orthogonal views.

Methods of Calibration

Although determination of absolute coronary dimensions requires correction for radiographic magnification, no universally accepted method exists for calibration (13). Several approaches calculate magnification from the known geometry of the radiographic imaging chain. Using a C-arm angiographic system, the heart is placed at the "isocenter," defined as the position in which the x-ray source to object distance (SOD) remains constant throughout the full arc of motion of the gantry. If the position of the image intensifier is also stationary, the magnification remains constant for any angle of view and can be readily calculated from the inverse square law. A variation of this method employs a metallic ball or other object of known size that is imaged at the isocenter position either before or after catheterization. Comparison of the diameter of this target object in the projected cinefilm with its known dimensions allows the operator to precisely determine the magnification factor.

More recently, quantitative methods have favored calibration using measurements of the diameter of the angiographic catheter (Fig. 13.2). This approach employs either manual tracing of the catheter borders or automated edge detection to determine the dimensions of the angiographic catheter. Since the operator can physically measure the nominal external diameter of the catheter, comparison of the apparent diameter with the actual dimensions enables fairly precise calculation of magnification. A refinement of this method employs metallic markers on the catheter placed exactly 1 cm apart. However, this method requires careful orthogonal biplane views with complex mathematical calculations to overcome the confounding effects of catheter foreshortening.

Border Detection Methods

Since most modern quantitative angiography systems employ automated computer methods to determine the vessel and catheter con-

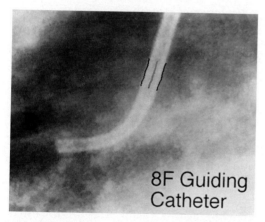

8F Guiding Catheter

Figure 13.2. Method of calibration for quantitative angiography. In this example the computer system identifies the center line of the angiographic catheter. Searching tangentially to the center line, the computer identifies borders of the angiographic catheter. Subsequently, the computer program averages diameter values along this segment of the catheter and compares these values to the known dimensions of the catheter. This process yields an accurate magnification factor enabling accurate determination of the absolute value of the vessel luminal diameter.

tours, the technique for border detection constitutes an important variable (14). Typically, the computer program or operator first determines the centerline of the interrogated vessel. Subsequently, at a series of points along the long axis of the vessel, the computer searches orthogonal to the centerline to generate a density versus distance curve. Next, the computer analyzes the density-distance curve to determine the location of the maximal change in image density (first derivative) or another mathematical descriptor of the vessel border. Finally, the computer applies a smoothing algorithm to convert the rough and sometimes jagged contour into a visually appealing outline.

Most QCA approaches have validated their contour detection scheme by imaging phantom vessels of known dimensions. Evaluation of phantom arteries has demonstrated that the first derivative of the density versus distance curve significantly underestimates actual vessel size, while the second derivative overestimates arterial dimensions. Accordingly, many QCA algorithms utilize a weighted average of the first and second derivatives (empirically determined) to approximate the vessel contour. Unfortunately, the absence of a universally accepted mathematical definition of the vessel border often prevents direct comparison of measurements obtained from different laboratories (PW Serruys, personal communication). The presence of side branches, overlying structures, and nonuniform vessel contours, can interfere with accurate determination of vessel contours. Accordingly, all current approaches to border detection permit and often require manual correction of computer-derived vessel contours.

Videodensitometric Stenosis Sizing

Coronary cineangiography is a two-dimensional projection of a three-dimensional structure. In an effort to more precisely assess the severity of coronary obstructions, an alternative approach to quantitative angiography employs computer density measurements of the degree of coronary opacification to determine percent stenosis (16). This method, commonly termed videodensitometry, compares the summated brightness values for regions of interest (ROI) placed over the stenosis, the reference segment, and "background" to calculate the relative degree of coronary narrowing. This approach yields a percent stenosis measurement, but not absolute coronary dimensions, because no method exists for calibrating the relationship between density and size. Theoretically, videodensitometric methods should accurately reflect the relative narrowing at the target stenosis regardless of the geometric shape of the obstruction. Ideally, this approach would enable precise determination of the percent stenosis from a single angiographic projection, obviating the need for orthogonal biplane views.

In actual practice, videodensitometric methods perform very poorly (17). The assumptions underlying videodensitometric stenosis sizing require a precise and reproducible relationship between the contrast concentration and the brightness of the contrast-containing artery. For radiographic imaging of iodinated contrast, this relationship consists of a logarithmic transfer function, known as the Lambert-Beer Law. However, the simple logarithmic relationship applies only to monochromatic radiation, a requisite not present in currently available angiographic x-ray systems (18). The markedly polychromatic characteristics of radiation in the catheterization laboratory produce an unpredictable curvilinear relationship between density and contrast concentration. Other important non-linearities confound the densitometric method, including scatter and veiling glare in the image intensifier and camera optics, respectively. If videodensitometric methods utilize cinefilm, a characteristic nonlinear density-exposure relationship of film (Hurter and Driffield curve) further impairs accuracy.

The mathematic assumptions underlying videodensitometry also require a known or uniform background density. In actual practice the background density overlying the coronary is unpredictable and includes superimposed structures ranging from lung to bone density. Accordingly, some investigators have tried to employ digital subtraction techniques to attempt to eliminate inhomogeneity of the background prior to densitometry. Unfortunately, temporal subtraction techniques introduce another large potential source of error, misregistration artifact produced by slight patient motion during the time between acquisition of the mask and contrast-containing frames. In clinical practice, videodensitometry performs so poorly that there exists virtually no correlation between measures of severity obtained from alternative angiographic projections (17). Accordingly, videodensitometry, although currently available on many brands of angiographic equipment, is an unreliable gauge of stenosis severity and should not be employed for clinical decision making.

Calculation of Stenosis Flow Reserve

Dimensional measurements, including minimum luminal diameter or cross-sectional area do not describe the precise physiologic consequences of coronary lesions. Many other factors, including stenosis geometry, lesion length, coronary pressure, blood viscosity, and extent of turbulent flow, will determine the actual pressure drop across a coronary obstruction. An important descriptor of the physiologic impact of a stenoses, termed coronary flow reserve (CFR), was introduced 20 years ago by Gould et al. (19). CFR is defined as the ratio of maximal coronary blood flow (CBF) following a hyperemic stimulus divided by the CBF under basal conditions. Typical values for CFR exceed 5:1 for normal coronaries, falling to nearly 1:1 for critical coronary lesions.

A novel approach to quantitative angiography, first proposed by Kirkeeide and Gould, applies sophisticated fluid dynamics equations to QCA, thereby calculating a predicted pressure drop across the lesion (20). The proponents of this method make several further assumptions about the normal intracoronary pressure and velocity to ultimately calculate a predicted or theoretic CFR ratio. However, many of the variables required for precise modeling of coronary flow cannot be measured in vivo from quantitative angiography. Although apparently well validated in vitro and in simple experimental animal studies, this method remains somewhat controversial. Prudence requires caution in applying this approach for clinical decision making.

Criticisms and Limitations of QCA

Although widely used in research, most practitioners do not employ formal quantitative angiography in clinical practice. Many important theoretic and practical limitations have impaired routine application of QCA to interventional practice. For each angiographic projection, QCA typically employs analysis of a single selected frame to determine MLD and percent stenosis. However, the visualization of a lesion and apparent severity of the stenosis varies considerably during the cardiac cycle. Accordingly, studies have demonstrated that interobserver variability in frame selection constitutes an important uncontrolled variable affecting measurement results (21).

Because coronary lesions are characteristically eccentric, accurate QCA requires at least two orthogonal views of each lesion. However, the presence of overlapping structures and the limitations of x-ray gantry movement preclude obtaining orthogonal views of many stenoses. There exist complex obstructions for which no angiographic views can reliably depict the anatomy of the stenosis. The presence of intraluminal thrombus constitutes an important confounding variable affecting the accuracy of QCA. The computer algorithms that determine the vessel borders assume a relatively circular arterial cross section. Presence of intracoronary thrombus distorts the density pattern within the vessel of obviating reliable computerized or manual border detection.

A complex, noncircular luminal cross-sectional profile may arise from mechanical coronary interventions, which produce complicated dissections in the vessel wall. The result may consist of a "hazy" or "double" lumen that is difficult to measure by any angiographic method (Fig. 13.3). Geometric distortion produced by the image intensifier represents another important limiting factor affecting accuracy. Typically, "pincushion" distortion produces spatially dependent variability in magnification across the imaging field. Thus a stenosis will appear smaller or larger if imaged at the edge, rather than the center, of the image intensifier.

Considerable variability and inaccuracy originate from the method used to calibrate for magnification. Most current methods use the angiographic catheter for calibration. The small size of the catheter, typically 2.33 to 3.33 mm, greatly magnifies any small error in contour tracing. Thus a slight imprecision in measuring catheter width results in a large error in the magnification correction. Furthermore, the position of the angiographic

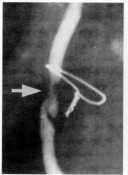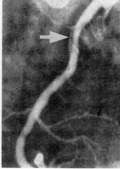

Figure 13.3. Two examples of lesions difficult to assess by quantitative angiography. The left panel illustrates a complex lesion with intracoronary thrombosis and dissection. In the right panel a linear dissection is apparent in the area previously treated by balloon angioplasty. Complex lesions such as these can confound any computerized edge-detection algorithm.

catheter may fall outside of the plane of the stenosis. Accordingly, the calibration will misrepresent the magnification correction required for the target lesion. Finally, the nominal dimensions of the catheter exhibit significant variability from individual manufacturers. Thus precise QCA requires specific knowledge of the catheter source and probably experimental testing of each catheter brand.

Because of the aforementioned methodologic problems, QCA should not be accepted as an absolutely precise method for stenosis sizing. A recent analysis of data obtained from measurement of identical lesions by different laboratories reveals surprisingly large interobserver variability (PW Serruys, personal communication). Thus serial measurements of a specific lesion in a single laboratory exhibit excellent reproducibility. However, studies performed in different laboratories cannot be directly compared without controlling for the equipment and operator technique.

DIGITAL ANGIOGRAPHY

Since its introduction to the cardiac catheterization laboratory in 1982, digital angiography has gradually gained acceptance as an important alternative to conventional video or film recording techniques (22–24). The increasing role for digital angiography reflects several inherent advantages provided by this relatively new imaging modality. Digital angiography offers immediate access to high-quality images during diagnostic catheterization—a feature that enables significant improvements in the speed and efficiency of the operator. In addition, the direct digital acquisition of angiographic images facilitates quantitative approaches to stenosis evaluation, including QCA and coronary flow reserve determination.

Basic Principles of Digital Angiography

The principles underlying digital recording of video-generated images are relatively sim-

ple. Current digital imaging systems employ a conventional television camera for image acquisition. Images are typically acquired simultaneously during cineangiography using a semisilvered mirror that divides the visible image formed on the output phosphor of the image intensifier into two parallel pathways. Digital angiography systems typically provide 80 to 90% of the light output to cine film and 10 to 20% to the video camera. This unequal division is necessary because of the relative insensitivity of the cine film emulsions to visible light in comparison to modern video cameras.

The video camera output consists of an analog signal in which the voltage level of the video signal is proportional to the brightness of each point in the raster line. Because computers work in binary numbers, the number of possible gray levels is determined by the number of bits available for analog-to-digital conversion. In cardiac digital angiography, this is typically 8 bits (1 byte), which in binary numbers, corresponds to 256 possible gray levels. The horizontal and vertical sampling rate of the analog-to-digital converter determines the *matrix size* of the digital image (Fig. 13.4). Most current systems generate 512 horizontal and 512 vertical samples, each referred to as a picture element, or pixel.

Some digital imaging systems now employ video cameras and monitors with 1024 line capability (high-line rate video) and digitize the video signal at 1024 × 1024 × 8 bit resolution. Because the output monitor displays 1024 scan lines, not 525, the unpleasant effects of visible raster lines are significantly reduced. Despite several important advantages, 1024 digital systems do not yield images with twice the spatial resolution of 525 line systems. This disparity occurs because the low radiation doses used for cardiac imaging result in an image significantly degraded by quantum statistical noise. Accordingly, not all the potential for increased resolution translates into a usable

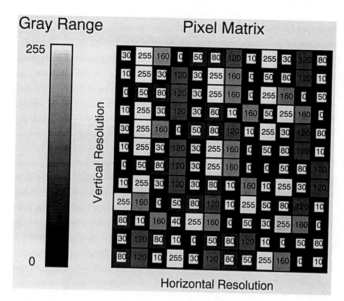

Figure 13.4. Illustration of the principles of analog-to-digital conversion of the image. In the left panel the continuous gray levels of an analog image are depicted. In the right-hand panel the digital image is conveyed as a series of discrete values ranging from 0 to 256. Higher numbers indicate areas of greater brightness, whereas lower numbers indicate a gray value approaching black. In digital imaging the number of rows and columns of discrete numeric elements is known as the pixel matrix. A larger number of pixels can record greater resolution, whereas a larger number of gray values increases dynamic range (better gray scale). The digitization process is required for computer analysis of any angiographic image.

improvement in image quality. In addition, high-line rate video cameras often generate more electronic noise than 525 line systems.

QCA from Digital Angiography

Digital angiography records images directly into a computer system, thus enabling QCA without the added step of film digitization (25). This feature reduces or eliminates several of the confounding variables that impair accuracy of film-based methods. Direct digital angiography obviates problems generated by the nonlinear film density versus exposure relationship and variability in the light source or optics of the film projector. Improvements in computer capability have enabled some newer digital systems to provide nearly instantaneous quantitative angiography—permitting assessment of stenosis severity during the interventional procedure. The ability to precisely measure coronary diameter during revascularization potentially facilitates device sizing and enables serial evaluation of the lesion during the procedure. Although intuitively useful, there exist no randomized studies documenting improvement in outcome when interventional procedures are guided using quantitative angiography.

QCA using digital angiography, rather than cineangiographic film, also has important disadvantages. Cardiac digital angiography most often consists of a 512×512 pixel acquisition with 8 bits (1 byte) gray scale per pixel. This matrix size is slightly below the optimum necessary to capture all the spatial information available from the best image intensifiers. At a 512×512 matrix, the digital system will generate 3.4 pixels per mm for a 15-cm (6-inch) field of view. However, a top-quality intensifier may resolve 4 to 5 line-pairs per mm and technically, at least two pixels are required to reproduce each line pair. Thus a 512×512 digital image probably slightly undersamples the available diagnostic information. Although this phenomenon has important scientific implications for QCA of digital angiography, clinical studies fail to document major differences between film-based and digital angiographic QCA.

Coronary Flow Reserve

Recognizing the limitations of stenosis sizing by angiography, investigative efforts began more than 20 years ago to assess the functional significance of coronary lesions by analysis of density-time curves (26). The first rudimentary equipment enabled measurement of voltage levels from analog video signals. With the development of advanced computers, these efforts shifted to digital angiography, a more facile approach, although the principles remained essentially the same. Typically, digital subtraction angiography (DSA) has been employed to remove unwanted background density from the angiographic images. A variety of computer analysis methods have been proposed for determining coronary flow reserve from digital angiography (27–31). Virtually all proposed algorithms rely on precise measurement of density-time curves for regions of interest within the coronary or myocardial perfusion bed.

Because CFR determination requires pharmacologic induction of reactive hyperemia, the method for increasing CBF is important. Initial studies employed injection of iodinated contrast media as the stimulus for hyperemia (28). However, this approach produces submaximal flow increases and a relatively brief (<20 sec) plateau of hyperemia. Intracoronary papaverine (8 to 12 mg) produces near maximal flow augmentation persisting at least 30 to 45 seconds (32). While papaverine is better suited for pharmacologic induction of hyperemia, this agent has never received FDA approval for intracoronary use, sometimes produces profound ECG changes, and in our experience may precipitate during contact with some contrast agents. Recently, some protocols have employed intracoronary adenosine to induce reactive hyperemia.

Regardless of the method used to produce hyperemia, the physiologic effects of contrast injection on the coronary circulation are an important variable that may confound application of DSA techniques. Following injection of contrast media, there is a triphasic response consisting of unaltered flow for a fraction of a cycle, followed by a transient 15 to 45% decrease in CBF during epicardial transit of contrast, followed by a hyperemic response that peaks within 15 to 30 seconds (33). Thus radiographic contrast, the indica-

tor used for densitometric measurements, substantially alters the precise variable, coronary flow, that DSA methods attempt to quantify.

Coronary Transit Time

Initial attempts to evaluate blood flow from videodensitometry employed a simple approach based on coronary transit time (26). Two regions of interest (ROI) are identified, one superimposed on the proximal coronary and a second over the distal vessel, and transit time is derived from density curves generated during passage of the contrast bolus. Velocity is calculated as distance between sampling points divided by transit time, and flow is determined from velocity multiplied by cross-sectional area. This simple epicardial transit-time approach is limited by several methodologic problems. The time interval for bolus passage between ROIs is very short— less than one cardiac cycle—and not easily resolvable by 30- to 60-frame-per-second angiography. Since only a portion of a single cycle is evaluated, the technique cannot account for the phasic nature of CBF. The spreading of the contrast bolus during passage through the coronary circulation obscures precise delineation of the transit time. Finally, the actual distance between ROIs is difficult to measure because epicardial vessels exhibit complex curvature and are rarely perpendicular to the x-ray beam.

An adaptation of transit-time method was reintroduced in the early 1980s by Vogel et al. (28) (Fig. 13.5). Initially, proponents of this approach measured a phenomenon termed myocardial contrast appearance time (MCAT), defined as the time interval between onset of ECG-triggered contrast injection and the point at which density in a myocardial ROI reached a certain percentage of maximum. DSA was performed using ECG-triggered end-diastolic imaging at one frame per cardiac cycle and iodinated contrast media employed to induce hyperemia. CFR was determined from the ratio of MCAT under

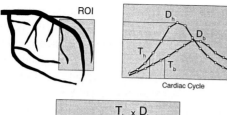

Figure 13.5. Schematic representation of the method of coronary flow reserve known as contrast myocardial appearance time. In the upper left the region of interest is generated over the perfusion bed of a contrast angiogram. At the upper right is a depiction of the time-density curves over several cardiac cycles. Curves are obtained under basal conditions and after induction of hyperemia using a coronary vasodilator. The bottom panel illustrates the mathematic calculation of coronary flow reserve. *Tb,* Contrast appearance time under basal conditions; *Th,* contrast appearance time under hyperemic conditions; *Db,* maximum density achieved during the basal contrast injection; *Dh,* maximum density achieved during the hyperemic contrast injection.

basal conditions divided by MCAT during hyperemia. It was hypothesized that MCAT would be shorter during induced hyperemia compared with the basal state and that a physiologically significant stenosis would blunt the decrease in MCAT normally observed following hyperemia.

Subsequent investigations revealed several limitations inherent to this approach. In an animal model the maximum ratio of basal to hyperemic MCAT never exceeded about 1.7:1, while simultaneous CFR by surgically implanted electromagnetic (EMF) probe exceeded 5:1. This disparity arises from a blunting of increased hyperemic flow velocity produced by augmentation of coronary cross-sectional area during drug-stimulated reactive hyperemia. Subsequently, proponents of the MCAT method modified the approach to calculate an index of relative flow that employed, not only MCAT, but also maximal density achieved (31). This modification was based on the premise that the increased myocardial density under hyperemic conditions represented increased volume of the

vasculature, while decreased MCAT represented increased velocity. By measuring and quantifying both phenomena (more rapid transit and increased density) the MCAT method yielded reasonably close agreement between CFR calculated by DSA in comparison with EMF in well-controlled animal studies (34).

Although used in a few centers, the MCAT method never found widespread acceptance. Cusma et al. demonstrated several important limitations, particularly the requirement to completely displace blood in the coronary with iodinated contrast to fulfill the theoretic requirements of the method (31). This can require more than 12 ml per second under hyperemic conditions and requires prophylactic pacing to prevent excessive bradycardia. Specialized equipment for ECG-gated end-diastolic image acquisition is required, and the method is sensitive to misregistration of contrast and mask frames, thus requiring excellent patient cooperation.

Alternative Methods

An alternate approach was initially proposed by Foerster et al. and subsequently investigated by our laboratory (27, 29). The approach is based on the physiologic principles of indicator dilution, known as the Stewart-Hamilton method. A known quantity of contrast is injected subselectively in the coronary, and density-time curves are generated for two ROIs, one superimposed on the epicardial coronary and a second over the nearby adjacent myocardium. Values for the myocardial ROI are subtracted from the coronary ROI to yield net density values for the epicardial vessel. The area under the time-density curve for this background-corrected coronary ROI is determined for both basal conditions and following induction of hyperemia. Flow is inversely related to the area under the curve and therefore, if identical ROIs are used, relative blood flow (CFR) is proportional to the ratio of the two curve areas (basal/hyperemic) multiplied by the ratio of the contrast doses (hyperemic/basal). Although theoretically sound, the indicator-dilution approach also failed to achieve widespread application. The method requires subselective contrast injection, ECG-triggered image acquisition and contrast injection, and good registration of subtracted images. These practical limitations precluded easy application in the clinical setting.

Limitations of DSA Methods

Since radiography is a silhouette technique, the density of each pixel reflects all underlying and overlying structures. Accordingly, mask-mode subtraction requires motion-free imaging to remove noniodinated structures from digital images for densitometric analysis. High-quality subtractions are easily achieved in the experimental laboratory in anesthetized, mechanically ventilated animals, but are substantially more difficult to accomplish in awake patients undergoing catheterization (35).

For most approaches, the phasic nature of CBF represents a significant confounding variable (36). Density-time curves derived from DSA are influenced by the phase of the cardiac cycle used for contrast injection. During diastole, when CBF is high, contrast injection will result in lower contrast density and rapid contrast passage, while injection during systole will yield higher density and less rapid transit. Thus most DSA methods require ECG-triggered injection of contrast media with a power injector. The necessity for ECG-triggered power injection undoubtedly contributes to reluctance to use these methods in clinical practice. Although no known misadventures have been published, it is difficult to dispute the perception that coronary power injection might represent a hazard.

The physics of radiographic imaging are also important in quantitative application of DSA. Because the relationship between iodine concentration and image density is logarithmic (Lambert-Beer law), pixel gray level values must be logarithmically trans-formed prior to subtraction (37). However, as previously discussed, the Lambert-Beer relationship is valid only for monochromatic radiation, a requisite not present for x-ray sources available in the catheterization laboratory.

Despite the success of DSA methods for calculation of CFR in well-designed animal studies, substantial difficulties impede clinical application (36). Most DSA methods determine the CFR ratio with the numerator representing hyperemic flow and the denominator basal flow. Reduced CFR can be produced by at least two phenomena, reduction in hyperemic flow secondary to epicardial stenoses or elevation of basal flow produced by factors unrelated to the specific lesion. The latter mechanism is often evident in the clinical setting. For example, following an acute MI, flow in the contralateral perfusion bed may be increased as a consequence of compensatory hyperkinesis. Left ventricular hypertrophy, tachycardia, or valvular disease may diminish CFR by augmenting resting CBF. The presence or absence of collateral circulation represents another independent variable. These phenomena make it extremely difficult to apply CFR measurements in clinical decision making. Importantly, these limitations to clinical application of coronary flow reserve apply equally well to other proposed methods for measurement, including Doppler flow.

New DSA Approaches

A relatively new approach to DSA assessment of coronary flow has been developed by Pijls et al. (35). This method avoids measuring CFR ratios as a means to evaluate the functional significance of coronary lesions. Instead, these investigators determine myocardial transit time during continuous maximal coronary vasodilation induced by infusion of dipyridamole. This approach prevents changes in vascular volume from influencing measurement of transit time. With the volume of distribution excluded as a variable, their data demonstrate a close relationship between absolute flow and mean transit time. Instead of yielding a measurement of CFR, this method generates a value representative of the maximal possible flow achievable for the analyzed vascular bed. This approach has the potential to measure an index of maximal flow for a specific stenosis before and after balloon angioplasty. In this clinical application the improvement in maximal flow can be assessed and related to outcome.

CORONARY INTRAVASCULAR ULTRASOUND

The recent development of coronary intravascular ultrasound provides the first practical alternative to angiography for clinical decision making during diagnostic and interventional catheterization (38–47). The cross-sectional orientation of intravascular ultrasound permits quantification of coronary lesions from a tomographic perspective. Accordingly, intravascular ultrasound provides measurements of reference vessel and lesional dimensions independent of lumen shape. Ultrasound scanners typically overlay an electronically generated distance scale within the image (Figs. 13.6 to 13.12). Because the velocity of sound in soft tissue represents a well-established constant, this internal calibration obviates the troublesome requirement of QCA to correct for radiographic magnification.

Although dimensional measurements represent an important contribution of intravascular ultrasound, the ability to image the soft tissues within the arterial wall represent a unique contribution. Intravascular imaging can characterize atheroma size, plaque distribution, and lesion composition during diagnostic or therapeutic catheterization. Technologic progress has enabled significant reduction in the size of intravascular devices, thereby enabling routine imaging of coronary target lesions before revascularization. Analysis of images obtained before and after intervention can determine the mechanism and extent of lumen enlargement. The ability of ultrasound to provide detailed preinterventional images of the atheromas has facilitated a lesion-specific approach to treatment of coronary stenoses. This rapidly

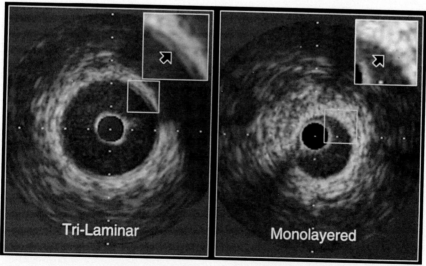

Figure 13.6. Two examples of normal coronary anatomy by intravascular ultrasound. In the left panel, a vessel with a tri-laminar structure is illustrated. This appearance is typical of approximately 40% of normal coronaries. In the magnified inset the arrow indicates a discrete intimal leading edge with a subjacent sonolucent zone. In the right panel a normal subject with a monolayered artery is illustrated. The magnified inset shows a single layer without an apparent intimal leading edge or sonolucent zone. In this case the intima is thinner than the axial resolution of the intravascular ultrasound device and is therefore not imaged.

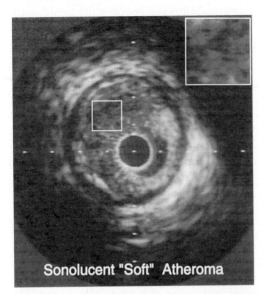

Sonolucent "Soft" Atheroma

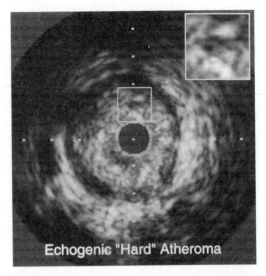

Echogenic "Hard" Atheroma

Figure 13.7. An example of a "soft" atherosclerotic plaque. The catheter is seen near the center of the image contained in a small lumen. In this case the catheter occupies more than three-fourths of the luminal area. The magnified inset shows an area of atherosclerotic plaque that is relatively sonolucent, indicating a high lipid content with minimal fibrosis.

Figure 13.8. Example of a "hard" coronary atheroma. The ultrasound catheter is recognized as the dark circle in the center of the image. The sonolucent zone represents the vessel media. The magnified inset shows a portion of the atherosclerotic plaque that is highly echogenic, indicating the presence of large amounts of fibrous tissue.

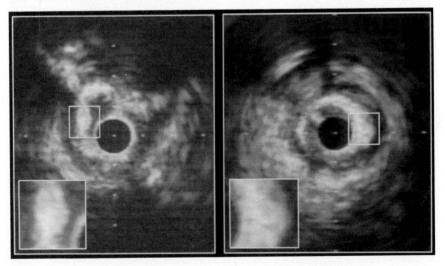

Figure 13.9. Two examples of extremely dense plaques. In both cases the atherosclerotic plaque components are highly echogenic, exceeding the brightness of the surrounding adventitia. These plaques are difficult to treat and require high-pressure balloon inflations for angioplasty, sometimes resulting in large arterial dissections.

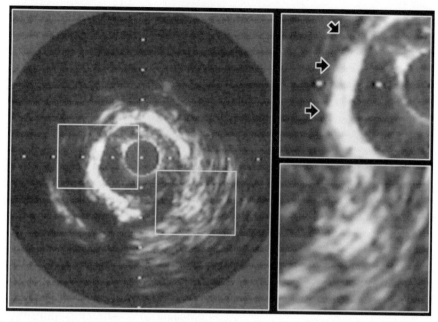

Figure 13.10. Example of a calcified coronary lesion. The magnified inset at the upper right shows a very echogenic plaque that obstructs penetration of ultrasound, thus "shadowing" the underlying structure of the vessel. The magnified inset at the lower right indicates an area of plaque without calcification.

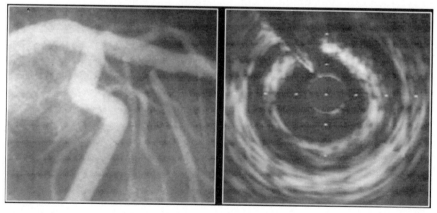

Figure 13.11. Example of false-negative coronary angiography. In the angiogram the left anterior descending coronary shows only slight luminal irregularities. In the right panel the intravascular ultrasound obtained from this segment of vessel shows extensive atherosclerosis. Studies have indicated that intravascular ultrasound is much more sensitive than angiography at detecting coronary atherosclerosis.

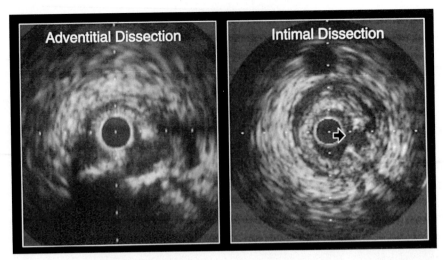

Figure 13.12. Two examples of coronary dissection following balloon angioplasty. In the left panel a large gap in the intima and media is seen at approximately 4 o'clock. This channel extends into the adventitia, indicating a deep dissection. In the right panel the dissection is confined to the atheroma and does not extend to the media or deeper structures.

evolving interventional strategy employs preangioplasty plaque morphology to determine the optimal type and size of device for revascularization.

Ultrasound Catheter Design

The initial devices available for intravascular ultrasound were relatively large, ranging from 4.3 to 5.5 Fr (1.43 to 1.67 mm), limiting examination to proximal and occasionally mid vessels imaged after revascularization. A new generation of smaller devices, 2.9 to 3.5 Fr in diameter (0.96 to 1.17 mm), offer improved image quality and better handling characteristics. Although current catheters provide improved mechanical properties, handling characteristics are distinctly inferior to the latest generation of angioplasty equipment. Two dissimilar technical approaches to transducer design have emerged, mechanically rotated devices and multielement electronic arrays. Currently, only a single commercial vendor offers a nonmechanical device, consisting of a 32-element array. To facilitate subselective coronary cannulation and catheter exchanges, all modern ultrasound devices provide a lumen for a movable guidewire. Most systems employ a monorail design to facilitate rapid catheter exchanges without the necessity for a long guidewire or a docking apparatus.

Multielement designs generally result in catheters with optimal flexibility and guidewire tracking. Although the multielement electronic array offers excellent handing characteristics, this approach has thus far yielded suboptimal image quality. A novel multielement device presently undergoing clinical testing incorporates an imaging transducer mounted proximal to a standard angioplasty balloon. However, this combined device exhibits substandard handling properties and a crossing profile that compares poorly with modern balloon catheters. Unfortunately, this device currently also yields relatively poor image quality and FDA approval has been delayed following an unfavorable recommendation by the advisory panel.

Several commercially available intravascular ultrasound systems employ mechanically rotated transducers. Three successive generations of catheters have resulted in devices with a maximum diameter as small as 2.9 to 3.5 Fr (0.96 to 1.17 mm). Compared with the multielement probes, mechanically rotated intravascular ultrasound catheters offer greater acoustic power and improved image quality. However, the catheter handling characteristics of mechanical intravascular devices remain somewhat inferior to the multielement array device. Current mechanical designs are small and flexible enough for routine coronary imaging, but require skill to successfully negotiate tortuous vessels.

Artifacts and Limitations

All current intravascular ultrasound devices generate artifacts that may adversely affect image quality, alter interpretation, or reduce quantitative accuracy. Mechanical transducers sometimes exhibit cyclical oscillations in rotational speed, a phenomenon known as nonuniform rotational distortion (NURD). This effect arises from differential mechanical drag on the catheter driveshaft during a portion of the rotational cycle. NURD is most evident in situations where the driveshaft is bent into a small radius of curvature by a tortuous vessel. Nonuniform speed variation produces readily visible distortion, recognized as circumferential stretching of a portion of the image with compression of the contralateral vessel wall. Historically, each successive reduction in catheter size initially exacerbated problems with rotational distortion. However, in each generation of devices, engineering improvements have eventually reduced the frequency and severity of NURD.

An additional image defect, transducer ring-down artifact, appears in virtually all medical ultrasound devices. Ring-down artifacts arise from acoustic oscillations in the piezoelectric transducer material resulting in high-amplitude ultrasound signals that preclude imaging within a few tenths of a millimeter of the surface. Inability to image structures immediately adjacent to the transducer results in an "acoustic" catheter size slightly larger than its physical size. The most recent designs use carefully chosen transducer and backing materials, specialized coatings, and electronic filtering to suppress ring-down artifacts.

An additional limitation of all intravascular imaging systems originates from the vulnerability of ultrasound techniques to geometric distortion produced by oblique imaging. When the ultrasound beam interrogates a plane not orthogonal to the vessel walls, an artery with a circular lumen appears elliptical in shape. This phenomenon increases the maximum, but not minimum luminal dimensions and can represent a significant confounding variable in some quantitative measurements. Under some circumstances, it is possible to recognize a nonorthogonal catheter position and manipulate the device to a more coaxial position. Fortunately, the small size of the coronary vasculature limits the degree of obliquity possible during ultrasound examinations, although the phenomenon is more troublesome for aortic or peripheral vascular studies.

Safety of Coronary Ultrasound

Although intravascular ultrasound requires intracoronary instrumentation, initial studies conducted during diagnostic catheterization demonstrated few serious untoward effects (43, 45, 46). Transient coronary spasm occurs in about 5% of patients, but usually responds rapidly to administration of intracoronary nitroglycerin. The imaging transducer can transiently occlude the coronary when advanced into tight stenoses or small distal vessels, but patients generally do not experience chest pain if the catheter is promptly withdrawn. In interventional practice, operators have employed coronary ultrasound immediately following virtually all types of procedures, including balloon angioplasty, atherectomy, rotablation, and stent deployment.

Despite the relative safety of coronary ultrasound, any intracoronary instrumentation carries the potential risk of intimal injury or acute vessel dissection. Virtually every invasive coronary device, including intravascular ultrasound catheters, has produced a documented or suspected vessel injury.

Accordingly, the prudent practitioner will approach any intracoronary instrumentation with reasonable and appropriate caution. Although many centers employ ultrasound during diagnostic catheterization, most laboratories limit credentialing for intravascular imaging procedures to personnel with interventional training. In the unlikely event of intimal disruption, this safety measure ensures that the necessary personnel and equipment are immediately available to initiate appropriate corrective action.

Morphologic Features

Careful in vivo studies report a distinctly laminar appearance to the normal vessel wall in many but not all normal subjects (see Fig. 13.6). Some normal subjects exhibit an intimal leading edge that poorly reflects ultrasound, a phenomenon that leads to *dropout* of ultrasound signals. Thus distinct laminations of the vessel wall are absent in more than 50% of the normal coronary sites, particularly in younger normal subjects (age <30). In those normal subjects with a distinct intimal leading edge the maximum intimal thickness averages 0.15 ± 0.07 mm, and most investigators consider the upper limit of normal as 0.25 to 0.30 mm.

Coronary atherosclerotic plaques typically appear as variably echogenic intraluminal encroachments overlying a thin, sonolucent subintimal band representing normal media (see Figs. 13.7 to 13.12). Coronary atheromas less echogenic than the vessel adventitia are often termed "soft" plaques, because in vitro studies demonstrate a high lipid content in these sonolucent lesions. Soft atheromas vary widely in echogenicity, ranging from plaques nearly as sonolucent as blood to more echogenic, highly textured lesions (see Figs. 13.7 and 13.8). Differences in the resolution and dynamic range of the differing ultrasound instrumentation undoubtedly contribute to the variability in appearance.

Some atherosclerotic vessels exhibit abnormal intimal thickening with markedly increased plaque echogenicity (see Fig. 13.9). Most authorities describe these more echogenic lesions as "hard" plaques because in vitro studies indicate the presence of significant fibrosis in tissues with a highly echogenic appearance. These hard plaques behave differently when approached with interventional devices, often requiring higher balloon pressures for effective dilation. In the most extreme examples of plaque echogenicity, an echo-dense portion of the lesion attenuates transmission of low-energy, high-frequency ultrasound, thus obscuring the underlying structures of the arterial wall (see Fig. 13.10). Studies performed in vitro demonstrate the presence of calcium in lesions that impede the penetration of ultrasound.

Calcified lesions exhibit considerable biomechanical rigidity and often require higher balloon pressures to achieve adequate luminal gain during angioplasty. Dense atherosclerotic atheromas that exhibit acoustic shadowing also resist plaque removal by directional atherectomy. The presence of extensive "shadowing" plaques can preclude measurement of total atheroma area, because ultrasound cannot visualize the full thickness of atheromas.

The lumen of the vessel is primarily sonolucent; however, higher-frequency transducers (>25 MHz) yield images with a distinctive pattern of echogenicity within the lumen. Moving blood appears as a faint, swirling pattern with finely textured echogenicity, although the precise blood elements responsible for this appearance are unknown. The faint, smokelike appearance of moving blood can prove invaluable in identifying vessel wall structures that communicate with the lumen, such as intramural dissection. Injection of iodinated contrast dramatically enhances the echogenicity of moving blood, presumably because of the presence of microbubbles within the medium. Following interventional procedures, contrast opacification can confirm the presence of a dissection plane in difficult-to-analyze cases.

ULTRASOUND: DIAGNOSTIC APPLICATIONS

Angiographically Unrecognized Disease

In patients undergoing diagnostic or therapeutic catheterization, coronary intravascular ultrasound commonly detects atherosclerotic abnormalities at sites containing no apparent lesion by angiography (see Fig. 13.11). The extraordinary extent of ultrasound abnormalities in angiographically normal vessels confirms the finding, previously reported from necropsy studies, that coronary disease is more diffuse than apparent by radiographic methods. The high prevalence of angiographically occult coronary disease includes the left main coronary artery. In a recent study intravascular imaging discovered unrecognized left main coronary artery narrowing in many patients undergoing routine left coronary interventions (48, 49).

Several phenomena explain the greater sensitivity of ultrasound in detection of coronary atherosclerosis. Angiography relies on luminal encroachment to identify diseased sites. However, in some cases, compensatory remodeling of the vessel wall preserves angiographic lumen size in atherosclerotic arteries, a phenomenon originally described by Glagov (see Fig. 13.11) (50). Adventitial enlargement obscures luminal encroachment by the atheroma, thus concealing the disease from angiography. Diffuse concentric atherosclerosis commonly yields false-negative angiography. In the diffusely diseased artery, the entire vessel is reduced in caliber and there exists no focal stenosis to produce a characteristic luminal narrowing.

Assessment of Ambiguous Lesions

Despite thorough radiographic evaluation using multiple projections, angiographers commonly encounter lesions of uncertain severity. Difficult-to-evaluate lesions typically include moderate stenoses in symptomatic patients, bifurcation lesions, and stenoses of the left main coronary artery. In such cases intravascular ultrasound provides a tomographic view of the lesion, enabling quantitation of stenosis independent of the radiographic projection (51). This approach is somewhat limited by the physical dimensions of ultrasound catheters, typically 0.95 to 1.17 mm. However, most important stenoses occur in vessels with a normal caliber of 2.5 mm or greater. Accordingly, for a 2.5- to 3.0-mm vessel, if ultrasound demonstrates a minimum luminal diameter less than the catheter size, the lesion will represent a diameter reduction at least 60 to 67% and an area of stenosis 84 to 90%. Most vessels with this degree of narrowing will warrant intervention.

Intravascular ultrasound can frequently provide valuable adjunctive information to clarify the extent and severity of ostial or bifurcation lesions. Ostial lesions are examined by placing the ultrasound catheter distal to the stenosis, disengaging the guiding catheter and performing a slow pullback of the ultrasound transducer to interrogate the ostium of the vessel. Examination of bifurcation lesions requires subselective placement of the transducer in the main trunk and each of the daughter branches. Accurate assessment of the extent of involvement of the bifurcation often provides essential data necessary for optimal planning of interventional procedures. The presence of disease in both daughter vessels may influence the need for a "double-wire" technique or may impact on the suitability of the vessel for stenting. Detection of ostial disease, particularly involvement of the LMCA, can have considerable impact on clinical decision making. In such cases the operator may elect surgical revascularization rather than proceed with a percutaneous interventional procedure.

Dimensional Measurements

A broad range of therapeutic decisions depends on assessment of coronary luminal dimensions. Practitioners routinely employ luminal measurements to evaluate the severity of stenoses, determine the size of the "normal" reference segment, and assess luminal gain achieved by the procedure. Accordingly, precise quantitation of vascular dimensions from a tomographic perspective represents an important clinical application of intravascular ultrasound. Because atherosclerotic coronaries are frequently complex and eccentric, a tomographic imaging technique such as ultrasound can yield measurements that differ significantly from quantitative angiography.

We compared angiographic and ultrasound dimension in patient subgroups stratified by the extent of eccentricity determined by ultrasound (46). A standardized index of eccentricity, the circular shape factor, determined the degree of deviation of the lumen cross section from a perfect circle. The planimetered cross-sectional area (CSA) was utilized to calculate a mean vessel diameter:

$$d = 2\sqrt{\frac{CSA}{\pi}}$$

The perimeter for a perfect circle of this diameter is $P = \pi d$ (where P = perimeter). An index of eccentricity, the circular shape factor (CSF) was defined as:

$$CSF = \left(\frac{\text{calculated perimeter}}{\text{observed perimeter}}\right)^2$$

This index yields a value of 1.0 for a perfect circle with smaller values indicating increasing eccentricity.

In these normal subjects CSF averaged 0.92 ± 0.02, demonstrating a nearly circular lumen shape in the patients without coronary disease, and the correlation between QCA- and ultrasound-derived diameter was close, $r = .92$, demonstrating concordance between planar and tomographic measurement. In approximately two-thirds of atherosclerotic vessels, the lumen was concentric in shape (CSF <.92) and the correlation between ultrasound and angiography was also close, $r = .93$. However, in the subgroup of patients with an eccentric lumen shape (CSF <.92) regression analysis demonstrated significant disagreement be-

tween angiographic and ultrasonic diameters, $r = .78$. This reduced correlation likely results from the irregular, noncircular cross-sectional profile of atherosclerotic arteries. These data demonstrate the potential superiority of a tomographic technique such as intravascular ultrasound in measurement of coronary dimensions for the complex, eccentric vessels commonly encountered in patients with atherosclerosis.

The differences between ultrasound and angiography observed in eccentrically diseased coronaries have important implications for quantitative assessment of lumen dimensions following balloon angioplasty. Both intravascular ultrasound and necropsy studies illustrate that mechanical coronary revascularization, particularly balloon angioplasty, distorts the vessel wall, producing complex fractures or dissections within the intima, media, or adventitia (8, 45, 46) (see Fig. 13.12). In this setting, measurements of the angiographic silhouette of the vessel lumen would predictably exhibit a limited correlation with dimensions obtained by a cross-sectional imaging method. In several studies of residual stenosis post-PTCA, comparisons by linear regression analysis of angiographic and ultrasonic measurements of minimum diameter have revealed a relatively poor correlation, generally in the range of $r = .40$ to $.60$.

Stenosis Severity

In current interventional practice, measurement of percent stenosis represents the standard approach to assessment of procedural success, typically expressed either as percent diameter or cross-sectional area reduction. However, this calculation requires measurement of both lesional and reference segment dimensions. Any inaccuracy in the sizing of either segment provides the opportunity to distort the postinterventional assessment of residual percent stenosis. Using linear regression analysis, several studies have revealed a strikingly poor correlation between ultrasound and angiography, typically approximately $r = .30$, for measurement of percent stenosis following coronary angioplasty. Analyses of these comparative studies have shown that disparities in percent stenosis determination arise from differences in both lesional and reference vessel measurements.

The relatively poor correlation between angiographic and ultrasonic dimensions following angioplasty raises provocative clinical and scientific issues. In certain patients, does "restenosis" represent a failure to adequately augment luminal area rather than the subsequent overexuberant proliferation of cellular elements? Can ultrasound assessment of the residual lumen predict acute post-interventional complications or identify patients with a high likelihood of poor long-term results? Although large-scale prospective trials will be required to answer these important clinical questions, preliminary retrospective studies demonstrate that ultrasound can successfully identify subsets of patients likely to manifest suboptimal long-term results. Several multicenter clinical trials, currently in the initial stages of organization, will examine whether such knowledge can favorably affect long-term outcome.

Reference Segment Disease

The diameter of the coronary reference segment plays a pivotal role in determining the choice and size of mechanical revascularization device. Recent ultrasound studies have documented that reference segments exhibit highly variable morphology ranging from extensive angiographically occult atherosclerosis to unexpected ectasia (52). Comparisons of the "normal" reference sites used to size angioplasty devices reveal only a moderate correlation, approximately $r = .70$, between angiographic and intravascular ultrasound measurements of luminal diameter. Several of these comparisons also demonstrate a relatively large standard error, typically exceeding 0.50 mm. This phenomenon presents a complex dilemma for the interventional practitioner who must select a specific device for the revascularization procedure. Is the "normal" reference segment diffusely diseased, truly normal, or even ectatic? Will a slightly larger device increase the lumen gain or induce a catastrophic acute complication?

There exist no prospective randomized data documenting a clear advantage for device sizing by intravascular ultrasound. However, preliminary data from our laboratory indicate that differences between ultrasound and angiographic "reference" diameters represent an important factor determining both initial results and long-term clinical outcomes (53). These data demonstrate that diffuse atherosclerosis reduces luminal diameter by more than 50% in approximately one-third of angiographically normal reference segments. In this subgroup of patients the operator selects a smaller interventional device than that employed for patients without reference segment disease. Intuitively, the systematic undersizing of interventional devices could significantly impair the success of percutaneous revascularization procedures.

Analysis of acute results in patients with a variable extent of reference segment narrowing demonstrates a reduced luminal gain and greater residual stenosis in the subgroup with significant reference disease. Furthermore, follow-up studies at 4 to 6 months indicate that these patients suffer from an increased incidence of recurrent adverse clinical events. Accordingly, precise ultrasound measurement of coronary dimensions at "normal" reference sites may emerge as the "gold standard" for interventional device sizing. Potentially, improved device sizing by intravascular ultrasound may impact on both the acute complication and recurrence rates for coronary lesions. However, this approach must contend with a critical confounding variable, coronary remodeling, in which the vessel adventitia expands outward during the early stages of atherosclerosis.

Wall Morphology After Intervention

The ability of ultrasound to provide images before, as well as after, angioplasty has enabled routine evaluation of the mechanism and extent of luminal enlargement. Intravascular ultrasound demonstrates a diverse spectrum of morphologic findings following balloon angioplasty that often include complex fractures or dissections in the vessel wall. The extreme distortion of lumen shape produced by balloon dilation represents the most adverse environment for angiographic quantitation of lesion severity. Theoretically, extravasation of contrast through narrow dissection channels within the intima, media, or adventitia of the vessel can enhance the apparent angiographic diameter of the vessel. In this setting, the angiographic appearance consists of a large, but "hazy" lumen, in which intravascular ultrasound reveals minimal balloon augmentation of lumen size.

Clinical studies of intravascular ultrasound document several distinct effects of balloon dilation. In some patients intimal fracture constitutes the sole or principal mechanism responsible for luminal enlargement. In these cases ultrasound can readily determine the depth of the dissection, which may range from superficial intimal disruption to extensive periadventitial tears. Plaque dissections typically consist of single fracture, but can occasionally comprise multiple tears. The typical site for dissection consists of a junction between hard and soft plaque elements. Experienced observers have noted that hard or calcified plaques require higher balloon pressures for successful dilation. Several ongoing studies will examine the relationship between the extent of dissection and long-term clinical outcome.

Although dissection represents the most common mechanism of luminal enlargement, intravascular imaging in some patients does not yield demonstrable evidence of plaque fracture after angioplasty. In such vessels ultrasound usually identifies an alternative mechanism responsible for balloon enlargement of the lumen, most often stretching of the vessel wall. Analysis of the intravascular images can confirm this dilation effect whenever ultrasound measurements of media-adventitia diameter at the lesion site increase substantially following the procedure. In certain cases stretching of the vessel wall constitutes the sole mechanism responsible for the luminal gain. In a few patients, luminal enlargement results primarily from an apparent reduction in the cross-sectional area of the atheromatous plaque. Whether this phenomenon represents true plaque compression or simply axial redistribution of atheroma remains controversial.

Analysis of ultrasound before and after angioplasty does not always demonstrate a single mechanism of luminal enlargement. In more than half of patients, ultrasound examination shows a combination of the three mechanisms—dissection, stretching, and compression. However, the acute and long-term implications of each of the various mechanisms of luminal enlargement remain uncertain. Preliminary data suggest that vessels exclusively enlarged by media-adventitia stretching are more susceptible to restenosis secondary to acute or chronic recoil. However, there exist no prospective data describing the relationship between these morphologic patterns and long-term prognosis. Several clinical trials will examine this issue during the next several years.

Some investigators have speculated that intravascular ultrasound would prove particularly valuable in identifying angioplasty-related acute complications or predict the likelihood of abrupt closure. However, no criteria exist to distinguish therapeutic from pathologic dissection by intravascular ultrasound. In occasional cases dissection planes may be difficult to differentiate from certain plaque features, particularly sonolucent, lipid-laden atheromas. A potentially important morphologic feature, the presence or absence of thrombus, has thus far eluded accurate ultrasound characterization. The acoustic properties of intraluminal thrombus are similar to blood—a phenomenon that makes it difficult to identify thrombi with certainty. Some investigators have explored advanced acoustic techniques such as backscatter analysis to characterize thrombus, but with limited success in vivo. Another new imaging modality, fiberoptic angioscopy, appears better suited for this diagnostic application.

Directional Coronary Atherectomy

In experienced laboratories, intravascular ultrasound imaging has proven particularly valuable in the guidance of directional coronary atherectomy. Most clinicians consider the location and distribution of the atheroma as important factors in the selection of patients for directional atherectomy. Both the design of the device and initial angiographic studies have suggested that eccentric plaque would represent the optimal target for atherectomy. However, recent comparative studies have shown that the apparent distribution of the atheroma by angiography correlates poorly with plaque location determined by

intravascular ultrasound. Accordingly, lesions that appear concentric by angiography are often highly eccentric when examined by ultrasound. Conversely, angiographically eccentric lesions are frequently concentric by ultrasound. The poor correlation for plaque distribution likely reflects the disadvantages of a silhouette imaging method (angiography) in comparison with a tomographic imaging technique (ultrasound).

In ultrasound-guided atherectomy, the operator uses assessment of plaque distribution by intravascular ultrasound to determine both the device size and orientation of atherectomy cuts (Fig. 13.13). However, successful application of this approach requires experience, patience, and careful planning. Although ultrasound provides an excellent view of the circumferential distribution of plaque, precise orientation of the intravascular image remains a difficult challenge. Accordingly, experienced ultrasound practitioners will carefully examine the target vessel segment prior to atherectomy to locate anatomic landmarks, particularly side branches. The operator subsequently uses

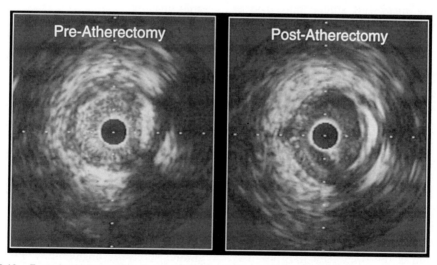

Figure 13.13.   Example of intravascular ultrasound before and after directional coronary atherectomy. In the left panel the preinterventional image shows a catheter occupying all of the lumen and surrounded by atherosclerotic plaque. At 3 o'clock there is an area of more echogenic plaque with shadowing of the underlying structures, thus indicating calcification. In the right panel the image postatherectomy shows approximately 80% of the plaque has been removed without deep injury to the artery. The calcified plaque remains unchanged.

these anatomic features to orient the intravascular ultrasound image. For example, an eccentric plaque in the left anterior descending coronary can be described as contralateral or ipsilateral to the septal perforators. Using this information, the operator can subsequently direct atherectomy cuts toward the appropriate side of the vessel.

The presence and extent of vessel wall calcification constitute important determinants of the efficacy of directional atherectomy. Traditionally, significant fluoroscopic calcification has constituted a contraindication to atherectomy. However, studies have confirmed that intravascular ultrasound reveals vessel calcification more frequently than fluoroscopy. Unlike radiographic methods, ultrasound can readily determine the circumferential location and depth of calcification. Vessels with extensive superficial calcification resist plaque removal by directional atherectomy, but arteries with extensive deep calcification can undergo successful atherectomy if ultrasound demonstrates only deep calcium. Conversely, vessels with little or no calcium on fluoroscopy may actually contain extensive superficial calcification, thus precluding successful atherectomy. During coronary atherectomy some experienced operators employ repeated examinations by ultrasound to guide the procedure, assisting determination of the extent of plaque removal and establishing the need for additional cuts.

Rotational Atherectomy

Utilization of the Rotablator, a high-speed, diamond-coated burr for percutaneous coronary revascularization, has increased rapidly following approval for human use by the Food and Drug Administration. Although experience remains limited, coronary intravascular ultrasound can significantly benefit clinical application of the Rotablator (54, 55). This device is particularly effective at removing superficial intimal calcium, precisely the type of lesion least suitable for directional coronary atherectomy. Accordingly, intravascular ultrasound evidence of the location and extent of calcification enables differentiation of lesions most suitable for rotablation from vessels more appropriate for directional atherectomy. Furthermore, the precise vessel sizing provided by ultrasound facilitates selection of the appropriately sized burr for rotational ablation.

Some initial clinical studies have suggested that the Rotablator may not be adequate as the sole treatment for some coronary lesions. In such cases intravascular ultrasound following the procedure can readily quantitate the size of the neolumen and characterize the morphology of the remaining atherosclerotic plaque. The operator can subsequently select the optimal technique and size of device used for further luminal enlargement. If little or no calcium remains following rotablation, directional atherectomy may be feasible. Conversely, the presence of extensive calcification will require the use of a larger Rotablator burr or adjunctive balloon angioplasty. Controlled trials of ultrasound-guided rotablation have not yet appeared, but anecdotal experience suggests that this will be a particularly effective niche for intravascular imaging.

Ultrasound Guidance of Stent Placement

The importance of coronary stenting has increased following publication of data demonstrating a reduction in the risk of restenosis with this therapy. However, studies have shown an increased risk of hemorrhagic complications following coronary stenting, presumably secondary to the aggressive anticoagulation and large sheath sizes required by most devices. Recent intravascular ultrasound studies have demonstrated failure to fully deploy coronary stents in a significant subset of patients in which the procedure was guided solely by angiography. Presumably, the porous nature of these stents results in the angiographic appearance of an enlarged lumen, even when some stent struts are not fully apposed to the vessel wall.

Some investigators have proposed that routine application of intravascular ultrasound to determine the adequacy of stent deployment could improve clinical outcome and reduce anticoagulation requirements. Employing ultrasound to assist stent deployment, a preliminary report from a single European center has reported a low stent thrombosis rate without vigorous anticoagulation. However, widespread application of this approach will require careful testing through prospective randomized trials.

New Coronary Ultrasound Devices

Important technical advances in intravascular imaging technology will likely emerge during the next few years. Industry engineers anticipate further reductions in the size of imaging catheters, and most authorities believe that an imaging guidewire will be feasible. A guidewire-sized ultrasound probe would enable simultaneous imaging during many revascularization procedure, regardless of the device. Very small devices would also enable imaging of virtually any coronary stenosis prior to treatment. Several investigators have demonstrated three-dimensional reconstruction of cross-sectional ultrasound images, but artifacts and other limitations have precluded any practical application of this technique.

Several industry and academic centers are jointly developing combination devices incorporating both diagnostic ultrasound imaging and therapeutic capability. An angioplasty balloon incorporating an ultrasound transducer has undergone extensive clinical testing (56). Other emerging devices include the combination of an ultrasound transducer within an atherectomy device and a cold laser combined with imaging probe. If combination devices provide practical assistance during interventional procedures, this technology will likely evolve as the future standard for revascularization procedures. Other imaging catheters under development incorporate a tip-mounted Doppler flow probe to allow simultaneous determinations of cross-sectional area and flow velocity. The impact of such a device remains uncertain, but it potentially offers the opportunity for simultaneous anatomic and functional assessment of coronary lesions.

SUMMARY

Determination of coronary dimensions and stenosis severity represents a fundamental requirement of modern interventional practice. The traditional approach to lesion assessment employs simple visual inspection of the angiogram to determine the extent and severity of luminal narrowing. However, visual methods are limited by large interobserver variability and poor correlation between apparent lesion severity and the physiologic effect of stenoses. Quantitative angiography provides more reproducible measurements of coronary dimensions, but is limited by difficulty in obtaining optimal angiographic projections and inability to portray the complex luminal shape of some atherosclerotic lesions. Attempts to quantify coronary flow reserve by digital angiography have also been thoroughly explored. However, such methods are severely limited by the cumbersome requirement for mask-mode subtraction and the limitations inherent in expressing coronary flow reserve as a ratio of hyperemic to basal flow.

Recent advances in microelectronic and piezoelectric technology have permitted development of miniaturized ultrasound devices capable of real-time tomographic intravascular imaging. The cross-sectional perspective of ultrasound appears ideally suited for precision measurements of luminal diameter and cross-sectional area. Ultrasound improves assessment of problem lesions, including ostial stenoses or disease at bifurcations, and permits identification of the morphologic characteristics of coronary plaques. Postprocedure, intravascular ultrasound often yields smaller luminal size measurements than QCA and indicates greater stenosis severity. These differences likely reflect augmentation of the apparent angiographic diameter by extraluminal contrast within cracks, fissures, or dissection planes. However, the clinical value of routine ultrasound imaging following mechanical revascularization has not been tested by randomized trials.

Thus there exists no universally accepted criteria for determination of the severity of a coronary stenoses, and no single method can provide optimal guidance of coronary interventions. Accordingly, the interventional practitioner must combine common sense with a fundamental understanding of the value and limitations of each of the quantitative methods to deduce the optimal course of action in approaching coronary stenotic lesions.

REFERENCES

1. Arnett EN, Isner JM, Redwood CR, Kent KM, Baker WP, Ackerstein H, Roberts WC. Coronary artery narrowing in coronary heart disease: comparison of cineangiographic and necropsy findings. Ann Intern Med 1979;91:350–356.

2. Grodin CM, Dydra I, Pastgernac A, Campeau L, Bourassa MG. Discrepancies between cineangiographic and post-mortem findings in patients with coronary artery disease and recent myocardial revascularization. Circulation 1974;49:703–709.

3. Isner JM, Kishel J, Kent KM. Accuracy of angiographic determination of left main coronary arterial narrowing. Circulation 1981;63:1056–1061.

4. Roberts WC, Jones AA. Quantitation of coronary arterial narrowing at necropsy in sudden coronary death. Am J Cardiol 1979;44:39–44.

5. Vlodaver Z, Frech R, van Tassel RA, Edwards JE. Correlation of the antemortem coronary angiogram and the post-mortem specimen. Circulation 1973;47:162–168.

6. Zir LM, Miller SW, Dinsmore RE, Gilber JP, Harthorne JW. Interobserver variability in coronary angiography. Circulation 1976;53:627–632.

7. White CW, Wright CB, Doty DB, Hirtza LF, Eastham CL, Harrison DG, Marcus ML. Does visual interpretation of the coronary arteriogram predict the physiologic importance of a coronary stenosis? N Engl J Med 1984;310:819–824.

8. Waller BF. "Crackers, breakers, stretchers, drillers, scrapers, shavers, burners, welders, and melters": the future treatment of atherosclerotic coronary artery disease? A clinical-morphologic assessment. J Am Coll Cardiol 1989;13:969–987.

9. Brown BG, Bolson E, Frimer M, Dodge HT. Quantitative coronary arteriography: estimation of dimensions, hemodynamic resistance, and atheroma mass of coronary artery lesions using the arteriograms and digital computation. Circulation 1977;55:329–337.

10. Selzer RH, Gagert CM, Azen SP, Siebes M, Lee P, Shircore A, Blankenhorn DH. Precision and reproducibility of quantitative coronary angiography with applications to controlled clinical trials. J Clin Invest 1989;83:520–526.

11. Reiber JHC, Serruys PW, Kooijman CJ, Wijns W, Slager CJ, Gerbrands JJ, Schuurbiers JCH et al. Assessment of short-, medium-, and long-term variations in arterial dimensions from computer-assisted quantitation of coronary cineangiograms. Circulation 1985;71:280–288.

12. Spears JR, Sandor T, Baim DS, Paulin S. The minimum error in estimating coronary luminal cross-sectional area from cineangiographic diameter measurements. Cathet Cardiovasc Diagn 1983;9:119–128.

13. Wollschlager H, Lee P, Zeiher A, Solzbach U, Bonzel T, Just H. Improvement of quantitative angiography of exact calculation of radiological magnification factors. Comput Cardiol 1985;483–486.

14. Kirkeeide RL, Fung P, Smalling RW, Gould KL. Automated evaluation of vessel diameter from arteriograms. Comput Cardiol 1982;215–218.

15. Deleted in proofs.

16. Nichols AB, Gabrieli CFO, Fenoglio JJ, Esser PD. Quantification of relative coronary arterial stenosis by cinevideo-densitometric analysis of coronary arteriograms. Circulation 1984;69:512–522.

17. Sanz ML, Mancini GB, LeFree MT, Nicholson JK, Starling MR, Vogel RA, Topol EJ. Variability of quantitative digital subtraction coronary angiography before and after percutaneous transluminal coronary angiography. Am J Cardiol 1987;60:55–60.

18. Shaw CG, Ergun DL, Myerowitz PD, Van Lysel MS, Mistretta CA, Zarnstorff, Crummy AB. A technique for scatter and veiling glare correction for video densitometric studies in digital subtraction videoangiography. Radiology 1982;142:209–215.

19. Kirkeeide RL, Gould KL, Hamilton GW. Physiologic basis for assessing critical coronary stenosis. Instantaneous flow response and regional distribution during coronary hyperemia as measures of coronary flow reserve. Am J Cardiol 1974;33:87–93.

20. Kirkeeide RL, Gould KL, Parsel L. Assessment of coronary stenoses by myocardial perfusion imaging during pharmacologic coronary vasodilation. VII. Validation of coronary flow reserve as a single integrated functional measure of stenosis severity reflecting all its geometric dimensions. J Am Coll Cardiol 1986;7:103–113.

21. Gurley JC, Nissen SE, Booth DC, Harrison M, DeMaria AN. Influence of operator and patient-dependent variables on the suitability of automated coronary arteriography. J Am Coll Cardiol 19(6):1237–1243.

22. Gurley JC, Nissen SN, Booth DC, Harrison MR, Grayburn PA, Elion JL, DeMaria AN. Comparison of simultaneously performed digital and film-based angiography in the assessment of coronary artery disease. Circulation 1988;78(6):1411–1420.

23. Gurley JC, Nissen SE. Digital coronary angiography: Is it ready to replace cine film? Cardio 1991;8(2):82.

24. Nissen SE, Pepine CJ, Block PC, Brinker J, Douglas JS, Johnson WL, Klinke WP et al. Cardiac angiography without cine film: erecting a "Tower of Babel" in the catheterization laboratory. J Am Coll Cardiol (in press).

25. Mancini GBJ, Simon SB, McGillem MJ, LeFree MT, Friedman HZ, Vogel RA. Automated quantitative coronary arteriography: morphologic and physiologic validation in vivo of a rapid digital angiographic method. Circulation 1987; 75:452–460.

26. Rutishauser W, Simon H, Stucky JP, Schaad N, Noseda G, Wellauer J. Evaluation of Roentgen densitometry for flow

measurement in models and in intact circulation. Circulation 1967;36:951–963.

27. Foerster JM, Link DP, Lanz BMT, Holcroft JW, Mason DT. Measurement of coronary reactive hyperemia during clinical angiography video dilution technique. Acta Radiol Diagn 1981;22:209–216.

28. Vogel RA, LeFree MT, Bates ER, O'Neil WW, Foster R, Kirlin P, Smith D et al. Application of digital techniques to selective coronary arteriography: use of myocardial appearance time to measure coronary flow reserve. Am Heart J 1983;7:153–164.

29. Nissen SE, Elion JL, Booth DC, Evans J, DeMaria AN. Value and limitations of computer analysis of digital subtraction angiography in the assessment of coronary flow reserve. Circulation 1986;73:562–571.

30. Whiting JS, Drury JK, Pfaff JM, Chang BL, Eigler NL, Meerbaum S, Corday E et al. Digital angiographic measurement of radiographic contrast material kinetics for estimation of myocardial perfusion. Circulation 1986; 73:789–798.

31. Cusma JT, Toggart EJ, Folts JD, Peppler WW, Hagiandreou NJ, Lee CS, Mistetta CA. Digital subtraction angiographic imaging of coronary flow reserve. Circulation 1987;74:461–472.

32. Wilson RF, White CW. Intracoronary papaverine: an ideal coronary vasodilator for studies of the coronary circulation in conscious humans. Circulation 1986;73:444–451.

33. Hodgson JMCB, Mancini JGB, Legrand V, Vogel RA. Characterization of changes in coronary blood flow during the first six seconds after intracoronary contrast injection. Invest Radiol 1985;20:246–252.

34. Hodgson JMcB, Legrand V, Bates ER, Mancini GB, Aueron FM, O'Neil WW, Simon SB et al. Validation in dogs of a rapid digital angiographic technique to measure relative coronary blood flow during routine cardiac catheterization. Am J Cardiol 1985;55:188–193.

35. Pijls NHJ, Uijen GJH, Hoevelaken A, Arts T, Aengevaeren WRM, Bos HS, Fast JH et al. Mean transit time for the assessment of myocardial perfusion by videodensitometry. Circulation 1990;81:1331–1340.

36. Nissen SE, Gurley JC. Assessment of the functional significance of coronary stenoses. Is digital angiography the answer? Circulation 1990;81:1431–1435.

37. Bursch J, Johs R, Heintzen P. Validity of Lambert-Beer law in roentgen densitometry of contrast material (urograaffin) using continuous radiation. In: Heintzen PH, ed. Roentgencine and videodensitometry. Stuttgart: Georg Thieme Verlag, 1971.

38. Bom N, Lancee CT, Van Egmond FC. An ultrasonic intracardiac scanner. Ultrasonics 1972;10:72–76.

39. Yock PG, Johnson EL, Linker DT. Intravascular ultrasound: development and clinical potential. Am J Card Imaging 1988;2:185–193.

40. Roelandt JR, Bom N, Serruys PW. Intravascular high-resolution real-time, two-dimensional echocardiography. Int J Card Imaging 1989;4:63–67.

41. Nissen SE, Gurley JC. Application of intravascular ultrasound for detection and quantitation of coronary atherosclerosis. Int J Card Imaging 1991;6(3-4):165–177.

42. Nissen SE, Grines CL, Gurley JC, Sublett K, Haynie D, Diaz C, Booth DC et al. Application of a new phased-array ultrasound imaging catheter in the assessment of vascular dimensions: in vivo comparison to cineangiography. Circulation 1990;81(2):660–666.

43. Hodgson J, Graham SP, Savakus AD, Dame SG, Stephens DN, Dhillion D, Brands D et al. Clinical percutaneous imaging of coronary anatomy using an over-the-wire ultrasound catheter system. Int J Card Imaging 1989;4:187–193.

44. Nissen SE, Gurley JC, DeMaria AN. Assessment of vascular disease by intravascular ultrasound. Cardiology 1990;77(5):398–410.

45. Tobis JM, Mallery J, Mahon D, Lehmann K, Zalesky P, Griffith J, Gessert J et al. Intravascular ultrasound imaging of human coronary arteries in vivo. Analysis of tissue characterizations with comparison to in vitro histological specimens. Circulation 1991;83(3):913–926.

46. Nissen SE, Gurley JC, Grines CL, Booth DC, McClure R, Berk M, Fischer C et al. Intravascular ultrasound assessment of lumen size and wall morphology in normal subjects and coronary artery disease patients. Circulation 1991; 84(3):1087–1099.

47. Pandian NG, Kreis A, Brockway B, Isner JM, Sacharoff A, Boleza E, Caro R et al. Ultrasound angioscopy: real-time, two-dimensional, intraluminal ultrasound imaging of blood vessels. Am J Cardiol 1988;62:113–116.

48. Hermiller JB, Buller CE, Tenaglia AN, Kisslo KB, Phillips HR, Bashore TM, Stack RS et al. Unrecognized left main coronary artery disease in patients undergoing interventional procedures. Am J Cardiol 1993;71(2):173–176.

49. De Franco AC, Tuzcu EM, Eaton G, Raymond RE, Franco I, Guyer A, Nissen SE. Detection of unrecognized LMCA disease by intravascular ultrasound in patients undergoing interventions: prevalence and severity. Circulation 1993; 88(4)I:411A.

50. Glagov S, Weisenberg E, Zarins CK et al. Compensatory enlargement of human coronary arteries. N Engl J Med 1987;316:1371–1375.

51. White CJ, Ramee SR, Collin TJ, Jain A, Mesa JE. Ambiguous coronary angiography: clinical utility of intravascular ultrasound. Cathet Cardiovasc Diagn 1992; 26(3):200–203.

52. Nissen SE, De Franco AC, Raymond RE, Franco I, Eaton G, Tuzcu EM. Angiographically unrecognized disease at "normal" reference sites: a risk factor for sub-optimal results after coronary interventions. Circulation 1993; 88(4)I:412A.

53. Nissen SE, Tuzcu EM, DeFranco AC, Franco I, Raymond RE, Elliot J, Lefkovits J et al. Intravascular ultrasound evidence of atherosclerosis at "normal" reference sites predicts adverse clinical outcomes following percutaneous coronary intervention. J Am Coll Cardiol (Special Issue) 1994;1A-484A:271A.

54. Mintz GS, Potkin BN, Keren G, Satler LF, Pichard AD, Kent KM, Popma JJ et al. Intravascular ultrasound evaluation of

the effect of rotational atherectomy in obstructive athero-sclerotic coronary artery disease. Circulation 1992; 86(5):1383–1393.

55. Tuzcu EM, Whitlow PL, DeFranco AC, Raymond RE, Elliot J, Lefkovits J, Guyer S et al. Comparison of DCA and rotab-lation by intravascular ultrasound: mechanism and extent of plaque removal. J Am Coll Cardiol (Special Issue) 1994;1A-484:301A.

56. Cacchione JG, Reddy K, Richards F, Sheehan H, Hodgson JM. Combined intravascular ultrasound/angioplasty bal-loon catheter: initial use during PTCA. Cathet Cardiovasc Diagn 1991;24(2):99–101.

14. Myocardial Revascularization as Therapy for Silent Ischemia

PAUL W. DIGGS and PETER F. COHN

Ischemic heart disease becomes clinically apparent when the heart's supply of oxygenated blood is insufficient to meet its metabolic demands at the time. Clinical syndromes range from acute myocardial infarction to episodes of silent (painless) myocardial ischemia. Appropriate management is based on manipulating those variables that affect myocardial oxygen supply and demand in the most innocuous manner possible. The physician's ultimate goal is to prevent morbidity and mortality. This chapter discusses the role of coronary revascularization, particularly percutaneous transluminal coronary angioplasty (PTCA), in the management of silent myocardial ischemia. Before considering how this treatment modality is being used to treat patients with this syndrome, a brief review of the pathophysiology and prognosis of the syndrome is warranted.

PATHOPHYSIOLOGY OF SILENT ISCHEMIA

Our understanding of the pathophysiology of coronary disease has grown significantly in the last decade. We now know that the atheromatous plaque is only one factor in a complex equation. Abnormalities of vasomotor tone and coagulability are also significant. The coronary vasculature is autoregulated with input from the neurohumoral system, as well as metabolic and physical factors. Additionally, the coronary arteries are richly innervated by the parasympathetic and sympathetic nervous system. The compressive force of the left ventricle, the left ventricular wall stress, and its architecture all affect flow in a purely physical manner. There is also some degree of inherent myogenic tone. Endothelial dysfunction, with resulting loss of ability to produce endothelium-derived relaxing factor (EDRF), has recently been appreciated as a major contributor to the development of abnormal vasoconstriction.

The myocardial ischemia that is a consequence of the factors described above may or may not be associated with anginal symptoms. The reasons for lack of anginal pain with the ischemic episodes are unclear (1). Coronary angioplasty has helped shed light on whether less myocardium is rendered ischemic during silent ischemia. Wohlgelernter et al. (2) reported no differences in the fall in left ventricular ejection fraction during silent as compared with painful ischemia produced by angioplasty (Fig. 14.1). A clear appreciation of the sequence of events during myocardial ischemia has also resulted from angioplasty studies. For example, Sigwart and colleagues (3) were among the first to use this procedure to shed additional light on the ischemic cascade. In 12 patients, a catheter was placed in the pulmonary artery, and a high-fidelity micromanometer was placed in the left ventricle via the transseptal approach. Figure 14.2 shows the sequence of events over the course of the first 30 seconds after occlusion. It was of interest that the relaxation parameters were the most sensitive of all the variables. (This confirmed earlier reports in experimental animals.) The authors concluded that "ischemia in conscious man is always characterized by a transition period during

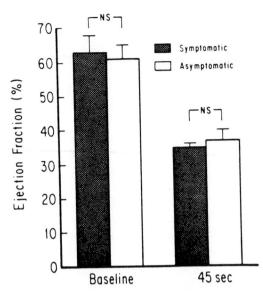

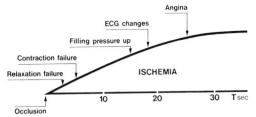

Figure 14.2. Appearance of events during transient coronary occlusion associated with PTCA. (From Sigwart U, Grbic M, Payot M, Goy J-J, Essinger A, Fischer A. In: Rutishauser W, Roskamm H, eds. Silent myocardial ischemia. Berlin: Springer-Verlag, 1984. Reproduced with permission.)

Figure 14.1. Comparison of global left ventricular ejection fraction responses to balloon inflation in patients who were symptomatic or asymptomatic during PTCA. There were no differences between the groups in ejection fraction values at baseline or at 45 seconds into inflation. T, ±1 SD. (From Wohlgelernter D, Jaffe CC, Cabin HS, Yeatman LA Jr, Cleman M. J Am Coll Cardiol 1987;10:491. Reproduced with permission.)

which it remains silent." Labovitz et al. (4) reported similar findings in their echocardiographic studies, as did Serruys et al. (5) using cine ventriculography. Recently, Tomai et al. (6) reported on the pathogenesis of the cardiac pain mechanism during coronary angioplasty. They concluded that the degree of stretching of the vessel wall could explain which inflations were painful.

PROGNOSIS IN SILENT ISCHEMIA

For an asymptomatic condition such as silent ischemia to be clinically important, it must have some association with patient outcome. The relationship of silent ischemia and adverse outcome has been addressed in the various clinical subsets of patients with coronary artery disease, that is, totally asymptomatic patients, postinfarction patients, and patients with angina (7). Within each clinically defined group there are subgroups of patients who are at very high risk and others

at very low risk for adverse outcome. Thus recent studies indeed indicate a strong association between silent ischemia and risk of adverse outcome, especially in the presence of multivessel coronary artery disease and left ventricular dysfunction. These studies may be divided into those involving exercise or other forms of stress-induced silent ischemia (8) and those relying on transient ischemia detected during the patient's daily life by Holter monitoring (9). Most of the latter episodes (70 to 90%) are without symptoms (10). In general, the greater degree of ischemia (as documented by perfusion defects, reduction in left ventricular ejection fraction, degree or duration of ST segment depression, etc.), the worse the prognosis (10).

GOALS OF THERAPY

Once one accepts the prognostic importance of silent ischemia, then therapy is a reasonable sequence, but one must have a clear understanding of the goals of therapy. The first and foremost objective of therapy is the prevention of death. However, other goals include minimizing periods of ischemia, ensuring adequate organ perfusion, and creating a minimum of adverse effects, as well as preserving lifestyle. The initial decision facing patients in every clinical subgroup is that of whether medical therapy is adequate or whether some form of revascularization should be attempted. There are certain categories that clearly require surgical therapy such as left main coronary artery stenosis and three-vessel coronary disease with reduced left ventricular systolic function. In addition, patients with stenosis of two vessels, where one of the affected arteries is the proximal portion of the left anterior descending, should probably be revascularized, especially if there is any decrease in the left ventricular ejection fraction. PTCA could play an important role in the management of many of these patients, but *all* patients must be evaluated according to their specific ischemic syndrome. Patient lifestyle and preference, as well as response to medical therapy, should be considered. Patients whose vigorous activity schedules are limited by anginal symptoms, objective indices of ischemia, or medication side effects may require more liberal consideration of revascularization.

MEDICAL THERAPY

The first step in the medical treatment of ischemic heart disease is risk-factor modification and lifestyle adjustment. Patients who smoke should quit; otherwise any form of therapy will be difficult. Any dyslipidemia should be aggressively treated. Patients with "normal" lipid levels will benefit from further lipid lowering. It is quite clear that the rigorous control of serum lipids will provide some degree of regression of the coronary atheroma. Increased physical activity should be encouraged, with a progressive exercise program. The benefits of exercise are twofold; improvement in the lipid profile and in conditioning. These measures should occur no matter what form of medical therapy is undertaken, and should not be ignored in the face of surgical therapy.

The first pharmacologic agent to consider is aspirin. It is accepted that rheologic factors must be modified and that antiplatelet therapy improves outcome. We routinely prescribe aspirin in the 80 to 325 mg range daily. The patient who suffers from gastrointestinal distress will find enteric-coated formulations available in this dosage.

Antiischemic agents can be given alone or in combination therapy (11). We begin with nitroglycerin, an inexpensive agent that should be the mainstay of therapy. Its actions include coronary vasodilation and a reduction in myocardial wall stress and preload. It also has some antiplatelet effects; however, it is not clear what the clinical significance of these are. The key point to remember is to avert the development of tolerance with a nitrate-free interval. This interval is usually governed by the symptom complex and should occur at a time when the patient would ordinarily be angina free. Given the cost considerations and the efficacy of this agent, it is certainly a first-line therapy.

Beta-blockers are the other first-line agents. There are a myriad of benefits to beta-blocker use. Their main effect is to reduce the myocardial oxygen demand via a reduction in the heart rate. By causing a greater diastolic interval, this may also allow greater coronary filling. These agents have also been shown to have an antiplatelet effect, the significance of which is again not known. There is an adverse effect on lipid levels with the use of these agents; however, they clearly benefit morbidity and mortality in spite of this. There are three features that separate agents of this class: presence of intrinsic sympathomimetic activity, lipophilicity, and cardioselectivity. Agents with intrinsic sympathomimetic activity allow less resting bradycardia, with beta-blockade only on activity. These agents do not provide survival benefit after myocardial infarction. Cardioselectivity is a measure of the relative specificity for the beta-1 receptor found in cardiac tissue; however, at full beta-blocking doses, this effect seems to be lost. These agents are negative inotropes and should be used with caution in patients with congestive heart failure. They should also be avoided in patients with greater than first-degree heart block. In appropriately selected patients they are the most efficacious class of drugs for relieving both painful and painless episodes of ischemia. They should be dosed as the patient maintains adequate blood pressure and organ perfusion.

The calcium channel blockers are the final class of anti-ischemics. They are a heterogenous group comprised of three prototypical drugs: nifedipine, diltiazem, and verapamil. These agents cause vasodilation, as well as a decrease in the myocardial oxygen demand. The most potent vasodilator and clinically least negatively inotropic is nifedipine; however, the opposite is true for verapamil, and diltiazem falls between the two. These agents are excellent antianginals, but they are less effective than the beta-blockers. They have not been as successful in post–myocardial infarction protection. Dosage should be the maximal tolerated as assessed by blood pressure and AV conduction. These agents are negative inotropes that also block the conduction system, and therefore caution should be exercised in patients with congestive failure or greater than first-degree heart block. Newer agents such as amlodopine and felodopine may allow use in the setting of congestive heart failure or low ejection fraction.

In translating this data to actual patient care, one must individualize and use patient profiling. Patients with significant congestive heart failure and angina may be managed with nitrates and aspirin only, or one of the newer calcium blockers. However, if this is not successful and revascularization therapy is not an option, beta-blockers may be attempted in a low dose with slow titration to effect. In the patient with normal ventricular function and chronic stable angina, aspirin, nitrates, and or beta-blockers would be the agents of first choice. Calcium channel blockers would also be useful in the patient who needed them to improve lifestyle or because beta-blockers are contraindicated. Patients with severe symptoms frequently require all three agents in combination. In the setting of combination therapy with beta and calcium blockers, one should be alert to the development of AV block or congestive heart failure.

Assessing response to therapy is a key part of the management of coronary disease. The primary variable to follow is the history. The patient with no symptom relief is clearly experiencing a failure of therapy, but what of the patient with frequent episodes of silent ischemia, with or without concomitant angina? This patient should experience an improvement in exercise tolerance and other objective measures of ischemia reduction. Repeat exercise testing is a convenient and easy-to-evaluate maneuver. The functional capacity, time to ST-segment depression, and magnitude of ST depression are all variables to evaluate; they allow objective quantification of the success of therapy and alert the physician to the need for a more invasive workup. Holter monitoring is another tool for follow-up. The variables to follow on the Holter monitor are the number and duration of episodes and the total minutes of ischemic ST depression. The Holter monitor allows assessment of therapy in the patient's native environment and therefore may be a less artificial method.

Improvement in prognosis following medical therapy has been difficult to establish, but in 1994 the Atenolol Silent Ischemia Study (ASIST) (12) provided such data in 306 patients randomized either to atenolol or placebo.

REVASCULARIZATION PROCEDURES

The proper role for PTCA and coronary artery bypass grafting (CABG) in the treatment of silent ischemia in still evolving. Five recent reports all suggest that PTCA can be safely done in patients with silent ischemia (13–17) (Table 14.1). Representative of these studies is that of Anderson et al. Of 6545 patients who had elective PTCA over a 7.5-year period, 114 (1.7%) never had symptoms of myocardial ischemia. Exercise-induced silent ischemia was documented in 94% of the patients (the other 6% did not undergo exercise tests for a variety of reasons). PTCA was successful in 87% and unsuccessful in 7% (who had no in-hospital cardiac events), with another 4% requiring emergency coronary artery surgery and yet another 2% having

15. The Calcified Lesion

ALAA E. ABDELMEGUID and PATRICK L. WHITLOW

THE SUBSTRATE

Intimal splitting and plaque fracture are frequently associated with percutaneous transluminal coronary angioplasty (PTCA). Indeed, plaque and intimal disruption with or without localized medial dissection are components of the major mechanism of successful PTCA (1). Although this sequence may be necessary in many cases for satisfactory enlargement of the arterial lumen, the degree of injury caused by the procedure is difficult to control. In some cases extensive dissection occurs, resulting in acute closure of the vessel. Morphologic and histologic assessment of atherosclerotic plaques suggests that certain plaque compositions are more, or less, susceptible to PTCA-induced dissection, and that the type and extent of disruption caused by balloon inflation are a function of the biomechanical properties of the atherosclerotic plaque itself (1–4).

Calcification is a widely accepted risk factor for decreased success and increased complications with PTCA in part because of the increased pressures required for dilation. Several studies demonstrated that dissections typically originate at regions where there is a transition between plaque and more "normal" vessel wall (3, 4). These inflection points result in a sudden increase in flexibility of the arterial segment (4). Using computer modeling to predict the interaction of plaque composition and stress distribution in the formation of intimal tears, Richardson et al. showed that regions of high circumferential stress correlate well with the site of intimal tears found at necropsy, and that high tensile stress within a diseased vessel segment occurs at

junctions between tissue types with different elastic properties, for example, regions of transition between plaque and normal wall or between areas of soft and calcific plaque (3). Biomechanical modeling studies of plaque also suggest that the presence of calcium is in part responsible for high shear forces during balloon inflation, substantially increasing the likelihood of dissection (3).

Therefore coronary artery calcification appears to be an important determinant of the arterial response to percutaneous coronary interventions. Moderate-to-heavy coronary calcification has been associated with a decreased success rate, as well as increased acute closure and complication rates during balloon angioplasty (5, 6).

Detection of Coronary Calcification

Fluoroscopy is the standard method for detection of coronary artery calcification, but while it indicates the presence of calcification within the vessel wall, it does not provide information regarding the amount or location of calcium within the plaque substance. Moreover, only 14 to 58% of patients with documented coronary artery disease have fluoroscopic calcification compared with 79% on pathologic examination (7–10), reflecting the low sensitivity of fluoroscopy in the detection of coronary artery calcification.

Recent advances in intravascular ultrasound (IVUS) imaging have renewed interest in the study of coronary artery calcification. This new imaging modality offers the potential for a detailed characterization of coronary artery calcification, as well as increased sensitivity for its detection. Mintz et al. showed that fluoroscopic calcification increases with increasing amounts of target lesion calcification (7). Fluoroscopy detected calcium in 74% of patients with multiquadrant target-lesion calcification and in 86% of patients with long multiquadrant calcification ≥6 mm in length. However, fluoroscopy missed all short multiquadrant calcifications <5 mm in length. Using IVUS, 52 to 83% of patients with documented coronary artery disease have been shown to have some coronary artery calcification (7–9). Recent IVUS studies showed a relationship between coronary artery calcification and coronary dissection (8). At the PTCA site, arterial dissection occurs more frequently in calcified plaques, whereas arterial expansion occurs more frequently in noncalcified plaques. The presence of calcium within the vessel wall appears to be significantly associated with both the location and the site of the dissection from the vessel wall (11, 12). These data suggest that localized calcium deposits have a direct role in causing dissection, presumably by increasing shear stresses and defining cleavage planes within the plaque.

THE APPROACH

At the Cleveland Clinic the traditional approach toward balloon angioplasty of calcified lesions has been modified by the recent availability of new transcatheter therapies that have lower complication rates compared with historical controls treated with conventional PTCA (13–16). The recent data provided by IVUS are helpful in guiding percutaneous interventions of calcified lesions: IVUS can differentiate target lesion calcification from calcification of contiguous arterial segments, document the progress of decalcification during rotational atherectomy or excimer laser ablation, and identify deep calcium deposits at the intimal medial border (7). Deep calcification in the absence of superficial calcification does not preclude the use of directional coronary atherectomy (DCA) and may actually protect against

severe medial injury. As more transcatheter therapies become available, IVUS may be routinely used to analyze target lesion composition and characterize the types of plaque to select among the various percutaneous modalities.

Percutaneous Transluminal Coronary Angioplasty (PTCA)

PTCA of calcified lesions often requires higher balloon inflation pressures, with the attendant risk of balloon rupture, vessel trauma, and balloon entrapment. The Rotablator is the first choice for heavily calcified lesions at the Cleveland Clinic, and the Rotablator or the excimer laser (ELCA) is frequently used for moderately calcified lesions. For mildly calcified focal stenoses with no other adverse angiographic characteristics, PTCA is frequently performed using a balloon that can withstand high inflation pressure (polyethylene terephthalate, PET, or Duralyn). The balloon is positioned with the distal one-third inflated in the lesion, so that less balloon material is trapped within the lesion in the event of balloon rupture, thus facilitating balloon withdrawal. At the Cleveland Clinic, PTCA of long calcified lesions (>10 mm) is rarely attempted because of the increased risk of ischemic complications and/or technical failure. The Rotablator and ELCA appear better suited for these lesions based on their ability to ablate hard, calcified atheromas and the high success rate of ELCA in excessively long lesions. Adjunctive PTCA is usually performed following the Rotablator or ELCA, but it does not have the same adverse effects as primary PTCA of calcified lesions, most likely because of the changes in plaque characteristics induced by ELCA or the Rotablator.

The Rotablator

Because of its high rotational speed, the Rotablator preferentially ablates inelastic, fixed, atheromatous tissue. Plaque-free wall segments are spared from mechanical trauma because their viscoelastic properties make them deflect around the rotating burr. Rotational atherectomy burrs can also traverse tortuous vessels because of the flexibility of the coaxial shaft.

In vitro experimental studies show that the residual lumen after rotablation is smooth and polished. The endothelium is denuded, various portions of the atheromatous plaque are ablated, damage to the media is minor, and extensive dissections are not present (17, 18). In vivo the appearance of a coronary artery and its lumen after rotablation is very different from its appearance after either balloon angioplasty or directional coronary atherectomy (19). IVUS images after using the Rotablator show a circular or near circular lumen, especially in areas of heavy calcification. The arc of calcium becomes smaller, and the interface between the residual atherosclerotic plaque and the lumen is smooth. Fissures and/or dissections are uncommon, occurring in less than one-half of patients, with significant tissue disruption occurring in less than one-third of patients. When dissections occur, they are typically superficial, located within an arc of calcium, and have limited axial and circumferential extension. This is in contrast to balloon angioplasty of calcified lesions in which dissections, frequently extensive, are the rule (12).

The Rotablator is our first choice for moderately to heavily calcified lesions. Usually a small burr size (1.75 mm) is used initially and gradually upsized to minimize microparticle embolization during burr passage. Passing the burr slowly with minimal forward pressure against the stenosis in runs ≤45 seconds is

thought to reduce spasm and minimize slow flow. The burr size is gradually increased in 0.25 to 0.365 mm increments. The rotablation procedure is terminated at a burr/artery ratio of ≈0.80 or when a residual stenosis of <20% is achieved. This is followed by adjunctive PTCA or DCA to achieve the largest, safest residual lumen. Using a single large burr as proposed by Zacca et al. works well with restenotic lesions, but may cause more complications in de novo stenoses (20). The sequential utilization of small to large burrs decreases plaque burden with each pass and may lower the risk of dissection, microembolism, and slow flow. When Stertzer et al. analyzed 23 lesions in which there was either a severe dissection, occlusion, or perforation, it was shown that in 61% of these cases burr sizes were skipped, and that in 26% of these cases a relatively large burr was used as the first device (21). The Rotablator is continuously rotated during advancement and withdrawal of the burr. The speed is not allowed to drop below 90% of the free-running speed, which could be an indication of excessive load being placed on the burr because of the rapid advancement. Once a dissection has been identified, rotablation is stopped to avoid its extension.

The majority of patients undergoing rotational atherectomy have lesions with complex morphology (type B2 or C) that are known to adversely affect PTCA results. Despite that, the angiographic success, complication profile, and restenosis associated with rotational atherectomy appear to compare favorably with PTCA (Table 15.1) (21–24). Lesion calcification does not appear to adversely affect

Table 15.1
Rotational Atherectomy: Acute Results

	N	Success (%)	Q-Wave MI (%)	Non–Q-Wave MI (%)	CABG (%)	Death (%)
Buchbinder 1991	745	94	0.8	4.6	1.4	0.0
Bertrand 1992	129	86	2.3	5.5	1.6	0.0
Stertzer 1993	302	95	3.3	11.0	1.2	0.0
Cowley 1993	1362	95	0.9	4.6	2.1	0.8

the procedural success rates of rotational atherectomy, and major complications (death, emergency CABG, and Q-wave MI) are similar for calcified compared with noncalcified lesions (13). Moreover, the degree of calcification itself does not seem to affect the success or complication rates of the Rotablator (25). In a series of 41 complex lesions, 74% with calcification and 72% with marked eccentricity, the Rotablator was successful in 98% of lesions (26). Whitlow et al. reported on 874 lesions in 745 patients treated with the Rotablator and found that lesion calcification did not have an adverse effect on angiographic success (14). Moreover, unlike PTCA, cumulative effects of angiographic risk factors on success were not apparent; in fact, type A, B1, B2, and C lesions had comparable angiographic success rates (97%, 94%, 95%, and 95%, respectively). Popma et al. found that angulation $\geq 45°$ was the only risk factor for procedural failure (angiographic failure, death, Q-wave MI, or emergency CABG) ($P < .005$; odds ratio 3.67) and that minor complications (recurrent ischemia, abrupt closure, and repeat PTCA) were related to proximal tortuosity ($P < .05$; odds ratio 3.36), bifurcation lesions ($P < .05$; odds ratio 2.31), and de novo lesions ($P < .001$; odds ratio 5.68). These results suggest that the technique may be the preferred method of revascularization in heavily calcified and complex lesions (27, 28).

Excimer Laser Coronary Angioplasty (ELCA)

Continuous-wave laser irradiation is ineffective against calcium; however, pulsed-wave laser devices may partially ablate calcium (29). Experience with ELCA in calcified lesions has been favorable. Stand-alone ELCA was successful in 72% (68 of 95) calcified lesions and in 96% (91 of 95) with adjunctive PTCA (15). Cook et al. also reported a success rate of 91% in moderately to heavily calcified lesions (16). One limitation of ELCA is related to its occasional inability to ablate heavily calcified plaque (30). In vitro

the ablation threshold for atherosclerotic plaque approximates 50 mjoule/mm^2 for a single fiber; however, this threshold is obtained at an ideal perpendicular orientation of plaque and fiber surface. In vivo, laser energy may hit plaques only at an oblique angle, thus not achieving ablation; moreover, the use of a low ratio of effective fiber surface to total catheter surface may contribute to failures in heavily calcified plaques. Buchwald et al. found that in a small number of patients, the ELCA catheter could not be advanced across the lesion despite the presence of a guidewire (30), pointing to the inability of ELCA to ablate heavily calcified lesions. Improved results may be obtained by starting with a small probe and lasing with higher than usual energy densities (50–60 mjoule/mm^2).

The ELCA is particularly useful in long calcified lesions (≥ 20 to 25 mm). Rotablator results are most effective on lesions < 25 mm, but are less productive when there is diffuse coronary artery disease (14, 31). Whitlow et al. reported on 874 lesions treated with the Rotablator and found that while the procedural success rate was similar for stenoses < 10 mm in length compared with lesions between 10 and 25 mm in length (95% versus 94%, respectively), the acute major complications (3.6% versus 6.0%, respectively) and the restenosis rates (36% versus 45%, respectively) were higher in patients with diffuse disease (14). In a much smaller population (42 patients) that underwent stand-alone rotablation, Tiersten et al. also found higher complication and restenosis rates with diffuse disease (31). Reisman et al. evaluated the use of rotational atherectomy in the treatment of long lesions (15 to 25 mm) and found that despite the high initial procedural success rate (92%), these lesions carry a higher rate of Q-wave MI (2.8%) when compared with shorter lesions (32). There was also a trend toward higher procedural complications and restenosis in patients with long lesions. Therefore rotational atherectomy is avoided in stenoses ≥25 mm in length unless the artery is severely calcified, and ELCA may be preferable for lesions >25 mm in length without heavy calcification.

Adjunctive PTCA

Adjunctive PTCA following rotational atherectomy or ELCA does not appear to be associated with the same adverse results as primary PTCA of calcified stenoses. In vivo studies showed that dissection planes caused by adjunct balloon angioplasty are located within the plaque (19), in contrast to standalone PTCA of calcified lesions where the dissection planes appear at the junction of calcified and noncalcified plaque (12). When adjunctive PTCA is used, indirect indices of plaque compliance (lesion stretch, acute gain, and elastic recoil) suggest that the responsiveness of the lesion is altered as a result of rotational atherectomy, verifying that ablation of the fibrocalcific plaque increases lesion compliance and permits more effective adjunctive PTCA (25). The relative safety and success of adjunctive PTCA are also partially related to the pattern of coronary artery calcification, which has been recently evaluated by IVUS: circumferential deposition of calcium tends to be greater than axial deposition; therefore short arterial segments with extensive (multiquadrant) circumferential calcification are more common than are long segments with single quadrant calcification. When this short segment is removed by the Rotablator or ELCA, adjunctive PTCA (or DCA) can be easily performed. Also the Rotablator might not only ablate plaque but also may cause or unmask weakness in the structural integrity of the residual calcific deposit. The Rotablator may also remove a thin layer of superficial calcium to expose noncalcified fibrotic or soft plaque. This modification of the characteristics of the calcified plaque allows successful application of adjunctive PTCA. At the Cleveland Clinic IVUS is frequently used to determine when to terminate rotablation or ELCA after completion of decalcification and when to start adjunctive PTCA or DCA. A trial is planned to determine whether attempting to achieve the largest safest residual lumen with rotablation (Rotablator) alone or following with adjunctive PTCA in vessels ≤3 mm is the best strategy in minimizing restenosis, presumably by decreasing the residual plaque burden and possibly decreasing deep wall injury.

Adjunctive Directional Coronary Atherectomy

DCA does not cut target lesion calcium well, and proximal vessel calcification impedes passage of the atherectomy device. Subsequently, the success rate of DCA in angiographically calcified lesions has been as low as 52% (33). Recent IVUS studies have been pivotal in increasing our understanding of the potential role of DCA in the treatment of calcified lesions. Fitzgerald et al. studied the influence of calcium distribution within plaque on tissue retrieval (quantified as tissue weights) by DCA using IVUS (11). Significantly less tissue was removed from superficially calcified lesions (located within the intima) compared with lesions with only deep calcification (located below the surface of the plaque at the medial border) or noncalcified lesions. Tissues extracted from noncalcified lesions were heavier than those from deeply calcified lesions. Thus the pattern of lesion calcification as detected by IVUS affects success with superficial calcium greatly reducing tissue retrieval. This is noteworthy because significant superficial calcification is most effectively approached by rotational atherectomy. However, the results are suboptimal in large arteries because the largest burr tip in human coronary interventions is 2.5 mm, and because rotational atherectomy is usually stopped at a burr:artery ratio of 0.7 to 0.8. Large arteries are ideally approached by DCA, which is limited in calcified lesions. In large vessels superficial calcification may be ablated with the Rotablator followed by more complete tissue extraction with DCA. Characterization of tissue calcification by IVUS may expand the role of DCA in the treatment of calcified lesions.

DCA has also proven to have an adjunctive role to the Rotablator (34). Rotational atherectomy appears to alter calcified plaque, rendering it susceptible to directional atherectomy. Adjunctive DCA may remove weakened calcified plaque or newly exposed noncalcified plaque, or both. Quantitative analysis shows that the total procedural gain in minimal lumen diameter after combined Rotablator and DCA is as large as the typical acute gain after DCA alone in noncalcified lesions. The acute gain attributed to adjunctive DCA is larger than that of adjunctive PTCA after rotational atherectomy. Furthermore, the cross-sectional area of the external elastic lamina does not increase after adjunctive DCA, indicating successful atherectomy and less Dotter effect as a mechanism for DCA after the Rotablator. Serial IVUS imaging shows that after the Rotablator removes 23% of the arc of calcium in calcified coronary arteries, adjunctive DCA can remove another 22% of the calcium arc, with distinct cuts into the calcified plaque and significant tissue retrieval and with the lumen showing the classical geometric distortion after DCA (34). This is different from stand-alone DCA where IVUS typically shows that the device cuts proximal to, distal to, and adjacent to calcium, but rarely into calcium.

SUMMARY

At the Cleveland Clinic moderately to heavily calcified lesions are treated with the Rotablator, and ELCA is reserved for the treatment of long, mildly calcified lesions ($\geq$20 to 25 mm). The type of adjunctive procedure depends on the size of the target vessel, with PTCA applied to vessels <3.0 mm in diameter and DCA applied to vessels $\geq$3.0 mm in diameter and with no contraindication for DCA. IVUS is frequently used to initially characterize coronary artery calcification and to monitor the progress of decalcification with the Rotablator or the laser.

The results of randomized trials are needed to establish the most suitable intervention, or combination of interventions, for the treatment of calcific coronary artery disease. At the present time, new devices appear more promising than PTCA in treating heavily calcified lesions.

REFERENCES

1. Waller BF, Orr CM, Pinkerton CA et al. Coronary balloon angioplasty dissections: "The good, the bad, and the ugly." J Am Coll Cardiol 1992;20:701–706.
2. Waller BF. Pathology of coronary balloon angioplasty and related topics. In: Topol EJ, ed., Textbook of interventional cardiology. Philadelphia: WB Saunders, 1990.
3. Richardson PD, Davies MJ, Born GVR. Influence of plaque configuration and stress distribution on fissuring of coronary atherosclerotic plaques. Lancet 1989;2:941–944.
4. Chin AK, Kinney TB, Rurik GW et al. A physical measurement of the mechanisms of transluminal angioplasty. Surgery 1984;95:196–201.
5. Ellis SG, Vandormael MG, Cowley MJ et al. Coronary morphologic and clinical determinants of procedural outcome with angioplasty for multivessel coronary disease: implications for patient selection. Circulation 1990;82:1193–1202.
6. Detre KM, Holmes DR, Holubkov R et al. Incidence and consequences of periprocedural occlusion. The 1985–1986 National Heart, Lung and Blood Institute PTCA registry. Circulation 1990;82:739–750.
7. Mintz GS, Douek P, Pichard AD et al. Target lesion calcification in coronary artery disease: an intravascular ultrasound study. J Am Coll Cardiol 1992;20:1149–1155.
8. Potkin BN, Keren G, Mintz GS et al. Arterial responses to balloon coronary angioplasty: an intravascular ultrasound study. J Am Coll Cardiol 1992;20:942–951.
9. Hoyne J, Mahon DJ, Jain A et al. Morphological effects of coronary balloon angioplasty in vivo assessed by intravascular ultrasound imaging. Circulation 1992;85:1012–1025.
10. Gianrossi R, Detrano R, Colombo A et al. Cardiac fluoroscopy for the diagnosis of coronary artery disease: a meta-analytic review. Am Heart J 1990;120:1179–1188.
11. Fitzgerald PJ, Muhlberger VA, Moes NY et al. Calcium location within plaque as a predictor of atherectomy tissue retrieval: an intravascular ultrasound study. Circulation 1992;86:I-516 (abstract).
12. Fitzgerald PJ, Ports TA, Yock PG. Contribution of localized calcium deposits to dissection after angioplasty. An observational study using intravascular ultrasound. Circulation 1992;86:64–70.
13. Leon MB, Kent KM, Pichard AD et al. Percutaneous transluminal coronary rotational angioplasty of calcified lesions. Circulation 1991;84:II-521 (abstract).
14. Whitlow PL, Buchbinder M, Kent K et al. Coronary rotational atherectomy: angiographic risk factors and their relation to success/complication. J Am Coll Cardiol 1992; 19:334A (abstract).
15. Levine S, Mehta S, Krauthamer D et al. Excimer laser coronary angioplasty of calcified lesions. J Am Coll Cardiol 1991;17:206A (abstract).

16. Cook SL, Eigler NL, Shefer A et al. Percutaneous excimer laser coronary angioplasty of lesions not ideal for balloon angioplasty. Circulation 1991;84:632–643.

17. Ahn SS, Auth DC, Marcus DR et al. Removal of focal atheromatous lesions by angioscopically guided high-speed rotary atherectomy. J Vasc Surg 1988;7:292–299.

18. Hanson DD, Auth DC, Vrocko R et al. Rotational atherectomy in atherosclerotic rabbit iliac arteries. Am Heart J 1988;115:160–165.

19. Mintz GS, Potkin BN, Keren G et al. Intravascular ultrasound evaluation of the effect of rotational atherectomy in obstructive atherosclerotic coronary artery disease. Circulation 1992;86:1383–1393.

20. Zacca NM, Kleiman NS, Rodriguez AR et al. Rotational ablation of coronary artery lesions using single, large burrs. Cathet Cardiovasc Diagn 1992;26:92–97.

21. Stertzer SH, Rosenblum J, Shaw RE et al. Coronary rotational ablation: initial experience in 302 procedures. J Am Coll Cardiol 1993;21:287–295.

22. Buchbinder M, Warth D, Zacca N et al. Multicenter registry of percutaneous coronary rotational ablation using the Rotablator. Circulation 1991;84:II-82 (abstract).

23. Cowley MJ, Warth D, Whitlow PL et al. Factors influencing outcome with coronary rotational ablation: multicenter results. J Am Coll Cardiol 1993;21:31A (abstract).

24. Bertrand ME, Lablanche JM, Leroy F et al. Percutaneous transluminal coronary rotary ablation with Rotablator (European experience). Am J Cardiol 1992;69:470–474.

25. Altmann DB, Popma JJ, Kent KM et al. Rotational atherectomy effectively treats calcified lesions. J Am Coll Cardiol 1993;21:443A (abstract).

26. Brogan WC, Popma JJ, Pichard AD et al. Rotational coronary atherectomy after unsuccessful coronary balloon angioplasty. Am J Cardiol 1993;71:794–798.

27. Popma JJ, Satler LF, Pichard AD et al. A quantitative analysis of factors affecting late angiographic outcome after rotational coronary atherectomy. J Am Coll Cardiol 1993; 21:31A (abstract).

28. Popma JJ, Satler LF, Pichard AD et al. Clinical and angiographic predictors of procedural outcome after rotational coronary atherectomy in complex lesions. J Am Coll Cardiol 1993;21:228A (abstract).

29. Isner JM. Pathology in cardiovascular laser therapy. In: Isner JM, Clarke RH, eds. Cardiovascular laser therapy. New York: Raven, 1989.

30. Buchwald AB, Werner GS, Unterberg C et al. Restenosis after excimer laser angioplasty of coronary stenoses and chronic total occlusions. Am Heart J 1992;123:878–885.

31. Tierstein PS, Warth DC, Haq N et al. High-speed rotational coronary atherectomy for patients with diffuse coronary disease. J Am Coll Cardiol 1991;18:1694–1701.

32. Reisman M, Cohen B, Warth D et al. Outcome of long lesions treated with high-speed rotational ablation. J Am Coll Cardiol 1993;21:443A (abstract).

33. Robertson GC, Hinohara T, Selmon MR et al. Directional coronary atherectomy. In: Topol EJ, ed. Textbook of interventional cardiology. Philadelphia: WB Saunders, 1990.

34. Mintz GS, Pichard AD, Popma JJ et al. Preliminary experience with adjunct directional coronary atherectomy after high-speed rotational atherectomy in the treatment of calcific coronary artery disease. Am J Cardiol 1993; 71:799–804.

16. The Eccentric Lesion

JOHN F. BRESNAHAN

The term "eccentric lesion" refers to a heterogeneous class of atherosclerotic plaque that differs both anatomically and functionally from concentrically distributed atherosclerotic disease. Eccentric lesions were identified early in the interventional experience as a "risk factor" for adverse procedural outcome with balloon angioplasty (1, 2). Other studies have suggested that eccentric lesions may be a predictor for late restenosis (3). More recent studies, however, have challenged the relative importance of eccentricity in the early and late outcome following balloon angioplasty (4–6).

In spite of the apparent controversy over the significance of eccentric lesions, most interventionists approach eccentric lesions with caution. The advent of the newer interventional devices has allowed more complex eccentric lesions to be treated with potentially greater margins of safety. In this chapter the pathophysiologic aspects and clinical interventional experience with eccentric lesions will be presented as a prelude to a discussion of the interventional approach to these lesions.

PATHOPHYSIOLOGY OF ECCENTRIC LESIONS

From a pathologic standpoint, an eccentric lesion is defined as an atherosclerotic plaque that does not involve the entire circumference of the vessel wall, thus leaving a segment relatively free of disease (7). Autopsy studies of coronary atherosclerosis have reported the incidence of eccentric lesions to range from 25 to over 70% (7–9). In a study of 500 consecutive coronary artery segments with narrowings of 76 to 95%, Waller found that 73% were eccentric with the disease-free segment of vessel wall comprising an average of 16.6% (range 2.3 to 32%) of the vessel circumference (7). For the most part the disease-free sections demonstrated relatively normal vessel architecture, with intact internal elastic laminae and normal medial thickness (Fig. 16.1).

From a functional standpoint, the disease-free portion of the vessel usually retains the capacity for normal or near normal vasoreactivity. Hence endogenous or administered vasoactive substances can produce significant changes in luminal cross-sectional area, with resultant alterations in coronary flow reserve and ischemic threshold. Several studies have, in fact, documented that changes in lumen caliber with vasoactive drugs (e.g., ergonovine, nitrates) are significantly greater for eccentric lesions when compared with concentric stenoses (10, 11).

The anatomic and behavioral differences of eccentric lesions have potentially important implications for interventional cardiology, particularly balloon angioplasty. There have been a number of mechanisms proposed whereby balloon angioplasty improves luminal cross-sectional area (12, 13). In eccentric stenoses, where the compliance of the nondiseased portion of the vessel is much higher than that of the adjacent atherosclerotic plaque, luminal improvement produced by balloon angioplasty is largely caused by stretching of the nondiseased portion of the vessel wall. There are several potentially adverse sequelae of this mechanism of luminal improvement. First of all, overstretching

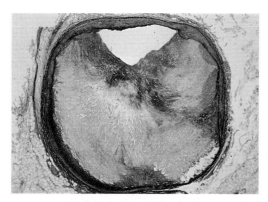

Figure 16.1.   An eccentric atherosclerotic plaque demonstrating a disease-free segment. Intimal and medial structure, and presumably function, are preserved. (Photograph courtesy of Dr. William D. Edwards.)

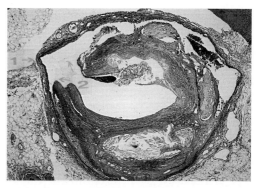

Figure 16.2.   Autopsy specimen from a patient following failed coronary angioplasty. Note thinning of media *(1)* from balloon stretching and extensive disruption and separation at the presumed plaque-normal segment junction *(2)*. (Photograph courtesy of Dr William D. Edwards.)

the nondiseased segment can lead to significant disruption at the plaque/nondiseased segment interface, creating a large intimal dissection (Fig. 16.2). Secondly, early elastic recoil of the stretched, nondiseased segment could result in suboptimal dilatation or even frank coronary spasm. A final concern relates to late restenosis. If the medial smooth muscle recovers its functional capacity after the initial stretch injury from balloon angioplasty, late recoil could result in loss of luminal cross-sectional area (12, 14).

CLINICAL STUDIES

The issues raised by the pathologic and physiologic studies mentioned above have not been directly addressed by any large study. Additionally, most of the concerns relate to balloon angioplasty and hence are probably not directly applicable to the newer interventional devices. Some insight into whether eccentric lesions are significant contributors to adverse early or late outcome may be gained by analyzing the published balloon angioplasty and new device experience.

Dissection and Abrupt Closure

Early reports from the NHLBI Registry and others indicated that lesion eccentricity was an important predictor of major dissec-

tion and acute closure with balloon angioplasty (12, 15). More recent studies have, however, suggested that eccentricity does not predispose to acute complication and should therefore no longer be considered a "risk factor" (4, 6). Possibilities cited for the discrepant results were improvements in catheter technology (e.g., perfusion balloon) and operator experience (4). These factors have certainly played a significant role, since patient selection criteria and improved management of dissections have reduced the need for emergency bypass procedures and other major clinical complications. Unfortunately, it is difficult to compare the studies relating to eccentricity since the definitions for eccentricity were not uniform and the studies were not specifically designed to assess the importance of eccentricity as a predictor of outcome. Hence it is possible that variables not evaluated could explain the apparent differences in conclusions. One such possibility is the degree of eccentricity, which was not addressed in any of these studies. In a study involving concentric laser catheters, the degree of eccentricity using quantitative coronary angiography proved to be the single most important procedural predictor of major acute complications (16).

Several of the new interventional devices offer the promise of reducing the incidence of dissection associated with eccentric stenoses. Of these devices, the directional atherectomy and the directional laser systems have design characteristics that are ideally suited for eccentric lesions. Rowe et al. found directional atherectomy to have a markedly reduced incidence of dissection in eccentric lesions in comparison with balloon angioplasty (17). Abrupt closure, however, was similar in both study groups. Similarly, a report from a multicenter study involving the directional atherectomy catheter indicated a very high primary success rate with a low incidence of acute complications in eccentric lesions (18). Concentric excimer laser catheter results with eccentric lesions have been comparable to balloon angioplasty (19); however, as noted above, highly eccentric lesions are associated with an increased incidence of acute complication (16). The directional laser catheter is currently under active investigation. Our preliminary experience with this device suggests that in uncomplicated eccentric lesions the incidence of dissection and acute closure is very low. There is limited information concerning the rotational atherectomy device (Rotablator) and stents in eccentric lesions. Preliminary reports with the rotational device indicated that it was employed without increased complications in a small series of patients with eccentric lesions (20). Stents, which are commonly used to manage dissection, are logical choices in situations where there is a high risk of dissection.

While some controversy exists, the preponderance of data would suggest that eccentric lesions are at increased risk for dissection and possibly also abrupt closure with balloon angioplasty. Those lesions with a high degree of eccentricity probably represent the subgroup at highest risk for complication and hence may be best managed with alternate technology. Directional atherectomy and possibly directional excimer laser angioplasty appear to be superior to balloon angioplasty in these lesions with regard to reducing the risk of major dissection.

Elastic Recoil

Elastic recoil following balloon angioplasty, defined as the difference between the inflated balloon size and final luminal diameter, can cause a suboptimal initial result and may also contribute to late restenosis (3). Early elastic recoil typically accounts for a 20 to 30% reduction in luminal cross-sectional area, but reports have ranged as high as 50% (21–23). Eccentric lesions, presumably because of the relatively elastic nondiseased segment, have been documented to have significantly higher amounts of recoil than concentric lesions following balloon angioplasty (21, 24, 25). Of the newer devices, directional atherectomy and stents appear to be associated with minimal recoil in comparison with balloon angioplasty (26). Laser and rotational atherectomy are used in conjunction with balloon angioplasty in the majority of cases, and hence the degree of recoil could conceivably approach that of balloon angioplasty. There is some suggestion, however, that recoil may be reduced with the rotational atherectomy device (27).

In the early angioplasty era coronary vasospasm was a significant concern, occurring in approximately 5% of cases. With the advent of potent calcium channel blockers, however, this problem has largely been eliminated. In comparing the complications in the 1977–1981 NHLBI Registry with the later 1985–1986 NHLBI Registry experience, Holmes et al. found that the most significant change was the decline in the incidence of coronary spasm (28). In addition, a recent study comparing spontaneous vasoconstriction in eccentric and concentric lesions following angioplasty in patients pretreated with calcium blockers found no significant differences between the two groups (29).

Restenosis

In theory, delayed elastic recoil, excessive "stretch" injury, and significant disruption at the plaque/nondiseased segment interface could predispose eccentric lesions to restenosis. Evidence in support of any of these concepts is, however, scant. In large angioplasty series that attempted to correlate lesion morphology with subsequent restenosis, only one found eccentricity to be significant (3, 4). In a recent study analyzing the impact of elastic recoil on restenosis, Ardissino et al. concluded that while elastic recoil negatively impacted on initial results, it had no additional influence on late restenosis (23). As the final angiographic stenosis has been shown to correlate with restenosis (4), it might be reasonable to postulate that the principal effect of eccentric lesions on restenosis is their propensity for early elastic recoil.

INTERVENTIONAL APPROACH TO ECCENTRIC LESIONS

From the preceding discussion, it is apparent that balloon angioplasty may not be the optimal technology of choice for all eccentric lesions because of potential problems with dissection and elastic recoil. Alternative devices, in particular directional atherectomy, directional excimer laser angioplasty, intracoronary stents, and rotational atherectomy, appear to offer significant advantages in some situations and thus may be safer and more effective in selected, highly eccentric, complex lesions.

The role of the interventional cardiologist is to match the appropriate technology to the individual case to obtain the optimal result. As no device, with the exception of stents, has as yet been proven conclusively to offer a significant restenosis advantage, the primary goal of therapy is to produce the best initial result at the lowest possible risk. In planning the interventional approach to eccentric lesions, the interventionist must consider a number of factors relating to the devices, the patient, and the lesions themselves.

Devices

The potential advantages of the newer interventional devices in treating eccentric lesions are mitigated somewhat by their structural characteristics and patient-related incapabilities. Unlike balloon catheters that can access the majority of coronary arterial segments, be employed in vessels of virtually any size, and treat lesions of almost any length, some of the newer devices have significant vessel size, location, and geometric constraints.

The directional atherectomy catheter is a bulky, relatively inflexible device; hence, its use is confined to larger vessels (greater than 3 mm) with little tortuosity proximal or distal to the stenosis. The aperture of the cutting chamber is either 5 or 9 mm, limiting use of the device in long lesions. Finally, the cutting blade is not capable of removing heavily calcified plaque. The directional atherectomy catheter is therefore best suited for eccentric lesions that are discrete, not heavily calcified, and located in predominantly straight, proximal segments in the left anterior descending, right coronary artery, or in vein grafts. The directional atherectomy catheter is also very useful for ostial or thrombus-containing stenoses (30).

The directional excimer laser catheter is of intermediate size and flexibility between that of balloon catheters and the directional atherectomy catheter and, hence, has a wider range of lesions in which it can be used. The catheter is capable of ablating calcified plaque and eccentric lesions of virtually any length. The currently available catheter is 1.8 mm in diameter and can be used in vessels of greater than 2.5 mm. Eccentric lesions in vessels larger than 3.0 mm will usually require adjunctive balloon angioplasty; the device is "steerable," however, and by turning the device 30 to 45 degrees and making multiple passes, a larger lumen can be achieved. The protruding protective tip of the device may not cross high-grade stenoses and consequently pretreatment of the lesions, with either a smaller (1.3 mm) concentric laser catheter or a balloon catheter may be necessary.

There are a variety of intracoronary stent designs currently under investigation, each with somewhat different characteristics. The Gianturco-Roubin (Cook) and the Palmaz-Schatz (Johnson & Johnson) stents have been approved for clinical use, and approval of other stents is anticipated in the near future. The balloon-mounted stents can be delivered to most arterial segments, excepting those where there is significant tortuosity. There is little data involving the use of stents as primary therapy for eccentric lesions; however, stents are exceptionally useful in treating dissections and in situations where there is excessive elastic recoil (31). The major limitations of stents are the small but significant incidence of subacute thrombosis and the possible need for anticoagulation therapy after stent placement. In addition, the utility of stents in small vessels (less than 3 mm), lesions containing significant thrombus, or at major branch points is also somewhat diminished.

The rotational atherectomy device should in theory be ideal for eccentric lesions since this device is reported to selectively remove noncompliant plaque while leaving normal tissue relatively unharmed. Recent studies have, in fact, reported excellent results in eccentric stenoses (27). Particular advantages for the rotational atherectomy device appear to be in calcific or otherwise rigid lesions, especially those with ostial locations, and in tortuous vessels that other non-balloon devices have difficulty traversing. Relative disadvantages of this device include the need for using multiple burrs and the high frequency of adjunctive balloon angioplasty. Additionally, in long or diffuse lesions, microemboli can potentially lead to non–Q-wave infarction or the no-reflow phenomenon (32).

Patient Factors

In any interventional procedure, a host of patient-related factors must be taken into consideration that, while not directly bearing on the lesion itself, influence technical feasibility and overall procedural risk. Vascular access can be a troublesome problem, but with balloon angioplasty it occurs relatively infrequently because of the flexibility and variety of guide catheter sizes and the ability to use the brachial, as well as the femoral, arteries. Directional atherectomy and, to a lesser extent, the other devices require larger, stiffer guiding catheters that limit their use in the arm or in tortuous or stenosed iliac vessels. Contrast media usage with directional atherectomy and with devices that require adjunctive balloon angioplasty tend to run much higher than when balloon angioplasty is used alone. Hence, in patients with significant impairment of renal function, the risk of acute renal failure may be increased. Stents often require anticoagulation therapy and thus are not appropriate in many patients with bleeding diatheses. Finally, consideration must be given to overall patient risk. Left ventricular function, severity of disease in the nontarget vessels, and the amount of myocardium jeopardized by the target lesion must be considered, in addition to lesion-related factors. A high-risk lesion in a high-risk patient should be approached with extreme caution, if at all.

Angiographic Factors

By far the most important factors influencing the technical approach to eccentric lesions are the lesion characteristics and the surrounding coronary anatomy. Lesion characteristics associated with an increased risk of procedural failure or complications with balloon angioplasty were compiled and classified by the ACC/AHA Task Force in 1988. The presence of multiple adverse characteristics further increases overall risk. Numerous reports have indicated that the newer interventional devices improve initial success rates and decrease complications in these complex lesions (19, 27, 30). As discussed previously, however, these devices have

Table 16.1
Angiographic Factors Associated With Reduced Procedural Success or Increased Risk of Complication With Balloon Angioplasty[a]

Calcification	Thrombus
Length	Bifurcation lesion
Proximal tortuosity	Acute bend

[a]Modified from AHA/ACC criteria.

structural and anatomic limitations, and hence these variables must also be factored into the decision regarding the technical approach to the complex, eccentric lesion. Table 16.1 lists the angiographic lesion characteristics that must be considered in conjunction with the device and patient factors in approaching eccentric lesions.

TECHNICAL APPROACH TO ECCENTRIC LESIONS: ONE INTERVENTIONALIST'S VIEWPOINT

The factors that must be considered when planning the interventional approach to an eccentric lesion are too numerous to permit construction of a simple algorithm. Additionally, the approach is also influenced by the availability of new technology, as some of the new devices have only very recently been approved for clinical use. In this section a personal viewpoint as to the technical strategies concerning the interventional management of eccentric lesions will be discussed.

The ideal angioplasty would result in a smooth luminal surface with a residual stenosis of less than 20%, no procedural or in-hospital complications, and no restenosis. With the possible exception of stents, no device has been proven to offer a major advantage over any other in terms of restenosis. While our understanding of restenosis is continuing to evolve, the stent and other experience suggests that the probability of restenosis may be minimized by reducing the final residual stenosis (4). Therefore the goal of any interventional procedure is to obtain the optimal initial result as described above. For eccentric lesions this entails assessing the lesion

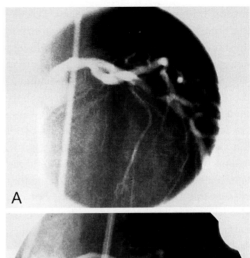

A

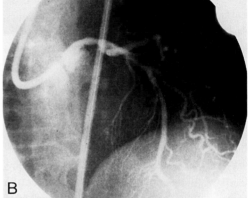

B

Figure 16.3. Highly eccentric atherosclerotic plaque prior to (**A**) and following (**B**) directional atherectomy.

and the patient for associated procedural risk factors and determining which device would provide the greatest degree of luminal improvement with the least procedural risk.

Uncomplicated Eccentric Lesions

In stenoses where eccentricity is the only risk factor, the technical approach to the lesion is dictated primarily by the degree of eccentricity and the size of the vessel. For lesions where the degree of eccentricity is mild to moderate, eccentricity is probably not associated with an increased incidence of adverse outcome with balloon angioplasty; therefore this approach is the most appropriate. In my opinion, however, lesions with a very high degree of eccentricity (Fig. 16.3) have a significantly increased risk of a major dissection, especially if the associated stenosis is severe. Under these circumstances, debulking the plaque and minimizing the injury to the nondiseased segment should produce a better primary result. For lesions greater than or equal to 3.0 mm, directional atherectomy is the device of choice. In a situation where there is difficulty advancing the device into the left main, circumflex, or around a bend, the short cutter can be very useful, even in lesions up to 10 mm in length. The directional laser catheter is the best choice for smaller vessels (between 2.3 and 3.0 mm), but can also be used in larger vessels with adjunctive balloon angioplasty if, for technical reasons, directional atherectomy cannot be used. In small vessels (less than 2.3 mm) balloon angioplasty is the best alternative, although small burr rotational atherectomy may be an excellent option.

Complex Eccentric Lesions

Lesions with multiple angiographic risk factors have been associated with relatively low primary success rates and high complication rates using balloon angioplasty. These lesions, which fall into the B2 or C AHA/ACC classification, are probably best treated, at least initially, with the newer interventional devices. The choice of the device is dependent on the particular combination of risk factors present and must be individualized for each patient. In many of these complex lesions, multiple devices will be needed. The technical approach to several complex eccentric lesions will be presented, emphasizing the theoretic and practical advantages of the different technologies.

Calcified Lesions

Calcified lesions are among the most troublesome facing the interventionalist. In general, these lesions tend to be brittle and, in response to mechanical dilation, fracture at the weakest point in the vessel circumference. In eccentric lesions this is usually at the plaque/normal segment interface and frequently produces a large dissection. With the

exception of rotational atherectomy, results with all of the newer interventional devices in calcified lesions have been suboptimal as well. Calcified lesions are difficult to cross with the bulky directional atherectomy device and are resistant to being cut by the rotating blade. Laser energy does not vaporize calcium, but rather fractures calcified plaque by shock-wave trauma (33). Ablation of calcified lesions requires high laser energy, and the disruption of the calcified plaque results in varying degrees of local vascular trauma.

The technical approach to calcified eccentric lesions is influenced by the degree of calcium in the lesion. For otherwise suitable vessels, our experience with directional atherectomy has been quite good if the degree of calcification is mild or, at most, moderate. In heavily calcified lesions rotational atherectomy is our initial device of choice to "soften up" the lesion, followed by directional atherectomy or balloon angioplasty, depending on the vessel size and lesion location. Stenting of the lesion is appropriate if there is significant recoil of the noninvolved segment or significant luminal disruption.

Long Eccentric Lesions

Long eccentric lesions (greater than 10 mm) are probably at higher risk for complication with balloon angioplasty because of the variability in plaque composition and density that may exist along the length of the stenosis. The "hard" and "soft" portions of the plaque may not respond uniformly to balloon pressure, potentially leading to dissection at the interface of these regions. The relatively normal segment in the eccentrically stenosed vessel adds yet another "hard"/"soft" interface. Debulking the plaque while protecting the normal segment may reduce the risk of dissection. The directional laser is best suited for this type of lesion since, unlike the directional atherectomy device, lesion length is not a design limitation. As a rule, balloon angioplasty using longer-than-standard balloon lengths is necessary as an adjunct. Single and multiple stents may also be needed if, despite debulking the lesion prior to balloon angioplasty, significant dissection occurs.

Eccentric Bifurcation Lesions

The management of lesions involving the orifices of both limbs of a major bifurcation is, under the best of circumstances, complex. When balloon angioplasty is employed, two separate catheter systems are generally required. "Plaque shifting" from one branch to the other can occur when sequential inflations are used, and overstretching the proximal segment with its attendant risk of dissection can occur when simultaneous inflations are performed. In our experience with the "kissing balloon" technique, satisfactory results were obtained in both limbs of the bifurcation in only two-thirds of patients. Plaque removal systems face a number of significant logistic constraints in treating bifurcation lesions because of their relatively large size. In addition, while the potential problem of plaque shifting is obviated, damage to the guidewire or system in the other branch of the bifurcation is a significant concern. By far the most important concern with plaque removal devices, however, is perforation.

The technical approach to highly eccentric bifurcation lesions is dictated by the location of the plaque in relation to the bifurcation point or "crotch" of the vessel (Fig. 16.4). Debulking plaque in this region is associated with an increased risk of perforation (34). Hence the eccentric bifurcation lesion with the most favorable anatomy is one where the bulk of the atheroma is situated away from the bifurcation point (Fig. 16.3). In these cases the directional laser is an excellent choice of device since the protruding sheath serves to protect not only the bifurcation point, but also the guidewire in the other branch. If the vessel is large, directional atherectomy can be similarly employed.

In eccentric lesions where the plaque is predominantly located around the bifurcation point (Fig. 16.3B), plaque removal devices

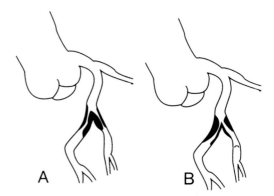

Figure 16.4. Diagram of a highly eccentric lesion at a bifurcation point. **A** demonstrates anatomy favorable for intervention while **B** depicts anatomy at high risk for complication.

should probably be avoided or, if used, significantly undersized relative to the vessel. Lesions with this anatomic configuration may also be predisposed to plaque shifting with balloon angioplasty and thus may have suboptimal success rates with this modality as well. This group of lesions are at higher procedural risk, and hence patient-related risk factors should also be carefully considered before deciding whether to proceed.

Eccentric Lesions at Bend Points

Highly eccentric lesions located at a significant bend in a vessel present a situation somewhat analogous to the bifurcation lesion above. Although there is little published data available about the results of the various technologies in these lesions, conventional wisdom has it that plaque removal devices may cause vessel perforation when the bulk of the lesion is located on the inner aspect of the bend (Fig. 16.5). Because of potential delivery problems with the directional atherectomy device, the directional laser is probably the catheter best suited for those situations where the plaque is located on the outer wall.

Balloon angioplasty is unquestionably the easiest device to perform in these lesions. There is a significant risk of dissection, however, because the inflated balloon tends to

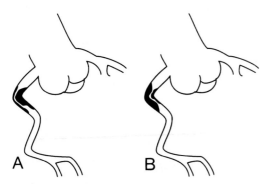

Figure 16.5. Eccentric bend point lesions. Anecdotal data suggests that **B** is at higher risk for complication with plaque removal devices.

straighten, resulting in uneven distribution of pressure on the vessel wall. This risk can be minimized by using undersized, highly compliant balloons, which tend to conform to the vessel curvature and straighten less than noncompliant balloons. Perhaps the best choice of device for eccentric lesions located on bends, regardless of plaque location, is the stent. Flexible stents such as the Gianturco-Roubin or the Wiktor stent can usually be negotiated around bends of moderate degree without great difficulty and may provide the best luminal result with the least risk of complication.

SUMMARY

Eccentric lesions have significantly different anatomic and functional characteristics from concentric lesions. The key to these differences lies in the relatively normal segment of arterial wall that is present in varying degrees in these stenoses. From an interventional standpoint, eccentric lesions are associated with an increased incidence of complications with balloon angioplasty, although there is considerable controversy about this issue. In all likelihood it is the degree of eccentricity and not its presence that determines risk; risk is probably significantly increased only in those lesions with a high degree of eccentricity. The highly eccentric lesion, particularly when coupled with other anatomic variables associated with adverse outcome, presents a challenge to the interventionalist. Newer interventional devices, in particular directional atherectomy, directional lasers, and stents have expanded the ability to treat these complex, high-risk lesions and improve the likelihood of a successful acute outcome. Rotational atherectomy may also be helpful in selected situations. By weighing the angiographic and patient-related factors and choosing the device or devices that will provide maximal improvement in luminal dimension with the least amount of damage to the near normal segment, procedural and possibly long-term success rates for these complex lesions can be optimized.

REFERENCES

1. Meier B, Gruentzig AR, Hollman J, Ischinger T, Bradford JM. Does length or eccentricity of coronary stenoses influence the outcome of transluminal dilatation? Circulation 1983;67:497–499.
2. Cowley MJ, Dorros G, Kelsey SF, Van Raden M, Detre KM. Emergency coronary bypass surgery after coronary angioplasty: The National Heart, Lung, and Blood Institute's Percutaneous Transluminal Coronary Angioplasty Registry experience. Am J Cardiol 1984;53(12):22C–26C.
3. Weintraub WS, Kosinski AS, Brown CL, King SB. Can restenosis after coronary angioplasty be predicted from clinical variables? J Am Coll Cardiol 1993;21(1):6–14.
4. Savage MP, Goldberg S, Hirshfeld JW, Bass TA, MacDonald RG, Margolis JR, Taussig AS et al. Clinical and angiographic determinants of primary coronary angioplasty success. M-Heart Investigators. J Am Coll Cardiol 1991;17(1):22–28.
5. Bourassa MG, Lesperance J, Eastwood C, Schwartz L, Cote G, Kazim F, Hudon G. Clinical, physiologic, anatomic and procedural factors predictive of restenosis after percutaneous transluminal coronary angioplasty. J Am Coll Cardiol 1991;18(2):368–376.
6. Ellis SG, Vandormael MG, Cowley MJ, DiSciascio G, Deligonul U, Topol EJ, Bulle TM, Multivessel Angioplasty Prognosis Study Group. Coronary morphologic and clinical determinants of procedural outcome with angioplasty for multivessel coronary disease: implications for patient selection. Circulation 1990;82:1193–1202.
7. Waller BF. The eccentric coronary atherosclerotic plaque: morphologic observations and clinical relevance. Clin Cardiol 1989;12:14–20.
8. Vlodaver Z, Edwards JE. Pathology of coronary atherosclerosis. Prog Cardiovasc Dis 1971;14:256.
9. Chopra P, Sethi U, Gupta PK, Tandon HD. Coronary artery stenosis. An autopsy study. Acta Cardiol 1983;38:183.
10. Kaski JC, Tousoulis D, Haider AW, Gavrielides S, Crea F, Maseri A. Reactivity of eccentric and concentric coronary stenoses in patients with chronic stable angina. J Am Coll Cardiol 1991;17:627–633.
11. Brown BG. Response of normal and diseased epicardial coronary arteries to vasoactive drugs: quantitative arteriographic studies. Am J Cardiol 1985;56:23–29.
12. Waller BF. The pathology of transluminal balloon angio-

plasty used in the treatment of coronary heart disease. Hum Pathol 1987;18:476.

13. Block PC. Mechanism of transluminal angioplasty. Am J Cardiol 1984;53:69C–71C.

14. Saner HE, Gobel FL, Salomonowitz E, Erlien DA, Edwards JE. The disease-free wall in coronary atherosclerosis: its relation to degree of obstruction. J Am Coll Cardiol 1985;6:1096.

15. Bentivoglio LG, Van Raden MJ, Kelsey SF, Detre KM. Percutaneous transluminal coronary angioplasty (PTCA) in patients with relative contraindications: results of the National Heart, Lung, and Blood Institute PTCA Registry. Am J Cardiol 1984;53(12):82–88.

16. Ghazzal ZM, Hearn JA, Litvack F, Goldenberg T, Kent KM, Eigler N, Douglas JS Jr et al. Morphological predictors of acute complications after percutaneous excimer laser coronary angioplasty. Results of a comprehensive angiographic analysis: importance of the eccentricity index. Circulation 1992;86(3):820–827.

17. Rowe MH, Hinohara T, White NW, Robertson GC, Selmon MR, Simpson JB. Comparison of dissection rates and angiographic results following directional coronary atherectomy and coronary angioplasty. Am J Cardiol 1990; 66:49–53.

18. Ellis SG, De Cesare NB, Pinkerton CA, Whitlow P, King SB, Ghazzel ZM, Kereiakes DJ et al. Relation of stenosis morphology and clinical presentation to the procedural results of directional coronary atherectomy. Circulation 1991;84(2):942–944.

19. Litvack F, Eigler NL, Margolis JR, Grundfest WS, Rothbaum D, Linnemeier T, Hestrin LB et al. Percutaneous excimer laser coronary angioplasty. Am J Cardiol 1990; 66:1027–1032.

20. Stertzer SH, Rosenblum J, Shaw RE, Sugeng I, Hidalgo B, Ryan C, Hansell HN et al. Coronary rotational ablation: initial experience in 302 procedures. J Am Coll Cardiol 1993; 21:287–295.

21. Hanet C, Wijns W, Michel X, Schroeder E. Influence of balloon size and stenosis morphology on immediate and delayed elastic recoil after percutaneous transluminal coronary angioplasty. J Am Coll Cardiol 1991;18:506–511.

22. Rensing BJ, Hermans WRM, Beatt KJ et al. Quantitative angiographic assessment of elastic recoil after percutaneous transluminal coronary angioplasty. Am J Cardiol 1990;66:1039–1044.

23. Ardissino D, Di Somma S, Kubica J, Barberis P, Merlini PA, Eleuteri E, De Servi S et al. Influence of elastic recoil on restenosis after successful coronary angioplasty in unstable angina pectoris. Am J Cardiol 1993;71:659–663.

24. Rensing BJ, Hermans WR, Strauss BH, Serruys PW. Regional differences in elastic recoil after percutaneous transluminal coronary angioplasty: a quantitative angiographic study. J Am Coll Cardiol 1991;17:34B–38B.

25. Hjemdahl-Monsen CE, Ambrose JA, Borrico S, Cohen M, Sherman W, Alexopoulos D, Gorlin R et al. Angiographic patterns of balloon inflation during percutaneous transluminal coronary angioplasty: role of pressure-diameter curves in studying distensibility and elasticity of the stenotic lesion and the mechanism of dilation. J Am Coll Cardiol 1990; 16(3):569–575.

26. Kimball BP, Bui S, Cohen EA, Carere RG, Adelman AG. Comparison of acute elastic recoil after directional coronary atherectomy versus standard balloon angioplasty. Am Heart J 1992;124:1459.

27. Brogan WC III, Popma JJ, Pichard AD, Satler LF, Kent KM, Mintz GS, Leon MB. Rotational coronary atherectomy after unsuccessful coronary balloon angioplasty. Am J Cardiol 1993;71:794–798.

28. Holmes DR Jr, Holubkov R, Vlietstra RE, Kelsey SF, Reeder GS et al. Comparison of complications during percutaneous transluminal coronary angioplasty from 1977 to 1981 and from 1985 to 1986: The National Heart, Lung, and Blood Institute Percutaneous Transluminal Coronary Angioplasty Registry. J Am Coll Cardiol 1988;12:1149–1155.

29. Fischell TA, Bausback KN. Effects of luminal eccentricity on spontaneous coronary vasoconstriction after successful percutaneous transluminal coronary angioplasty. Am J Cardiol 1991;68(5):530–534.

30. Hinohara T, Rowe MH, Robertson GC, Selmon MR, Braden L, Leggett JH, Vetter JW et al. Effect of lesion characteristics on outcome of directional coronary atherectomy. J Am Coll Cardiol 1991;17:1112–1120.

31. Haude M, Erbel R, Issa H, Meyer J. Quantitative analysis of elastic recoil after balloon angioplasty and after intracoronary implantation of balloon-expandable Palmaz-Schatz stents. J Am Coll Cardiol 1993;21:26–34.

32. Teirstein PS, Warth DC, Haj N, Jenkins NS, McCowan LC, Aubanel-Reidel P, Morris N et al. Methods: high-speed rotational coronary atherectomy for patients with diffuse coronary artery disease. J Am Coll Cardiol 1991; 18(7):1694–1701.

33. Bresnahan DR. Lasers in cardiovascular disease. In: Holmes DR Jr, Vlietstra RE, eds. Interventional cardiology. Philadelphia: LA Davis, 1989.

34. Bittl JA, Ryan TJ Jr, Keaney JF Jr, Tcheng JE, Ellis SG, Isner JM, Sanborn TA. Coronary artery perforation during excimer laser coronary angioplasty. The Percutaneous Excimer Laser Coronary Angioplasty Registry. JACC

17. The Long Lesion

A. Treatment of the Long Lesion

JOEL A. SHAPIRO, NEAL L. EIGLER, and
FRANK LITVACK

BACKGROUND

Percutaneous transluminal angioplasty (PTCA) is presently in its second decade of experience. During the early period it became rapidly apparent that the success of primary angioplasty was dependent on lesion characteristics (1–3). Progressive lesion length was identified as a factor inversely related to primary success rate. This continues to be a significant factor despite advances in balloon catheter design (4). In addition, experience with lesion length in excess of 10 mm has been associated with increased risk for complications leading to increased morbidity and mortality, as described most recently by Sharma et al. (5) Ellis et al. (6) described lesion length two or more times the luminal diameter as a predictor for acute closure and increased repeat PTCA, myocardial infarction, and death.

Characterization of lesion morphology to attempt to predict the risk associated with PTCA has been addressed. Based on work from the mid 1980s, the American College of Cardiology/American Heart Association Task Force fractionated lesions into three risk groups: type A, type B, and type C based on multiple lesion characteristics (7, 8). Lesion length was an important parameter of stratification. Type A lesions with the lowest risk and highest success rate included lesions less than 10 mm in length. Type B lesions were assigned intermediate risk and success rate and included lesion length between 10 and 20 mm. Highest risk and lowest success rate was designated to type C lesions and included lesions greater than 20 mm in length.

Beyond its impact on primary success and complications, multiple studies have described the involvement of lesion morphology as a risk factor in luminal narrowing following angioplasty. Among the angiographic factors significantly associated with restenosis is increasing lesion length (3, 9–14). In addition, some studies have cited progressive increase in lesion length following repeated balloon angioplasties despite no significant change in the reference or stenosis diameters (14). There is therefore a need to address optimum methodology in respect to lesion length since it not only is a problem for primary intervention but also is a complicating factor of intervention for restenosis lesions.

One approach that is presently being explored involves the concept of lesion debulking with an advanced interventional device such as excimer laser, rotational atherectomy, or directional coronary atherectomy followed by adjunct balloon angioplasty. The theoretic advantage of removing some of the plaque burden prior to balloon angioplasty is appealing. The question of which device is optimal for debulking has not yet been established. Each device will be discussed below.

PERCUTANEOUS TRANSLUMINAL CORONARY ANGIOPLASTY

Balloon angioplasty continues to be the most ubiquitous form of intracoronary intervention. Recent studies continue to suggest that increasing lesion length adversely affects outcome, although results with longer balloons are somewhat encouraging. Savage et al. (15) prospectively evaluated 826 patients enrolled in the Multi-Hospital Eastern Atlantic Restenosis Trial (M-HEART) and concluded that primary coronary angioplasty success was not related to stenosis length. Hirshfeld et al. (9) using a subset of the same patient group described the probability of restenosis after angioplasty as predominantly determined by the characteristics of the lesion being dilated. Increasing length was associated with increased probability of restenosis. Ghazzal et al. (16) described the PTCA of lesions longer than 20 mm. The treatment of a cohort of 181 consecutive patients between January 1986 and December 1989 with standard (20-mm) balloon angioplasty demonstrated that primary success with PTCA could be achieved at a good rate (85.8%). The risk of arterial complications and emergency surgery utilizing standard balloon length, however, was increased.

Zidar et al. (17) described the treatment of long coronary lesions using standard length and long angioplasty balloon catheters. One group of patients, with either short lesions or long lesions (greater than 10 mm), was treated with standard length balloons from April 1986 to July 1989. Another group of patients with long lesions was treated with long balloons from July 1990 to July 1991. They described higher success rates (97.8%) and lower complication rates with the long balloons (similar to the historical control group of short lesions treated with standard balloon PTCA). Long balloons may afford a good primary success rate with a decreased complication rate compared with standard length balloon angioplasty (18). PTCA balloon lengths of 30 and 40 mm are now routinely available. At present there are multiple hypotheses for the success of long balloons. Increased balloon length may afford a more gradual transition in arterial wall stretch. Having the shoulders of the balloon beyond the lesion margins may provide decreased sheer force at the end-

points of the lesion. More even dispersion of pressure may also occur with the long balloons.

Long, diffusely diseased lesions are often associated with other complicating morphologic features. Ellis et al. (19) described the marked increase in complication rates associated with lesions that incorporated two type B characteristics (type B2). Of particular note, moderate-length lesions (20 mm) in conjunction with moderate angulation (45 degrees) were associated with low primary success rates and high (20.5%) rates of complication when "standard" length balloons were used. Savas et al. (20) described a high success rate and modest complication rate in 69 lesions with the combination of length greater than 20 mm and location on bends greater than 45 degrees. They suggested that this might be attributable to increased conformability of long balloons relative to conventional balloons. Subsequent reduction in the straightening of the natural arterial bend was felt to limit tissue injury and dissection and therefore lower the rate of complication. Despite the excitement in the potential application of long balloons to long lesions, relatively few studies are available at this time. Cates et al. (21) have described the use of extremely long (80-mm) balloons in diffusely diseased vessels with lesions greater than 40 mm in length. Good primary results with a low complication rate were seen in their initial small cohort of patients.

EXCIMER LASER CORONARY ANGIOPLASTY

Excimer laser coronary angioplasty has been successfully performed in an extensive number of complex lesions, including very long lesions. Importantly, it has been determined that increased lesion length is not predictive of complications with excimer laser coronary angioplasty (22). The registry report of the first consecutive 3000 patients treated with excimer laser coronary angioplasty demonstrated no significant difference in success or complication rates with respect to lesion length (23). Twenty percent of the lesions treated were greater than 20 mm in length. No significant differences in success rates or major complications were seen between lesions under 10 mm, 10 to 19 mm, 20 to 29 mm, and greater than 30 mm in length. In addition, no significant difference was found between selected complex lesions and simple lesions. Procedural success (final stenosis less than 50% and no in-hospital Q-wave MI, CABG, or death) was 90% and did not differ for the first 2000 versus the last 1000 patients treated. Of note, coronary perforation occurred in 1.2% of patients (1% of lesions), but significantly dropped to 0.4% in the last 1000 patients (0.3% of lesions). Adjunct balloon angioplasty was performed in 79% of the patients. The registry data has demonstrated that the excimer laser procedure can be safely and effectively applied to a variety of complex lesions that are considered less than ideal for PTCA, including long lesions and type B2 lesions.

ROTATIONAL ATHERECTOMY

High-speed rotational atherectomy using the Rotablator was used by Teirstein et al. (24) in a small cohort of patients who were felt not to be well suited for balloon angioplasty. Three-quarters of the patients had diffuse coronary artery disease, defined as stenosis greater than 10 mm in length. Procedural success was achieved in only 70% of the patients with long lesions as opposed to 92% of the patients with lesions shorter than 10 mm. Small non–Q-wave myocardial infarction occurred in 19% of the patients and was associated with longer lesions. Restenosis defined as greater than 50% narrowing on follow-up angiography (at a mean time of 6.2 months) was 22% for the lesions shorter than 10 mm and 75% for the lesions greater than 10 mm. This study therefore suggests that high-speed rotational atherectomy has a decreased probability for primary success and an increased immediate and delayed morbidity associated with longer lesions. Of note, the recent multicenter reg-

istry trial of this device included lesions greater than 15 mm as a relative contraindication.

DIRECTIONAL CORONARY ATHERECTOMY

Directional coronary angioplasty was designed to remove portions of a plaque using a side-cutting catheter system. Since directional atherectomy involves significant differences in technique and lesion accessibility compared with balloon angioplasty, new operators gained preapproval experience through a training program. Guidelines for case suitability were separated into four levels of complexity. Diffuse lesions were described as level III, that is, "challenging for DCA" (25).

Increased lesion length (greater than 20 mm) has been described as associated with decreased primary success (74%) and increased complication rate (10.8%) (26). Although not characterized relative to lesion length, adjunctive balloon angioplasty can provide an additional primary gain in luminal diameter (27) as described for excimer laser debulking and rotational atherectomy debulking.

INTRACORONARY STENT

The use of primary stent implantation was explored by Kimura et al (28). The cohort consisted of 275 patients, one-third of whom received stent implantation and two-thirds of whom underwent balloon angioplasty. The lesion morphology was approximately 20 mm in length within vessels of approximately 3 mm in diameter. Early stenosis exacerbation dominated in the balloon angioplasty group, whereas late loss of diameter was greater in the stent population. Overall, the reduction in restenosis rate of the stent group was dependent on a larger lumen obtained during the procedure. In addition, intracoronary stent implantation holds great promise as an adjunct modality to various of the aforementioned interventional techniques. In general, stents are 15 to 20 mm in length and as such have been relegated to lesions of this category. Extensive data on stents in long lesions are not available.

SUMMARY

One of the problems with assessing comparative studies on long-lesion intervention has been the absence of good historical controls. Because of increasing operator experience, advancement of PTCA balloon catheter design, and the introduction of advanced interventional devices, the results of PTCA on long lesions have improved over the early experience. Randomized prospective studies to determine which factors have contributed to this improvement are not yet available. The most effective therapy for long lesions is presently undetermined and may well involve a combination of techniques. Promising interventional modalities include conventional and long balloon PTCA, excimer laser coronary angioplasty (ELCA), rotational atherectomy, directional atherectomy, and intracoronary stent implantation. There is insufficient data at this time to unequivocally support one technology over the other. Such determination will require the completion of randomized trials with a substantial enrollment of subjects.

REFERENCES

1. Meier B, Gruentzig AR, Hollman J et al. Does length or eccentricity of coronary stenosis influence the outcome of transluminal dilatation? Circulation 1983;67:497–499.
2. Ischinger T, Gruentzig AR, Meier B et al. Coronary dissection and total coronary occlusion associated with percutaneous transluminal coronary angioplasty: significance of initial angiographic morphology of coronary stenoses. Circulation 1986;74:1371–1378.
3. Vandormael MG, Deligonul U, Kern MJ et al. Multilesion coronary angioplasty: clinical and angiographic follow-up. J Am Coll Cardiol 1987;10:246–252.
4. Myler RK, Shaw RE, Stertzer SH et al. Lesion morphology and coronary angioplasty: current experience and analysis. J Am Coll Cardiol 1992;19:1641–1652.
5. Sharma SK, Israel DH, Kamean JL et al. Clinical, angiographic, and procedural determinants of major and minor coronary dissection during angioplasty. Am Heart J 1993;126(1):39–47.
6. Ellis SG, Roubin GS, King SB III et al. Angiographic and clinical predictors of acute closure after native vessel coronary angioplasty. Circulation 1988;77:372–379.
7. Ryan TJ, Faxon DP, Gunnar RP, and the ACC/AHA Task Force. Guidelines for percutaneous transluminal coronary angioplasty. J Am Coll Cardiol 1988;12:529–545.
8. Ryan TJ, Faxon DP, Gunnar RP, and the ACC/AHA Task Force. Guidelines for percutaneous transluminal coronary angioplasty. Circulation 1988;78:486–502.

9. Hirshfeld JW Jr, Schwartz JS, Jugo R et al. Restenosis after coronary angioplasty: a multivariate statistical model to relate lesion and procedure variables to restenosis. J Am Coll Cardiol 1991;18:647–656.
10. Yamaguchi T. Risk factors for later restenosis after successful coronary angioplasty: Mitsui Memorial Hospital experience. J Cardiol 1991;21(1):43–52.
11. Rensing BJ, Hermans WR, Beatt KJ et al. Angiographic risk factors of luminal narrowing after coronary balloon angioplasty using balloon measurements to reflect stretch and elastic recoil at the dilatation site. Am J Cardiol 1993; 69(6):584–591.
12. Lallemant R, Bauters C, Leroy F et al. L'angioplastie coronaire des lesions multitronuclaires. Apropros de 1,664 procedures. Resultats immediats et a 6 mois. Arch Mal Coeur Vaiss 1992;85(6):815–822.
13. Rensing BJ, Hermans WR, Vos J et al. Luminal narrowing after percutaneous transluminal coronary angioplasty. A study of clinical, procedural, and lesional factors related to long-term angiographic outcome. Circulation 1993; 88(3):975–985.
14. Bauters C, Lablanche JM, Leroy F et al. Morphological changes of coronary stenosis after repeated balloon angioplasties: a quantitative angiographic study. Cathet Cardiovasc Diagn 1991;24(3):158–160.
15. Savage MP, Goldberg S, Hirshfeld JW et al., and the M-Heart Investigators. Clinical and angiographic determinants of primary coronary angioplasty success. J Am Coll Cardiol 1991;17:22–28.
16. Ghazzal ZMB, Weintraub WS, Ba'albaki NA, Carlin SF, Morris DC, Liberman H, Douglas JS et al. PTCA of lesions longer than 20 mm: initial outcome and restenosis. Circulation 1990;82(Suppl):III-509 (abstract).
17. Zidar J, Tenaglia A, Jackman J et al. Improved acute results for PTCA of long coronary lesions using long angioplasty balloon catheters. J Am Coll Cardiol 1992;19:34A (abstract).
18. Brymer JF, Khaja F, Kraft PL. Angioplasty of long or tandem coronary artery lesions using a new longer balloon dilatation catheter: a comparative study. Cathet Cardiovasc Diagn 1991;23:84–88.
19. Ellis SG, Vandormael MG, Cowley MJ et al., and the Multivessel Angioplasty Prognosis Group. Coronary morphologic and clinical determinants of procedural outcome with angioplasty for multivessel coronary artery disease: implications for patient selection. Circulation 1990; 82:1193–1202.
20. Savas V, Puchrowicz S, Williams L et al. Angioplasty outcomes using long balloons in high-risk lesions. J Am Coll Cardiol 1992;19:34A (abstract).
21. Cates CU, Knopf WD, Lembo NJ et al. The 80-mm balloon: the first 95-vessel cumulative experience. J Am Coll Cardiol 1995 (in press) (abstract).
22. Ghazzal ZMB, Hearn JA, Litvack F et al. Morphological predictors of acute complications after percutaneous excimer laser coronary angioplasty. Circulation 1992; 86(3):820–827.
23. Litvack F, Eigler N, Margolis J et al., and the ELCA investi-

gators. Percutaneous excimer laser coronary angioplasty: results of the first consecutive 3000 patients. J Am Coll Cardiol 1994;23:323–329.

24. Teirstein PS, Warth DC, Haq N et al. High-speed rotational coronary atherectomy for patients with diffuse coronary artery disease. J Am Coll Cardiol 1991;18(7):1694–1701.

25. Cowley MJ, DiSciascio G. Experience with directional coronary atherectomy since pre-market approval. Am J Cardiol 1993;72:12E–20E.

26. Baim DS, Hinohara T, Holmes D et al., and the US Directional Atherectomy Investigator Group. Results of directional coronary atherectomy during multicenter preapproval testing. Am J Cardiol 1993;72:6E–11E.

27. Gordon PC, Kugelmass AD, Cohen DJ et al. Balloon postdilitation can safely improve the results of successful (but suboptimal) directional coronary atherectomy. Am J Cardiol 1993;72:71E–79E.

28. Kimura T, Nosaka H, Yokoi H et al. Serial angiographic follow-up after Palmaz-Schatz stent implantation: comparison with conventional balloon angioplasty. J Am Coll Cardiol 1993;21(7):1557–1563.

B. Approach to Long Lesions

KEITH E. DAVIS, RILEY D. FOREMAN, and
MAURICE BUCHBINDER

Long stenoses in diffusely diseased, atherosclerotic coronary vessels remain a challenging problem for percutaneous revascularization. Advances in angioplasty technique, operator experience, and catheter-based technology has fueled exponential growth in the utilization of PTCA. These factors have resulted in a dramatic increase in the overall success rate from 65% in early published reports to well over 90% in current series (1–3). Long coronary lesions have also benefitted from these improvements and particularly from the introduction of innovative, interventional devices that have expanded the capabilities of percutaneous intervention.

SUCCESS AND COMPLICATIONS WITH CONVENTIONAL ANGIOPLASTY

The influence of lesion length on PTCA outcome has been recognized since the initial report from the NHLBI registry when "nondiscrete" lesion morphology was found to be a significant predictor of adverse events (4). Meir and Gruentzig found that eccentric lesions greater than 5 mm in length were associated with a 24% complication rate compared with 12% for shorter, concentric lesions (5). Furthermore, analysis of the 1985–1986 NHLBI registry identified diffuse and multiple discrete lesions to be a significant morphologic predictor of procedural occlusion, which occurred in 8.5% of those with diffuse disease versus 3.3% of those with single, discrete lesions (6). In a subsequent retrospective analysis of 4772 procedures between 1982 and 1986, Ellis et al. identified lesion length twice the vessel diameter or greater as one of seven independent preprocedural predictors of acute closure (7).

The ACC/AHA Task Force report designated lesion length of 1 to 2 cm as a type B lesion characteristic (predictive of moderate success, 60 to 80%; moderate risk) and lesion length of greater than 2 cm a type C characteristic (low success, <60%; high risk) (8). The relative accuracy of the predicted procedural success based on the ACC/AHA classification has been supported in a series of 552 patients from the Thoraxcenter on cases performed in 1991 and 1992 using conventional PTCA techniques (Table 17B.1).

Length greater than 20 mm was associated with an increased failure rate with an odds ratio of 3.0, and the combination of "functional occlusion" (i.e., TIMI 1 flow), calcification, and length greater than 20 mm was strongly predictive of procedural failure (9). However, midlength, type B lesions (10 to 19 mm) have been associated with significantly higher success rates and lower complication

Table 17B.1
Relation of ACC/AHA Morphology Score to Results of Balloon Angioplasty in 1991 to 1992

	A	B	B1	B2	C
Total no. of lesions	164	569	323	246	39
Success	94.5%	88.8%	90.4%	86.6%	56.4%
Failure[a]	1.2%	3.7%	5.3%	1.6%	12.8%

[a]Failure rates caused by immediate complications (abrupt occlusion, surgery, or death).

rates than predicted by the type B designation in some series. Ten percent of the 1000 lesions dilated in the M-HEART (Multi-Hospital Eastern Atlantic Restenosis Trial) were 10 to 19 mm in length with a procedural success rate of 93% (10).

One of the difficulties encountered when comparing data on long lesions is the differentiation of those with long lesions from those with diffuse disease involving the entire vessel with associated long, high-grade lesions. Goudreau et al. reviewed 98 patients undergoing PTCA for diffuse disease and subdivided them into three groups: group I (40 patients) had greater than 50% narrowing of the entire vessel, group II (39 patients) had a narrowing greater than 20 mm, and group III (19 patients) had greater than three lesions per vessel. The overall angiographic success was 93% for all groups combined. Seven of the eight complications (death, MI, or CABG) occurred in the group I patients yielding a 17.5% complication rate for this subset of patients. Only one complication was experienced in the group II patients, suggesting that diffuse atherosclerosis with significant involvement of the entire vessel has a markedly adverse effect on procedural outcome (11).

LONG BALLOONS

Recently, long balloons measuring 30 to 60 mm have been introduced with considerable success in long lesions. In a study evaluating the utility of these new balloons Brymer et al. randomized 44 patients with tandem lesions or lesions measuring 15 to 25 mm in length to undergo PTCA using standard-length (20-mm) versus long (30-mm) balloons. The long-balloon group required fewer inflations and demonstrated a lower incidence of intimal dissection. Dissection was present in four of 22 patients undergoing PTCA with long balloons compared with 12 of 22 undergoing PTCA with standard-length balloons. The overall procedural success was 95% in both groups (12). Savas et al. reported their experience in 109 lesions greater than 20 mm in

length (average 38 mm) treated with long balloons. They reported an overall success rate of 90%, with major complications occurring in only 2% (13). In a review of their experience Zidar et al. at Duke University reported a 97.8% success rate in 90 lesions greater than 10 mm long dilated with 30- to 40-mm balloons. This compared with an 89.9% success rate for a similar group of patients dilated using standard-length balloons. The dissection and acute closure rates were significantly lower for those treated with long balloons (14).

Additional balloon design innovations may prove applicable to the treatment of long lesions. In a review of 100 consecutive coronary arteriograms, it was found that 50% of the arteries analyzed demonstrated significant tapering of 0.5 mm or greater over the length of the artery measured from a point 10 mm proximal to 10 mm distal to a targeted lesion. PTCA was performed on lesions in 94 such tapered coronary segments using 25-mm-long balloons with a 0.5-mm taper. PTCA was successful in 98% with only two arteries demonstrating significant dissection. In this series there were no abrupt closures or requirement for emergency CABG (15).

RESTENOSIS

As the capability to successfully dilate longer lesions improves, one might expect restenosis rates to increase commensurate with the more complex anatomy. Although the data remains unsettled, reports suggest that longer lesions are unfortunately associated with an increased restenosis rate. However, in a review of PTCA procedures at Emory from 1982 to 1985, lesion length was not found to be a significant predictor of restenosis (16). In a series of 98 patients with diffuse disease undergoing PTCA, Goudreau et al. reported a clinical restenosis rate of only 31% with a mean follow-up of 29 months. On the other hand, Bourassa et al. reported a 58% angiographic restenosis rate for lesions greater than 10 mm compared with 32% in lesions less than 10 mm (17). In the M-HEART Trial the restenosis rate for lesions 7.1 to 28 mm was 48.5% compared with 33% for lesions less than 4.6 mm (18). In a series of lesions treated with long balloons at Duke University, angiographic follow-up demonstrated a restenosis rate of 57%. However, it was noted that the mean restenotic lesion length was only 7 mm compared with an original mean lesion length of 17.6 mm (14).

NEW INTERVENTIONAL DEVICES

Rotablator

As an extension to long balloons, second-generation devices have also been used in longer lesions very effectively. Indeed, the Rotablator has been used with excellent success in patients with lesions greater than 10 mm in length (Fig. 17B.1). In the Rotablator multicenter registry, procedural success was achieved in 92% of patients with 143 lesions 1.5 to 2.5 cm long. These longer lesions were associated with a non–Q-wave MI rate of 6.2% and a Q-wave MI rate of 2.8%. This compares with 4.0% and 0.7%, respectively, for lesions less than 10 mm. Lesions that were 11 to 15 mm in length were successfully treated in 97% when combined with balloon angioplasty with a non–Q-wave MI rate of 5.5% (19). In a recent review of single-center experience Stertzer et al. reported a 94.6% success rate in lesions greater than 10 mm with a low, 4% major complication rate. The overall restenosis rate in this series was 38%

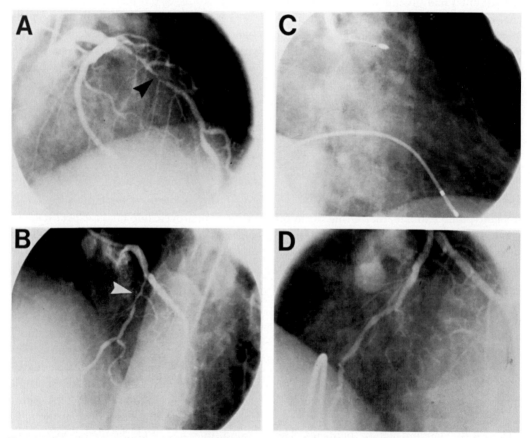

Figure 17B.1. Successful rotational atherectomy of a long, diseased segment of the LAD. **A.** RAO projection demonstrating the lesion. **B.** LAO projection demonstrating the length of the LAD lesion. **C.** RAO projection with 1.75-mm burr in artery and temporary pacemaker in place in right ventricle. **D.** Postprocedure LAO projection with no significant residual stenosis at the lesioned segment.

for type B and C lesions (20). Other reports suggest that restenosis rates may be somewhat higher with longer lesions (19, 21). Of note is that during the FDA-sponsored investigational trials with the Rotablator, lesions greater than 25 mm were excluded because of concerns regarding potential increased incidence of "slow flow." Slow flow has been observed in up to 9.5% in an analysis of 286 treated lesions with 33% and 9% of these developing non–Q-wave and Q-wave infarctions, respectively. Compromised distal vascular beds, large plaque burden, and long burr times were predictive of "slow flow" (22). Our experience with the Rotablator has also shown that the "slow flow" phenomena is seen primarily in patients with long lesions combined with diffuse disease, small caliber, and limited distal run-off.

Laser

Similarly, excimer laser, approved for use in coronary artery lesions greater than 20 mm in length, has been used with good success in long lesions. Indeed, the procedural results with excimer laser in coronary angioplasty have been shown to be somewhat independent of lesion length with an overall success rate of 91% when combined with balloon PTCA. The complications rates were likewise similar in all groups with Q MI in 1.6% and CABG in 4.6%. Of the 1179 lesions treated, only 7% were type A while 30% were type C (23). The ELCA investigators reported an 89% success rate in lesions greater than 20 mm long (with PTCA as an adjunct in 69%.) This compared with a procedural success rate of 75% for lesions greater than 20 mm treated with balloon alone. Laser was associated with perforation in 1.5% and occlusion in 4.1% (24). As with balloon PTCA and rotational atherectomy, somewhat higher restenosis rates have been observed in longer lesions. Overall restenosis rates of 46% have been reported, increasing to 59% in lesions greater than 10 mm in length (25).

Directional Coronary Atherectomy

Although DCA is primarily indicated for lesions less than 10 mm in length because of the limitation imposed by the length of the cutting window, the device has been used successfully in lesions greater than 10 mm in length. However, while the major complication rate was only 3.1% in 65 restenotic lesions greater than 10 mm in length treated with DCA, it increased to 12.5% in 32 de novo lesions greater than 10 mm. The overall success rates were 95% and 84%, respectively, when combined with PTCA (26). In 19 patients with lesions greater than 20 mm in length, success was achieved in 79%, but CABG was required in 10.5%, and the restenosis rate was 62.5% (27). Mooney et al. reported encouraging results when looking primarily at LAD lesions in 3-mm or larger vessels with lesion length greater than 10 mm. Procedural success rate was 99% with an abrupt closure rate of 4.6% and emergency surgery rate of 1.0% (28).

In our laboratory a novel application of DCA in longer lesions has been as an adjunct to rotational atherectomy in larger-diameter, calcified vessels previously considered unsuitable for DCA. To date our preliminary results have been good, and encouraging results have also been reported in a preliminary study of 10 patients treated with this approach (29). It appears that initial treatment with the Rotablator improves vessel compliance allowing the DCA catheter to cross the lesion and excise atheroma from otherwise inaccessible vessels.

Stents

Stents have not played a major role in the treatment of longer lesions because of potentially increased thrombotic complications occurring with the use of multiple stents (30, 31). However, a preliminary study suggests that restenosis rates are not affected by lesion length in vessels treated with a single Palmaz-Schatz stent. Restenosis occurred in 30% of lesions with a mean length of 6.8 mm and a range of 1.2 to 27.6 mm. Twenty-five percent of the 221 lesions treated were 8.7 to 27.6 mm in length (32). Despite the encouraging restenosis rates with single stents, restenosis rates of 63% have been seen with use of multiple stents (33–35).

In a series of 66 patients with long lesions, stents were incorporated into the treatment plan by combining long-balloon angioplasty with adjunctive stenting for unsatisfactory results following balloon dilatation. Angiographic success was achieved in 99% with adjunctive stenting required in 17%. The complication rate was low with one death and three myocardial infarctions (36).

RECOMMENDED APPROACH TO LONG LESIONS

One's approach to long lesions must be tailored to fit the specific lesional and clinical characteristics present. The impact of restenosis rates, especially in lesions greater than 20 mm, must also enter into the decision, as well as the informed consent. Long, compliant lesions that allow passage of the balloon are generally treated with long-balloon angioplasty, especially in larger caliber vessels. If significant flow-limiting dissection occurs, we attempt to treat the dissection with a carefully placed, single stent. Long lesions that are calcified, noncompliant, uncrossable, or undilatable with balloon PTCA are generally treated with the Rotablator and adjunctive balloon PTCA. Lesions that are very long (greater than 25 to 30 mm), calcified, and involve relatively straight segments may also be approached with laser-assisted, long-balloon angioplasty. Tortuous vessels with long lesions are usually approached with rotablation or long-balloon angioplasty because of the risk of perforation with the laser. However, the Rotablator should not be used in the presence of significant thrombus.

SUMMARY

As the utilization of second-generation interventional devices becomes more widespread, it is anticipated that the application of the various devices will become better defined. At present, the zeal to dilate long, complex stenoses is tempered somewhat by restenosis, despite the increasing ability to achieve procedural success with acceptably low complication rates. The development of solutions to the problem of restenosis will undoubtedly result in more widespread acceptance and utilization of percutaneous intervention in increasingly complex cases, especially those with long lesions and diffuse disease.

REFERENCES

1. Gruentzig A, Senning A, Siegenthaler W. Nonoperative dilatation of coronary artery stenosis. N Engl J Med 1979;301:61–68.
2. Faxon DP, Kelsey SF, Ryan TJ, McCabe CH, Detre K. Determinants of successful percutaneous transluminal coronary angioplasty: report from the National Heart, Lung, and Blood Institute Registry. Am Heart J 1984;108:1019–1023.
3. Detre K, Holubkov R, Kelsey S, Cowley M, Kent K, Williams D, Myler R et al. Percutaneous transluminal coronary angioplasty in 1985–1986 and 1977–1981. The National Heart, Lung, and Blood Institute Registry. N Engl J Med 1988;318(5):265–270.
4. Cowley MJ, Dorros G, Kelsey SF, Van Raden M, Detre KM. Acute coronary events associated with percutaneous transluminal coronary angioplasty. Am J Cardiol 1984;53(12):12C–16C.
5. Meier B, Gruentzig A, Hollmam J, Ischinger T, Bradford J. Does length or eccentricity of coronary stenoses influence the outcome of transluminal dilatation? Circulation 1983;67:497.
6. Detre KM, Holmes DR Jr, Holubkov R, Cowley MJ, Bourassa MG, Faxon DP, Dorros GR et al. Incidence and consequences of periprocedural occlusion. The 1985–1986 National Heart, Lung, and Blood Institute Percutaneous Transluminal Coronary Angioplasty Registry. Circulation 1990;82(3):739–750.
7. Ellis SG, Roubin GS, King SB III, Douglas JS Jr, Weintraub WS, Thomas RG, Cox WR. Angiographic and clinical predictors of acute closure after native vessel coronary angioplasty. Circulation 1988;77(2):372–379.
8. ACC/AHA Task Force. Guidelines for percutaneous transluminal coronary angioplasty. J Am Coll Cardiol 1988; 12:529–545.
9. MacLeod D, Maas A, Domburg R, Brand M, Serruys P, Feyter P. Angiographic predictors of the immediate outcome of coronary balloon angioplasty. J Am Coll Cardiol 1993;21:340A.

10. Savage MP, Goldberg S, Hirshfeld JW, Bass TA, MacDonald RG, Margolis JR, Taussig AS et al. Clinical and angiographic determinants of primary coronary angioplasty success. M-HEART investigators. J Am Coll Cardiol 1991; 17(1):22–28.

11. Goudreau E, DiSciascio G, Kelly K, Vetrovec GW, Nath A, Cowley MJ. Coronary angioplasty of diffuse coronary artery disease. Am Heart J 1991;121:12–19.

12. Brymer JF, Khaja F, Kraft PL. Angioplasty of long or tandem coronary artery lesions using a new longer balloon dilatation catheter: a comparative study. Cathet Cardiovasc Diagn 1991;23(2):84–88.

13. Savas V, Puchrowicz S, Williams L, Grines C, O'Neill B. Angioplasty outcome using long balloons in high-risk lesions. J Am Coll Cardiol 1992;19:34A.

14. Zidar J, Tenaglia A, Jackman J, Fortin D, Frid D, Tcheng J, Royal S et al. Improved acute results for PTCA of long coronary lesions using long angioplasty balloon catheters. J Am Coll Cardiol 1992;19:34A.

15. Banka VS, Baker HA III, Vemuri DN, Voci G, Maniet AR. Effectiveness of decremental diameter balloon catheters (tapered balloon). Am J Cardiol 1992;69:188–193.

16. Ellis S, Roubin G, King S, Douglas J. Importance of stenosis morphology in the estimation of restenosis after elective percutaneous transluminal coronary angioplasty. Am J Cardiol 1989;63:30–34.

17. Bourassa MG, Lesperance J, Eastwood C, Schwartz L, Cote G, Kazim F, Hudon G. Clinical, physiologic, anatomic and procedural factors predictive of restenosis after percutaneous transluminal coronary angioplasty. J Am Coll Cardiol 1991;18(2):368–376.

18. Hirshfeld JW Jr, Schwartz JS, Jugo R, MacDonald RG, Goldberg S, Savage MP, Bass TA et al. Restenosis after coronary angioplasty: a multivariate statistical model to relate lesion and procedure variables to restenosis. J Am Coll Cardiol 1991;18(3):647–656.

19. Reisman M, Cohen B, Warth D, Fenner J, Gocka I, Buchbinder M. Outcome of long lesions treated with high-speed rotational ablation. J Am Coll Cardiol 1993;21:443A.

20. Stertzer S, Rosenblum J, Shaw R, Sugeng I, Hidalgo B, Ryan C, Hansell H et al. Coronary rotational ablation: initial experience in 302 procedures. J Am Coll Cardiol 1992; 21:287–295.

21. Tierstein P, Warth D, Haq N, Jenkins N, McCowan L, Aubanel-Reidel P, Morris N et al. High-speed rotational coronary atherectomy for patients with diffuse coronary artery disease. J Am Coll Cardiol 1991;18:1694–1701.

22. Ellis S, Franco I, Satler L, Whitlow P. Slow reflow and coronary perforation after rotablator therapy—incidence: clinical, angiographic and procedural predictors. Circulation 1992;86:I-652.

23. Holmes D, Bresnahan J, Bell M, Litvak F. Lesion morphology and outcome after laser angioplasty. A prospective evaluation: Excimer Laser Angioplasty Registry. J Am Coll Cardiol 1993;21:288A.

24. Hartzler G, Litvak F, Margolis J, Leon M, Cumins R, Goldenberg T. Adjunctive excimer laser coronary angioplasty improves primary PTCA results for lesions greater than 20 mm in length. J Am Coll Cardiol 1992;19:48A.

25. Bittl JA, Sanborn TA, Tcheng JE, Siegel RM, Ellis SG. Clinical success, complications and restenosis rates with excimer laser coronary angioplasty. The Percutaneous Excimer Laser Coronary Angioplasty Registry. Am J Cardiol 1992;70(20):1533–1539.

26. Hinohara T, Rowe MH, Robertson GC, Selmon MR, Braden L, Leggett JH, Vetter JW et al. Effect of lesion characteristics on outcome of directional coronary atherectomy. J Am Coll Cardiol 1991;17(5):1112–1120.

27. Robertson G, Selmon M, Hinohara T, Rowe M, Leggett J, Braden L, Simpson J. The effect of lesion length on outcome of directional coronary atherectomy. Circulation 1990;82:III-623.

28. Mooney M, Mooney J, Nahhas A, Lesser J, Madison J. Directional atherectomy in long lesions: improved acute results. Cathet Cardiovasc Diagn 1993;29:83.

29. Mintz GS, Pichard AD, Popma JJ, Kent KM, Satler LF, Leon MB. Preliminary experience with adjunct directional coronary atherectomy after high-speed rotational atherectomy in the treatment of calcific coronary artery disease. Am J Cardiol 1993;71(10):799–804.

30. Doucet S, Fajadet J, Gaillard J, Cassagneau B, Robert G, Marco J. Predictors of thrombotic occlusion following coronary Palmaz-Schatz stent implantation. Circulation 1992;86:I-113.

31. Agrawal S, Hearn J, Liu M, Cannon A, Bilodeau L, Iyer S, Baxley W et al. Stent thrombosis and ischemic complications following coronary artery stenting. Circulation 1992; 86:I-113.

32. Wong C, Rocha-Singh K, Tierstein P, Schatz R. Lesion length does not influence restenosis following placement of single Palmaz-Schatz coronary stents. Circulation 1992; 86:I-512.

33. Ellis SG, Savage M, Fischman D, Baim DS, Leon M, Goldberg S, Hirshfeld JW et al. Restenosis after placement of Palmaz-Schatz stents in native coronary arteries. Initial results of a multicenter experience. Circulation 1992;86(6):1836–1844.

34. Haude M, Erbel R, Straub U, Dietz U, Meyer J. Short- and long-term results after intracoronary stenting in human coronary arteries: monocentre experience with the balloon-expandable Palmaz-Schatz stent. Br Heart J 1991; 66(5):337–345.

35. Fajadet J, Coucet S, Gaillard J, Cassagneau B, Robert G, Marco J. Predictors of restenosis after Palmaz-Schatz implantation. Circulation 1992;86:I-531.

36. Cannon A, Hearn J, Bilodeau L, Iyer S, Agrawal S, Dean L, Baxley W et al. Long balloon angioplasty and adjuvant stenting for long type B and C lesions. Circulation 1992;86:I-511.

C. Treating Long Lesions with PTCA

VICKY SAVAS

Andreas Gruentzig initially included short lesions measuring less than 5 mm in length as one of the indications for percutaneous transluminal coronary angioplasty (PTCA). Since then, indications for PTCA have dramatically expanded.

In 1987 the American College of Cardiology/American Heart Association Task Force risk-stratified lesions based on PTCA results in the mid 1980s vis-a-vis several morphologic features. With respect to lesion length, type A are less than 10 mm in length, are found to be of low risk, and meet with a high success rate when treated with PTCA. Type B lesions measure 10 to 20 mm and are of moderate risk and success rate, whereas type C lesions exceed 20 mm in length and are found to be of high risk and low success when treated with PTCA (1). The poor outcome of long, type C lesions when treated with PTCA led to the American College of Physicians Task Force recommendations against percutaneous revascularization (2). Others similarly found that increased lesion length paralleled the increase in complication rates (3–5). Ellis et al. found that lesion length of ≥2 luminal diameters was a predictor for acute closure resulting in urgent CABG, myocardial infarction, or repeat angioplasty (6). Despite these results, there remains a strong interest in treating diffuse disease percutaneously, principally because these patients typically are at increased risk for surgical revascularization. Not infrequently, patients with diffuse disease have compromised left ventricular function, are elderly, and/or diabetic. Moreover, the diffusely diseased segments are often heavily calcified, making these vessels suboptimal targets for placement of grafts. Endarterectomy combined

with coronary artery bypass grafting (CABG) is sometimes used as an alternative, but the marked increase in morbidity and mortality compared with CABG alone makes this method less attractive (7), particularly in those patients with the following risk factors: age greater than 70 years, ejection fraction less than or equal to 0.30, and repeat surgery. Some studies have shown a 16% perioperative mortality if one risk factor is present compared with 3.0% in the absence of any of these risk factors. The mortality rate increases as the number of risk factors increases (8).

Female gender and diabetes mellitus are also known to be associated with an increased surgical risk. Although a more recent study suggests a lower mortality rate in this subset of patients, they still represent a greater risk than those patients who are free of these risk factors (9). With improved technique and marked evolution in equipment, more recent studies suggest improved results when treating diffuse disease with PTCA (10, 11).

TECHNICAL APPROACH

Guide Catheter

It is common for long, diffuse disease to incorporate arterial bends. This in combination with other complex lesion morphology may create difficulties when attempting to cross the diseased segment with angioplasty equipment, including wires and balloons, necessitating adequate guide catheter support or "backup." Generally, adequate "backup" can be achieved with a standard Judkins guide catheter; however, deep engagement or alternatives such as an Amplatz or Voda guide may be necessary.

Guidewire

Even with excellent guide support, one may encounter difficulties crossing diffusely diseased segments, particularly when the segments are heavily calcified or when they involve secondary branches or tortuous segments. In these situations diffusely diseased regions may be more effectively crossed with a steerable, tapered core wire (Hyperflex, Reflex, Silk). Unfortunately, this type of wire is often radiopaque, and identification of dissections and focal regions of stenosis may be compromised, particularly in smaller arteries (diameter less than 2 mm) or in the presence of heavy calcification. This problem may be circumvented by using a steerable, radiolucent wire (Phantom) or by exchanging the radiopaque wire with one that is radiolucent. The latter can be quickly and easily achieved while the balloon catheter remains across the lesion. This technique will ensure luminal access.

By virtue of their length, diffusely diseased segments are more likely to incorporate natural arterial bends; therefore one must be cognizant of the "pseudolesion" phenomenon. These temporary "narrowings" may be created when a tortuous coronary artery segment is artificially straightened with an angioplasty wire. The mechanism is felt to be caused by arterial wall invaginations at critical points along the vessel to accommodate "excess" length along a shorter linear distance. This author has found an increased incidence of this phenomenon with stiffer wires and balloon shafts. Removal of the guidewire allows the vessel to return to its original configuration with complete resolution of the pseudolesions (Fig. 17C.1). These narrowings can be distinguished by their characteristic wedge shape and their occurrence at bend points or in extremely tortuous segments. It is crucial to recognize this phenomenon since treatments likely to be considered such as additional balloon inflations, intracoronary urokinase, or use of stents are unnecessary and may place the patient at additional risk.

Balloon Length

Recently, some investigators have found that treating long lesions with long balloons appears to lower the acute complication rate compared with conventional length, 20-mm balloons (10, 11) (Fig. 17C.2). The improved

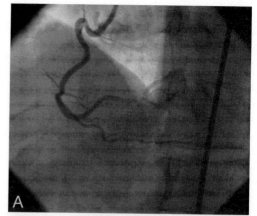
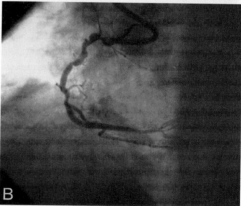
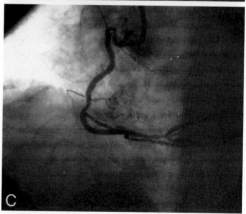

Figure 17C.1. Pseudolesion. **A.** Initial angiogram of right coronary artery. **B.** Multiple pseudolesions created by guidewire. **C.** Resolution of pseudolesions after removal of guidewire.

results seen with long balloons may be multifactorial. First, overlapping the balloon across the entire length of the diseased segment, particularly at the normal artery-

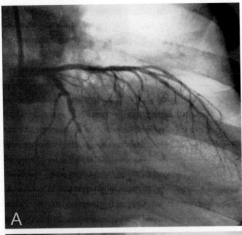

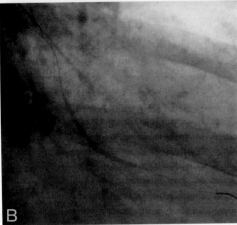

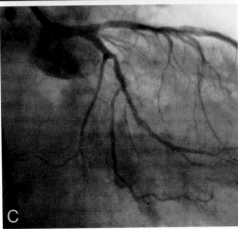

Figure 17C.2. **A.** Obtuse marginal branch with long stenosis. **B.** Long-balloon inflation. **C.** Post-PTCA angiogram.

plaque edge interface, appears to lower the dissection rate. Using a conventional-length balloon (20 mm in length), which is long relative to lesion length, type A lesions (less than 10 mm in length) are predictably low risk. It is hypothesized that the PTCA outcome of long, type C lesions is improved when a balloon that is longer than that of the lesion is used. When the balloon length exceeds the lesion length by a ratio ≥1, there may be a more gradual transition of arterial wall stretch and more even dispersement of pressure (Fig. 17C.3). Second, using a balloon longer than the lesion avoids multiple, fragmented dilatations across the diseased segment. Finally, since long lesions are more likely to eventually incorporate an arterial bend, a longer balloon affords superior conformability compared with a short balloon (10). Less straightening of a natural bend lowers vessel trauma and tissue injury.

Despite the apparent advantages afforded by the use of long balloons, one must be aware of their potential disadvantages. First, it is not uncommon for the artery to taper

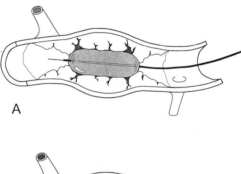

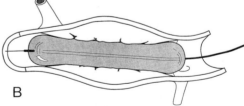

Figure 17C.3. **A.** Conventional length balloon is shorter than the stenosis. Inflation results in dissections, particularly at plaque edge-normal artery interface. **B.** Balloon length exceeds stenosis length by a ratio ≥1 resulting in lower dissection rate.

across a 40-mm segment. This is true particularly when that segment of the primary vessel gives rise to a large side branch or multiple, small branches. For example, the proximal-to-mid left anterior descending artery tapers dramatically as it gives rise to two or three major diagonal branches. Side branches themselves frequently taper as their myocardial territory becomes limited by bordering branches. When faced with the situation of tapered segments, one must size the balloon cautiously. If the balloon is sized according to the larger lumen of the proximal segment, it will be oversized for the distal portion of the segment and lead to a marked increase in dissections. Sizing to the distal portion of the segment will cause undersizing of the proximal portion and inadequate dilatation; however, this is a more desirable outcome compared with an increased complication rate. One alternative to this potential hazard of the long balloon would be the use of a long, tapered balloon.

An additional complication more likely to occur with long balloons is inadvertent placement of the balloon tip within the "hinge" point of a vessel. During the cardiac cycle there is coronary artery motion. The artery will bend and stretch at critical points along its path. Placing the balloon tip in these regions counters the natural torsion, increasing tissue trauma and injury. One need not be concerned with placement of the balloon midmarker in the middle of the lesion as with conventional length balloons, but instead focus on avoiding placement of the balloon tip within the "hinge" points or alternatively completely overlapping these regions with the balloon.

Balloon Material

Studies have found conflicting results on the outcome of dilating lesions with different balloon materials. Inconsistent findings may be the result of differences in operator experience, inflation technique, and lesion selection. Intuitively, some interventionalists re-

main concerned with compliant balloon material. Unlike soft, noncalcified focal lesions laden with lipid pools, long lesions are typically hard and calcified. The diffusely diseased segments are more likely to require higher inflation pressures. There is some concern that use of high pressures in compliant balloons will result in unintentional increase in balloon size, with balloon-to-artery oversizing resulting in an increase in major complication rates. Final recommendations regarding choice of balloon material in long, diffusely diseased segments await prospective, randomized trials.

Inflation Strategy

Recent interest has focused on outcome based on balloon inflation strategy. This author found that inflating the balloon using a "fast" versus "slow" strategy had no significant effect on acute outcome with respect to residual lesion or major complication rates (unpublished data). However, that study may have been limited by inadequate differential in rates of inflation. It is the feeling of this author that slow inflation is preferable to a more rapid strategy. Specifically, the balloon is inflated to 2 to 3 atm. This pressure is held constant even if the "waist" remains. In fact, it is more desirable to inflate below the pressure in which there is a loss of waist on the first one or two inflations. Inflation duration should be a minimum of 2 minutes. In doing so, it is felt that the artery has time to gently "mold" to the balloon. This technique may avoid "overshooting" or snapping and tearing the vessel as is seen with a rapid inflation to the point of loss of waist.

If the waist persists, additional inflations with gradual increases in pressure are used, increasing the pressure by 1 or 2 atm every 30 to 60 seconds. This is done under fluoroscopic visualization. Once the waist gives way, the pressure is decreased by 1 to 2 atm. Although efficient use of time is important to every interventionalist, saving 2 or 3 minutes by using a more rapid inflation technique mod-

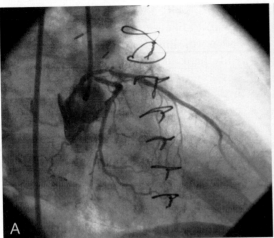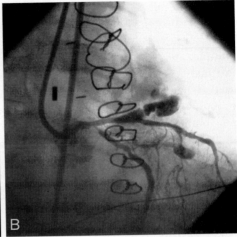

Figure 17C.4. **A.** Left anterior descending artery with subtle bend in mid region. **B.** Angiogram immediately following excimer laser revealing large perforation at bend site.

estly decreases total case time while perhaps markedly increasing major complications, which may lead to even longer cases requiring cutting, "tacking-up," or stenting potentially avoidable dissections.

Despite use of the techniques described above, dissections and poor outcomes may still occur. Specifically, dense calcification, particularly when inconsistently distributed along the stenotic region, appears to be associated with an increased complication rate. This poor outcome has led to interest in the use of debulking agents such as the excimer laser and Rotablator. However, proper case selection for these devices demands awareness of their limitations. If the diseased segment incorporates tortuosity or bends, the excimer laser beam will become malaligned with respect to the arterial lumen, resulting in dissections and perforations (Fig. 17C.4).

Although the Rotablator can negotiate tortuosity and bends more safely than the excimer laser, its wire technology lags behind traditional PTCA wires, particularly with respect to steerability.

REFERENCES

1. Ryan TJ, Faxon DP, Gunnar RM et al. Guidelines for percutaneous transluminal coronary angioplasty. A report of the American College of Cardiology/American Heart Association Task Force on assessment of diagnostic and therapeutic cardiovascular procedures (Subcommittee on percutaneous transluminal coronary angioplasty). Circulation 1988;78:486–502.

2. Ryan TJ, Klocke FJ, Reynolds WA. Clinical competence in percutaneous transluminal coronary angioplasty. A statement for physicians from the ACP/ACC/AHA Task Force on clinical privileges in cardiology. Circulation 1990;81:2041–2046.

3. Meier B, Gruentzig AR, Hollman J et al. Does length or eccentricity of coronary stenoses influence the outcome of transluminal dilatation? Circulation 1984;67:497–499.

4. Bredlau CE, Roubin GS, Leimgruber PP et al. In-hospital morbidity and mortality in patients undergoing elective coronary angioplasty. Circulation 1985;72:1044–1052.

5. Hall DP, Gruentzig AR. Influence of lesion length on initial success and recurrence rates in coronary angioplasty. Circulation 1984;70(Suppl II):II-176.

6. Ellis SG, Roubin GS, King SB III et al. Angiographic and clinical predictors of acute closure after native vessel coronary angioplasty. Circulation 1988;77:372–379.

7. Livesay JJ, Colley DA, Hallman GL et al. Early and late results of coronary endarterectomy. J Thorac Cardiovasc Surg 1986;92:649–660.

8. Brenowitz J, Kayser K, Johnson D. Triple-vessel coronary artery endarterectomy and reconstruction: results in 144 patients. J Am Coll Cardiol 1988;11:706–711.

9. Sommerhaug RG, Wolfe SK, Reid DA. Early clinical results of long coronary arteriotomy, endarterectomy and reconstruction combined with multiple bypass grafting for severe coronary artery disease. Am J Cardiol 1990; 66:651–659.

10. Savas V, Grines CL, Puchrowicz S et al. Angioplasty using long balloons in high-risk coronary lesions. Am J Cardiol (in press).

11. Tenaglia AN, Zidar JP, Jackman JD et al. Treatment of long coronary artery narrowings with long angioplasty catheters. Am J Cardiol 1993;71:1274–1277.

EDITORS' SUMMARY

Device	Comments
20-mm balloon	No role. Although this has not been tested in moderate- to large-scale randomized trial, results with long balloons appear clearly superior.
30- to 40-mm balloons	Probably the "gold standard" for cost-effective treatment, if there is one (with exceptions as noted below).
Excimer laser	Provides results equal to that of long balloons, probably not better (see recent AMRO trial). Especially indicated for long and severe stenoses that do not have features placing them at high risk with this form of therapy (e.g., marked angulation, bifurcation [for the concentric lasers]).
Holmium laser	Probably as good as the excimer laser in this situation, except perhaps for moderately calcified lesions (neither is good for severe calcification).
Rotablator	Indicated only for moderate to severe calcification in conjunction with long lesions (early data suggested a high rate of complications in this setting, but technique modifications may have changed this).
Directional atherectomy	Role is very limited. Occasionally may be useful for the eccentric lesion in a large vessel, especially if the lesion has been pretreated (without pretreatment the dissection rate is very high).
TEC	Consider only for diffusely diseased vein grafts.
Stents	As restenosis rates appear to be greater when multiple stents are overlapped (at least for the Palmaz-Schatz design—the only design at present shown to successfully impact the problem of restenosis), stenting should perhaps be limited to treatment of dissection resulting from primary therapy. This may not be true when longer Palmaz-Schatz stents become available, nor in large saphenous vein grafts (where data for the use of multiple stents is not nearly as ominous).

18. The Angulated Lesion

A. Treatment of the Angulated Lesion

JOHN A. BITTL

Although coronary angioplasty is a useful treatment for a wide range of lesion types, the treatment of angulated lesions with balloon dilatation (1–5) or with excimer laser angioplasty (6, 7) is associated with a high risk of vessel dissection, abrupt closure, and ischemic complications. A strategy for angulated lesions can be formulated, however, on the provisional use of perfusion balloon angioplasty, directional atherectomy, or intracoronary stenting if complications arise. Advanced interventional techniques thus provide a "safety net" for treating the complications commonly encountered during angioplasty of angulated lesions.

Although the techniques discussed in this chapter may be generalized to other lesion types inherently involving angulation such as bifurcation lesions, ostial lesions, or anastomotic vein graft lesions, the specific approach to these lesion morphologies are covered in other sections in this textbook. The purpose of this chapter is to define an angioplasty strategy for angulated lesions lying within native coronary arteries.

THE ANGULATED LESION

Flow disturbances within angulated arterial segments and at branch points predispose to the development of atherosclerosis (8, 9) and impairment of endothelial function (10). Thus angulated lesions are common. Coronary le-

sions in bends ≥45° comprise up to 45% of lesions selected for balloon angioplasty (1–5), 25% of lesions treated with directional atherectomy (11), 20% of lesions treated with rotational atherectomy (12), and 13% of lesions treated with coronary stenting (13). Patients who undergo balloon angioplasty for angulated lesions have the same baseline clinical variables (age, sex, etc.) as those who undergo angioplasty for lesions in straight segments (4).

OUTCOME OF BALLOON ANGIOPLASTY FOR THE ANGULATED LESION

Angulated lesions treated with angioplasty have worse outcomes than straight lesions. The risk of dissection for angulated lesions treated with angioplasty is approximately twice that for straight lesions (1–5). The tendency for the inflated balloon to straighten may promote intimal disruption because of uneven distribution of stresses along the vessel wall. This accounts for the observation that dissections originate within the atherosclerotic plaque itself and at the ends of the dilating balloon (1–4). In a case-matched study the success rate for lesions in a bend ≥45° was 70%, whereas the success rate for lesions in a straight segment was 89% (4). Angulated lesions treated with angioplasty also have higher rates of restenosis than straight lesions. In one study, in which the rate of restenosis was 41% for angulated lesions and 28% for straight lesions, lesion angulation was identified as the strongest independent predictor of restenosis from a large series of preprocedural variables (14).

Figure 18A.1. Method of angle measurement and balloon positioning. **A.** In an end-diastolic view, free from foreshortening, the arterial centerline is drawn for a 20-mm segment centered on the stenosis. The angle between the proximal and distal segments is measured. **B.** The dilating balloon is positioned across the lesion and into the straight segment. (Modified from Ellis SG, Topol EJ. Am J Cardiol 1990;66:932–937 with permission.)

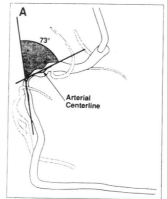
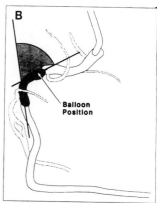

TECHNICAL CONSIDERATIONS FOR ANGIOPLASTY OF ANGULATED LESIONS

Assessment of Angulation

Assessment of coronary artery angulation must be made in a nonforeshortened end-diastolic projection (Fig. 18A.1). Visual assessment is frequently used, but is less accurate than the semiquantitative method in which 10-mm arterial centerlines originating at the stenosis are drawn and used to calculate the angle between the proximal and distal segments (4). A handheld protractor may be useful to measure the angle (2). Some investigators measure the angle of the noninflated balloon catheter positioned across the stenosis (2). In spite of multiple methods available for measuring angulation, there is large variability in the assessment of the degree of angulation. Thus lesions associated with bends ≥45° are simply classified as "angulated," and lesions ≥90° are commonly classified as "severely angulated."

Patient and Lesion Selection

The selection of patients with angulated lesions for angioplasty is based on the severity of angulation, as well as the risk of cardiovascular collapse and the likelihood of a successful approach to the angulated lesion with advanced interventional devices if abrupt vessel closure occurs. Although some studies have suggested that highly angulated lesions (>60°) do not have a higher rate of complica-

tion than moderately angulated lesions (45° to 60°) (4), other studies have reported the highest risk for lesions in angles ≥90° (5).

Lesions located in the "shepherd's crook" of the dominant right coronary artery deserve special attention (Fig. 18A.2). This is so because abrupt vessel closure at this site is frequently associated with cardiogenic shock from acute right ventricular failure and inferoseptal left ventricular dysfunction. Thus angioplasty of the proximal right coronary lesion complicated by abrupt closure is a strong predictor of procedural *death* (15). If an angulated lesion is associated with other risk factors for abrupt closure such as the presence of thrombus (2, 16, 17), alternative therapies such as elective bypass surgery should be considered.

Technique of Angioplasty for the Angulated Lesion

Although the treatment of the angulated lesion often begins with conventional balloon dilatation, it may evolve into a complex intervention with perfusion balloon catheters, directional atherectomy, or coronary stenting. Thus the strategy for the successful treatment of the angulated lesion benefits from anticipating the results of balloon dilatation and need for advanced interventional approaches. The femoral sheath, coronary guiding catheter, and guidewire should be selected to accommodate all possible devices that may

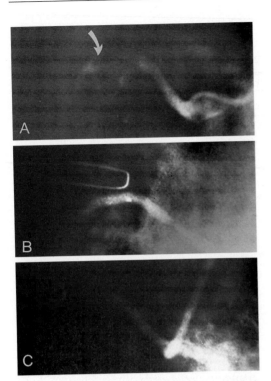

Figure 18A.2. Proximal right coronary artery lesion. **A.** An eccentric and ulcerated lesion is identified in the proximal right coronary artery associated with a filling defect *(arrow)*. After intracoronary urokinase and balloon inflation **(B),** the artery became totally occluded **(C),** necessitating insertion of an intraaortic balloon pump and emergency coronary artery bypass surgery.

be required for treatment of an angulated lesion.

The initial dilating balloon should be chosen to have an inflated diameter that approximates the diameter of the normal reference segment of the vessel. Although use of oversized balloons increases the risk of dissection (18), intentional undersizing of balloons does not appear to reduce the risk of dissection for angulated lesions (4). The balloon should be dilated with the lowest pressure that allows full expansion. Although no formal analysis of the relation between inflation pressure and dissection of angulated lesions has been reported, it seems reasonable to minimize forcible balloon straightening and barotrauma to the angulated site by avoiding high balloon pressures. The relation between balloon length and risk of dissection in angulated lesions has not been rigorously evaluated. For lesions immediately adjacent to but not directly in a bend, it seems prudent to use a 20-mm balloon whose proximal or distal segment can dilate the lesion without stressing the angulated segment. For longer lesions directly involving the angulated segment (19), it seems reasonable to cover the involved stenotic segment and the adjacent segments with 30-mm or 40-mm balloons to avoid the concentration of excessive stress at the edges of the stenosis (Fig. 18A.1).

The type of balloon material may influence the likelihood of dissection. The risk of dissection may be lower with balloons constructed of polyethylene teraphthalate (PET) than other materials (4). Comparative studies have shown that PET balloons straighten a 90° acrylic model of the coronary artery by only 36° to 43°, whereas polyolefin balloons straighten the model by 57° to 63° (4).

Rotational atherectomy has been used successfully in angulated lesions. In a recent report 23 of 116 lesions (20%) treated with rotational atherectomy were associated with vessel angulation ≥45° (12). Although guidewire fracture occurred in three of 116 lesions, it is not clear whether vessel angulation was responsible for the mechanical failure (12). Technical refinements in rotational atherectomy have reduced the incidence of guidewire fracture, making treatment of angulated lesions with rotational atherectomy safer.

Excimer laser angioplasty (Fig. 18A.3) should not be performed with standard concentric catheters for lesions located in angles of ≥45° because of the risk of perforation caused by radial, rather than coaxial, application of laser energy (6, 7). Similarly, the transluminal extraction atherectomy (20) does not seem suitable for lesions in angulated segments because of inherent device rigidity.

The development of significant dissection or abrupt vessel closure complicating angio-

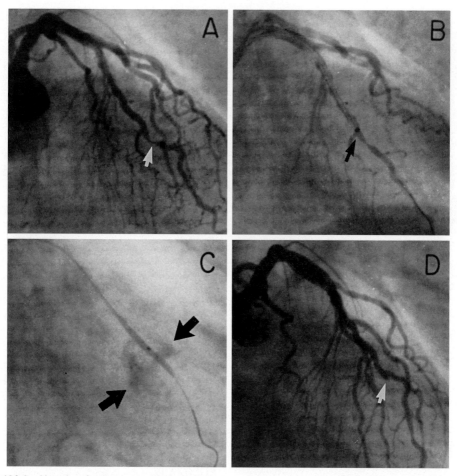

Figure 18A.3. Vessel perforation caused by excimer laser angioplasty of an angulated lesion. **A.** A lesion in the mid-segment of the left anterior descending artery is associated with an angle of 60° *(white arrow).* **B.** Although the guidewire and laser catheter have apparently straightened the segment *(black arrow),* vessel perforation ensues after application of laser energy leading to contrast extravasation **(C)** *(black arrows).* Prolonged balloon inflation **(C)** completely seals the perforation, leaving a mild luminal irregularity and no further evidence of extravasation **(D)** *(white arrow).* (Modified from Bittl JA, Sanborn TA, Abela GS, Isner JM. J Intervent Cardiol 1992;5:275–291 with permission.)

plasty of an angulated lesion requires the use of additional interventional therapies such as perfusion balloon catheter, directional atherectomy, or coronary stenting. These additional therapies often require "extra-support" coronary guidewires and oversized femoral sheaths and guiding catheters for delivery. Although the primary use of perfusion balloon angioplasty may reduce the incidence of dissection (21), the provisional use of perfusion balloon angioplasty is also helpful if a severe dissection has occurred. An adequate test of

the efficacy of a perfusion balloon for the treatment of dissection entails inflation for approximately 20 minutes if myocardial ischemia is absent or mild.

If angioplasty of an angulated lesion produces a focal dissection and the target vessel is not calcified, salvage directional atherectomy is often successful (22, 23). This requires placement of a 10 Fr femoral sheath and use of a 10 Fr guiding catheter. Although the previously positioned sheath and guiding catheter can be exchanged over a long coro-

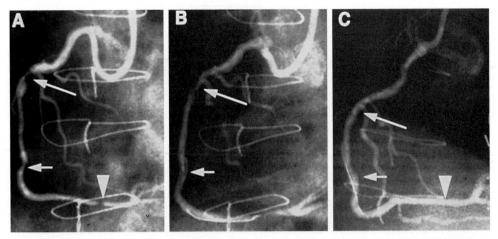

Figure 18A.4. Angulated lesion treated with coronary stenting. An angulated lesion **(A)** *(upper arrow)* and two straight lesions *(middle and lower arrows)* are treated with the balloon angioplasty, leaving a significant residual stenosis and dissections **(B)** *(arrows)*, which necessitated the insertion of two Gianturco-Roubin stents **(C)** *(upper and middle arrows)* with good result.

nary guidewire (or preferably over a pair of 0.018-inch extra-support guidewires) without sacrificing wire position in the coronary artery, planned use of the 10 Fr system will obviate the need for lengthy exchanges. The risk of perforation is theoretically increased, however, during directional atherectomy of deep wall dissections or of eccentric lesions arising from the inner angle of the angulated segment (24).

Coronary stenting has revolutionized the treatment of angulated lesions (Fig. 18A.4). Although the more rigid Palmaz-Schatz slotted-tube stent may not conform as easily to angulated lesions as other stent designs, the slotted-tube stent has been successful for lesions involving moderate degrees of angulation. In the BENESTENT study, 13% of patients treated with the Palmaz-Schatz stenting had angulated lesions (13). The more conformable Gianturco-Roubin flexible-coil stent has been extensively evaluated as a treatment for vessel dissection and abrupt vessel closure for a wide range of lesion morphologies (25, 26). Appropriate planning for this device involves placement of an 8 Fr sheath and use of an 8 Fr guiding catheter with 0.086-inch inner lumen diameter and a configuration

providing adequate "back-up" for target vessels ≤3.5 mm. For vessels >3.5 mm, however, a 9 Fr guiding catheter is required. Adequate planning for insertion of the flexible coil stent also requires use of an 0.018-inch extra-support guidewire and pretreatment with heparin, dextran, dipyridamole, and aspirin.

SUMMARY

The angulated lesion remains a significant challenge in interventional cardiovascular medicine, but responds successfully to the device of anticipation. Although the risk of dissection and abrupt vessel closure after balloon angioplasty may be minimized by accurate balloon sizing and careful balloon inflation, a successful outcome is often achieved by anticipating and successfully implementing additional treatments such as perfusion balloon angioplasty, directional atherectomy, and coronary stenting.

REFERENCES

1. Ischinger T, Grüntzig AR, Meier B, Galan K. Coronary dissection and total coronary occlusion associated with percutaneous transluminal coronary angioplasty: significance of initial angiographic morphology of coronary stenoses. Circulation 1986;74:1371–1378.
2. Ellis SG, Roubin GS, King SB III et al. Angiographic and clinical predictors of acute closure after native vessel coronary angioplasty. Circulation 1988;77:372–379.

3. Ellis SG, Vandormael MG, Cowley MJ et al. Coronary morphologic and clinical determinants of procedural outcome with angioplasty for multivessel coronary disease: implications for patient selection. Circulation 1990;82:1193–1202.

4. Ellis SG, Topol EJ. Results of percutaneous transluminal coronary angioplasty of high-risk angulated stenoses. Am J Cardiol 1990;66:932–937.

5. Meckel CR, Ahmed W, Ferguson JJ et al. Angiographic predictors of severe dissection during balloon angioplasty: a report from the Hirulog Angioplasty Study. Circulation 1993;90:I-64 (abstract).

6. Bittl JA, Ryan TJ Jr, Keaney JF Jr et al. Coronary artery perforation during excimer laser coronary angioplasty. 1993;21:1158–1165.

7. Holmes DR Jr, Reeder GS, Ghazzal ZMB et al. Coronary perforation after excimer laser coronary angioplasty: the Excimer Laser Coronary Angioplasty Registry experience. J Am Coll Cardiol 1994;23:330–335.

8. Fuster V, Badimon JJ, Badimon L. Clinical-pathological correlations of coronary disease progression and regression. Circulation 1992;86(Suppl III):III-1–III-11.

9. Zarins CK, Giddens DP, Bharadvaj BK, Sottiuir VS, Mabon RF, Galgov S. Carotid bifurcation atherosclerosis: quantitative correlation of plaque localization with flow velocity profiles and wall shear stress. Circ Res 1983;53:502–514.

10. McLenachan JM, Vita J, Fish DR et al. Early evidence of endothelial vasodilator dysfunction at coronary branch points. Circulation 1990;82:1169–1173.

11. Adelman AG, Cohen EA, Kimball BP et al. A comparison of coronary atherectomy with coronary angioplasty for lesions of the proximal left anterior descending coronary artery. N Engl J Med 1993;329:228–233.

12. Safian RD, Niazi KA, Strzlelecki M et al. Detailed angiographic analysis of high-speed mechanical rotational atherectomy in human coronary arteries. Circulation 1993;88:961–968.

13. Serruys P, de Jaegere P, Kiemeneij F et al. A comparison of balloon-expandable–stent implantation with balloon angioplasty in patients with coronary artery disease. N Engl J Med 1994;331:489–495.

14. Ellis SG, Roubin GS, King SB III, Douglas JS Jr, Cox WR. Importance of stenosis morphology in the estimation of restenosis risk after elective percutaneous transluminal coronary angioplasty. Am J Cardiol 1989;63:30–34.

15. Ellis SG, Myler RK, King SB III et al. Causes and correlates of death after unsupported coronary angioplasty: implications for use of angioplasty and advanced support techniques in high-risk settings. Am J Cardiol 1991;68:1447–1451.

16. de Feyter PJ, van den Brand M, Jaarman G, van Domburg R, Serruys PW, Suryapranata H. Acute coronary artery occlusion during and after percutaneous transluminal coronary angioplasty: frequency, prediction, clinical course, management, and follow-up. Circulation 1991;83:927–936.

17. Myler RK, Shaw RE, Stertzer SH et al. Lesion morphology and coronary angioplasty: current experience and analysis. J Am Coll Cardiol 1992;19:1641–1652.

18. Roubin GS, Douglas JS Jr, King SB III et al. Influence of balloon size on initial success, acute complications, and restenosis after percutaneous transluminal coronary angioplasty: a prospective randomized study. Circulation 1988;78:557–565.

19. Cannon AD, Roubin GS, Hearn JA, Iyer SS, Baxley WA, Dean LS. Acute angiographic and clinical results of long balloon percutaneous transluminal coronary angioplasty and adjuvant stenting for long narrowings. Am J Cardiol 1994;73:635–641.

20. Popma JJ, Leon MB, Mintz GS et al. Results of coronary angioplasty using the transluminal extraction catheter. Am J Cardiol 1992;70:1526–1532.

21. Ohman EM, Marquis J-F, Ricci DR et al. A randomized comparison of the effects of gradual prolonged versus standard primary balloon inflation on early and late outcome: results of a multicenter clinical trial. Circulation 1994;89:1118–1125.

22. McCluskey ER, Cowley M, Whitlow PL. Multicenter clinical experience with rescue atherectomy for failed angioplasty. Am J Cardiol 1993;72:42E–46E.

23. Harris WO, Berger PB, Holmes DR Jr, Garratt KN, Bresnahan JF, Bell MR. "Rescue" directional coronary atherectomy after unsuccessful percutaneous transluminal coronary angioplasty. Mayo Clin Proc 1994;69:717–722.

24. Hinohara T, Rowe MH, Robertson GC et al. Effect of lesion characteristics on outcome of directional coronary atherectomy. J Am Coll Cardiol 1991;17:1112–1120.

25. Sutton JM, Ellis SG, Roubin GS et al. Major clinical events after coronary stenting: the multicenter registry of acute and elective Gianturco-Roubin stent placement. Circulation 1994;89:1126–1137.

26. Roubin GS, Cannon AD, Agrawal SK et al. Intracoronary stenting for acute and threatened closure complicating percutaneous transluminal coronary angioplasty. Circulation 1992;85:916–927.

B. Current Approaches to Percutaneous Treatment of the Angulated Coronary Stenosis

STEPHEN G. ELLIS

BACKGROUND AND EARLY PTCA RESULTS

It is recognized that flow disturbances associated with changes in coronary artery direction predispose to atheroma buildup, and perhaps as many as 10% of significant stenoses requiring treatment occur at bend points (1, 2). Such data, and clinical practice in this regard, are hampered somewhat by the need to assess vessel angulation in nonforeshortened views and at end-diastole, both of which are not always routinely available.

Balloon angioplasty, as it was practiced in the early and mid 1980s with relatively bulky, stiff, and short (≤20-mm) balloons, was noted in several series to be associated with a heightened risk of complications when attempted at bend-associated lesions compared with nonbend sites (3–5). For example, we studied 100 consecutive patients with bend lesions treated with PTCA between 1986 and 1989 and compared results with those seen in 344 consecutive contemporaneous patients without bend lesions (5). Procedural success was diminished (70% versus 89%, $P <.001$) and major ischemic complications increased (13% versus 3.5%, $P <.001$) in the patients with bend lesions. Complications were virtually always caused by angiographically apparent dissection (present in 46% of treated bend lesions versus 8% of nonbend lesions; $P <.001$). In that study it appeared that PET balloons, more axially flexible than other balloons available at the time, provided better results.

Comparison of results between different angiographic laboratories and different angioplasty operators must be done carefully, because definitions, measurement technique, and operator technique differ. While randomized trials with core angiographic laboratories are perhaps ideal, such data is not available for device evaluation for treatment of angulated lesions in numbers sufficient to draw meaningful conclusions. Much of the data that follows does, however, come from a single core angiographic laboratory, thereby increasing one's confidence in comparisons to a certain degree.

NEWER BALLOON ANGIOPLASTY APPROACHES

In the 1990s balloon technology has improved, and the use of longer (>20-mm) balloons in this setting has been emphasized.

The 1991 MAPS study provides somewhat more recent data regarding PTCA performed in this setting just prior to the widespread availability of long balloons (6). In 52 lesions the success rate (<50% stenosis by calipers in the view showing the lesion at its worst and no major ischemic complications) was 83%, largely the result of residual 50 to 70% stenoses (mean residual diameter stenosis = 34 ± 16%). Major ischemic complications were infrequent (1.9%) (6). By way of reference, balloon-treated, nonangulated lesions had a 92% success rate ($P = .03$), a 0.4% complication rate ($P = NS$), and a mean residual stenosis of 33 ± 15% ($P = NS$). Possibly because of less satisfactory initial results (in some series) or via other mechanisms, bend lesions have been associated with a greater likelihood of restenosis (7).

The use of longer balloons to reduce focal wall stress has been advocated, perhaps first in print by Savas and colleagues (8). They reported an 88% procedural success rate and major complications in only 1% of 69 consecutive patients with angulated (>45°) lesions treated with 40-mm-long angioplasty balloons.

The 1993 Cleveland Clinic experience with long balloons, generally used with the lowest possible pressure needed to achieve a "reasonable" result, in angulated lesions is also representative of current balloon results. Procedural success was achieved in 89% of lesions (compared with 94% of nonangulated lesions, $P <.001$). Interestingly, lesions with 45° to 59° angulation had a 93% success rate, compared with 77% for lesions with greater angulation ($P = .002$). In the latter group there was a 21% incidence of major ischemic complications.

NEWER DEVICES

Directional Atherectomy

As currently configured, this device has little or no role to play in the treatment of angulated stenoses. Probably because of its bulk and rigidity, dissections are frequently produced. In the core angiographic multicenter experience (9), procedural success was achieved in only 69% of lesions, final diameter stenosis was no better than that achieved with balloon technique (33% despite an average 12.6 cuts), and emergency bypass surgery was required in 14.3%.

Rotational Atherectomy

By virtue of its flexibility and capacity to ablate tissue, and thus perhaps decrease the chances of major dissection, Rotablator treatment of angulated stenoses has potential merit. Extreme caution should be urged, however, in two specific circumstances: (a) in treatment of lesions where the bulk of the atheroma lies on the inside of the curve, as the "differential cutting" often will not protect against perforation of the outer, relatively nondiseased edge of the vessel, and (b) in treatment of actively "flexing" lesions. In the core angiographic multicenter experience (10), perforation was seen in 5% of all angulated lesions, especially those that actively flexed between systole and diastole (19% of 16 lesions) and those that were eccentric as described (14% of 14 lesions). Excluding these, perforation was noted in none of 29 lesions treated, all of which were successfully treated (but one required bailout stenting for abrupt closure).

Excimer Laser

Somewhat similarly, because of its ablative potential, the use of concentric excimer laser in bend lesions should be avoided as there is risk of perforation. A greater than fivefold increased risk of perforation in this setting has been described by Bittl and colleagues (11). At the Cleveland Clinic we have not had sufficient experience with directional laser in this setting to be able to draw much in the way of conclusions. We have been somewhat disturbed by the relatively frequent production of unexpected dissections in the vicinity of,

but not at, the lesion treated with this technique, as has been reported (12).

Stents

At present the role of elective stenting in this setting is evolving and not fully proven. Because of the heightened risk of complications (particularly for lesions with >60° bend) and possible restenosis with nonstent technology, as well as a diminishing role for warfarin with stenting (13), it can now be cogently argued that any angioplasty candidate with an angulated lesion in a ≥3.0-mm artery should have elective Palmaz-Schatz stent placement. Angulated lesions do not seem to have an increased risk of restenosis compared with nonangulated lesions when treated with this slotted-tube stent (14). However, as we achieve "optimal" stent results in only about 90% of our stent placements and subject the remaining patients to the risk and cost of long-term anticoagulation with warfarin (15, 16), a posture of "fallback stenting" (use only with an unsatisfactory result with another technology) is also reasonable. In any event, patients should be queried beforehand for risk of bleeding, and guide catheters should be chosen to give enough power and coaxial support to deliver a stent if needed. Coil stents should be reserved for fallback or bailout only when slotted-tube stents cannot be delivered, as there is no good current evidence that coil stents reduce the risk of restenosis (17). Clearly, at this time stenting has no role for either the lesion beyond severe tortuosity or that in an artery <2.8 mm because of inaccessibility and risk of subacute thrombosis, respectively.

Transluminal Extraction Catheter

Very limited data exist on the use of this flexible, yet front-cutting device in native vessels with angulated stenoses. Its front-cutting attributes will likely increase the risk of perforation in a manner somewhat analogous to other ablative devices, and at present we would not advocate its use in this setting.

SUMMARY

Even with improved balloon technology, angulated lesions, particularly those associated with bends of $\geq 60°$, are at considerably increased risk of dissection-induced closure. Newer techniques of rotational atherectomy, directional laser, and primary stenting may have a role in the treatment of selected angulated lesions. Ablative techniques are considerably limited by the risk of perforation in this setting, however.

These facts should be carefully considered when a patient is considered for percutaneous revascularization, although the presence of such a lesion should not necessarily preclude such treatment. If the decision to proceed is made, the operator must be ready to deal with the heightened risk of dissection-induced ischemia and, for most patients, be well positioned to place a bailout stent expeditiously.

REFERENCES

1. Zarins CK, Giddens DP, Bharadvaj BK, Sottiurai VS, Mabon RF, Galgov S. Carotid bifurcation atherosclerosis: quantitative correlation of plaque localization with flow velocity profiles and wall shear stress. Circ Res 1983; 53:502–514.

2. Ellis S, Alderman EL, Cain K, Wright A, Bourassa M, Fisher L, and the participants of the Coronary Artery Surgery Study (CASS). Morphology of left anterior descending coronary territory lesions as a predictor of anterior myocardial infarction: a CASS registry study. J Am Coll Cardiol 1989;13:1481–1491.

3. Ischinger T, Gruentzig AR, Meier B, Galan K. Coronary dissection and total coronary occlusion associated with percutaneous transluminal coronary angioplasty: significance of initial angiographic morphology of coronary stenoses. Circulation 1986;74:1371–1378.

4. Ellis SG, Roubin GS, King SB, Douglas JS, Weintraub WS, Thomas RG, Cox WR. Angiographic and clinical predictors of acute closure after native vessel coronary angioplasty. Circulation 1988;77:372–379.

5. Ellis SG, Topol EJ. Results of percutaneous transluminal coronary angioplasty of high-risk angulated stenoses. Am J Cardiol 1990;66:932–937.

6. Ellis SG, Cowley MJ, Whitlow PL, Vandormael M, Lincoff AM, DiSciascio G, Dean LS et al for the MAPS study group. Markedly improved results with percutaneous transluminal coronary revascularization of patients with multivessel disease between 1986–87 and 1991. J Am Coll Cardiol 1993 (submitted for publication).

7. Ellis SG, Roubin GS, King SB, Douglas JS, Cox WR. Importance of stenosis morphology in the estimation of restenosis risk after elective percutaneous transluminal coronary angioplasty. Am J Cardiol 1989;63:30–34.

8. Savas V, Puchrowicz S, Williams L, Grines CL, O'Neill WW. Angioplasty outcome using long balloons in high-risk lesions. J Am Coll Cardiol 1992;19:34A.

9. Ellis SG, De Cesare NB, Pinkerton CA, Whitlow P, King SB III, Ghazzal ZMB, Kereiakes CJ et al. Relation of stenosis morphology and clinical presentation to the procedural results of directional coronary atherectomy. Circulation 1991;84:644–653.

10. Ellis SG, Popma JJ, Buchbinder M, Franco I, Leon MB, Kent KM, Pichard AD et al. Relation of clinical presentation, stenosis morphology and operator technique to the procedural results of rotational atherectomy and rotational atherectomy–facilitated angioplasty. Circulation 1994; 89:882–892.

11. Bittl JA, Ryan TJ, Keaney JFJ, Tcheng JE, Ellis SG, Isner JM, Sanborn TA for the Percutaneous Excimer Laser Coronary Angioplasty Registry. Coronary artery perforation during excimer laser coronary angioplasty. J Am Coll Cardiol 1993;21:1158–1165.

12. Leon MB, Bonner RF. Recent trends and future directions in laser angioplasty. In: Topol EJ, ed. Textbook of interventional cardiology. Philadelphia: WB Saunders, 1993.

13. Colombo A, Hall P, Almagor Y, Maiello L, Gaglione A, Nakamura S, Borrione M et al. Results of intravascular ultrasound–guided coronary stenting without subsequent anticoagulation. J Am Coll Cardiol 1994:335A.

14. Ellis SG, Savage M, Fischman D, Baim DS, Leon M, Goldberg S, Hirshfeld JW et al. Restenosis after placement of Palmaz-Schatz stents in native coronary arteries: initial results of a multicenter experience. Circulation 1992;86:1836–1844.

15. Schatz RA, Penn IM, Baim DS, Nobuyoshi M, Colombo A, Ricci DR, Cleman MW et al for the STRESS investigators. STent REStenosis Study (STRESS): analysis of in-hospital results. Circulation 1993;88:I-594.

16. Serruys PW, Macaya C, de Jaegere P, Kiemeneij F, Rutsch W, Heyndrickx G, Emanuelsson H et al on behalf of the Benestent study group. Interim analysis of the Benestent trial. Circulation 1993;88:I-594.

17. Gianturco-Roubin U.S. Multicenter Investigator Group, unpublished data.

EDITORS' SUMMARY

1. If the vessel is large enough and the patient suitable, always be prepared to place a bailout stent (good guide support; know the bleeding risk of your patient).

2. While ablative techniques may be helpful, be certain that you know the circumstances where the risk of perforation is increased.

3. Overall approach to device choice:

	Eccentric Outer/ Actively Flexing	≥60 Degrees	Neither
First choice	Long balloon	Slotted-tube stent[a]	Long balloon
Other reasonable choices	Slotted-tube stent[a]	Rotablator	Rotablator, slotted-tube stent[a]
Coil stents	Bailout[b]	Bailout[b]	Bailout[b]
DCA	No	No	No
DELCA	Perhaps	Perhaps	Perhaps
ELCA	No	No	No
Rotablator	Definitely not	As above	As above
Standard length (20-mm) balloon	No	No	No
Slotted-tube stent	As above	As above	As above
TEC	No	No	No

[a]Assuming artery >2.8 to 3.0 mm.

[b]Slotted-tube stent preferred if it can be delivered.

19. The Bifurcation Lesion

ARTUR M. SPOKOJNY and TIMOTHY A. SANBORN

Percutaneous transluminal coronary angioplasty (PTCA) of bifurcation lesions entails a higher risk and greater challenge than usual because of potential occlusion of side branches (1). In the early days of angioplasty these lesions were considered contraindications to PTCA. The incidence of side-branch occlusion following angioplasty of lesions in the parent vessel was 14% with ostial disease, compared with 1% in normal side branches (1). Other reports also indicate that worsening or occlusion of side branches was seen in 27% of cases, but in only 4% when significant ostial disease was absent (2). Interestingly, late repeat angiography showed that most of these acutely closed branches recanalized.

The first approach to treatment of bifurcation lesions using a protecting branch technique required placement of two guide catheters and two angioplasty balloons simultaneously and frequently resulted in prolonged procedure time with an increase in complications (2). Newer advances in technology such as larger lumen guiding catheters, smaller balloon shafts, and improved wire technology allowed the use of a single guiding catheter. Today, monorail and fixed balloon-on-the-wire systems allow much easier deployment of the balloon with a markedly reduced procedure time. Over time the complication rate in bifurcation lesions has significantly dropped from 15% to 3.8% (1–6). Newer modalities such as directional or rotational atherectomy, as well as excimer laser with an eccentric fiber array, have been proposed as alternatives to balloon angioplasty (7–9).

MECHANISM OF SIDE-BRANCH OCCLUSION

Most commonly, side-branch occlusion occurs because of a "snowplow" effect. During angioplasty of the lesion in the parent vessel presumably atherosclerotic plaque or thrombotic material is pushed inside the side branch, compromising or occluding the origin. Other potential mechanisms include spasm caused by either device-related mechanical irritation or possibly release of vasoactive substances (Table 19.1). In our experience spasm occurs more often during atherectomy and laser procedures and usually responds well to intracoronary nitroglycerin. In refractory spasms the use of diluted, intracoronary, calcium channel blocker or papaverin has been advocated (4). Also, propagating dissection originating in the parent vessel can cause branch occlusion. In acute myocardial infarction with high thrombus load within the lesion, when revascularization is attempted via direct angioplasty, distal embolization can result in branch occlusion.

GENERAL CONSIDERATIONS

Several methods can minimize the risk of side-branch occlusion. Newer advances in technology made it possible to use more than one balloon catheter within a single guiding catheter. The most common approach is to advance two wires side by side, one in the parent vessel and the other to protect or allow access to the side branch. With two guidewires in place, the following strategies can be considered: the use of bare guidewire to protect side branch, and the use of two balloons

Table 19.1
Mechanism of Side-Branch Occlusion

"Snowplow" effect, shifting of atherosclerotic and thrombotic material
Spasm
Propagation dissection
Embolization

("kissing balloon") with either sequential inflations or simultaneous inflations.

The use of monorail catheters greatly facilitates bifurcation angioplasty, especially when the sequential approach is used. It reduces time because of faster exchange. Often the same balloon catheter can be used for both lesions if the parent vessel and side branch are of the same size. When both target vessels are of different sizes, a variant of this approach has been used. Instead of using a bare wire, a fixed balloon-on-the-wire system is advanced into the side branch. This way the parent vessel can be dilated with any balloon, and after completion the side branch can be dilated or vice versa. The disadvantage of this strategy is lack of access to the side branch in case of failure, where either a larger balloon size or other salvage modality such as atherectomy or laser is indicated. Therefore we do not recommend the use of fixed-wire systems in important or large side branches.

There has been a lot of discussion of whether the sequential or simultaneous inflation strategy is better. The sequential approach is more cost-effective when side branch dilatation does not become necessary or both branches are of the same size. On the other hand, not infrequently material shifts back and forth between the parent and side branch, necessitating the "kissing-balloon" approach. However, simultaneous inflation of two balloons has a higher incidence of dissection and disruption, especially if the combined cross-sectional areas of both balloons exceed the cross-sectional area of the parent vessel (5). A strategy being recommended that uses the "best of both worlds" is to leave a deflated balloon across one lesion while the other is dilated. The deflated balloon acts as a temporary stent and minimizes closure and/or "snowplowing" (4, 5).

Which strategy is the best? Much depends on the actual nature of the lesion, its anatomy, and the presence of thrombus or calcium (Fig. 19.1). However, despite adequate sizing there is a relatively high incidence of elastic recoil and dissection. In addition, careful manipulation is necessary to avoid entangling the two wires around each other and preventing the advancement of a balloon catheter. Therefore some interventionalists recommend advancing both wires simultaneously up to the target area before crossing the lesions (4). The newer modalities in percutaneous revascularization, directional atherectomy (DCA) and excimer laser, seem to yield better results than conventional balloon angioplasty. However, in contrast to PTCA, DCA and excimer laser are not suitable for all lesions. Extreme tortuosity of the proximal segment will hamper delivery of these devices to the lesion. DCA and excimer laser are contraindicated in lesions in an angulated segment and DCA is contraindicated in a vessel smaller than 2.5 mm in diameter. While presence of significant calcification decreases the success rate for DCA, excimer laser might yield a far better result than any other modality.

In addition, the most common bailout devices such as perfusion balloons or stents are of limited value because only one branch can be protected. Prolonged inflation will invariably cause ischemia by occluding the other branch. Deployment of a stent might salvage one branch but impede access to the other branch. Stenting is an acceptable alternative if the side branch is not suitable for grafting.

USE OF DCA IN BIFURCATION LESIONS

Directional atherectomy, despite the large size of the device, has been very effective in treating bifurcation lesions (Fig. 19.2). Initially, directional atherectomy in the presence of a second guidewire was absolutely

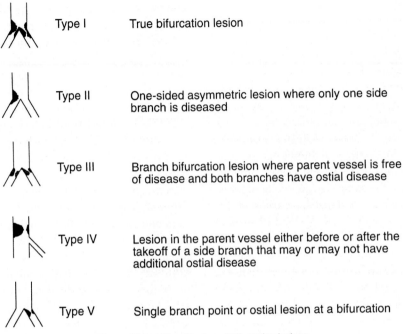

Figure 19.1. Classification of bifurcation lesions.

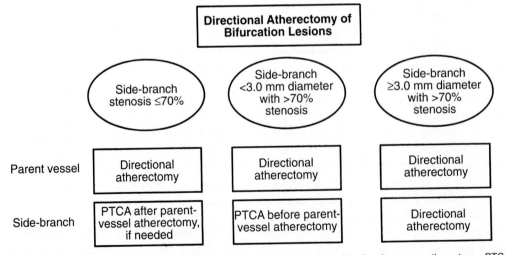

Figure 19.2. Recommended algorithm for treatment of bifurcation lesions using directional coronary atherectomy. *PTCA*, Percutaneous transluminal coronary angioplasty.

contraindicated because of the inherent danger of entrapping in the housing or cutting the adjacent wire. The use of nitinol wires (Microvena) allows the use of a cutting device without risking damage to the protecting guidewire. However, this wire is much more difficult to use and is less torque-responsive than conventional wires. Also, there is a higher risk of intimal trauma because of added stiffness in the tip. Thus the following strategies can be used:

1. Double wiring, by treating the ostium of the side branch with conventional PTCA first and then treating the parent vessel with DCA after removing the guidewire from the side branch. Treatment of the side branch first is preferable.
2. Advancing two exchange-length nitinol wires side by side and treating both parent vessel and side branch with DCA. With newer, shorter, and lower profile atherocaths such as the 5- and 9-mm EX devices, tortuosity can be navigated better and even the branches taking off on a slight angle can be successfully treated with DCA.
3. In general, the risk of side branch occlusion with the use of DCA is less than with conventional PTCA since debulking will reduce shifting or snowplowing (8, 9).

If necessary, one can successfully advance a low-profile monorail catheter into a side branch without having to remove the atherocath, when a large, 11 Fr guide is used. A detailed algorithm of these various strategies can be found in Figure 19.3.

USE OF EXCIMER LASER IN BIFURCATION LESION

Until recently laser treatment of bifurcation lesions was contraindicated because of the increased incidence of dissection and side branch occlusion. Because of the potential risk of laser damage to a parallel guidewire, a protecting wire could not be used previously. In limited application, excimer laser can be used to debulk eccentric plaques without affecting the side branch. Excimer laser may be especially effective in calcified lesions for which neither conventional balloon angioplasty nor DCA will yield a good result (7). Newer catheters with eccentrically arranged fibers allow directed delivery of laser energy similar to DCA, since only part of the circum-

ference of the artery is affected. With this technique a parallel guidewire to protect side branches can be used (10). More recently, a "flush and bathe" technique has been advocated. Within the artery, while ablating the lesion, crystalloids (e.g., saline) replace blood and contrast and allow significant reduction in dissection and improvement in acute outcome (11).

BAILOUT FOR FAILED BALLOON ANGIOPLASTY

Should conventional balloon angioplasty fail as a result of either elastic recoil or localized dissection, DCA has been shown to be very successful. By debulking the eccentric flap or removing the recoiled tissue, a good final result has been achieved. In our laboratory salvage DCA was used in seven cases of failed bifurcation angioplasty with a good result. None of the patients required CABG, and only one patient had a significantly elevated CPK without lasting EKG changes. One should note that in this situation the goal is to debulk the lesion just enough to obtain an adequate result. Aggressive oversizing and extensive cutting in this situation might result in perforation or severe dissection. In extensive and spiral dissections DCA is contraindicated. Thus DCA has proven itself to be an excellent tool as a salvage procedure after failed PTCA.

SPECIFIC CONSIDERATION

Nonsymmetric Lesions (Types II and IV)

Most commonly, nonsymmetric lesions are encountered in a major vessel (e.g., left anterior descending or circumflex coronary artery) with close proximity to a major side branch (e.g., diagonal or marginal branch). In general, these side branches are not at risk for occlusion unless the ostium itself is diseased or there is a large thrombus burden in the parent vessel, as in an acute MI in which case thrombotic material is "snowplowed" into the side branch.

Small side branches with a diameter less

than 1.5 mm, which are unsuitable for bypass surgery, usually do not require protection. Even if compromised, there have been no reports of serious side effects (2). Protection is not necessary when the ostium of the side branch is free of disease or less than 50% narrowed. Not infrequently, a worsening of the ostium is observed; only rarely does a total occlusion occur. In most cases the patient remains asymptomatic and no further intervention is required since the additional narrowing often resolves. If, however, the patient has chest pain or EKG changes indicating ischemia or the ostium is more than 80% narrowed, especially in a large branch, angioplasty of the ostium is advisable and can be done easily.

In large side branches with ostial lesions greater than 50%, it is generally recommended to advance a second wire into the side branch for protection. If occlusion of the side branch occurs, a second balloon can be advanced to open the side branch (5). Often the presence of a wire across the ostium will prevent a complete occlusion and further therapy is not necessary.

In a truly asymmetric lesion with very little involvement of the contralateral branch, DCA and eccentric laser seem to yield a better result than conventional balloon angioplasty. In this situation a second guidewire is rarely needed. Since force is extended circumferentially with balloon inflation and preferentially stretches the uninvolved side rather than the lesion, debulking seems to be preferable. As outlined above, the use of a protective wire depends mainly on the size of the branch and the severity of ostial stenosis.

Symmetric Lesions (Type I and III)

True bifurcation lesions are rare (1.3%); however, they present a vexing problem in obtaining adequate results (2). Despite the use of proper techniques, the success rate has been reported to be only 89% as compared with 96% in other nonbifurcation lesions (2). If conventional balloon therapy is used, the double-wire technique should be used. If the parent vessel is larger than both bifurcating branches, proper sizing becomes increasingly difficult. Either the proximal vessel is undersized or the distal vessel is oversized. One solution is to use the kissing-balloon technique in which two smaller balloons, when sized for the branches, roughly equal the size of the larger proximal vessel if inflated simultaneously. However, a higher incidence of dissection and failure has been observed (1). In addition, the restenosis rate is usually higher than in comparable lesions in different locations. Newer balloon technology such as the recently released tapered balloons might be appropriate in this situation. However, if branches are larger than 2.5 mm, strong consideration should be given to use of DCA as first-line therapy. It is important to evaluate the accessibility of the target area, that is, the presence of tortuosity of the proximal vessel, calcification, and other factors hampering the use of DCA.

Branch Point or Ostial Lesion (Type V)

Even though these lesions are not really bifurcation lesions since only one branch is involved, there are lot of similar features. Ostial branch stenosis is isolated in 61% of the patients and associated with a bifurcation stenosis in 39%. Despite a balloon-to-artery ratio of 1.05:1, angiographic success was 74% in ostial branch stenoses versus 91% in nonostial stenosis (4). The complication rate is higher (13%) for ostial lesions versus 5% for nonostial lesions, and there is more elastic recoil and a higher dissection rate (4). Accordingly, the restenosis rate appears to be higher in these lesions. DCA and excimer laser appear to have a higher success rate and lower complication rate (6, 8, 9). Lesions in branches with diameter's larger than 2.5 mm respond well to DCA. If diameters are smaller than 2.5 mm, PTCA still can be applied; however, high pressures and a slightly oversized balloon are necessary to obtain an adequate result.

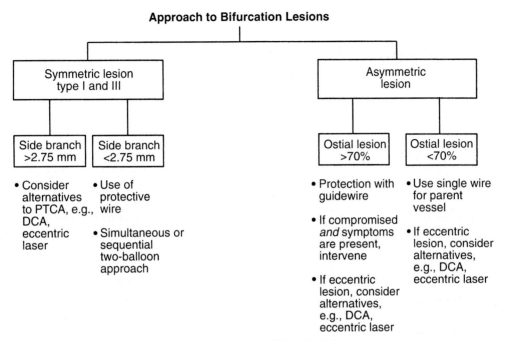

Figure 19.3. Approach to bifurcation lesions.

SUMMARY

Bifurcation lesions are challenging; however, new advances in technology allow safe and successful treatment. In large vessels DCA seems to be the modality of choice; in smaller vessels a successful outcome can be achieved with the proper strategy using conventional PTCA. In selected cases such as calcified lesions excimer laser is the therapy of choice. Newer technologies such as the Rotablator appear to be promising in treating calcified and tortuous lesions. However, size is limited and more clinical experience is needed to evaluate its use for bifurcation lesions.

REFERENCES

1. Weinstein JS, Baim DS, Sipperly ME et al. Salvage of branch vessels during bifurcation lesion angioplasty. Cathet Cardiovasc Diagn 1991; 22:1–6.

2. Meier B, Gruentzig AR, King SB III et al. Balloon angioplasty of coronary bifurcation lesions. Cathet Cardiovasc Diagn 1991;22:167–173.

3. Myler RK, Shaw RE, Stertzer SH et al. Lesion morphology and coronary angioplasty: current experience and analysis. J Am Coll Cardiol 1992;19:1641–1652.

4. Mathias DW, Mooney JF, Lange HW et al. Frequency of success and complications of coronary angioplasty of a stenosis at the ostium of a branch vessel. Am J Cardiol 1991;67:491–495.

5. Renkin J, Wijns W, Hanet C et al. Angioplasty of coronary bifurcation stenoses: immediate and long-term results of the protecting branch technique. Cathet Cardiovasc Diagn 1991;22:167–173.

6. Pinkerton CA, Slack JD. Complex coronary angioplasty: a technique for dilatation of bifurcation stenosis. Angiology 1985:543–548.

7. Bittl JA, Sanborn TA, Tcheng JE et al. Clinical success, complications and restenosis rates with excimer laser coronary angioplasty. The Percutaneous Excimer Laser Coronary Angioplasty Registry. Am J Cardiol 1992; 70:1533–1539.

8. Hinohara T, Rowe MH, Robertson GC et al. Effect of lesion characteristics on outcome of directional coronary atherectomy. JACC 1991:1112–1120.

9. Altman DB, Popma JJ, Pichard AD et al. The impact of directional atherectomy on adjacent branch vessels. Am J Cardiol 1993;72:351–353.

10. Bittle JA, Sanborn TA, Abela GS, Isner JM. Wire-guided excimer laser coronary angioplasty: instrument selection, lesion characterization, and operator technique. J Interven Cardiol 1992;5:275–291.

11. Tcheng JE, Wells LD, Phillips HR et al. Development of a new technique for reducing pressure pulse generation during 308-nm excimer laser coronary angioplasty. Cathet Cardiovasc Diagn 1995;34:15–22.

20. The Lesion With Thrombus

A. The Lesion With Intracoronary Thrombus— An Approach

DAVID R. HOLMES JR. and GUY S. REEDER

The importance and frequency of coronary arterial thrombus has been well documented in the pathophysiology of the acute ischemic syndromes of acute myocardial infarction and unstable angina. Angioscopy has documented thrombus in the vast majority of those studied. Angiography, although clearly not as sensitive, may often identify coronary thrombus.

There are a variety of settings in which the thrombus occurs: (a) in patients with unstable angina, even if it is not evident at angiography, thrombus is usually present; (b) during acute myocardial infarction, thrombus is almost universal and is recognized by persistent staining of contrast in a totally occluded vessel; (c) in some patients angiographically visible thrombus is seen at or just distal to a high-grade stenosis (this is usually in the setting of unstable angina and represents a significant thrombus burden); (d) in patients with acute occlusion secondary to a catheterization procedure, thrombus and dissection often coexist; or (e) in some patients there is extensive thrombus formation throughout a large segment of the vessel. This is most commonly the right coronary artery or a vein graft. Depending on the clinical setting in which the thrombus occurs and the specific angiographic features, the treatment strategy will vary.

The importance of coronary arterial thrombus for the interventional cardiologist has also been increasingly well recognized. An initial series in 1985 by Mabin et al. evaluated the outcome of percutaneous transluminal coronary angioplasty (PTCA) in 238 patients. Patients with chronic occlusion and those receiving thrombolytic therapy were excluded from this analysis. The angiograms were reviewed for the presence of predilatation thrombus defined as (a) the presence of an intraluminal filling defect or lucency surrounded by contrast material seen in multiple angiographic views; (b) absence of calcification within the defect, and (c) persistence of contrast within the lumen (Fig. 20A.1, A–C). Using these criteria, there were 15 patients (6%) with intracoronary thrombus prior to PTCA. The patients with thrombus had a higher incidence of prior infarction and infarction within the preceding month, although none of them had an evolving acute infarction. There was a striking difference in outcome. Despite treatment with antiplatelet agents (dipyridamole 75 to 100 mg t.i.d. or q.i.d. and also aspirin), as well as heparin 5000 to 10,000 units at the time of the procedure, complete occlusion requiring emergency coronary bypass graft surgery occurred during or immediately after PTCA in 11 (73%) of the 15 patients with intracoronary thrombus and in only 18 (8%) of the patients without angiographic evidence of coronary thrombus. The occlusion was at or immediately adjacent to the stenosis/thrombus in all patients, and dissection was not present angiographically. In patients without thrombus, typically if occlusion occurred, it was the result of dissection. The authors concluded that they had

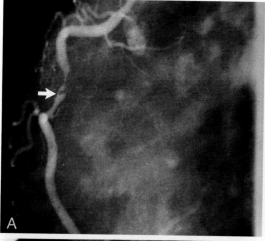
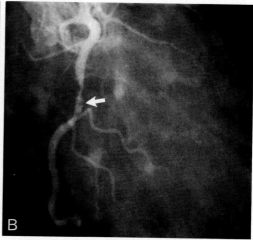
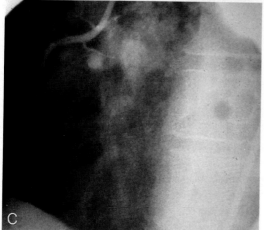

Figure 20A.1. **A.** Left anterior oblique view of right coronary artery, showing severe stenosis in the proximal region and a filling defect consistent with intracoronary thrombus immediately downstream *(arrow)*. **B.** Right anterior oblique view documenting filling defect just distal to high-grade stenosis *(arrow)*. **C.** Angiogram taken during attempted dilation. After initial success, total occlusion developed at the stenosis, with faint visualization of the distal vessel. (By permission from Mabin TA, Holmes DR Jr, Smith HC et al. J Am Coll Cardiol 1985;5:198–202.)

identified a "small but important subset of patients" at increased risk. Given the ever-increasing emphasis on early dilatation in these patients, the authors had indeed identified a high-risk group of patients. It has evolved, however, into a large and not a small group.

Since that time, there have been multiple other series. A follow-up study by Sugrue et al. in 1986, in a subsequent group of 297 consecutive patients without acute myocardial infarction, documented improvement in outcome. However, 24% of patients with angiographic thrombus still had complete occlusion either during or immediately after the procedure compared with a 13% incidence of complete occlusion in patients without preexisting thrombus. Similar trends have been

seen in other series, and the problem remains that preexisting coronary thrombus continues to identify a group of patients at increased risk for acute closure.

Even when thrombus is not visible angiographically, but is present by inference as in patients with very unstable angina, acute complication rates are increased compared with that of patients with stable angina. In these patients angiography may not be sensitive enough to identify thrombus. This insensitivity has been previously well described in patients with unstable angina. In the setting of unstable angina, dilatation success rates are usually slightly lower than in patients with stable angina. In this setting, failure of dilatation usually results in complications, for example, complete occlusion compared with failure of dilatation in a stable patient population in whom the failure may be uncomplicated.

Thrombus continues to be a risk factor for adverse events for interventional procedures. Reeder assessed the continued effect over a 7-year period from 1984 to 1991. The study population included patients undergoing single-lesion dilatation for the first time during those 7 years. Only patients being treated with conventional PTCA were studied. The primary analysis was focused on assessing whether preexisting coronary thrombus remained an independent predictor for angioplasty failure. Of 2699 patients meeting the study criteria, 1121 (42%) had angiographic evidence of intracoronary thrombus. Several characteristics were found on univariate testing to be associated with angioplasty failure, including history of congestive heart failure ($P = .004$), new onset of angina or worsening anginal pattern ($P = .003$), severe predilatation stenosis ($P = .0001$), acute infarction ($P = .0001$), angiographic thrombus ($P = .0001$), multivessel disease ($P = .0001$), and left main dilatation ($P = .0005$). Using multivariate analysis, the only factors associated with procedural failure were thrombus, history of congestive heart failure, and multivessel disease. The study was arbitrarily divided into three time periods to assess the importance of thrombus over time. Multivariate analysis documented that the risk of angioplasty failure in the setting of coronary arterial thrombus was unchanged from 1984 to 1991.

Table 20A.1
Approach to the Patient With Intracoronary Thrombus

- Optimize anticoagulants/antiplatelet agents
- Thrombolytic therapy
- Optimize results of PTCA
  Timing of intervention
  Selection of catheters
- New technology

Given the continued problem with treatment of patients with coronary arterial thrombus, there has been substantial interest in optimizing the results of interventional procedures. There are several tiers of approaches (Table 20A.1). Most of these approaches have not been rigorously tested in scientifically controlled trials.

OPTIMIZE ANTICOAGULATION/ ANTIPLATELET AGENTS

Antiplatelet agents and heparin anticoagulation both play an essential role during interventional procedures, particularly in those patients at increased risk of acute closure. Aspirin was originally studied as an agent to decrease restenosis rates; although it was negative in this regard, pretreatment with aspirin reduced acute closure in the catheterization laboratory. Given the importance of white (or platelet) thrombus in unstable angina documented by angioscopy, this makes sense. Currently, prior to dilatation, aspirin should be administered. Usually, one adult aspirin is given as part of the preinterventional orders. If the patient arrives in the catheterization laboratory without having received aspirin, four chewable aspirin are administered. In Europe intravenous acetylsalicylic acid is also available. Aspirin should be continued indefinitely. If aspirin cannot be used, ticlopidine should be administered at least for the short term and is probably equally as effective.

The dose of heparin administered at the time of interventional procedures has increased substantially. Early manuscripts documented the use of 5000 to 10,000 units. With the widespread availability of Activated Clotting Time (ACT) machines, doses have increased because of the realization that in some patients empiric use of doses in the early studies may have been inadequate. We currently administer 15,000 units of heparin at the beginning of the procedure and follow sequential ACTs with boluses given to maintain an ACT >300 to 350 seconds. Several studies have now documented that an ACT <300 seconds is associated with increased complication rates. There is some suggestion that an ACT of >350 seconds may even be better. Other assessments use activated clotting time differential (the difference between the standard ACT and a heparinized ACT) or ACT index (ACT/U/kg/hour). In any case, measurement of the degree of anticoagulation during the procedure is a powerful predictor of procedural success or, alternatively, adverse outcomes.

Typically, in patients with coronary arterial thrombus, a continuous heparin drip is started during the procedure, usually at 1000 units/hour. Following the procedure, the heparin may be discontinued to allow for sheath removal but then is resumed. During this time, activated partial thromboplastin time (APTT) is monitored to document effect, which is usually kept >70 to 80 seconds. Typically, the heparin is continued for approximately 48 hours. During the procedure heparin (2500 units) may also be administered directly down the coronary artery. Data on this approach are very limited.

Dextran has also been used because of its antithrombotic effects and its effect on decreasing platelet adhesion. Early during the initial development of dilatation, most routine cases received dextran empirically with an infusion started approximately 1 hour prior to the procedure and continued through the procedure and afterward for 1 to 2 hours for a total of 500 to 1000 cc. A small randomized study in patients undergoing PTCA in 1984 documented no difference in outcome irrespective of whether dextran was administered. Use of routine dextran after this decreased in many laboratories. With the development and widespread use of intracoronary stents, there has been enhanced use of dextran. Most stent protocols include the same regimen of dextran used during the early days of angioplasty, although there are no well-controlled data. The use of dextran has been felt to be particularly important dur-

ing the period immediately after stent implantation when the heparin is decreased to allow for sheath removal. Dextran may also be used empirically in patients with intracoronary thrombus. It must be remembered that anaphylaxis can occur with 10% dextran-40. Often steroids are given prophylactically or a test dose of dextran is administered. More recently, because of the potential for side effects and lack of documented efficacy, the use of dextran has declined again.

New therapeutic advances should make treatment of the patient with acute ischemic syndromes and coronary arterial thrombus safer and more effective. Specific antithrombins such as hirudin and hirulog are in clinical evaluation. These are direct thrombin inhibitors in contrast to heparin, which requires antithrombin III as a cofactor, which has no affinity to clot bound heparin, and which is bound or inactivated by several plasma proteins. In a pilot study of patients with unstable angina, there was increased inhibition of thrombin activation and more evidence of culprit-vessel clot lysis with hirudin than with heparin. This effect must be watched carefully; in the GUSTO IIa trial of recombinant hirudin versus heparin for acute coronary syndromes, there was an excess in hemorrhagic stroke with hirudin (1.5%) versus heparin (0.8%) ($P = .11$). In patients receiving thrombolytic therapy plus hirudin, the incidence of hemorrhagic stroke was highest at 3.6%. A similar increase in hemorrhagic stroke was also seen in TIMI-9a. Both of these studies stopped prematurely and then resumed using a lower dose of hirudin and heparin. The subsequent doses used have been found to be safe. Very careful titration of doses may be required to decrease the incidence of bleeding. Hirudin has also been compared with heparin in a randomized trial of patients undergoing PTCA for treatment of stable angina (HELVETICA).

Antiplatelet antibodies have also been tested. The EPIC trial has now been reported. In this trial a monoclonal antibody directed against the platelet glycoprotein IIb/IIIa was tested in high-risk angioplasty. In this prospective, double-blinded, randomized trial 2099 patients received either a bolus and an infusion of placebo, a bolus or drug followed by placebo infusion, or a bolus and an infusion of the drug. All patients received aspirin and heparin. The primary endpoint was a composite at 30 days of death, nonfatal myocardial infarction, coronary bypass surgery or repeat percutaneous intervention for acute ischemia, insertion of a stent because of procedural failure, or placement of an intraaortic balloon pump. A primary endpoint occurred in 12.8%, 11.4%, and 8.3%, respectively, of the placebo, bolus drug plus placebo, and bolus drug plus infusion drug ($P = .009$, a 35% reduction). There was no difference in mortality but a striking difference in need for subsequent emergency repeat PTCA ($P < .001$, 4.5% versus 0.8%). There was, however, a substantial excess of bleeding with the active drug—7% of placebo-treated patients had major bleeding compared with 14% of bolus and infusion of drug. Other platelet receptor antibodies are being evaluated.

THROMBOLYTIC THERAPY

Given the documented efficacy of thrombolytic therapy for acute myocardial infarction, there has been interest in this approach in patients with unstable angina and presumably also coronary arterial thrombus. The results of this approach have been mixed. The largest trial of intracoronary thrombolytic therapy has been the TAUSA trial. A pilot study for this trial had documented that low-dose urokinase reduced angiographic thrombus formation following PTCA for rest ischemia in unstable angina. The full trial of 469 patients was recently reported. During the first phase of this trial, 250,000 units of intracoronary urokinase were administered (150,000 units prior to PTCA and 150,000 units after PTCA) in patients with unstable angina. In the second phase of the study,

500,000 units were used (250,000 units prior to PTCA and 250,000 units after PTCA). The endpoints for this randomized study were angiographic thrombus, acute closure, and in-hospital events of recurrent ischemia, infarction, or coronary bypass graft surgery. There was no statistically significant difference in angiographic thrombus between patients treated with placebo and those treated with intracoronary urokinase. In addition, the incidence of acute closure was actually increased at 6.9% in the urokinase group versus 1.7% in the placebo-treated patients. The mechanism of acute closure was thrombotic in 45% and secondary to dissection in 40%.

Based on this randomized trial, routine prophylactic treatment of patients with unstable angina using intracoronary urokinase may not be indicated. There still are patients with a significant amount of intracoronary thrombus in whom intracoronary lytic therapy may be administered. Typically, urokinase is used although both rt-PA and streptokinase have been administered. For urokinase, typically 500,000 units are administered; for rt-PA 50 mg are used; and for streptokinase 500,000 units are given. Administering the drug in close proximity to the thrombus with a subselective infusion catheter optimizes the local effect in the segment to be treated.

In some patients a more prolonged infusion is administered for 24 or up to 72 hours. This is typically used in vein grafts with thrombotic occlusion but also may be used in the native coronary artery (Fig. 20A.2, *A–E*). For this infusion urokinase is most commonly used. Multiple sidehole perfusion catheters currently available are positioned across the segment with thrombus. Urokinase is then administered by continuous infusion at 50,000 U/hour after an initial bolus. The guiding catheter may be kept in the ostium, particularly if a vein graft is being treated, or may be withdrawn to the descending thoracic aorta. In the former case urokinase is also administered at 50,000 U/hour through the guiding catheter or, in the latter case, saline

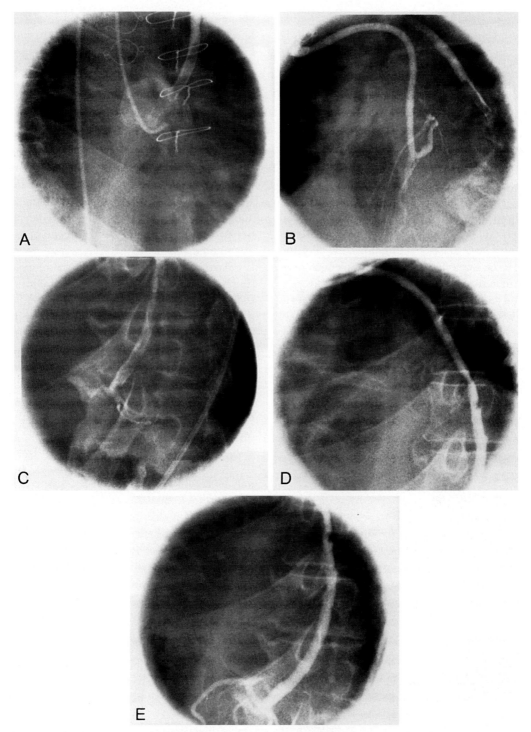

Figure 20A.2. **A**. Right anterior oblique view of a long saphenous circumflex bypass graft with persistent contrast staining and a large amount of thrombus. **B.** Left anterior oblique view of the same graft with a long filling defect. **C.** After initial infusion of urokinase, there is some more flow into the distal part of the vein graft and some filling of the distal grafted vessel. **D.** After 24 hours of urokinase infusion, flow has been restored (left anterior oblique view). There is still moderate stenosis present within the graft. **E.** Flow now is well seen at 24 hours into the native grafted vessels.

can be used to keep the lumen clear. Guide catheter damping should be particularly avoided if there is a prolonged infusion of the native coronary artery. Nursing care of these patients can be problematic because of the need for continuing infusions and the requirement that the patient be fully immobilized. Vascular access bleeding in our experience is quite common. Following treatment repeat angiography is required to document effect.

OPTIMIZE RESULTS OF PTCA

Optimizing the results of PTCA is essential, particularly in high-risk lesions. In patients with a large amount of thrombus, the decision may be made to treat with intravenous heparin and aspirin and delay dilatation for several days (Fig. 20A.3). There is limited data to support this, but it does make intuitive sense. Several days, however, may be required, which increases the cost of this approach substantially, particularly if the patient requires intensive care unit hospitalization.

At the time of dilatation, matching the balloon size with the artery to be treated is very important. Undersizing and leaving behind a significant residual stenosis may result in sta-

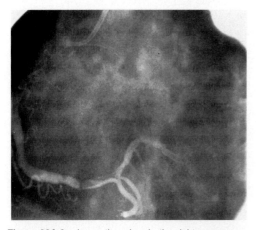

Figure 20A.3. Large thrombus in the right coronary artery immediately beyond a severe stenosis. Persistence of contrast within the vessel raises the possibility of extensive thrombus. In this setting, if the clinical situation is stable, consideration should be given to pretreatment with heparin for several days to decrease the thrombus burden.

sis and set the stage for acute closure. Prolonged inflations, often with perfusion balloons, are used frequently. With prolonged inflations the initial angiographic result is often improved, although the restenosis rates are typically not affected.

An essential part of the strategy is a period of watchful waiting after PTCA. Typically, we would wait for 10 minutes, sometimes with the dilatation wire across the lesion but more often after it has been withdrawn. During this 10 minutes the ACT is checked to document adequate anticoagulation and supplemental heparin is given if needed. At the end of the 10 minutes, repeat angiography is performed. If renarrowing has occurred, or if radiolucent filling defects are seen to be accumulating, then repeat dilatation is performed, either for a longer time or sometimes with a slightly larger balloon (either by increasing the pressure in a compliant balloon or changing balloon size). Intracoronary heparin may be given, as well as intravenous dextran. Following repeat dilatation, another 10-minute period of observation is mandated. If the same sequence of events recurs, the cycle of repeat dilatation can be performed. Alternatively, intracoronary thrombolytic therapy may be administered and may be effective. It is important to treat any outlet stenosis in the vascular bed to decrease stasis. If part of the problem is recoil, decreased flow and then more thrombus, treatment with another device (e.g., directional coronary atherectomy or intracoronary stenting) may be very helpful. If the problem is recurrent thrombus, in general, intracoronary stents should not be used.

Following successful treatment, anticoagulation and antiplatelet therapy should be maintained aggressively, although that may increase the potential for vascular access site bleeding.

NEW TECHNOLOGY

Given the problems of conventional dilatation for treatment of thrombus-containing lesions, there has been interest in new technology. Some of these approaches are often useful in selected patients; others have no role to play.

Atherectomy

Three types of atherectomy catheters are currently in use: (a) rotational atherectomy, (b) transluminal extraction catheter, and (c) directional coronary atherectomy. Rotational atherectomy should not be used in soft, thrombus-containing lesions. Its mechanism of action is differential ablation of hard fibrous tissue compared with more normal elastic arterial wall. The TEC catheter is used infrequently, but may be helpful for treating long thrombotic vein graft lesions. By extracting the thrombus, distal embolization may be decreased, although it is still common in treatment of vein graft disease. Directional coronary atherectomy has been the most commonly used. In an initial multicenter report, with thrombus-containing lesions, directional coronary atherectomy resulted in marked improvement in angiographic lumen and a significantly decreased acute closure rate compared with historical cohorts of patients treated with conventional PTCA. In the setting of a large vessel with a bulky lesion and coronary thrombus, we continue to use directional atherectomy to optimize the initial result and decrease the potential for acute closure.

Laser

At the present time laser systems for use in the coronary arteries are ablative and designed to treat plaque, not thrombus. The most common systems use an excimer laser with a wavelength of 308 nm. There is a limited amount of information on the use of this laser system in lesions containing thrombus. In the Excimer Laser Coronary Angioplasty Registry (Advanced Interventional Systems, Irvine, CA), 141 lesions with associated thrombus have been treated. The success rate in these 141 lesions was 85%; 1.5% of patients developed Q-wave myocardial infarc-

tion, 3.8% required coronary bypass graft surgery, and 4.6% had sustained occlusion. How this would compare with conventional dilatation in a similar subset of patients is not clear. However, there is no particular conceptual reason that excimer laser would be more effective for coronary thrombus.

A second system is the holmium laser angioplasty system (Eclipse Surgical Technologies, Inc., Palo Alto, CA). This is a mid-infrared holmium/YAG laser that can ablate tissue in a blood media by a predominant photothermal effect compared with excimer laser. The 2-micron wavelength is absorbed by water, both in atherosclerotic plaque and in intracoronary thrombus. This laser may therefore offer some specific advantages in the treatment of thrombus-containing lesions. This laser has been used clinically during acute myocardial infarction in a small number of cases, as well as in patients with unstable angina with excellent results. Future randomized trials will be needed to directly compare excimer laser with holmium laser angioplasty.

Stents

Specific stents are now approved for acute and threatened closure after PTCA. In general, they are most effective in large vessels with an intimal dissection. In this setting thrombus may also be playing a role. For primary thrombotic acute closure, however, stents have not been used as they may be inherently somewhat thrombogenic. If stents are placed in the setting of coronary thrombus to optimize the result, it is strongly suggested that intracoronary lytic therapy be administered.

SUMMARY

Identification of the importance of coronary arterial thrombus as a marker for an active lesion with the potential for adverse outcome from interventional cardiology procedures has led to continued new approaches to the problem. Selection of the optimal approach involves consideration of clinical circumstances, the location and specific angio-

Table 20A.2
Thrombus-Containing Lesions

Clinical Setting	Treatment
Acute myocardial infarction	
Native coronary artery	Conventional PTCA
Vein graft	Lytic therapy, then PTCA
	TEC, then PTCA
	Laser angioplasty
Acute occlusion after PTCA	
Thrombus present	Redilate with or without slight oversizing, optimize anticoagulation, intracoronary lytic therapy after PTCA.
Dissection and thrombus	Perfusion balloon, early stent decision, may need lytic therapy after stent, DCA for localized dissection.
Unstable angina	
No visible thrombus	Conventional PTCA, new technology depending on lesion characteristics and operator experience, DCA, laser. No lytic therapy.
Visible thrombus	Depending on size, may pretreat with prolonged heparin or occasionally thrombolytic therapy, then conventional PTCA. New technology, for example, DCA, plays an important role in selected angiographic subsets. Avoid rotational atherectomy.

graphic characteristics of the lesion and the thrombus, and the techniques available (Table 20A.2). Careful attention to anticoagulation and antiplatelet agents before, during, and after the procedure is essential. New therapeutic drugs such as specific antithrombins and platelet receptor antibodies should play an increasingly important role. Intracoronary thrombolytic therapy may also be used in selected cases, although as routine prophylaxis it is not indicated. Equally careful attention must be paid to optimizing the result of PTCA. Following treatment a period of observation to assess the stability of the lesion is mandatory. Finally, new technology, for instance, directional atherectomy, may be optimal in selected patients to enhance initial outcome.

SUGGESTED READINGS

Ambrose JA, Sharma S, Torre S et al. Thrombolysis and angioplasty in unstable angina (TAUSA) trial. Circulation 1993;88:1113 (abstract).

Bergelson B, Jacobs A, Cupples A, Ruocco N Jr, Kyller G, Ryan T, Faxon D. Prediction of risk for hemodynamic compromise during percutaneous transluminal coronary angioplasty. Am J Cardiol 1992;70:1540–1545.

Buchalter M, Been M, Williams D, Adams P, Reid D. The occurrence of early sudden coronary artery occlusion following angioplasty may be predicted from the clinical characteristics of the patient and their coronary lesion morphology. Jpn Heart J 1992;33:295–302.

de Feyter P, van den Brand M, Jaarman G, van Domburg, Serruys P, Suryapranata H. Acute coronary artery occlusion during and after percutaneous transluminal coronary angioplasty. Circulation 1991;83:927–936.

de Marchena E, Mallou S, Posada JD et al. Direct holmium laser–assisted balloon angioplasty in acute myocardial infarction. Am J Cardiol 1993;71:1223–1225.

de Marchena E, Mallou S, Topaz O et al. Unstable angina treated with laser angioplasty. J Am Coll Cardiol 1993; 21:196AA.

Detre K, Holmes D Jr, Holubkov R, Cowley M, Bourassa M, Faxon D, Dorros G et al. Incidence and consequences of periprocedural occlusion. Circulation 1990;82:739–750.

Ellis S, Roubin G, King S III, Douglas J Jr, Weintraub W, Thomas R, Cox W. Angiographic and clinical predictors of acute closure after native vessel coronary angioplasty. Circulation 1988;77:372–379.

Harrington RA, Leimberger JD, Berdan L et al. The ACT index: a method for stratifying likelihood of success and risk of acute complications in coronary intervention. Circulation 1993;88:1111 (abstract).

Hermans W, Foley D, Rensing B, Rutsch W, Heyndrickx G, Danchin N, Mast G et al. Usefulness of quantitative and qualitative angiographic lesion morphology and clinical characteristics in predicting major adverse cardiac events during and after native coronary balloon angioplasty. Am J Cardiol 1993;72:14–20.

Holmes DR, Klein LW, Litvack F. Lesion morphology and acute outcome after excimer laser angioplasty: a prospective evaluation (in press).

Laskey M, Deutsch R, Hirshfeld J Jr, Kussmaul W, Barnathan E, Laskey W. Influence of heparin therapy on percutaneous transluminal coronary angioplasty outcome in patients with coronary arterial thrombus. Am J Cardiol 1990; 65:179–182.

Mabin TA, Holmes DR Jr, Smith HC, Vlietstra RE, Bove AA, Reeder GS, Chesebro JH et al. Intracoronary thrombus: role in coronary occlusion complicating percutaneous transluminal coronary angioplasty. J Am Coll Cardiol 1985; 5:198–202.

Maraganore JM, Bourdin P, Jablonski J, Ramachandran KL. Design and characterization of hirulogs: a novel class of bivalent peptide inhibitors of thrombin. Biochemistry 1990;29:7095–7101.

Mooney M, Mooney J, Goldenberg I, Almquist A, Van Tassel R. Percutaneous transluminal coronary angioplasty in the setting of large intracoronary thrombi. Am J Cardiol 1990; 65:427–431.

Myler R, Shaw R, Stertzer S, Bashour T, Ryan C, Hecht H, Cumberland D. Unstable angina and coronary angioplasty. Circulation 1990;82:II-88–II-95.

Pitney MR, Kelly SM, Owen KJ et al. Activated clotting time differential is a superior method of monitoring anticoagulation following coronary angioplasty. Circulation 1993;88:1110 (abstract).

Reeder GS, Bryant SC, Suman VJ, Holmes DR. Intracoronary thrombus: still a risk factor for PTCA failure? Cathet Cardiovasc Diagn 1995;34:191–195.

Sugrue D, Holmes D Jr, Smith H, Reeder G, Lane G, Vlietstra E, Bresnahan J et al. Coronary artery thrombus as a risk factor for acute vessel occlusion during percutaneous transluminal coronary angioplasty: improving results. Br Heart J 1986;56:62–66.

Swanson KT, Vlietstra RE, Holmes DR et al. Efficacy of adjunctive dextran during PTCA. Am J Cardiol 1984; 54:447–448.

Topol E. Integration of anticoagulation, thrombolysis, and coronary angioplasty for unstable angina pectoris. Am J Cardiol 1991;68:136B–141B.

Topol EJ et al. A randomized trial of intravenous heparin versus recombinant hirudin for acute coronary syndromes. Circulation 1994;90:1631–1637.

Topol EJ, Fuster V, Califf RM et al. Recombinant hirudin for unstable angina pectoris. A multicenter randomized angiographic trial. Circulation 1994;89:1557–1566.

Topol EJ, Leya F, Pinkerton CA, Whitlow PL, Hofling B, Simonton CA, Masden RR et al. (CAVEAT study group). A comparison of directional atherectomy with coronary angioplasty in patients with coronary artery disease. N Engl J Med 1993;329:221–227.

Vaitkus P, Herrmann H, Laskey W. Management and immediate outcome of patients with intracoronary thrombus during percutaneous transluminal coronary angioplasty. Am Heart J 1992;124:1–8.

B. Management of the Coronary Lesion with Associated Thrombus

JOHN S. DOUGLAS, JR.

In our early experience with balloon angioplasty, it became apparent that lesion-associated thrombus was a predictor of complications, including further thrombus propagation at the angioplasty site, distal thromboembolization, or more commonly abrupt closure a few minutes or hours later. Subsequently, many studies have shown that the presence of thrombus was an important predictor of angioplasty success and complications (1–10). It is not clear whether the thrombus itself or the underlying unstable plaque surface is the principal cause of these adverse events. Commonly, thrombus dissolution reveals plaque ulceration. Instrumentation of thrombus-containing lesions would be expected to expose variable amounts of clot-bound thrombin and subintimal collagen, both potent initiators of thrombosis.

Thrombus may be recognized angiographically by the presence of discrete intraluminal filling defects, or a less specific hazy appearance, or suspected when lesion surfaces are irregular or have overhanging edges or an unusual abrupt leading or trailing contour. Using angioscopic techniques for diagnosis of thrombus, the most sensitive method available clinically, White and colleagues reported that the presence of thrombus was associated with a greater than fivefold increase in major complications of death, myocardial infarction, or coronary bypass surgery (12.2% versus 2.1%, $P = 0.4$) and more recurrent ischemia manifest by abrupt occlusion, repeat PTCA, or recurrent angina (25.7% versus 10.4%, $P = 0.3$) (11). The presence of thrombus has also been associated with a higher restenosis rate, but this is apparently because of increased reocclusion rather than accentuated intimal proliferation (12). While it is clear that angiography is relatively insensitive compared with percutaneous angioscopy in the diagnosis of intracoronary thrombus, experienced operators recognize thrombus more frequently by incorporating "softer" angiographic criteria with clinical intuition. This ability to make an educated guess is part of the art of medicine that denotes an experienced operator.

Most patients with intracoronary thrombus have unstable angina or recent myocardial infarction, and the patients with the greatest likelihood of angioplasty complications are those with considerable thrombus and persisting ischemic symptoms while on medical therapy. We found that most patients with these findings could be stabilized eventually on aspirin, heparin, and intravenous nitro-

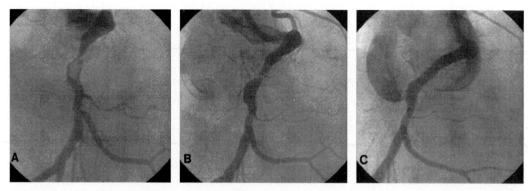

Figure 20B.1. A 57-year-old female smoker with a 3-day history of unstable angina was found to have normal left ventricular function, a normal left coronary artery, and severe stenosis of the right coronary artery. **A.** Right anterior oblique view with a large thrombus just distal to the lesion. She was stabilized on intravenous heparin, nitroglycerin, and aspirin, and repeat angiography 6 days later **(B)** revealed persisting severe stenosis but complete resolution of thrombus. Balloon angioplasty yielded an excellent result **(C),** and the patient was discharged the following day with no complications. In our experience intravenous heparin for 5 to 7 days is an excellent strategy for management of large intracoronary thrombi. (From Douglas JS Jr et al. J Am Coll Cardiol 1988;11:238.)

glycerin, and that intervention was much safer after 5 to 7 days of this therapy (Fig. 20B.1), even if some thrombus remained (13). Importantly, in a few patients the residual lesions after prolonged heparin were noncritical and no intervention was required. Similar results were reported by Laskey and colleagues, who observed that treatment of patients with intracoronary thrombus with intravenous heparin for a mean of 5.8 days was associated with higher angiographic success (94% versus 61%, $P < 0.5$), and significantly reduced postprocedural abrupt closure (6% versus 33%, $P < .05$) compared with patients treated with no heparin or with heparin for less than 24 hours (14).

Some investigators have performed balloon angioplasty in spite of intracoronary thrombus with relatively favorable results. Mooney et al. used oversized balloons (balloon/artery ratio of 1.2) to treat lesions with intracoronary thrombi, occupying at least 50% of the lumen diameter, with procedural success in 92%, and 7% required bypass surgery (15). Although this direct approach may be favored by third-party payers who attempt to restrict hospital days, it could prove to be more expensive because of the need to treat more complications and to per-

form procedures that would be unneeded if sufficient time were allowed for spontaneous thrombolysis to occur (13, 16).

Thrombolytic agents have been administered via intracoronary or intravenous infusion before and after PTCA or as a bolus to treat intracoronary thrombus, but the optimal strategy is unclear (17–20). Williams et al. in an observational study compared intravenous tissue plasminogen activator, intracoronary urokinase, and intravenous heparin for treatment of intracoronary thrombus and reported more complete and rapid thrombus resolution with TPA (20). Prolonged intracoronary infusions are technically demanding, uncomfortable for the patient, and have some inherent risk of coronary artery trauma. We generally attempt to avoid the use of thrombolytic agents because of the attendant serious bleeding complications and because of the observation that stable-appearing large thrombi subjected to thrombolytic therapy not infrequently change shape and occlude flow, necessitating an urgent attempt at angioplasty. The results of thrombolytic therapy for treatment of large thrombi, in our experience, parallel those of the Thrombolysis and Angioplasty in Unstable Angina (TAUSA) Trial, which showed that use of urokinase was deleterious, leading to more frequent ischemic complications (21). If, however, an unstable patient with intracoronary thrombus proves refractory to aggressive non-invasive medical therapy, angioplasty frequently can be accomplished successfully utilizing intracoronary thrombolytic agents if needed to reduce thrombus burden. In this case prolonged balloon inflations are frequently used, and better antiplatelet agents and more potent thrombin inhibitors, strategies of the immediate future, would be welcomed.

In a small experience, we and others have had favorable initial experience with delivery of urokinase directly to the thrombotic lesion using a new, local, drug-delivery device, the Dispatch catheter (Scimed Life Systems, Maple Grove, MN). In a recent report, six patients were successfully treated with complete dissolution of angiographic intracoronary thrombus by local infusion of limited amounts of urokinase (21a). These preliminary observations are quite encouraging.

The transluminal extraction catheter (TEC) has not been widely applied in native coronary lesions, but may play a role in selected patients. In native coronary arteries, however, TEC atherectomy has been associated with major complications (death, MI, and CABG) in 11% of patients (22). In our experience, and in that of Ellis and colleagues (23), directional atherectomy can be applied effectively in the presence of thrombus or after thrombolytic therapy (Fig. 20B.2) for appropriate anatomic features (marked eccentricity), but some investigators have noted more frequent need for coronary bypass surgery when directional atherectomy was carried out in the presence of thrombus (10.3% versus 3.9%, $P = .03$) (24). Use of the excimer laser in the presence of thrombus has been associated with thromboembolic complications in 25% of patients, abrupt closure in 17%, and a reduced clinical success (25). Recent reports from the NACI registry indicate that intracoronary thrombus was independently associated with major complications during new

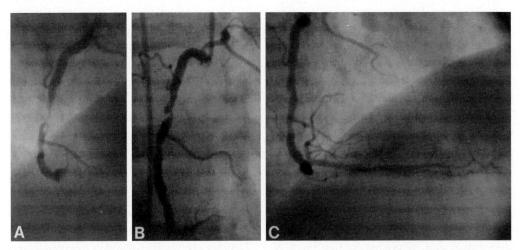

Figure 20B.2. A 50-year-old male with known coronary artery disease was hospitalized with prolonged chest pain and minimal EKG changes. **A.** Coronary arteriography showed severe stenosis of the right coronary artery with a moderate-sized thrombus (right anterior oblique view). Because of persisting chest pain, intracoronary urokinase 750,000 units was administered over 90 minutes with resolution of chest pain and improved coronary flow. **B.** After 4 days of intravenous heparin, coronary arteriography revealed a very eccentric stenosis with no obvious thrombus (right anterior oblique view). Directional atherectomy with a 7 Fr device was successful and free of complications. Histology showed moderately cellular fibrous connective tissue with attached partially organized thrombus. By using a combination of thrombolytic therapy and heparin for 4 days, intervention in the presence of obvious thrombus was avoided and a lesion-specific approach was possible.

device intervention (9% versus 3% if thrombus was absent, $P < .001$) (26).

The following comments summarize strategies currently applied in treatment of intracoronary thrombus associated with native coronary lesions at Emory University Hospital.

NATIVE CORONARY ARTERY LESION: SMALL OR SUSPECTED THROMBUS

In patients with irregular lesion surface, angiographic lucency, or small filling defects, the timing and selection of interventional strategy are dependent on clinical stability and estimated consequences of abrupt closure. If symptoms are occurring at rest in an accelerating pattern, we maximize medical therapy (aspirin, intravenous nitroglycerin, beta blockers, calcium channel blockers, intravenous heparin) and defer intervention for at least 48 hours if possible. The larger the artery and the more adverse the consequences of abrupt closure, the longer we prefer to wait. Prophylactic use of thrombolytic agents is not recommended based on our experience at Emory and the recently reported TAUSA trial (21). Perfusion balloons are frequently used to achieve 10- to 20-minute inflations, and directional atherectomy is often selected to treat bulky or ulcerated lesions, recognizing an increased rate of creatine kinase release with this strategy (27). Heparin is continued for 24 to 48 hours postprocedure. In patients whose symptoms are not markedly unstable and in those who have already been stabilized on heparin, postponement of intervention is less critical, especially in low-risk patients. We do not favor use of the transluminal extraction catheter or excimer laser in this setting, and avoid use of rotational atherectomy and stents when thrombus is suspected. We do use intracoronary urokinase adjunctively (250,000 to 1,000,000 units over 30 to 90 minutes) or the TEC to treat obvious intracoronary thrombus that cannot be adequately managed with prolonged balloon inflations.

NATIVE CORONARY ARTERY LESION: LARGE THROMBUS

Larger intracoronary thrombi, most often observed postinfarction and in smokers, are usually managed with 5 to 7 days of intravenous heparin, based on our favorable experience with this strategy (13) (see Fig. 20B.1). Rarely, large thrombi have been aspirated into a guide catheter when quite proximal or entangled and removed by wrapping a guidewire and balloon-on-a-wire. Obviously, improved means of catheter-based thrombectomy are needed, and preliminary reports of new thrombectomy devices are encouraging (28). Prohibitively long intracoronary infusions of thrombolytic agents can be required to lyse large thrombi, but we have used 250,000 to 1,000,000 units of urokinase over 3 hours, or intravenous TPA 80 to 100 units over 4 hours to achieve at least partial thrombolysis when ischemia could not be managed by other means. If thrombolytic agents alone are successful in stabilizing ischemic symptoms and coronary flow, heparin is continued for 3 to 5 days before repeat angiography and possible angioplasty (see Fig. 20B.2). Thrombolytic agents clearly speed up clot lysis (20), but, systematically administered, expose the patient to the risk of serious bleeding complications and increased ischemic complications if emergency angioplasty becomes necessary (21). The recent availability of the Dispatch catheter for local intracoronary delivery of drug has provided a promising alternative method for treatment of intracoronary thrombus. Infusion of 150,000 units of urokinase over 30 minutes was reported to achieve complete dissolution of angiographic thrombus in a small series of patients (21a). If there is a large amount of thrombus and persisting ischemia, we have elected to intervene surgically if an important vessel such as a large LAD was involved, and in a few postinfarction patients we have used the TEC device followed by balloon angioplasty or DCA.

Lesion-associated thrombus is common in saphenous vein grafts and may present difficult management problems. If thrombus was recently formed, as in acute myocardial infarction, primary balloon angioplasty is usually effective without the need for thrombolytic therapy (29–31). However, in most patients presenting for intervention, intragraft thrombus has been present for days and brief infusions of thrombolytic therapy are relatively ineffective. Patients in some cases can be stabilized on heparin and treated with Coumadin for 30 to 60 days before intervention, allowing thrombus to lyse spontaneously or organize (16). Alternatively, intragraft infusions of thrombolytic agents can be administered for 8 to 24 hours with frequent successful reduction in thrombus burden (18, 19). Use of prolonged heparin and/or thrombolytic agents to achieve clot lysis has the potential advantage of permitting stenting if clot lysis is relatively complete, and this strategy appears to have the best chance for long-term patency. Recently, investigators have reported experience in vein grafts with the transluminal extraction catheter, which permits aspiration of thrombus and atheroma (31, 32), and this is usually followed up with balloon angioplasty or directional atherectomy.

Unfortunately, with both prolonged thrombolytic therapy and TEC, complications are relatively common. Prolonged intragraft infusion of thrombolytic agents has resulted in intracranial and intramyocardial hemorrhage and thromboembolic myocardial infarction (34–36). Recent data from the NACI registry indicates that use of the TEC in saphenous vein grafts with thrombus resulted in coronary embolization in 17%, and the mortality of patients with coronary emboli was 35% (32). In a recently published, single-center experience with TEC in 158 saphenous vein graft lesions, 28% had thrombus, distal embolization occurred in 12%, no reflow occurred in 9%, death occurred in 2%, and the 6-month restenosis rate was 69%. These rather sobering data should lead one to apply this strategy conservatively, if at all (33).

The following comments summarize current management strategies applied in thrombotic saphenous vein graft lesions at Emory University.

SAPHENOUS VEIN GRAFT LESIONS: LIMITED THROMBUS

When evaluating saphenous vein graft lesions for intervention, the angioplasty operator must first consider possible consequences of thromboatheroembolism, realizing that the entire lesion and accompanying thrombus may be fragmented and dislodged. If the risk of major atheroembolism is acceptable (i.e., the lesion mass and thrombus are small), early intervention may be appropriate. An overriding issue, however, is the availability of the Palmaz-Schatz stent, a most effective strategy currently not approved for use in saphenous vein grafts in the United States. When this stent is available, we believe the preferred strategy would be a maneuver to eliminate thrombus (such as intragraft or local thrombolytic therapy or prolonged anticoagulation), followed by stenting of the lesion and subsequent Coumadin anticoagulation. Until this stent is approved for use, we favor balloon angioplasty or, in cases of ostial or eccentric lesions, directional atherectomy, realizing the restenosis rate will be 50% or higher on long-term follow-up.

SAPHENOUS VEIN GRAFT LESION: EXTENSIVE THROMBUS

Intervention in thrombus-laden grafts should be undertaken only after careful study of potential risks and benefits. It is rarely appropriate to subject patients to the risk of prolonged selective thrombolytic therapy or TEC atherectomy, given the significant procedural risks incurred and the high restenosis rates expected following manipulation of older saphenous vein grafts. In some patients, however, the presence of patent grafts to major coronary arteries or other factors make reoperative surgery unattractive, and intervention in the presence of graft thrombus may be selected over more conservative measures when ischemia cannot be controlled (Fig. 20B.3). In this setting it is not clear whether prolonged intragraft thrombolytic therapy or TEC atherectomy is preferable (see discussion above).

While it is clear that intracoronary thrombus is a significant predictor of adverse outcome with coronary interventional procedures, it is possible in most patients to select strategies that maximize safety and long-term efficacy. Availability of more potent anti-platelet agents, thrombin inhibitors, catheter-based techniques for clot lysis (37), and thrombectomy (28) may permit more optimal therapy in this difficult subgroup in the future.

REFERENCES

1. Mabin T, Holmes D, Smith H et al. Intracoronary thrombus: role in coronary occlusion complicating percutaneous transluminal coronary angioplasty. J Am Coll Cardiol 1985;5:198–202.

2. Sugrue D, Holmes D, Smith H et al. Coronary artery throm-

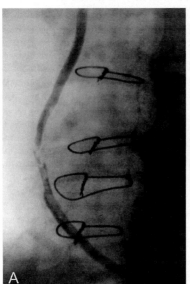
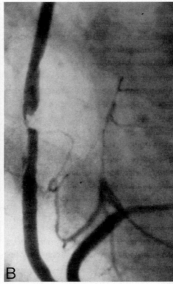
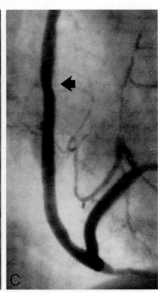
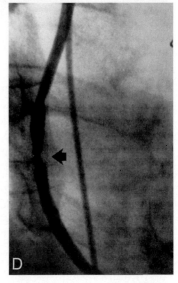

Figure 20B.3. Unstable angina in a 59-year-old male 10 years following coronary bypass surgery led to coronary arteriography **(A)**, which revealed severe stenosis and a large amount of thrombus in a saphenous vein graft which supplied the right and circumflex coronary arteries (frontal view). Grafts to the left anterior descending, diagonal, and anterior obtuse marginal coronary arteries were widely patent. The inferior left ventricular wall was hypokinetic. Because of poor flow in the stenotic graft and persisting ischemic chest pain, urokinase 250,000 units was infused over approximately 60 minutes with improvement in flow and diminished thrombus. **B.** After 5 days of intravenous heparin, coronary arteriography showed a very severe eccentric stenosis in the saphenous vein graft (right anterior oblique view). **C.** A 4.0-mm Palmaz-Schatz stent was placed with excellent angiographic result and no complications. **D.** Follow-up angiography 6 months later showed only mild narrowing, and the patient was asymptomatic. By utilizing thrombolytic therapy plus prolonged intravenous heparin, it was possible to make use of a metal stent to achieve good 6-month patency in this thrombus-laden graft.

bus as a risk factor for acute vessel occlusion during percutaneous transluminal coronary angioplasty: improving results. Br Heart J 1986;56:62–66.

3. Deligonul U, Gabliani G, Caralis D et al. Percutaneous transluminal coronary angioplasty in patients with intracoronary thrombus. Am J Cardiol 1988;62:474–476.

4. Arora R, Platko W, Bhadwar K, Simpfendorfer C. Role of intracoronary thrombus in acute complications during percutaneous transluminal coronary angioplasty. Cathet Cardiovasc Diagn 1989;16:226–229.

5. Ellis SG, Roubin GS, King SB III et al. Angiographic and clinical predictors of acute closure after native vessel coronary angioplasty. Circulation 1988;77:372–379.

6. Ellis SG, Vandormael MG, Cowley MJ et al. Coronary morphologic and clinical determinants of procedural outcome with angioplasty for multivessel coronary disease: implications for patient selection. Circulation 1990; 82:1193–1202.

7. Myler RK, Shaw RE, Stertzer SH et al. Lesion morphology and coronary angioplasty: current experience and analysis. J Am Coll Cardiol 1992;19:1641–1652.

8. Tenaglia AN, Fortin DF, Frid DJ et al. A simple scoring system to predict PTCA abrupt closure. J Am Coll Cardiol 1992;19:139A.

9. Ellis SG, Cowley MJ, Vetrovec GW. Is the ACC/AHA angioplasty lesion classification scheme obsolete? Circulation 1992;86(Suppl I):I-785.

10. Tan KH, Sulke N, Taub N et al. Lesion morphological determinants of coronary balloon angioplasty success and complications: time for a reappraisal. J Am Coll Cardiol 1994;222A.

11. White CJ, Ramee SR, Collins TJ et al. Angioscopically detected coronary thrombus correlates with adverse PTCA outcome. Circulation 1993;88(Suppl I):I-596.

12. Violaris AG, Herrman JP, Melkert R et al. Does local thrombus formation increase long-term luminal renarrowing following PTCA? A quantitative angiographic analysis. J Am Coll Cardiol 1994;139A.

13. Douglas JS Jr, Lutz JF, Clements SD et al. Therapy of large intracoronary thrombi in candidates for percutaneous transluminal coronary angioplasty. J Am Coll Cardiol 1988;11:238.

14. Laskey MAL, Deutch E, Hirshfeld JW Jr et al. Influence of heparin therapy on percutaneous transluminal coronary angioplasty outcome in unstable angina pectoris. Am J Cardiol 1990;65:1425–1429.

15. Mooney MR, Mooney JF, Goldenberg IF et al. Percutaneous transluminal coronary angioplasty in the setting of large intracoronary thrombi. Am J Cardiol 1990; 65:427–431.

16. Kolansky DM, Shapiro TA, Laskey WK. Prolonged heparin therapy for occlusive intracoronary thrombus. Cathet Cardiovasc Diagn 1993;30:150–152.

17. Evans DJ, Pacheco T, Grambow D et al. Bolus versus prolonged intracoronary urokinase infusion: a therapeutic quagmire? J Am Coll Cardiol 1994;185A.

18. Chapekis AT, George BS, Candela RJ. Rapid thrombus

dissolution by continuous infusion of urokinase through an intracoronary perfusion wire prior to and following PTCA: results in native coronaries and patent saphenous vein grafts. Cathet Cardiovasc Diagn 1991;23:89–92.

19. Pitney MR, Cumpston N, Mews GC et al. Use of twenty-four-hour infusions of intracoronary tissue plasminogen activator to increase the application of coronary angioplasty. Cathet Cardiovasc Diagn 1992;26:255–259.

20. McKendall GR, Berman MS, Sharaf BL, Lee B, Williams DO. Comparison of the effectiveness of intravenous heparin, intravenous rt-PA, and intracoronary urokinase for treatment of intracoronary thrombus. J Am Coll Cardiol 1993;21:137A.

21. Torre SR, Ambrose JA, Sharma SK et al. Adjuvant intracoronary urokinase worsens the procedural outcome for PTCA of complex lesions in unstable angina: results of the thrombolysis and angioplasty in unstable angina (TAUSA) trial. J Am Coll Cardiol 1994;105A.

21a. McKay RG, Fram DB, Hirst JA, Kiernan FJ, Primiano CA, Rinaldi MJ et al. Treatment of intracoronary thrombus with local urokinase infusion using a new, site-specific drug delivery system: The Dispatch Catheter. Cathet Cardiovasc Diagn 1994;33:181-188.

22. Gitlin JB, Sutton JM, Casale PN et al. Transluminal extraction catheter atherectomy in bypass grafts vs. native vessels: are there significant differences? J Am Cardiol 1994;220A.

23. Ellis SG, DeCesare NB, Pinkerton CA et al. Relation of stenosis morphology and clinical presentation to the procedural results of directional coronary atherectomy. Circulation 1991;84:644–653.

24. Emmi R, Movsowitz H, Manginas A et al. Directional coronary atherectomy in lesions with coexisting thrombus. Circulation 1993;88(Suppl I):I-596.

25. Estella P, Ryan TJ, Landzberg JS et al. Excimer laser-assisted coronary angioplasty for lesions containing thrombus. J Am Coll Cardiol 1993;21:1550–1560.

26. O'Neill WW, Sketch MH Jr, Steenkiste A, Detre K et al. New device intervention in the treatment of intracoronary thrombus: report of the NACI Registry. Circulation 1993; 88(Suppl I):I-595.

27. Waksman R, Scott NA, Douglas JS Jr et al. Distal embolization is common after directional atherectomy in coronary arteries and vein grafts. Circulation 1993; 88:(Suppl I)I-299.

28. Fajadet J, Bar O, Jordan C et al. Human percutaneous thrombectomy using the new hydrolyser catheter: preliminary results in saphenous vein grafts. J Am Coll Cardiol 1994;220A.

29. Grines CL, Booth DC, Nissen SE et al. Mechanism of acute myocardial infarction in patients with prior coronary artery bypass grafting and therapeutic implications. Am J Cardiol 1990;65:1292–1296.

30. Kavanaugh KM, Topol EJ. Acute intervention during myocardial infarction in patients with prior coronary bypass surgery. Am J Cardiol 1990;65:924–926.

31. Kahn JK, Rutherford BD, McConahay DR et al. Usefulness

of angioplasty during acute myocardial infarction in patients with prior coronary artery bypass grafting. Am J Cardiol 1990;65:698–702.

32. Moses JW, Tierstein PS, Sketch MH Jr, Siegel RM, Yeh W et al. Angiographic determinants of risk and outcome of coronary embolus and myocardial infarction (MI) with the transluminal extraction catheter (TEC): a report from the New Approaches to Coronary Intervention (NACI) Registry. J Am Coll Cardiol 1994;220A.

33. Safian RD, Grines CL, May MA, Lichtenberg A, Juran N, Schreiber TL et al. Clinical and angiographic results of transluminal extraction coronary atherectomy in saphenous vein bypass grafts. Circulation 1994;89:302–312.

34. Bedotto JB, Ruthford BD, Hartzler GO. Intramyocardial hemorrhage due to prolonged intracoronary infusion of urokinase into a totally occluded saphenous vein bypass graft. Cathet Cardiovasc Diagn 1992;25:52–56.

35. Gurley JC, MacPhail BS. Acute myocardial infarction due to thrombolytic reperfusion of chronically occluded saphenous vein coronary bypass grafts. Am J Cardiol 1991; 68:274–275.

36. Margolis JR, Mogensen L, Mehta S et al. Diffuse embolization following percutaneous transluminal coronary angioplasty of occluded vein grafts: the blush phenomenon. Clin Cardiol 1991;14:489–493.

37. Chasteney EA, Ravichandran PS, Furnary AP et al. Laser thrombolysis for bypass graft thrombosis. J Am Coll Cardiol 1994;374A.

21. The Ostial Lesion

A. Aorto-Ostial Stenoses

JAMES D. BOEHRER and ERIC J. TOPOL

Coronary ostial lesions, defined as stenoses within 3 mm of the aortic root, are rare manifestations of coronary disease found in from 0.13 to 2.7% of patients in angiographic series (1, 2). The incidence reported in autopsy series is higher (3), reflecting the inherent difficulties encountered in the angiographic detection of these stenoses. The etiology of ostial lesions is varied. In the past, syphilis was a major etiologic consideration (4). Presently, atherosclerosis is the most common etiology (1) with a particularly high incidence in patients with homozygous familial hypercholesterolemia (5, 6). Other reported causes of ostial lesions include Takayasu's arteritis (7, 8), radiation therapy (9, 10), and cannulation of coronary artery ostia during aortic valve surgery (11, 12). Most recently, ostial atherosclerosis induced by guiding catheter trauma during coronary angioplasty has been reported (13–17).

Many interventional series have considered aorto-ostial (right coronary artery, left main coronary artery, and saphenous vein graft) lesions together with branch ostial (left anterior descending and circumflex) lesions. Although frequently grouped together for analysis, each of these types of ostial stenosis differ regarding technical requirements, initial success rates, procedural complications, and long-term results. In this chapter, percutaneous coronary intervention for all types of ostial stenoses will be considered with particular attention to the unique approach and results for each location.

In general, coronary intervention for ostial stenoses is associated with a lower rate of primary success, a higher rate of procedural complications, and a higher rate of restenosis compared to nonostial stenoses. Once successfully crossed with the device, unique anatomic features of ostial lesions often lead to difficulty in achieving an optimal result. Histologic data from pathologic series (18), and more recently from atherectomy specimens (19), show that ostial lesions are frequently heavily calcified, fibrotic, and sclerotic. In addition, there may be more elastic recoil at ostial sites because of highly elastic tissue in the adjacent aortic wall. That is, these lesions frequently may behave more like aortic wall than coronary artery.

Complications necessitating emergency bypass surgery appear to be more frequent with angioplasty of coronary ostial lesions. An increased rate of acute complications may be explained by guiding catheter trauma, which creates added injury at the site of the ostial angioplasty. Finally, the ostial location inherently engenders a large territory of myocardium at risk. As a result, acute closure is more likely to result in significant ischemia, which in turn prompts emergency bypass grafting.

The reasons for the high restenosis rates observed at ostial lesions are not fully understood. One highly likely explanation is an incomplete result caused by calcification, fibrosis, or dense plaque accumulation. The recent availability of intravascular ultrasound (IVUS) has demonstrated that angiographically normal or mildly stenosed ostia may contain significant plaque burden (Fig. 21A.1). Guide catheter trauma, which has been documented to cause ostial lesions (13–17), may play an important role in re-

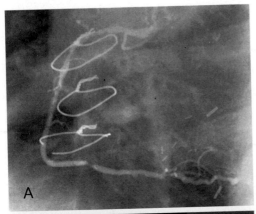

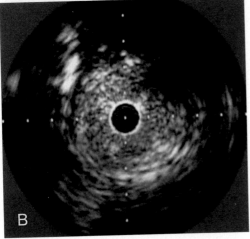

Figure 21A.1. Intravascular ultrasound of the right coronary ostium. **A.** Cineangiogram of right coronary revealing an apparently normal ostium. **B.** Intravascular ultrasound performed to evaluate a distal lesion in the vessel revealed unsuspected ostial stenosis. This image from the ostium of the vessel reveals 75% area stenosis.

stenosis by increasing the injury to the treated site. Other possible factors include increased shear forces associated with the ostial location and increased late recoil caused by the elastic nature of the aortic wall (18).

Because of the suboptimal results reported with balloon angioplasty of ostial lesions, there is a great deal of interest in alternative percutaneous therapies for these lesions. Much of the data reported to date have appeared only in abstract form. Despite the preliminary nature of these data, the reports parallel the findings with balloon angioplasty of ostial lesions. Specifically, although initial angiographic success appears improved with some of the new devices, major complications are relatively frequent, and restenosis, where reported, is high.

Since rates of success, complications, and restenosis can be expected to be different for right coronary, vein graft, left coronary, or branch ostial lesions, each lesion type will be discussed separately.

RIGHT CORONARY ARTERY OSTIAL LESIONS

Angioplasty

To date, the right coronary artery ostial lesion is the best studied and serves as a prototype for the other ostial lesions. A summary of reported experiences in the treatment of right coronary ostial stenoses is presented in Table 21A.1 (19–23). The first reported series of

Table 21A.1
Summary of Experiences With Right Coronary Ostial Stenosis

Author (Reference)	Device	N	Initial Success (%)	Complications (%)	Angiographic Restenosis (%)	Clinical Restenosis (%)
Topol (20)	Balloon	53	42 (79)	5/53 (9.4) CABG	16/42 (38)	20/42 (48)
Whitlow	Directional atherectomy	50	43 (86)	3/50 (5.7) CAGB	10/22 (45)	NA
Popma (19)	Directional atherectomy	7	6 (86)	0 (0)	1/6 (17)	NA
Popma (21)	Rotational atherectomy	45	44 (98)	1/45 (2.2)	NA	NA
Bernardi (22)	Rotational atherectomy	106	99 (93)	3/106 (2.8) CABG 2/106 (1.9) Death	30/59 (51)	(39)
Eigler (23)	Laser	124	110 (89)	7/124 (5.6) CABG 0/124 (0) Death	16/46 (35)	NA

N, Number of patients with right coronary ostial stenosis; *NA*, not available for right coronary artery ostial lesions; *CABG*, emergency coronary artery bypass grafting.

right coronary artery ostial lesions was a multi-center experience published in 1987 (20). In this report of 53 patients, the procedure was successful in 42 (79%), and five (9.4%) required emergency bypass surgery. At an average of 12.5 months of follow-up, 20 of the 42 patients with an initially successful procedure had a clinical recurrence of angina. Sixteen of these had angiographically documented restenosis. Repeat angioplasty was performed in six, and elective bypass surgery in eight patients. Thus, including the five patients who went to emergency surgery, 13 of 53 or one-quarter of the patients had bypass surgery during follow-up. This report of poor results with balloon angioplasty of right coronary ostial lesions has been widely cited and has led to a great deal of interest in the use of new technologies to treat these lesions. Subsequent reports have suggested that the more recent results with balloon angioplasty may be better than this first report. Bedotto et al. reported an 85% angiographic success rate with no emergency bypass operations and no myocardial infarctions in their 55-patient series (24). At follow-up 31% required a repeat procedure and 20% had class III or IV angina. Vallbracht reported an 83.3% success rate in a 60-patient series of right coronary, vein graft, and branch ostial lesions. The rate of emergency bypass surgery was lower in patients with ostial lesions compared with controls (5% versus 10%, NS). Restenosis occurred in 26.5% (25). Thus recent reports suggest that the results of balloon angioplasty using newer equipment may be better than previously reported.

To maximize the likelihood of success and minimize the incidence of acute complications, several technical factors are important when approaching the right coronary artery ostium. First, it is critical to minimize trauma to the ostium during the procedure. Proper guiding catheter selection is most important in this regard. Unconventional guiding catheters are sometimes required to obtain access to the vessel without overly deep cannulation of the ostium. Amplatz and multipurpose catheters, which tend to "deep seat" the right coronary ostium, should be avoided. For normal right coronary takeoffs, an appropriately sized Judkins right catheter is usually adequate. Short right coronary curves may be useful for downgoing takeoffs while shepherd's crook or hockey stick catheters are usually suitable for upgoing takeoffs. Prior to dilatation of the ostial lesion, the guiding catheter may be partially withdrawn from the ostium. If necessary, one may first inflate the balloon that anchors the dilatation catheter while the guide is gently disengaged (Fig. 21A.2). Such manipulations should be minimized to avoid ostial trauma.

High inflation pressures are often required to obtain complete balloon expansion. In the multicenter experience with right coronary artery lesions, the average inflation pressure required to achieve full balloon inflation was nearly 10 atm. Thirty-nine percent of lesions required more than 12 atm for successful dilatation (20). Our practice therefore is to use balloons constructed of materials designed to withstand high inflation pressures, such as polyethylene terephthalate (PET), and to size the balloon 1:1 with the normal reference segment.

Directional Atherectomy

Coronary atherectomy permits the removal of tissue and results in larger residual coronary dimensions in nonostial lesions (26, 27). It was theorized therefore that atherectomy of ostial lesions might yield improved initial and long-term results. Experience with atherectomy of right coronary ostial lesions to date has shown an initial success rate that is comparable to angioplasty (Table 21A.1). Popma et al. reported successful atherectomy of right coronary ostial lesions in six of seven patients with no ischemic complications (19). A recent review of the multicenter registry for patients undergoing directional atherectomy of right coronary ostial lesions found 50 such patients treated between 1987 and 1991 (P.L. Whit-

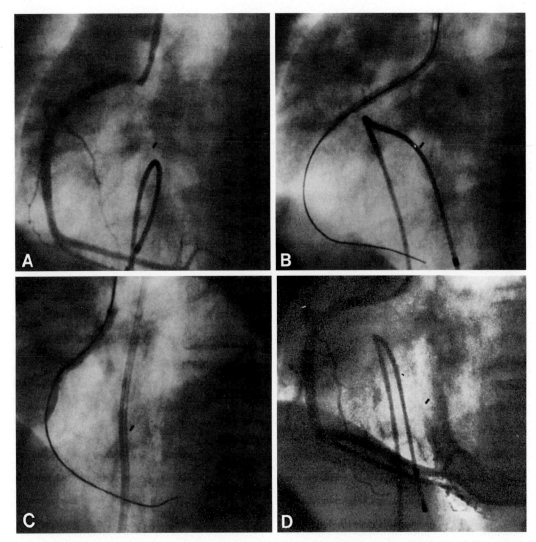

Figure 21A.2. Successful dilation of right coronary artery ostial stenosis. **A.** Left anterior oblique view of discrete, high-grade ostial lesion. **B.** Attempt at dilation of this lesion was not successful when the balloon was inflated within the guide catheter. **C.** With backing out of the guide catheter and proper seating of the dilation catheter, full balloon inflation was achieved. **D.** Relief of the ostial stenosis, as demonstrated here, was associated with a reduction in the translesional gradient from 74 to 10 mm Hg. (From Topol EJ, Ellis S, Fishman-Rosen J, Leimgruber P, Myler RK, Stertzer SH, O'Neill WW et al. J Am Coll Cardiol 1987;9:1214–1218 with permission.)

low, unpublished data). Directional atherectomy was initially successful in 43 (86%). Three patients (6%) required emergency CABG, and restenosis occurred in 10 of 22 patients undergoing follow-up angiography. Kerwin recently reported a series of 15 patients with right coronary artery ostial stenosis treated with directional atherectomy with a 93% success rate and a 7% clinical restenosis rate (28).

Technical problems associated with atherectomy are similar to those experienced with coronary angioplasty (19). Lack of guiding catheter support can be a particular problem in view of the large device profile. In the registry series, six of eight unsuccessful procedures failed because of inability to position the device across the stenosis or because of guiding catheter failure. For right coronary ostial lesions a Judkins right "short tip" DVI guide is preferred (29). Frequently, predilatation with a standard balloon catheter is required to pass the device. The SCA-EX atherectomy device with its flexible distal tip may be easier to pass across a right coronary ostial stenosis (28) and is reported to obtain similar amounts of tissue when compared with the original (SCA-1) catheter (30).

The presence of fluoroscopic calcification has been identified as a predictor of lower success rates for atherectomy (31). Thus atherectomy of heavily calcified right coronary artery ostial lesions should be avoided. Current investigation has focused on the role of intravascular ultrasound both in determining the extent of calcification prior to intervention and in evaluating residual plaque burden after atherectomy (32). Ultrasound may be particularly useful for assessing the residual plaque burden of right coronary ostial lesions because there are inherent difficulties in angiographic visualization.

Rotational Atherectomy

The multicenter registry for the Rotablator includes 106 patients who underwent rotational atherectomy for isolated right coronary artery stenoses (22). Adjunctive PTCA was performed in only 13 of these 106 patients. Primary success was achieved in 99 (93%). Two patients (1.9%) died, three (2.8%) required emergency CABG, and six (5.7%) had a non–Q-wave myocardial infarction. Specific lesion characteristics were not predictive of angiographic success or clinical complications. Six-month angiographic follow-up was available for 59 of the 106 patients. Thirty of these patients (51%) had restenosis. The clinical restenosis rate, which included patients who did not undergo repeat angiography but who were asymptomatic at follow-up, was 39%. The Washington Hospital Center has reported success in 44 of 45

(98%) of right coronary ostial stenoses treated with the Rotablator (21).

Rotational atherectomy has some technical advantages in the approach to right coronary ostial lesions. Once the guidewire successfully crosses the lesion, the device need not be separately positioned at the ostium. It merely needs to be passed along the guidewire and debulks the lesion as it is advanced. Furthermore, calcium is not an impediment to plaque removal. Compared with directional atherectomy, the technique requires smaller guiding catheters (8 and 9 Fr) and may be used to treat smaller vessels. Figure 21A.3 illustrates a right coronary ostial stenosis before and after treatment with rotational atherectomy. Our practice is to start with small burr sizes (1.5 to 1.75 mm) and to subsequently use a larger burr if appropriate. After the burr is rotating at greater than 180,000 rpm, the abrasive tip is advanced over the guidewire. It is important to maintain this speed of rotation to preserve differential cutting. If resistance is encountered, the burr is withdrawn and then readvanced in a "pecking" fashion. Adjunctive balloon angioplasty is frequently performed. It has been suggested that rotational atherectomy should be the procedure of choice for heavily calcified right coronary ostial lesions. (21). Lesions with the angiographic appearance of thrombus or severely angulated lesions should not be approached with the Rotablator.

Excimer Laser

The multicenter experience of the Excimer Laser Coronary Angioplasty (ELCA) registry with aorto-ostial stenoses has recently been reported (23). This experience included 124 patients with ostial right coronary lesions. Interestingly, at the time of writing, this is the largest reported experience with right coronary ostial stenoses with any device, *including* balloon angioplasty. Acute success with ELCA for right coronary ostial lesions was 110 of 124 lesions (89%). Seven patients (6%) required emergency

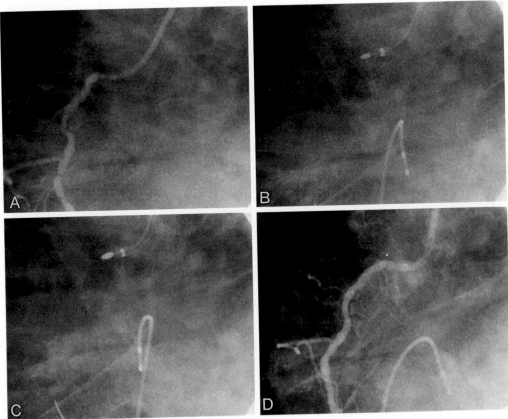

Figure 21A.3.   Successful rotational atherectomy of heavily calcified right coronary ostium. **A.** Severely calcified 80% ostial stenosis in the LAO projection. **B.** Rotablator burr (1.75 mm) in the RCA ostium. **C.** Rotablator burr (2.15 mm) in the RCA ostium. **D.** Ten percent final residual stenosis after rotational atherectomy. (From Topol EJ, ed. Textbook of interventional cardiology. 2nd ed. Philadelphia: WB Saunders, 1994 with permission.)

bypass surgery. There were no Q-wave infarctions or deaths. Four patients had non–Q-wave myocardial infarctions. At angiographic follow-up in 46 of the 90 eligible patients the restenosis rate was 34.8%. Six-month follow-up was obtained in all 111 eligible patients. Seven patients required bypass surgery, 14 had a repeat intervention, two had a myocardial infarction, and none died; 52% of patients were angina free. This experience compares favorably with the long-term results of angioplasty reported by the multicenter series (20).

Excimer laser coronary angioplasty has technical advantages as well. Once the guidewire is passed, the laser is advanced across the ostial lesion. Since the laser fiber is small, there may be less interruption of coronary flow during treatment compared with other devices (33). The technique used by the ELCA registry investigators included the use of relatively high fluences of 50 to 60 mJ/mm². Initial passes were made with a 1.3-mm concentric catheter with the device being advanced across the lesion at a rate of approximately 1 mm/sec. Multiple (one to five) passes were made. If the residual stenosis was greater than 30%, a larger (2.0 or 2.2 mm) laser catheter or adjunctive balloon angioplasty was employed. Another technique described was the reangulation of the guiding catheter to redirect the laser catheter and establish a wider lumen. Improved laser catheters, including the new excimer directional laser catheter, may lead to improved "debulking" of ostial lesions compared with the concentric excimer laser catheters (34, 35).

There does not appear to be a specific ostial lesion type that responds best to laser treatment. In a morphologic analysis of 175 ostial lesions treated with laser, no baseline morphologic feature, including eccentricity, calcification, and presence of thrombus, was predictive of primary success or complications (36). Disadvantages of the technique include the need for expensive equipment and the requirement for adjunctive balloon angioplasty in the majority of patients.

Stents

Small numbers of right coronary ostial lesions treated with stents have been reported in the literature. There is one report of Palmaz-Schatz stenting for ostial lesions (37), including only four right coronary lesions. Technical considerations for the stenting of ostial lesions will be discussed subsequently with regard to the treatment of ostial vein graft lesions. It has been our practice to reserve stents in the right coronary ostium for acute or threatened closure or multiple restenoses.

LEFT MAIN OSTIAL LESIONS

Left main ostial stenoses are rare targets for percutaneous intervention. The ELCA registry demonstrated that patients with left main ostial stenosis treated with percutaneous laser therapy have a significantly worse late outcome compared with patients with ostial right coronary or saphenous vein graft disease. The procedure was initially successful in 24 of 26 patients without any death or requirement for emergency bypass surgery. Two patients had a non–Q-wave myocardial infarction. Of 24 patients in the series with 6-month follow-up, 64% had angiographically documented restenosis, one-half had an adverse event during follow-up, and only one-third remained functional class 0, I, or II.

Similar data are not available for balloon angioplasty or other devices used to treat ostial left main disease. Although the risk of bypass surgery and repeat bypass surgery (38) is higher in patients with left main stenosis, it appears that surgical therapy in this group of patients may be more likely to result in good long-term outcome.

If coronary bypass surgery is not an alternative, percutaneous therapy may be performed with caution. Consideration should be given to the use of prophylactic intraaortic balloon counterpulsation or percutaneous bypass in patients with unprotected left main stenosis with or without depressed left ventricular systolic function.

OSTIAL VEIN GRAFT LESIONS

Balloon Angioplasty

Angioplasty of proximal saphenous vein graft lesions is plagued by a very high rate of restenosis. Douglas reported an angiographic restenosis rate of 62% (31 of 50) for these lesions in a compilation of patients from different series (39). The Mid America Heart Institute reported an initial success rate of 85% in a series of 25 saphenous vein graft and 35 right coronary artery ostial lesions with 31% of patients requiring repeat intervention for restenosis in an average 19-month follow-up (24). In an analysis of vein graft interventions using both balloon angioplasty and new devices, ostial location was a strong predictor of late cardiac events (40).

Technical considerations for the angioplasty of ostial vein graft lesions are similar to those involved with angioplasty of right coronary ostial stenoses. Although ostial vein graft lesions are infrequently calcified, they are often very resistent to dilitation caused by fibrotic tissue. Balloons constructed to withstand high inflation pressures are recommended. Although some authors have recommended oversizing balloons for the treatment of vein graft lesions, it is our practice to start with one-to-one sizing.

Directional Atherectomy

In view of the poor results of balloon angioplasty for ostial vein graft lesions, many have advocated the use of directional atherectomy. Robertson et al. reported an 81% acute success rate for 21 saphenous vein graft lesions (41). Long-term results, however, appear to be disappointing. In a series of 11 patients who underwent directional atherectomy of 12 ostial vein graft stenoses at the Mayo Clinic (42), the procedure was successful in all. Ten of the 11 patients had repeat coronary angiography within 6 months. Angiographic restenosis was found in 6 (55%) of 11 treated lesions. Over a longer follow-up (11.5 ± 9.5 months) seven patients had repeat intervention, two patients had repeat CABG, and two patients died.

The second coronary angioplasty versus excisional atherectomy trial (CAVEAT II) has randomized 305 patients with saphenous vein graft disease to atherectomy or angioplasty (43). Of the entire group, 56 patients in the trial had ostial lesions. Twenty-nine were randomized to atherectomy and twenty-seven to angioplasty. Results of this trial, which should be available soon, will provide a comparison of the two procedures for ostial vein graft lesions.

Excimer Laser Coronary Angioplasty

The excimer laser coronary angioplasty registry series (23) reported on 56 ostial vein graft lesions. Acute success was obtained in 54 of 56 patients (91.5%). No patient died or required emergency bypass surgery, and only one patient had a Q-wave myocardial infarction. Another series of excimer laser reported a 100% success rate for the treatment of 64 ostial saphenous vein graft lesions (44). Techniques of laser therapy for ostial vein graft lesions are similar to those previously discussed for ostial right coronary lesions.

Stents

Stents may have a role in the therapy of ostial saphenous vein graft lesions. While the biliary stent is not FDA approved for use in coronary arteries, recent studies demonstrating reduced restenosis rates with these stents in vein grafts are encouraging. This patient group appears to have a high rate of late clinical events both with and without restenosis (45, 46). Figure 21A.4 illustrates the treatment of an ostial vein graft lesion with a biliary stent.

The use of stents at ostial locations has several theoretic advantages. First, the ostial location entails high flow through a large seg-

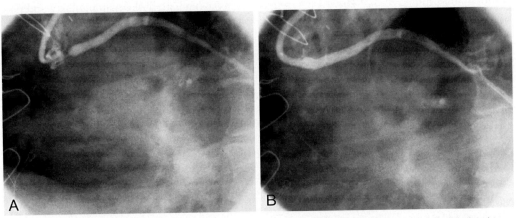

Figure 21A.4. Stenting of an ostial vein graft lesion. **A.** Severe ostial stenosis of a saphenous vein graft to the obtuse marginal branch. **B.** After deployment of a PS204 stent.

ment of the vessel. These are the two most important characteristics for avoiding stent thrombosis. Second, stents may be particularly useful in preventing elastic recoil at ostial locations. For these reasons, the use of intracoronary stents for the treatment of ostial lesions deserves careful study.

Teirstein reported Palmaz-Schatz stenting for 28 ostial lesions (37), including aorto-ostial and branch ostial lesions. There was an 89% primary success rate. Although there were no acute closures, two patients had subacute closure leading to myocardial infarction and one died as a result. Of 17 patients undergoing 6-month follow-up angiography, six had restenoses.

There are several important technical considerations when using stents to treat ostial coronary lesions. Delivery of the stent to the appropriate location is critical. The recent consensus among experienced stent operators is to leave a small "tail" (1 to 2 mm) of the stent in the aorta to be certain the diseased segment is fully covered. To date, this practice has not been associated with embolic complications. The use of a half (disarticulated) Palmaz-Schatz stent with a length of only 7 mm has been reported in two patients (47). Intravascular ultrasound is very helpful in confirming appropriate stent expansion and location (32, 48). Once the stent is deployed in an ostial location, it is important to avoid deformation of the stent by manipulations of the guiding catheter. Therefore it is recommended that guide catheter manipulation be minimized after stent deployment and that final angiographic assessment be performed using a diagnostic catheter.

BRANCH OSTIAL LESIONS

Though frequently grouped together with aorto-ostial lesions in studies of ostial lesions, the approach to non–aorto-ostial (branch ostial) lesions is technically different, and initial success and complication rates are different as well. For example, there is evidence to suggest that atherectomy of non–aorto-ostial lesions has a higher success rate and a lower complication rate compared with atherectomy of aorto-ostial lesions. Robertson and colleagues at Sequoia Hospital reported a success rate of 92% for 75 non–aorto-ostial lesions compared with 78% in 41 aorto-ostial lesions ($P = .06$) (41); 4.9% of patients with aorto-ostial lesions required emergency bypass surgery compared with none of the patients with branch ostial lesions. Success rates reported for individual locations were as follows: left anterior descending, 95%; circumflex, 86%; diagonal, 71%; left main, 78%; and saphenous vein graft, 81%. An important message from this analysis is that it may be misleading to group aorto-ostial and non–aorto-ostial lesions together when evaluating a new technique for the therapy of ostial lesions.

Atherectomy Versus Angioplasty: CAVEAT I

The coronary angioplasty versus excisional atherectomy trial (CAVEAT) included 73 patients with ostial left anterior descending lesions who were randomized to therapy with either balloon angioplasty or directional atherectomy (27). Treatment of an ostial LAD lesion with atherectomy is illustrated in Figure 21A.5. The results of angioplasty and atherectomy for these 73 patients are shown in Table 21A.2. For comparison, the results for the treatment of nonostial LAD lesions are also shown. Success rates, as quantified by the angiographic core laboratory and defined as <50% residual stenosis, were identical for the two procedures (86.5% and 86.7% for atherectomy and angioplasty, respectively). The incidence of myocardial infarction, emergency bypass surgery, and death was also similar for the two procedures. By logistic regression analysis there was no significant difference between atherectomy and balloon angioplasty for the treatment of ostial LAD lesions in terms of initial success, acute complications, or restenosis. However, in the

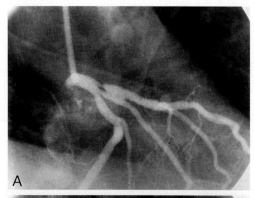

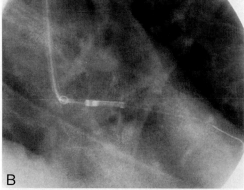

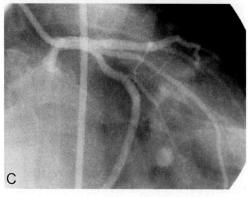

Figure 21A.5. Atherectomy of ostial LAD lesion. **A.** Eighty percent ostial LAD stenosis in RAO projection. **B.** Atherectomy device (7 Fr) cutting at the lesion. **C.** Final angiographic result. (From Topol EJ, ed. Textbook of interventional cardiology. 2nd ed. Philadelphia: WB Saunders, 1993 with permission.)

Table 21A.2
CAVEAT Experience With Ostial LAD Lesions Compared With Nonostial LAD Lesions

	Ostial LAD		Nonostial LAD	
	DCA (%)	PTCA (%)	DCA (%)	PTCA (%)
N	40	33	250	237
Success				
no	5 (13.5)	4 (13.3)	22 (9.0)	50 (22.0)
yes	32 (86.5)	26 (86.7)	221 (91.0)	177 (78.0)
Restenosis				
no	16 (51.6)	14 (53.3)	93 (49.2)	52 (32.4)
yes	15 (48.4)	12 (46.2)	96 (50.8)	100 (65.8)
Acute complications				
Death	0 (0.0)	0 (0.0)	0 (0.0)	2 (0.8)
MI	3 (7.5)	2 (6.1)	20 (8.0)	7 (3.0)
CABG	2 (5.0)	1 (3.0)	4 (1.6)	5 (2.1)

CAVEAT, Coronary angioplasty versus excisional atherectomy trial; *LAD*, left anterior descending; *DCA*, directional coronary atherectomy; *PTCA*, percutaneous transluminal coronary angioplasty; *MI*, myocardial infarction; *CABG*, emergency coronary artery bypass grafting.

treated by both procedures. There was no significant difference in the rate of procedure success, acute complications, or restenosis. These findings contrast sharply with the findings for the treatment of aorto-ostial lesions as reviewed above and underscore the point that aorto-ostial lesions and branch ostial lesions should be considered separately.

Rotablator

Rotablator series have included branch ostial lesions with a very high rate of initial success (21, 49). Popma and colleagues reported an initial success rate of 30 out of 31 (97%) for left anterior descending ostial lesions and 21 out of 22 (95%) for circumflex ostial lesions (21). Adjunctive balloon angioplasty was performed in 85% of the procedures in this series.

Technical considerations for rotational atherectomy of branch ostial lesions are similar to those described for rotablation of right coronary artery ostial stenoses. The technique is particularly useful for calcified lesions. One unique consideration for branch ostial lesions is the potential for embolization of debris down the uninvolved artery. This can lead to "no reflow" phenomena in both the

nonostial location of the proximal left anterior descending lesion, there was an advantage of atherectomy over angioplasty with regard to restenosis and initial success.

In a further analysis, ostial LAD lesions were compared with nonostial LAD lesions circumflex and left anterior descending distribution with resultant serious ischemia.

CURRENT APPROACH AND CONCLUSIONS

Balloon angioplasty of ostial stenoses is associated with a lower initial success rate, higher rates of procedural complications, and a high rate of restenosis. Although many new technologies have been advocated for the treatment of these lesions, it remains to be demonstrated that any are truly superior to balloon angioplasty. Rotational atherectomy, directional atherectomy, excimer laser, and stenting all hold potential promise since the effect of debulking or more extensive luminal expansion are desirable features of ostial intervention.

Our current approach at the Cleveland Clinic is to use the Rotablator plus adjunctive balloon for calcified ostial lesions, particularly those of the right coronary artery, and directional atherectomy for noncalcified lesions. De novo stenting for native coronary ostial lesions is increasingly being used in select patients and may prove to be particularly well suited for ostial vein graft lesions. Intravascular ultrasound is most helpful at the putative "end of the intervention" to monitor the extent of luminal expansion and to press on if the result is not fully adequate. Hopefully, ongoing research will serve to better define the most appropriate therapeutic strategy for this challenging lesion subgroup.

REFERENCES

1. Pritchard CL, Mudd JG, Barner HB. Coronary ostial stenosis. Circulation 1975;52:46–48.
2. Thompson R. Isolated coronary ostial stenosis in women. J Am Coll Cardiol 1986;7:997–1003.
3. Rissanen V. Occurrence of coronary ostial stenosis in a necropsy series of myocardial infarction, sudden death, and violent death. Br Heart J 1975;37:182–191.
4. Scharfman WB, Wallach JB, Angrist A. Myocardial infarction due to syphilitic coronary ostial stenosis. Am Heart J 1950;40:603–613.
5. Roberts W, Ferrans V, Levy R, Fredrickson D. Cardiovascular pathology in hyperlipoproteinemia. Am J Cardiol 1973;31:557–570.
6. Ribeiro P, Shapiro L, Gonzales A, Thompson G, Oakley C. Cross-sectional echocardiographic assessment of the aortic root and coronary ostial stenosis in familial hypercholesterolemia. Br Heart J 1983;50:432–437.
7. Chun P, Jones R, Robinowitz M, Davia J, Lawrence P. Coronary arterial stenosis in Takayasu's arteritis. Chest 1980;78:330–331.
8. Martin de Dios R, Pey J, Cazzaniga M et al. Coronary arterial stenosis and subclavian steal in Takayasu's arteritis. Eur J Cardiol 1981;12:229–234.
9. Handler CE, Livesey S, Lawton PA. Coronary ostial stenosis after radiotherapy: angioplasty or coronary artery surgery? Br Heart J 1989;61:208–211.
10. Nakhjavan FK, Yazdanfar S, Friedman A. Percutaneous transluminal coronary angioplasty for stenosis of the ostium of the right coronary artery after irradiation for Hodgkin's disease. Am J Cardiol 1984;53:341–342.
11. Silver MD, Wigle ED, Trimble AS et al. Iatrogenic coronary ostial stenosis. Circulation 1972;146:989–994.
12. Midell AI, DeBoer A, Bermudez G. Postperfusion coronary ostial stenosis: incidence and significance. J Thorac Cardiovasc Surg 1976;72:80–85.
13. Wilson VE, Bates ER. Subacute bilateral coronary ostial stenoses following cardiac catheterization and PTCA. Cathet Cardiovasc Diagn 1991;23:114–116.
14. Waller BF, Pinkerton CA, Foster LN. Morphological evidence of accelerated left main coronary artery stenosis: a late complication of percutaneous transluminal balloon angioplasty of the proximal left anterior descending coronary artery. J Am Coll Cardiol 1987;9:1019–1023.
15. Bashore TT, Hanna ES, Edgett J, Geiger J. Iatrogenic left main coronary artery stenosis following PTCA or valve replacement. Clin Cardiol 1985;8:114–117.
16. Graf RH, Verani MS. Left main coronary artery stenosis: a possible complication of transluminal coronary angioplasty. Cathet Cardiovasc Diagn 1984;10:163–166.
17. Hamad N, Pichard A, Oboler A, Lindsay J. Left main coronary artery stenosis as a late complication of percutaneous transluminal coronary angioplasty. Am J Cardiol 1987;60:1183–1184.
18. Stewart JT, Ward DE, Davies MJ, Pepper JR. Isolated coronary ostial stenosis: observations on pathology. Eur Heart J 1987;8:917–920.
19. Popma JJ, Dick RJL, Haudenschild CC, Topol EJ, Ellis SG. Atherectomy of right coronary ostial stenoses: initial and long-term results, technical features and histologic findings. Am J Cardiol 1991;67:431–433.
20. Topol EJ, Ellis SG, Fishman J et al. Multicenter study of percutaneous transluminal angioplasty for right coronary artery ostial stenosis. J Am Coll Cardiol 1987;9:1214–1218.
21. Popma JJ, Brogan WC, Pichard AD et al. Rotational atherectomy of ostial stenoses. Am J Cardiol 1993;71:436–438.
22. Bernardi MM, Cleman MW, Whitlow PL. Treatment of right coronary artery ostial stenosis with rotational atherectomy: results of a multi-center registry. Circulation 1993;88(4):I-546.
23. Eigler NL, Weinstock B, Douglas JS, Goldenberg T,

Hartzler G, Holmes D, Leon M et al. Excimer laser coronary angioplasty of aorto-ostial stenoses: results of the excimer laser coronary angioplasty (ELCA) registry in the first 200 patients. Circulation 1993;88:2049–2057.

24. Beddotto JB, McConahay DR, Rutherford BD, Giorgi LV, Johnson WL, Shimshak TM, Hartzler GO. Balloon angioplasty of aorta coronary ostial stenoses revisited. Circulation 1991;84(Suppl II):II-251.

25. Vallbracht C, Althen D, Kneissl GD, Kadel C, Hartmann A, Kober G, Kaltenbach M. Conventional PTCA in ostial lesions is better than its reputation. Eur Heart J 1993; 14:247.

26. Muller DW, Ellis SG, Debowey DL, Topol EJ. Quantitative angiographic comparison of the immediate success of coronary angioplasty, coronary atherectomy and endoluminal stenting. Am J Cardiol 1990;66:938–942.

27. Topol EJ, Leya FL, Pinkerton CA, Whitlow PL, Hofling B, Simonton CA, Masden RR et al. A comparison of directional atherectomy with coronary angioplasty in patients with coronary artery disease. N Engl J Med 1993; 329(4):221–227.

28. Kerwin PM, McKeever LS, Marek JC, Hartmann JR, Enger EL. Directional atherectomy of aorto-ostial stenoses. Cathet Cardiovasc Diagn 1993;(Suppl I):17–25.

29. Whitlow PL. Guiding catheters for directional coronary atherectomy. Cathet Cardiovasc Diagn 1993;(Suppl I):72–75.

30. Selmon MR, Hinohara T, Robertson GC, Vetter JW, Sheehan DJ, McAuley BJ, Gress JP et al. Use of the new low-profile directional coronary atherectomy SCA-EX devices. Circulation 1993;88(Suppl I):I-496.

31. Hinohara T, Rowe MH, Robertson GC, Selmon MR, Braden L, Leggett JH, Vetter JW et al. Effect of lesion characteristics on outcome of directional coronary atherectomy. J Am Coll Cardiol 1991;17(5):1112–1120.

32. Nakamura S, Mahon DJ, Yang J, Zelman R, Moore D, Tobis JM. Intravascular ultrasound imaging before and after directional coronary atherectomy (DCA). Circulation 1993; 88(Suppl I):I-502.

33. Lawson CS, Cooper IC, Webb-Peploe MM. Initial experience with excimer laser angioplasty for coronary ostial stenoses. Br Heart J 1993;69:255–259.

34. Leon MB, Henson KD, Javier SP, S MG, Greenberg AO, Sweet LC, Bucher TA et al. Early results with directional laser angioplasty in unfavorable coronary lesions. Circulation 1993;88(Suppl I):I-23.

35. Ghazzal ZMB, Litvack F. Rothbaum DA, Shefer A, King SB. The directional laser catheter: quantitative angiographic core lab analysis from the first five centers. Circulation 1993;88(Suppl I):I-23.

36. Weinstock BS, Eigler NL, Litvack F. Excimer laser angioplasty of aorto-ostial stenosis in 175 patients: acute and follow-up results and core lab analysis. J Am Coll Cardiol 1993;21:289A.

37. Teirstein P, Stratienko AA, Schatz RA. Coronary stenting for ostial stenoses: initial results and six-month follow-up. Circulation 1991;84(Suppl II): II-251.

38. Loop FD, Lytle BW, Cosgrove DM, Woods EL, Stewart RW, Golding LAR, Goormastic M et al. Reoperation for coronary atherosclerosis: changing practice in 2509 consecutive patients. Ann Surg 1990;212:378–385.

39. Douglas JS. Angioplasty of saphenous vein and internal mammary artery bypass grafts. In Topol EJ, ed. Textbook of interventional cardiology. Philadelphia: WB Saunders, 1990.

40. Hong MK, Chuang YC, Prunka N, Satler LF. Predictors of early and late cardiac events in patients undergoing saphenous vein graft angioplasty with PTCA and new device modalities. Circulation 1993;88(Suppl I):I-601.

41. Robertson GC, Simpson JB, Vetter JW, Selmon MR, Doucette JW, Sheehan DJ, McAuley BJ et al. Directional coronary atherectomy for ostial lesions. Circulation 1991; 84(Suppl II):II-25.

42. Garratt KN, Bell MR, Berger PB, Bresnahan JF, Higano ST. Directional coronary atherectomy of saphenous vein graft ostial lesions. Circulation 1991;84(Suppl II)II-26.

43. Caveat II Investigators. The coronary angioplasty versus excisional atherectomy trial (CAVEAT) II: preliminary results. Circulation 1993;88(Suppl I):I-594.

44. Tcheng JE, Bittl JA, Sanborn TA et al. Treatment of aorto-ostial disease with percutaneous excimer laser coronary angioplasty. Circulation 1992;86(Suppl I):I-512.

45. Fenton S, Fischman D, Savage M, Schatz R, Goldberg S. Long-term angiographic and clinical outcome after implantation of balloon-expandable stents in saphenous vein grafts: a report from the core angiographic laboratory. Circulation 1993;88(Suppl I):I-308.

46. Piana RN, Kugelmass AD, Moscucci M, Cohen DJ, Gordon PC, Senerchia C, Kuntz RE. Angiographic and clinical outcome of endoluminal stenting for stenotic saphenous vein grafts—single center experience. Circulation 1993; 88(Suppl I):I-308.

47. Nordrehaug JE, Priestley K, Chronos N, Buller N, Sigwart U. Implantation of half Palmaz-Schatz stents in short aorto-ostial lesions of saphenous vein grafts. Cathet Cardiovasc Diagn 1993;29:141–143.

48. Goldberg SL, Colombo A, Almagor Y, Maiello L, Gaglione A, Nakamura S, Tobis JM. Can intravascular ultrasound improve coronary stent deployment? Circulation 1993; 88(Suppl I)(4):I-597.

49. Goudreau E, Cowley MJ, DiSciascio G, DeBotis D, Vetrovec GW, Sabri N. Rotational atherectomy for aorto-ostial and branch-ostial lesions. J Am Coll Cardiol 1993;21:31A.

B. The Ostial Lesion: Clinical Aspects, Interventional Devices, and Case Studies

NEAL EIGLER and FRANK LITVACK

Although advances in the technology and technique of percutaneous transluminal coronary angioplasty (PTCA) have improved its safety and efficacy, certain coronary lesion morphologies are relatively poor candidates for balloon dilatation (1, 2). One such morphology, the ostial stenosis, has been associated with a reduced acute succes rate, more frequent complications, and a high rate of restenosis. Newer types of interventional devices, including lasers, atherectomy, and stents, now play an important role in treating these patients. This chapter is organized to present a concise review of the clinical aspects of the ostial lesion and the results of various angioplasty devices. Additionally, we will comment on their application, with attention focused on technique and procedural judgment. Finally, we will describe several illustrative cases with an emphasis on either avoiding or treating threatened complications so that the reader may profit from our experience.

CLINICAL FEATURES OF OSTIAL STENOSIS

Stenosis of the coronary and vein graft ostia (within 3 mm from the origin) is a morphologic class of lesions that differ from disease of other coronary segments with respect to patient demographics, histopathology, etiology, and response to the mechanical injury following balloon angioplasty. Aorto-ostial stenosis of the right and left coronary arteries is a rare condition seen in 0.8 to 1.3% of coronary arteriograms performed for suspected coronary artery disease (3, 4). A substantial majority of patients (81 to 86%) have multivessel coronary disease. The subgroup of patients with isolated ostial stenosis, however, tends to be exclusively younger women, 30 to 50 years old, with a low incidence of risk factors for coronary disease and a short, progressive history of angina. In one such instance the obstruction was documented to be a lipid-rich, fissured, atherosclerotic plaque with fresh obstructive thrombus (5). Patient subsets undergoing angioplasty of an aorto-ostial stenosis have a higher proportion of women and tend to be older than when disease is located in other segments (6, 7). Aorto-ostial lesions have been described as having simultaneously rigid and elastic characteristics based on the response to balloon angioplasty (8). This apparent paradox may be explained by the presence of older fibrotic lesions, which frequently contain dense calcific deposits in continuity with the plentiful, multilayered elastic fibers of the aortic wall. Higher balloon inflation pressures are required to overcome the intrinsic rigidity of the stenosis, and compression of the adjacent elastic structures results in spring-back or recoil once the balloon is deflated. For the same reason, recoil frequently limits angioplasty success for ostial stenosis of saphenous vein grafts. Stenosis at the proximal anastomosis of vein grafts has also been attributed to the acute angulation of the graft from the aortic root causing a slitlike lumen or an unduly large aortotomy (9, 10). Even less frequently, aorto-ostial lesions may not be atherosclerotic in origin, but may be the result of the healing response to vascular injury following thoracic irradiation for malignancy or inflammatory changes following coronary bypass surgery, or may be associated with chronic inflammatory diseases such as syphilitic aortitis or nonspecific aortitis.

Stenosis of the origin of the left anterior descending, left circumflex, or other branch coronary artery more closely resembles the atherosoclerotic lesions of the major coronary segments with respect to age and gender distribution. Technical failure of angioplasty has been primarily attributed to elastic recoil (11). This again may be a consequence of more plentiful elastic fiber content present because of increased shear stress at bifurcations (12).

The criteria for selecting patients with ostial disease for revascularization is now fundamentally no different from selecting any other patient for angioplasty. The vast majority of the patients with ostial disease are technically approachable by one device or another. The first question to be asked is—

does the patient really require revascularization? The only demonstrated beneficial outcome of angioplasty in these lesions is to alleviate symptoms; treating minimally symptomatic patients, even those with extensive manifest ischemia, has yet to be proven beneficial and remains controversial. Fibrocalcific aorto-ostial disease is often chronic, and the plaques are stable with a low propensity for abrupt occlusion. Such patients can often be successfully medically managed for long periods until their symptoms progress. Patients with significant left main disease severe multivessel disease, or depressed left ventricular function are often best managed with bypass surgery. Thus symptomatic and intractable patients with isolated ostial disease are probably best suited for catheter-based intervention.

Rather than declare a device or strategy superior for a given lesion, the sections below indicate that a skilled operator may be able to perform successful angioplasty with any of several devices. It is more important to anticipate the specific limitations of each device with respect to anatomic and procedural variables.

Before discussing individual devices, there are important considerations for choosing guiding catheters and guidewires. The immediate proximity of the stenotic lesion to the tip of the guide catheter in aorto-ostial disease deserves special consideration. Ideally, the guide should not be capable of deeply intubating the ostia because this will become an injured surface, ripe for further traumatic dissection. As such, support for crossing the stenosis is accomplished by other means, including using the intrinsic stiffness of the guide catheter, bracing the opposite aortic wall or aortic cusp, ensuring the guide catheter is coaxial with the vessel lumen, and using stiff-shaft guidewires (e.g., high-torque floppy, extra-support; ACS) for added trackability. Other considerations include catheter damping with reduced coronary perfusion and use of the guide catheter to enlarge and control the quantity of plaque debulking. A guide catheter without side holes will predictably impede flow in aorto-ostial disease. Guide-catheter side holes, whether factory-made or carefully punched in the laboratory by the operator, are a must. Not only do they enhance perfusion, they also permit runoff after contrast injection and serve as a blow-off relief exit for the high-pressure jet of contrast injection into the small volume of the coronary lumen and thus may prevent some dissections or even some vessel ruptures.

BALLOON ANGIOPLASTY

Despite the widespread recognition that balloon angioplasty of aorto-ostial stenosis has a relatively lower success and higher complication rate, there is only minimal literature documentation. In the only published series Topol et al. (8) described 53 patients undergoing PTCA of the right coronary ostia at three high-volume centers between 1981 and 1986. Acute success was low at 79%. Technical failure was attributed to the frequent presence of calcified, unexpandable lesions, elastic recoil, and poor guide-catheter support; 9.4% required emergency bypass surgery predominantly caused by propagating intimal dissection. Follow-up of initially successful patients revealed clinical recurrence in 48%, and in the subgroup with repeat angiography the restenosis rate was 73%. Six-month follow-up events included bypass surgery in 19% and repeat PTCA in 14%. The authors warned that angioplasty was suboptimal treatment for right coronary ostial disease and that bypass surgery should be considered the treatment of choice.

No study has specifically addressed success, complications, or restenosis at the ostia of saphenous vein grafts; however, the overall primary success rate of PTCA at all vein graft sites ranges from 78 to 94%, and restenosis rates of 48 to 68% have been reported (13–15). These disappointing results led to a reduced use of PTCA for aorto-ostial stenosis and constitute the rationale for testing second-generation interventional devices, including laser, atherectomy, and stents. Alternatively, these data may also reflect balloon angioplasty as practiced prior to 1988 before the widespread use of high-pressure and perfusion balloons. Preliminary results of a recent series of 55 patients, which included those with right coronary and vein graft ostial lesions at one referral center, showed that improved acute results may be achievable with PTCA alone (16). Although angiographic success was described in 85% and there were no major ischemic complications, a substantial proportion of patients (31%) required a repeat revascularization procedure during follow-up.

Even less is known about balloon angioplasty of stenosis at the ostium of the major left coronary primary branch vessels. One preliminary report with follow-up angiographic results compared 30 patients with left anterior descending ostial stenosis with 142 patients with stenosis elsewhere in the LAD (17). Using a loss of 50% of the original gain as the definition of recurrence, they reported that ostial lesions had a 63% restenosis rate compared with 38% for the other locations. These authors concluded that, despite similar immediate angioplasty results, ostial LAD stenosis has a significantly higher restenosis rate.

Balloon angioplasty of ostial stenosis in a more distal branch vessel is also associated with lower success and higher complication rates. Mathias et al. (11) described 106 patients with 109 ostial branch stenoses out of a group of 1274 consecutive patients undergoing PTCA. The distribution of ostial branch lesions included a diagonal in 58, a posterior descending in 21, and an obtuse marginal or ramus branch in 40. In most the lesions involved only the origin of the branch vessel, but in 39% the stenosis included the bifurcation. Despite using slightly oversized balloons, the angiographic success rate of 74% for the ostial branch stenoses was significantly less compared with 91% for nonostial

locations. The lower success rate was directly attributed to elastic recoil. Moreover, the major complication rate was 13% versus 5% for non-ostial disease, a significant increase. Double-wire and double-balloon techniques were useful for preserving side-branch patency; however, they did not appear to improve the technical success of the dilated ostial branch or to prevent ischemic complications. Clinical follow-up was available in all 88 successful patients at a mean of 7.8 months. Only 22% required repeat angiography, and 72% were asymptomatic or improved. Repeat PTCA was performed in 12, and only two patients required bypass surgery and two suffered a myocardial infarction. Thus, once successfully dilated, branch ostial stenoses appear to have recurrence and adverse-event rates similar to angioplasty at other nonostial locations.

Comment. Balloon angioplasty probably should not be considered as "stand-alone" treatment for aorto-ostial stenosis because it does not address the problem of recoil and is less effective in calcified lesions. On the other hand, balloon angioplasty is an important adjunctive strategy for each of the other devices. Balloon angioplasty may be employed prior to using another device to predilate the lesion and thus to assist in the passage of a larger-profile device such as a directional atherectomy catheter or a stent. PTCA is now more frequently used following debulking with a laser or with atherectomy devices when the stenosis may be more pliable and less resilient. The goal of using adjunctive balloon angioplasty is to achieve the largest acute gain in lumen dimensions to offset the consequences of late loss from intimal proliferation and chronic recoil.

Balloon angioplasty with a perfusion balloon is often a successful, single-modality treatment for ostial disease of the LAD or circumflex arteries, albeit these lesions still represent a high risk if acute closure compromises the left main coronary. Despite the hemodynamic advantages of a perfusion balloon, obstruction of the major, uninvolved branch of the left coronary may result in a large ischemic burden and the inability to achieve prolonged balloon inflation.

Lastly, a new type of balloon with longitudinal cutting blades on the balloon surface has been developed (Barath Cutting Balloon, IVT). Balloon expansion results in radially directed intimal and medial incisions, the goal of which is to interrupt the fibrous cap of the atheroma and the elastic components of the nondiseased arc of vessel wall in eccentric stenoses. Clinical trials are now under way, and the acute results, including those of rigid, undilatable lesions and ostial branch stenoses, appear promising (18).

EXCIMER LASER ANGIOPLASTY

The strategy of debulking the stenotic mass prior to balloon dilatation makes intrinsic sense for treating the dual rigidity and elastic characteristics of the aorto-ostial lesion. In theory, ablation of fibrocalcific plaque will render it more pliable to balloon expansion and perhaps less susceptible to developing lumen-compromising dissection. Moreover, recoil may be reduced because less tissue is displaced to achieve a given balloon diameter.

Excimer laser coronary angioplasty (ELCA) has been reported to be effective therapy for patients with anatomy deemed suboptimal for PTCA, including patients with aorto-ostial stenosis (19, 20). A prospective multicenter registry report documented improved acute success and a low incidence of major complications in 209 stenoses in the first 200 consecutive patients with aorto-ostial stenosis treated with the LAIS concentric excimer laser catheter system (6). These patients constituted 9.5% of the total patients treated with ELCA in these centers. The mean age was 65 ± 9 years, and almost half of the patients (47%) were women. The distribution of stenotic locations was the left main coronary in 26, the right coronary in 124, and vein grafts in 59

cases. The left main was protected by a patent bypass graft in all but six cases. Procedural success, defined as achieving a ≤50% stenosis in the absence of major in-hospital complications, was 90% and was not affected by lesion location (left main, right coronary, and vein graft—92%, 89%, and 90%, respectively). Adjunctive PTCA was performed in 72%. Univariate and multivariate logistic regression analysis of demographic and angiographic variables showed that the only predictor of procedure failure was female gender.

The vessels treated tended to be large in size with a mean reference normal diameter of 3.3 ± 1.0 mm, and stenoses were generally short in length averaging 3.5 ± 2.8 mm. Quantitative angiography documented an improvement in percent diameter stenosis from 76 ± 14% to 36 ± 15% ($P < .01$). The acute gain in diameter was 1.3 ± 0.6 mm, increasing from 0.8 to 2.1 mm. The majority of the gain (1.0 ± 0.6 mm) resulted from laser angioplasty, and the lumen diameter on average was the same diameter of the laser catheter. Adjunctive PTCA yielded an additional 0.5 ± 0.5 mm gain. The resultant lumen was, however, significantly smaller than the nominal diameter of the inflated balloon (2.1 versus 3.1 mm; $P < .001$). These data suggest that there may be less acute recoil after tissue ablation but that recoil still occurs after adjunctive PTCA.

Major in-hospital complications occurred in 3.9%. There were no deaths, Q-wave myocardial infarction was infrequent, occurring in one patient (0.5%), and bypass surgery was required in seven (3.4%) of the cases. Less severe complications included non–Q-wave MI (defined as any diagnostic elevation of CK) in 6.3% and dissection extending beyond the lesion in 3.9%. There were two (1.0%) perforations, neither of which required additional therapy.

Six-month angiographic follow-up, available in 51%, documented an average diameter stenosis of 1.7 ± 1.0 mm or 46 ± 26%. Restenosis defined as a greater than 50%

diameter stenosis occurred in 39%. Restenosis was more common for the left main at 64% than for the right coronary or vein grafts, each with a 35% incidence. Restenosis was less likely when residual stenosis at the completion of the procedure was ≤35%, with an incidence of 28% compared with 53% (P <.05).

Clinical events at follow-up were available in 100% of initially successful cases. Death was reported in 2.7%, bypass surgery in 6.5%, and myocardial infarction in 2.2%; repeat angioplasty was performed in 16.2%. An adverse event during follow-up was more than twice as likely in the group of patients treated for stenosis of the left main, with an incidence of 50% compared with 21% for the right coronary and vein graft patients.

These results indicate a high frequency of adverse outcomes in patients with left main disease. Such patients are also at higher risk to undergo repeat bypass surgery. Loop et al. (21) reported that the surgical mortality in 80 consecutive patients exceeded 20%, an increase in relative risk of 6.9-fold compared with other patients undergoing repeat CABG. Moreover, long-term survival was also significantly diminished with a relative risk of 2.0. Despite these risks, surgical treatment has a high likelihood of providing sustained improvement and should presently be considered as the method of first choice for primary and repeat revascularization in patients with ostial left main stenosis.

Nearly identical results with respect to patient selection, acute outcome, and follow-up are now available for the first 173 patients with aorto-ostial stenosis similarly treated with another excimer laser system (Spectranetics) (22) (J.E. Tcheng, personal communication). This multicenter registry also reports a success rate of 90% with adjunctive PTCA required in 75%. Death occurred in three patients, two of which had left main involvement; bypass surgery was required in 4% during hospitalization; there were no Q-wave or non–Q-wave myocardial infarctions; and one

patient had a significant perforation. Unstable angina and calcification were multivariate predictors of procedural failure. At present there are no series of laser-treated patients with ostial stenosis of LAD, circumflex, or branch vessels, but several case examples are provided later in this chapter. Furthermore, there are no studies directly comparing laser to PTCA.

Comments and Technique. Taken together, these data indicate that a therapeutic strategy of debulking and dilating, using excimer laser in combination with balloon angioplasty, is acutely effective and safe for patients with aorto-ostial coronary stenosis. Acute complications, six-month clinical events, angiographic restenosis, and functional status are substantially poorer in the group with left main disease. Thus ELCA may be considered as an alternative to bypass surgery in carefully selected patients with isolated aorto-ostial stenosis of the right coronary artery and saphenous vein grafts.

The aorto-ostial lesion is one of the best uses of excimer laser angioplasty. Although perhaps not as efficient at ablating calcified plaque as high-speed rotational atherectomy, small-diameter laser catheters with densely packed fiber optics tuned to high energy density nearly always cross the lesion. For example, the model 1.3 mm Z (LAIS) at an energy of 60 mJ/mm^2, pulsed at 20 Hz, will cross all but the most heavily calcified stenoses. Many recalcitrant stenoses will yield by increasing the energy density to 70 mJ/mm^2 or by increasing the pulse rate to 30 Hz. Initial passage of the stenosis is usually quite rapid, and care should be taken not to advance the pulsing laser uncontrollably beyond the lesion. Once crossed, the catheter can be exchanged for a larger-diameter system if more tissue ablation is desired.

The use of multiple passes and reangulation of the guide catheter was first applied for lasing aorto-ostial lesions. The path traversed by the catheter can be altered by adjusting the

Figure 21B.1. Schematic of 1.8 mm in diameter directional excimer laser catheter (LAIS, model DLC). Features include the following: an eccentric guidewire lumen; a fiberoptic bundle located adjacent to the guidewire, a protective plastic tip that shields the opposite wall from fiber contact; an eccentric radiopaque marker for alignment of the laser bundle with the atheroma; a torque transmission control knob that rotates the tip for proper orientation.

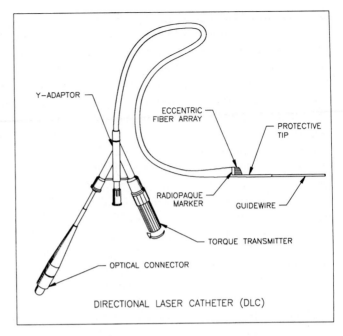

orientation of the guide catheter with respect to the diseased lumen, thereby creating a larger area of ablation. This requires a guide catheter that maintains a stable position and that can be advanced or withdrawn to angle the tip superiorly or inferiorly and the ability to apply torque for clockwise or counterclockwise rotation. Judkin's catheters are frequently inadequate, but because of their safety and controllability, they should be considered when guide-catheter difficulty is not anticipated. Left Amplatz and hockey-stick shapes are often chosen for the right coronary and left-sided bypass grafts. A multipurpose shape is frequently the best for coaxial alignment with a right-sided bypass graft.

Ischemia related to catheter obstruction is usually very brief and microembolization with its sequelae are infrequent. Thus long lesions, vein grafts, and patients with poor ventricular function frequently are candidates for laser ablation. All but the most eccentric of aortoostial stenoses can be successfully treated with the concentric type of laser catheters as long as the catheter diameter remains $\leq\frac{2}{3}$ of or 1.0 mm smaller than the adjacent normal coronary segment. Oversizing the catheter can predispose to dissection and perforation. With careful patient selection, the incidence of perforation should be less than 1%. Newer directional catheters may be particularly advantageous for highly eccentric lesions or for affecting more tissue removal with multiple passes (Fig. 21B.1).

Ostial stenosis of the LAD or circumflex can be approached with concentric excimer catheters but only with the greatest of care. Concentric catheters may be used safely if the passage from the left main to the stenosis is fairly straight. This requires performing multiple angiographic views to visualize any tortuosity of the left main bifurcation. The concentric catheters tend to preferentially ablate along the outer curvature of a bend. If the outer curvature happens to involve the carina of the bifurcation, then a perforation is much more likely. Extra downsizing of catheters is required. This problem with bifurcation lesions applies to all types of concentric ablation devices whether laser or rotational atherectomy. One potential solution is to use the newer directional type laser catheter. The

LAIS 1.8-mm DLC system is particularly well suited for the bifurcation lesion since the leading protective hooded tip can protect the wall of the outer curvature and the carina from the laser energy (Fig. 21B.2). This device offers another advantage in that a second guidewire can be placed to protect important side branches.

Results of using the directional laser catheter are available on 43 patients from five medical centers (Ghazzal, personal communication). The stenosis location distribution was the right coronary artery in 24, saphenous vein grafts in six, left main in two, and branch ostial stenosis in eleven and included four at the LAD ostium. Stenosis morphology included marked eccentricity in 33% and moderate to heavy calcification in 47%. Procedure success was achieved in 86% with the mean stenosis improving from 68% at baseline to 49% after laser to 27% after adjunctive balloon angioplasty. There were no deaths. In-hospital bypass surgery was required in two patients, one of which suffered a Q-wave myocardial infarction. There was a single uncomplicated perforation. Coronary dissection was unusual, occurring in only three patients. At present, these results should be considered preliminary and no follow-up data is available. The data suggests, however, that directional excimer laser coronary angioplasty may be a feasible alternative for patients with eccentric calcified stenosis of the ostial lesions or branch point lesions.

DIRECTIONAL ATHERECTOMY

Small numbers of patients having directional side-cutting atherectomy (DVI) of aorto-ostial stenosis in native coronaries and vein grafts have been reported. Robertson et al. (23) described their single-center experience in 41 patients with aorto-ostial and 75 patients with ostial disease primarily at the origin of the LAD and circumflex arteries. They noted a lower procedural success rate for aorto-ostial lesions compared with ostial lesions of

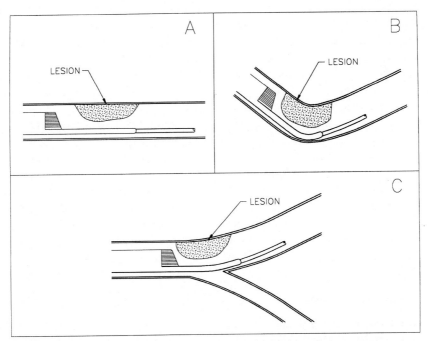

Figure 21B.2. Schematic of lesion morphologies that can be treated with the directional excimer laser catheter. **A.** Eccentric stenosis, ostial or nonostial. **B.** Eccentric stenosis located on a bend. **C.** Lesions involving a bifurcation or ostial branch stenosis.

the major left coronary branches (78% versus 92%). Aorto-ostial patients had a 4.9% incidence of acute occlusion and 4.9% required emergency bypass surgery. Success rates were lower and complications more frequent in patients with calcification. Non–aorto-ostial lesions had a more benign course: there were no cases of acute reocclusion or bypass surgery. Restenosis at six-month follow-up was 42% in non–aorto-ostial native disease and 73% in ostial vein grafts (24). There were insufficient numbers to evaluate native aorto-ostial restenosis.

Comments and Technique. Directional atherectomy should be avoided in fluoroscopically calcified arteries. Failure to retrieve tissue often signifies a hard lesion, and the degree of calcification may become apparent only following intravascular ultrasonic examination. Predilatation of fibrotic lesions is often required to allow passage of the atherectomy device. Patients with tortuous vessels, poor peripheral vascular access, and coronary vessels smaller than 3 mm in diameter are not good candidates for directional atherectomy. Excellent guide catheter support and position are prerequisites for attempting aorto-ostial lesions. This is important for avoiding catheter-induced dissection from overaggressive engagement. Also, poor guide support may be responsible for the cutting device to be unstable and spring from the ostium, risking systemic embolization of partially removed tissue. We believe that directional atherectomy is an excellent method to treat ostial stenosis of the LAD and the circumflex arteries as long as the above caveats are kept in mind. It can also be successfully used in aorto-ostial cases, but fewer patients will meet the selection criteria.

ROTATIONAL ATHERECTOMY

High-speed rotational coronary atherectomy (Heart Technology, Inc.), which ablates fibrocalcific plaque using a high-speed burr, has also been used in patients with ostial stenosis of native coronary arteries. In a single-center report, Popma et al. (7) described 105 patients (44% women, mean age 66) with lesions distributed in the left main in seven, LAD in 31, circumflex in 22, and the right coronary artery in 45. Rotational atherectomy was performed with burrs ranging from 1.25 to 2.50 mm in diameter. Adjunctive PTCA was performed in 85%.

Moderate to dense lesion calcification was present in 74%; stenoses were graded as eccentric in 70%, and the mean lesion length was 4.1 mm. The reference segment diameter of 2.6 ± 0.5 mm was smaller than in series with other second-generation devices. Minimal lumen diameter increased from 0.7 ± 0.4 to 1.5 ± 0.4 mm after rotational atherectomy, further improving to 2.0 ± 0.4 mm after PTCA. Procedural success was obtained in 97% of patients without procedure related death, or Q-wave MI. Two patients required emergency bypass surgery. Less severe complications included non–Q-wave MI, defined by a CK-MB fraction increased ≥5 times the upper limit of normal, in 8%. Coronary dissection was documented in 17%; spasm, thrombus, and side branch occlusions were each seen in 3%.

At a mean follow-up of 5.4 months, 34% had recurrent symptoms, and angiographic restenosis was observed in 23 of 73 eligible patients (32%). Adverse follow-up events included bypass surgery in seven, repeat coronary angioplasty in 11, and death in four.

Comments and Technique. High-velocity rotational atherectomy is very successful at ablating densely calcified stenoses. As with excimer laser, the strategy of debulking before dilating appears to be more successful than conventional balloon angioplasty. Importantly, when performing rotational atherectomy, the operator should consider the consequences of microembolization and be prepared to deal with it. Long lesions, noncalcified lesions, and degenerated vein graft lesions should be avoided. Right coronary ostial lesions supplying the AV node artery should be attempted after inserting a well-functioning temporary transvenous pacemaker. Transient complete heart block is a commonly occurring nuisance but invariably not a severe problem in these patients. Patients with poor left ventricular function (LVEF <30%) should be considered with extra caution since they may not tolerate protracted ischemia caused by spasm or microembolization. The 0.009-inch guidewire may be difficult to maneuver across a tight, tortuous, or eccentric stenosis. This may require using a more conventional wire first, followed by crossing the lesion with a low-profile catheter or balloon, and then exchanging for the rotational atherectomy guidewire. A 9 Fr guiding catheter should be selected so that upsizing from a small diameter burr can be more easily accomplished. As with laser, multiple passes with a large burr can be performed after reangulating the guide catheter from its initial coaxial position. This may help to create a lumen larger than the burr size. A test injection should be performed after each pass, and further ablative passes should not be performed in the presence of dissection, extravasation, or vessel closure. As with excimer laser, vessel perforation is a potential risk and the same precautions and case selection criteria apply.

STENTS

The application of stents for treating ostial stenosis is conceptually appealing because, more so than any other device, they solve the problem of acute elastic recoil. Preliminary data with elective placement of the Palmaz-Schatz stent in ostial lesions at one center in the first 41 patients suggest encouraging results (R. Schatz, personal communication). The distribution of target lesions was the ostium of the LAD in 8, the left circumflex in 2, the right coronary in 9, and saphenous vein grafts in 22 patients. In 71%, the stent was implanted for a de novo stenosis. One-third of the lesions were calcified, stenoses averaged

4.7 mm in length, and the normal vessel diameter was 3.2 mm. Three patients with lesions longer than 10 mm received tandem stents; the ostial lesion was treated with a single stent in the remainder, and six patients received an additional stent at another lesion location.

All stents were successfully implanted with good angiographic results. The postdeployment diameter was as large as the normal segment averaging 3.3 mm and thus leaving no residual stenosis. The procedural success rate was reduced to 93% because two patients suffered subacute thrombosis, both after anticoagulants were discontinued for untoward reactions. One of these patients died of cardiac causes, and a second patient died in the hospital of progressive renal failure and sepsis. Three patients had significant bleeding or vascular access complications. Follow-up angiography at six months, available in 95% of eligible patients, showed a recurrence rate of 28% with a minimal lumen diameter averaging 2.8 mm. Restenosis appeared to be more common for ostial lesions of saphenous vein grafts than for native coronaries (35% versus 19%).

Comments and Technique. At this juncture with a relatively small clinical experience, elective placement of the Palmaz-Schatz stent in carefully selected patients with ostial stenosis can be performed with excellent procedural success rates. There is insufficient experience with other stents to warrant any comment about efficacy or safety. Although there are insufficient data to document an impact on restenosis, it is reasonable to assume that, if there are benefits, they will be similar to those demonstrated in the BENESTENT and STRESS randomized trials of elective, native coronary placement and that the growing experience with the lower incidence of restenosis after stenting vein grafts will compare with rates reported for any other device.

Our experience with electively stenting aorto-ostial stenosis had been largely confined to the implantation of Palmaz-Schatz stents into saphenous vein grafts. This is usually a straightforward procedure if one adheres to a few obvious but easy-to-neglect rules. Ostial graft stenoses are seldom calcified and may be longer than their coronary counterparts. It is not unusual to exceed the length of a single, 15-mm coronary stent. Stenting vein grafts may require expansion up to 6.0 mm in diameter. This will result in the stent shortening by approximately 2 mm. Thus tandem stents are often required to expand the entire length of the stenosis. Unlike stenting the body of a vessel where the most distal stent is deployed first, it is most crucial to properly place the proximal stent precisely at the ostium and then to subsequently deliver a second stent through the lumen created by the first.

The importance of selecting the proper guide catheter, already stressed in this chapter, cannot be overemphasized. The guide must be able to align coaxial with the ostium and provide adequate support to advance the bulky stent delivery system across the stenosis. The guide catheter must be sufficiently maneuverable so that it can be torqued or backed out of the ostium during stent delivery and subsequent postdelivery stent expansion with a conventional balloon. The guide position should be stable enough not to uncontrollably engage the freshly stented ostium because of the risk of snagging a stent strut and thus making further attempts to dilate the stent hazardous. There must be adequate contrast flow around the bulky stent delivery system to clearly outline the junction of the ostium with the aorta. For these reasons, we often start with a 9 Fr left Amplatz 1 or 2 shape for left-sided bypass grafts or a 9 Fr multipurpose shape for right coronary grafts. Thin-walled, large-lumen 8 Fr guides work well in many cases, but at the first sign of difficulty one should switch to the larger-diameter guides. Although any floppy-tipped, 0.014-inch angioplasty wire will usually suffice, we often choose a floppy-tipped, extra-support wire (ACS, Temecula, CA) to enhance trackability of the high-profile stent delivery system.

Baseline angiography should be performed with attention to clearly defining the junction between the ostium and the aorta with the least foreshortening. Where possible, adjacent stationary objects such as surgical clips should be projected in the vicinity of the ostium and the precise relationship between the object and the ostium studied to use as a template when adequate contrast opacification of the ostium is impossible. Intravascular ultrasound can be of enormous value for defining the true location of the ostia, which may be assumed to be in error if the angiographic projection is foreshortened. Fluoroscopic localization of the ultrasonic crystal when it is imaging the true ostia can be used to adjust the radiographic projection for the optimal orthogonal view.

Predilatation with a 2.5-mm balloon is prerequisite. If full balloon expansion is not achievable, this indicates an extremely fibrous orifice. In such cases debulking with laser or rotational atherectomy may be helpful in making the lesion more pliable. Prior to inserting the stent, the relationship of the stent ends to the proximal and distal radiopaque markers should be carefully studied. The stent delivery system should be advanced until the entire balloon is within the vein graft before the protective sleeve is withdrawn into the guide catheter. Care must be taken that, if the balloon has been advanced too far, it be retracted in a fixed relationship with the guide catheter rather than risk reentry of the stent into the guide catheter tip, which may embolize the stent. Stent delivery should err on leaving a small portion of the stent extending into the ascending aorta. Keeping in mind the stent diameter versus length relationship, more stent should extend into the aorta when a diameter of 5 to 6 mm is desired. This is important because placing the stent distal to the true ostium may result in discrete restenosis occurring precisely at the unstented ostium.

Once deployed, we usually inflate the delivery balloon for a second brief inflation to ensure expansion of the midportion of the stent. We then withdraw the balloon so that the distal half remains in the stent and perform a third "trumpeting" inflation with the relatively compliant delivery balloon to flare the proximal end of the stent. The balloon is then removed with care not to engage the guide catheter. Postdeployment dilatation should be performed with extreme care. The introduction of 4.5- to 6.0-mm peripheral balloons may be difficult if the blunt catheter nose snags on any part of the partially expanded stent, or if the guide catheter is withdrawn and not coaxial with the ostium. Whenever possible, the stent should be expanded so there is no remaining stenosis visible. Our practice is to create the best possible angiographic appearance and then perform intravascular ultrasound to ensure that all portions of the stent are expanded and that the struts are in contact with the vascular wall. High-pressure, noncompliant balloons often work best for "punching out" a partially expanded stent. Preprocedure, periprocedure, and postprocedure compliance with antiplatelet and anticoagulation protocols are as important as they are when stenting other locations.

Recent experience with stent restenosis shows that, in addition to intimal proliferation, there may be chronic recoil of the stent, particularly in the aorto-ostial location. This may be caused by the force of scar contraction on the relatively flimsy coronary type of stent. Stronger versions of the stent, including models designed for biliary tract applications, may have advantages in this regard.

Less experience is available with elective stenting of coronary aorto-ostial stenosis. The right coronary ostia is often densely calcified or its proximal portion tortuous with a "shepherd's crook" configuration, making positioning and expansion difficult. The left main is only occasionally of sufficient length to accept a full 15-mm stent. For these reasons stronger and shorter stent models are now being developed. Ostial lesions of the LAD and circumflex are difficult targets for elective stenting. Positioning the stent leaves no room for error. If distal by even 1 to 2 mm, the lesion may be missed, and if too proximal by the smallest of margins, the adjacent major branch will be jeopardized or put into "stent jail." For these reasons we do not believe that elective permanent stenting is an acceptable definitive procedure for treating stenosis precisely at the bifurcation of the left main, but may be acceptable if the lesion starts 1 to 3 mm distal to the bifurcation.

"Bailout" stenting in the setting of threatened or manifest acute closure caused by spiral dissection, whether as definitive treatment or as a bridge to bypass surgery, can be a lifesaving procedure. Stenting almost always immediately restores brisk flow to the ischemic myocardium. For very long dissections (>25 mm) we recommend placing the most distal stent first if possible. Next, the most proximal stent can be placed in the ostial position. Lastly, any gap between the two stents should be treated with a third stent. Since the incidence of subacute stent thrombosis is at least fourfold greater than with elective placement and can be expected to occur in about 25% of cases of manifest closure, it is wise to keep these patients in the hospital for 7 to 10 days when they are at high risk for this potentially catastrophic event.

Case Examples

The conclusion of this chapter contains six brief case reports from our experience with ostial stenosis. The cases were specifically chosen to emphasize the recognition, management, and avoidance of major ischemic complications.

CASE #1

A 41-year-old male with severe angina has an unclassified metabolic disorder consisting of short stature with extensive calcification of multiple organs, including the cardiovascular system. Angiography showed extensive

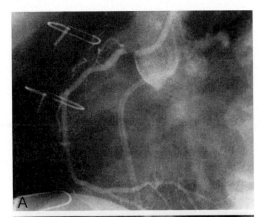

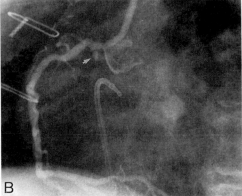

Figure 21B.3. Case #1. **A.** Pretreatment LAO right coronary angiogram showing a densely calcified, subtotal aorto-ostial stenosis. **B.** After multipass "stand-alone" excimer laser angioplasty with concentric catheter system. In addition to the marked improvement in lumen diameter there is a contained perforation *(arrow)* in the region of the lesion. The guide catheter was upsized from 8 to 9 Fr between the pretreatment and posttreatment views.

"eggshell" calcification of the entire ascending aorta and a densely calcified, 10-mm-long, subtotal stenosis of the ostial right coronary artery. Bypass surgery was performed with a single RIMA graft placed to the right coronary artery. The aortic root could not be cannulated for cardiopulmonary bypass or for placement of vein grafts. Shortly after surgery his angina recurred and progressed to refractory rest pain. The entire length of the RIMA graft was occluded and he was referred for excimer laser angioplasty of the ostial right coronary stenosis (Fig. 21B.3).

Because of the small size of the aorta, a JR 3.5 was the only acceptable guide catheter. After crossing the lesion with a 0.018-inch, extra-support, floppy-tip wire, a 1.3-mm LAIS catheter at 45 mJ/mm^2 was successfully advanced across the lesion. Although improved, there was substantial residual stenosis prompting upsizing to a 2.0-mm diameter catheter. In an attempt to further enlarge the lumen, the guide catheter was manipulated to give different angles of entry of the laser catheter into the right coronary ostium. After five additional passes there was noted a small area of contrast extravasation outside the artery through the floor of the lesion. The residual stenosis was improved with a diameter of 2.6 mm, and there were no hemodynamic sequelae of the perforation. At 9 months the patient was asymptomatic, and follow-up angiography revealed a widely patent artery with a mild 30% ostial stenosis.

This case, although successful, shows the limitation of performing multiple passes in an attempt to further debulk the lesion. Fortunately, this resulted in a contained perforation that spontaneously sealed, aided perhaps by the obliteration of the pericardial space after bypass surgery. This type of complication is also possible with high-speed rotational atherectomy. In retrospect, with the lesion improved to within 1.0 mm of the

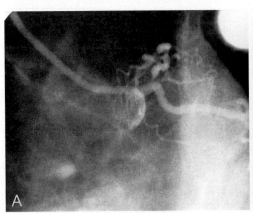

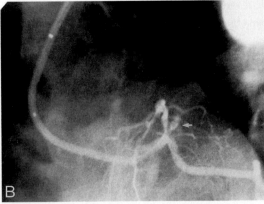

Figure 21B.4. Case #2. **A.** Pretreatment LAO/caudal projection of left coronary artery with ostial stenosis of the LAD. Note angulation of the origin of the LAD from the left main coronary. **B.** Following passage of 2.0-mm diameter concentric excimer laser catheter there is a perforation originating at the bifurcation *(arrow)*. The guide catheter was upsized to 9 Fr.

reference segment diameter, the ablation procedure should be stopped and adjunctive balloon angioplasty performed to achieve the largest acute gain.

CASE #2

A 59-year-old female with crescendo angina and severe stenosis at the origin of a 2.5-mm diameter LAD had recently diagnosed carcinoma of the breast and was concurrently undergoing radiation therapy. The lesion was first crossed with a 1.3-mm laser catheter at 60 mJ/mm², resulting in improvement but with a residual 60% narrowing. The laser catheter was upsized to a 2.0 mm, and a single pass at 45 mJ/mm² was performed. Perforation at the bifurcation was noted with contrast dissecting into the surrounding periadventitia (Fig. 21B.4). After several prolonged inflations with a perfusion balloon, there was no further leak visualized and the patient remained hemodynamically stable. Because of intracoronary filling defects she was main-

tained on heparin and brought back the next day for a relook. She remained asymptomatic and repeat angiography showed a widely patent lumen with no evidence of perforation. At 6 months she had redeveloped class II angina, which was controlled medically. Follow-up angiography showed restenosis of 65% beginning 8 mm distal to the origin of the LAD.

This case illustrates a second setting for perforation. The LAO caudal projection demonstrates that the entrance into the LAD from the left main involves an abrupt turn. This was successfully negotiated by the small, 1.3-mm laser catheter. The 2.0-mm catheter was too large for the vessel (less than 1.0-mm clearance) even if the path contained no tortuosity. The bend point preferentially caused tissue ablation along the outer curvature with perforation of the carina between the LAD and circumflex. The correct procedure would have been to switch to balloon angioplasty after passage of the small laser catheter. Even though the lumen was insufficient, the smaller laser may have

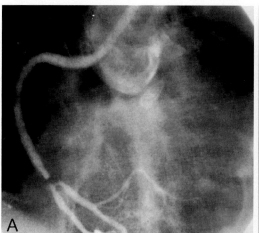

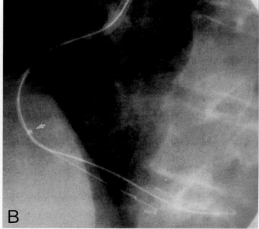

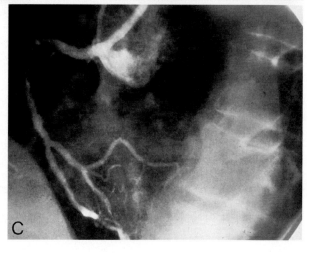

Figure 21B.5. Case #3. **A.** Pretreatment LAO/cranial view of right coronary artery. There is a very eccentric stenosis involving the bifurcation of the posterior descending branch. **B.** Guidewires have been placed into both branches, and the directional excimer laser catheter has been advanced over the guidewire that enters the upper branch *(arrow)*. The tip marker is aligned so that the laser fibers are oriented at the eccentric atheroma mass and so the protective tip (not visible) will shield the region of the vascular carina. **C.** After excimer/adjunctive balloon angioplasty showing a widely patent bifurcation.

successfully ablated tissue and limited the elastic recoil expected in this location. The abrupt change in direction at the ostium of the LAD would have been problematic for each of the second-generation devices, although this case may also have been successfully performed with directional or high-speed rotational atherectomy. Tamponade of the perforation site with a balloon is often successful at sealing the leak. Delayed cases of pericardial tamponade have been described, so it is important to stop anticoagulation as soon as the clinical situation will allow and closely follow the patient for several days.

CASE #3

A 71-year-old male with a recent inferior myocardial infarction successfully treated with thrombolysis. Angiography showed a subtotal, highly eccentric bifurcation lesion involving the ostia of the posterior descending and continuation of the right coronary artery (Fig. 21B.5). Guidewires were placed separately in the two major branches. A 1.8-mm, directional laser catheter (LAIS) was advanced and positioned using biplane fluoroscopy such that the eccentrically arranged ablation surface would contact the bulk of the atheroma and the plastic hood on the opposite side of the catheter would protect the region of the vascular carina. After one pass the eccentric lesion was largely ablated, but there remained significant residual narrowing at the origin of the posterior descending branch. Both branches were successfully treated with adjunctive PTCA without apparent acute recoil. Follow-up angiography at 10 months showed no restenosis.

This case illustrates a new way to treat branch ostial stenosis combined with a bifurcation lesion. Concentric laser catheters are contraindicated in this situation for two reasons that predispose to perforation or dissection: first, the lesion is highly eccentric, and second, it involves a bifurcation with a highly acute angle between the branches. Ablation of the atheroma may have contributed to the absence of recoil observed in this case.

CASE #4

A 71-year-old male with limiting, effort-related angina had clinically successful, multipass, directional excimer laser/adjunctive balloon angioplasty of a densely calcified, highly eccentric, right coronary ostial stenosis. Although a 2.2-mm diameter lumen was documented by quantitative angiography of the LAO views, there was persistent lucency in the region of the lesion felt to be consistent with remaining eccentric plaque. After 6 months he redeveloped symptoms and angiography showed a recurrence (Fig. 21B.6).

Repeat directional excimer laser angioplasty followed by dilatation with a 3.5-mm balloon was performed with identical angiographic results obtained in the prior procedure. Intravascular ultrasound revealed a 180° rim of calcification with a residual 60% obstructive plaque and a 1.6-mm diameter lumen. Angiography in an RAO/cranial view showed an eccentric plaque that recurred despite full balloon expansion suggestive of recoil of the noncalcified wall. A 3.5-mm Palmaz-Schatz coronary stent was placed in the ostium and further expanded with a 4.0-mm PET balloon. Intravascular ultrasound showed that the stent had created a 3.7-mm diameter circular lumen and repeat angiography showed no residual stenosis. The patient was discharged on day 5 without thrombotic or vascular complications and has remained angina free.

This case shows the potential value of intravascular ultrasound imaging, which provided additional information sufficient to alter treatment and convert a marginally acceptable result into an exceptional result. Moreover, it shows that, once debulked with laser, residual atheroma mass in the form of eccentric calcific plaque may not give way to subsequent balloon angioplasty, especially if the thinner, more pliable arc of vessel wall elastically expands and subsequently recoils. If further debulking is not possible, placement of a permanent stent will predictably solve the problem of recoil.

CASE #5

An 82-year-old male with intractable angina, severe triple-vessel disease, poor left ventricular function, and moderate azotemia. He was deemed not to be a surgical candidate. Angiography revealed a dominant right coronary artery with a 90%, 15-mm-long stenosis. The LAD had a separate origin from the aorta with an 80% ostial, highly eccentric narrowing (Fig. 21B.7). Successful excimer laser and adjunctive balloon angioplasty were performed on the right coronary artery with a 30% residual stenosis. A 9 Fr AL-2 side-hole guide catheter was positioned to sit just outside the LAD ostium. A single pass was made with a 1.8-mm directional excimer laser catheter (LAIS model DLC) at 55 mJ/mm² with improvement leaving a 1.8-mm stenotic diameter. Because the vessel was thought to exceed 3.0 mm in diameter, a 2.2-mm concentric laser catheter tuned to 45 mJ/mm² passed through the lesion. Repeat injection showed acute occlusion associated with an angiographically visible, 40-mm-long, spiral dissection that appeared to stop at a 2.0-mm diameter diagonal branch. Prolonged inflation with a perfusion balloon was unsuccessful at restoring patency. A Palmaz-Schatz stent was placed at the distal extent of the dissection with no effect on flow. A second stent was placed at the ostium, but the region between the two stents was

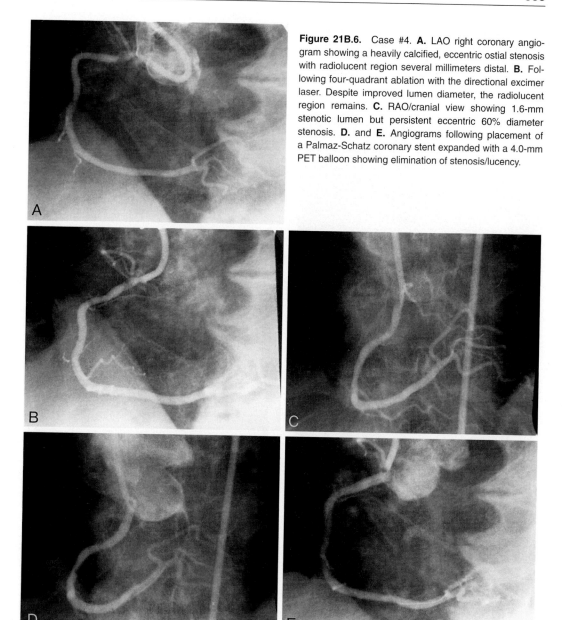

Figure 21B.6. Case #4. **A.** LAO right coronary angiogram showing a heavily calcified, eccentric ostial stenosis with radiolucent region several millimeters distal. **B.** Following four-quadrant ablation with the directional excimer laser. Despite improved lumen diameter, the radiolucent region remains. **C.** RAO/cranial view showing 1.6-mm stenotic lumen but persistent eccentric 60% diameter stenosis. **D.** and **E.** Angiograms following placement of a Palmaz-Schatz coronary stent expanded with a 4.0-mm PET balloon showing elimination of stenosis/lucency.

still occluded with a large flap. A third stent was placed to span the gap between the first two, resulting in immediate patency with restoration of TIMI grade 3 flow. The stents were postdilated with a 4.0-mm PET balloon with further improvement resulting in a slightly overdilated appearance. The patient developed acute renal failure, but subsequently recovered and has been angina free for more than 6 months.

This case illustrates the extraordinary value of multiple stent placement to solve acute closure caused by

extensive dissection. This type of dissection may have been avoided by performing balloon angioplasty after first successfully debulking the eccentric ostial lesion with the directional laser system.

CASE #6

A 71-year-old man with previous bypass surgery and refractory rest angina. He had poor left ventricular function with an ejection fraction of approximately 20% and severe azotemia with a creatinine of 5.0. He was turned down for repeat surgery. There was a subtotal stenosis at the ostia of a 12-year-old saphenous vein to the LAD, which also supplied the inferior wall via collaterals (Fig. 21B.8). Five millimeters distal to the ostia there was a

second area of narrowing immediately after an 80° bend. The severity of each lesion was also documented by intravascular ultrasound, which showed a lumen the same size as the catheter (approximately 1.2 mm in diameter). After predilating with a 2.5-mm balloon, a 3.5-mm Palmaz-Schatz stent was deployed at the ostium and subsequently postdilated to 4.0 mm. Although it required 14 atm to expand the presumed fibrous lesion, the angiographic result was excellent with no residual stenosis.

The choice of stenting in this case was made because of several factors. Stenting of vein grafts has the lowest reported rates of distal embolization and restenosis of any angioplasty procedure. In our view this makes it the procedure of choice for patients who are not candidates for CABG, with depressed LV function, undergoing revascularization of a bypass graft that supplies the majority of the remaining viable myocardium.

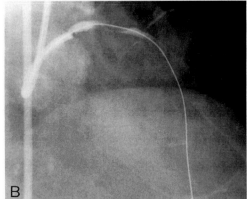

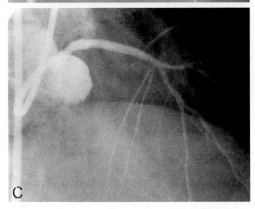

Figure 21B.7. Case #5. **A.** Pretreatment RAO projection of eccentric ostial LAD stenosis. LAD arises from its own separate origin. **B.** Following excimer laser angioplasty with upsized 2.2-mm catheter there is acute occlusion caused by spiral dissection. **C.** Restoration of patency after placing three contiguous Palmaz-Schatz coronary stents.

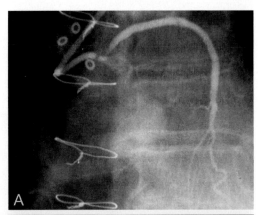

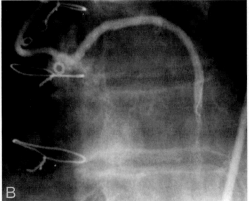

Figure 21B.8. Case #6. **A.** Pretreatment frontal projection of saphenous vein graft to the LAD. There is severe ostial narrowing with a tandem stenosis on a hinge point 5 mm from the ostium. **B.** Following deployment of a single, Palmaz-Schatz, 15-mm coronary stent.

REFERENCES

1. Ellis SG, Roubin GS, King SB, Douglas JS, Wentraub WS, Thomas RG, Cox WR. Angiographic and clinical predictors of acute closure after native vessel coronary angioplasty. Circulation 1988;77:372-379.

2. Ellis SG, Vandormael MG, Cowley MJ, DiSciascio G, Deligonul U, Topol EJ, Bulle TM. Multivessel angioplasty prognosis study group: coronary morphological and clinical determinants of procedural outcome with angioplasty for multivessel coronary disease. Circulation 1990; 82:1193–1202.

3. Thompson R. Isolated coronary ostial stenosis in women. J Am Coll Cardiol 1986;5:997–1003.

4. Miller AH, Honey M, El Sayed H. Isolated coronary ostial stenosis. Cathet Cardiovasc Diagn 1986;12:30–34.

5. Stewart JT, Ward DE, Davies MJ, Pepper JR. Isolated coronary ostial stenosis: observations on the pathology. Eur Heart J 1987;8:917–920.

6. Eigler N, Weinstock B, Douglas JS, Goldenberg T, Hartzler G, Holmes D, Leon M et al. for the ELCA investigators. Excimer laser coronary angioplasty of aorto-ostial stenosis: results of the excimer laser coronary angioplasty (ELCA) registry in the first 200 patients. Circulation 1993;88:2049–2057.

7. Popma JJ, Brogan WC, Pichard AD, Satler LF, Kent KM, Mintz GS, Leon MB. Rotational coronary atherectomy of ostial stenosis. Am J Cardiol 1993;71:436–438.

8. Topol EJ Ellis SG, Fishman J, Leimgruber P, Myler RK, Stertzer SH, O'Neill WW et al. Multicenter study of percutaneous transluminal angioplasty for right coronary artery ostial stenosis. J Am Coll Cardiol 1987;9:1214-1218.

9. Spray TL, Roberts WC. Changes in saphenous veins used as aortocoronary bypass grafts. Am Heart J 1977; 94:500–516.

10. Dorros G, Johnson WD, Tector AJ, Schmai TM, Kalush SL, Janke L. Percutaneous transluminal coronary angioplasty before initial and repeat coronary artery bypass grafting in the coronary artery surgery study (CASS) registry population. Am J Cardiol 1984;53:112C–115C.

11. Mathias DW, Fishman Mooney J, Lange HW, Goldenberg IF, Gobel FL, Mooney MR. Frequency of success and complications of coronary angioplasty of a stenosis at the ostium of a branch vessel. Am J Cardiol 1991;67:491–495.

12. Saltissi S, Webb-Pebloe MM, Coltart DJ. Effect of variation in coronary artery anatomy on distribution of stenotic lesions. Br Heart J 1979;42:186–191.

13. Block PC, Cowley MJ, Kaltenbach M, Kent KM, Simpson J. Percutaneous angioplasty of stenoses of bypass grafts or of bypass graft anastomotic sites. Am J Cardiol 1984; 53:666–668.

14. Platko WP, Hollman J, Whitlow PL, Franco I. Percutaneous transluminal angioplasty of saphenous vein graft stenosis: long-term follow-up. J Am Coll Cardiol 1989;14:1645–1650.

15. Cote G, Myler RK, Stertzer SH, Clark DA et al. Percutaneous transluminal angioplasty of stenotic coronary artery bypass grafts: 5 years' experience. J Am Coll Cardiol 1987;9:8–17.

16. Bedotto JB, McConahay DR, Rutherford BD, Giogi LV, Johnson WL, Shimshak TM, Hartzler GO. Balloon angioplasty of aorta coronary ostial stenoses revisited. Circulation 1991;84(Suppl II):II-251.

17. Whitworth HB, Pilcher GS, Roubin GS, Gruentzig AR. Do proximal lesions involving the origin of the left anterior descending artery (LAD) have a higher restenosis rate after coronary angioplasty (PTCA)? Circulation 1985;72:III-398.

18. Eigler N, Forrester J. Non-pharmacologic device prevention of restenosis. In: Topol E, ed. Textbook of interventional cardiology. 2nd ed. New York: WB Saunders, 1993.

19. Cook SL, Eigler NL, Shefer A, Goldenberg T, Forrester JS, Litvack F. Percutaneous excimer laser coronary angioplasty of lesions not ideal for balloon angioplasty. Circulation 1991;84:632–643.

20. Bittl JA, Sanborn TA. Excimer laser–facilitated coronary angioplasty. Relative risk analysis of acute and follow-up results in 200 patients. Circulation 1992;86:71–80.

21. Loop FD, Lytle BW, Cosgrove DM, Woods EL, Stewart RW, Golding LAR, Goormastic M et al. Reoperation for coronary atherosclerosis: changing practice in 2509 consecutive patients. Ann Surg 1990;212:378–385.

22. Tcheng JE, Bittl JA, Sanborn TA, Siegel RM, Ginsburg R, Power JA, Cohen ED et al. Treatment of aorto-ostial disease with percutaneous excimer laser coronary angioplasty. Circulation 1992;86:I-512.

23. Robertson GC, Simpson JB, Vetter JW, Selmon MR, Doucette JW, Sheehan DJ, McAuley BJ et al. Directional coronary atherectomy for ostial lesions. Circulation 1991; 84:II-251.

24. Hinohara T, Robertson GC, Selmon MR, Vetter JW, Rowe MH, Braden LJ, McAuley BJ et al. Restenosis after directional coronary atherectomy. J Am Coll Cardiol 1992; 20:623–632.

C. The Potential Approaches and Technical Problems of Treating The Ostial Lesion

MICHEL E. BERTRAND, EUGENE McFADDEN, CHRISTOPHE BAUTERS, JEAN MARC LABLANCHE, and PHILIPPE QUANDALLE

Over the last 15 years interventional cardiologists have sought to treat increasingly complex lesions with traditional balloon coronary angioplasty and with the newer interventional techniques designed to overcome some of the limitations of balloon dilatation. The ACC/AHA task force provided a useful classification that identified subclasses of lesions with particular characteristics associated with a decreased likelihood of primary success, or with a higher rate of acute complication (1). Ostial location was one such characteristic. In this review we outline the potential approaches to the treatment of ostial lesions, present the reported experience with these different strategies, and discuss the particular technical problems encountered.

CLASSIFICATION OF OSTIAL LESIONS

The technical difficulties and potential complications related to the dilation of ostial lesions are intimately related to the anatomic location of the lesions. Ostial lesions can be classified into three subclasses. This review will focus on aorto-ostial and ostial coronary lesions.

Aorto-Ostial Lesions

These include right coronary ostial lesions and aorto-ostial lesions located at the proximal anastomosis of a saphenous vein graft. There have been several reports of angioplasty of isolated left main ostial coronary lesions. However, when unprotected by patent bypass grafts, these lesions are not, except in exceptional circumstances, an indication for coronary angioplasty (2, 3). Finally, although rarely encountered, ostial lesions may occur at the origin of an internal mammary graft (4, 5).

Ostial Coronary Lesions

Ostial coronary lesions, located at the junction between the left main coronary artery and the left anterior descending or circumflex arteries, are more frequently encountered. Although theoretically only lesions that include the origin of the left anterior descending or the origin of the circumflex coronary arteries should be classified as ostial, several reports have included in this category lesions that are located near the origin of these vessels. Dilation of such "near-ostial" or "very proximal" lesions shares some but not all of the potential difficulties encountered with true ostial lesions.

Branch Ostial Lesions

Lesions at the junction of a major epicardial vessel and a secondary branch are also frequently encountered. The most common locations are at the junction of the left anterior descending coronary and the first or second diagonal branch or at the junction of the right coronary artery and its two major distal branches. These lesions may be isolated or may occur in conjunction with a lesion in the parent vessel, in which case the dual problem of an ostial lesion and that of a bifurcation lesion need to be taken into consideration.

HISTOPATHOLOGIC CHARACTERISTICS

It is particularly important to carefully consider the pathologic aspects of these lesions. Some clearly result from an aortitis, cardiovascular syphilis, a frequent disease in the past characterized by an obliterative endarteritis leading to obstruction of the ostia of the coronary arteries. The muscular and elastic tissues of the media are infiltrated by the spirochetes and the subsequent inflammatory reaction results in an accumulation of vascular fibrous tissue. This particular etiology is rare in the Western world today (6); however, ostial lesions related to other specific arteritis such as Takayashu's syndrome, Reiter's syndrome, or Beçhet's disease may be, albeit infrequently, encountered. Ostial lesions have also been described in familial forms of hypercholesterolemia, after aortic valve replacement, and after therapeutic mediastinal irradiation as, for example, in Hodgkin's disease (6–8). In such cases where the disease is predominantly located in the aortic wall, a small protuberance centered around the obstructed ostia of the vessel is frequently seen on angiography; this may render selective angiography of the involved vessel extremely difficult.

The most commonly encountered lesions are those related to atherosclerotic involvement of the origin of the coronary vessels and those related to the implantation of coronary artery bypass grafts. These lesions are characterized by their rigidity; they are poorly distensible because of their large elastic fiber content. Popma et al. studied the histopathologic characteristics of tissue fragments removed by atherectomy from right coronary ostial stenoses (9). The major lesion components were fibrocellular (39 ± 14%) or sclerotic (28 ± 14%) tissue. Lipid-rich components were infrequent (10%), and thrombus was rarely observed. Similar histopathologic findings have been observed in ostial lesions at the proximal anastomosis and the adjacent proximal part of a saphenous vein graft. These lesions are mainly comprised of fibrogranulomatous tissue, which is, in essence, scar tissue that results from the healing process after suture of the graft to the aortic wall. These histopathologic characteristics may in part account for the difficulties encountered by the interventional cardiologist when treating such lesions, which are often difficult to dilate with a balloon, even at high pressures, or which, alternatively, demonstrate immediate elastic recoil.

REPORTED RESULTS WITH CONVENTIONAL BALLOON DILATION AND NEWER ALTERNATIVES

Balloon Angioplasty

One of the earlier reported studies was that by Topol et al. (10) who described the multicenter experience (Emory University, The San Francisco Heart Institute, and The University of Michigan) of balloon angioplasty of right coronary artery ostial (<3 mm from the ostium) stenoses. The series included 53 patients; technical success, defined as a residual stenosis of <50% and a transstenotic gradient <15 mm Hg, was achieved in 42 patients (79%). Distinctive technical features included the use of high-pressure balloon inflation pressures (9.8 ± 4 atm) and the need for unconventional guide catheters in almost half the patients. Five patients (9.4%) underwent emergency bypass surgery related to a dissection that in three patients resulted in

abrupt closure. Of the 42 patients with initial success, 20 developed recurrent angina and angiographic restenosis was confirmed in 16 of these patients. The other four patients had noninvasive evidence of reversible ischemia in the inferior wall suggestive of restenosis. Repeat coronary angioplasty was performed in six patients and a further restenosis occurred in three patients. This study was somewhat disappointing and characterized by a relatively low rate of success (79%) and a high risk of major complications leading to emergency bypass operation in 9.4% of cases.

Recent reports have been more encouraging. Bedotto et al. (11) reported a small series of patients who underwent angioplasty for aorto-ostial lesions. They encountered no acute complications, although the primary success rate was still inferior to that of angioplasty performed at other types of lesions (Table 21C.1). Vallbracht et al. recently reported their experience with conventional balloon angioplasty in 60 patients with aorto-ostial or ostial-coronary lesions (12). They found that the procedural success rate (81.6%) was similar to that of matched nonostial lesions. Follow-up angiography, performed in 80% of patients, showed restenosis at 34% of ostial and 26% of nonostial lesions (P = ns).

In another recent report, Mathias et al. reported on the results of angioplasty procedures performed at branch ostial lesions

Table 21C.1
Balloon Angioplasty Results With Ostial Lesions

Author/ Reference	Lesions/ Patients	Location	Success (%)	Complications[a] (%)
Topol (10)	53/53	A-O, RCA	79	9.4
Bedotto (11)	60/55	A-O	85	0
Vallbracht (12)	60/60	A-O/OC	83	5
Mathias (13)	119/106	BO	74	13

[a]Death, acute myocardial infarction, emergency coronary artery bypass surgery.
A-O, aorto-ostial; BO, branch ostial; OC, ostial coronary; RCA, right coronary artery.

(n = 119). These authors defined a branch ostial stenosis as a stenosis occurring in the proximal 3 mm of a major branch vessel. The lesions were isolated in 61% of cases and associated with a lesion in the parent vessel in 39%. Angiographic success (residual stenosis <50%) was achieved at 74% of ostial lesions compared with a 91% success rate for control nonostial lesions (13). The mean balloon-to-artery ratio for the ostial lesions was 1.05:1. The complication rate (13%) was also significantly higher for ostial lesions than for nonostial (5%) lesions.

Directional Coronary Atherectomy

In 1991 Popma et al. (9) presented seven cases of right coronary ostial stenosis treated by atherectomy. Procedural success was achieved in six of seven patients, but in the remaining patient a 6 Fr atherectomy catheter could not be positioned across the stenosis as the 9.5 Fr guide catheter provided insufficient backup. The minimal luminal diameter increased from 0.4 to 3.2 ± 0.8 mm, and the percent diameter stenosis was reduced from 61 ± 5% to 14 ± 16%. At 6-month follow-up only one patient had developed restenosis. The marked increase in minimal lumen diameter after directional atherectomy highlights the major interest of this technique, namely, the ability to obtain a greater acute gain than with traditional balloon angioplasty. Even if the greater gain in lumen diameter results in a proportionately greater late loss in lumen diameter, the end result may be better, particularly in vessels with a large reference diameter. Kerwin et al. recently reported their experience with directional atherectomy in the treatment of aorto-ostial stenosis (14). They performed directional atherectomy in 23 patients, 15 of whom had stenoses <3 mm from the origin of the right coronary artery. The other eight had lesions at or within 3 mm of the origin of a saphenous vein graft. Primary success was obtained in 96% of patients; there were no acute complications. Brogan et al. (15) reported the impact of new

Table 21C.2
Directional Coronary Atherectomy Results With Ostial Lesions[a]

Author/ Reference	Lesions/ Patients	Location	Success (%)	Complications[b] (%)
Popma (9)	7/7	A-O, RCA	86	0
Kerwin (14)	23/23	A-O	96	0
Brogan (15)	58/NR	A-OC	97	2
Ghazzal (16)	162/162	A-O	88	2.3
Robertson (17)	NR/75	OC/BO	92	0
Robertson (17)	41/NR	A-O	78	5
Garrett (18)	12/11	A-O:SVG	100	0
Hinohara (19)	21/NR	A-O:OC	71	NR

[a]Some of the reports cited are serial studies from the same groups.
[b]Death, acute myocardial infarction, emergency coronary artery bypass surgery.
A-O, Aorto-ostial; BO, branch ostial; NR, not reported; OC, ostial coronary; RCA, right coronary artery; SVG, saphenous vein graft.

devices on the treatment of ostial lesions: directional atherectomy was successful in 97% of 58 cases, which comprised both aorto-ostial and branch ostial lesions. Table 21C.2 (9, 14–19) shows the pooled data from six studies of directional atherectomy as treatment for ostial lesions. Overall primary success rates and complication rates were comparable to those reported for nonostial lesions. The restenosis rate is difficult to estimate because of the lack of systematic angiographic follow-up, but does not, overall, appear to be less than that reported with conventional balloon angioplasty. Hinohara et al. reported an angiographic (>50% stenosis) rate of restenosis of 25% for aorto-ostial lesions in native coronary arteries, a 42% restenosis rate for the combined group of ostial coronary and branch ostial lesions, and a 73% rate of restenosis for saphenous vein graft ostial lesions (20).

High-Speed Rotational Coronary Atherectomy

High-speed rotational atherectomy with the Rotablator was introduced in an attempt to overcome some of the limitations of balloon angioplasty. On the basis of observational studies, rotational atherectomy appears to be

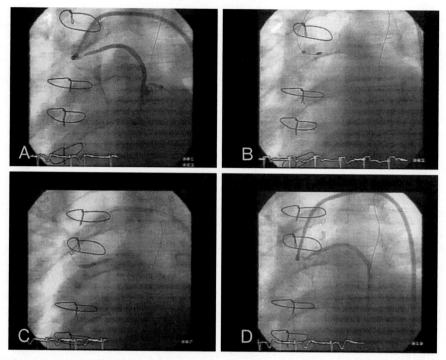

Figure 21C.1. Lesion of the ostium of a saphenous vein graft. Balloon angioplasty failed and two balloons blew up at >14 atm. Then a rotational abrasion with a 2-mm burr was performed, leading to a modification of the compliance of the lesion. The procedure was successfully completed with a 2.5-mm balloon. *1.* Before treatment. *2.* Rotary ablation. *3.* Adjunctive balloon angioplasty. *4.* Final result.

particularly useful in treating lesions that are rigid and nondistensible such as those that are calcified. Rotational atherectomy alone usually results in a significant residual stenosis because of the small size of the burrs that can be introduced into the coronary circulation. However, this predilation, which abrades the plaque, appears to alter the compliance of the plaque and allows a satisfactory angiographic result to be obtained by adjunctive balloon angioplasty. Observational studies suggest that this technique may be useful for treating ostial lesions. Figure 21C.1 shows a typical example of a tight narrowing of the aortic anastomosis of a saphenous vein graft. Two attempts at balloon dilatation led to rupture of the balloons at high pressure without any significant alteration in lesion severity. A 2-mm burr was used to abrade the lesion, and subsequent balloon dilatation resulted in a satisfactory angiographic result.

Table 21C.3
High-Speed Rotational Coronary Atherectomy Results With Ostial Lesions[a,b]

Author/ Reference	Lesions/ Patients	Location	Success (%)	Complications[c] (%)
Brogan (15)	101/NR	A-O/OC	97	2
Kent (21)	147/NR	A-O/OC	93	5.4
Goudreau (22)	31/31	A-O/OC	97	3

[a]Most patients had adjunctive balloon angioplasty.
[b]Some of the reports cited are serial studies from the same groups.
[c]Death, acute myocardial infarction, emergency coronary artery bypass surgery.
A-O, Aorto-ostial; *OC,* ostial coronary; *NR,* not reported.

Table 21C.3 (15, 21, 22) summarizes the pooled results of three reports of ostial lesions treated with the Rotablator. Primary success was obtained in 96% of cases. Major complications occurred in less than 2% of cases; emergency coronary artery bypass grafting was performed in 1.8% of cases; acute myocardial infarction occurred in 0.3%; and death occurred in 0.01%. However, overall restenosis rates were high, reaching 50% in the series reported by Kent (21). Thus the primary benefit of this technique in the treatment of ostial lesions appears to be as a tool to predilate calcified or fibrotic lesions and thus enable an angiographically acceptable result to be obtained with subsequent balloon angioplasty.

Excimer Laser

Douglas et al. (23) reported their preliminary experience in 16 patients with ostial lesions treated by excimer laser angioplasty; primary success defined as a residual stenosis <50% without major in-hospital complications (Q-wave myocardial infarction, emergency coronary artery bypass grafting, or death) was achieved in 15 of the 16 patients (93.8%). Percent lesion severity decreased from $77 \pm 10\%$ preprocedure to $40 \pm 19\%$ postlaser and to $23 \pm 12\%$ after complementary balloon angioplasty. In this first trial, excimer laser angioplasty appeared promising in the treatment of ostial lesions, including those with moderate to heavy calcifications. In Table 21C.4 the pooled results of six reports are presented (15, 23–27). The

procedure was successful in 93% of cases with few major complications (death, 0.15%; acute myocardial infarction, 1.2%; emergency coronary bypass grafting, 1.4%).

Recently, the results of the excimer laser registry concerning 200 patients with aorto-ostial stenoses were published (25): An adjunctive PTCA was performed in 72% of cases. A procedural success was achieved in 90% of cases. Major complications occurred in 3.9% (death, 0%; Q-wave MI, 0.5%; bypass surgery, 3.4%). Six-month angiographic follow-up, available in 51% of eligible patients, documented restenosis in 39%. Clinical events at follow-up were death, 2.7%; bypass surgery, 6.5%; myocardial infarction, 2.2%; and repeat angioplasty, 16.2%. Finally, directional excimer laser angioplasty appears particularly useful in the treatment of ostial lesions that are calcified but, as with rotational atherectomy, adjunctive balloon angioplasty is frequently required and the restenosis rate appears to be high.

Stents

The use of balloon-expandable stents produces in the vast majority of cases an excellent immediate angiographic result. However, the trauma induced by stent implantation appears to provide a potent stimulus for subsequent restenosis. In addition, subacute stent thrombosis remains a problem. The achievement of a better immediate result may, however, result in a better long-term outcome in spite of the more marked late loss in lumen diameter, particularly in large vessels. Teirstein et al. (Table 21C.5) reported a series of 28 patients who underwent Palmaz-Schatz stent implantation for aorto-ostial (n = 12) or ostial coronary (n = 16) stenoses (28). Acute success was achieved in 89% of patients. Two patients developed sub-acute stent closure that was related to premature discontinuation of anticoagulation. Both developed Q-wave myocardial infarction, and one died. Restenosis was documented angiographically in 35% of patients.

Table 21C.4
Excimer Laser Coronary Angioplasty Results With Ostial Lesions[a,b]

Author/ Reference	Lesions/ Patients	Location	Success (%)	Complications[c] (%)
Brogan (15)	16/NR	A-O/OC	94	6
Douglas (23)	16/16	A-O	94	0
Tcheng (24)	138/138	A-O	94	2
Eigler (25)	114/114	A-O	96	3
Bittl (26)	47/NR	A-O	87	5
Weinstock (27)	175/175	A-O	86	4.1

[a]Most patients had adjunctive balloon angioplasty.
[b]Some of the reports cited are serial studies from the same groups.
[c]Death, acute myocardial infarction, emergency coronary artery bypass surgery.
A-O, Aorto-ostial; OC, ostial coronary; NR, not reported.

Table 21C.5
Coronary Stent Results With Ostial Lesions

Author/ Reference	Lesions/ Patients	Location	Success (%)	Compli- cations[a] (%)
Brogan (15)	11/NR	A-O/OC	91	0
Teirstein (28)	28/28	A-O/OC	89	7

[a]Death, acute myocardial infarction, emergency coronary artery bypass surgery, related to the procedure or to subacute stent thrombosis.
A-O, Aorto-ostial; OC, ostial coronary; NR, not reported.

Table 21C.6
Transluminal Extraction Catheter Results With Ostial Lesions[a]

Author/ Reference	Lesions/ Patients	Location	Success (%)	Compli- cations[b] (%)
Brogan (15)	19/NR	A-O/OC	95	0
Popma (30)	15/NR	NR	93	NR

[a]Most patients had adjunctive balloon angioplasty.
[b]Death, acute myocardial infarction, emergency coronary artery bypass surgery, related to the procedure or to subacute stent thrombosis.
A-O, Aorto-ostial; OC, ostial coronary; NR, not reported.

Different types of stents are now available. The aorto-ostial lesions may require special considerations. These lesions located in the ostium of a saphenous vein graft are usually short and often create unusual angles and bends between the aorta and the graft. In this particular case it could be useful, as published by Nordrehaug (29), to implant a half Palmaz-Schatz stent (length of 7 mm). This device is obtained in cutting the 15-mm Palmaz-Schatz stent at the point of articulation. Reducing stent length can also reduce the restenosis risk, which is very high in that type of lesion. Usually, these stenoses are made of a very hard, undilatable, fibrous material, and it could be useful to use the Wallstent from Medinvent, which is resistant to radial compression. However, this prosthesis, which is autoexpandable, is more difficult to implant in that particular site. (Editors

note: There is far from uniform agreement regarding this issue.) The excellent visibility under fluoroscopy of the Wiktor stent could justify its use, but the arrangement of the wires and the poor radial strength resistance can be inconvenient.

In summary, stent implantation is very promising and if the problems related to stent thrombosis can be solved, this technique will be a useful adjunct in the management of ostial lesions.

Transluminal Extraction Catheter Atherectomy

This technique appears to have a promising role in the treatment of lesions that have a large component of thrombus, particularly lesions that are located in old saphenous vein grafts. Popma et al. reported on 51 patients who underwent transluminal extraction atherectomy (Table 21C.6). Fifteen had ostial lesions; primary angiographic success was achieved in 14 patients (30). As with rotational atherectomy and excimer laser coronary angioplasty, the procedure most often needed adjunctive balloon angioplasty.

TECHNICAL CONSIDERATIONS

Guiding Catheter Selection

The first and one of the most important problems is identifying a suitable guide catheter. When the lesion is characterized by a small protuberance with the coronary orifice at the center, it can be extremely difficult to achieve adequate guide catheter support. It is important to avoid deep-seating of the catheter into the artery, to prevent guide catheter–induced ostial trauma. The choice of guide catheter is based on the principle that coaxial alignment should be maintained, as far as possible, between the tip of the guide and the proximal vessel segment. Many of these lesions thus require the use of unconventional guide catheters. For right coronary ostial lesions, the classic Judkins guide is usually adequate. In a significant minority of cases it may, however, be necessary to choose an Amplatz, Arani, Multipurpose, or El Gamel catheter, depending on the anatomic variations in aortic root width and in the angle of takeoff of the right coronary artery. The same considerations apply to the choice of catheter for right coronary graft ostial stenoses. For left anterior descending ostial stenoses, the classic left Judkins catheters are usually adequate, although on occasion when the left main stem is short, a short-tip catheter may be advantageous. For left circumflex ostial stenoses the additional backup provided by an Amplatz curve may be useful. Finally, for posteriorly located bypass grafts, El Gamel, left coronary bypass, or left Amplatz curves may be needed. In addition, it is often preferable to use catheters with side holes.

Device Stability

A common problem relates to the stability of the balloon, or other device, on the lesion. Frequently, the balloon tends to slip out of the coronary ostium or alternatively to slip back into the artery during balloon inflation—the so-called "watermelon-seed effect." This problem may be overcome by using a long balloon but with the obvious consequence of increasing the surface exposed to the trauma of balloon inflation. Furthermore, it is necessary to inflate the balloon at the point where the guide catheter engages the artery. Of course, the ideal situation is to withdraw the guide catheter from the ostium just before or during balloon inflation to avoid inflation of the balloon within the guide catheter. In practice, this can be extremely difficult.

Other devices pose particular technical difficulties. During high-speed rotational atherectomy of true ostial lesions, the relationship between the burr and the guide catheter is somewhat difficult to handle. One should avoid high-speed rotation in the distal part of the guide catheter; however, if the latter is retracted from the ostium, there is often inadequate backup to maintain the continuous pressure required to advance the burr

through the lesion. It may be advantageous to deliberately undersize the burr.

The same problem of backup is encountered with directional atherectomy. It is useful to have two experienced operators to coordinate retraction of the guide catheter and simultaneous advancement of the cutter. When coronary stent placement is attempted, it is critical to position the stent correctly to avoid protrusion into the aorta. The technical difficulties that result from the lack of stability predispose to a higher than average risk of failure to deploy the stent correctly and to the hazard of systemic embolization. In this respect, it may be advantageous to use a stent that is easily visualized on fluoroscopy such as the Wiktor stent.

Treatment Strategy and Device Selection

As outlined above, the acute and long-term results of percutaneous revascularization at ostial stenoses have varied markedly in reported studies. In the absence of randomized studies, the treatment strategy that we suggest depends on our personal experience and on the cumulative results of published experience. Unfortunately, few studies have included systematic angiographic follow-up; therefore the impact of newer alternatives to balloon angioplasty on restenosis rates cannot be judged accurately.

Advances in our understanding of the process of restenosis have demonstrated that there is a close relation between the acute result and the coronary lumen diameter at late follow-up angiography, irrespective of the device used. Baim's group, in a study of the late outcome after coronary stenting or coronary atherectomy, showed that the late loss in lumen diameter after intervention was associated with the immediate postprocedure lumen diameter, with the acute gain, and with the postprocedure percent stenosis, but not with the coronary location or with the particular device employed (31). Thus for aorto-ostial and ostial coronary lesions, which are generally located in vessels with a large absolute reference diameter, it appears logical to attempt to achieve the maximum possible acute gain.

The choice of a device and the strategy employed to achieve the optimal initial result largely depends on the morphologic characteristics of the lesion. The important characteristics to consider are the presence or absence of calcification, the presence of associated thrombus, and the degree of eccentricity.

Calcified lesions should probably be treated by rotational atherectomy, or by excimer laser angioplasty, in association with adjunctive balloon angioplasty. At present, the most commonly used technique to assess the degree of calcification is visual assessment on angiography; the use of intravascular ultrasound may provide a more precise assessment of the degree of calcification that may lead to further refinements in therapy. Eccentric lesions located in a large vessel that are not calcified, or only mildly calcified, may be best treated by directional atherectomy. Lesions with a large component of thrombus may respond best to transluminal extraction atherectomy, usually completed by balloon angioplasty. In concentric noncalcified focal stenoses, there is no clear evidence that any of these new techniques are superior to balloon angioplasty. In such cases it would appear reasonable to perform balloon angioplasty and to consider the use of another device as a second option. Finally, when elastic recoil is the major problem, the use of intracoronary stents needs to be further investigated.

In summary, ostial lesions are complex and often difficult to treat. However, with the new devices available, immediate procedural success rates are high, and the risk of major complications is relatively limited and comparable with the risk when more conventional lesions are dilated. The major problem relates to the high risk of restenosis. In our personal experience we have frequently performed several repeat percutaneous revascularization procedures in such patients. It is perhaps not surprising that some of the patients eventually choose to eschew the well-intentioned efforts of the invasive cardiologist and either continue to suffer in silence or seek the advice of our cardiac surgical colleagues.

REFERENCES

1. Ryan TJ, Faxon DP, Gunnar RM, Kennedy JW, King SB III, Loop FD, Peterson KL et al. Guidelines for percutaneous transluminal coronary angioplasty. A report of the American College of Cardiology/American Heart Association Task Force on Assessment of Diagnostic and Therapeutic Cardiovascular Procedures (Subcommittee on Percutaneous Transluminal Coronary Angioplasty). Circulation 1988; 78:486–502.
2. O'Keefe JH, Hartzler GO, Rutherford BD, McConaghey DR, Johnson WL, Giorgi LV, Ligon RW. Left main coronary angioplasty: early and late results of 127 acute and elective procedures. Am J Cardiol 1989;64:144–147.
3. Eldar M, Schulhoff N, Herz I, Frankel R, Feld H, Shani J. Results of percutaneous transluminal angioplasty of the left main coronary artery. Am J Cardiol 1991; 68:255-256.
4. Vivekaphirat V, Yellen FS, Foschi A. Percutaneous transluminal coronary angioplasty of a stenosis at the origin of the left internal mammary artery graft. Cathet Cardiovasc Diagn 1988;15:176–178.
5. Almagor Y, Thomas J, Colombo A. Balloon-expandable stent implantation of a stenosis at the origin of the left internal mammary artery graft: a case report. Cathet Cardiovasc Diagn 1991;24:256–258.
6. Miller GA, Honey M, El-Sayed H. Isolated coronary ostial stenosis. Cathet Cardiovasc Diagn 1986;12:30–34.
7. Verdiere C, Drobinski G, Evans JI, Cahen C, de Gennes JL, Thomas D. Sténoses ostiales coronaires droites dans l'hypercholesterolémie homozygote. Diagnostic coronorographique et echocardiographique. Presse Med 1984; 13:1770–1776.
8. Nakhjavan FK, Yazdanfar S, Friedman A. Percutaneous transluminal coronary angioplasty for stenosis of the ostium of the right coronary artery after irradiation for Hodgkin's disease. Am J Cardiol 1984;53:341–342.
9. Popma JJ, Dick RJ, Haudenschild CC, Topol EJ, Ellis SG. Atherectomy of right coronary ostial stenoses: initial and long-term results, technical features and histologic findings. Am J Cardiol 1991;67:431–433.
10. Topol EJ, Ellis SG, Fishman J, Leimgruber P, Myler RK, Stertzer SH, O'Neill WW et al. Multicenter study of percutaneous transluminal angioplasty for right coronary artery ostial stenosis. J Am Coll Cardiol 1987;9:1214–1218.
11. Bedotto JB, McConahay DR, Rutherford BD, Giorgi LV, Johnson WL, Shimshack TM, Hartzler GO. Balloon angioplasty of aorta coronary ostial stenoses revisited. Circulation 1991;84(Suppl II):251 (abstract).
12. Vallbracht C, Althen D, Kneissl GD, Kadel C, Hartmann A, Kober G, Kaltenbach M. Conventional PTCA in ostial

lesions is better than its reputation. Eur Heart J 1993; 14(Suppl):247 (abstract).

13. Mathias DW, Fishman Mooney J, Lange HW, Goldenberg IF, Gobel FL, Mooney MR. Frequency of success and complications of coronary angioplasty of a stenosis at the ostium of a branch vessel. Am J Cardiol 1991;67:491–495.

14. Kerwin PM, McKeever LS, Marek JC, Hartmann JR, Enger EL. Directional atherectomy of aorto-ostial stenoses. Cathet Cardiovasc Diagn 1993;29(Suppl 1):17–25.

15. Brogan WC, Popma JJ, Pichard AD, Kent KM, Satler LF, Mintz GS, Keller MB et al. A lesion-specific approach to new device therapy in ostial lesions. J Am Coll Cardiol 1993; 21:233 (abstract).

16. Ghazzal ZMB, Douglas JS, Holmes DR, Ellis SG, Kereiakes DJ, Simpson JB, King SB, and the Directional Atherectomy Multicenter Investigational Group. Directional coronary atherectomy of saphenous vein grafts: recent multicenter experience. J Am Coll Cardiol 1991;17:219A (abstract).

17. Robertson GC, Simpson JB, Vetter JW, Selmon MR, Doucette JW, Sheehan DJ, McAuley BJ et al. Directional coronary atherectomy for ostial lesions. Circulation 1991; 84(Suppl II):251A (abstract).

18. Garrett KN, Bell MR, Berger PB, Bresnahan JF, Higano ST. Directional coronary atherectomy of saphenous vein graft ostial lesions. Circulation 1991;84(Suppl II):26A (abstract).

19. Hinohara T, Rowe MH, Robertson GC, Selmon MR, Braden L, Leggett JH, Vetter JW et al. Effect of lesion characteristics on outcome of directional coronary angioplasty. J Am Coll Cardiol 1991;17:1112–1120.

20. Hinohara T, Robertson GC, Selmon MR, Vetter JW, Rowe MH, Braden LJ, McAuley BJ et al. Restenosis after directional coronary atherectomy. J Am Coll Cardiol 1992; 20:623–632.

21. Kent KM, Stertzer S, Bass T, Cowley M. High-speed rotational ablation in patients with ostial lesions. Circulation 1992;86(Suppl I):513A (abstract).

22. Goudreau E, Cowley MJ, DiSciascio G, deBotis D, Vetrovec G, Sabri N. Rotational atherectomy for aorto-ostial and branch ostial lesions. J Am Coll Cardiol 1993;21:31A (abstract).

23. Douglas JS, Ghazzal ZMB, Ba'albaki HA, Miller SJ, King SB. Excimer laser coronary angioplasty of ostial lesions: acute success and complications. Cathet Cardiovasc Diagn 1991;23:75 (abstract).

24. Tcheng JE, Bittl JA, Sanborn T, Siegel RM, Ginsburg R, Power JA, Cohen ED et al., and the PELCA Registry. Treatment of aorto-ostial disease with percutaneous excimer laser coronary angioplasty. Circulation 1992;86(Suppl I):512A (abstract).

25. Eigler NL, Douglas JS, Margolis JR, Hestrin L, Litvack FI, and the ELCA Investigators. Excimer laser coronary angioplasty of aorto-ostial stenosis: results of the ELCA registry. Circulation 1993;88:2049–2057.

26. Bittl JA, Sanborn TA, Tcheng JE, Siegel RM, Ellis SG, for the Percutaneous Excimer Laser Coronary Angioplasty Registry. Clinical success, complications and restenosis rates with excimer laser coronary angioplasty. Am J Cardiol 1992;70:1533–1539.

27. Weinstock BS, Eigler NL, Litvack FI, and the ELCA investigators. Excimer laser angioplasty of aorto-ostial stenosis in 175 patients: acute and follow-up results and core lab analysis. J Am Coll Cardiol 1993;21:289A (abstract).

28. Teirstein P, Stratienko AA, Schatz RA. Coronary stenting for ostial stenoses: initial results and six-month follow-up. Circulation 1991;84(Suppl II):250A (abstract).

29. Nordrehaug JE, Priestley K, Chronos N, Buller N, Sigwart U. Implantation of half Palmaz-Schatz stents in short aorto-ostial lesions of saphenous vein grafts. Cathet Cardiovasc Diagn 1993;29:141–143.

30. Popma JJ, Leon MB, Mintz GS, Kent KM, Satler LF, Garrand TJ, Pichard AD. Results of coronary angioplasty using the transluminal extraction catheter. Am J Cardiol 1992; 70:1526–1532.

31. Kuntz RE, Safian RD, Carrozza JP, Fishman RF, Mansour M, Baim DS. The importance of acute luminal diameter in determining restenosis after coronary atherectomy or stenting. Circulation 1992;86:1827–1835.

EDITORS' SUMMARY

1. Not all ostial locations behave the same.
2. Guide catheter positioning is especially difficult; it needs to be stable, coaxial, but not too deep in its intubation.
3. Recoil is a problem to virtually all lesions, but rigidity is primarily a problem for aorto-ostial lesions.
4. Limited data are available on which to base treatment decisions.
5. Suggested role of treatment interventions

	Native Aorto-Ostial Lesions (RCA, LMT)	Graft Aorto-Ostial Lesions	Proximal LAD and Circumflex Ostial Lesions	Distal Native Branch Ostial Lesions
Usual preferred treatment	Rotablator[a]	Palmaz-Schatz stent (? with or without Coumadin); DCA	Rotablator[a]	PTCA; DELCA[a]
PTCA	Limited by recoil and rigidity; poor initial result often translates to high likelihood of restenosis	Limited by recoil and rigidity; poor initial result often translates to high likelihood of restenosis	Recoil is more a problem than rigidity; LMT occlusion limits long inflations	Somewhat limited by recoil
DCA	Frequent Ca limits; may have a role after debulking-compliance change by Rotablator or laser	Await CAVEAT II results	May have a role but CAVEAT I, CCAT results disappointing	Inadequate data; possibly increased risk of perforation
Rotablator[a]	Often preferred except when slow reflow (poor LV function, long lesions) or perforation (angulated lesion with eccentric inner lesion or considerable flexing) a major concern; burr size limits debulking	Burrs are too small to adequately debulk; emboli a major concern	Initial debulking likely; allows better final result with adjunctive PTCA	Increased risk of dissection and perforation
Stenting[b]	Specifically useful for ≥3.0- to 3.5-mm vessels; may require debulking for full stent expansion	If adequate runoff is present may be best choice	Proximity to LMT and still possible subacute thrombosis limit stent use	Primary vessel or side branch occlusion (stent jail) severely limits role
(D)ELCA[a]	May be best initial choice when Rotablator contraindicated; catheter size limits debulking except with DELCA; perforation still a worry	Somewhat limited in debulking compared with other strategies	Occasional, unpredictable perilesion dissection limits role here	Perhaps treatment of choice, but perforation and dissection still a concern
TEC	No role	Has a role for debulking when thrombus, diffuse disease present	No role	No role

[a]Adjunctive therapy (e.g., PTCA) usually required.

[b]Available stents vary considerably in their resistance to recoil. Consideration of this issue may be particularly important in stenting ostial lesions.

DCA, Directional coronary atherectomy; DELCA, directional excimer laser coronary angioplasty; LAD, left anterior descending coronary artery; LCX, left circumflex coronary artery; LMT, left main trunk; RCA, right coronary artery; TEC, transluminal extraction catheter.

22. The Simple De Novo Lesion

A. Single-Vessel Dilation

CONRAD SIMPFENDORFER

BACKGROUND

During the past 10 years we have witnessed an exponential growth in the number of percutaneous transluminal coronary angioplasty (PTCA) procedures performed in the United States and Europe (1, 2). Reasons given for this rapid growth are expanded indications, including multivessel PTCA, as a result of improved technology and operator experience. Although many centers, including our own, have reported a growing proportion of patients with multi-vessel disease, single-vessel angioplasty in patients with either single or multi-vessel disease continues to be the most common procedure in patients undergoing PTCA. At the Cleveland Clinic Foundation in 1994, of 2103 coronary angioplasties, 62% involved single-vessel, single-lesion procedures.

Two recent publications describe angioplasty practice patterns in the United States. Using a large, private-insurance claims database, Topol et al. described a group to 2101 patients who underwent coronary angioplasty from 1988 through 1989 (3). Only 4% of the patients had multivessel coronary angioplasty during the index procedural hospitalization. This study showed no difference among geographic regions or between hospitals with and hospitals without cardiology training programs. Hannan et al., using the New York State Coronary Angioplasty Registry, reported on 5827 patients receiving PTCA from January 1991 through June 1991 in thirty-one hospitals in New York State.

The large majority of patients (85.4%) had single-vessel PTCA, whereas 13% had two-vessel and only 0.9% had three-vessel angioplasty (4).

These data demonstrate that despite the rapid growth in the number of PTCA procedures, most patients still undergo single-vessel angioplasty. In this chapter I review several aspects of single-vessel dilation such as guide catheters, choice of balloon, dilation techniques, and early and late clinical results.

GUIDE CATHETER CHOICE

Improvements in guide catheter technology (torque control, firmness, resistance to kinking, soft atraumatic tips, and friction-free inner lining) associated with the extremely low profiles of standard balloon catheters have made crossing a coronary stenosis much easier. For most simple de novo coronary lesions, the standard Judkins left and right configurations are adequate. The current trend in coronary angioplasty is toward smaller size guide catheters. The original 9.4 Fr guide catheters have been replaced by less traumatic 8 Fr catheters, with internal diameters of 0.084 to 0.086 inch. These 8 Fr guide catheters may be superseded by even smaller catheters (Table 22A.1). Several patient series have demonstrated the feasibility of PTCA using 7 Fr and 6 Fr guide catheters that are now commercially available (5, 6).

Advantages of a small guide catheter include (a) less coronary pressure dampening, particularly in the right coronary artery; (b) less vascular complications, especially in patients with peripheral vascular disease in whom larger catheters can produce limb

Table 22A.1
Guide Catheters—6 Fr and 7 Fr

Catheter	Shaft Size	Internal Diameter (inches)	Manufacturer
Sherpa	6 Fr	0.057	Medtronic
Petite Brite Tip	6 Fr	0.062	Cordis
Sherpa	7 Fr	0.070	Medtronic
Marathon	7 Fr	0.070	Baxter
Super 7	7 Fr	0.070	USCI
Proformer	7 Fr	0.071	Mansfield
Sherpa Peak Flow	7 Fr	0.072	Medtronic
Brite Tip	7 Fr	0.072	Cordis
Tri-Guide	7 Fr	0.072	SciMed
Power Base	7 Fr	0.072	ACS
Lumax	7 Fr	0.073	Cook
Guidezilla	7 Fr	0.074	Schneider

ischemia; and (c) the possibility of a shorter hospital stay or earlier ambulation because of smaller arterial puncture. Some drawbacks of the smaller systems include (a) inability to insert equipment such as perfusion balloons, two-balloon systems simultaneously, or stents; and (b) limitations in the degree of vessel opacification. In my experience smaller guide catheters are clearly advantageous in women who have small proximal right of left coronary arteries and in women with small body habitus, in whom an 8 Fr guide catheter could result in limb ischemia. I have also used it in markedly obese patients, in whom hemostasis after sheath removal is potentially a problem. Guide catheter support is surprisingly good with 7 Fr guide catheters.

In my opinion, a 6 Fr has no advantage over a 7 Fr guide catheter, and it has a clear disadvantage in that it reduces vessel opacification when a balloon catheter is in place, unless a balloon-on-a-wire system is used. I have reserved the use of 6 Fr guide catheters for patients with straightforward restenotic lesions who are having a diagnostic angiogram with a 6 Fr system and for patients having angioplasty through a radial artery approach. In these patients, using a balloon-on-a-wire or an ultra-low-profile over-the-wire system can be used with adequate opacifica-

tion of the distal coronary artery. I do not see smaller guide catheters as a major determinant of shorter hospitalizations. At present 64% of our patients undergoing single-vessel PTCA with an 8 Fr system are discharged the day after the procedure. It is usually the patient's clinical condition that determines a longer hospitalization. No clear rationale exists for the use of guide catheters smaller than 6 Fr or for the use of diagnostic catheters for coronary angioplasty.

COMPLIANT OR NONCOMPLIANT BALLOONS?

Compliance, or "stretch," refers to the change in balloon diameter with change in inflation pressure, also called balloon distension. Each balloon material has a different distension rate with increasing inflation pressures.

The original balloons were made of polyvinyl chloride (PVC). In addition to PVC the following balloon materials, listed in decreasing rate of compliance, are available: polyolefin copolymer (POC), polyethylene (PE), Duralyn, and polyethylene terephthalate (PET). For the patient with a simple de novo lesion, balloon material is probably not an important factor in balloon selection. Published data would suggest little or no effect of balloon material on either coronary dissection or clinical complication rate (7, 8).

A noncompliant PET balloon has a potential advantage in lesions expected to require high inflation pressures such as seen in elderly patients or in patients with a long history of angina or coronary calcification. A compliant POC balloon has the potential for excessive "dog-boning" at higher inflation pressures with overstretching of the normal artery adjacent to the lesion. The lower burst pressure of PVC and PE balloons makes them less favorable for these lesions. How often are high inflation pressures needed? Kahn et al. reported that 86% of stenoses responded to a maximal pressure of 8 atm or less and 97% responded to 10 atm

Table 22A.2
Long Balloons

Balloon	Balloon Length (mm)	Balloon Material	Rated Burst Pressure (atm)	Compatible Wire (in)	Manufacturer
Over-the-wire					
Slider Long	30–40	P.E.	12	0.014–0.018	Mansfield
Evergreen	30	P.E.	8	0.014	Medtronic
Edge	30–40	P.E.-600	8	0.014	ACS
Pinkerton	30–40	P.E.-600	8	0.018	ACS
Force	30–40	PET	12	0.018	USCI
Predator-XL	30–40	Duralyn	10	0.014	Cordis
Olympix	30–40	Duralyn	10	0.018	Cordis
Trakstar	30–40	Duralyn	10	0.014	Cordis
Long-Cobra	30–40	POC	9	0.018	SciMed
Mystic	30–40	Thalane	12	0.014	Schneider
Monorail					
MC Rail	30–40	Thalane	12–14	0.014	Schneider
RX Streak	30–40	PE-600	8	0.010–0.014	ACS
RX Elipse	30–40	PE-600	8	0.014	ACS
On-the-wire					
Long ACE	40	POC	8	—	SciMed
Perfusion					
Rx Perfusion	30	PE-600	8	0.018	ACS
Rx Flowtrack Long	30–40	PE-600	8	0.018	ACS

or less (9). No clinical or angiographic variables appeared to be useful in predicting stenosis that did not yield to usual inflation pressures. Because of its good conformability (tendency not to straighten out arterial curves), PET balloons could have an advantage in dilating angled lesions (10).

Compliant balloons such as POC allow the operator to achieve a range of balloon diameters by varying the inflation pressure. This ability is advantageous in patients in whom estimating the artery diameter correctly is difficult. It also allows a single balloon to be used to dilate lesions in arteries of different diameters. In this regard, PE and POC balloons maintain a better wrap around the catheter, with less "winging" after repeat inflations, compared with PVC and PET balloons. With more patients undergoing treatment for multiple lesions, attention should be given to the properties of balloons after deflation in the coronary arteries. The ongoing multicenter randomized study of Compliance Related Acute Complications (CRAC) should provide answers regarding the efficacy and safety of different angioplasty balloon materials.

LONG BALLOONS AND PROLONGED INFLATIONS

Angioplasty catheters with balloon lengths of 30 to 40 mm are now commercially available and have performance characteristics similar to the regular-length balloons. Research supports their use in long lesions (more than 10 mm), tandem lesions, and lesions on bends (Table 22A.2).

Bymer et al. reported on 44 patients with long lesions (15 to 25 mm) or tandem lesions close enough to be encompassed by a 30-mm balloon. They assigned patients to treatment with either standard 20- or 30-mm balloons. Those treated with long balloons required fewer inflations, had fewer moderate or severe intimal dissections, and had shorter procedure times (11).

Tenaglia et al. analyzed 89 patients with long lesions (more than 10 mm) treated with long balloons at Duke University over a 1-year period. Procedural success was 97%, abrupt closure occurred in 6%, and major dissections occurred in 11% (12). These results compare favorably with historical results in patients with long stenoses treated with regular-length balloons.

Today's angioplasty practice frequently includes patients with unstable, acute ischemic syndromes. In general, these lesions carry a high complication rate, usually because of some element of complexity such as eccentricity or thrombus. Prolonged inflations of 10 to 20 minutes using autoperfusion balloon catheters appear to yield excellent angiographic and clinical results. Reports from a randomized trial comparing prolonged inflations (up to two dilations of 15 minutes each) with standard inflations (up to four dilations of 1 minute each) show that patients assigned to prolonged dilations had a higher success rate, less severe residual stenosis by quantitative angiography, and a lower rate of major dissections. This initial improvement in angiographic appearance did not lead to a reduc-

tion in restenosis or clinical events during follow-up (13).

New, low-profile, autoperfusion balloon catheters can be used as the primary and single device in a majority of these cases (Figs. 22A.1 and 22A.2). General application of this technique is limited by angiographic exclusions such as vessels less than 2.5 mm in diameter, lesions longer than 30 mm, and lesions with major side branches (Table 22A.3).

RESULTS

Despite important technologic developments, single-vessel dilation is by far the most common indication for coronary angioplasty at the present time. It is well known that patients with single-vessel disease enjoy a favorable prognosis with medical treatment. For PTCA

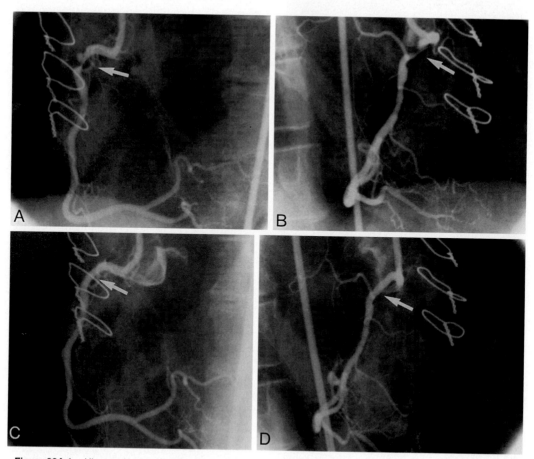

Figure 22A.1. Ulcerated lesion involving the proximal right coronary artery, before (**A** and **B**) and after (**C** and **D**) a 10-minute inflation with a perfusion balloon.

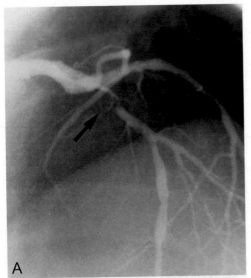

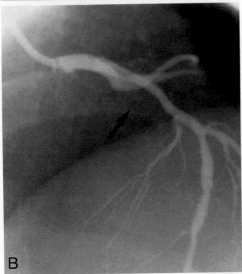

Figure 22A.2. Eccentric lesion in the proximal left anterior descending coronary artery, cranial view. Before (**A**) and after (**B**) a 10- and 15-minute inflation at 5 atm.

to become the treatment of choice, it should combine ease, low morbidity, and high success rates.

Early Results

In 1988 we analyzed the clinical and angiographic characteristics determining primary success in 2677 consecutive patients who underwent elective single-vessel PTCA. Although the study included patients undergoing angioplasty between 1980 and 1987, the primary success defined as angiographic success in the absence of myocardial infarction, emergency bypass surgery, or death was 93%. All subgroups had success rates of more than 90%, with the exception of patients with calcified lesions (84%) or totally occluded vessels (79%) (14).

That same year the combined ACC-AHA task force characterized lesions as type A, B, or C, with PTCA success rates of more than 85%, 60 to 85%, and less than 60%, respectively (15). Ellis et al. modified the ACC-AHA classification, reporting results for 1986 to 1987 at four centers. In this study success and complication rates were 92% and 4%, respectively, for type A lesions, 84% and 4% for type B1 lesions; 76% and 10% for type B2 lesions, and 61% and 21% for type C lesions (16). Myler et al. questioned the accuracy of these classifications based on the fact that they preceded significant improvements in catheter technology. Reporting on 533 consecutive patients with 1000 lesions in 1990 to 1991, angioplasty success and complication rates were achieved in 99% and

Table 22A.3
Perfusion Balloons

Balloon	Balloon Length (mm)	Balloon Diameter (mm)	Shaft Diam. Prox/Distal (Fr)	Crossing Profile X 3 mm (in)	Flow Rates (cc/min)	Max Wire (in)
Stack Perfusion	20	2.0–4.0	3.9/4.5	0.058	60	0.018
Stack 40-S Perfusion	20	2.0–4.0	3.9/3.9	0.053	40	0.018
Stack Perfusion Long	25	2.5–4.0	3.9/4.5	0.058	55	0.018
ACS RX Perfusion	20–30	2.0–4.0	3.7/4.2	0.055	60	0.018
ACS RX Flowtrack	20–40	2.0–4.0	2.3/3.5	0.050	36–40	0.018

1.2%, respectively, for type A lesions; 95% and 1.5% for type B1 lesions; 89.5% and 2.3% for type B2 lesions, and 90% and 2% for type C lesions (17). In 1993 at the Cleveland Clinic procedural success (PTCA alone) was achieved in 100% of type A lesions, 98.7% of B1 lesions, 91.5% of B2 lesions, and 80.7% of C lesions, implying that this schema, while perhaps in need of a revision, still has diagnostic merit.

Late Results

Two reports from the Cleveland Clinic Foundation describe long-term results for PTCA in patients with single-vessel left anterior descending disease. Kramer et al. reported on 781 patients with isolated left anterior descending disease treated with either bypass surgery (368 patients) or PTCA (413 patients) between 1980 and 1984. The overall cardiac survival rate was 99% for the PTCA group compared with 98.5% for the surgical group, and the rate of survival without myocardial infarction was 96.5% and 96% for the PTCA and surgical groups, respectively. The PTCA group required significantly more repeat revascularization procedures during follow-up, so the 5-year, postdischarge, event-free survival was 93% in the surgical group but only 72% in the PTCA group (18).

Frierson et al. reported on 537 consecutive patients who underwent angioplasty for proximal left anterior descending disease from 1984 to 1987. The procedure was clinically successful in 96% of the patients, with an in-hospital mortality rate of 0.4%, a myocardial infarction rate of 2.2%, and a bypass surgery rate of 3%. At a mean follow-up of 44 months, 19% required additional revascularization for recurrent left anterior descending stenosis. The actuarial 5-year cardiac survival rate was 97%; freedom from death and myocardial infarction was 94%; and freedom from cardiac death, myocardial infarction, bypass surgery, and repeat left anterior descending PTCA was 77%. Follow-up angiography in 76% of the patients found a 39.6% angio-graphic restenosis rate. At follow-up 76% of patients were free of angina (19).

A second Cleveland Clinic study compared multivessel to single-vessel angioplasty in sex- and age-matched groups. Of the 569 patients undergoing single-vessel PTCA, 41% had multivessel disease. At a mean follow-up of 44 months, clinical events included 5.3% mortality, 4.8% myocardial infarction, 15.5% bypass surgery, and 19.9% repeat PTCA. The 5-year actuarial survival rate free of myocardial infarction or bypass surgery was 74% (20).

These observational studies suggest that simple PTCA can provide excellent long-term results with a low risk of cardiac death and myocardial infarction in patients with single-vessel angioplasty, but that the need for further interventions is frequent.

COMPARATIVE RANDOMIZED STUDIES

Despite the widespread use of PTCA, most information concerning its success has been derived from observational studies. In patients with single-vessel disease, only two reports have prospectively evaluated results of PTCA compared with medical or surgical treatment.

The recently published ACME (Angioplasty Compared to Medicine) trial, randomly assigned 212 patients with stable angina, a markedly positive stress test, and single-vessel disease to PTCA or medical therapy. In-hospital events for the PTCA group included a clinical success rate of 80% and a myocardial infarction rate of 4%, and 2% of the patients required bypass surgery. The principal finding was that at 6-month follow-up, PTCA offered earlier and more complete relief of angina than medical therapy (64% versus 46%) and was associated with better performance on exercise testing (21).

Of the several ongoing trials designed to compare the long-term effects of coronary angioplasty and coronary bypass surgery, the RITA (Randomized Intervention Treatment of Angina) trial is the only study to include patients with single-vessel disease. Of the 493 patients randomized to PTCA who had the procedure, 267 (54%) had angioplasty of a single artery. At a median follow-up of 2.5 years, the combined endpoints of death or myocardial infarction did not differ between treatment groups (8.6% for the surgical group compared with 9.8% for the PTCA group). Surgically treated patients enjoyed better relief of angina, required fewer antianginal drugs, and required fewer additional myocardial revascularization procedures. At 2 years of randomization 36% of the patients undergoing single-vessel PTCA had an event or required a subsequent procedure, compared with only 11% for the entire surgical group (22). This is a preliminary report and a detailed subgroup analysis is expected to be presented at a later date. Goy et al. recently reported on a randomized trial designed to compare PTCA with left internal mammary grafting in 134 patients with isolated proximal left anterior descending artery stenosis. At a median follow-up of 24 months the rates of cardiac death and myocardial infarction did not differ between the groups. Clinical and functional status improved similarly in both groups; however, there were significantly more repeat interventions in the PTCA group (34% versus 3%) (23).

SUMMARY

Despite technologic advances and rapid growth in the number of PTCA procedures, single-artery dilation continues to be by far the most common indication for PTCA at the present time. With today's armamentarium it is possible to approach the majority of lesions with a high success rate and few complications. Long-term results indicate excellent myocardial infarction–free survival rates that are comparable with surgical groups. However, the need for repeat revascularization procedures continues to be a limiting factor of this treatment modality.

For the patient with a simple de novo lesion, the need for new devices is limited. The two recent randomized trials comparing coronary angioplasty with directional atherectomy demonstrated that at present atherectomy offers no obvious advantage over balloon angioplasty. It is possible that additional experience in performing more aggressive atherectomy may lead to the identification of specific lesions that are more effectively approached with this technique (24).

Two recently completed randomized trials of elective coronary stenting show that at 6 months the need for repeat revascularization was reduced with stenting, as compared with standard angioplasty (25, 26). There are potential refinements of coronary stenting, including the use of stents coated with anti-thrombotic agents and deployment of stents with intravascular ultrasound guidance, potentially precluding the need for aggressive anticoagulation that may soon make elective stenting the preferred method of revascularization.

REFERENCES

1. Hartzler GO. PTCA in evolution: Why is it so popular? Cleve Clin J Med 1990;57:121–124.
2. Serruys PW, Breeman A. Coronary angioplasty: clinical application. Neth J Cardiol 1991;4:146–154.
3. Topol EJ, Ellis SG, Cosgrove DM et al. Analysis of coronary angioplasty in the United States with an insurance claims data base. Circulation 1993;87:1489–1497.
4. Hannan EL, Arani DT, Johnson LW, Kemp HG, Lukacik G. Percutaneous transluminal coronary angioplasty in New York State. Risk factors and outcomes. JAMA 1992; 268:3092–3097.
5. Villavicencio R, Meier B, Pande AK, Urban P, Sztajzel J, De La Serna F. Coronary angioplasty with 7F guiding catheters. Am Heart J 1991;122:1519–1521.
6. Feldman R, Glemser E, Kaizer J, Standley M. Coronary angioplasty using new 6 French guiding catheters. Cathet Cardiovasc Diagn 1991;23:93–99.
7. Mooney MR, Fishman Mooney J, Longe TF, Brandenburg RO. Effect of balloon material on coronary angioplasty. Am J Cardiol 1992;69:1481–1482.
8. Raymenants E, Bhandari S, Desmet W et al. The impact of balloon material and lesion characteristics on the incidence of angiographic and clinical complications of coronary angioplasty. Cathet Cardiovasc Diagn 1994;32:303–309.
9. Kahn JK, Rutherford BD, McConahay DR, Hartzler GO. Inflation pressure requirements during coronary angioplasty. Cathet Cardiovasc Diagn 1990;21:144–147.
10. Ellis SG, Topol EJ. Results of percutaneous transluminal coronary angioplasty of high-risk angulated stenoses. Am J Cardiol 1990;66:932–937.
11. Brymer JF, Khaja F, Kraft PL. Angioplasty of long or tandem coronary artery lesions using a new longer balloon dilatation catheter: a comparative study. Cathet Cardiovasc Diagn 1991;23:84–88.
12. Tenaglia AN, Zidar JP, Jackman JD et al. Treatment of long coronary artery narrowings with long angioplasty balloon catheters. Am J Cardiol 1993;71:1274–1277.

13. Ohman EM, Marquis JF, Ricci DR et al. A randomized comparison of the effects of gradual prolonged versus standard primary balloon inflation on early and late outcome. Results of a multicenter clinical trial. Circulation 1994;89:1118–1125.

14. Tuzcu EM, Simpfendorfer C, Badhwark et al. Determinants of primary success in elective percutaneous transluminal coronary angioplasty for significant narrowing of a single major coronary artery. Am J Cardiol 1988; 62:873–875.

15. Ryan TJ, Faxon DP, Gunnar RP, and the ACC/AHA Task Force. Guidelines for percutaneous transluminal coronary angioplasty. J AM Coll Cardiol 1988;12:529–545.

16. Ellis SG, Vandormael MG, Cowley MJ et al., and the Multivessel Angioplasty Prognosis Group. Coronary morphologic and clinical determinants of procedural outcome with angioplasty for multivessel coronary disease: implications for patient selection. Circulation 1990;82:1193–1202.

17. Myler RK, Shaw RE, Stertzer SH et al. Lesion morphology and coronary angioplasty: current experience and analysis. J Am Coll Cardiol 1992;19:1641–1652.

18. Kramer JR, Proudfit WL, Loop FD, Goormastic M, Zimmerman K, Simpfendorfer C. Late follow-up of 781 patients undergoing percutaneous transluminal coronary angioplasty or coronary artery bypass grafting for an isolated obstruction in the left anterior descending coronary artery. Am Heart J 1989;118:1144–1153.

19. Frierson JH, Dimas AP, Whitlow PL et al. Angioplasty of the proximal left anterior descending coronary artery: initial success and long-term follow-up. J Am Coll Cardiol 1992;19:745–751.

20. Hollman J, Simpfendorfer C, Franco I, Whitlow P, Goormastic M. Multivessel and single vessel coronary angioplasty: a comparative study. Am Heart J 1992;124:9–12.

21. Parisi AF, Folland ED, Hartigan P, on behalf of the Veterans Affairs ACME investigations. A comparison of angioplasty with medical therapy in the treatment of single vessel coronary artery disease. N Engl J Med 1992;326:10–16.

22. RITA trial participants. Coronary angioplasty versus coronary artery bypass surgery: the randomized intervention treatment of angina (RITA) trial: Lancet 1993; 341:573–580.

23. Goy JJ, Eeckhout E, Burnand B et al. Coronary angioplasty versus left internal mammary artery grafting for isolated proximal left anterior descending artery stenosis. Lancet 1994;343:1449–1453.

24. Holmes DR, Topol EJ, Adelman AG, Cohen EA, Califf RM. Randomized trials of directional coronary atherectomy: implications for clinical practice and future investigation. J Am Coll Cardiol 1994;24:431–439.

25. Serruys PW, de Jaegere P, Kiemenen F et al. A comparison of balloon-expandable-stent implantation with balloon angioplasty in patients with coronary artery disease. N Engl J Med 1994;331:489–495.

26. Fischman DL, Leon MB, Baim DS et al. A randomized comparison of coronary-stent placement and balloon angioplasty in the treatment of coronary disease. N Engl J Med 1994;331:496–501.

B. Primary Stenting for the De Novo Native Coronary Artery Stenosis

PAUL S. TEIRSTEIN

Recent reports describe increased procedural success, decreased angiographic restenosis, and improved 1-year clinical outcome when Palmaz-Schatz stents are deployed in native coronary artery stenoses. These benefits have created a potential indication for the Palmaz-Schatz coronary stent as a primary therapy for the de novo native coronary artery stenosis. Like any important clinical decision, the relative benefits of stenting must be weighed against the relative risks, morbidity, and cost.

ADVANTAGES OF CORONARY STENTING

Improved Procedural Angiographic Outcome

In the STent REStenosis Study (STRESS), 409 patients with de novo lesions of native coronary arteries ≥3.0 mm in diameter were randomized to either Palmaz-Schatz stent implantation (n = 207) or balloon angioplasty (n = 202) (1–4). The STRESS core laboratory quantitative angiographic review reported an angiographic success rate (<50% diameter stenosis) of only 92.6% in the balloon angioplasty group compared with 99.5% in the stent group ($P < .001$). The stent patients had less elastic recoil (13% versus 24%, $P < .0001$) and fewer intimal dissections (6% versus 36%, $P < .0001$). The improved angiographic results in this study were largely because of the stent's profound impact on acute luminal gain compared with balloon angioplasty (5). This increase in acute gain increases the likelihood of a predictably excellent angiographic result. Furthermore, the excellent angiographic results following Palmaz-Schatz stent deployment appear independent of the underlying lesion morphology. Angiographic features such as lesion eccentricity, moderate angulation, ulceration, or the presence of moderate calcification do not adversely affect procedural success (6) as has been well described following balloon angioplasty (7–9).

Reduced Angiographic Restenosis Rates

Results from the United States non-randomized, multicenter trial were highly suggestive of a decreased angiographic restenosis rate following Palmaz-Schatz stenting of de novo lesions requiring a single stent. The core laboratory, quantitative analysis of 4- to 6-month follow-up angiograms found a restenosis rate ($\geq$50% diameter stenosis) of only 14% for de novo lesions (10–12) compared with historic controls of 30 to 56% (13–15). This decrease in angiographic restenosis also translated into improved clinical outcome at 1 year. Clinical events at follow-up (including procedural complications) were low. Fully 87% of patients were free of major events (myocardial infarction, death, repeat coronary angioplasty, or bypass surgery) at 1 year (12). In the STRESS trial the impact of stenting on clinical restenosis was also significant. The need for target lesion revascularization at 180 days was only 10.2% after stenting compared with 15.4% after balloon angioplasty, $P = .05$ (3).

Results from the European multicenter randomized Benestent trial also indicate a restenosis benefit following coronary stenting. In the Benestent trial 520 patients with de novo coronary artery stenoses were randomized to either Palmaz-Schatz stenting or balloon angioplasty. Restenosis ($\geq$50% diameter stenosis at follow-up) occurred in 22% of the stent group compared with 32% of the balloon angioplasty group ($P <.05$) (16, 17). Mean minimal luminal diameter at follow-up was also larger in the stent group (1.83 mm versus 1.67 mm, $P <.05$).

The improved angiographic restenosis rate after Palmaz-Schatz stent deployment appears to be the result of the improved initial acute luminal gain achieved following stent-

ing (5, 18–21). Although absolute luminal renarrowing (late loss) is increased following stenting, the immediate poststent deployment luminal diameter (acute gain) is sufficiently large to compensate for this renarrowing, and the net luminal improvement at 6-month follow-up is larger than that obtained following balloon angioplasty.

DISADVANTAGES OF CORONARY STENTING

The above benefits of coronary stenting must be weighed against the risks of subacute stent thrombosis, bleeding complications, the requirement for a prolonged hospitalization, and increased costs.

Stent Thrombosis

Subacute stent thrombosis has proven to be the Achilles heel of coronary stenting. Despite an intense anticoagulation regimen, the 1988–1991 United States multicenter trial of the Palmaz-Schatz stent documented a subacute stent thrombosis rate of approximately 5% for elective stent placement (22, 23). Clinical and angiographic factors found to be associated with stent thrombosis include reference vessel diameters <3.2 mm, angiographic presence of periprocedural thrombus, stent placement as a "bailout" following failed angioplasty, the presence of a luminal dissection following stent deployment, bleeding complications that require interruption of the anticoagulation regimen, and a platelet count >350,000 (22). Stent thrombosis is usually a devastating clinical problem. The overwhelming majority of stent thromboses occur during the first 2 weeks following stent deployment, and almost one-half occur after discharge from the hospital. The clinical presentation is almost always acute myocardial infarction associated with complete thrombotic occlusion of the stent. Death, myocardial infarction, and the need for emergency bypass surgery occur in 2%, 45%, and 81% of patients with stent thrombosis, respectively (22, 23).

Naturally, procedural complications also occur following balloon angioplasty. In the randomized STRESS trial, acute or subacute vessel closure occurred in 1.5% of balloon angioplasty patients versus 3.4% of stent patients, P = NS (3, 4). The incidence of myocardial infarction (5.0 versus 5.4 P = NS) and death (1.5% versus 0%, P = NS) were also similar, but there was a trend toward an increased need for emergency bypass surgery in the balloon angioplasty group (4% versus 2.4%, P = NS). Thus the overall risk of procedural complications following stenting was nearly equivalent to the risks following balloon angioplasty with stent patients having a trend toward slightly higher risk of vessel closure and slightly lower need for emergency bypass surgery.

Two methods of combatting stent thrombosis have arisen since 1992. In the first, Colombo and others have found that high-pressure (>16 to 18 atm) ultrasound-guided (to assure strut apposition to the arterial wall and minimal cross-sectional area in the stent >90% of the adjacent reference vessel) stent placement with aspirin and ticlopidine alone yields stent thrombosis in <1 to 2% of patients. In the second, heparin-coated Palmaz-Schatz stents have been used, also without long-term heparin and Coumadin. In the BENESTENT II pilot study of 202 patients this also looked promising (Tables 22B.1, 22B.2, and 22B.3), although it is difficult to separate the effects of the coating and that from high-pressure postimplant balloon inflation.

Bleeding Complications

The anticoagulation regimen approved in the United States when stents were released includes preprocedural aspirin, persantine, and intravenous heparin, as well as an intravenous infusion of low–molecular weight dextran. Following the procedure oral warfarin is initiated and continued for 1 month. This intense anticoagulation regimen results in significant bleeding complications. The

Table 22B.1
BENESTENT II Pilot—Protocol

Part	No. of Pts.	Heparin	Coumadin	ASA	Ticlopidine
I	51	6 hr	+	+	+
II	50	12 hr	+	+	+
III	51	36 hr	+	+	+
IV	50	0	−	+	+

Table 22B.2
BENESTENT II Pilot—Acute Results

Part	IVUS Used %	>12 Atm %	Procedural Success %	Subacute Thrombosis %	Hosp Days
I	10	43	100	0	7.4
II	3	76	98	0	6.1
III	20	65	100	0	7.0
IV	0	78	100	0	3.0
BENESTENT I	0	0	93	3.5	8.5

Table 22B.3
BENESTENT II Pilot—Restenosis

	MLD-Pre (mm)	MLD-Post (mm)	MLD-F/U (mm)	% Restenosis
BII Pilot (stents)	1.11	2.76	2.12	13
BI (stents)	1.07	2.12	1.85	22

need for transfusion or surgical repair of the femoral access site was 7.9% in the United States multicenter trial (24). In the randomized STRESS trial, bleeding complications (transfusion or surgical repair) were more common in the stent group (7.3%) versus balloon angioplasty patients (4.0%), P = .14 (3, 4). While the majority of these complications were not life threatening, the impact of bleeding complications on patient morbidity should not be minimized. Femoral access site and gastrointestinal bleeding add significantly to the cost and ordeal of the angioplasty procedure.

The recent elimination of the routine use of heparin for several days and also Coumadin has also dramatically reduced bleeding complications. Quality-controlled data from large numbers of patients are presently difficult to obtain, but, for instance, no patient in phase IV of the BENESTENT II pilot required vascular surgery compared with 9.7% in the BENESTENT I trial.

Procedural Costs

Procedural costs are increased following Palmaz-Schatz stenting because of (a) an increased need for equipment during the stent procedure, (b) an increased length of hospital stay required to achieve adequate anticoagulation, and (c) increased bleeding complications requiring the need for blood transfusions, endoscopy, and surgical repair of the access site. In one non-randomized study comparing coronary stenting with balloon angioplasty, in-hospital charges were 202% higher in patients undergoing stenting (25, 26). Data with contemporary anticoagulation is not yet available.

SHOULD STENTS BE USED AS A PRIMARY THERAPY FOR THE DE NOVO NATIVE CORONARY ARTERY STENOSIS?

From the above analysis it is obvious that the pros and cons of coronary stenting for the primary de novo lesion are complex. The data are somewhat conflicting. The very significant advantages of stenting are somewhat mitigated by the very significant complications, increased length of hospital stay, and costs of this technique. Although the restenosis rate following Palmaz-Schatz stent deployment is clearly lower, it can be argued that a patient undergoing two balloon angioplasty procedures (an initial procedure and then a subsequent procedure to treat restenosis) would still endure an overall shorter length of hospital stay, less risk of bleeding complications, and costs similar to that of a single stent procedure. If one assumes a 30% risk of restenosis following an initial balloon angioplasty procedure and a 40% restenosis risk following a second procedure to treat restenosis (27–30), the risk of a given patient requiring three angioplasty procedures is only 12%,

similar to the requirement for repeat revascularization following stent placement (31).

This author has taken a practical approach to this clinical dilemma. I favor routine balloon angioplasty for the simple, straightforward ACC/AHA type A lesion. One can treat this simple lesion using balloon angioplasty and expect an extremely high rate of procedural success (>95%) with few complications. Most patients treated in this manner will be discharged from the hospital after a single night's stay. Balloon angioplasty for this lesion subtype is usually a relatively straightforward procedure that is easy for the patient to endure. When and if this patient returns with a restenosis, repeat balloon angioplasty can be expected to be similarly straightforward and the patient is usually treated and discharged after a single night of hospitalization. If, however, the target lesion contains angiographic features predictive of decreased success and/or increased complications such as severe ulceration or eccentricity, moderate angulation (<45°) or calcification, lesion length >10 mm (but <15 mm), or preexisting dissection, I strongly consider stenting as a primary therapy. Stenting these lesion subtypes provides a predictably excellent angiographic result independent of the underlying complex morphology. Here, stenting has the advantage of higher procedural success rates with fewer complications. When the additional advantage of improved late outcome is considered, the risk:benefit ratio swings in favor of Palmaz-Schatz stent placement in patients with these complex lesion subtypes.

Several important caveats must be considered prior to stent deployment. Importantly, the clinical trials described above relate only to lesions in relatively large diameter (>3 mm) vessels. Target stenoses in smaller diameter vessels were excluded. Similarly excluded were lesions in the left main coronary artery, ostial in location, involving large side branches, within heavily calcified vessels, and patients with extremely poor left ventricular function. Stent deployment in patients with these clinical and anatomic characteristics will likely be associated with lower success and higher complication rates. It is imperative to avoid elective stenting of target lesions within vessels <3 mm in diameter because of the clear increased risk of stent thrombosis in small diameter vessels. It is also important to note that the above clinical trials all utilized the Johnson and Johnson Palmaz-Schatz balloon-expandable coronary stent. This slotted, stainless steel, tubular design is quite different from numerous other stent designs currently under investigation (i.e., coil, woven, tantalum, nitinol). Presently, there are no data to indicate a lower restenosis rate or improved late clinical outcome following elective deployment of these other stent designs, and there is no indication for use of these stent designs as a primary therapy for the de novo native artery stenosis (32).

Finally, it should be noted that the above risk-benefit analysis is strongly influenced by the risk of stent thrombosis and the increased risk of bleeding complications, cost, and morbidity associated with the intense anticoagulation required for stenting. If future stents and treatment protocols virtually eliminate stent thrombosis and the need for systemic anticoagulation, the risk:benefit ratio would likely swing dramatically in favor of coronary stenting.

REFERENCES

1. Fischman D, Savage M, Leon M, Schatz R, Baim D, Penn I, Detre K et al. for the STRESS investigators. Acute and late angiographic results of the STent REStenosis Study (STRESS). J Am Coll Cardiol 1994;1A:60A (abstract).
2. Schatz RA, Penn IM, Baim DS, Nobuyoshi M, Colombo A, Ricci DR, Cleman MW et al. for the STRESS investigators. STent REStenosis Study (STRESS): analysis of in-hospital results. Circulation 1993;88:I-594 (abstract).
3. Leon MB, Fischman D, Schatz RA, Baim DS, Penn I, Nobuyoshi M, Colombo A et al. Analysis of early and late clinical events from the STent REStenosis Study (STRESS). J Am Coll Cardiol 1994;1A:60A (abstract).
4. Fischman DL, Leon MB, Baim DS, Schatz RA, Savage MP, Penn I, Detre K et al. for the Stent Restenosis Study investigators. A randomized comparison of coronary-stent placement and balloon angioplasty in the treatment of coronary artery disease. N Engl J Med 1994; 331:496–501.
5. Kuntz RE, Safian RD, Levin MJ, Reis GJ, Diver DJ, Baim DS. Novel approach to the analysis of restenosis after the use of three new coronary devices. J Am Coll Cardiol 1992;19:1493–1499.
6. Rocha-Singh KJ, Fischman DL, Savage MP, Goldberg S, Teirstein PS, Schatz RA. Influence of angiographic lesion characteristics on early complication rates after Palmaz-Schatz stenting. J Am Coll Cardiol 1993;21:292A (abstract).
7. Ryan TJ, Faxon DP, Gunnar RM, Kennedy JW, King SB III, Loop FD, Peterson KL et al. Guidelines for percutaneous transluminal coronary angioplasty. A report of the American College of Cardiology/American Heart Association Task Force on Assessment of Diagnostic and Therapeutic Cardiovascular Procesures (Subcommittee on Percutaneous Transluminal Coronary Angioplasty). J Am Coll Cardiol 1988;12:529–545.
8. Ellis SE, Vandormael MG, Cowley MJ, DiSciascio G, Deligonul U, Topol EJ, Bulle TM, the Multivessel Angioplasty Prognosis Study Group. Coronary morphologic and clinical determinants of procedural outcome with angioplasty for multivessel coronary disease—implications for patient selection. Circulation 1990;82:1193–1202.
9. Ellis SG, Roubin GS, King SB III, Douglas JS Jr, Weintraub WS, Thomas RG, Cox WR. Angiographic and clinical predictors of acute closure after native vessel coronary angioplasty. Circulation 1988;77:372–379.
10. Teirstein PS, Schatz RA, Leon M, Goldberg S, Ellis S, Baim D, Stratienko AA et al. Should patients with discrete, de novo coronary stenoses undergo stenting as a primary procedure? Risk vs benefit. J Am Coll Cardiol 1991;17:280A (abstract).
11. Savage M, Fischman D, Leon M, Schatz R, Teirstein P, Baim D, Gebhardt S et al. Efficacy of coronary stents in the treatment of refractory restenosis following balloon angioplasty. J Am Coll Cardiol 1993;32:33A (abstract).
12. Savage MP, Fischman DL, Schatz RA, Teirstein PS, Leon MB, Baim D, Ellis SG et al. for the Palmaz-Schatz stent study group. Long-term angiographic and clinical outcome after implantation of a balloon-expandable stent in the native coronary circulation. J Am Coll Cardiol 1994; 24:1207–1212.
13. Topol EJ, Leya F, Pinkerton CA, Whitlow PL, Hofling B, Simonton CA, Masden RR et al. for the CAVEAT study group. A comparison of directional atherectomy with coronary angioplasty in patients with coronary artery disease. N Engl J Med 1993;329:221–227.
14. The Multicenter European Research Trial with Cilazapril After Angioplasty to Prevent Transluminal Coronary Obstruction and Restenosis (MERCATOR) study. Does the new angiotensin converting enzyme inhibitor Cilazapril prevent restenosis after percutaneous transluminal coronary angioplasty? Results of the MERCATOR study: a multicenter, randomized, double-blind placebo-controlled trial. Circulation 1992;86:100–110.

15. Hirshfeld JW Jr, Schwartz JS, Jugo R, MacDonald RG, Goldberg S, Savage MP, Bass TA et al. Restenosis after coronary angioplasty: a multivariate statistical model to relate lesion and procedure variables to restenosis. J Am Coll Cardiol 1991;18:647–656.

16. Serruys PW, Macaya C, de Jaegere P, Kiemeneij F, Rutsch W, Heyndrickx G, Emanuelsson H et al. Interim analysis of the Benestent trial. Circulation 1993;88:I-594 (abstract).

17. Serruys PW, de Jaegere P, Kiemeneij F, Macaya C, Rutsch W, Heyndrickx G, Emanuelsson H et al. for the Benestent Study Group. A comparison of balloon-expandable–stent implantation with balloon angioplasty in patients with coronary artery disease. N Engl J Med 1994;331:489–495.

18. Ellis S, Fischman D, Hirshfeld J, Savage M, Goldberg S, Erbel R, Cleman M et al. Mechanism of stent benefit to limit restenosis following coronary angioplasty: regrowth vs. larger initial lumen? Circulation 1990;82(Suppl):III-540 (abstract).

19. Kuntz RE, Gibson CM, Nobuyoshi M, Baim DS. Generalized model of restenosis after conventional balloon angioplasty, stenting and directional atherectomy. J Am Coll Cardiol 1993;21:15–25.

20. Kuntz RE, Baim DS. Defining coronary restenosis. Newer clinical and angiographic paradigms. Circulation 1993; 88:1310–1323.

21. Kuntz RE, Safian RD, Carrozza JP, Fishman RF, Mansour M, Baim DS. The importance of acute luminal diameter in determining restenosis after coronary atherectomy or stenting. Circulation 1992;86:1827–1835.

22. Shaknovich A, Rocha-Singh K, Teirstein P, Lieberman S, Moses J. Subacute stent thrombosis in Palmaz-Schatz (PS) stents in native coronary arteries: time course, acute management and outcome. U.S. multicenter experience. Circulation 1992;86:(Suppl):I-113. (abstract).

23. Rocha-Singh K, Shaknovich A, Wong SC, Teirstein PS. Management of subacute stent thrombosis. 1992; (Suppl):I-114 (abstract).

24. Schatz RA, Baim DS, Leon M, Ellis SG, Goldberg S, Hirshfeld JW, Cleman MW et al. Clinical experience with the Palmaz-Schatz coronary stent. Initial results of a multicenter study. Circulation 1991;83:148–161.

25. Dick RJ, Popma JJ, Muller DW, Burek KA, Topol EJ. In-hospital costs associated with new percutaneous coronary devices. Am J Cardiol 1991;68:879–885.

26. Cohen DJ, Kuntz RE, Freidrich SP, Gordon PC, Breall JA, Ho KK, Weinstein MC et al. Cost-effectiveness of directional atherectomy, stenting, and conventional angioplasty in single-vessel disease: a decision-analytic model. J Am Coll Cardiol 1993;21:227A (abstract).

27. Teirstein PS, Hoover CA, Ligon RW, Giorgi LV, Rutherford BD, McConahay DR, Johnson WL et al. Repeat coronary angioplasty: efficacy of a third angioplasty for a second restenosis. J Am Coll Cardiol 1989;13:291–296.

28. Quigley PJ, Hlatky MA, Hinohara T, Rendall DS, Perez JA, Phillips HR, Califf RM et al. Repeat percutaneous transluminal coronary angioplasty and predictors of recurrent restenosis. Am J Cardiol 1989;63:409–413.

29. Black AJR, Anderson VH, Roubin GS, Powelson SW, Douglas JS, King SB III. Repeat coronary angioplasty: correlates of a second restenosis. J Am Coll Cardiol 1988; 11:714–718.

30. Moscucci M, Piana RN, Kuntz RE, Kugelmass AD, Carrozza JP Jr, Senerchia C, Baim DS. Effect of prior coronary restenosis on the risk of subsequent restenosis after stent placement or directional atherectomy. Am J Cardiol 1994; 73:1147–1153.

31. Shaknovich A, Lieberman SM, Moses JW. Clinical and angiographic outcomes of native coronary stenting with single Palmaz-Schatz (PS) stents. Update of U.S. multicenter experience. J Am Coll Cardiol 1993;21:29A (abstract).

32. Ellis SG, Verlee PN, Muller DWM. Comparison of outcome after coil vs. slotted-tube stainless steel coronary stent implantation to prevent restenosis—lessons from a single group experience. J Am Coll Cardiol 1993;21:292A (abstract).

EDITORS' SUMMARY	
Balloon angioplasty	The primary form of therapy because of simplicity and low cost
DCA	May be justified for proximal LAD lesions on the basis of decreased restenosis (CAVEAT I)
Stents	May be justified for lesions in vessels ≥3.0 mm to reduce stenosis—but at the risk of excess initial cost
Rotablator	No role
Laser	No role
TEC	No role

23. The Restenotic Lesion

A. Therapeutic Strategies for the Restenotic Lesion

MICHAEL P. SAVAGE, SHELDON GOLDBERG,
DAVID L. FISCHMAN, ANDREW ZALEWSKI,
and PAUL WALINSKY

Despite the continued improvements in the technique and primary results of coronary angioplasty over the past 15 years, restenosis has endured as a vexing clinical problem. The inability to overcome restenosis can be attributed to our imprecise understanding of its pathogenic mechanisms and the lack of an experimental model applicable to the human situation. The failure of numerous pharmacologic and mechanical interventions tested in isolation also points to the probable multifactorial nature of this complex biologic process involving platelet-thrombus deposition, residual obstruction from the primary dilatation, delayed elastic recoil, and vascular smooth muscle cell proliferation. Patients with restenosis and recurrent myocardial ischemia are usually managed by a second angioplasty procedure. However, the potential for lesion recurrence is not diminished by repeat angioplasty procedures. Therefore approximately 20% of patients with restenosis treated by a second angioplasty will require coronary bypass surgery, suffer an acute myocardial infarction, or die during short-term follow-up (1, 2). In response to this tenacious clinical problem, a variety of new technologies for transcatheter revascularization have been developed.

REPEAT BALLOON ANGIOPLASTY

Compared with the primary results of angioplasty for de novo lesions, repeat balloon dilation of restenotic lesions is associated with a higher success rate and a lower complication rate. In a series from Emory University the primary success rate was significantly higher for second angioplasty procedures (97%) than for initial angioplasty procedures (85%) (3). Similar results were observed in the National Heart, Lung, and Blood Institute registry (1). Death, myocardial infarction, or emergency bypass surgery occurred in only 3% of second PTCA procedures compared with 9.5% of initial PTCA procedures. In contrast to the favorable results of acute procedural outcome, the likelihood of lesion recurrence is not lessened by repeat angioplasty. The overall restenosis rate following a second balloon angioplasty for a previously dilated stenosis is 35% (4).

The long-term efficacy of conventional balloon angioplasty is significantly diminished in patients with recurrent restenosis, that is, restenosis of the same lesion following two or more prior PTCA. Teirstein et al. studied 74 patients who underwent a third angioplasty for a second restenosis (5). Initial procedural success was achieved in 93% of patients. However, during a mean follow-up of 18 months, 43% of patients developed clinical restenosis. An additional subset of 15 patients underwent a fourth angioplasty procedure with a subsequent clinical restenosis rate of 53%. Similar findings were observed in the Cleveland Clinic series, which included 46 patients who underwent a successful third

Table 23A.1.
Risk Factors Associated With Recurrent Restenosis Following Repeat Coronary Angioplasty

Two or more prior restenoses of the same lesion
Interprocedural interval <3 months
Multiple lesions dilated
Native LAD location
Venous bypass graft lesion
Presence of diabetes mellitus

angioplasty of the same site (2). The clinical restenosis rate in this cohort with two prior recurrences was 48%. Therefore restenosis of a given lesion that has occurred on more than one occasion is associated with a high likelihood of clinical failure if treated by another balloon angioplasty.

Risk factors associated with an increased likelihood of recurrent restenosis following repeat PTCA are summarized in Table 23A.1. Patients with two or more restenoses of the same lesion appear to be at particularly high risk of recurrence with subsequent balloon dilation procedures. Another important predictive factor, which has been noted in virtually all series of repeat PTCA, is the time interval between procedures (2–10). A short interval of less than 3 months between the first and second procedures is associated with a high likelihood of recurrent restenosis. A similar relationship between a short interprocedural interim and subsequent restenosis is also seen in patients undergoing a third PTCA procedure following multiple restenoses (2, 5). Restenosis following repeat angioplasty also appears to be influenced by the lesion location. Lesions situated in the native left anterior descending coronary artery or in venous bypass grafts are at increased risk of recurrent restenosis compared with other sites (5, 9, 11). In contrast, with the exception of diabetes, patient-related factors have not consistently correlated with restenosis risk after repeat PTCA. The long-term efficacy of redilating a restenosed lesion is independent of gender, smoking, or serum-lipid status.

PHARMACOLOGIC INTERVENTIONS

With rare exception, drug trials of postangioplasty restenosis have been based on study populations with de novo lesions. While most pharmacologic interventions have failed to modify restenosis, it is unclear whether the negative results observed with de novo lesions can be extrapolated to restenotic lesions. One prospective randomized trial evaluated the effect of high-dose corticosteroids for the prevention of recurrent restenosis following repeat PTCA (12); 102 patients were enrolled with angiographic follow-up obtained in 53%. There was no difference in restenosis between the steroid treated group (methylprednisolone 125 mg intramuscularly prior to PTCA followed by prednisone 60 mg daily for 1 week) and a control group, 59% versus 56%, respectively. Because of the salutary effects of heparin sulfate as an inhibitor of vascular smooth-muscle proliferation and as an antithrombin agent, we conducted a pilot study of long-term, low-dose heparin in the prevention of recurrent restenosis after repeat coronary angioplasty (13). The study population consisted of 46 patients, who were considered high risk for recurrent restenosis because of three or more angioplasties of the same site, the presence of multiple lesions, and/or left anterior descending location. Porcine heparin sulfate (5000 units) was administered subcutaneously every 12 hours for 3 months. A clinical restenosis rate of 26% was observed in this select, high-risk, patient population.

ATHEROMA DEBULKING

The concept that the long-term outcome of angioplasty would be improved by removing rather than dilating the atheroma has spawned the development of several ingenious devices. Plaque debulking may be achieved by excision (directional and extraction atherectomy), pulverization (rotational atherectomy), or vaporization (laser angioplasty). Although these technologies are useful for the primary revascularization of morphologically unfavorable lesions, their impact on the problem of late restenosis has been disappointing.

In two recently completed randomized trials of de novo native coronary lesions, directional atherectomy failed to improve long-term outcome over conventional balloon angioplasty (14, 15). Results from large observational studies suggest that the treatment of recurrent lesions by directional atherectomy is associated with a pattern of restenosis similar to conventional angioplasty. Hinohara and colleagues reported restenosis rates in native coronary arteries of 31% for de novo lesions, 28% for lesions treated with one prior angioplasty, and 47% for lesions treated with two or more prior angioplasties (16). Corresponding restenosis rates for saphenous vein grafts in this study were 53% for de novo lesions, 58% for lesions treated with one prior angioplasty, and 82% for lesions treated with two or more prior angioplasties. Thus directional atherectomy has limited efficacy as a treatment for multiple, recurrent restenoses. Similar to balloon angioplasty, recurrence rates following atherectomy of restenotic lesions correlate with the interprocedural time interval (Fig. 23A.1). The restenosis rate for lesions with a duration of <120 days after prior PTCA was significantly higher (56%) than for lesions with a duration of ≥120 days (19%).

Rotational atherectomy and excimer laser angioplasty both appear to have selective, niche applications in the primary treatment of unfavorable lesions. Rotational atherectomy has been successfully used in calcified and ostial lesions. Excimer laser ablation, used adjunctively with balloon angioplasty, is helpful in the treatment of ostial stenoses and for long diffuse lesions (Fig. 23A.2). Unfortunately, data from uncontrolled studies indicate that the restenosis rates with both of these devices are relatively high (17, 18). Thus, although both the Rotablator and excimer laser appear to improve the outcome of angioplasty in select cases, they are not indicated as a routine strategy for either the prevention or treatment of restenosis.

CORONARY STENTS

Intravascular stents have been proposed as a means of overcoming two major limitations of balloon angioplasty—acute vessel closure and late restenosis. Initial enthusiasm for this technology was dampened by reports of relatively high rates of thrombosis for the self-expanding Wallstent (19). Subsequent reports on the balloon-expandable coil stent (Gianturco-Roubin) and the balloon-expandable slotted tube stent (Palmaz-Schatz) have demonstrated the utility of these prostheses in the management of coronary dissection associated with abrupt or threatened closure (20, 21). In addition, the Palmaz-Schatz stent has shown particular promise in the management of restenosis. When expanded by a conventional balloon beyond its elastic limit, the Palmaz-Schatz stent possesses considerable radial hoop strength. Because of its radial noncompliance, this device pro-

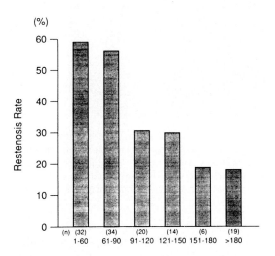

Figure 23A.1. Restenosis after successful atherectomy as a function of the time interval between prior angioplasty and atherectomy. (With permission from Hinohara T et al. J Am Coll Cardiol 1992;20:623–632.)

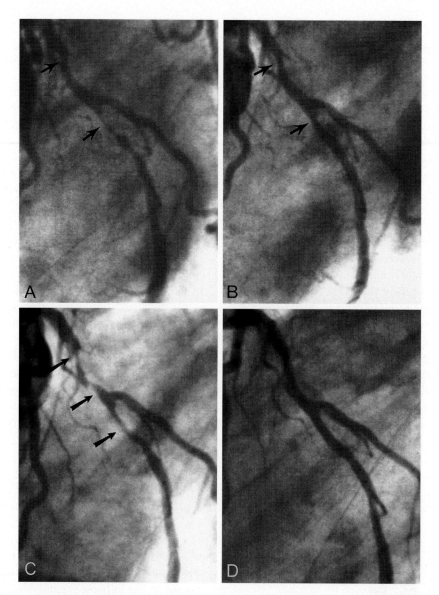

Figure 23A.2. Use of excimer laser angioplasty for a recurrent lesion with elastic recoil and repeated restenoses. **A.** Serial stenoses of the left circumflex coronary artery *(arrows)* in a 66-year-old diabetic man with unstable angina. **B.** Result after balloon angioplasty demonstrating partial residual obstruction caused by elastic recoil. **C.** Angiogram demonstrating diffuse restenosis after three PTCA procedures performed within a 3-month period. **D.** Improved primary result after laser-assisted debulking and balloon dilation. Patient has remained asymptomatic with a negative stress test more than one year after laser angioplasty.

vides an effective intravascular scaffold that is capable of resisting elastic recoil and that results in a wide, smooth initial lumen. The mechanism by which stents appear to reduce restenosis may be attributed to the enhanced acute gain that is achieved in comparison with conventional balloon angioplasty, rather than to a reduction of the late loss from intimal hyperplasia.

As reported by Ellis et al., the most important risk factors for restenosis following Palmaz-Schatz implantation are the use of multiple overlapping stents and a prior history of restenosis of the stented lesion (22). Because of the disappointingly high rates of restenosis with multiple stents, we currently recommend elective stenting with this device only for lesions that can be spanned by a single, 15-mm stent. The long-term clinical outcome and quantitative angiographic results from the core laboratory of the Palmaz-Schatz stent investigator group have been reported (23). Three hundred consecutive patients were followed after elective implantation of single Palmaz-Schatz stents in the native coronary circulation with angiographic restudy at 6 months and clinical follow-up at 1 year. There were no acute in-laboratory closures in any of the 300 patients. However, subacute stent thrombosis occurred in 14 patients (4.7%) after 5 ± 3 days. Absolute minimal lumen diameter (MLD) increased from 0.80 ± 0.39 mm at baseline to 1.65 ± 0.51 mm after balloon dilation and increased significantly further to 2.55 ± 0.49 mm after stent placement. At follow-up there was a 0.85-mm late loss in lumen diameter with a final MLD at 6 months of 1.70 ± 0.71 mm. Restenosis, defined as a $\geq 50\%$ diameter stenosis at follow-up, occurred in only 14% of de novo lesions and in 39% of lesions that had been previously dilated. Most importantly, stent implantation was associated with an excellent long-term clinical outcome. Clinical events (both acute and late) for all 300 patients after 1 year included death in 0.7%, myocardial infarction in 4%, bypass grafting in 8%, and repeat PTCA in 13%. Freedom from *any* adverse clinical event was 87% in the de novo group and 77% in the prior PTCA group. Efficacy of the Palmaz-Schatz stent in the treatment of discrete, de novo lesions of saphenous vein bypass grafts has also been reported (24). The clinical utility of elective coronary stenting compared with conventional balloon angioplasty in preventing restenosis of de novo lesions in native coronary arteries has recently been confirmed by prospective randomized trials (STRESS and BENESTENT).

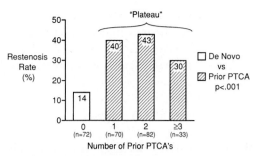

Figure 23A.3. Restenosis after Palmaz-Schatz stent implantation. Angiographic restenosis rates are plotted for de novo lesions and for lesions with one, two, and three or more prior PTCA procedures. Note that for previously dilated lesions, restenosis does not progressively increase as a function of the number of prior PTCA procedures (suggesting a restenosis "plateau" for stents).

A parallel prospective trial of coronary stenting for de novo vein graft stenoses is also in progress (SAVED).

Because stent restenosis is more common in lesions that have been previously subjected to balloon angioplasty, the role of elective stenting in the treatment of the restenotic lesion has not been established. In contrast to other interventional therapies, it is noteworthy that coronary stenting is associated with a unique "restenosis plateau" (Fig. 23A.3). For recurrent lesions that have been dilated previously, the restenosis risk associated with stenting does *not* increase as a function of the number of prior angioplasty procedures. Restenotic lesions that had recurred after one, two, and three or more prior PTCA procedures are associated with stent restenosis in 40%, 43%, and 30%, respectively (23). Taken together, these results suggest that the clinical utility of coronary stenting is most apparent when employed either "up front" in the treatment of de novo lesions or as an option "down the line" for lesions that recur after multiple prior procedures.

APPROACH TO THE PATIENT WITH RESTENOSIS

Following successful PTCA, close clinical surveillance of patients is routinely carried out for the first 6 months during the high-risk period for restenosis. Most important is the assessment of the patient's functional status and the presence of anginal symptoms. However, one cannot rely solely on the presence or absence of angina in the assessment of restenosis. Even in patients with preexistent angina prior to PTCA, clinically significant restenosis may occur without recurrence of the prior symptoms. Therefore we routinely perform exercise stress testing at 6 months following angioplasty even in asymptomatic patients. Early stress testing in the post-procedural period is indicated if any of the following are present: presence of an equivocal primary angiographic result, incomplete revascularization, recent myocardial infarction, or participation in high-risk occupations or athletic activities.

With close follow-up and prompt management of recurrent symptoms, acute myocardial infarction is an uncommon clinical presentation of restenosis. Within 12 months after successful coronary angioplasty, 1 to 5% of patients will suffer an acute myocardial infarction following hospital discharge. Aspirin (325 mg daily) has been demonstrated to reduce the risk of acute myocardial infarction during late clinical follow-up after successful PTCA, even though aspirin does not reduce the overall incidence of angiographic restenosis. Therefore we generally prescribe one enteric-coated aspirin and sublingual nitroglycerin to be taken as needed for a minimum of 6 months postprocedure. Except for patients with variant angina, calcium channel blockers neither reduce the angiographic restenosis rate nor improve late clinical outcome after successful angioplasty.

In approaching a patient with suspected or documented restenosis, the physician must weigh a variety of therapeutic options, including medical management, repeat balloon angioplasty, use of a new interventional device, and surgical revascularization. In the individual patient the decision-making process must integrate a variety of clinical and anatomic factors. These include the patient's age, occupation, general activity level, the severity of anginal symptoms, and objective documentation of ischemia by noninvasive studies. Therapy will also be influenced by the extent of the patient's underlying coronary disease, the relative completeness of revascularization and the status of left ventricular function. In patients in whom a repeat revascularization procedure is clinically indicated, it is particularly important to assess that patient's relative risk of recurrent restenosis with repeat balloon angioplasty. In patients assessed to be at high risk for recurrent restenosis with conventional balloon dilation alone, we would more strongly consider alternative modes of revascularization. Table 23A.1 summarizes the various clinical and anatomic factors associated with an increased risk of recurrent restenosis after repeat PTCA.

We generally recommend repeat myocardial revascularization for patients with recurrent angina associated with restenosis and for asymptomatic patients if there is significant myocardial ischemia by physiologic testing and a high-grade restenosis. However, it should be pointed out that the role of repeat revascularization for patients with asymptomatic restenosis is controversial. Prospective studies have demonstrated that one-fourth to one-half of all patients with angiographic restenosis are asymptomatic. Asymptomatic patients with a positive stress test and angiographic restenosis are at increased risk for late recurrence of angina (25). Repeat angioplasty is generally effective in preventing late recurrence of angina and in improving the abnormal stress test results. On the other hand, patients with proven restenosis who are asymptomatic and have negative stress tests have a generally benign clinical course during long-term follow-up (25). In light of their excellent prognosis, asymptomatic patients with a negative stress test are best managed conservatively, and myocardial revascularization can be deferred unless symptoms later recur.

In patients with restenosis where additional percutaneous revascularization is indicated, one must weigh the option of repeat balloon angioplasty against the various new transcatheter techniques. In making this decision, we reexamine the cine angiograms from the initial PTCA procedure noting the overall quality of the result achieved during the primary dilation. It is also important to distinguish between a first episode of restenosis and recurrent restenosis since repeat balloon angioplasty is less likely to yield a successful long-term outcome in the latter circumstance. The most common scenario is that of an initial episode of restenosis after balloon angioplasty of a de novo lesion, where the primary procedure was uncomplicated and yielded a good angiographic result. In this circumstance, we usually opt for a second balloon angioplasty with the rationale that the primary success rate is high, the complication rate is low, and the restenosis risk is comparable to the first procedure. When restenosis is suspected on the basis of clinical findings, we perform repeat PTCA during the same sitting as the diagnostic catheterization if the expected anatomic findings are confirmed.

This approach minimizes the number of invasive procedures required, reduces the length of hospital stay, and is cost-effective.

In patients with a first episode of restenosis, we strongly consider alternative transcatheter technologies when the primary result of the initial PTCA was suboptimal because of either an intimal dissection or elastic recoil. Since the likelihood of restenosis correlates with the degree of residual stenosis, we often use a debulking device to treat a restenotic lesion that displayed significant elastic recoil during the initial procedure (see Fig. 23A.2). The rationale is that by partially debulking the atheroma, relative elastic recoil will be minimized, and a more ideal large lumen will be achieved. Selection of laser angioplasty or one of the atherectomy devices can be based on the specific anatomic findings including lesion morphology, lesion length, tortuosity, and vessel size. Elastic recoil can also be effectively opposed by placement of a coronary stent (21). Intravascular stents are particularly valuable when elastic recoil is associated with an intimal dissection flap (Fig. 23A.4). Use of a stent in the setting of an intimal dissection does not diminish its resteno-

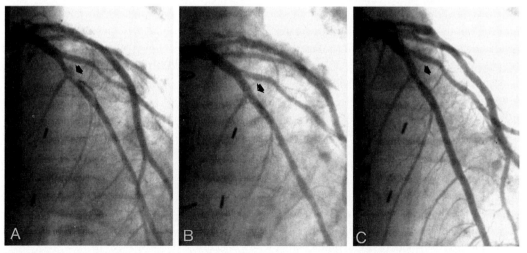

Figure 23A.4. Use of intracoronary stent for restenosis associated with an intimal tear. **A.** Control angiogram—from a 63-year-old man with recurrent angina after three prior balloon angioplasties of the left anterior descending coronary artery—demonstrating severe intimal flap at site of prior dilatations *(arrow)*. **B.** Result after stent placement. **C.** Follow-up angiogram at 6 months demonstrating continued patency.

sis efficacy. On the other hand, debulking devices are often contraindicated in the presence of a complex intimal tear because of the potential for acute complications such as coronary perforation.

The management of patients with more than one restenosis of the same lesion (i.e., recurrent restenosis) is especially problematic. Use of a third balloon angioplasty procedure to treat a second episode of restenosis will result in yet another recurrence of restenosis in more than 40% of patients. Clinical restenosis following a fourth balloon angioplasty on the same lesion exceeds 50%. Available data indicate that directional atherectomy and other debulking devices do not significantly improve the long-term outcome of patients with recurrent restenosis. In light of the increased chance of clinical failure if another angioplasty is attempted, the alternative of coronary artery bypass surgery should be strongly considered when faced with the need for a third or fourth revascularization procedure for the same stubborn lesion. Therapeutic decisions must be individualized after consultation between the patient and physician on the benefits and risks of alternative options. Patients with restenosis of multiple lesions or with recurrent restenosis of the proximal LAD, especially when the interprocedural intervals are brief, would be appropriate for referral to bypass surgery.

Of all interventional techniques, coronary artery stenting has demonstrated the greatest promise as an alternative therapy for recurrent restenosis. The utility of this device for multiple restenosis can be attributed to the apparently unique "restenosis plateau" associated with stenting (see Fig. 23A.3). In contrast to balloon angioplasty and directional atherectomy where restenosis is significantly higher after multiple prior recurrences than after the first episode of recurrence, stent restenosis does not progressively increase as a function of the number of prior angioplasty procedures. To better determine the role of

intracoronary stenting in the management of restenosis refractory to conventional PTCA, we studied the late clinical outcome of 40 consecutive patients treated with single Palmaz-Schatz stents for lesions that had recurred after *3 or more* prior PTCA (26). Follow-up coronary angiography was performed in 36 patients (90%) at a mean of 6.2 months, and quantitative coronary analysis was performed at a core laboratory. Angiographic restenosis occurred in 10 of 36 stented sites (28%). Clinical events at 1-year follow-up included no deaths, myocardial infarction in one (2.5%) patient caused by stent thrombosis, coronary bypass surgery in two (5%) patients, and repeat angioplasty in four (10%) patients. At 1-year follow-up after stent placement, 85% of patients (34 of 40) remained free of any adverse clinical event. Therefore coronary stenting may be the preferred therapeutic option for patients with refractory restenosis.

SUMMARY

Restenosis after successful PTCA continues to pose a major clinical challenge for the interventional cardiologist. Although the primary prevention of restenosis has been evaluated in numerous prospective randomized trials, treatment of the restenotic lesion has not been rigorously subjected to controlled studies. Therefore clinical decision making must rely on available observational data, risk stratification of the likelihood of recurrent restenosis, and the physician's expertise in a variety of transcatheter techniques. Among these, slotted tubular stents appear especially promising both in the prevention of initial restenosis and in the treatment of recurrent restenosis. Further prospective studies will be required to define the optimal role of the newer interventional devices in the management of restenosis.

REFERENCES

1. Williams DO, Gruentzig AR, Kent KM, Detre KM, Kelsey SF, To T. Efficacy of repeat percutaneous transluminal coronary angioplasty for coronary restenosis. Am J Cardiol 1984;53:32C–35C.
2. Dimas AP, Grigera F, Arora RR et al. Repeat coronary angioplasty as treatment for restenosis. J Am Coll Cardiol 1992;19:1310–1314.

3. Meier B, King SB III, Gruentzig AR, Douglas JS, Hollman J, Ischinger T et al. Repeat coronary angioplasty. J Am Coll Cardiol 1984;4:463–466.

4. Califf RM, Ohman EM, Frid DJ, Fortin DF, Mark DB, Hlatky MA et al. Restenosis: the clinical issues. In: Topol EJ, ed. Textbook of interventional cardiology. Philadelphia: WB Saunders, 1990.

5. Teirstein PS, Hoover CA, Ligon RW, Giorgi LV, Rutherford BD, McConahay DR et al. Repeat coronary angioplasty: efficacy of a third angioplasty for a second restenosis. J Am Coll Cardiol 1989;13:291–296.

6. Black AJ, Anderson V, Roubin GS, Powelson SW, Douglas JS Jr, King SB III. Repeat coronary angioplasty: correlates of a second restenosis. J Am Coll Cardiol 1988; 11:714–718.

7. Quigley PJ, Hlatky MA, Hinohara T, Rendall DS, Perez JA, Phillips HR et al. Repeat percutaneous transluminal coronary angioplasty and predictors of recurrent restenosis. Am J Cardiol 1989;63:409–413.

8. Glazier JJ, Varricchione TR, Ryan TJ, Ruocco NA, Jacobs AK, Faxon DP. Factors predicting recurrent restenosis after percutaneous transluminal coronary balloon angioplasty. Am J Cardiol 1989;63:902–905.

9. Deligonul U, Vandormael M, Kern MJ, Galan K. Repeat coronary angioplasty for restenosis: results and predictors of follow-up clinical events. Am Heart J 1989;117:997–1002.

10. Bauters C, Lablanche JM, McFadden EP, Leroy F, Bertrand ME. Clinical characteristics and angiographic follow-up of patients undergoing early or late repeat dilation for a first restenosis. J Am Coll Cardiol 1992;20:845–848.

11. DeFeyter PJ, Van Suylen RJ, DeJaegere PPT, Topol EJ, Serruys PW. Balloon angioplasty for the treatment of lesions in saphenous vein bypass grafts. J Am Coll Cardiol 1993;21:1539–1549.

12. Stone GW, Rutherford BD, McConahay DR, Johnson WL, Giorgi LV, Ligon RW, Hartzler GO. A randomized trial of corticosteriods for the prevention of restenosis in 102 patients undergoing repeat coronary angioplasty. Cathet Cardiovasc Diagn 1989;18:227–231.

13. Savage M, Delacourt P, Nardone D et al. Subcutaneous heparin to prevent recurrent restenosis after repeated coronary angioplasty. Cathet Cardiovasc Diagn 1991; 23:75 (abstract).

14. Topol EJ, Leya F, Pinkerton CA et al. A comparison of directional artherectomy with coronary angioplasty in patients with coronary artery disease. N Engl J Med 1993; 329:221–227.

15. Adelman AG, Cohen EA, Kimball BP et al. A comparison of directional atherectomy with balloon angioplasty for lesions of the left anterior descending coronary artery. N Engl J Med 1993;329:228–233.

16. Hinohara T, Robertson GC, Selmon MR et al. Restenosis after directional coronary atherectomy. J Am Coll Cardiol 1992;20:623–632.

17. Teirstein PS, Warth DC, Haq N et al. High-speed rotational coronary atherectomy for patients with diffuse coronary artery disease. J Am Coll Cardiol 1991;18:1694–1701.

18. Bittl JA, Sanborn TA. Excimer laser–facilitated coronary angioplasty: relative risk analysis of acute and follow-up results in 200 patients. Circulation 1992;86:71–80.

19. Serruys PW, Strauss BH, Beatt KJ et al. Angiographic follow-up after placement of a self-expanding coronary artery stent. N Engl J Med 1991;324:13–17.

20. Roubin GS, Cannon AD, Agrawal SK, Macander PJ, Dean LS, Baxley WA, Breland J. Intracoronary stenting for acute and threatened closure complicating percutaneous transluminal angioplasty. Circulation 1992;85:916–927.

21. Fischman DL, Savage MP, Leon MB et al. Effect of intracoronary stenting on intimal dissection after balloon angioplasty: results of quantitative and qualitative coronary analysis. J Am Coll Cardiol 1991;18:1445–1451.

22. Ellis SG, Savage M, Fischman D. Restenosis after placement of Palmaz-Schatz stents in native coronary arteries. Initial results of a multicenter experience. Circulation 1992;86:1836–1844.

23. Savage M, Fischman D, Schatz RA et al. Long-term angiographic and clinical outcome after implantation of a balloon-expandable stent in the native coronary circulation. J Am Coll Cardiol 1994;24:1207–1212.

24. Fenton S, Fischman DL, Savage MP et al. Long-term clinical and angiographic outcome after implantation of balloon-expandable stents in aortocoronary saphenous vein grafts. Am J Cardiol 1994;74:1187–1191.

25. Hernandez RA, Macaya C, Iniguez A, Alfonso F, Goicolea J, Fernandez-Ortiz A, Zarco P. Midterm outcome of patients with asymptomatic restenosis after coronary balloon angioplasty. J Am Coll Cardiol 1992;19:1402–1409.

26. Savage M, Fischman D, Leon M et al. Efficacy of coronary stents in the treatment of refractory restenosis following balloon angioplasty. J Am Coll Cardiol 1993; 21(Suppl A):33A (abstract).

B. The Restenotic Lesion— Use of New Devices

MASAKIYO NOBUYOSHI and TAKESHI KIMURA

Despite significant improvements in technique and equipment, restenosis remains a major limitation of percutaneous transluminal coronary angioplasty (PTCA). With the advent of new devices, marked reduction of restenosis had been expected. However, initial enthusiasm encountered disappointment when it was realized that the new devices were not free from the restenotic process.

The primary mechanism of restenosis has been reported to be proliferation of smooth muscle cells and subsequent secretion of matrix substances (1). Recently, it has been learned that restenosis in a significant proportion of patients resulted from suboptimal initial results. Ellis et al., using computer assisted quantitative coronary angiography, reported that in complex lesion subsets, procedural success rate was significantly lower than that generally believed (2). Although we have not yet found a solution to initial hyperplasia, we do have some mechanical solutions to suboptimal intimal result. Most of the suboptimal angioplasty results are caused by dissection, recoil, and the undilatable nature of the lesion. Intracoronary stenting and directional coronary atherectomy (DCA) are effective in preventing and treating dissection and recoil. Rotational atherectomy is extremely effective in treating undilatable, heavily calcified lesions. With the combined use of these three new devices, we can achieve improved acute results in a significant proportion of patients.

We generally accept the hypothesis that the bigger the better (3). Our current approach is to achieve the best possible final angiographic result in a given lesion morphology. We do not have different strategies for treating de novo lesions versus restenotic lesions. For example, in an ideal situation for coronary stenting, we do not have any reason to wait until restenosis occurs. In several series of stenting and directional coronary atherectomy, de novo lesions have consistently lower restenosis rates as compared with restenotic lesions (4, 5). There are three possible mechanisms for the higher restenosis rates when treating restenotic lesions. Firstly, the initial injury from the first PTCA and the presence of intimal hyperplasia might have an unfavorable influence on the second procedure. Secondly, the original lesion that actually restenosed might be more prone to aggressive intimal hyperplasia. Finally, lesions that are less ideal for stenting or atherectomy might be prevalent in restenotic lesions. In any case, we believe that the first step in reducing the overall restenosis rate is

to achieve the best possible luminal result at the time of the initial intervention.

Recently, several observational studies of the Palmaz-Schatz stent and directional coronary atherectomy demonstrated improved long-term results compared with historical controls (4–6). Two randomized trials comparing the Palmaz-Schatz stent and balloon angioplasty (BENESTENT trial and STRESS trial) demonstrated restenosis rates favoring the Palmaz-Schatz stent. The CAVEAT trial comparing directional coronary atherectomy and balloon angioplasty demonstrated marginal reduction in angiographic restenosis. Both directional coronary atherectomy and the Palmaz-Schatz stent are suitable for discrete lesions in large-sized arteries. Both of these technologies are often effective in treating eccentric and complex lesions unsuitable for balloon angioplasty. In spite of the aforementioned evidence favoring these two new devices over balloon angioplasty, the selection of patients for directional coronary atherectomy or the Palmaz-Schatz stent has not yet been clarified. To evaluate initial and follow-up outcomes, analysis of a single-center experience of the Palmaz-Schatz stent (298 patients, 309 lesions) and DCA (195 patients, 210 lesions) is ongoing in our center. Exclusion criteria were saphenous vein graft treatment and bailout use for abrupt closure. Baseline patient demographics were different in that the stent group included significantly more multivessel disease (57% versus 43%; $P < .05$), poor LV (12% versus 4%; $P < .05$), and class III and IV angina (52% versus 28%; $P < .001$). Baseline lesion characteristics such as lesion length, vessel size, and minimal lumen diameter (MLD) before the procedure were similar for the two groups. The stent group included more restenotic lesions (44% versus 31%; $P < .05$) and less LAD lesions (44% versus 56%; $P < .05$). Aggressive strategy to achieve the largest final MLD possible was generally adopted by both groups. In the atherectomy group a 7 Fr device was used in 93% of lesions, and in the stent group postdilatation was performed with a final balloon

Table 23B.1.
Initial Result of the Palmaz-Schatz Stent and Directional Atherectomy

	Stent (%)	Atherectomy (%)	P Value
Procedure success	98	91	<.001
Acute closure	0.3	1.9	NS
Subacute closure	1.3	0	NS
Death/QMI/CABG	1.9	1.0	NS
Bleeding	3.4	2.1	NS

CABG, Coronary artery bypass grafting; *QMI,* Q-wave myocardial infarction.

Table 23B.2.
Follow-Up Result of the Palmaz-Schatz Stent and Directional Atherectomy

	Stent	Atherectomy	P Value
N of lesions with FU	237	110	
Intervals to FU angio (days)	182 ± 42	137 ± 47	P <.001
MLD pre (mm)	0.83 ± 0.36	0.90 ± 0.36	NS
MLD post (mm)	2.91 ± 0.38	2.61 ± 0.45	P <.001
MLD FU (mm)	2.13 ± 0.61	1.86 ± 0.66	P <.001
% DS ≥50% at FU	13%	24%	P <.05

DS, Diameter stenosis; *FU,* follow-up; *MLD,* minimal lumen diameter.

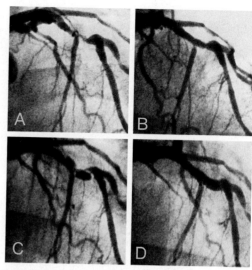

Figure 23B.1. **A.** Before atherectomy LAD lesion. **B.** After atherectomy angiogram showing 20 to 30% residual stenosis. **C.** Ulcerated restenosis 3 months later. **D.** After Palmaz-Schatz stent implantation. Overdilated appearance was noted.

size of 3.6 ± 0.4 mm for a vessel size of 3.2 ± 0.6 mm. Results are shown in Tables 23B.1 and 23B.2. Although both forms of treatment could be performed with acceptable complication rates, stenting achieved significantly higher procedural success rates and larger postprocedure MLD. Despite a longer mean follow-up interval, the stent group maintained a larger MLD at follow-up. This is still an ongoing study, and more patient enrollment and longer follow-up intervals are required. However, we feel that by using stents, it is much easier to achieve a larger final MLD without increasing risks. Figure 23B.1 shows a patient in whom directional coronary atherectomy was performed as an initial option and the Palmaz-Schatz stent was implanted for recurrence.

Therefore at this time we favor Palmaz-Schatz stent implantation for prevention of restenosis if lesion morphology is ideal for stenting. Indications for stent implantation are not as straightforward in cases of ostial lesions, bifurcational lesions, calcified lesions,

small arteries, and lengthy lesions. For ostial lesions and bifurcational lesions with sufficient vessel size, we usually try directional atherectomy first. A bifurcation lesion is shown in Figure 23B.2. For moderate to heavy calcification, our first choice of treatment is rotational atherectomy followed by balloon angioplasty. Reported incidence of restenosis after rotational atherectomy is similar to that of balloon angioplasty (7). However, rotational atherectomy is currently the only device that could "successfully" treat heavily calcified lesions. Combined use of rotational atherectomy and the Palmaz-Schatz stent is expected to improve the long-term result of heavily calcified lesions. Figure 23B.3 shows a patient in whom rotational atherectomy was initially performed and in whom, at the time of stenosis, the Palmaz-Schatz stent was implanted. For small-sized arteries and lengthy lesions, we are generally reluctant to use stents. For these lesions conventional balloon angioplasty is still the treatment of choice. Use of long balloons (often slightly oversized)

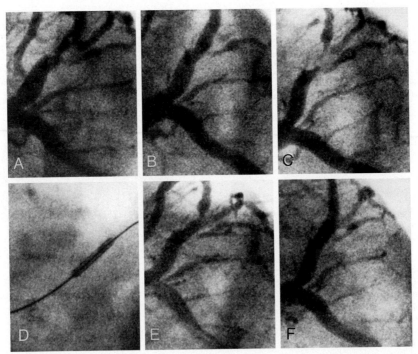

Figure 23B.2. A. Before atherectomy bifurcation LAD lesion. **B.** After atherectomy. The second diagonal branch was occluded. **C.** Restenosis 6 months later. **D.** Before stent implantation, atherectomy of the second diagonal branch was performed. **E.** After atherectomy. **F.** After Palmaz-Schatz stent implantation. The second diagonal branch was patent.

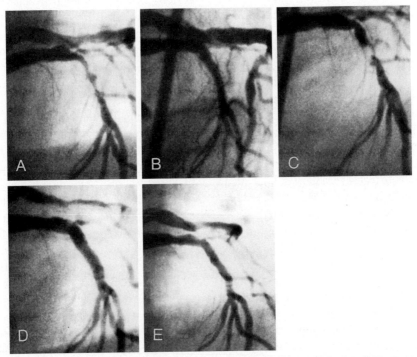

Figure 23B.3. A. Before rotational atherectomy. The LAD lesion was a moderately calcified long lesion. **B.** After rotational atherectomy and adjunctive balloon angioplasty. **C.** Focal restenosis 3 months later. **D.** After Palmaz-Schatz stent implantation. **E.** One-year follow-up angiogram revealing fully patent LAD.

might be effective in modifying stenosis morphology. Currently, stent implantation and directional atherectomy for small arteries and lengthy lesions result in unfavorable long-term outcomes. Use of multiple overlapping stents was associated with an unacceptably high incidence of restenosis (4). We generally perform stent implantation for these types of lesions only after two or three prior balloon angioplasties. However, with future modification of stent designs, these types of lesions might be successfully treated with acceptable long-term results.

REFERENCES

1. Nobuyoshi M, Kimura T, Ohishi H et al. Restenosis after percutaneous transluminal coronary angioplasty: pathologic observation in 20 patients. J Am Coll Cardiol 1991; 17:433–439.
2. Ellis SG, Vandormael MG, Cowley MJ, Deligonul U, Topol EJ, Bulle TM. Coronary morphologic and clinical determinants of procedural outcome with angioplasty for multivessel coronary disease: implications for patient selection. Circulation 1990;82:1139–1202.
3. Kuntz RE, Gibson M, Nobuyoshi M, Baim DS. Generalized model of restenosis after conventional balloon angioplasty, stenting and directional atherectomy. J Am Coll Cardiol 1993;21:15–25.
4. Ellis SG, Savage M, Fischman D, et al. Restenosis after placement of Palmaz-Schatz stents in native coronary arteries: initial results of a multicenter experience. Circulation 1992;86:1836–1844.
5. Hinohara T, Robertson GC, Selmon MR. Restenosis after directional coronary atherectomy. J Am Coll Cardiol 1992; 20:623-632.
6. Kimura T, Nosaka H, Yokoi H, Iwabuchi M, Nobuyoshi M. Serial angiographic follow-up after Palmaz-Schatz stent implantation: comparison with conventional balloon angioplasty. J Am Coll Cardiol 1993;21:1557–1563.
7. Stertzer SH, Rosenblum J, Shaw RE, et al. Coronary rotational ablation: initial experience in 302 procedures. J Am Coll Cardiol 1993;21:287–295.

C. The Restenotic Lesion

JAMES E. TCHENG

The problem of restenosis following percutaneous coronary revascularization persists despite an enormous effort to limit its occurrence. Because of the large number of patients being treated with percutaneous revascular-

ization and the high rate of clinical events during follow-up, the management of restenosis has far-reaching implications on the quality, quantity, delivery, and cost of health care. Even given our incomplete understanding of the pathophysiology of restenosis, it is therefore incumbent on clinicians to develop logical management approaches to this problem. The purpose of this chapter is to synthesize the available information and provide a framework and rationale for managing the patient with restenosis following percutaneous coronary revascularization.

Since "an ounce of prevention is worth a pound of cure," it is worth briefly discussing efforts invested to date in reducing or eliminating restenosis (1, 2). While a complete review of all such studies is well beyond the scope of this chapter, there are two strategies that appear promising. The first is the use of agents that block the platelet integrin glycoprotein IIb/IIIa during coronary intervention. In the EPIC trial, a 12-hour treatment with c7E3 Fab (Centocor, Malvern, PA) was associated with a 35% reduction in 30-day clinical events and a 23% reduction in death, myocardial infarction, and target vessel revascularization at 6 months (3, 4). Comparable reductions in event rates were also found in the STRESS and Benestent investigations of the Palmaz-Schatz coronary stent (Johnson and Johnson, Warren, NJ) (5, 6). These trials documented a statistically significant difference in minimal luminal diameter at follow-up angiography, correlating improved clinical outcomes with reduced angiographic restenosis. Despite these major advances, however, it is anticipated that these strategies will have a modest overall effect on reducing the vexing problem of restenosis and that they do not eliminate the necessity for a rational and balanced approach to the patient with restenosis.

THE PROBLEM

What is restenosis? Today, restenosis remains an evolving concept (7). While clinical decision making is best accommodated by a dichotomous definition of restenosis, it is quite clear that the biologic process is not a "yes or no" phenomenon, but instead occurs along a continuous spectrum. In fact, renarrowing occurs to some extent in all patients. It is the extent of the renarrowing, placed in the context of the patient's clinical situation, that determines whether "restenosis" has occurred. Information obtained from the clinical history, provocative testing, and the cardiac catheterization laboratory should be integrated. While there are numerous published definitions of angiographic restenosis (1, 8), none currently encompass the breadth of angiographic, clinical, and functional information sufficiently to present a unified definition (7).

The angiographic vessel renarrowing that serves as the pathophysiologic basis for clinical restenosis encompasses several phenomena. Renarrowing that occurs in the first several days or so implies an inadequate initial result, vigorous elastic recoil, or abrupt closure. True abrupt closure most often occurs following severe vessel disruption with plaque dissection; thrombosis often contributes to this complication. On the other hand, early renarrowing (without abrupt closure) may be asymptomatic; this is typically caused by elastic recoil rather than thrombosis.

Following this early renarrowing phase, further loss of luminal diameter is caused by a combination of vessel remodeling, elastic recoil, and/or fibrointimal proliferation. It is this delayed renarrowing that results in clinical "restenosis." Depending on the definition and the study, this process can be expected to occur in up to 50% of patients within a 1- to 6-month time frame. Serial angiographic studies actually document slight overall regression (i.e., improvement in the minimal luminal diameter) of treated lesions over the first 30 days following angioplasty (9, 10). This is followed by a gradual loss in minimal luminal diameter up to 6 months, with most of the angiographic renarrowing occurring in the

first 3 to 4 months. After 1 year, further luminal encroachment is unusual.

Even with a reasonably complete understanding of the angiographic time course of restenosis, the clinical management of the patient remains largely empirical. Clinically, the time frame for recurrence of symptoms corresponds with angiographic renarrowing, with the majority of patients with recurrent symptoms presenting in a 1- to 3-month time frame. The next most frequent picture of angiographic restenosis is the absence of symptoms; as many as 15 to 20% of patients with angiographic renarrowing do not redevelop angina. Presentation of restenosis as an acute myocardial infarction or sudden death is distinctly unusual (11); restenotic lesions are more fibromuscular than native lipid-laden plaques and are less susceptible to rupture (and thrombosis) than de novo lesions. Acute myocardial infarction during the posthospitalization phase, when it does occur, is usually caused by thrombosis of a new lesion site.

Complicating the development of a straightforward management algorithm are several factors. The frequency of multivessel disease in the typical angioplasty population is well appreciated; residual or recurrent symptoms following incomplete revascularization may be the result of preexisting (untreated) lesions rather than restenosis. The symptoms of angina are not 100% sensitive nor specific for coronary ischemia. Finally, coronary disease tends to be progressive, with a substantial proportion of recurrent symptoms being caused by the development of new lesions rather than restenosis of an angioplasty site, even within the classic 6-month window (12).

How does one then establish the diagnosis of restenosis? While repeat angiography is the most appropriate single study to establish the presence of arterial renarrowing, routine follow-up angiography (given the expense, risk, and discomfort of catheterization) is best viewed as a research tool. Routine functional

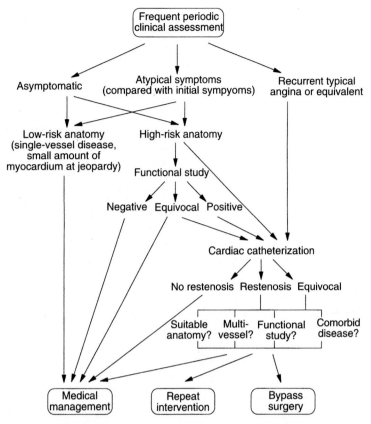

Figure 23C.1. Patient surveillance following coronary intervention. Clinical, demographic, anatomic, angiographic, functional, psychologic, and socioeconomic factors must be considered in determining the optimal patient-care strategy. This customized approach to patient care requires refinement whenever new, relevant patient data is identified.

testing also cannot be recommended because of the inadequate positive and negative predictive accuracy, as well as the expense and risk, of these studies. At the present time, since there is compelling evidence that the incidence of clinical events (besides recurrent angina) resulting from renarrowing of the target lesion is extremely low, it appears that the most practical and pragmatic approach is one that emphasizes a high level of clinical surveillance and evaluation (Fig. 23C.1). Patients who develop recurrent symptoms should undergo repeat cardiac catheterization to establish the anatomic basis of their symptoms. Those with atypical or different symptoms may be evaluated with provocative functional testing to determine if there is any myocardium at jeopardy; often these patients

will need functional testing anyway when coronary angiography is equivocal. Finally, those patients with a large amount of myocardium at jeopardy (especially multivessel disease and lesions involving the proximal left anterior descending) may deserve a more aggressive approach to their disease. In these patients the threshold for repeat functional testing and/or cardiac catheterization should be low to impart the maximum potential mortality benefit.

MANAGING THE PATIENT WITH RESTENOSIS

As noted previously, one of the most difficult aspects of managing the patient with restenosis is deciding who qualifies as having developed this diagnosis. The lack of consensus about unequivocal angiographic definitions with clear-cut clinical relevance, coupled with the relative paucity of data about mortality benefit, dictates that most of the recommendations remain empirical and inferential. The elements that need to be synthesized include clinical status, results of angiographic and functional studies, and consideration of the degree of myocardium at jeopardy.

A logical approach to the patient with restenosis is to consider the treatment objectives defined at the time of the initial coronary intervention. In the patient undergoing direct angioplasty during myocardial infarction, data exist showing that angioplasty confers a mortality benefit (13). Besides this situation, the primary benefit appears to be relief of the symptoms of angina (including anginal equivalents). Repeat intervention in the patient with recurrent symptoms and documented angiographic restenosis would thus be appropriate, with the objective to improve the patient's symptom complex (14). The fact that a second procedure does not appear to induce more aggressive restenosis also supports this approach (15–17). In fact, by this approach the second intervention might be considered an expected part of an overall percutaneous revascularization strategy. The obvious and unfortunate component of this is that the patient has to undergo multiple procedures.

The role of provocative functional testing is to add ancillary information to the overall management approach. Importantly, routine follow-up testing cannot be recommended because of the well-recognized limitations in predictive accuracy. Also, an early positive functional study does not have the same predictive value postintervention as it does in the de novo situation. Nonetheless, there are several scenarios where such information might be useful. In patients with atypical symptoms or symptoms different from those prior to angioplasty, negative functional studies may be used to support a decision to defer invasive catheterization. In patients with an equivocal follow-up angiogram, functional testing may be necessary to aid in the decision to proceed to repeat revascularization. The one group of patients in whom routine repeat testing might prove useful comprises those with a large portion of myocardium at jeopardy. Even in the absence of symptoms, it would seem reasonable to identify such patients early in the course of restenosis so that repeat revascularization can be accomplished before the development of a detrimental clinical ischemic outcome.

Should a patient be suspected of having restenosis, complete left heart catheterization with coronary arteriography is indicated. While the majority of patients will have developed restenosis of the originally treated lesions, the proclivity for development of new lesions cannot be underestimated. In patients with known multivessel disease, complete catheterization is particularly vital since percutaneous revascularization strategies typically do not achieve complete revascularization; catheterization will help identify whether there were significant lesions not originally approached. Cardiac catheterization may also provide an explanation in those situations where the initial intervention afforded only partial or incomplete relief. In summary, the detailed anatomic information provided by repeat catheterization will help decide whether to manage the patient medically, retreat the original target lesion(s), revascularize new territories, or refer the patient for elective coronary artery bypass surgery (18).

TECHNICAL CONSIDERATIONS

Several factors should be considered in deciding whether to proceed to repeat angioplasty. The overall experience with repeat balloon angioplasty is generally gratifying. Success rates approach 98 to 99%, the rate of emergency bypass surgery is similar (if not lower) than that associated with a first procedure, restenosis is not any more frequent after a second procedure, and relief of anginal symptomatology can generally be anticipated, especially when the first procedure afforded relief (15–17). Thus a percutaneous approach to the patient with a restenotic lesion appears to have the same (or better) benefit-to-risk ratio as an initial procedure.

The enthusiastic endorsement of repeat angioplasty must be tempered by several factors. In the patient in whom the initial angioplasty was complicated by severe hypotension, ventricular dysrhythmias, abrupt closure, myocardial infarction, or other serious sequelae, the technical approach should be rethought to determine whether alternative strategies (such as perfusion balloon catheter angioplasty, intraaortic balloon pump placement, or percutaneous cardiopulmonary support) might mitigate complications. Interval development of serious, life-threatening comorbidity might predicate a more conservative approach. Patients with multivessel disease that cannot be completely revascularized, especially when relief of angina was initially incomplete, should be considered for coronary bypass surgery.

In approaching the restenotic lesion, recall of the initial procedural parameters may augment the ability of the interventionalist to more efficiently and effectively treat the patient (Table 23C.1). Knowledge of equipment that worked (guidewires, guide catheters, devices) and those that failed will im-

Table 23C.1.
Treatment of the Restenotic Lesion

- Expect similar benefits and risks as at initial coronary intervention
- Review procedure details from initial intervention
  - Choose guide catheter providing proper alignment and support
  - Select additional devices based on previous procedure
- Consider modifying balloon inflation parameters
  - Use ideal to minimally oversized balloon
  - Apply lower or higher balloon pressure
  - Use prolonged balloon inflations
- Consider alternative technologies
  - Use atherectomy or ablation to remove tissue
  - Deploy stent to prevent recoil
  - Use adjunctive balloon angioplasty to maximize result
- Consider pharmacologic manipulation
  - Treat with platelet glycoprotein IIb/IIIa blocker

prove the cost-effectiveness of the procedure and reduce procedure duration. A different technical approach (larger or longer balloon, longer inflation duration) has intellectual appeal in trying to improve short- and long-term outcomes, although improvements have not been documented. Whether new devices will be important in reducing the incidence of a second restenosis is unknown. Debulking devices (both devices that excise and ablate) and intracoronary stenting, especially when combined with adjunctive balloon angioplasty, will usually improve the luminal result compared with balloon angioplasty alone (19). Special situations (such as restenosis at a previous stent implantation site) may dictate a particular approach (20). Since data support achieving as open a final luminal result as possible in trying to modulate restenosis (21), adjunctive treatment should be considered in the appropriate anatomic and morphologic settings. Again, however, this approach has not been studied in a randomized trial specifically designed to address this problem.

The patient who develops a third (or greater) restenosis event presents a different dilemma. Two opposing schools suggest either that the lesions "burn out" after repeated angioplasty (justifying further interventional attempts) or that such lesions have an inherent tendency for restenosis (suggesting that further angioplasty is futile) (22). Currently, there is no clear consensus; repeat angioplasty is probably worth considering, but alternatives, particularly coronary bypass surgery, may afford a better long-lasting outcome.

SUMMARY

Restenosis following coronary intervention remains a serious and expensive limitation of percutaneous revascularization. Surveillance following coronary angioplasty should be pragmatic and practical and should feature close clinical follow-up, with routine functional testing and/or cardiac catheterization reserved only for specific circumstances. The best treatment would be prevention;

several treatments appear promising, but no approach eradicates this persistent problem. Substantial further effort will be required to conquer this limitation. In the interim the clinician and the patient must be prepared for the development of restenosis and must redouble treatment efforts when it occurs.

REFERENCES

1. Fortin DF, Tcheng JE, Hillegass WB, Phillips HR III. Clinical management of restenosis. In: Roubin GS, Califf RM, O'Neill WW, Phillips HR III, Stack RS, eds. Interventional cardiovascular medicine: principles and practice. New York: Churchill Livingstone, 1994.

2. Franklin SM, Faxon DP. Pharmacologic prevention of restenosis after coronary angioplasty: review of the randomized clinical trials. Coronary Artery Dis 1993; 4:232–242.

3. The EPIC Investigators. Use of a monoclonal antibody directed against the platelet glycoprotein IIb/IIIa receptor in high-risk coronary angioplasty. The EPIC investigation. N Engl J Med 1994;330:956–961.

4. Topol EJ, Califf RM, Weisman HF et al. Randomized trial of coronary intervention with antibody against platelet IIb/IIIa integrin for reduction of clinical restenosis: results at six months. The EPIC Investigators. Lancet 1994; 343:881–886.

5. Fischman DL, Leon MB, Baim DS et al. A randomized comparison of coronary-stent placement and balloon angioplasty in the treatment of coronary artery disease. N Engl J Med 1994;331:496–501.

6. Serruys PW, De Jaegere P, Kiemeneij F et al. A comparison of balloon-expandable-stent implantation with balloon angioplasty in patients with coronary artery disease. N Engl J Med 1994;331:489–495.

7. Kuntz Re, Baim DS. Defining coronary restenosis. Newer clinical and angiographic paradigms. Circulation 1993; 88:1310–1323.

8. Califf RM, Fortin DF, Frid DJ, Harlan WR III et al. Restenosis after coronary angioplasty: an overview. J Am Coll Cardiol 1991;17:2B–13B.

9. Serruys PW, Luitjen H, Beatt KJ et al. Incidence of restenosis after successful coronary angioplasty: a time-related phenomenon. A quantitative angiographic study in 342 patients at 1, 2, 3 and 4 months. Circulation 1988; 77:361–371.

10. Nobuyoshi M, Kimura T, Nosaka H et al. Restenosis after successful percutaneous transluminal coronary angioplasty: serial angiographic follow-up of 229 patients. J Am Coll Cardiol 1988;12:616–623.

11. Meier B. Long-term results of coronary balloon angioplasty. Annu Rev Med 1991;42:47–59.

12. Joelson JM, Most AS, Williams DO. Angiographic findings when chest pain recurs after successful percutaneous transluminal coronary angioplasty. Am J Cardiol 1987; 60:792–795.

13. Grines CL, Browne KF, Marco J et al. A comparison of immediate angioplasty with thrombolytic therapy for acute myocardial infarction. The Primary Angioplasty in Myocardial Infarction study group. N Engl J Med 1993; 328:673–679.

14. Meier B, King SB III, Gruentzig AR et al. Repeat coronary angioplasty. J Am Coll Cardiol 1984;4:463–466.

15. Quigley PJ, Hlatky MA, Hinohara T. Repeat percutaneous transluminal coronary angioplasty and predictors of recurrent restenosis. Am J Cardiol 1989;63:409–413.

16. Weintraub WS, Ghazzal ZM, Douglas JS Jr et al. Initial management and long-term clinical outcome of restenosis after initially successful percutaneous transluminal coronary angioplasty. Am J Cardiol 1992;70:47–55.

17. Dimas AP, Grigera F, Arora RR et al. Repeat coronary angioplasty as treatment for restenosis. J Am Coll Cardiol 1992;19:1310–1314.

18. Weintraub WS, Ghazzal ZM, Cohen CL et al. Clinical implications of late proven patency after successful coronary angioplasty. Circulation 1991;84:572–582.

19. Whitlow PL, Franco I. Indications for directional coronary atherectomy. Am J Cardiol 1993;72:21E–29E.

20. Baim DS, Levine MJ, Leon MB, Levine S, Ellis SG, Schatz RA, for the U.S. Palmaz-Schatz Stent investigators. Management of restenosis within the Palmaz-Schatz coronary stent (the U.S. multicenter experience). Am J Cardiol 1993;71:364–366.

21. Baim DS, Kuntz RE. Directional coronary atherectomy: How much lumen enlargement is optimal? Am J Cardiol 1993;72:65E–70E.

22. Bauters C, McFadden EP, Lablanche JM, Quandalle P, Bertrand ME. Restenosis rate after multiple percutaneous transluminal coronary angioplasty procedures at the same site. A quantitative angiographic study in consecutive patients undergoing a third angioplasty procedure for a second restenosis. Circulation 1993;88:969–974.

EDITORIAL SUMMARY

Restenosis lesions are unfortunately common. They are usually particularly amenable to repeat interventions. The approach to restenotic lesions involves several considerations.

1. The lesions are usually subtotal; even in patients in whom the initial lesion was a chronic total occlusion, when restenosis occurs, it is usually subtotal and can be easily crossed with the guidewire.

2. Success rates are usually higher than with de novo lesions. This is a self-selection process as only those lesions that were initially successful can develop restenosis. Patients in whom the initial procedure failed for technical reasons (e.g., undilatable lesions or tortuosity that prevented access) would never have developed restenosis. In addition, the lesion itself may be easier to cross with some devices. In the early directional coronary atherectomy experience, the presence of a restenotic lesion was associated with significantly higher success rates than that of de novo lesions. In addition, restenotic lesions with directional atherectomy usually do not require predilation.

3. The mechanisms of restenosis for the initial lesion should be studied. The initial film should be evaluated if at all possible. If restenosis occurred because the initial result was suboptimal, then attempts should be made to change the subsequent procedure with more optimally sized balloons or different devices to improve the result. Often if conventional dilation technology is to be used again, the balloon size is slightly increased by either 0.25 or 0.5 mm.

4. Selection of the specific catheter-based treatment for a restenotic lesion is largely empiric. As yet, there have been no randomized trials of new devices in restenotic lesions, although one is currently planned using a specific stent configuration. Often a new device or alternative device either is used to optimize the initial result because the patient and/or physician want to try something new or, based on the results of trials, is used in other patient subsets. It must be remembered that repeat conventional dilation may give equivalent results and is frequently performed.

5. Complications of repeat procedures may be somewhat less common in part because of the self-selection process referred to above (#2). Also, the underlying neointimal hyperplasia may respond more uniformly to repeat treatment. A specific subset of patients are those with stent restenosis. Repeat PTCA can be carried out usually with a very high success rate and without complication. Most of these patients have very stable results and can be dismissed without any anticoagulant therapy.

6. Restenosis remains a problem with restenotic lesions. In general, restenotic rates are lower with de novo lesions. It may be that the very first treatment has the best chance for long-term excellent outcome. Even though repeat restenosis occurs, it affects a smaller and smaller absolute number of patients.

The number of repeat dilations that either can or should be performed in patients with restenosis varies. If the goal of the patient is to avoid surgery or if there is not a surgical option, then multiple repeat procedures on the same lesion can be performed. From a practical standpoint, often after the third restenosis, the patient is interested in exploring other alternatives such as coronary bypass graft surgery. The time to restenosis may be important in this regard. If there is a decreasing interval between the treatment and subsequent restenosis from the second to the third procedure, and if the results of each treatment are truly optimal, then subsequent interventional procedures will probably also have suboptimal long-term results. However, if the time interval between procedure and restenosis is increasing, that is often considered a positive sign. In this setting the patient may elect for an additional repeat percutaneous procedure.

24. The Chronic Occlusion

A. Chronic Total Occlusion

NOWAMAGBE A. OMOIGUI and STEPHEN G. ELLIS

The term chronic total occlusion is used to identify coronary stenoses with complete luminal compromise of at least 3 months' duration. The 3-month benchmark used by the American College of Cardiology (1) is an arbitrary dichotomous threshold that tries to capture the essence of the problem—that older occlusions are much less likely to be successfully recanalized using conventional catheter-based techniques. However, the precise point in time when an occlusion becomes clinically chronic has never been convincingly clarified by reproducible data. Chronicity may be attained in days to weeks rather than months.

Indeed, it is difficult to date occlusions. The two most widely used methods are the dates of documented territory-specific myocardial infarction or diagnostic coronary angiography, both of which have obvious limitations. Furthermore, although there is a correlation between occlusion age and histology, their relationship in the natural history of total occlusions is neither consistent nor precise, but varies from individual to individual. It may well be that a continuous rather than dichotomous approach to chronicity is preferable.

Occlusions can be classified on the basis of anatomy or clinical setting. The *anatomic* approach broadly separates functional from total occlusions. A *functional* occlusion (99%) is one in which faint, delayed, distal opacification (without visually apparent luminal continuity) is present as a result of enlarged vasavasorum or intraluminal microchannels resulting in apparent stenosis severity less than 100% with TIMI 1 or 2 flow. Some functional occlusions are actually severe (>95%) subtotal stenoses. On the other hand, true *total* occlusions are not associated with distal anterograde opacification. The *clinical* approach separates occlusions in the setting of acute myocardial infarction from those identified during evaluation in other clinical settings (Table 24A.1).

Total occlusions of *all* varieties were initially considered a contraindication to coronary angioplasty in the 1979 NHLBI guidelines for the procedure. In time, however, patients with interval occlusion while awaiting angioplasty for previously documented subtotal stenoses were treated, followed subsequently by patients with short-length (ostensibly recent) occlusions (2, 3). Experience has confirmed that acute occlusions (with relatively young, soft, and less-organized thrombus) are more amenable to guidewire penetration and recanalization than chronic occlusions (4–7).

Unfortunately, the literature on total occlusions has been confusing. Subacute occlusions have been lumped with more chronic occlusions in a number of analyses. Some authors have combined functional with total occlusions, while duration of occlusion varies from study to study (Table 24A.2). Results vary with inclusion and exclusion criteria, thus limiting reliability and reproducibility.

Table 24A.1.
Total Coronary Occlusion: Clinical and Pathologic Features[a]

	Acute Occlusion of Mild Stenosis	Slowly Progressive Occlusion of Severe Stenosis
Symptoms	Acute infarction	Change in anginal status: usually
Histology	Ruptured fibrous cap overlying soft plaque; large occlusive clot	Laminated organized thrombus Underlying fibrocalcific matrix
Spontaneous recanalization (clot lysis)	Occasional; more likely as time passes	Rare
Collaterals	Rare intracoronary collaterals	Occasional bridging collaterals from dilated vasavasorum/neovascularization
	Occasional intercoronary collaterals if preexisting high-grade stenosis	Intercoronary collaterals are common
Probability of primary PTCA success	Excellent	Low (depending on angiographic characteristics)

[a]Modified from Freed MS. Total occlusion. In: Freed MS, Grines CL, eds. Manual of interventional cardiology. Birmingham, MI: Physician's Press, 1992.

Table 24A.2.
Outcomes of Conventional Angioplasty in Chronic Total Coronary Occlusions—Summary of Experience From Large Series[a]

Reference	22a	22	32	25	25b	23
Sample size	484[c]	905[c]	480[c]	354[c]	500	2907[b,c]
Occlusion age in months						
Mean	8	12	NR	2	2	7
Visible collaterals	74%	NR	NR	40%	100%	76%
Prior infarction	NR	NR	55%	63%	47%	49%
Primary success	NR	72%	69%	66%	67%	68%
Emergency CABG	NR	1%	NR	3%	1%	2%
Infarction	NR	1%	2%	4%	1%	2%
In-hospital death	NR	1%	1%	2%	2%	1%
Mean follow-up in months	24	NR	36	32	NR	28
Recurrence	77%	NR	54%	59%	NR	64%
Restenosis	56%	NR	38%	45%	NR	46%
Reocclusion	21%	NR	16%	14%	NR	17%
Long-term improvement if primary success	NR	69%	60%	NR	NR	68%[d]

[a]Modified from Meier B. Chronic Total Occlusion, In Topol EJ (ed): Textbook of Interventional Cardiology. Philadelphia: WB Saunders, 1994.

[b]Pooled data includes smaller series.

[c]Includes functional occlusions.

[d]Includes repeat angioplasty.

NR, not reported.

DEFINITION, HISTOLOGY, AND PATHOPHYSIOLOGY

For simplicity we define chronic total occlusion as any total occlusion occurring outside the setting of acute myocardial infarction (see Table 24A.1). Extensive collateralization distal to the occlusion may provide the flow-equivalent of a 90% stenosis (8).

A total occlusion has several components, notably an underlying plaque with overlying thrombus at potentially different stages of organization (9). There may be a single internal luminal thrombus or multiple meristematic layers with a mature fibrocellular matrix and/or calcification. Successful uncomplicated intervention is predicated on passage of a guidewire or device through the most recent occlusive thrombus or an intraluminal channel that opens into the true distal lumen (Fig. 24A.1).

An appearance of spontaneous recanalization of a total occlusion may occur via

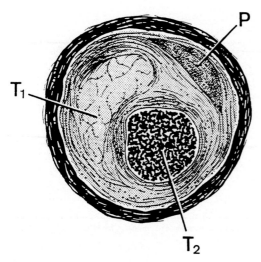

Figure 24A.1. Schematic diagram of a cross section of a totally occluded coronary artery segment. There are thrombotic foci (T_1, T_2) of different ages indicating a first plaque (P) fissure with an organized and heavily fibrosed thrombus (T_1) and a more recent one causing the final complete occlusion (T_2). The extent of fibrosis of the most recent thrombus is the decisive factor in determining the chance of successful balloon recanalization. (From Meier B. Chronic total occlusion. In Topol EJ, ed. Textbook of interventional cardiology. Philadelphia: WB Saunders, 1994.)

several mechanisms—clot lysis (10), intraarterial arterialization (11), vasovasoral dilatation, or combinations thereof. The distal coronary bed may be perfused by anterograde or retrograde collaterals. Angiography is most reliable in broadly distinguishing total occlusions with no anterograde flow from recanalized total occlusions. It is unreliable in discerning the mechanism of recanalization and cannot always identify a severe subtotal occlusion (with or without collaterals) that was never completely occluded. On occasion, copious vasovasora may create the false impression of a moderately severe stenosis, misleading the operator altogether. This possibility may be reduced by evaluating occlusions with multiple angulated views.

The significance of collaterals (8, 12–16) is that they may prevent or limit cell necrosis. It has been estimated that a coronary wedge pressure of ≥45 mm Hg generally implies the presence of enough distal flow to prevent ischemia during stress (17). On the other hand, a well-collateralized chronic total occlusion (CTO) may be associated with angina secondary to increased oxygen demands, while maintaining long-term viability in an area of "hibernating" (18) or "stunned" myocardium (19).

GOALS OF INTERVENTION

As in other circumstances where intervention is contemplated, the rationale must be clearly understood in the context of competing therapeutic alternatives—multimodal medical therapy or surgery (1). Symptom relief (enhancing quality of life) and prognosis are the major strategic objectives. Occlusion angioplasty may achieve this by relieving exertional and rest angina, increasing exercise capacity, and improving left ventricular contractile reserve, while potentially limiting remodeling. The target vessel becomes available to provide collaterals to other vascular territories in the setting of multivessel disease and myocardial infarction "at a distance." Typically, however, these objectives are met with different degrees of success. Overall left ventricular function, in particular, tends to improve only modestly (20–26).

THE THREAT

A strategic approach to CTO must enhance acute success, limit complications, and maintain long-term patency at acceptable costs in the context of broader clinical objectives such as symptom relief and freedom from myocardial infarction, bypass surgery, or death. A fundamental prerequisite for outlining such a strategy, however, is an appreciation of the threat.

Chronic occlusions constitute 10 to 15% of all percutaneous interventions (22). They have long been associated with significant technical difficulty, resulting principally from uncertainty about the path of the true coronary lumen and resistance of the organized thrombus or fibrocellular matrix to guidewire probing (23). Inability to cross with a guide-wire has generally been correlated with failure. It has been estimated that 25% of CTOs cannot be crossed with a guidewire. Approximately 50% can be canalized with a floppy wire, while another 25% will require intermediate or standard-stiffness wires (24, 25). Other causes of failure include inability to track a balloon (or other device) over the wire and failure to reduce stenosis by dilation or other modality (22, 26). The problem of subintimal passage of a guidewire is by no means trivial. Balloon inflation or device deployment in this setting may be associated with extensive dissection, collateral compromise, and/or increased risk of coronary rupture.

In spite of greater radiation exposure, procedure time, and material costs (27), success rates (42 to 72%, mean 68%) (23) have been lower than with angioplasty of subtotal stenoses, which are typically in excess of 90% (7). In addition, since total occlusions of shorter duration and favorable anatomy tend to be selected for treatment because of a higher likelihood of success, the 68% figure may represent an overestimate. On the plus side, acute complication rates are generally lower in the setting of unsuccessful attempts at occlusion PTCA (26). Clinically silent reocclusion may occur in up to 5 to 10% of procedures. While non–Q-wave infarctions are not infrequent, true Q-wave infarction is rare, although derecruitment of collaterals may contribute to this problem. The estimated 10% incidence of distal embolization is usually free of lethal implications. Emergency surgery rates average less than 1%. Reported mortality rates of 1 to 2%, however, are not trivial (see Table 24A.2).

Because failure is much more common during occlusion angioplasty than non-occlusive intervention, overall complication rates may not be dissimilar (26). Furthermore, the evolution of more pliable guidewires for nonocclusive angioplasty in the last 10 years may have rendered this form of PTCA less prone to complications, whereas firm steerable wires continue to be used for CTOs. Where complications have occurred, guide catheter trauma, distal embolization, proximal propagation of dissection, major side-branch closure, and concurrent intervention at sites other than the CTO have been implicated (23). Guidewire entrapment and arrhythmias have been observed. Contrast load tends to be high.

Collaterals are potentially recruitable during *late* reocclusion of previously total occlusions (27a). In earlier experience, periinterventional infarction was considered a distinct rarity because one cannot make a previously closed artery worse. More recent data, however, illustrates the fact that collateral inflow can on occasion be compromised, thereby increasing the likelihood of infarction (or sudden death) in the setting of acute reclosure (28, 29). Distal vasoconstriction (resulting from alterations in coronary vasomotor autoregulation) after successful recanalization may also limit flow (30). If unstable angina is the clinical substrate of intervention, complications may be more likely (31).

Maintenance of patency once the vessel is recanalized constitutes another major problem. These lesions have a tendency to subacute closure (symptomatic and asymptomatic) as well as high restenosis rates (22A, 22B, 25, 32, 33, 40a). Lack of success frequently leads to bypass surgery. The mean incidence of reocclusion and restenosis is about 64% (43 to 77%). Of these, complete reocclusion occurs in 17% while nonocclusive restenosis comprises 46% of cases (see Table 24A.2). Fortunately, major clinical events are uncommon, perhaps the result of rerecruited collaterals. Treatment options include medical therapy, repeat recanalization, PTCA, or bypass surgery depending on symptoms, overall risk profile, and patient-valued outcomes.

There is a high incidence of prior infarction and LV dysfunction among patients with CTO (25, 32). Therefore measures designed to achieve complete revascularization, limit disease progression, enhance collateral recruitment in the event of reocclusion and decrease restenosis are likely to be proportionally more crucial in these patients than in others with less impaired reserve. Taken together with the formidable technical challenges, these factors make the presence of a chronic total occlusion a strong point in favor of elective surgical revascularization. However, long-term results when PTCA is successful have given it a place in management (33a, 33b).

LESSONS AND INSIGHTS FROM 15 YEARS OF OCCLUSION ANGIOPLASTY

A number of lessons and insights have emerged from 15 years of clinical and pathologic experience. The most obvious benefit of successful CTO angioplasty is a significant decrease in subsequent bypass surgery rates (25, 25a). Two-thirds of successful cases were free of angina at 4 years in the Emory series (32). Event-free 5-year survival was 86.4% in successful cases compared with 76.3% (P <.01) among unsuccessful cases in an interim report from Frankfurt (33a), but the incidence of myocardial infarction and death was similar at 7 years in the Mayo experience (25). Because net clinical gain tends to be modest, it is prudent to limit risks and costs. Patients, lesions, equipment, operators, and institutions should match. Combining intervention with the diagnostic study helps to reduce costs (27). Perhaps most important is the need for the operator to know when to quit.

A combination of anatomic features and duration of occlusion allows fairly reliable estimates of probability of success (22, 25, 26, 32, 34–38). Anatomic predictors of success include the absence of bridging collaterals, the presence of a tapered angiographic occlusion morphology with an entry port, and short occlusion length. These factors are synergistic. For example, a 1-year-old occlusion with a long occluded segment (occlusive gap) identifies a lesion that should probably not be attempted. However, occlusion length has been difficult to ascertain retrospectively,

rendering this variable imprecise in prediction models and inconsistent from study to study. While an occlusive gap of less than 10 to 15 mm is clearly desirable, longer gaps have been successfully tackled in the right setting (39). A tapering morphology may be favorable for occlusion angioplasty because small-lumen recanalized areas or loose fibrous tissue penetrates the occluded segment and thus forms a route for guidewire passage (40). The advantage of a nonangulated vessel segment is evident.

Other predictors include degree of calcification and the presence of a side branch at or within 1 cm of the CTO site (because of the tendency of guidewires to track preferentially into adjacent side branches). In our experience this is a problem only if the side branch originates at the point of occlusion. Extreme tortuosity, angioplasty in the setting of unstable angina, number of diseased vessels, vessel and lesion location, the absence of distal antegrade filling, and vessel diameter less than 3 mm have also been reported (Table 24A.3). One group reported a relatively high 13% dissection rate in the right coronary artery (35). Interventions when diffuse proximal disease is present or those within 1 cm of the left main trunk may not be advisable.

Table 24A.3.
Occlusion Angioplasty: Predictors of Acute Success

Favorable	Unfavorable
Absent bridging collaterals	Presence of bridging collaterals
Tapered entry configuration	Flush total occlusion
Short occlusion gap	Long or unknown occlusive gap
(<10 to 15 mm)	Occlusion >3 months
Occlusion <4 weeks	Absence of antegrade filling
Functional occlusion	Presence of side branch at or
	within 1 cm of occlusion
	Moderate/severe calcification
	Moderate/severe tortuosity
	Severe angulation
	Vessel diameter <3 mm
	Diffuse proximal disease
	Location:
	Within 1 cm of LMCA trunk
	In the RCA
	In vein grafts

As previously emphasized, a relatively short duration of occlusion (<2 months) is a powerful predictor of success. The window of best opportunity is typically within the first 4 weeks after total occlusion. The presence of thrombus at the site of CTO is favorable (perhaps indicating a relatively recent event). The Emory group also reported that a functional rather than total occlusion is associated with higher success and lower reocclusion rates (32). This pattern of behavior suggests that *functional occlusions should be considered separately from total occlusions.*

One limitation in the assessment of restenosis after CTO angioplasty has been the relatively poor angiographic follow-up rates. This is further confounded by the difficulty of differentiating an estimated 10% (or greater) occurrence of silent early reocclusion from late restenosis (23). It has, however, been observed that the presence of clot in the lesion may predict higher restenosis rates and that restenosis follows a time course similar to subtotal angioplasty. In one study restenosis reached a plateau after the tenth month (32). A less than ideal result, the presence of good collaterals, the persistence of collateral pressure (in spite of collateral disappearance), and location in the left anterior descending or circumflex arteries may also contribute to restenosis (34), while the absence of multivessel disease is favorable. *However, it is important to recognize that an excellent angiographic angioplasty result in this setting still poses a high risk for restenosis* (34a).

In a provocative quantitative angiographic pooled analysis of 3549 lesions in 2950 patients from four major restenosis trials (with 92% follow-up), restenosis occurred in 44.67% of total occlusion angioplasties and 32.65% of nontotal occlusion (NTO) interventions. When reocclusions were specifically evaluated, there was an 18% rate among CTOs and a 4.7% rate among NTOs. Excluding reocclusions from analysis, restenosis rates among CTOs and NTOs were similar. The authors speculated

that there may be a subset of CTO patients with an intrinsic hematologic or lesion propensity to acute thrombosis (40a). This observation may have implications for future treatment strategies.

It has generally been advisable to perform CTO angioplasty first when contemplating staged multivessel PTCA and to restrict intervention to the culprit lesion in acute coronary syndromes. Total occlusions in vein grafts should be approached cautiously (or avoided) because of the high risk of distal embolization. Microvascular obstruction may result in a diffuse myocardial blush (41). However, prolonged intragraft infusions with urokinase have been used as a prelude to definitive angioplasty and should be considered if intervention is clinically indicated.

In a multicenter study Hartman et al. administered 100,000 to 360,000 units/hour of urokinase for 24 to 36 hours, or until vein graft recanalization, to 107 predominantly white, male smokers with prior infarction and a mean age of 61 years. Average graft age was 9 years, and occlusions were deemed to be ≤6 months old. Urokinase was given for 25 ± 11 hours in a total dose of 4.1 ± 5.5 million units. Fibrinogen nadir was 250 ± 89 mg/dL. Adjunctive PTCA was performed in 88% of cases. Primary success (defined as TIMI 2 to 3 flow) occurred in 76 of 107 cases (71%) and was not related to graft age. Death occurred in 7%, CVA in 3%, emergency bypass surgery in 4%, and Q-wave infarction in 5% of patients. Elevated CK-MB was observed in 17%, while 12% had chest pain. Bleeding complications occurred in 8% of cases (2% intracranial, 2% retroperitoneal, and 4% groin). With 51% angiographic follow-up, 41% overall patency was noted. Six-month patency was 67% if initial TIMI flow was 3 and 30% if TIMI flow was 2 (42). Anecdotal experience suggests that CTOs with otherwise advantageous features in internal mammary grafts are amenable to intervention with good long-term outcome (43).

THE TOOL BOX

Three broad principles govern the tactical approach to intervention—power, mobility, and protection. Within this context the operator must avoid surprises (by knowing the anatomic and clinical terrain) and be capable of concentrating superior technology against the weakest element in the lesion.

In anticipation of a highly resistant lesion over a range of aortic root sizes, proximal vessel sizes, and tortuosities, *guide catheter* selection is based on the principle of maximum backup support for guidewire and subsequent balloon (or other device) advancement. While standard Judkins catheters are usually adequate for the left anterior descending artery, an Amplatz configuration is ideal for the left circumflex and the right coronary arteries. Deep-seating of Judkins or multipurpose catheters may be necessary, but could also provide a substrate for dissection. Unusual coronary takeoffs may require less commonly used catheters such as the El-Gamal, Arani, or hockey stick.

Perhaps more than in other interventional setting, coaxial *guidewire* power ("pushability"), stability, torque control, and trackability are critical. These attributes must be balanced against the need to protect the vessel from injury by using flexible wires whenever possible. Radiopaque wires with diameters of 0.010, 0.012, 0.014, 0.016, 0.018, 0.025, 0.035, and 0.038 inch and a range of stiffness from *floppy* to *intermediate* to *standard* have been used. The capacity to extend to exchange-length is an important ancillary quality, but magnet-assisted exchange may become a viable option in the future.

A steerable, low-profile, high–tensile-strength, *balloon-dilatation system* with the capacity to grow and perform distal contrast injections would be ideal for occlusion angioplasty. Unfortunately, these characteristics are unlikely to be simultaneously present in currently available balloons. *On-the-wire* and *over-the-wire* systems should be available at 20-, 30-, and 40-mm lengths. Longer bal-

Table 24A.4.
The Tool Box

Conventional	New Technology
Standard guiding catheters	Laser-based devices:
Conventional guidewires:	Excimer laser
(0.010 to 0.038 inch)	LASTAC bare argon
Floppy	Rotational drills:
High torque, Entre, Lumisilk	ROTACS (low speed)
Intermediate	Special guidewires:
Standard	Magnum (0.021 inch)
Standard balloons:	Cragg (open-ended)
Over-the-wire	Terumo (glide)
On-the-wire	Omniflex fixed-wire balloon
Undefined role (evolving):	Probe catheter
Rotablator	Balloonless infusion
Transluminal extraction	catheter
device	Vibrational oscillating wire
Stents	
Thrombolytic agents	
Limited role:	
Simpson AtheroCath	

loons, however, decrease the ease of initial crossing and should therefore probably be discouraged. The inability to exchange balloons (to allow sizing up, for example) while maintaining guidewire position is a disadvantage of the fixed-wire systems, although they generally tend to have lower profiles. Deployment in parallel with a free guidewire may be helpful (44). Although potentially cumbersome, an alternative approach is with monorail balloons. Other tools are listed in Table 24A.4. They include low-profile infusion and probing catheters, shaft-enforced tip-deflecting catheters (Omniflex), Cragg open-ended wires, ball-tip recanalization wires (Magnum-Meier), glidewires (Terumo), laser catheters, and rotational and vibrational wire systems (45–56).

SPECIAL WIRES AND NON–GUIDEWIRE-DEPENDENT SYSTEMS

The *Magnum wire* (Schneider) has a 0.021-inch solid steel shaft with a flexible distal segment and a terminal ball-tip 1 mm in diameter. A success rate of 62% in conventional wire failure has been described. However, its apparent superiority to conventional wire in one randomized trial (51) was not confirmed in a subsequent study (52). The Magnarail, Magnum, and Mega balloons are probably the only balloon catheters with a compatible lumen. Details of technique for using this wire have been reviewed in detail elsewhere (23). In our hands it has been successful in 20 to 25% of cases in which other techniques have failed.

The open-ended *Cragg wire* is a 0.035-inch guidewire with a detachable core (50). This allows variability in stiffness and contrast injections as deemed necessary by the operator. The core is compatible with 0.025-inch or smaller wires, allowing combinations with other tools as the situation dictates.

Rotational wires are of the low-speed (<200 rpm—ROTACS) and high-speed (≤100,000 rpm—Kensey) varieties. The Kensey type stalled in early development (55). ROTACS has a 1.3 to 1.8-mm ball-tip and is a battery motor–driven, over-the-wire catheter comprising stainless steel helical coils and a movable outer plastic sleeve. It may be used with or without the motor (36). It is typically deployed through an 8 Fr guide catheter, over a conventional wire up to the proximal end of the CTO. The guidewire is then removed and forward pressure applied in rotational or static modes. The sleeve can be repositioned as needed to splint the system and enhance pushability. After crossing the lesion, the guidewire is reinserted and the system exchanged for a conventional balloon.

Although a preliminary report of ROTACS revealed a low, device-specific success rate (20%), a subsequent publication of its utility for CTOs in 200 patients resistant to conventional techniques was more encouraging (36). In this difficult lesion subset, overall success was 58%. The Magnum wire was successful in 45% of conventional guidewire failures, and ROTACS was successful in 30 cases in which the magnum wire had failed. There were no procedural deaths, bypass surgery was performed in three patients, and one patient died suddenly at 5 days. Success was 91% and 72% in lesions 1 to 3 months and 4 to 6

months old, respectively. In comparison with the 20% success rate typical of conventional techniques, ROTACS was successful in 55% of 6 to 12-month old CTOs. (Lesions older than 1 year were recanalized 8% of the time.) There was a 30% incidence of asymptomatic dissections. Distal embolization was documented in three patients. The nonocclusive restenosis rate at 4 months was 38%, with reocclusion in an additional 19%.

The *Terumo glidewire* comes in angled and nonangled configurations (56). Its titanium-nickel alloy core is covered with a hydrophilic polymer coating. It is resistant to kinking and highly pushable. Based on a strong track record in peripheral vascular work, it was introduced into coronary use. Available in 0.016, 0.018, 0.035, and 0.038-inch sizes, reports suggest that it may be successful in 30 to 65% of conventional guidewire failures. Its generally poor visibility, shapability, and steerability, however, contrast with its unique gliding capability, and high subintimal dissection rates have been observed. The availability of a gold-tipped option in the 0.016 and 0.018-inch categories, a Cragg-compatible 0.025-inch wire and an exchange-length version will substantially expand the role of this interesting wire.

In a recent report, a reciprocating wire oscillating at 100 to 500 Hz (thus transmitting vibrations through the free end of the wire to the lesion) was used to successfully treat three CTOs (9 months to 9 years old) without dissection (57). This represents the first documented application of *vibrational angioplasty*.

The Argon laser-heated hot-tip wire is now of historical interest. The LASTAC bare argon, thermal laser device (UV Medical, Inc.) was reportedly successful in 63% of 41 guidewire failures (58). The laser fiber is positioned just beyond a balloon catheter tip 2 mm proximal to the CTO. The balloon is inflated to bring the laser fiber into coaxial alignment with the vessel. A couple of laser emissions are then used to create a channel, after which the fiber is exchanged for a conventional wire and routine PTCA performed. Complications documented in premarket approval data include perforation (1.3%), infarction (2.5%), emergency bypass surgery (1.3%), and death (1.9%).

Investigation of the bare excimer laser guidewire has begun. The shapable, 0.018-inch, exchangeable *Spectranetics* wire may be promising (59), but the prototype ACS 0.021-inch, deflectable-tip, nonexchangeable wire has been associated with frequent dissections and occasional perforations (N. Eigler, personal communication, 1994). Laser systems triggered by spectral analysis of target tissue are far from clinical application (61). In general, these devices are expensive, not strikingly advantageous, fraught with unique complications (e.g., perforation), and therefore unlikely to enter common usage. Early work suggests that perhaps 50% of selected occlusions that cannot be crossed using conventional technique may be crossed with the bare laser wire, but that proper technique is difficult and time-consuming (P. Serruys, personal communication, 1995.)

OTHER GUIDEWIRE-DEPENDENT SYSTEMS

A guidewire-dependent system is one that relies on prior successful guidewire crossing for its subsequent deployment. Conventional balloon angioplasty has been discussed. Directional, rotational, and extractional atherectomy are of limited applicability, although experience continues to accrue and the role of the Rotablator, for example, may be better defined in the near future. Preliminary data from the Multicenter Rotablator Registry revealed 91% success rate without major complications (61a). Its A and C wires can be deployed through a perfusion catheter after prior canalization with a less flexible wire. It may be useful in debulking nondilatable, noncompliant (usually calcified) lesions with the potential drawback of distal embolization. On the other hand, the transluminal extrac-

tional catheter (TEC) may conceptually be of value in safely debulking thrombus.

Stents require prior dilatation, are intrinsically thrombogenic, and are not appropriate for all vessel sizes. No obvious advantage accrued when stenting was used to improve results of conventional occlusion angioplasty in one report (62). In a more recent series, however, 85% of patients were asymptomatic at 8.8 months, with a 6-month angiographic restenosis rate of 24%, when Palmaz-Schatz stents were placed in vessels ≥3.0 mm diameter after prior successful occlusion angioplasty resulted in residual stenoses >20% (63).

In a pilot series, stand-alone excimer laser PTCA (ELCA) was infrequently successful (24%), usually requiring adjunctive balloon dilation (76%). There was an 8% reocclusion rate after 24 hours (64). The large multicenter ELCA registry report (53) was limited to patients in whom a guidewire *had crossed*. Laser success was 83% while procedural success was 90%. Adjunctive balloon angioplasty was required in 74% of cases. Major complications occurred in 2% of cases, but even more striking was the 2.5% coronary perforation rate. There are as yet no data on the Holmium laser in this setting.

The excellent success rate of stand-alone balloon angioplasty after guidewire crossing (90 to 95%) suggests that the role of laser is limited to uncommon situations in which primary balloon dilatation has failed because of either failure to cross or failure to dilate. Even in such situations, however, severely angulated segments should be avoided.

PRACTICAL TIPS (TABLE 24A.5)

Integral to technique are the aforementioned principles of case selection and familiarity with the strengths and weaknesses of available tools. Standard principles of preprocedural anticipation apply. Surgical backup should be evaluated on a case-by-case basis because of the real (although uncommon) likelihood of complications. In selecting tools

Table 24A.5.
Flow Chart: Suggested Approach to Occlusion Angioplasty

1. Evaluate extent and viability of myocardium subserved by occluded vessel.
2. Consider degree of symptom and quality-of-life improvement that may result from intervention and patient opinion regarding alternative therapy.
3. Assess technical difficulty of lesion in the context of operator experience and available tools. Anticipate potential problems/complications and plan accordingly. Determine need for surgical backup.
4. Initial procedure:
   Ensure adequate aspirinization/heparinization
   Obtain/clarify angiographic roadmap
   Choose guiding catheter for *maximum* support
   Consider adjunctive intracoronary thrombolysis if TIMI grade 0 flow at baseline
      (Lower threshhold for use in vein grafts)
   Use conventional guidewires with step-up approach:
      Floppy to intermediate to standard
      (Reassess procedure before proceeding to standard wire)
   Consider splinting flexible wire with:
      Perfusion catheter/balloon
      Cragg open-ended wire
5. If usual wire fails to cross:
   Reassess entire procedure again
      Consider Terumo wire
      Consider Magnum wire
      Consider ROTACS without motor unit
      Consider ROTACS with motor unit
      Consider vibrational angioplasty wire
6. If wire crosses, confirm location with contrast injection in at least two orthogonal projections; then proceed with dilation/other strategy.
7. If wire crosses, but balloon fails to cross:
   Consider low-profile, noncompliant balloon (e.g., Sleek)
   Consider more trackable wire (exchange through perfusion catheter)
   Reassess procedure: consider excimer-laser, investigational laser, or Rotablator
8. If balloon fails to dilate:
   Consider less compliant balloon at higher pressure
   Reassess procedure; consider excimer-laser (or Rotablator)
9. If lesion successfully treated:
   Evaluate angiographic result—Is bigger better? Consider stent in larger vessels?
   Optimize results with intravascular ultrasound/QCA? Assess collaterals?
   Administer long-term adjunctive therapy—aspirin, heparin, coumadin?

and tactics, the operator should be sensitive to costs.

Angiographically defining the vessel and lumen pathway is an essential prerequisite. Side-by-side freeze frames of the CTO and its collateral-dependent donor artery are invaluable. Another approach is simultaneous angiography of the occluded vessel and its contralateral collateral-dependent artery via selective engagement through a second peripheral vascular access (64a). While the LAO-cranial view may help direct the guidewire away from diagonals, the RAO helps to avoid septals and RV marginals. The Lateral view places the LAD in profile and may also help avoid RV marginals. Modification of fluoroscopy views during the procedure can substantially reduce operator radiation dose. The LAO view (particularly when angulated) should be used sparingly (65).

A generally accepted approach to guidewire selection is gradual step-up of stiffness and thickness. This comes at the cost of decreased steerability and increased risk of trauma. For example, one might begin with a 0.014-inch, high-torque, floppy wire, stepping up to an intermediate before selecting a standard wire. Some operators begin up front with an extrasupport 0.018-inch wire. Patience and persistence are crucial—using multiply shaped tips and advancing only when the wire tip is free. Improved transition wires (e.g., Reflex M) may be helpful when other wires tend to prolapse down a nearby branch vessel. In the event of failure with conventional 0.014 to 0.018-inch wires, we often will try (and have succeeded with) an 0.010-inch intermediate wire under the assumption that it may better find a small entryway and is clearly less traumatic than larger options. If a standard wire is used to establish a distal bridgehead, one might consider exchanging it for a floppy after intraluminal passage is confirmed.

It cannot be overemphasized that the guide-wire tip should always be free in co-axial and rotational axes. For usual guide-wires, "screw-in" torque and "wedging" within the lesion are unsound practices and may lead to guidewire entrapment, fracture, or occasionally the need for surgical retrieval. Frequent contrast injections help to confirm course. To establish safe, distal, wire positioning, at least two orthogonal views should be obtained. Contrast may also be given through a balloon, exchange, or perfusion catheter (or Cragg wire). When a balloon is advanced over the wire, initial inflations may proceed over a range of 2 to 12 atm for 30 to 180 seconds.

Guidewire pushability can be enhanced markedly by using an infusion catheter, Cragg convertible wire (50), conventional balloon, or 4 Fr probe exchange catheter (PEC) for support (46), which is positioned 1 to 2 cm from the guidewire tip to prevent proximal buckling and helps direct the force of pushing coaxially. It may be followed by an ultra-low-profile, probing, balloon-on-wire catheter (47) or a thin-shaft, balloon-over-wire (48). Only through experience can one acquire the correct feel for safe degrees of resistance to wire passage. Some operators prefer the 2- to 2.5-mm Omniflex balloon-on-wire system, alongside of which they then pass a conventional guidewire before exchanging for a larger balloon (44, 49). It is worth reemphasizing that the Terumo wire is poorly visible and tends to either cross the lesion or dissect

the artery. The Magnum wire requires more forceful pushing than conventional wires. Another approach is the use of the pliable distal tip of a sheath introducer to dotterize the lesion.

After crossing the lesion with a wire, failure to pass a balloon or dilate with a high-pressure balloon may necessitate the use of alternative technology such as the Rotablator (after A or C wire exchange) or laser. Acute closure is treated using standard methods—prolonged inflations, perfusion balloon, and stenting. However, serious ischemic complications are unusual.

On completion of the procedure, some operators have suggested that the status of collaterals should be ascertained angiographically. We do not do this routinely.

ADJUNCTIVE THERAPY

Thrombolytics

The use of thrombolytics as an adjunct to CTO angioplasty may have merit. Underlying lesion morphology is better appreciated after debulking associated thrombus, but any large-scale use of thrombolytics for this indication should be tempered by the understanding that adequate intracoronary dosages may approach the systemic doses associated with intracranial hemorrhage. Furthermore, impact on restenosis has not been rigorously assessed. Studies using either t-PA (5 to 10 mg/hour for 6 hours) or urokinase (100 to 200,000 units/hour for 8 to 24 hours) have shown increases in TIMI flow grade (≥ 1 grade in 29%) (66) and PTCA success rates of 56 to 90% (66, 67). Intracoronary thrombolysis with 0.2 to 0.4 mg/minute t-PA for 60 to 90 minutes in native vessel CTO resulted in a decreased mean stenosis severity (99 $\pm$ 3% to 94 $\pm$ 6%), an increased TIMI flow grade, and a 94% PTCA success rate in another study (68). In a dose-ranging study, relatively lower doses of urokinase were effective in an interim report (69), but no randomized comparisons of specific agents have been performed. A modified approach to intracoronary thrombolysis using proximal balloon occlusion may enhance safety and efficiency (70). There are no data on the use of ultrasonic techniques to lyse clot in this setting.

Heparin, Coumadin, and Aspirin

Aspirin and heparin are standard medications during any form of angioplasty, but no study has unequivocally demonstrated the benefits of prolonged anticoagulation *after* CTO angioplasty. None of these agents have reduced restenosis rates in unselected patients, for example. However, it is not uncommon for experienced operators to prescribe 24 hours of IV heparin followed by warfarin for 1 month (PT 16 to 18) and 160 to 325 mg/day soluble aspirin indefinitely. More potent agents like Hirudin and Integrelin may gain a place in future therapy. A major problem, however, is to predict which patients will reocclude and therefore require focused aggressive antithrombotic treatment.

FOLLOW-UP

The relatively high prevalence of multivessel disease, prior partial infarction, and LV dysfunction in these patients renders conventional noninvasive testing somewhat limited in predictive value. Early angiographic follow-up after CTO angioplasty may be reasonable on the premise that a totally reoccluded CTO is unlikely to remain patent in the long run after a second intervention. However, whether early treatment of restenosis before late reocclusion will impact long-term patency is unknown, particularly since it is unclear whether early reocclusion, restenosis, and late reocclusion are parts of the same continuum or distinct endpoints to which different patient subsets are prone (40a). Vascular thrombus imaging and systemic tests of clot activation may eventually prove to be helpful. A careful balancing of costs and expected utility should guide decision making in this difficult setting.

FUTURE APPROACHES

Three-dimensional, digital, biplane, angiographic reconstruction of vessel segments to improve guidewire passage across occlusive gaps is feasible and in the early stages of development (71). Forward-looking, intravascular, ultrasound imaging may emerge in the future and help distinguish clot from atheroma and calcium, while identifying small-lumen, recanalized pathways. It might also render debulking technologies more feasible. Retrograde recanalization of resistant femoral occlusions via a popliteal approach has been performed in the periphery (72). Whether such an approach (via bypass grafts) will ever gain a place in coronary intervention remains to be seen.

SUMMARY

Chronic total occlusions are not uncommon. They are technically challenging and constitute a frequent cause of referrals for bypass surgery. Against a background of prior myocardial infarction and left ventricular dysfunction, clinical events are common among these patients. Although of low risk, occlusion angioplasty is by no means a no-risk undertaking. Long-term patency rates are modest. When successful, however, occlusion angioplasty is associated with a decrease in bypass surgery rates and acceptable degrees of freedom from angina. With careful case selection, the current tools and techniques can result in higher primary success rates with minimal complications and long-term patency at reasonable costs.

REFERENCES

1. Ryan TJ, Bauman WB, Kennedy JW et al. ACC/AHA guidelines for percutaneous transluminal coronary angioplasty: a report of the American College of Cardiology/American Heart Association Task Force on Assessment of Diagnostic and Therapeutic Cardiovascular Procedures (Committee on Percutaneous Transluminal Coronary Angioplasty). J Am Coll Cardiol 1993;22(7):2033–2054.
2. Savage R, Hollman J, Gruentzig AR, King SB III, Douglas J, Tankersley R. Can percutaneous transluminal coronary angioplasty be performed in patients with total occlusion. Circulation 1982;66:II-330 (abstract).
3. Heyndriniks GR, Serruys PW, Brand M, Vandormael M, Reiber JHC. Transluminal angioplasty after mechanical recanalization in patients with chronic occlusion of coronary artery. Circulation 1983;66:II-5 (abstract).

4. Holmes DRJ, Vlietstra RE, Reeder GS, Bresnahan JF, Smith HC, Bove AA, Schaff HV. Angioplasty in total coronary artery occlusion. J Am Coll Cardiol 1984;3:845–849.

5. Kereiakes DJ, Selmon MR, McAuley BJ, McAuley DB, Sheehan DJ, Simpson JB. Angioplasty in total coronary artery occlusion: experience in 76 consecutive patients. J Am Coll Cardiol 1985;6:526–533.

6. Ferguson DW, Kouba CR, Little MM, Osborne JL, White CW, Kioschos JM. Combined intracoronary streptokinase and percutaneous coronary angioplasty for reperfusion of chronic total coronary occlusion. J Am Coll Cardiol 1984; 4:820–824.

7. Detre K, Holubkov R, Kelsey S et al., and the co-investigators of the National Heart, Lung and Blood Institute's Percutaneous Transluminal Coronary Angioplasty Registry. Percutaneous transluminal coronary angioplasty in 1985–1986 and 1977–1981. The Heart, Lung, and Blood Institute Registry. N Engl J Med 1988;318:265–270.

8. Flameng W, Schwarz F, Haehrlein FW. Intraoperative evaluation of the functional significance of coronary collateral vessels in patients with coronary disease. Am J Cardiol 1978;42:187–192.

9. Dick RJL, Haudenschild CC, Popma JJ, Ellis SG, Muller DW, Topol EJ. Directional atherectomy for total coronary occlusions. Coronary Artery Dis 1991;2:189–199.

10. Schwartz H, Leiboff RH, Bren GB et al. Temporal evolution of the human coronary circulation after myocardial infarction. J Am Coll Cardiol 1984;4:1088–1093.

11. Roberts WC, Virmani R. Formation of new coronary arteries within a previously obstructed epicardial coronary artery (intraarterial arteries): a mechanism for occurrence of angiographically normal coronary arteries after healing of acute myocardial infarction. Am J Cardiol 1984; 54:1361–1362.

12. Schwartz F, Flameng W, Ensslen R, Sesto M, Thorman J. Effect of coronary collaterals on left ventricular function at rest and during stress. Am Heart J 1978;95:570–577.

13. Rogers WJ, Hood WP, Mantle JA et al. Return of left ventricular function after reperfusion in patients with myocardial infarction: importance of subtotal stenoses or intact collaterals. Circulation 1984;69:338–349.

14. Saito Y, Yasuno M, Ishida M et al. Importance of collaterals for restoration of left ventricular function after intracoronary thrombolysis. Am J Cardiol 1985;55:1259–1263.

15. Nitzberg WD, Nath HP, Rogers WJ et al. Collateral flow in patients with acute myocardial infarction. Am J Cardiol 1985;56:729–736.

16. Cohen M, Rentrop KP. Limitation of myocardial ischemia by collateral circulation during sudden controlled coronary artery occlusion in human subjects: a prospective study. Circulation 1986;74:469–476.

17. Meier B, Leuthy P, Finci L et al. Coronary wedge pressure in relation to spontaneously visible and recruitable collaterals. Circulation 1987;75:906–913.

18. Rahimtoola SH. The hibernating myocardium. Am Heart J 1989;117:211–221.

19. Braunwald E, Kloner RA. The stunned myocardium: prolonged, postischemic ventricular dysfunction. Circulation 1982;66:1146–1149.

20. Melchior JP, Doriot PA, Chatelain P, Meier B, Urban P, Finci L, Rutishauser W. Improvement of left ventricular contraction and relaxation synchronism after recanalization of chronic total coronary occlusion by angioplasty. J Am Coll Cardiol 1987;9:763–768.

21. Serruys PW, Umans V, Heyndrickx GR et al. Elective PTCA of totally occluded coronary arteries not associated with myocardial infarction: short- and long-term results. Eur Heart J 1985;6:2–12.

22. Stone G, Rutherford B, McConahay D, Johnson W Jr, Giorgi L, Ligon R, Hartzler G. Procedural outcome of angioplasty for total coronary artery occlusion: analysis of 971 lesions in 905 patients. J Am Coll Cardiol 1990; 15:849–856.

22a. Ellis SG, Shaw RE, Gershony G, Thomas R, Roubin GS, Douglas JS, Topol EJ et al. Risk factors, time course and treatment effect for restenosis after successful percutaneous transluminal coronary angioplasty of chronic total occlusion. Am J Cardiol 1989;63:897–901.

22b. DiSciascio G, Vetrovec GW, Cowley MJ, Wolfgang TC. Early and late outcome of percutaneous transluminal coronary angioplasty for subacute and chronic total coronary occlusion. Am Heart J 1986;111:833–839.

23. Meier B. Chronic total occlusion. In: Topol EJ, Ed. Textbook of interventional cardiology. 2nd ed. Philadelphia: WB Saunders, 1994.

24. Safian RD, McCabe CH, Sipperly ME, McKay RG, Baim DS. Initial success and long-term follow-up of percutaneous transluminal coronary angioplasty in chronic total occlusion versus conventional stenoses. Am J Cardiol 1988;61:23G–28G.

25. Bell MR, Berger PB, Bresnahan JF, Reeder GS, Bailey KR, Holmes DR Jr. Initial and long-term outcome of 354 patients following coronary balloon angioplasty of total coronary artery occlusions. Circulation 1992;85:1033–1011.

25a. Warren RJ, Black AJ, Valentine PA, Manolas EG, Hunt D. Coronary angioplasty for chronic total occlusion reduces the need for subsequent coronary bypass surgery. Am Heart J 1990;120:270–274.

25b. Haine E, Urban P, Dorsaz PA et al. Outcome and complications of 500 consecutive chronic total occlusion angioplasties. J Am Coll Cardiol 1993;21:138A.

26. Ruocco NAJ, Ring ME, Holubkov R, Jacobs AK, Detre KM, Faxon DP, and the co-investigators of the National Heart, Lung, and Blood Institute Percutaneous Transluminal Coronary Angioplasty Registry. Results of coronary angioplasty of chronic total occlusions (The National Heart, Lung, and Blood Institute 1985–1986 Percutaneous Transluminal Coronary Angioplasty Registry). Am J Cardiol 1992;69:69–76.

27. Bell MR, Berger PB, Menke KK, Holmes DR Jr. Balloon angioplasty of chronic total coronary artery occlusions: What does it cost in radiation exposure, time, and materials. Cathet Cardiovasc Diagn 1992;25:10–15.

27a. Moles VP, Meier B, Urban P et al. Instantaneous recruitment of reversed coronary collaterals that had been dormant for six years. Cathet Cardiovasc Diagn 1992; 26:148–151.

28. Avanindra J, Frantz D, Sapin P. Myocardial ischemia during balloon angioplasty of chronic totally occluded vessels: role of collaterals. Coronary Artery Dis 1992;3:933–938.

29. Burger W, Kadel C, Keul H, Vallbracht C, Kaltenbach M. A word of caution: reopening chronic coronary occlusions. Cathet Cardiovasc Diagn 1992;27:35–39.

30. Leung WH. Coronary vasoconstriction after angioplasty of total occlusions: relation to change in coronary perfusion pressure. J Am Coll Cardiol 1993;22:1635–1640.

31. Plante S, Laarman G, de Feyter PJ, Samson M, Rensing BJ, Umans V, Suryapranata H et al. Acute complications of percutaneous transluminal coronary angioplasty for total occlusion. Am Heart J 1991;121:417–426.

32. Ivanhoe RJ, Weintraub WS, Douglas JSJ, Lembo NJ, Furman M, Gershony G, Cohen CL et al. Percutaneous transluminal coronary angioplasty of chronic total occlusions. Primary success, restenosis, and long-term clinical follow-up. Circulation 1992;85:106–115.

33. Finci L, Meier B, Favre J, Righetti A, Rutishauser W. Long-term results of successful and failed angioplasty for chronic total coronary arterial occlusion. Am J Cardiol 1990; 66:660–662.

33a. Kadek C, Burger W, Hartmann et al. Long-term follow-up in 686 patients with attempted reopening of chronic coronary occlusions. Circulation 1993;88(4):II-2722.

33b. Seggewib H, Streck S, Everlein M et al. Successful recanalization of chronically occluded infarct-related arteries in patients with single-vessel disease results in reduction of cardiac events. Circulation 1994;90:I-435.

34. Meier B. "Occlusion angioplasty": light at the end of the tunnel or dead end. Circulation 1992;85:1214–1216.

34a. Ellis SG, Shaw RE, King SB III et al. Restenosis after excellent angiographic angioplasty result for chronic total coronary artery occlusion—implications for newer percutaneous revascularization devices. Am J Cardiol 1989; 64:667–668.

35. Stewart JT, Denne L, Bowker TJ, Mulcahy DA, Williams MG, Buller NP, Sigwart U et al. Percutaneous transluminal coronary angioplasty in chronic coronary artery occlusion. J Am Coll Cardiol 1993;21:1371–1376.

36. Kaltenbach M, Hartmann A, Vallbracht C. Procedural results and patient selection in recanalization of chronic coronary occlusions by low-speed rotational angioplasty. Eur Heart J 1993;14:826–830.

37. Maiello L, Colombo A, Gianrossi R, Mutinelli M, Bouzon R, Thomas J, Finci L. Coronary angioplasty of chronic occlusions: factors predictive of procedural success. Am Heart J 1992;124:581.

38. Tan KH, Sulke N, Taub NA, Watts E, Karani S, Sowton E. Determinants of success of coronary angioplasty in patients with a chronic total occlusion: a multiple logistic regression model to improve selection of patients. Br Heart J 1993;70:126–131.

39. Taylor MA, Vetrovec GW. Angioplasty of a totally occluded right coronary artery. Cathet Cardiovasc Diagn 1992; 25:61–65.

40. Katsuragawa M, Fujiwara H, Miyamae M, Sasayama S. Histologic studies in percutaneous transluminal coronary angioplasty for chronic total occlusion: comparison of tapering and abrupt types of occlusion and short and long occluded segments. J Am Coll Cardiol 1993;21:604–611.

40a. Violaris AG, Melkert R, Umans VA. Long-term luminal renarrowing following coronary angioplasty of chronic total occlusions—a quantitative angiographic analysis of 3,549 lesions. Circulation 1993;88(4):II-2797.

41. Margolis JR, Mogensen L, Mehta S et al. Diffuse embolization following percutaneous transluminal coronary angioplasty of occluded vein grafts: the blush phenomenon. Clin Cardiol 1991;14:489–493.

42. Hartmann JR. A 1994 update (personal communication) to Hartmann JR, Mckeever LS, Enger EL et al. Recanalization of chronically occluded bypass grafts with prolonged urokinase infusion site trial (ROBUST). Circulation 1993; 88(4):II-2717.

43. Mehan VK, Meier B, Urban P. Balloon recanalization of a chronically occluded left internal mammary artery graft. Br Heart J 1993;70(2):195–197.

44. Hopp HW, Franzen D, Deutsch HJ, Kux A, Hilger HH. New option for balloon recanalization of total coronary occlusions. Cathet Cardiovasc Diagn 1991;24:226–230.

45. de Swart JBRM, van Gelder LM, van der Krieken AM, El Gamal MIH. A new technique for angioplasty of occluded coronary arteries and bypass grafts, not associated with acute myocardial infarction. Cathet Cardiovasc Diagn 1987;13:419–423.

45a. Little T, Pichard AD, Lindsay J. Probe angioplasty of total coronary occlusion using an intracoronary probing catheter. Cathet Cardiovasc Diagn 1989;17:218–223.

46. Kiemeneij F, Suwarganda JSM, van der Wieken LR. Probe exchange catheter used for angioplasty of total coronary artery occlusions. Cathet Cardiovasc Diagn 1990;19:289–293.

47. Little T, Rosenberg J, Seides S, Lee B, Lindsay J, Pichard AD. Probe angioplasty of total coronary occlusion using the probing catheter technique. Cathet Cardiovasc Diagn 1990;21:124–127.

48. Gilchrist IC, Clemson BS. Angioplasty of occluded coronary arteries: use of thin shaft balloon over-the-wire system without pre-dilatation. Cathet Cardiovasc Diagn 1990; 21:121–123.

49. Hamm CW, Kupper W, Kuck K, Hofmann D, Bleifeld W. Recanalization of chronic, totally occluded coronary arteries by new angioplasty systems. Am J Cardiol 1990; 66:1459–1463.

50. Vassanelli C, Turri M, Morando G et al. Open-ended guidewire: new technique for balloon angioplasty of chronically occluded coronary arteries. Cathet Cardiovasc Diagn 1989;17:224–227.

51. Pande AK, Meier B, Urban P, de la Serna F, Villavicencio R, Dorsaz PA, Favre J. Magnum/Magnarail versus conventional systems for recanalization of chronic total coronary occlusions: a randomized comparison. Am Heart J 1992;123:1182–1186.

52. Haerer W, Schmidt A, Eggeling T et al. Angioplasty of chronic total coronary occlusions. Results of a controlled randomized trial. J Am Coll Cardiol 1991;17(2):113A.

53. Holmes DR Jr, Forrester JS, Litvack F et al. Chronic total obstruction and short-term outcome: The Excimer Laser

Coronary Angioplasty Registry experience. Mayo Clin Proc 1993;68:5–10.

54. Searching for therapeutic niches for new coronary interventional devices: the unyielding nature of chronic occlusions. Mayo Clin Proc 1993;68:83–85 (editorial).

55. Kensey KR. The Kensey catheter: What have we learned to date? J Invasive Cardiol 1991;3:25–31.

56. Gray DF, Sivananthan UM, Verma SP et al. Balloon angioplasty of totally and subtotally occluded coronary arteries: results using the hydrophilic Terumo Radifocus guidewire M (Glidewire). Cathet Cardiovasc Diagn 1993;30:293–299.

57. Rees MR, Michalis LK. Vibrational angioplasty in chronic total occlusions. Lancet 1993;342:999–1000.

58. Plokker HW, Mast EG, Margolis J. Laser coronary angioplasty systems: a realistic appraisal. J Myocardial Ischemia 1992;4:11.

59. Sanborn TA, Spokojny AM, Bergman GW et al. A 0.018" excimer laser guidewire to recanalize chronic total occlusions and guide conventional catheters. Circulation 1993;88(4):II-2716.

60. Deleted in proofs.

61. Laufer G, Wollenek G, Hohla K et al. Excimer laser-induced simultaneous ablation and spectral identification of normal and atherosclerotic arterial tissue layers. Circulation 1988;78:1031–1039.

61a. Omoigui N, Booth J, Reisman M, Franco I, Whitlow P. Rotational atherectomy in chronic total occlusions. J Am Coll Cardiol 1995;97A.

62. Bilodeau L, Iyer SS, Cannon AD et al. Stenting as an adjunct to balloon angioplasty for recanalization of totally occluded coronary arteries: clinical and angiographic follow-up. J Am Coll Cardiol 1993;21:292A.

63. Almagor Y, Borrione M, Maiello L et al. Coronary stenting after recanalization of chronic total occlusions. Circulation 1993;88(4):II-2713.

64. Werner GS, Buchwald A, Unterberg C, Voth E, Kreuzer H, Wiegand V. Recanalization of chronic total coronary arterial occlusions by percutaneous excimer-laser and laser-assisted angioplasty. Am J Cardiol 1990;66:1445–1450.

64a. Grollier G, Commeau P, Foucault JP, Potier JC. Angioplasty of chronic totally occluded coronary arteries: usefulness of retrograde opacification of the distal part of the occluded vessel via the contralateral coronary artery. Am Heart J 1987;114:1324–1328.

65. Pitney MR, Allan RM, Giles RW et al. Modifying fluoroscopy views reduces operator radiation exposure during coronary angioplasty. Circulation 1993;88(4):II-3497.

66. Grines CL, Ajluni S, Savas V et al. Prolonged urokinase infusion for chronic total native coronary occlusions. J Am Coll Cardiol 1992;19(3):33A.

67. Vaska KJ, Whitlow PL. Selective tissue plasminogen activator infusion for chronic total occlusions of native coronary arteries failing angioplasty. Circulation 1991;84(4):II-250.

68. Ruocco NA, Currier JW, Jacobs AK, Ryan TJ, Faxon DP. Experience with low-dose intracoronary recombinant tissue-type plasminogen activator for nonacute total occlusions before percutaneous transluminal coronary angioplasty. Am J Cardiol 1991;68:1609–1613.

69. Zidar F, Schreiber T, Jones D et al. A prospective randomized trial of prolonged urokinase infusion for chronic total occlusion (CTO) in native coronary arteries. Circulation 1993;88(4):II-2718.

70. Busch U, Renner U, Weingartner F et al. Balloon occlusive lysis of thrombotic graft occlusion: speedy, safe and efficient. Circulation 1993;88(4):II-2719.

71. Morioka CA, Whiting JS, Eigler NL. Three-dimensional guidance system to aid in the revascularization of chronic total occlusions. Circulation 1993;88(4):II-2715.

72. Bajwa T, Schmidt DH. Retrograde popliteal recanalization of chronic total femoral occlusions in failed antegrade angioplasty: demonstration of improved primary success and enhanced long-term benefit. Circulation 1993;88(4):II-0527.

B. The Chronic Occlusion

URS KAUFMANN and BERNHARD MEIER

Chronic total occlusions have been a target for coronary angioplasty since its very beginning. The initial patients of Andreas Gruentzig with this indication were those who had silently occluded their coronary artery while waiting for angioplasty planned on a nontotal lesion. Their primary success rate was 62% (1). To date total occlusions account for approximately 10% of all coronary angioplasty procedures worldwide (2–4). The procedure is usually restricted to patients with documented or presumed recent occlusion and to acute occlusions during evolving myocardial infarction (5). A fresh and soft thrombus is an easy obstacle for a metallic guidewire, which makes acute occlusions less of a technical challenge than chronic occlusions.

Recanalization of totally occluded coronary arteries is a tempting procedure on the one hand because it is associated with a reduced acute and chronic risk. On the other hand, it is often frustrating, since even in the most experienced centers success rates rarely exceed 75%. A number of equipments specially designed for recanalization procedures such as the Magnum wire, or technical alternatives such as rotational atherectomy or laser angioplasty, have been used with variable success to open up occluded arteries, but have only moderately improved the efficiency of the technique. Total occlusions are by definition complex lesions. Success rates and clinical results depend on operator experience, bearing on case selection, clinical judgement, and knowledge of available angioplasty equipment, as well as technical skills.

WHY IS RECANALIZATION OF AN OCCLUDED ARTERY REASONABLE?

The decision to attempt to recanalize an occluded coronary artery is based on a projection of difficulties (in particular, duration and length of occlusion) balanced against the potential benefit for the patient. Indications may be wide if the recanalization attempt is part of the diagnostic coronary angiogram, since a failure is less costly and imposes most often only a somewhat longer procedure on the patient. Indications are intermediate if the patient is still hospitalized, but they should be restrictive if the patient has to travel or interrupt gainful activities to undergo the procedure. The intervention is far less costly and invasive than coronary bypass surgery. Hence, recanalization procedures need not be restricted to patients selected and ready for surgery should angioplasty prove impossible.

Expected Benefit

Improvement of clinical symptoms, disappearance of silent ischemia (6), improvement of left ventricular function (7), a marked decrease in need for bypass surgery (8–10), and the favorable local risk pattern (11) provide the rationale and ethical basis for percutaneous recanalization attempts. A further incentive is that even improved survival (9) could be documented in patients with successful recanalization.

Immediate improvement of regional wall motion is rarely observed after restoration of antegrade flow (6, 12). There is evidence that myocardium may be stunned (13) and/or hibernating (14) rather than dead for an

extended period. Such abnormalities may take weeks or months to resolve, which suggests that the "erectile" effect of reestablished blood flow and pressure (15) plays an insignificant role since it should be operative at once.

Overall, the average left ventricular improvement after recanalization of chronic total coronary occlusions is not overwhelming and is likely to escape detection by crude assessment of global left ventricular ejection fraction (6, 16). If improvement of left ventricular function was the primary goal, recanalization attempts would not be worthwhile.

Decision Criteria

The chance of success of a recanalization attempt depends largely on the histologic aspects of the lesion. An occluded coronary arterial segment almost always consists of an atherosclerotic plaque and variable forms of thrombi, which may constitute a major or a minor part of the luminal obstruction. There may be a single clot of uniform structure and age or layers of clots of disparate structures and ages associated with fibrointimal proliferation. Its texture is crucial for success or failure of coronary angioplasty, since the recanalization equipment should be passed through this thrombus. The older and the more fibrosed a clot, the smaller the chance to cross it safely. Obviously, a fresh, soft thrombus represents an ideal target to cross with a guidewire. Occlusions older than 6 months usually carry a very low chance of success, probably because most of the lesion consists of fibrosis or even calcific deposits impossible to be crossed with a guidewire. A spontaneously recanalized lesion, whether by lysis of a clot with formation of several new channels through the thrombus (intraarterial arteries 17), by dilation of the *vasa vasorum*, or by a combination of these mechanisms, may also be impossible to pass with a guidewire.

A total occlusion that is well collateralized is functionally equivalent to a 90% stenosis

(12). Myocardial viability is preserved, but clinically apparent ischemia during periods of increased oxygen demand are typical.

The presence of collaterals is an important predictor of successful recanalization. On the one hand, the quality of the artery distal to the occlusion can be assessed; on the other hand, collaterals usually imply that the concerned myocardium is alive. Collaterals are quite common in patients with long-standing coronary artery disease and subtotal stenosis. Although the degree of myocardial preservation during the initial period of acute coronary occlusion depends on already functional collaterals or on collaterals that are instantly recruitable, the myocardium subtended by collaterals is rarely completely infarcted (18–24). Some of the regional wall motion abnormality is usually caused by persisting chronic and repeated hypoxia, making the collateralized region an excellent candidate for revascularization, even in the absence of symptoms. However, when the occlusion occurred consecutively to plaque rupture in a large vessel with only mild, preexisting stenosis without collaterals, complete functional loss occurs. In such a situation revascularization is unlikely to improve the patient's situation.

A further reason why the presence of collaterals may be helpful to decide whether a occluded artery should be recanalized is the potential for reversed collateral flow from the recanalized artery to the artery supplying the initial collateral flow. This may be the rationale for recanalizing an occluded right coronary artery before dilating a significant stenosis of the left anterior descending coronary artery providing collaterals to the right coronary artery. The risk of an acute occlusion of the left anterior descending coronary artery will be much lower if sufficient collateral flow has been secured through the recanalized right coronary artery.

In multivessel disease the intricacy of recanalizing a chronic occlusion should be considered. Two chronic occlusions may be too time consuming with a few exceptions. A single additional nontotal lesion appears to be reasonable for a single session. If the vessel with the additional lesion provides collaterals to the occluded vessel, the recanalization should be done first and one should only proceed with the second vessel if the dilated vessel is reliably patent. Occasionally, patients with a chronic occlusion of the right coronary artery are accepted for angioplasty of the left anterior descending or the left circumflex coronary artery disregarding the occluded vessel (25–27). Although published results of pertinent series are acceptable, the increased risk of such interventions (particularly those on the left anterior descending coronary artery) has to be underscored.

Angiographic Criteria

Balloon recanalization attempts of chronic total coronary occlusions are more likely to be successful if a vessel stump is visible. With an occlusion that is flush at the orifice of the vessel or tapering into a small side branch, there is nowhere to probe for the occluded lumen.

Short lesions have a better prognosis than long ones. The longer the occluded segment, the more difficult it is to cross the lesion.

The presence of bridging collaterals from the proximal segment to the segment distal to a total occlusion is a strong predictor of an unsuccessful recanalization attempt (Fig. 24B.1). They should be considered as markers of old occlusions with minimal chances to cross.

RESULTS

Acute Results

Compared with angioplasty of nonoccluded coronary arteries, recanalization carries a lower risk of major complications, but is limited by lower success rates and at least equally high or higher recurrences rates.

Reported success rates range from 42% to 72% (3, 8, 9, 11, 16, 28, 29–41) with a mean of 68% in about 3000 pooled patients. Some

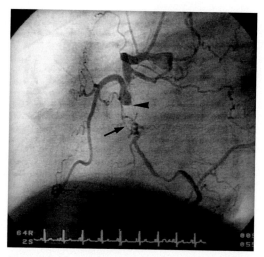

Figure 24B.1. Bridging collaterals in an old occlusion of the right coronary artery. The arrowhead indicates the site of occlusion. Tortuous but well-developed "bridging" collaterals *(arrow)* provide complete and prompt filling of the distal artery with contrast medium.

recent reports with better results can only partially be ascribed to a learning curve, since most of them include functional occlusions that are associated with a higher technical success (3, 9, 37). In fact, improvements resulting from a learning curve seem to occur with single-operator experience (40) but not in institutions with several operators (3), probably because large volume centers tend to treat more complex cases.

Predictors for Success

Most studies describe duration of occlusion as a key factor for success.[a] The chance of success seems to decline rapidly during the first 4 weeks after the occlusion (33). Success rates of 0% (36), 11% (9), and 55% (34), respectively, have been documented in three studies looking at occlusions presumed older than 6 months. For this reason recanalization of occlusions older than 6 months should be attempted only if the lesion has an angiographically favorable aspect and if there is a strong clinical indication.

---

[a] References 11, 16, 28, 29–34, 36, 38, 40, 41.

The length of the occlusion is the next important factor for success, although it has been less well documented in retrospective studies. The prognostic importance of occlusion length has been established in two reports (28, 40), but it is a matter of common sense and of experience that long occlusions are technically more difficult and yield a high risk for subintimnal passage of the guidewire. The presence of a stump or tapered segment as an entry port is another favorable criteria (9, 40), since it helps to find the true lumen. The negative influence of bridging collaterals has been explained above (40). Chronically occluded venous bypass grafts are usually considered to be associated with low short- and long-term success rates, but only anecdotal information is available (42–46). Some authors recommend the use of adjuvant intracoronary thrombolytics for recanalization of occluded vein grafts (44–46). Successful recanalization of a chronically occluded internal mammary artery bypass graft has also been described (47). It should have long-term results comparable to those in a native coronary artery.

Complications

MORTALITY

The acute risk of recanalization consists less in the consequences of acute reocclusion of the coronary artery, since the involved myocardial area is usually protected by collaterals, than in the instrumentation of proximal coronary arteries, especially the left main stem. Lethal outcome after recanalization has been reported for the first time only in 1990 (37). Looking at nine reports with a total of about 3000 patients (9, 16, 28, 29, 33, 35, 37, 41), we found a mean in-hospital mortality of 1%, with figures ranging from 0 to 2%.

Dissection of a coronary ostium, occlusion of a side branch proximal to the target occlusion, immobilization of retracted thrombi, or air injection might all occur in a procedure that is often considered to be an easy case. There is also a theoretical risk of tamponade secondary to a vessel perforation or rupture, but so far the reported cases of coronary perforation all had a benign course (48, 49). The exact incidence of major complications with recanalization procedures is unclear. Some authors report surprisingly high mortality rates with occlusion angioplasty, but a close look at the details shows that not all deaths were directly related to the recanalization attempts. Plante et al. (50) report a 20% incidence of serious complications in a group of 46 unstable patients, but in fact only two of them were clearly attributable to the recanalization attempt itself. The group of Kaltenbach reports three cases with fatal complications after recanalization (51), but two of them were caused by arrhythmia while the opened artery was patent at necropsy. A third patient died in cardiogenic shock, but had an open vessel at control angiography before death. In another report (52) they describe a case of sudden death five days after successful recanalization using the low-speed rotational atherectomy device. In this case the autopsy revealed thrombotic occlusion of the attempted segment.

In the Geneva experience of 500 occlusion angioplasties, 10 deaths occurred (41). Four patients died after a recanalization attempt in the setting of cardiogenic shock. In two patients, a left main-stem dissection occurred necessitating emergency surgery that had a fatal outcome. Two patients died suddenly before discharge. One patient died from anaphylactic shock after protamine injection (53) and one from septicemia. In summary, serious complications are rare with recanalization of occluded arteries since acute occlusion has usually no consequences, but one should remember that serious accidents related to coronary manipulation do occur even under these circumstances.

NEED FOR EMERGENCY SURGERY

Since recanalization angioplasty concerns myocardial tissue almost always supplied by collaterals, emergency surgery should hardly ever be necessary. In fact, the only indications for emergency bypass surgery are an occlusion of an important vessel proximal to the occlusion, damage to a left main, or a significant deterioration of collateral inflow into the vessel to be recanalized. The need for emergency bypass surgery is indicated between 0% and 4% and is less than 1% on the average. The five emergency operations of the Geneva series (1%) (41) became necessary because of left main dissection (2), aortic dissection (1) (54), or extensive damage to the distal vessel hampering collateral inflow (2).

INFARCTION

Acute reocclusion of a chronically occluded vessel should not cause a significant infarction. In fact, no reported Q-wave infarct has so far been unequivocally attributed to reclosure of a recanalized coronary artery, although some groups reported infarction rates as high as 18% (16). In the Geneva experience, five Q-wave infarctions occurred (1%) (41). Three were caused by occlusion of a proximal vessel and two by angioplasty of additional sites. Mild elevation of the CK were more frequent, indicating that subendocardial infarctions can occur.

Distal embolization represents another occasional and mostly bland complication of recanalization attempts that may cause a limited infarction. It was described in 10% of successful procedures in a study paying particular attention to such incidents (28). There were no clinical sequelae in these patients.

EXTENSIVE DISSECTION

Creation of a subintimal channel during the attempt to pass the occlusion is a frequent event that cannot be predicted or avoided. It usually has no consequences clinically since the intraluminal pressure caused by collaterals will promptly paste the flap back to the wall. In rare cases such a dissection has been documented to significantly impair collateral flow to the distal part of the artery

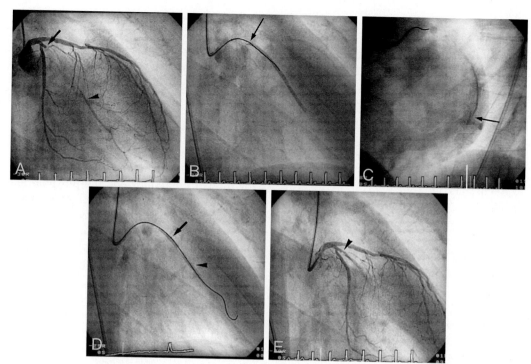

Figure 24B.2. Unsuccessful recanalization attempt of a totally occluded marginal branch of the left circumflex coronary artery. Demonstration of subintimal passage of the guidewire. **A.** Preintervention angiogram (right anterior oblique view). The stump of the proximal marginal branch of the left circumflex coronary artery *(arrow)* is shown. The distal part of the coronary artery is partially filled through collaterals from the distal circumflex and the left anterior descending coronary artery *(arrowhead)*. **B.** The occlusion could not be crossed with a 0.021-inch (0.53-mm) Magnum wire (Schneider), therefore a Magnum wire without ball-tip was tried. The wire crossed the occluded site, but opacification of a long dissection pouch suggested subintimal passage of the wire (arrow points to the subintimal entry). **C.** This left anterior oblique view demonstrates contrast medium flowing from the dissection pouch into the true lumen (arrow points to the reentry site). **D.** A 2.5-mm Magnarail balloon catheter (Schneider) was advanced to the site of occlusion and inflated *(arrow)*. The compression of the inner lumen of the balloon catheter causes some contrast medium to flow distally, staining the dissection area *(arrowhead)*. **E.** Despite several attempts to tack up the dissection flap by multiple inflations, immediate reocclusion occurred after retrieval of the guidewire. The marginal branch was less well filled with contrast, probably because of compression of collateral flow by the dissection. There were no signs of ischemia.

(41). Once such a false lumen has been created, the guidewire will almost invariably return into the dissection channel and a successful angioplasty becomes virtually impossible, even with a special device like a Magnum wire (Fig. 24B.2). Occasionally the true lumen can be reentered more distally and the layer between the true and the false lumen split with a balloon inflation, but usually the procedure has to be stopped at that point, since further manipulations will only increase the risk of damaging proximal parts of the vessel.

Recurrence

Recurrence (angiographically documented restenosis or reocclusion) is more frequent after successful recanalization of total occlusions than after angioplasty of nonoccluded arteries (35). We found recurrence rates ranging from 43 to 77%, average 64%, in a compilation of six reports (9, 16, 28, 29, 33, 35, 37, 41) describing the long-term angiographic outcome of roughly 1500 patients. This is twice as high as the average restenosis rate of 28% reported in a compiled cohort of almost 10,000 cumulated patients from a variety of reports with coronary angioplasty for mixed indications (55). It has to be emphasized that complete reocclusions of recanalized lesions occur only in an average of 18%, the remaining 46% being restenoses. Nonoccluded arteries with significant restenosis after recanalization can usually be redilated with high success rates and few complications, since they still benefit from the protection of collaterals on standby (56, 57).

Recurrence rates are likely to be overestimated. Since a routine control angiogram is unlikely to be done in patients who had few symptoms and a low-risk situation before angiography, only patients with marked recurrent ischemia will be restudied. Low restudy rates introduce a bias toward the unfavorable outcome, since restenosis or reocclusion is much more likely to occur in symptomatic patients. Moreover, in as many as 10% of all patients significant restenosis or reocclusion caused by dissection, thrombus, or elastic recoil might occur in the hours following recanalization; these should be regarded as unsuccessful procedures rather than restenosis. In many patients, however, these early recurrences will be detected only at the time of angiographic restudy and classified as restenosis or late reocclusions.

Finally, recurrence leading to a second angioplasty does not mean that the patient's quality of life was not improved. Long-term improvement, including repeat angioplasty, can be found in 60 to 80% of all patients treated successfully (9, 16, 28, 29, 33, 37).

PREDICTORS OF RECURRENCE

A number of factors unfavorably influencing outcome after recanalization can be identified. Suboptimal results are more likely to result in restenosis after recanalization than after angioplasty of nonoccluded arteries, because of the mechanism of angioplasty, as well as the fact that behind the occlusion one often finds a complex and long lesion associated with fresh and active thrombosis. This decreases the effective residual luminal di-

ameter, which in turn favors restenosis (9, 35, 58).

The competitive pressure exerted by collaterals increases the risk for restenosis. Collateral flow is likely to reduce the driving pressure across the dilated stenosis even after successful recanalization. The decrease of flow might favor parietal thrombosis and restenosis.

Recent occlusions and occlusions affecting the left circumflex and the proximal left anterior descending coronary artery have been reported to have a higher restenosis risk (49). Conversely, restenosis seems to be less frequent with lesions of the right coronary artery in clinically stable patients with single-vessel disease (39).

There is no difference in the timing of restenosis between angioplasty of occluded and nonoccluded arteries. With the exception of subacute reocclusions, which more often go clinically unrecognized than that of nonoccluded arteries, restenosis occurs within the first 6 months. The mechanisms to be held responsible are smooth muscle cell proliferation (59, 60) on top of organized thrombi (61) and, exceptionally, additional plaque formation (62). Since these mechanisms take time, significant restenoses are rare within the first month provided good initial patency.

MANAGEMENT OF RECURRENCE

Although restenosis and reocclusion are usually benign clinical events in the case of previously occluded coronary arteries, recurrence of symptoms or significant ischemia requires further interventions such as repeat angioplasty and bypass surgery in a number of patients. In fact, reinterventions are performed in up to 30% of patients after successful recanalization, compared with about 20% after angioplasty of nonoccluded arteries (34).

While bypass surgery is often chosen after a failed attempt to recanalize an occluded artery, especially if other major coronary arteries are diseased, recurrence is more often managed with reangioplasty or medical treatment. There is a general consensus that nonoccluded but restenosed arteries should be treated by repeat angioplasty and that they have an excellent chance to remain patent. The policy for recurrence of complete occlusion depends on the angiographic aspect and the importance of the concerned myocardial area. Since a second recanalization may be more difficult than the first one and carries a substantial risk of further reocclusion, it should be done only if the reocclusion is short and has a favorable pattern and if there is a clear clinical indication for a second attempt. Otherwise, either medical treatment or bypass surgery should be recommended.

TECHNICAL ASPECTS

Material Selection

The choice of material differs widely worldwide when it comes to performing total occlusion angioplasty. Conventional angioplasty material, devices developed specifically for recanalization procedures, and so-called alternative devices have been used with variable success.

Many operators use conventional over-the-wire systems, usually avoiding the highly flexible, "high-torque floppy" guidewires commonly used in nontotal occlusion angioplasty (28, 63–65). Splinting or stabilizing the tip of the guidewire by either the balloon catheter itself or a single-lumen catheter (e.g., perfusion or probing catheter (66, 67)) is often used to optimize axial push and torque transmission. Monorail systems (68) are chosen because of the easy exchange process, but with the the guidewire cannot be exchanged. Fixed-wire systems have been reported to be efficient in total occlusions, such as the Probe catheter (USCI), which can be stabilized by a probing catheter, or the Omniflex catheter (Medtronic), whose sturdy guidewire tip provides better axial push transmission than most other fixed-wire systems (64).

Other operators rely on systems specially developed for recanalization of totally occluded arteries, like the Magnum or the ROTAC systems described below. Alternative transluminal techniques (new devices) have so far failed to improve success rates or long-term results in occlusion angioplasty, most often because they need a guidewire to be inserted before the specific technology can be applied to the diseased site.

Angioplasty Technique

Before attempting a recanalization, the operator has to carefully scrutinize the diagnostic angiogram, with special attention to length of the occlusion and anatomy of the distal vessel. One should also be aware of any particular aspect of the proximal segments at risk for damage during manipulation of the guiding catheter or angioplasty material. Injections of contrast medium into the donor vessel during the recanalization attempt may be useful, but require a second arterial access in case of contralateral collaterals (69, 70).

Guiding-catheter position and backup stability are crucial in occlusion angioplasty, since more push has to be applied on the guidewire than in nontotal lesion angioplasty to cross the diseased segment. There is the choice between large, stiff catheters, which might be stable but potentially dangerous for the coronary ostium during extensive manipulation, and softer, low-profile catheters, which have to be stabilized by deep intubation into the proximal arterial segment but are less likely to cause ostial dissection. In our laboratory routine occlusion angioplasty is done with a Magnum system through a soft-tip, 7 Fr catheter (Pink Power, Schneider), while nonocclusion angioplasty is more often performed through 5 or 6 Fr catheters.

There is no special technique to cross an occluded arterial segment or to avoid subintimal passage of the guidewire. The J-tipped guidewire should gently probe the occlusion site to find the spot of least resistance, theoretically the site of recent thrombosis. Once the occlusion has been crossed, the guidewire should freely progress down the distal part of the coronary artery. If not, subintimal passage or position in a small side branch should be suspected, the guidewire pulled back, and the crossing procedure repeated. The balloon catheter or the probing catheter is then advanced into the stenosis. A contrast injection should be done very carefully to avoid worsening of the dissection if the injection is subintimal, either through the balloon catheter lumen or through the guiding catheter if a Monorail system is used to confirm the position in the correct lumen. If the distal lumen cannot be shown, the balloon should not be inflated because its position is probably incorrect.

In case of a dissection despite correct position of the guidewire, an attempt can be done to stabilize the dissecting flap by inflating the balloon more distally until the false lumen is tacked up. One of the problems with this technique is that the distal lumen is often smaller and thus the balloon oversized, creating new extensive dissection in a previously healthy segment.

After successful recanalization it is usually worth waiting for 5 minutes to make sure the result is stable, as a dissection may look harmless during the first minutes but cause reocclusion shortly thereafter. Another useful functional assessment of the recanalization procedure is to check disappearance of collaterals. Persistence of collaterals can indicate early failure or poor result with a high risk of early reocclusion. The demonstration of the disappearance of collaterals is more difficult in case of ipsilateral collaterals. In this case a good result can be assumed if the contrast meets precisely in the midportion of a previously collateral vessel (watershed phenomenon).

SPECIAL DEVICES AND OCCLUSION ANGIOPLASTY

Besides conventional balloon angioplasty equipment, specially designed devices and so-called alternative technologies have been used to recanalize chronically occluded coronary arteries.

Hydrophilic Wire

The glidewire (Terumo) minimizes friction forces thanks to its hydrophilic coating and is well suited to pass tortuous and tightly stenosed segments in peripheral arteries. The coronary version of the Terumo wire has been reported to be efficient to cross total coronary artery occlusions, but there are no comparative data available (71, 72).

Open-Ended Wire

Vassanelli et al. have described the successful use of a guidewire with a removable core that allows adjustments in stiffness and contrast medium injections (73).

Magnum Wire

In patients with completely occluded coronary arteries, without antegrade flow and not associated with acute myocardial infarction, primary success of recanalization angioplasty can be increased by 10 to 20% using a Magnum wire compared with conventional systems (65, 74, 75).

The Magnum wire combines a solid steel wire shaft of 0.021 inch (0.53 mm), a flexible distal coiled tip, and an olive-shaped ball tip of 1 mm diameter. It was initially designed for balloon recanalization of chronic total coronary occlusions (63, 65), but has since proved useful for routine coronary angioplasty as well (76). For recanalization angioplasty, the Magnum wire provides an excellent pushability and the advantage of the blunted, larger ball tip, which prevents to some extent from passing the wire tip under a plaque. In routine angioplasty the ball tip quite easily tracks along diffusely diseased distal arteries and the solid steel core provides a highly stable backup to advance the balloon catheter.

Because of the larger profile of the Magnum wire, balloon catheters with a larger inner lumen like the Magnum, Magnarail, or Magnarail-Speedy catheters, available with inflated diameters ranging from 2 to 6 mm, have to be used. The Magnarail system combines the advantage of the Magnum wire and the Monorail system (65), namely, the easy and rapid exchange of balloon catheters, and the possibility of faked distal injection through the short wire lumen. Magnum systems can be introduced through any 7 Fr or larger coronary guiding catheter.

RECANALIZATION TECHNIQUE WITH A MAGNUM SYSTEM (FIG. 3)

In contrast with conventional angioplasty, a firm push is necessary to cross a tight lesion with a Magnum system. Guiding catheter

backup is important, and one should choose a catheter allowing for deep intubation to obtain a stable position. In our laboratory Amplatz left catheters are often chosen to attempt a recanalization of the left circumflex or the right coronary arteries with a Magnum wire, since conventional Judkins shapes may offer unsufficient backup. With soft-tip guiding catheters advancement of the guiding catheter over the balloon catheter placed in the distal coronary artery allows for safe and atraumatic deep intubation. Figure 24B.3

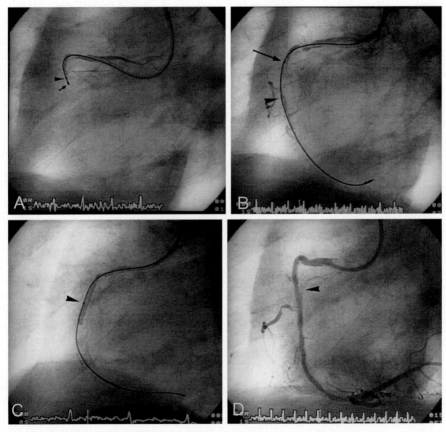

Figure 24B.3.   Recanalization of a chronic total occlusion of the proximal portion of a right coronary artery using a Magnum wire splinted by a probing catheter (Schneider). **A.** The right coronary artery ostium has been intubated with a 7 Fr Amplatz left II guiding catheter (Schneider). A 0.021-inch (0.53-mm) Magnum guidewire (arrow points to the ball tip) is placed in the stump of the occluded proximal artery. A probing catheter (tip marker indicated by arrowhead) is advanced to the tip of the Magnum guidewire to improve axial push strength. **B.** The occlusion has been passed with the guidewire. The probing catheter has been advanced into the occlusion site (tip marker indicated by arrow). Injection of contrast medium through the guiding catheter allows faint opacification of a distal lumen and side branches, confirming that the wire is in the correct lumen. The dye passes through the short Monorail guidewire lumen (faked distal injection). **C.** Dilatation of the right coronary occlusion with a 3.0-mm Magnarail balloon (Schneider). The midballoon marker is shown by an arrowhead. **D.** Final injection showing a widely patent lumen despite some wall irregularities *(arrowhead)* at the site of occlusion, probably caused by local dissection.

illustrates the major steps for recanalization of a chronic occlusion with a Magnum system. Magnum wires are available with pre-shaped J tips, or straight tips to be custom shaped with the fingertip or an instrument. Reaching the occlusion is rarely a problem since the Magnum wire provides superb steerability.

In the majority of the cases, splinting of the distal flexible portion by a catheter is necessary to obtain an optimal push and to be able to cross the occlusion. This can be obtained either with the balloon catheter, preferably a Monorail type, or a cheaper single-lumen probing catheter (65). Use of such a probing catheter can be reasonable for economic reasons if the lesion does not look promising, but its cost will add to the cost of the balloon catheter in case of successful angioplasty. Using a catheter just at the tip of the wire also provides the possibility to inject contrast medium distally to check the correct position of the ball tip either in the occlusion stump or in the distal lumen once the occlusion has been crossed. For these reasons, it is a waste of time to try to pass an occlusion only with a bare wire and inadequate to give up without having reinforced the distal part of the Magnum wire with a catheter.

Although the blunted ball tip of the Magnum wire offers some protection against subintimal passage, once such a false channel is created, the Magnum wire will readily reenter the false channel and worsen the dissection. In such a situation, changing to a conventional wire may allow one to find the correct lumen. Conversely, the Magnum wire may find the right way through an occlusive dissection created by a conventional wire.

The Magnum wire is not difficult to use but requires some caution. Its stiffness is attractive because it provides pushability and tracking stability, but is also potentially dangerous if inadequately pushed against a protruding plaque or onto the wall of an ostial segment. The 1-mm ball tip sometimes renders the assessment of the distal runoff diffi-cult. It is almost never a problem to pull the wire back to do a contrast medium injection and to readvance it afterwards, since the ball tip will follow the largest lumen and impact gently on the vessel wall. Exchange of the wire is not possible with the Magnum wire, as it is not possible with any Monorail equipment, but the Magnum wire is very resistant to kinking and need for exchange is quite rare. Another potential disadvantage of the Magnum system is the somewhat large profile of the deflated balloon catheters, which is compensated by the superior trackability of the system. In fact, it is seldom a problem to pass the lesion with the correctly sized balloon without predilatation once the Magnum wire is correctly positioned. If necessary, exchange of the balloon catheter is rapidly and easily done over the strong and stable guidewire. Nylon balloons (Magnarail-Speedy) offer the sleekest profile.

SUMMARY

Chronic total occlusion of a coronary artery is a common finding in patients undergoing coronary angiography for a variety of indications. If the expected benefits are reasonably clear in patients with clinical or demonstrable ischemia, the potential benefit derived from a recanalization is less evident in asymptomatic patients. The probability of further progression of the atherosclerotic disease is clearly higher in these patients than in the general population. In at least part of these patients, protection through collaterals of areas threatened in the future seems to constitute an good reason to attempt recanalization in a large vessel with well-developed collaterals. On the other hand, the low primary success numbers, the high recurrence rate, and the overall modest clinical improvement warrant moderation on the side of the interventional cardiologist. Occlusion angioplasty should remain cost-effective and of low risk. Sophisticated and expensive alternative technologies have so far found no justification in routine recanalization, but further development and research of more effective strategies are important. Conventional equipment is easier and faster to handle and finally not less effective, although, even with conventional means, occlusion angioplasty consumes more time, radiation, and material than angioplasty of nonoccluded coronary arteries (77). The Magnum wire together with a Monorail type catheter is easy to use and relatively cheap, especially if compared with the use of several conventional wires. It has proved to be superior to conventional systems in a randomized study. It is the first choice system for recanalization in our view.

Finally, the risk of occlusion angioplasty should not be underestimated, and recanalization procedures should not be left to beginners. As with all therapies applied to patients with no or few symptoms and a low vital risk, the "primum non nocere" remains an important dogma to be remembered before starting a recanalization attempt.

REFERENCES

1. Meier B. Chronic total coronary occlusion angioplasty. Cathet Cardiovasc Diagn 1989;17:212–217.

2. Detre K, Holubkov R, Kelsey S, Cowley M, Kent W, Williams D, Myler R et al., and the co-investigators of the National Heart, Lung, and Blood Institute's Percutaneous Transluminal Coronary Angioplasty Registry: Percutaneous transluminal coronary angioplasty in 1985–1986 and 1977–1981. The Heart Lung, and Blood Institute Registry. N Engl J Med 1988;318:265–270.

3. Bell MR, Berger PB, Bresnahan JF, Reeder GS, Bailey KR, Holmes DR Jr. Initial and long-term outcome of 354 patients following coronary balloon angioplasty of total coronary artery occlusions. Circulation 1992;85:1003–1011.

4. Dick RJL, Haudenschild CC, Popma JJ, Ellis SG, Muller DW, Topol EJ. Directional atherectomy for total coronary occlusions. Coronary Artery Dis 1991;2:189–199.

5. Meyer J, Merx W, Schmitz H, Erbel R, Kiesslich T, Dörr R, Lambertz H et al. Percutaneous transluminal coronary angioplasty after intracoronary streptokinase in evolving

6. Melchior JP, Doriot PA, Chatelain P, Meier B, Urban P, Finci L, Rutishauser W. Improvement of left ventricular contraction and relaxation synchronism after recanalization of chronic total coronary occlusion by angioplasty. J Am Coll Cardiol 1987;4:763–768.

7. Singh A, Murray RG, Chandler S, Shiu MF. Myocardial salvage following elective angioplasty for total coronary occlusion. Cardiology 1987;74:474–478.

8. Finci L, Meier B, Righetti A, Rutishauser W. Long-term results of successful and failed angioplasty for chronic total coronary arterial occlusion. Am J Cardiol 1990; 66:660–662.

9. Ivanhoe RJ, Weintraub WS, Douglas JS Jr, Lembo NJ, Furman M, Gershony G, Cohen CL et al. Percutaneous transluminal coronary angioplasty of chronic total occlusions: primary success, restenosis, and long-term clinical follow-up. Circulation 1992;85:106–115.

10. Warren RJ, Black AJ, Valentine PA, Manolas EG, Hunt D. Coronary angioplasty for chronic total occlusion reduces the need for subsequent coronary bypass surgery. Am Heart J 1990;120:270–274.

11. Melchior JP, Meier B, Urban P, Finci L, Steffenino G, Noble J, Rutishauser W. Percutaneous transluminal coronary angioplasty for chronic total coronary arterial occlusions. Am J Cardiol 1987;59:535–538.

12. Flameng W, Schwartz F, Hehrlein FW. Intraoperative evaluation of the functional significance of coronary collateral vessels in patients with coronary artery disease. Am J Cardiol 1978;42:187–192.

13. Braunwald E, Kloner RA. The stunned myocardium: prolonged, postischemic ventricular dysfunction. Circulation 1982;66:1146–1149.

14. Rahimtoola SH. The hibernating myocardium. Am Heart J 1989;117:211–221.

15. Vogel WM, Apstein CS, Briggs LL, Gaasch WH, Ahn J. Acute alterations in left ventricular diastolic chamber stiffness. Role of the "erectile" effect of coronary arterial pressure and flow in normal and damaged hearts. Circ Res 1982;51:465–478.

16. Serruys PW, Umans V, Heyndrickx GR, van den Brand M, de Feyter PJ, Wijns W, Jaski B et al. Elective PTCA of totally occluded coronary arteries not associated with acute myocardial infarction: short-term and long-term results. Eur Heart J 1985;6:2–12.

17. Roberts WC, Virmani R. Formation of new coronary arteries within a previously obstructed epicardial coronary artery (intraarterial arteries): a mechanism for occurrence of angiographically normal coronary arteries after healing of acute myocardial infarction. Am J Cardiol 1984; 54:1361–1362.

18. Schwartz F, Flameng W, Ensslen R, Sesto M, Thorman J. Effect of coronary collaterals on left ventricular function at rest and during stress. Am Heart J 1978;95:570–577.

19. Hamby RI, Antablian A, Schwartz A. Reappraisal of the functional significance of the coronary circulation. Am J Cardiol 1976;38:305–309.

20. Rogers WJ, Hood WP, Mantle JA, Baxley WA, Kirklin JK, Zorn GL, Nath HP. Return of left ventricular function after reperfusion in patients with myocardial infarction: importance of subtotal stenoses or intact collaterals. Circulation 1984;69:338–349.

21. Saito Y, Yasuno M, Ishida M, Suzuki K, Matoba Y, Emura M, Takahashi M. Importance of collaterals for restoration of left ventricular function after intracoronary thrombolysis. Am J Cardiol 1985;55:1259–1263.

22. Nitzberg WD, Nath HP, Rogers WJ, Hood WP, Whitlow PL, Reeves R, Baxley WA. Collateral flow in patients with acute myocardial infarction. Am J Cardiol 1985;56:729–736.

23. Schwartz H, Leiboff RH, Bren GB, Wasserman AG, Katz RJ, Varghese PJ, Sokil AB et al. Temporal evolution of the human coronary circulation after myocardial infarction. J Am Coll Cardiol 1984;4:1088–1093.

24. Cohen M, Rentrop KP. Limitation of myocardial ischemia by collateral circulation during sudden controlled coronary artery occlusion in human subjects: a prospective study. Circulation 1986;74:469–476.

25. Teirstein P, Giorgi L, Johnson W, McConahay D, Rutherford

B, Hartzler G. PTCA of the left coronary artery when the right coronary artery is chronically occluded. Am Heart J 1990;119:479–483.

26. De Bruyne B, Renkin J, Col J, Wijns W. Percutaneous transluminal coronary angioplasty of the left coronary artery in patients with chronic occlusion of the right coronary artery. Am Heart J 1991;122:415–422.

27. Buffet P, Danchin N, Marc MO, Feldmann L, Juillere Y, Anconina J, Selton-Suty C et al. Results of percutaneous transluminal coronary angioplasty of either the left anterior descending or left circumflex coronary artery in patients with chronic total occlusion of the right coronary artery. Am J Cardiol 1993;71:382–385.

28. Kereiakes DJ, Selmon MR, McAuley BJ, McAuley DB, Sheehan DJ, Simpson JB. Angioplasty in total coronary artery occlusion: experience in 76 consecutive patients. J Am Coll Cardiol 1985;6:526–533.

29. Dervan JP, Baim DS, Cherniles J, Grossman W. Transluminal angioplasty of occluded coronary arteries: use of a movable guidewire system. Circulation 1983;68:776–784.

30. Holmes DR Jr, Vlietstra RE, Reeder GS, Breshnahan JF, Smith HC, Bove AA, Schaff HV. Angioplasty in total coronary artery occlusion. J Am Coll Cardiol 1984;3:845–849.

31. Holmes DR Jr, Vlietstra RE. Angioplasty in total coronary arterial occlusion. Herz 1985;10:292–297.

32. Kober G, Hopf R, Reinemer H, Kaltenbach M. Langzeitergebnisse der transluminalen koronaren Angioplastie von chronischen Herzkranzgefässverschlüssen. Z Kardiol 1985;74:309–316.

33. DiSciascio G, Vetrovec GW, Cowley MJ, Wolfgang TC. Early and late outcome of percutaneous transluminal coronary angioplasty of subacute and chronic total coronary occlusion. Am Heart J 1986;111:833–839.

34. Safian RD, McCabe CH, Sipperly ME, McKay RG, Baim DS. Initial success and long-term follow-up of percutaneous transluminal coronary angioplasty in chronic total occlusions versus conventional stenoses. Am J Cardiol 1988;61:23G–28G.

35. Ellis SG, Shaw RE, Gershony G, Thomas R, Roubin GS, Douglas JS, Topol EJ et al. Risk factors, time course and treatment effect for restenosis after successful percutaneous transluminal coronary angioplasty of chronic total occlusion. Am J Cardiol 1989;63:897–901.

36. LaVeau PJ, Remetz MS, Cabin HS, Hennecken JF, McConnell SH, Rosen RE, Cleman MW. Predictors of success in percutaneous transluminal coronary angioplasty of chronic total occlusions. Am J Cardiol 1989;64:1264–1269.

37. Stone GW, Rutherford BD, McConahay DR, Johnson WL Jr, Giorgi LV, Ligon RW, Hartzler GO. Procedural outcome of angioplasty for total coronary artery occlusion: an analysis of 971 lesions in 905 patients. J Am Coll Cardiol 1990;15:849–856.

38. Jost S, Nolte CWT, Simon R et al. Angioplasty of subacute and chronic total coronary occlusions: success, recurrence rate, and clinical follow-up. Am Heart J 1991;122:1509–1514.

39. Ruocco NA, Ring ME, Holubkov R, Jacobs AK, Detre KM, Faxon DP, and the co-investigators of the National Heart, Lung, and Blood Institute Percutaneous Transluminal Coronary Angioplasty Registry. Results of coronary angio-

plasty of chronic total occlusions (the National Heart, Lung, and Blood Institute 1985–1986 Percutaneous Transluminal Coronary Angioplasty Registry). Am J Cardiol 1992; 69:69–76.

40. Maiello L, Colombo A, Gianrossi R, Mutinelli MR, Bouzon R, Thomas J, Finci L. Coronary angioplasty of chronic occlusions: factors predictive of procedural success. Am Heart J 1992;124:581–584.

41. Haine E, Urban P, Dorsaz PA, Meier B. Outcome and complications of 500 consecutive chronic total occlusion angioplasties. J Am Coll Cardiol 1993;21:138A (abstract).

42. De Feyter PJ, Serruys P, van den Brand M, Meester H, Beatt K, Suryapranata H. Percutaneous transluminal angioplasty of a totally occluded venous bypass graft: a challenge that should be resisted. Am J Cardiol 1989; 64:88–90.

43. Finci L, Meier B, Steffenino GD. Percutaneous angioplasty of totally occluded saphenous aortocoronary bypass graft. Int J Cardiol 1986;10:76–79.

44. Sievert H, Köhler KP, Kaltenbach M, Kober G. Re-opening long-segment occlusions of aorto-coronary vein bypasses: short and long-term results. Dtsch Med Wochenschr 1988;113:637–640.

45. Hartmann J, McKeever L, Teran J, Bufalino V, Marek J, Brown A, Goodwin M et al. Prolonged infusion of urokinase for recanalization of chronically occluded aortocoronary bypass grafts. Am J Cardiol 1988;61:189–191.

46. Marx M, Armstrong WP, Wack JP, Bernstein RM, Brent B, Francoz R, Gregoratos G. Short-duration, high-dose urokinase for recanalization of occluded saphenous aortocoronary bypass grafts. AJR 1989;153:167–171.

47. Mehan VK, Meier B, Urban P. Balloon recanalisation of a chronically occluded left internal mammary artery graft. Br Heart J 1993;70:195–197.

48. Meier B. Benign coronary perforation during percutaneous transluminal coronary angioplasty. Br Heart J 1985; 54:33–35.

49. Meier B. Total occlusion. In Faxon DP, ed. Practical angioplasty. New York. Raven Press, 1993.

50. Plante S, Laarman GJ, de Feyter PJ, Samson M, Rensing BJ, Umans V, Suryapranata H et al. Acute complications of percutaneous transluminal coronary angioplasty for total occlusion. Am Heart J 1991;121:417–426.

51. Burger W, Kadel C, Keul HG, Vallbracht C, Kaltenbach M. A word of caution: reopening chronic coronary occlusions. Cathet Cardiovasc Diagn 1992;27:35–39.

52. Kaltenbach M, Hartmann A, Vallbracht C. Procedural results and patient selection in recanalization of chronic coronary occlusion by low-speed rotational angioplasty. Eur Heart J 1993;14:826–830.

53. Neidhart PP, Meier B, Polla BS, Schifferli JA, Morel DR. Fatal anaphylactoid response to protamine after percutaneous transluminal coronary angioplasty. Eur Heart J 1992;13:856–858.

54. Moles VP, Chappuis F, Simonet F, Urban P, de la Serna F, Pande AK, Meier B. Aortic dissection as complication of percutaneous transluminal coronary angioplasty. Cathet Cardiovasc Diagn 1992;26:8–11.

55. Meier B. Restenosis after coronary angioplasty: review of the literature. Eur Heart J 1988;9(Suppl C):1–6.

56. Carlier M, Finci L, Meier B. Coronary collateral flow reversal. Heart Vessels 1991;6:112–115.

57. Moles VP, Meier B, Urban P, Pande AK. Instantaneous recruitment of reversed coronary collaterals that had been dormant for six years. Cathet Cardiovasc Diagn 1992; 26:148–151.

58. Ellis SG, Shaw RE, King SB III, Myler RK, Topol EJ. Restenosis after excellent angiographic result for chronic total coronary artery occlusion—implications for newer percutaneous revascularization devices. Am J Cardiol 1989;64:667–668.

59. Austin GE, Ratliff NB, Hollman J, Tabei J, Phillips DF. Intimal proliferation of smooth muscle cells as an explanation for recurrent coronary artery stenosis after percutaneous transluminal coronary angioplasty. J Am Coll Cardiol 1985;6:369–375.

60. Essed CE, van den Brand M, Becker AE. Transluminal coronary angioplasty and early restenosis. Fibrocellular occlusion after wall laceration. Br Heart J 1983; 49:393–396.

61. Steele PM, Chesebro JH, Stanson AW, Holmes DR Jr, Dewanjee MK, Badimon L, Fuster V. Balloon angioplasty. Natural history of the pathophysiological response to injury in a pig model. Circ Res 1985;57:105–112.

62. Waller BF, McManus BM, Gorfinkel J, Kishel JC, Schmidt ECH, Kent KM, Roberts WC. Status of major epicardial coronary arteries 80 to 150 days after percutaneous transluminal coronary angioplasty. Analysis of 3 necropsy patients. Am J Cardiol 1983;51:81–84.

63. Meier B, Carlier M, Finci L, Nukta E, Urban P, Niederhauser W, Favre J. Magnum wire for balloon recanalization of chronic total coronary occlusions. Am J Cardiol 1989; 64:148–154.

64. Hamm CW, Kupper W, Kuck KH, Hofmann D, Bleifeld W. Recanalization of chronic, totally occluded coronary arteries by new angioplasty systems. Am J Cardiol 1990;66:1459–1463.

65. Pande AK, Meier B, Urban P, de la Serna F, Villavicencio R, Dorsaz PA, Favre J. Magnum/Magnarail versus conventional systems for recanalization of chronic total coronary occlusions: a randomized comparison. Am Heart J 1992; 123:1182–1186.

66. De Swart JBRM, Van Gelder LM, Van der Krieken AM, El Gamal MIH. A new technique for angioplasty of occluded coronary arteries and bypass grafts, not associated with acute myocardial infarction. Cathet Cardiovasc Diagn 1987;13:419–423.

67. Meier B. Magnarail probing catheter: new tool for balloon recanalization of chronic total coronary occlusions. J Invas Cardiol 1990;2:227–229.

68. Finci L, Meier B, Roy P, Steffenino G, Rutishauser W. Clinical experience with the Monorail balloon catheter for coronary angioplasty. Cathet Cardiovasc Diagn 1988; 14:206–212.

69. Grollier G, Commeau P, Foucault JP, Potier JC. Angioplasty of chronic totally occluded coronary arteries: usefulness of retrograde opacification of the distal part of the occluded vessel via the contralateral coronary artery. Am Heart J 1987;114:1324–1328.

70. Sherman CT, Sheehan D, Simpson JB. Simultaneous cannulation: a technique for percutaneous transluminal coronary angioplasty of chronic total occlusions. Cathet Cardiovasc Diagn 1987;13:333–336.

71. Rees MR, Sivananthan MU, Verma SP. The use of the Terumo glidewires in the treatment of chronic coronary artery occlusions. Circulation 1991;84(Suppl II):II-519.

72. Freed MS, Boatman JE, Siegel N, Safian RD, O'Neill WW, Grines CL. Use of glidewire improves recanalization rates of resistant total coronary artery stenoses. J Am Coll Cardiol 1993;21:290A (abstract).

73. Vassanelli C, Turri M, Morando G, Menegatti G, Zordini P. Open-ended guidewire: new technique for balloon angioplasty of chronically occluded coronary arteries. Cathet Cardiovasc Diagn 1989;17:224–227.

74. Meier B. Magnum system for coronary angioplasty. In: Vogel JHK, King SB III, eds. The practice of interventional cardiology. 2nd ed. St Louis: Mosby–Year Book, 1993.

75. Seggewiss H, Fassbender D, Gleichmann U, Schmidt HK, Vogt J. Recanalization of occluded coronary arteries. Dtsch Med Wochenschr 1992;117:1543–1549.

76. Nukta ED, Meier B, Urban P, Muller T, Dorsaz PA, Favre J. Magnum system for routine coronary angioplasty: a randomized study. Cathet Cardiovasc Diagn 1992; 25:272–277.

77. Bell MR, Berger PB, Menke KK, Holmes DR Jr. Balloon angioplasty of chronic total coronary artery occlusions: what does it cost in radiation exposure, time, and materials? Cathet Cardiovasc Diagn 1992;25:10–15.

C. The ROTACS Approach to the Chronic Occlusion

MARTIN KALTENBACH and ANDREAS HARTMANN

Percutaneous transluminal coronary angioplasty (PTCA) has become a standard procedure for the treatment of high-grade stenosis of coronary arteries. The continuous development of the method since its introduction by Gruentzig in 1977 (1) has led many investigators to apply PTCA to more complex or multiple lesions. Early attempts of transluminal angioplasty in totally occluded coronary arteries were made in patients who had progressed from subtotal stenosis at the time of the diagnostic angiogram to complete occlusion at the time of the scheduled angioplasty procedure (2).

Total coronary occlusions are found in 10 to 20% of patients undergoing coronary angioplasty (3–5). The aims of recanalization are the relief of symptoms, a lessening of myocardial ischemia, and possible improvement of prognosis. A reduction in the number of episodes with angina and a superior medium-term outcome as compared with untreated patients have been found in patients with successfully recanalized chronic occlusions (6, 7).

Success rates in several series of patients with total chronic occlusions of coronary arteries treated by transluminal angioplasty ranged from 40 to 70% (3, 8–13). Recent studies have reported a higher success rate. However, some of them did not differentiate total from functional occlusions, and the duration of occlusion was less than 3 months in the majority of patients (4, 14–16).

Several authors have emphasized that the duration of occlusion has a strong influence on the success rate (11, 17). In occlusions of more than 2 months' duration success rates of 42% and 44% were reported (9, 11). In lesions older than 6 months the success rate declined to less than 20% (6, 10). In general lower success and complication rates have been reported for the recanalization of chronic total coronary occlusions as compared with angioplasty of subtotal stenosis (4, 18).

The crucial point in the recanalization of chronic total coronary occlusion is the passage of the obstructed vessel segment. Several devices such as high-speed rotating drills, certain laser systems, and atherectomy catheters can only be employed if the occlusion has first been traversed with a guidewire. We have developed and described a low-speed rotational angioplasty catheter (ROTACS) for application in chronic total coronary occlusion as an addition to conventional guidewire techniques (19, 20).

INDICATION AND PATIENT SELECTION

Signs of ischemia attributed to the myocardium distal to the occlusion were considered an indication for an attempt to recanalize a total chronic coronary occlusion. Prerequi-

sites were preserved myocardial contraction on ventriculography, angina pectoris, and/or signs of ischemia on the exercise ECG, on a [201]thallium myocardial scintigram, or on a radionuclide ventriculogram during exercise.

Two hundred consecutive patients (18 female, 182 male; age 55 ± 9 years) were included in a study evaluating the efficacy of low-speed rotational angioplasty (21). In all patients the total occlusion had been documented on a previous angiogram performed in our hospital or—in the majority—performed in the referring institution. If in a previous attempt a large dissection had occurred, a time for healing of at least 4 weeks was required before the procedure.

A reliable estimate of the age of the occlusion was possible in 98 of 200 lesions because of a clinical event (e.g., acute myocardial infarction) or because of a previous angiogram. Mean age of the occlusions was 12 ± 26 months (range 1 to 192 months, median 6 months, interquartile range 4 to 9 months). In 21 of 98 lesions (21%) the age of the occlusion was between 1 and 3 months; 36 of 98 (36%) occlusions were in the age range of 4 to 6 months; 29 of 98 (29%) occlusions were 7 to 12 months old; and 12 of 98 (13%) were older than 12 months. The total occlusions were localized in the right coronary artery in 107 of 200 (54%) cases, in the left anterior descending coronary artery in 57 of 200 (28%) cases, and in the circumflex branch of the left coronary artery in 24 of 200 (12%) cases. Twelve total occlusions of venous aorto-coronary bypass grafts were treated (12 of 200, 6%).

THE LESION

Chronic coronary occlusions are considered to consist of arteriosclerotic tissue and a thrombus. The morphology of the occlusion and the distribution of its various components often determine the result of the angioplastic procedure. Although the proximal part of the occlusion may appear angiographically as a suitable "stump," the internal structure of the occlusion is unknown. It may ideally consist of a small, fresh central thrombus as a path of least resistance surrounded by the firmer fibrocellular tissue of the plaque (22). In this instance recanalization within the true lumen is likely to be successful, depending on the age and the degree of fibrous organization of the occluding thrombus. However, in the alternate pathologic scenario plaque rupture has been found to be an important cause of coronary occlusion. A thin, fibrous layer may be covering deposits of intramural fatty cellular debris. Under these circumstances the recanalization device may enter the intramural, subintimal layers following a preexisting dissection as easily as the thrombotic formation within the true lumen (22).

THE DEVICE

The slowly rotating ROTACS catheter (Osypka, Grenzach, Germany; Oscor, Palm Harbour, FL) is made of several, helical, stainless steel coils to combine high flexibility of the shaft with maximum torque control. The tip of the steel catheter consists of an olivelike rounded tip with a diameter ranging from 1.3 to 1.9 mm (Fig. 24C.1). Rotation is achieved by a sterile, battery-driven, electric motor with a speed of up to 200 rpm. A shielding catheter made of polyethylene tubing covers the rotating inner catheter and protects the proximal vessel wall from the rotating catheter. The movable shielding catheter also gives one the opportunity to change the stiffness of the catheter end. The closer the shielding catheter is advanced toward the olive-shaped tip of the inner catheter, the higher the stiffness of the distal end. The rotating catheter is introduced through a conventional 8 Fr guiding catheter and advanced to the proximal part of the occlusion either directly or over a conventional guidewire. The guidewire is removed prior to the procedure of rotational angioplasty. After removal of the guidewire, the free lumen can be used for the injection of contrast agent during the procedure.

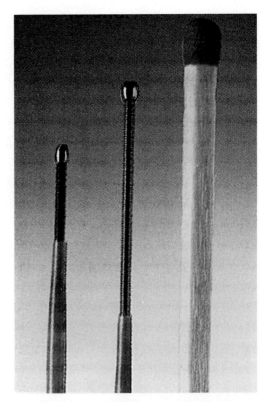

Figure 24C.1. Low-speed rotational angioplasty (ROTACS) catheter for coronary application with an olivelike, rounded tip (diameters ranging from 1.3 to 1.6 mm). The design of the catheter permits injection of contrast medium and insertion of a guidewire through a central lumen. The shielding catheter covers the rotating inner catheter and protects the proximal vessel wall from the rotating catheter.

PROCEDURE

Coronary angiography was performed via the brachial or femoral artery confirming the presence of a total coronary occlusion before and after an intracoronary injection of 0.3 mg nitroglycerine. In all patients an 8 Fr guiding catheter was inserted, and an attempt to pass the occlusion with a conventional guidewire was made. These attempts included the use of floppy, intermediate, and stiff guidewires (3-mm wire—ACS 0.014 inch, Schneider 0.012 inch, or Datascope 0.014 inch) and bracing the guidewire with a balloon catheter, a recanalization catheter, or a ROTACS catheter. In several occlusions we were informed

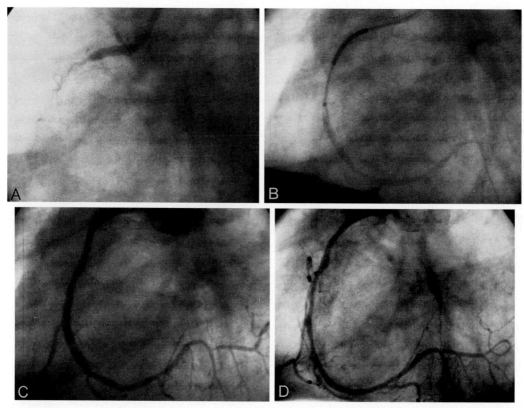

Figure 24C.2.   A. Occlusion of the right coronary artery 12 months after an inferior myocardial infarction. **B.** Passage of the rotational catheter (ROTACS) through the occlusion. Injection of contrast agent through the lumen of the catheter shows filling of the distal part of the vessel. **C.** Acute result after complete passage of the low-speed rotational catheter (ROTACS) through the obstruction and additional dilatation of the right coronary artery with a 3-mm balloon catheter. **D.** Follow-up angiography after 4 months shows a patent vessel with wall irregularities.

about a previous attempt performed with the Magnum wire. A patient was excluded from the study when it was possible to cross the occlusion solely with the guidewire or with a guidewire stiffened by a balloon catheter or a recanalization catheter.

In the 200 included patients passage through the occlusion was not possible with conventional guidewire techniques as listed above. The ROTACS catheter was inserted and advanced to the proximal end of the occlusion. Usually, the catheter was introduced over a conventional guidewire, occasionally without a wire. The correct placement of the tip of the catheter was documented by injection of contrast agent through the lumen of the catheter after removal of the guidewire (Fig.

24C.2). Passage of the occlusion was then attempted first without rotation and, if unsuccessful, while rotating the catheter up to 200 rpm. In long occlusions the proper localization of the catheter was reconfirmed during passage by repetitive injections of 0.5 to 1.0 ml of contrast medium through the lumen.

After successful passage of the occlusion and documentation by contrast injection that the catheter had arrived in the free lumen of the distal part of the vessel, the 3-mm guidewire was inserted and the ROTACS catheter was removed. Injection of contrast medium through the guiding catheter now confirmed *orthograde* flow through the newly formed channel. With the guidewire in place the occluded area of the coronary vessel was subsequently dilated with conventional balloon catheters. In several patients additional stenosis located separately from the occlusion had to be dilated. Patients were given 1.5 g of ASA prior to the procedure. Heparin (200 U/kg) as injected intraarterially at the beginning of the procedure. Throughout the intervention the guiding catheter was perfused with heparin 2000 U/hour. Initially, it was observed that coronary spasm tended to occur in the vessel distal to the occlusion after successful recanalization, requiring repetitive, intracoronary injections of nitroglycerine. Therefore continuous, intracoronary infusion of nitroglycerine 1 mg/hour was included in the pharmacologic regimen. Follow-up therapy after the procedure consisted of ASA 100 mg/day, calcium antagonists (usually gallopamil 50 mg t.i.d.), and long-acting nitrates (usually ISDN 20 g t.i.d.). All patients gave informed consent of follow-up angiography 4 months after the procedure.

RESULTS

Angiographic Results

Of the 200 patients with total chronic coronary occlusions inaccessible by conventional techniques, recanalization was achieved in 116 by low-speed rotational angioplasty (21). In the first 10 coronary occlusions three were successfully reopened. The success rate subsequently increased to 50% and in patients numbered 50 to 200 to 60%.

The recanalization rate for occlusions localized in different coronary arteries were determined as 56% (32 of 57) for the left anterior descending coronary artery, 55% (59 of 107) for the right coronary artery, and 75% (18 of 24) for the circumflex branch of the left coronary artery. The success rate in occluded bypass grafts was 58% (7/12).

There was a distinct correlation between success rate and age of the occlusion. As mentioned above, a reliable determination of the age of the occlusion was feasible in 98 patients. Recanalization was achieved in

19 of 21 (91%) occlusions of 4 weeks' to 3 months' duration. In occlusions of 4 to 6 months' duration 26 of 36 (72%) lesions were treated successfully. Occlusions 7 to 12 months of age were recanalized in 16 of 29 (55%) patients. For occlusion of more than 12 months' duration, the success rate dropped to 1 out of 12 (8%).

The channel of 1 to 1.5 mm diameter formed after the passage of the rotational catheter through the occluded vessel segment was visualized angiographically, and it usually showed smooth contours. The channel was dilated further by additional balloon angioplasty. The result of a successful recanalization by slow rotational angioplasty combined with subsequent conventional angioplasty was a reduction of the obstruction to 30 to 40% of the linear vessel diameter.

Functional Results

Functional results depend largely on indication. If reopening of arteries is performed in patients with large transmural infarctions in the postocclusional myocardium, only little functional improvement can be anticipated. Therefore in general the indication is restricted to patients with signs of ischemia in the postocclusional myocardium. Good contraction or at least some contraction in the postocclusional myocardium in the ventriculogram is required. The patient has to show subjective and/or objective signs of ischemia provoked during ergometry: typical angina or ischemic patterns on the electrocardiogram, the thallium scintigram, or the radionuclide ventriculogram.

Most patients experience subjective improvement and relief of angina as determined by exercise testing after recanalization of chronic occlusions. Improvement of left ventricular function was demonstrated by analysis of global and regional wall motion (23). Regional wall motion as a parameter of left ventricular function was analyzed from ventriculograms and revealed an improvement of left ventricular relaxation.

In 20 consecutive patients treated by low-speed rotational angioplasty (ROTACS), functional results were evaluated by repeat radionuclide ventriculography. In 40% of the patients improvement of resting ejection fraction was >5%; in 61% of the patients the increase of ejection fraction during exercise exceeded 5%; and 83% of the patients showed symptomatic improvement during repeat exercise testing (24).

ACUTE COMPLICATIONS

There was one in-hospital death (0.5%) in this series. The patient died suddenly 5 days after successful recanalization of an occlusion of the right coronary artery. At autopsy an acute thrombotic reocclusion at the recanalization site was found. In two out of 200 patients immediate surgical intervention was required. In both patients occlusions in the proximal part of the left anterior descending coronary artery less than 1 cm distant from the left main stem were approached. The vessel wall dissection, which developed in the occlusion of the left anterior descending coronary artery, showed retrograde progression and resulted in an impairment of blood flow to the previously unaffected circumflex branch of the left coronary artery. In another patient with an unsuccessful attempt to recanalize the left anterior descending coronary artery, dissection was caused by the guiding catheter in the left main stem without impairment of blood flow. In both cases immediate bypass surgery prevented myocardial infarction. As a result of these complications no further lesions located closely to the left main stem were treated by rotational angioplasty.

Asymptomatic dissections in the occluded vascular regions occurred in several patients. In some of these cases it was the investigators' impression that it was not a catheter-induced dissection but rather a preexisting intimal flap guiding the catheter into the vessel wall. At times the dissection caused some pain, which was not typical anginal and occurred without signs of ischemia.

In three patients embolization of thrombotic material into the distal part of the vessel occurred during the insertion and inflation of the balloon catheter following the recanalization. Two patients with embolization in the right coronary artery remained asymptomatic. In one patient a myocardial infarction occurred after embolization from a totally occluded aortocoronary venous bypass. The graft was occluded after the second bypass operation, and the attempt at recanalization was considered the last therapeutic option. Recanalization was performed successfully. After ROTACS application a good *antegrade* flow was established. However, additional balloon angioplasty led to embolization from the previously occluded bypass site into the left anterior descending coronary artery causing a transmural infarction. Complications relating to the brachial or femoral approach were similar to those of conventional PTCA.

FOLLOW-UP

In 99 of 116 patients (85%) with successfully recanalized chronic total coronary occlusions, follow-up angiography was performed 4 months after the initial procedure. The recanalized occlusion remained open in 80 of 99 (81%) patients. Reocclusion was found in 19 of 99 (19%). A second recanalization was attempted in a few cases. The success rate of these attempts, however, proved to be very low and second recanalizations were consequently only rarely carried out. Out of the 80 patients with open vessels on follow-up angiography, 50 (62%) required no further angioplasty while 30 patients (38%) had restenosis. In 28 of 30 cases (93%) this restenosis was treated successfully by conventional PTCA. Thus long-term patency was found in 78 of 99 (78%) of the patients with acute success.

In conclusion, this new technique seems to expand the option of nonsurgical revascularization in patients with chronic total coronary occlusions. It is advisable to attempt passage first with a conventional guidewire. If this fails, the ROTACS can be used without the motor. After failure of this approach the passage is attempted using rotation with the motor unit. With this stepwise application of more and more sophisticated techniques in a "stand-by" fashion, the technical and financial expense can be kept as low as possible.

REFERENCES

1. Grüntzig A. Transluminal dilatation of coronary artery stenosis. Lancet 1978;1:263.
2. Kober G, Reinemer H, Kaltenbach M. Vorkommen und Vorhersehbarkeit der Progredienz hochgradiger Koronargefäßstenosen zu Verschlüssen. Z Kardiol 1984; 73:674–678.
3. Safian RD, McCabe CH, Sipperly ME, McKay RG, Baim DS. Initial success and long-term follow-up of percutaneous transluminal coronary angioplasty in chronic total occlusions versus conventional stenosis. Am J Cardiol 1988;61:23G–28G.
4. Stone GW, Rutherford BD, McConahay DR, Johnson WL, Giorgi LV, Ligon RW, Hartzler GO. Procedural outcome of angioplasty for total coronary artery occlusion: an analysis of 971 lesions in 905 patients. J Am Coll Cardiol 1990; 15:849–856.
5. Baim DS, Ignatius EJ. Use of coronary angioplasty: results of a current survey. Am J Cardiol 1990;15:526–533.
6. Melchoir JP, Meier B, Urban P, Finci L, Steffenino G, Noble J, Rutishauser W. Percutaneous transluminal coronary angioplasty for chronic total coronary arterial occlusion. Am J Cardiol 1987;59:535–538.
7. Finci L, Meier B, Favre J, Righetti A, Rutishauser W. Long-term results of successful and failed angioplasty for chronic total coronary arterial occlusion. Am J Cardiol 1990; 66:660–662.
8. Dervan JP, Baim DS, Cherniles J, Grossman W. Transluminal angioplasty of occluded coronary arteries: use of a movable guidewire system. Circulation 1983;68:776–784.
9. Kober G, Hopf R, Reinemer H, Kaltenbach M. Langzeitergebnisse der transluminalen koronaren Angioplastie von chronischen Herzkranzgefäßverschlüssen. Z Kardiol 1985;309–316.
10. Kereiakes DJ, Selmon MR, McAuley BJ, McAuley DB, Sheehan DJ, Simpson JB. Angioplasty in total coronary artery occlusion: experience in 76 consecutive patients. J Am Coll Cardiol 1985;6:526–533.
11. Serruys PW, Umans V, Heyndrickx GR, van den Brand M, De Feyter PJ, Wijns W, Jaski B et al. Elective PTCA of totally occluded coronary arteries not associated with acute myocardial infarction: short-term and long-term results. Eur Heart J 1985;6:2–12.
12. DiSciascio G, Vetrovec GW, Cowley MJ, Wolfgang TC. Early and late outcome of percutaneous transluminal coronary angioplasty of subacute and chronic total coronary occlusion. Am Heart J 1986;111:833–839.
13. Stewart JT, Denne L, Bowker TJ, Mulcahy DA, Williams MG, Buller NP, Sigwart U et al. Percutaneous transluminal coronary angioplasty in chronic coronary artery occlusion. J Am Coll Cardiol 1993;21:1371–1376.
14. Bell MR, Berger PB, Bresnahan JF, Reeder GS, Bailey KR,

Holmes DR. Initial and long-term outcome of 354 patients after coronary balloon angioplasty of total coronary artery occlusions. Circulation 1992;85:1003–1011.
15. Ruocco N, Ring ME, Holubkov R, Jacobs AK, Detre KM, Faxon DP, and the Co-investigators of the National Heart, Lung and Blood Institute Percutaneous Transluminal Coronary Angioplasty Registry. Results of coronary angioplasty of chronic total occlusions (the National Heart, Lung and Blood Institute 1985–1986 Percutaneous Transluminal Angioplasty Registry). Am J Cardiol 1992;69:69–76.
16. Ivanhoe RJ, Weintraub WS, Douglas JS, Lembo NJ, Furman M, Gershony G, Cohen CL et al. Percutaneous transluminal coronary angioplasty of chronic total occlusions—primary success, restenosis and long-term clinical follow-up. Circulation 1992;85:106–115.
17. Holmes DR, Vlietsra RE, Reeder GS, Bresnahan JF, Smith HC, Bove AA, Schaff HV. Angioplasty in total coronary artery occlusion. J Am Coll Cardiol 1984;3:845–849.
18. Meier B. Total coronary occlusion: a different animal? J Am Coll Cardiol 1991;17:50B–57B.
19. Kaltenbach M, Vallbracht C. Rotationsangioplastik—ein neues Katheterverfahren. Fortschr Med 1987;21:412–414.
20. Kaltenbach M, Vallbracht C, Hartmann A. Recanalization of chronic coronary occlusions by low-speed rotational angioplasty (ROTACS). J Intervent Cardiol 1991;4:155–165.
21. Kaltenbach M, Hartmann A, Vallbracht C. Procedural results and patient selection in recanalization of chronic coronary artery occlusions by low-speed rotational angioplasty. Eur Heart J 1993;14:826–830.
22. Sanborn TA. Recanalization of arterial occlusions: pathologic basis and contributing factors. J Am Coll Cardiol 1989;7:1558–1560.
23. Melchior JP, Doriot PA, Chatelain P, Meier B, Urban P, Finci L, Rutishauser W. Improvement of left ventricular contraction and relaxation synchronism after recanalization of chronic total coronary occlusion by angioplasty. J Am Coll Cardiol 1987;9:763–768.
24. Gyöngyösi M, Klepzig H, Vallbracht C, Maul FD, Standke R, Hör G, Kaltenbach M. Myokardfunktion vor und nach Wiedereröffnung eines chronischen Koronarverschlusses. Z Kardiol 1992;81:591–595.

D. Percutaneous Revascularization of Chronic Total Occlusions

ALAA E. ABDELMEGUID and PATRICK L. WHITLOW

Angioplasty of chronic total occlusions continues to be a challenge for interventionalists. Despite many technical innovations, the primary success rate remains much lower (1–5) and the incidence of restenosis much higher

(6, 7) than that for percutaneous transluminal coronary angioplasty (PTCA) of subtotal coronary occlusions. Moreover, these procedures are associated with long periods of exposure to fluoroscopy and high equipment cost because of the use of multiple guide catheters, angioplasty balloon catheters, and guidewires (8). PTCA of chronic total occlusions, first described in 1982 (9) accounts for ≥10% of patients in the most recent NHLBI PTCA Registry (1). The primary success for these procedures is around 50% (1–5), and even with proper training and careful patient selection, a primary success rate of only ≈70% may be achieved (3, 10) compared with >90% in PTCA of subtotal occlusions. Similarly, the restenosis rate is >50% compared with the 30 to 40% for subtotal stenoses (6, 11).

Many patients with occlusions do not have complete transmural infarction in the involved zone because of the presence of collateral vessels (12). This is the rationale for revascularization of chronic total occlusions. Collateral flow may be sufficient to meet resting myocardial demands; however, it is frequently insufficient to meet the increased demands of exercise, since a well-collateralized chronic total occlusion is functionally equivalent to a 90% stenosis (13). The myocardium in the area served by the totally occluded artery may have been "hybernating" for an extended period, and restoration of blood flow might lead to improvement in ventricular function. Viable myocardial tissue may be present if there is (a) angina pectoris in the absence of other significant coronary artery lesions, (b) absence of Q waves on the ECG, (c) the preservation or inducibility of left ventricular wall motion, and (d) reversibility of perfusion defects. Successful angioplasty of occluded vessels in selected patients results in significant symptomatic improvement (14) and may also lead to improvement of LV function (4, 14) and avoidance of bypass surgery (15, 16). Continued efforts to improve the short- and long-term

Table 24D.1.
Angiographic Determinants of Success for PTCA of Chronic Total Occlusions

Functional versus total occlusion
Duration of occlusion
Tapered occlusion morphology
Estimated length of nonvisualized segment of the occluded artery
Absence of bridging collateral vessels
Multivessel disease
Presence of calcium in the lesion

results of PTCA of chronic total occlusions are warranted.

THE SUBSTRATE

The ability to cross the lesion without subintimal dissection and restenosis are the two important factors that ultimately determine the success of PTCA of chronic total occlusions. Both factors are related to the nature of the underlying lesion. Several angiographic characteristics of chronic total occlusions have been associated with success of PTCA in this setting (Table 24D.1). The importance of these characteristics can be explained by their histologic correlates.

Histologically, the occluded segment is composed of loose or dense fibrous tissue, atheroma, small vascular channels, and calcified tissue (17). Occlusions of short duration often consist solely of fresh thrombus, whereas organization and calcification occurs in the later stages. In an attempt to explain how the angiographic characteristics affect success, Karutsagawa et al. examined the histologic-angiographic relation of chronic total occlusions in human hearts (17). In each occluded segment there were small vascular channels, some extending from proximal to distal lumen (recanalization), while others extended to a small side branch or vasa vasorum (no recanalization). In a clinical setting, if the guidewire, balloon catheter, or both enter the recanalized vascular channel, angioplasty would likely be successful. However, if they enter a vascular channel that extends to a small side branch or vasa vasorum, a subintimal false lumen may be formed and perforation may occur. If the guidewire and catheter pass through a false lumen and return to the distal true lumen, dilatation may result in extensive dissection, and acute reclosure may complicate the procedure.

Small-lumen recanalized channels and surrounding loose fibrous tissue are frequently present in a tapering occlusion. The average diameter of the recanalized lumen is $200\mu m$, which is slightly smaller than currently available guidewires. In short occlusions these small-lumen recanalized channels penetrate the occluded segment and are surrounded by a mass of loose fibrous tissue, which may help the crossing of the guidewire through the recanalized lumen. In long, occluded segments, however, there is usually no recanalization, and loose fibrous tissue is dispersed in the occluded segment, making the guidewire crossing much more difficult.

Many favorable angiographic determinants coexist. A short, occluded segment is usually seen in coronary arteries with a tapering occlusion and is usually associated with small recanalized lumen. A short, abrupt occlusion is associated with loose fibrous tissue penetrating the occluded segment. Thus a tapering occlusion, a short, occluded segment, or both are favorable for angioplasty because of the presence of a vessel stump, a short segment, and favorable histologic features.

Clinically, the determinants of successful PTCA in chronic total occlusions (see Table 24D.1) can be explained by the histologic observations discussed previously. Of these determinants, the first four have been strongly correlated with the procedural success rate (3–5, 9, 15, 16).

The presence of functional occlusion, defined as antegrade faint and late opacification of the vessel segment beyond the occlusion with or without visible continuity of the artery, is associated with a higher success rate than in a total occlusion, which is defined as the absence of antegrade filling distal to the occlusion. This is likely related to the higher incidence of a large recanalization channel and/or residual lumen inside the functional occlusion that can accommodate a guidewire.

An inverse relationship between the duration of occlusion and success of PTCA has been reported by many investigators. This may be related to the fact that the duration of the occlusion determines the consistency of the lesion. Several studies showed that the primary success rate is substantially lower if the duration of the occlusion is more than 2 months (4, 5). However, other studies have denied any important predictive value of duration of occlusion (2, 3, 18). The difference in these conclusions is probably related to the difficulty in ascertaining the exact duration of occlusion in many patients. In our experience a duration of occlusion of >6 months has been one of the important predictors of success in PTCA of chronic total occlusions.

The length of the occluded segment can be assessed from the filling of the distal part of the vessel from collaterals. Kereiakes et al. showed that the outcome of PTCA is significantly influenced by the length of the nonvisualized segment. PTCA of occluded segments <1.5 cm in length was successful in 78% of cases versus 42% when the length of the "missing" segment was >1.5 cm (5). This is probably related to the histology of the occlusion as it relates to lesion length in this setting.

Tapered occlusion morphology may facilitate the procedure by guiding the wire or the perfusion catheter (3). Great difficulty usually occurs when side branches arise from the most distal end of the visibly occluded segment. When an abrupt occlusion is present, the main lumen is occluded just distal to the branching point of a side branch, and the lumen extends smoothly into the side branch. As a result, no vessel stump is seen. In addition, recanalization is rare with an abrupt type of chronic total occlusion because the guide-

Table 24D.2.
Potential Complications of PTCA of Chronic Total Occlusions

Dissection of the vessel proximal to the dilatation site
Perforation of the vessel wall
Dissection of the vessel wall
Occlusion of side branches beyond the lesion by embolization
Guidewire fracture by entrapment in the occlusion
Myocardial infarction, arrhythmias, death

wire easily enters the side branch but not the occluded segment.

COMPLICATIONS OF PTCA OF CHRONIC TOTAL OCCLUSIONS

The risk of major hemodynamic complications during PTCA for chronic total occlusions is uncertain, and the need for surgical backup for such procedures is controversial. Recanalization of a chronic total occlusion is usually considered safe because the target vessel is already blocked, and the complication rates reported by most centers have been low (3, 14, 19). A recent report examined 100 consecutive cases of PTCA of chronic total occlusions and confirmed the low overall incidence of procedural complications (19). However, there was one death, eight patients had extensive coronary dissections accompanied by acute myocardial ischemia, and 26 patients underwent elective bypass surgery. Thus, although the complication rate is relatively low, it is not zero, and claims that the procedure is safe must be treated with caution. Table 24D.2 enumerates the potential complications associated with PTCA of chronic total occlusions. Complications related to proximal extension of a dissection flap or to guide-induced dissection of the proximal vessel can have serious consequences. Indeed, the only death reported in a recent series resulted from a proximal extension of a dissection after attempted recanalization of the proximal LAD (19). Extensive dissection of the previously occluded artery itself may occur and may be associated with acute myocardial ischemia

from interruption of established collateral channels, although this is unlikely to cause serious hemodynamic disturbance and any infarct will probably be small.

RESTENOSIS

While the primary success rate of PTCA of chronic total occlusions has increased by advances in both operator experience and in angioplasty technology (3), the high restenosis rate after PTCA of chronic total occlusions persists. Angina recurs in 25 to 48% of the cases (2–5, 18), and the reported incidence of restenosis depends on the definition of restenosis and on the completeness of angiographic follow-up (2, 4, 6). Ellis et al. showed that a residual stenosis of >30% after PTCA and recanalization of a proximal LAD were significant predictors of restenosis (6, 11). A residual stenosis of ≤10% after PTCA of chronic total occlusions was associated with a 30% restenosis rate within 6 months, and a residual stenosis of 11 to 20% increases that restenosis rate to 39%. Another study also found that restenosis was related to a higher degree of post-PTCA narrowing (2). Ellis et al. also demonstrated that restenosis does not appear to reach a plateau at 6 months as is the case in PTCA of nonocclusive stenoses (6, 11). Furthermore, they showed that treatment with aspirin, dipyridamole, or warfarin did not influence long-term results.

TECHNIQUE

The most common reason for failure of PTCA in chronic total occlusions is the inability to cross the stenosis with the guidewire or dilatation catheter. For successful recanalization of the total occlusion, it is essential that the guide catheter provide maximal backup support for guidewire and balloon advancement. Standard Judkins catheters are generally used for dilatation of chronic total occlusions of the left anterior descending, and left Amplatz guiding catheters for occlusions of the circumflex coronary artery. Hockey stick and left Amplatz guides are frequently successfully used for right coronary occlusions. Firm support provided by deep guide engagement of the coronary artery may frequently be necessary when the Judkins catheter is used.

A 0.014-inch floppy or intermediate wire is recommended initially, and a standard wire may be used with caution only if adequate support of the floppy or intermediate guidewires with balloon or exchange catheters is unsuccessful. If the 0.014-inch floppy and intermediate wires fail, 0.016- or 0.018-inch wires, which have more body, are utilized. The 0.018-inch Glidewire Gold (Terumo/Meditech, Watertown, MA) is frequently successful when other wires fail. The occluded segment is probed while ensuring that the guidewire is in line with the major axis of the vessel. The guidewire should not be rotated more than 360° in either direction because of the possible risk of wire fracture. If the 0.014- and 0.018-inch floppy and intermediate wires and the Glidewire fail, then a 0.010-, 0.014-, or 0.018-inch standard wire may be used, but at an increased risk of subintimal passage. Once the occluded segment has been crossed, the guidewire is rotated around its axis to ensure that the tip is free and that the wire is intraluminal rather than intramural. Successful passage of the guidewire into the distal lumen of the vessel is suggested fluoroscopically by easy advancement of the wire into branches and free motion of its tip.

Orthogonal views should be obtained to ensure that the guidewire is located in the main vessel and not in a side branch. The collateral circulation provides a "road map" that can be very useful in PTCA of chronic total occlusions (20). This road map provides information on the length of the occlusion and delineates the course of the vessel beyond the lesion. Knowledge of the anatomy of the distal vessel may facilitate crossing the area of the stenosis with the wire and may reduce the risk of perforation.

When the wire tip position is confirmed to be intraluminal, it is advanced as far distally as possible, and an appropriately sized bal-

loon is advanced over the wire across the occlusion. Crossing with a 1.5-mm balloon is attempted if a larger balloon cannot cross. Alternatively, the balloon is removed, and a fixed-wire balloon is attempted because of the small profile of these catheters. The predilatation balloon is then exchanged for the balloon size appropriate for the involved vessel. At the Cleveland Clinic the patients are heparinized for 24 hours after PTCA of chronic occlusions in an attempt to reduce the risk of abrupt closure, even though there are no firm data to support the use of heparin after PTCA in this setting.

NEW TECHNIQUES

Many new techniques are under evaluation to increase the primary success of angioplasty of total coronary occlusions and potentially reduce the restenosis rate (Table 24D.3).

Guidewires

The Magnum Wire, Schneider, Inc., Minneapolis, MN (Fig. 24D.1). The Magnum wire is a 0.021-inch steel wire with a floppy tip equipped with a 1-mm-diameter, olive-shaped tip that provides pushability. The olive tip may frequently be forced through an occlusion without subintimal passage or side-branch cannulation. Its stiffness requires an

Table 24D.3.
New Technologies for Revascularization of Chronic Total Occlusions

1. Guidewires
     The Magnum wire
     The Glidewire
2. Guidewire-supporting devices
     The Hollow wire
     The Probing catheter
3. Laser angioplasty
     Excimer laser coronary angioplasty (ELCA)
     LASTAC
4. Atherectomy devices
     ROTACS
     Other atherectomy devices
5. Stents
6. Adjunctive intracoronary thrombolysis
     Tissue plasminogen activator
     Urokinase

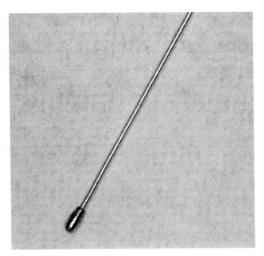

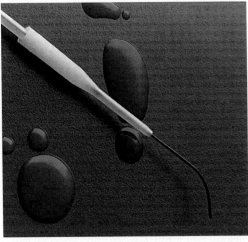

Figure 24D.1. Magnum wire: Specially designed wire with olive-shaped tip to cross total occlusions without subintimal passage. (Courtesy of Schneider, Inc., Minneapolis, MN.)

Figure 24D.2. Angled Glidewire with lubricious coating to enhance passage through a chronic total occlusion. (Courtesy of Mansfield/Boston Scientific Corporation, Watertown, MA.)

adequate guiding-catheter support for its advancement. Once across the occlusion, this wire provides a particularly stable rail for balloon advancement. One disadvantage of using the Magnum wire is the relatively large profile of the compatible balloon catheter compared with that of the sleeker balloons that can be used with usual PTCA guidewires. The blunt tip of the Magnum wire may slip underneath a plaque less often than the sharp tip of a conventional wire, but once a subintimal passage is created by an initially used conventional wire or by the Magnum wire itself, the Magnum wire will readily reenter this false channel and more powerfully advance in it than a conventional wire. In such situations a conventional wire is subsequently used to probe for the correct lumen. Therefore it is felt that if a decision to use the Magnum wire is made, the Magnum should be used as the initial choice rather than following failure of a conventional wire. On the other hand, the use of a conventional wire after failure of the Magnum system is reasonable.

The Magnum wire has been reported to yield a slightly higher success rate because of superior pushing power and a more blunt approach that reduces the risk of subintimal passage. Preliminary data from a randomized study suggest a higher success rate with the Meier-Magnum system (67% versus 45%) (21). However, Jacksch et al. obtained a success rate of 66% using a conventional guidewire compared with 40% using the Magnum wire (22). At the Cleveland Clinic, conventional wires have yielded results that are not inferior to the Magnum wire, and they remain our first choice. More studies and further experience with the Magnum wire are needed before its definitive role in PTCA of chronic total occlusions is established.

The Glidewire, Mansfield, Boston Scientific Corporation, Watertown, MA (Fig. 24D.2). The Glidewire is comprised of an elastic titanium-nickel alloy core and a hydrophilic polymer-coated polyurethane cover that imparts extreme flexibility, pushability, kink-resistance, and decreased surface tension when wet. The distal 3 cm of the wire are soft and flexible to facilitate atraumatic passage during crossing attempts. The disadvantages of this wire include limited visibility, inability to shape its tip, difficulty in steering it out of side branches, and the inability to extend it to exchange length. However, because of its lubricious surface and pushability, we sometimes use this wire when floppy wires fail to cross a total occlusion. In such cases a supporting catheter (PTCA balloon, Tracker, Hollow wire, or Probing Catheter) is tracked over the conventional wire to the point of occlusion, and the conventional wire is then exchanged with the Glidewire. This maneuver circumvents most of the previously mentioned disadvantages of the Glidewire. Freed et al. used the Glidewire to treat 59 total occlusions that failed conventional guidewire crossing and obtained favorable results (23). Successful lesion crossing was obtained in 54% of the cases. Coronary artery dissection occurred in 36% of successfully crossed occlusions, but there were no coronary artery perforations.

The Jagwire (Mansfield, Boston Scientific Corporation, Watertown, MA). The Jagwire is another wire specifically designed to cross chronic total occlusions. The body of the wire is 0.016 inches and provides a stable rail for maximum push of a balloon catheter. The distal 2 cm of the wire is radiopaque, 0.025 inches, and covered with a slippery hydrophilic polymer (the same polymer as the Glidewire). The improved radiodensity and pushability of the wire may provide an advantage in some chronic total occlusions that cannot be successfully crossed with other techniques. The 0.025-inch distal tip of the wire prevents pulling the wire back out of a PTCA balloon, but the advantages of this unique design are likely beneficial in selected cases. Large series of patients treated with this wire have not yet been reported, but the technology is new and promising.

Guidewire-Supporting Devices

Hollow Wires (USCI, Billerica, MA) and the Craig Wire (Medi-tech, Boston Scientific Corporation, Watertown, MA). The open-ended USCI guidewire is constructed with a stainless-steel coil wire covered by a Teflon overjacket, which provides catheter-like support to the spring to allow the device to be used like a catheter and a wire. The Sos openended guidewire is 0.035 or 0.038 inch in outer diameter and has an integral lumen (inner diameter: 0.018 or 0.021 inch, respectively) with a distal opening. A removable tapered core wire (outer diameter: 0.012 or 0.015 inch) is inserted in the inner lumen to add support to the system allowing the whole system to be steered toward the lesion. The core wire can be replaced with a 0.014- or 0.016-inch steerable guidewire. Through this wire, a conventional PTCA wire is passed to cross the lesion. Alternatively, the 0.038-inch hollow Craig wire can be loaded with traditional PTCA guidewires. Hollow wires are more maneuverable and flexible than a balloon catheter, and can be used to record distal pressure and to inject contrast into the distal vessel (24). If the attempts of passing the occlusion fail, a balloon catheter can be spared, reducing the cost of the procedure.

The Probing Catheter (USCI, Billerica, MA). This catheter is designed for use with a guidewire or a fixed-wire Probe balloon catheter, and is similar in principle to a hollow wire. It consists of a 4 Fr polyethylene shaft with an inside diameter of 0.039 inch. The Probing catheter is loaded with a preshaped guidewire and is then advanced to the tip of the guiding catheter. Using contrast medium injected through the guiding catheter, the guidewire is maneuvered to the total occlusion and attempts are made to cross it. If additional support is required, the Probing catheter itself is advanced to the occlusion and additional attempts are made to cross it. A stiffer wire may be used to cross difficult stenoses. Successful passage of the wire may be confirmed by contrast injection through the Probing catheter itself. After crossing the occlusion with the guidewire, the Probing Catheter is advanced to directly contact the occlusion at the entry site of the guidewire into the occlusion. The guidewire and the inner catheter are then removed, and a Probe balloon catheter is then advanced through the Probing catheter emerging into the stenosis at the site previously occupied by the guidewire. Alternatively, the Probing catheter may be exchanged for a low-profile, over-the-wire balloon while maintaining access across the stenosis with an exchange length wire. Used with a fixed wire balloon, this system combines the steerability of a guidewire system and the ultra-low profile of a fixed-wire balloon catheter. Although the stiffness of the Probing catheter is useful in supporting the dilatation system, it may increase the risk of dissection of the vessel. The Probing catheter also enables the Probe to be used in tortuous vessels without wrapping the balloon. Contrast injection through the Probing catheter after crossing the occlusion is helpful in verifying the intraluminal position of the wire and defining the coronary anatomy distal to the obstruction. Using this technique, Little et al. reported a success rate of 67% in a group of 13 patients, including six in whom other dilating systems failed to cross the occlusion (25).

Tracker Catheter (Target Therapeutics; San Jose, CA).   This 0.018- or 0.025-inch inner-lumen, end-hole catheter is extremely flexible and allows passage of any traditional PTCA wire or the Glidewire. This catheter is more flexible and less traumatic than the Probing catheter, but may provide less pushability in a straight arterial segment (especially the proximal LAD).

Laser Coronary Angioplasty

Excimer Laser Coronary Angioplasty (ELCA). With ELCA, prior passage of a wire into the distal part of the artery is necessary to avoid the risk of vessel perforation. Although attempts to guide the excimer laser by spectroscopy to differentiate between normal and atherosclerotic tissue have been made, this technique has not yet reached the stage of clinical application.

This technique may improve the immediate and long-term results of angioplasty of chronic total occlusions through ablation of the obstructive atherosclerotic tissue. However, this has not yet been validated in clinical applications; and laser angioplasty, as of today, offers no additional benefit over conventional techniques. Buchwald et al. reported their experience using excimer laser angioplasty in 56 patients with chronic total occlusions and reported an angiographic success rate of 70% and a restenosis rate of 47% (26). Procedural failures were caused by unsuccessful attempts to cross the occlusion with the guidewire in 82% of unsuccessful cases. However, in three patients, the laser catheter could not be advanced across the lesion after successful passage of the guidewire. This was related to the presence of heavy calcification, which requires higher laser energy for ablation. Although the study was not randomized, their results also suggest that restenosis after excimer laser angioplasty of chronic total occlusions is not markedly different from reported results of conventional balloon angioplasty. Preliminary reports from the AMRO trial (ELCA versus PTCA), in which a high proportion of patients had chronic occlusions, seem to confirm this impression that over-the-wire ELCA does little to improve clinical outcome in this setting.

However, early experience with an excimer laser wire (Spectrametics, Colorado Springs, CO), designed specifically to cross total occlusions, suggests that it may allow successful treatment of perhaps 50% of selected, previously uncrossable, total occlusions (P. Serruys, personal communication).

Argon-Laser Transluminal Angioplasty Catheter (LASTAC).   The LASTAC system generates, transmits, and controls continuous-wave argon-laser energy to vaporize plaque tissue. Unlike the excimer laser, the LASTAC does not require initial guidewire crossing. The LASTAC multilumen balloon catheter is introduced over a conventional guidewire and through a coronary guide catheter using standard percutaneous techniques. The multilumen balloon catheter is advanced over a conventional coronary guidewire and is positioned approximately 1 mm from the lesion and inflated. The guidewire is removed and exchanged for the optical laser fiber. The laser is positioned beyond the balloon catheter tip to within 2 mm of the occlusion. Prior to lasing, the balloon is inflated to ensure coaxial alignment between the fiber tip and major axis of the vessel. The procedure involves several consecutive exposures of emitted laser energy over 1 to 5 seconds. Once a laser channel is created, the fiber is reexchanged for an angioplasty guidewire and routine PTCA is performed.

Mast et al. successfully treated 18 of 30 (60%) total occlusions with the LASTAC system with no major ischemic complications (27). Over 150 chronic total occlusions have been treated with LASTAC with a similar overall success rate (60%) (28).

Atherectomy Devices

Low-Speed Rotational Atherectomy (ROTACS) (Fig. 24D.3). This over-the-wire catheter is comprised of several stainless steel coils in a helical configuration, a movable polyethylene sleeve, and a 1.3- to 1.8-mm olive-shaped ball tip. Low-speed rotational atherectomy is performed using a slow rotation (100 to 200 rpm) and is usually followed by conventional balloon angioplasty.

The ROTACS system is advanced over a conventional coronary guidewire into the proximal end of the occlusion. The guidewire

is then removed, the device activated, and continuous forward pressure is applied to the catheter as it rotates at 200 rpm. The central lumen of the catheter is used to deliver contrast injections and assess progress. If the device fails to cross the occlusion, the movable plastic sleeve is advanced distally to increase stiffness and pushability. Once the catheter has crossed the occlusion, the guidewire is reinserted, and the ROTACS is exchanged for a conventional PTCA catheter.

Using the ROTACS, Kaltenbach reported a success rate of 55% in 152 cases of chronic total occlusions, with more than half being >6 months old (29). There was one MI, two emergency CABGs, and a 54% incidence of restenosis. Danchin et al. recently reported on 70 patients with chronic total occlusions randomized to ROTACS or conventional PTCA (30). Primary success was achieved in 85% of patients treated with the ROTACS versus 42% for patients treated with PTCA alone. These preliminary results suggest that the ROTACS can be used to recanalize chronic total occlusions and might be superior to PTCA in this setting. Additional studies are needed to further evaluate the role of ROTACS in revascularization of chronic total occlusions.

High-Speed Rotational Atherectomy. The role of other atherectomy devices in the revascularization of chronic total occlusions remains to be defined. At the Cleveland Clinic, the Rotablator has occasionally been used in the treatment of chronic total occlusions, and cases of total occlusions have been

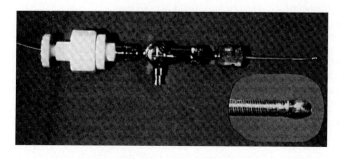

Figure 24D.3. ROTACS: Rotating wire introduced through the hemostatic valve with insert of magnified view of the wire tip. (Courtesy of Vallbracht C, Liermann D, Prignitz I, Beinborn W, Landgraf H, Paasch C, Roth FJ et al. Am J Cardiol 1988; 62:935–940.)

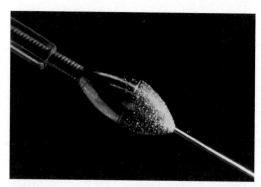

Figure 24D.4. Rotablator: Magnified view of the Rotablator burr, sheath, and drive shaft over a 0.009-inch guidewire. (Courtesy of Heart Technology, Inc., Redmond, WA.)

reported in the Heart Technology Registry (Fig. 24D.4). The role of transluminal extraction atherectomy (TEC) in the treatment of recent total occlusions is currently under investigation.

Stents

The rationale for using stents in chronic total occlusions is related to the prevailing view that obtaining the largest, safest postintervention diameter may be the best way to combat restenosis.

Maiello et al. presented their experience of intracoronary stenting with the Palmaz-Schatz stent after successful revascularization of chronic total occlusions in a limited number of patients (31). The only restenosis reported occurred in an asymptomatic patient who had two stents implanted. They suggested that the reduced rate of restenosis is the result of a larger arterial lumen. This may be due to the reduction of platelet deposition because of less blood flow turbulence or due to the relatively larger amount of myointimal proliferation needed to cause restenosis when the lumen is greater. However, one disadvantage of stents in this situation is the associated thrombogenicity of both chronic total occlusions and current stent materials, which could lead to a high incidence of early and late reocclusion. This is compounded by the fact that multiple stents are usually needed for long chronic total occlusions (>15 mm),

and this may increase the risk of restenosis. In such cases a multistaged approach may be useful. In the first procedure it would be reasonable to reopen the occluded artery to achieve the smallest final stenosis. If restenosis occurs and the length of the new stenosis is short, an intracoronary stent might be placed. This approach can limit the use of multiple stents.

Whether restenosis and reocclusion can be reduced by the use of stents remains to be established, and prospective randomized studies are needed to clarify the indications for coronary stenting after PTCA of chronic total occlusions.

Adjunctive Thrombolytics

Vaska and Whitlow reported their experience in a small number of patients with chronic total occlusions in whom PTCA wires failed to cross the lesions and were subsequently treated with intracoronary t-PA (32). There were no deaths, MI, or emergency CABG. Adjunctive PTCA was performed in all patients with a 90% success rate. This preliminary study suggested that selective t-PA infusion for chronic total occlusions resistant to PTCA alone was effective in restoring vessel patency and allowing successful balloon dilatation in the majority of cases. Similar results were obtained by Cecena who used prolonged urokinase infusion in native coronary arteries with chronic total occlusions after failed angioplasty and who reported a 90% successful reperfusion rate with no death, MI, or emergency CABG (33). Larger trials are needed to determine the ultimate utility of intracoronary thrombolytic infusion for chronic total occlusions.

SUMMARY

In conclusion, PTCA of chronic total occlusions is associated with a low incidence of serious complications. However, the primary success and restenosis rates are less favorable than for conventional stenoses. At the Cleveland Clinic percutaneous revascularization of chronic total occlusions is attempted when the angiographic characteristics are favorable. The duration of occlusion, its length, the presence of a stump, and the absence of bridging collaterals are integrated into the judgment of the suitability of chronic total occlusions for percutaneous revascularization. The patient's current symptoms, limitation of activity, and amount of myocardium at risk should be also taken into consideration, and if bypass surgery is justified, a percutaneous attempt is indicated, provided the anatomy is favorable.

Given the frequent presence of chronic total occlusions in patients with advanced coronary artery disease, the overall use of percutaneous revascularization would be enhanced significantly by better devices to cross, dilate, and maintain the long-term patency of such lesions. Such advances may lead to a more liberal approach toward revascularization of chronic total occlusions.

REFERENCES

1. Detre K, Holubkov R, Kelsey S et al. Percutaneous transluminal coronary angioplasty in 1985–1986 and 1977–1981: The National Heart, Lung, and Blood Institute Registry. N Engl J Med 1988;318:265–270.

2. DiSciascio G, Vetrovec GW, Cowley MJ et al. Early and late outcome of percutaneous transluminal coronary angioplasty for subacute and chronic total coronary occlusion. Am Heart J 1986;111:833–839.

3. Stone GW, Rutherford BD, McConahay DR et al. Procedural outcome of angioplasty for total coronary artery occlusion—an analysis of 971 lesions in 905 patients. J Am Coll Cardiol 1990;15:849–856.

4. Melchior JP, Doriot PA, Chatelain P et al. Improvement of left ventricular contraction and relaxation synchronism after recanalization of chronic total coronary occlusion by angioplasty. J Am Coll Cardiol 1987;9:763–768.

5. Kereiakes DJ, Selmon MR, McAuley BJ et al. Angioplasty of total coronary artery occlusion: experience in 76 consecutive patients. J Am Coll Cardiol 1985;6:526–533.

6. Ellis SG, Shaw RE, Gershony G, et al. Risk factors, time course and treatment effect for restenosis after successful percutaneous transluminal coronary angioplasty of chronic total occlusion. Am J Cardiol 1989;63:897–901.

7. Leimgruber PP, Roubin GS, Hollman J et al. Restenosis after successful coronary angioplasty in patients with single-vessel disease. Circulation 1986;73:710–717.

8. Bell MR, Berger PB, Menke KK et al. Balloon angioplasty of chronic total coronary artery occlusions: What does it cost in radiation exposure, time, and materials? Cathet Cardiovasc Diagn 1992;25:10–15.

9. Laarman G, Plante S, de Feyter PJ. PTCA of chronically occluded coronary arteries. Am Heart J 1990;119:1153–1160.

10. Haine E, Urban P, Dorsaz PA, Meier B. Outcome and complications of 500 consecutive chronic total occlusion coronary angioplasties. J Am Coll Cardiol 1993;21:138A (abstract).

11. Ellis SG, Shaw RE, King SB et al. Restenosis after excellent angiographic angioplasty result for chronic total coronary artery occlusion. Implications for newer percutaneous revascularization devices. Am J Cardiol 1989; 63:667–668.

12. Dervan JP, McKay RG, Baim DS. Assessment of the relationship between distal occluded pressure and angiographically evident collateral flow during coronary angioplasty. Am Heart J 1987;114:491.

13. Flameng W, Schwarz F, Hehrlein FW. Intraoperative evaluation of the functional significance of coronary collateral vessels in patients with coronary artery disease. Am J Cardiol 1978;42:187–192.

14. Finci L, Meier B, Favre J et al. Long-term results of successful and failed angioplasty for chronic total coronary arterial occlusion. Am J Cardiol 1990;66:660–662.

15. Bell MR, Berger PB, Bresnahan JF et al. Initial and long-term outcome of 354 patients after coronary balloon angioplasty of total coronary artery occlusions. Circulation 1992;85:1003–1011.

16. Ivanhoe RJ, Weintraub WS, Douglas JS et al. Percutaneous transluminal coronary angioplasty of chronic total occlusions. Circulation 1992;85:106–115.

17. Katsuragawa M, Fujiwara H, Miyamae M, Sasayama S. Histologic studies in percutaneous transluminal coronary angioplasty for chronic total occlusion: comparison of tapering and abrupt types of occlusion and short and long occluded segments. J Am Coll Cardiol 1993;21:604–611.

18. Safian RD, McCabe CH, Sipperly ME et al. Initial success and long-term follow-up of percutaneous transluminal coronary angioplasty in chronic total occlusions versus conventional stenoses. Am J Cardiol 1988;61:23G–28G.

19. Stewart JT, Denne L, Bowker TJ et al. Percutaneous transluminal coronary angioplasty in chronic coronary arterial occlusion. J Am Coll Cardiol 1993;21:1371–1376.

20. Grollier G, Commeau P, Foucault JP et al. Angioplasty of chronic totally occluded coronary arteries: usefulness of retrograde opacification of the distal part of the occluded vessel via the contralateral coronary artery. Am Heart J 1987;114:1324–1328.

21. Pande AK, Meier B, Urban P et al. Magnum/Magnarail versus conventional systems for recanalization of chronic total occlusions: a randomized comparison. Am Heart J 1992;123:1182–1186.

22. Jacksch R, Papadakis E, Rosanowski C, Toker Y. Comparison of 3 different techniques in reopening chronic coronary artery occlusion. Circulation 1992;86:I-781 (abstract).

23. Freed MS, Boatman JE, Siegel N, Safian RD, O'Neill WW, Grines CL. Use of the glidewire improves recanalization rates of resistant total coronary artery stenoses. J Am Coll Cardiol 1993;290A (abstract).

24. Vassanelli C, Turri M, Morando G, Menegatti G, Zardini P. Open-ended guidewire: new technique for balloon angioplasty of chronically occluded coronary arteries. Cathet Cardiovasc Diagn 1989;17:224–227.

25. Little T, Pichard AD, Lindsay J. Probe angioplasty of total coronary occlusion using an intracoronary Probing catheter. Cathet Cardiovasc Diagn 1989;17:218–223.

26. Buchwald AB, Werner GS, Unterberg C, Voth E, Kreuzer H, Wiegand V. Restenosis after excimer laser angioplasty of

coronary stenoses and chronic total occlusions. Am Heart J 1992;123:878–885.

27. Mast EG, Plokker HWM, Ernst JMPG et al. Percutaneous recanalization of chronic total coronary occlusions: experience with the direct Argon laser–assisted angioplasty system (LASTAC). Herz 1990;15:241–244.

28. Plokker HW, Mast EG, Margolis J et al. Laser coronary angioplasty systems: a realistic appraisal. J Myocardial Ischemia 1992;4:11.

29. Kaltenbach M, Vallbracht C, Hartmann A. Recanalization of chronic coronary occlusions by low-speed rotational angioplasty (ROTACS). J Interven Cardiol 1991;4:155–165.

30. Danchin N, Juilliere Y, Cassagnes J et al. Randomized multicenter study of low-speed rotational angioplasty versus standard angioplasty for chronic total coronary occlusion. Circulation 1992;86:I-782 (abstract).

31. Maiello L, Colombo A, Almagor Y et al. Coronary stenting with a balloon-expandable stent after recanalization of chronic total occlusions. Cathet Cardiovasc Diagn 1992; 25:293–296.

32. Vaska KJ, Whitlow PL. Selective tissue plasminogen activator infusion for chronic total occlusions of native coronary artery failing angioplasty. Circulation 1991;84:II-250 (abstract).

33. Cecena FA. Prolonged urokinase infusion in native coronary arteries with chronic total occlusions after failed angioplasty. Circulation 1992;86:II-781 (abstract).

EDITORIAL SUMMARY

- With success a reduction in ischemia, a modest improvement in ventricular function, an enhanced safety of contralateral vessel treatment, and possibly an improvement in survival can be expected.
- Likelihood of success is highly dependent on the following:
  - Duration of occlusion (rarely bother to try if >6 months unless all other aspects are favorable)
  - Length of occlusion
  - Presence of bridging collaterals (a very bad sign)
  - "Funnel" into occlusion
  - Side branch at site of occlusion
- To cross, be patient and progress through wires of increasing stiffness. (Be sure tip freely rotates before advancing; check position with ipsilateral or contralateral contrast injections.)
- Role of special wires and devices (e.g., Magnum wire, ROTACS, laser) remains to be clarified.
- Risk of complications is not nil. (Watch out for guide catheter trauma.)
- Risk of restenosis is high. (Long-term patency after restenosis, but not reocclusion, can be acceptable with repeat treatment.)
- Optimizing result may be beneficial in reducing restenosis, but this needs to be investigated further. (Consider IVUS-assisted debulking or stenting in suitable vessels.)

25. The Focal Vein Graft Lesion

STEVEN W. WERNS, DAVID W.M. MULLER, and ERIC R. BATES

The randomized clinical trials of coronary artery bypass graft surgery (CABG) have demonstrated both improvement of anginal symptoms and increased survival in certain subsets of patients with coronary artery disease (CAD) (1). Both the progression of disease in the native coronary circulation and the development of stenosis or occlusion in bypass grafts contribute to an annual incidence of recurrent ischemic symptoms of up to 6% during the first 7 years after CABG (2). The risks of reoperation have resulted in a growing role for percutaneous interventions in the treatment of patients with previous CABG. The goal of this chapter is to review the various percutaneous treatments of saphenous vein bypass graft disease and to propose a treatment algorithm based on reported success and complication rates.

PATHOGENESIS OF SAPHENOUS VEIN GRAFT DISEASE

The Cleveland Clinic reported that the 10-year survival of patients with an internal mammary artery (IMA) bypass graft was significantly better than the survival of patients with only saphenous vein bypass grafts (3). The survival advantage of the IMA graft most likely reflects the approximately 95% 10-year patency rate of IMA grafts, compared with the approximately 50% 10-year patency rate of saphenous vein grafts (3). Occlusion of the IMA graft is related primarily to surgical technique because the IMA is relatively resistant to atherosclerosis. Conversely, saphenous vein grafts are susceptible to acute thrombosis, intimal hyperplasia, and atherosclerosis.

The pathogenesis of saphenous vein graft (SVG) disease has been reviewed in detail by Cox et al. (4) and can be classified as acute (<1 month), subacute (1 to 12 months), intermediate (1 to 5 years), and long-term (>5 years). Acute thrombosis is the cause of SVG occlusion in the majority of occlusions during the first month after surgery (5). Several clinical trials have been performed to determine the effects of antiplatelet agents on the early patency of SVGs. A Mayo Clinic study demonstrated improved early patency in patients treated with aspirin plus dipyridamole (6). Angiography within 1 month after CABG demonstrated occlusion of the SVG distal anastomoses in 3% (10/351) of SVGs in the treated group compared with 10% (38/362) of SVGs in the control group. A Veterans Administration (VA) Cooperative Study (7) reported similar results.

Subacute occlusion of vein grafts (i.e., occlusion that occurs between 1 month and 12 months after CABG) has been attributed to fibrointimal hyperplasia, with or without concomitant thrombosis (4). Although the pathogenesis of intimal hyperplasia remains uncertain, several clinical trials have shown that antiplatelet therapy reduces the frequency of subacute occlusion. Both the Mayo Clinic and VA studies demonstrated that treatment with aspirin conferred a higher 1-year patency rate in SVGs that were patent within 1 month after CABG (8, 9).

SVGs are susceptible to progressive atherosclerosis, and despite some morphologic differences between SVG and coronary artery atherosclerosis, the end result is the same: plaque ulceration precipitating thrombosis and acute occlusion (10, 11). The VA Cooperative Study of CABG for Stable Angina reported cumulative SVG patency rates of 64% 5 years after CABG (146 patients evaluated) and 50% 10 years after CABG (67 patients evaluated) (12). The Montreal Heart Institute reported the angiographic findings in 82 patients 10 years after CABG (13). There were 132 patent SVGs 1 year after surgery, but 10 years after CABG 39 were totally occluded and 43 additional grafts had atherosclerotic lesions. Thirty of the 43 stenotic SVGs had a stenosis of at least 50%.

SVG DISEASE AND LIPIDS

In the Montreal Heart Institute study, multivariate analysis demonstrated that the plasma concentrations of LDL apoprotein B and HDL cholesterol were the best predictors of SVG atherosclerosis (13). The Cholesterol-Lowering Atherosclerosis Study (CLAS) examined the effect of therapy with colestipol plus niacin on atherosclerosis in patients with previous CABG and a baseline serum cholesterol between 185 and 350 mg/dL (14, 15). Coronary angiography was performed before and 2 years after randomization in 162 patients (80 in the drug group and 82 in the placebo group). New lesions were seen in the SVGs of 18% of the subjects in the drug group and 30% of the subjects in the placebo group ($P = .04$), with new total occlusions in 5% of the drug group and 10% of the placebo group (14). A subgroup of 103 subjects was maintained on active treatment or placebo and underwent coronary angiography 4 years after randomization. New lesions in SVGs were detected in significantly fewer of the drug-treated patients (16%) than in the placebo-treated patients (38%), with new total occlusions in 14% of the drug-treated patients versus 19% of the placebo-treated patients (15). Since the mean interval between CABG and enrollment in CLAS was 3.3 years, the results support the concept that late development of stenoses in SVGs is a manifestation of atherosclerosis that can be modified by treatment of lipids.

NATURAL HISTORY OF SAPHENOUS VEIN GRAFT DISEASE

Campos et al. (16) recently reported a series of patients who underwent angiographic follow-up a mean of 6 years and 11 years after coronary artery bypass graft (CABG) surgery. One hundred thirty-one SVGs were angiographically normal or minimally diseased (<35% diameter narrowing) 6 years post-CABG. Only 53% of those grafts remained free of significant stenosis 5 years later. Twenty-one percent were totally occluded, and 8% had a stenosis of 70% to 99%.

The Cleveland Clinic published a retrospective analysis of 723 patients with SVG disease who did not undergo PTCA or reoperation for at least 1 year after the catheterization (17). The clinical outcome was compared with that of 573 patients without SVG disease. For patients with an operation-to-catheterization interval of <5 years, the presence of SVG stenoses did not influence late outcome. For patients with an operation-to-catheterization interval of ≥5 years, a stenosis of 20 to 99% in an SVG to the left anterior descending coronary artery (LAD) was associated with decreased survival. It is noteworthy that there was a 30% 2-year mortality after catheterization for patients with a stenotic LAD graft, compared with only 3% for patients with a 50 to 99% stenosis in the native LAD and no LAD graft. Disease of circumflex or right coronary grafts did not influence late outcome.

THE ROLE OF PERCUTANEOUS INTERVENTION IN PATIENTS WITH PRIOR CABG

When SVG disease is diagnosed in patients with recurrent angina after CABG, several factors influence the choice of reoperation versus percutaneous revascularization for relief of symptoms. An important consideration is that reoperation is associated with increased mortality rates. At Emory University Hospital, for example, the in-hospital mortality rate was 7.2% for the 1400 patients who underwent reoperation between 1980 and 1990 (18). Additional considerations that may favor percutaneous procedures over reoperation include the risk of damaging patent grafts, the lack of suitable conduits, a small ischemic region, and clinical factors such as age, impaired left ventricular function, and comorbid medical conditions (e.g., lung disease, cancer).

The interventional cardiologist can employ a variety of percutaneous approaches in the treatment of SVG disease: balloon angioplasty, directional atherectomy, extraction atherectomy, laser angioplasty, endoluminal stents, and thrombolytic drugs. The age of the graft and the location and morphology of the lesion determine the appropriate treatment(s). Reported success and complication rates are quoted in the discussion below.

PTCA FOR VEIN GRAFT DISEASE

Success and Complication Rates

The results of balloon angioplasty of SVG stenoses have been reported in numerous publications. The high-volume centers have reported excellent success rates, for example, 90% at Emory University (599 patients) (18), the Cleveland Clinic (98 patients) (19), and the Thoraxcenter (454 patients) (20); and 85% (119 patients) at the San Francisco Heart Institute (21). DeFeyter et al. (22) tabulated the results of eight clinical series that reported success rates by site of stenosis. The success rate was slightly lower for proximal lesions, 86% (n = 216), compared with distal lesions, 90% (n = 226), and stenoses of the graft body, 93% (n = 162). As discussed below, new devices such as directional atherectomy or excimer laser have been advocated to achieve higher success rates for treatment of aorto-ostial SVG stenoses.

The overall major complication rates after PTCA of selected SVG stenoses have been relatively low. Death occurred in <1% of cases, myocardial infarction (MI) in approximately 4%, and urgent bypass surgery in <2% (22). Higher complication rates, however, have been associated with PTCA of older or totally occluded SVGs. In the Cleveland Clinic experience, there was a 15% incidence of cardiac complications in patients who were more than 3 years post-CABG, while the rate of cardiac complications was 0% in patients ≤3 years post-CABG (19). The higher rate of MI in older SVGs is probably because of a greater likelihood of distal embolization of thrombotic material into the native circulation, prompting some operators to advocate an infusion of urokinase before an elective PTCA of an SVG stenosis (this approach remains unproven to yield superior results) (23).

The Mayo Clinic reported the histopathologic findings of six SVGs that had undergone PTCA (24). Multiple, small, intramural coronary artery branches were obstructed by embolic atheromatous debris in one patient who died after treatment of a 6-year-old, totally occluded SVG with streptokinase and PTCA. Thus emergency bypass surgery may not relieve myocardial ischemia caused by distal emboli after PTCA of SVGs. Nevertheless, the hospital mortality rate was only 6.5% for 46 patients with previous CABG who underwent reoperation after unsuccessful PTCA at Emory University (25). The rate of nonfatal Q-wave MI after urgent reoperation was 33%.

PTCA of SVGs for Treatment of Unstable Angina

Figure 25.1 illustrates a successful PTCA of a stenotic SVG in a patient with unstable angina. Morrison et al. (26) recently reported a series of 75 consecutive patients with unstable angina who underwent PTCA of SVGs that were an average of 8 years old. The angiographic success rate was 94%, and the clinical success rate, defined as hospital discharge without major complications, was 93%. The incidence of non–Q-wave myocardial infarction was, however, 3%. Ten of the patients were in cardiogenic shock during

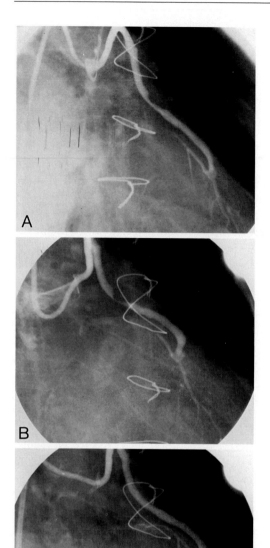

Figure 25.1. A. A 78-year-old woman underwent cardiac catheterization in February 1994 for evaluation of stable angina 4 years after CABG. There was approximately 60% stenosis of the SVG to a diagonal branch of the LAD. **B.** The patient was hospitalized for treatment of unstable angina in June 1994. Repeat catheterization showed progression of the stenosis to 90%. **C.** Successful PTCA of the SVG was performed using a 4.0-mm balloon.

PTCA, and all of them had successful procedures and were discharged from the hospital. The 30-day mortality rate of 3% compared favorably with the predicted 18% mortality for repeat CABG, but there was a 27% mortality after a follow-up period that ranged between 5 months and 3 years. The high initial success rate supports the conclusion that PTCA of SVGs is an effective palliative treatment in patients with unstable angina, but the long-term mortality rate suggests that repeat CABG should be considered after the patient has been stabilized.

Total Occlusions

Relatively high rates of distal emboli and MI have been reported after PTCA of SVG total occlusions (27, 28). Both initial and long-term success was achieved in only one of the 15 total occlusions attempted at the Thoraxcenter from 1980 to 1988 (27). The total occlusion was successfully crossed with both the guidewire and balloon in 14 of the patients, but initial angiographic success was achieved in only nine patients, and early reocclusion occurred in all but one patient. Distal emboli were observed in six of the patients, and MI was diagnosed in seven.

Excluding patients who presented with acute MI, 83 patients underwent PTCA of totally occluded bypass grafts at the Mid America Heart Institute between 1981 and 1991 (28). The results for mammary artery grafts (n = 3) and saphenous vein grafts (n = 80) were not reported separately. The mean duration of graft occlusion was estimated to be 31 days (range 1 to 180). After PTCA, TIMI grade 3 flow was achieved in 56 patients, and TIMI 2 flow in an additional five patients. Distal embolization was observed in nine cases, four of which resulted in elevation of the creatine kinase and/or closure of the distal artery. There were only two deaths, one after distal embolization of an SVG to the left anterior descending coronary artery and the other after elective CABG 3 days after PTCA. A repeat cardiac catheterization was performed in 37 of the 61 patients with a successful PTCA. Reocclusion of the graft was present in 17 (46%), and restenosis was found in 10 (27%). During the long-term follow-up of the 81 patients discharged from the hospital, the rates of freedom from repeat PTCA or CABG were 54% at 1 year and 34% at 3 years. Thus there is a low, sustained patency rate and a frequent need for reintervention after PTCA of totally occluded SVGs.

Hartmann et al. (29) have advocated the adjunctive use of extended, local infusion of

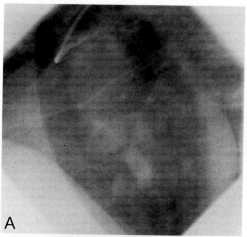

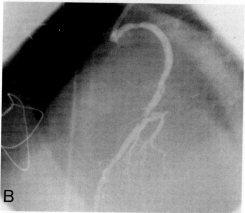

Figure 25.2. **A.** Total occlusion of an LAD SVG before overnight infusion of urokinase. **B.** After overnight infusion of urokinase, repeat angiography demonstrated graft patency and a ruptured plaque in the body of the SVG.

urokinase to recanalize chronically occluded SVGs. Forty-seven grafts were treated with urokinase at rates of 100,000 U/hour to 250,000 U/hour, divided equally between a 7 Fr angiographic catheter and an Sos wire advanced into the occlusion. The total dose of urokinase ranged from 0.7 to 9.8 million units over 7.5 to 77 hours (mean 31 hours). After PTCA and termination of the infusion, the TIMI flow grades were grade 3 in 29 cases (62%) and grade 2 in 8 cases (17%). Complications occurred in 15 patients: 10 patients (22%) developed a significant hematoma, and two patients developed a Q-wave MI. Angiographic follow-up was obtained in 20 successfully treated patients (14 with recurrent symptoms and six who were asymptomatic). Seven (35%) of the 20 grafts were totally occluded, and two of the 13 patent grafts were treated with PTCA for restenosis. Successful recanalization of a totally occluded SVG after infusion of urokinase is illustrated in Figure 25.2.

Restenosis After PTCA

The primary limitation of PTCA of SVGs is restenosis. Unlike the 6-month window for restenosis after PTCA of native arteries, it appears that restenosis of SVGs occurs up to 1 year after PTCA. The rate of restenosis varies with the site of PTCA and SVG age. Some, but not all, series have reported lower restenosis rates of distal anastomotic stenoses than of proximal and midgraft stenoses (Table 25.1) (30–34). The discrepancy is most likely related to the age of the stenosis at the time of PTCA. In the Cleveland Clinic series, for example, restenosis after PTCA of a distal anastomosis was less frequent in young compared with older SVGs (19). Douglas (18) reported the long-term follow-up of 599 patients after successful PTCA. The restenosis rates were 32% for SVGs dilated within 6 months after surgery; 43% for SVGs between 6 and 12 months old; 61% for 1- to 5-year-old SVGs; and 64% for SVGs older than 5 years.

Table 25.1.
Restenosis Rates After SVG PTCA

Authors (Ref.)	% F/U	Graft Site		
		Proximal	Body	Distal
Douglas(30)	NR	79% (11/14)	62% (40/65)	20% (10/51)
Cote (31)	70	33% (3/9)	24% (5/21)	15% (2/13)
Dorros (32)	57	60% (3/5)	43% (3/7)	31% (4/13)
Pinkerton (33)	92	33% (1/3)	60% (3/5)	40% (6/15)
Reeves (34)	94	64% (7/11)	63% (20/32)	36% (5/14)
Total		55% (46/84)	53% (80/150)	28% (37/130)

F/U, Follow-up; *NR*, not reported.

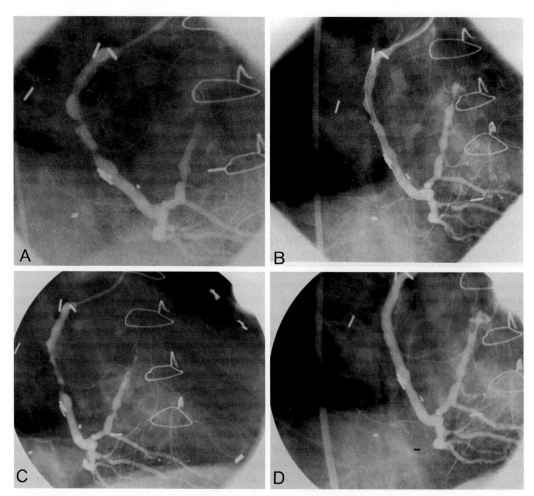

Figure 25.3.   A. A diffusely diseased RCA SVG before PTCA. **B.** Successful PTCA of the SVG was performed using a 4.0-mm balloon. **C.** Angiography 8 months later demonstrated restenosis of the SVG. **D.** Two Palmaz-Schatz biliary stents were successfully placed and dilated with a 5.0-mm balloon.

As discussed below, stenting of older SVGs may reduce the restenosis rate after PTCA, although there is a high probability of repeat intervention for treatment of progressive disease at other sites (35).

ENDOLUMINAL STENTING OF VENOUS BYPASS GRAFTS

A relatively recent development in the treatment of stenotic SVGs is the implantation of endoluminal stents (Fig. 25.3) (35–37). DeScheerder et al. (36) reported the results of 69 patients who underwent implantation of a total of 136 stents in 74 SVGs at four hospitals in The Netherlands and Belgium. The Medinvent Wallstent (Medinvent, Lausanne, Switzerland) was used in the first 26 patients, followed by the Medinvent Biogold stent in subsequent patients. Stent implantation was successful (<50% diameter stenosis) in all patients. Distal embolization was treated with intragraft infusion of thrombolytic drugs in two patients. Acute thrombotic events occurred in-hospital in seven patients. Bleeding complications occurred in 23 patients: two had fatal intracranial hemorrhages, one had a retroperitoneal hematoma, two had gastric bleeding, and 18 had hematomas at puncture sites. Follow-up angiography was performed at a mean of 4.9 months in 53 of the 59 patients who did not have major in-hospital complications. Restenosis, defined as diameter stenosis >50%, occurred in 25 of the 53 patients (47%), including total occlusion in three patients. Nineteen of the patients with restenosis underwent either repeat CABG (n = 7) or percutaneous intervention (n = 12) for recurrent angina.

Piana et al. (35) reported the results of stenting 200 SVG lesions in 150 patients. A total of 200 Palmaz-Schatz stents were implanted (146 coronary and 54 biliary). Deployment was successful in 197 of the 200 attempts (98.5%), reducing the mean diameter stenosis from 74 to 1%. Complications included 12 non–Q-wave MIs, two strokes, and two nonemergent CABGs, but only one death and no Q-wave MIs. Vascular complications were common: surgical repair was necessary in 14 of 164 procedures (8.5%), and an additional 23 patients (14%) required transfusion alone. Angiographic follow-up data were available for a cohort of the first 93 consecutive patients, which comprised 94 of 120 stented lesions (78%). Restenosis, defined as diameter stenosis ≥ 50%, was present in 17% of the lesions, which compares quite favorably with the published restenosis rates after PTCA. The estimated 2-year rate of target vessel failure was 34%, defined as late MI in the distribution of the vessel or a second revascularization (percutaneous or surgical) of the vessel. Hopefully, the low restenosis rate observed by Piana et al. (35) will be confirmed by an ongoing randomized trial of PTCA versus the Palmaz-Schatz stent for treatment of SVG stenoses. Nevertheless, the estimated 2-year rate of a second revascularization procedure over a follow-up period of 2 years after stent insertion was 49%, primarily for treatment of progressive disease at other sites.

Treatment of SVG stenoses with biliary stents was explored after the phase II studies of the Palmaz-Schatz coronary stent ended. The stainless steel filaments of the biliary stents are thicker (0.0040 inch or 0.0055 inch) than the filaments of the coronary stents (0.0025 inch), making the biliary stents more radiopaque and providing greater radial compressive force (37a). Also, the biliary stents are available in several lengths (10 mm, 15 mm, and 20 mm) and can be expanded to 9 mm, while the Palmaz-Schatz coronary stent is currently available in one length (15 mm) and its expansion limit is 5 mm. A disadvantage of the biliary stent is that it is more rigid and has a higher profile than the coronary stent and there is no protective sheath. Therefore successful deployment requires good guiding catheter support, adequate predilation of the stenosis, and hand-crimping of the stent on the delivery balloon.

Recently, Wong et al. (37a) published a comparative analysis of clinical and angiographic outcomes after SVG stenting with Johnson and Johnson coronary and biliary stents. Deployment of coronary stents was attempted in 110 patients with 146 SVG stenoses, and deployment of biliary stents was attempted in 124 patients with 163 SVG stenoses. Similar success and complication rates were observed. Deployment was unsuccessful in only three patients, two in the coronary stent group and one in the biliary stent group. The in-hospital complication rates for the coronary stent group were two deaths (1.9%), two Q-wave MIs (1.9%), no emergency CABG, and 16 non–Q-wave MIs (15%). For the biliary stent group, the complication rates were one death (0.8%), no Q-wave MIs, one emergency CABG (0.8%), and 13 non–Q-wave MIs (11%). Vascular repair was performed in 19 patients (8.4%), and transfusion was required in 55 patients (25%). The 6-month event-free survival rates were 77% for the coronary stent group and 80% for the biliary stent group ($P = .56$).

Stents may be especially useful for the treatment of aorto-ostial stenoses, which have a high rate of restenosis after conventional PTCA or directional atherectomy. Zampieri et al. (38) reported the successful stenting of five aorto-ostial SVG stenoses, with no cases of restenosis observed at follow-up angiography. However, in a series of 20 aorto-ostial SVG stenoses treated with Palmaz-Schatz coronary stents, restenosis occurred in seven grafts (35%) (38a). Successful treatment of aorto-ostial lesions may require "device synergy," using laser or atherectomy to debulk the lesion and allow full expansion of a stent.

Intracoronary ultrasound (IVUS) imaging has become an important tool in the deployment of stents in both native arteries and SVGs (39, 39a, 40). IVUS was performed after stenting in a series of 63 consecutive patients who underwent insertion of Palmaz-Schatz stents in native coronary arteries (40). Based on the IVUS observations, 80% of the lesions were judged to be underdilated and were treated with further dilation with larger balloons and/or higher inflation pressures. The angiographic minimum lumen diameter was 3.12 mm before IVUS and 3.61 mm after additional inflations were performed guided by the IVUS images. Mudra et al. (39a) reported the use of the Oracle Micro PTCA catheter, which is a combined intravascular ultrasound and PTCA balloon catheter (Endosonics Corp, Rancho Cordova, CA), to deploy Palmaz-Schatz coronary stents. Stent placement was successful in 18 of the 20 patients studied. Compared with angiography, IVUS revealed a smaller minimum lumen diameter within the stent. Additional inflations based on the IVUS observations resulted in a 40% increase in the minimum stent cross-sectional area. The studies suggest that IVUS imaging is useful during deployment of intracoronary stents to detect underexpansion of the stent and to choose an appropriately sized balloon to maximize the lumen within the stent. A catheter that combines IVUS and a noncompliant, high-pressure PTCA balloon might be especially useful for dilation after deployment of a stent.

Treatment of coronary and SVG stenoses with stents is evolving rapidly. Studies are in progress to determine whether high-pressure inflations with noncompliant PTCA balloons and IVUS-guided deployment of stents can obviate the need for aggressive anticoagulation, thereby reducing the risk of hemorrhage and vascular complications. Also, IVUS-guided stent deployment might decrease the incidence of subacute thrombosis or restenosis by reducing the frequency of inadequate stent expansion. Preliminary reports indicate that antiplatelet therapy alone (aspirin combined with ticlopidine) is associated with a low incidence of subacute thrombosis when optimal stent implantation is achieved using high balloon inflation pressures (40a, 40b), and that IVUS may not be necessary when stents are implanted using high balloon pressures (40b). Studies are in progress to compare aspirin versus ticlopidine without anti-coagulation after stenting (40c). Also, the stent designs that are under investigation may increase the feasibility of stenting long stenoses or diffusely diseased SVGs.

ATHERECTOMY OF VENOUS BYPASS GRAFTS

Directional Coronary Atherectomy (DCA)

Cowley and DiSciascio (41) reviewed the early use of DCA for SVG disease. The reported success rates have varied between 87% and 97%, and the major complication rates have ranged from 0 to 3.8% (41). High success rates can be expected for stenoses located in the SVG body, and DCA may be preferable for eccentric or complex lesions that are not well suited for PTCA. Distal anastomotic stenoses pose several technical problems: the size disparity of the graft and native vessel, bends at the point of insertion, and the need for shorter guide catheters (90 or 95 cm) to reach distal lesions. Aorto-ostial stenoses, which are notorious for their poor response to PTCA, are considered to be the most challenging location for DCA. Engagement of the guiding catheter and maintenance of coaxial alignment with the graft can be especially difficult with left coronary grafts that have horizontal or superiorly angled origins from the aorta. Cowley (41) suggested the use of a diagnostic angiographic catheter and exchange-length angioplasty guidewire to facilitate cannulation of ostial graft lesions. The use of stiffer angioplasty guidewires and predilation with a small PTCA balloon may facilitate crossing aorto-ostial stenoses with the DCA catheter. Given the technical challenges, it is not surprising that lower success rates and higher complication rates have been reported for DCA of aorto-ostial SVG lesions. A unique complication was reported by Kahn and Hartzler (42): the retrieval of suture fragments.

Hinohara et al. (43) reported high rates of restenosis after DCA of SVG stenoses. Angiographic follow-up data were obtained for 57 of 64 SVG stenoses successfully treated with DCA. The overall rate of restenosis, defined as >50% stenosis, was 63%. The restenosis rate was 73% for 11 ostial stenoses, compared with 61% for 46 lesions of the SVG body. After DCA of stenoses in the SVG body, the restenosis rate was lower for de novo lesions (52%; n = 23) than for restenotic lesions (70%; n = 23). Stephan et al. (44) reported the results of DCA for 54 ostial SVG stenoses. Based on an angiographic follow-up rate of 56%, the overall restenosis rate was 74%.

A lower rate of restenosis was observed in a series of patients treated at Beth Israel Hospital in Boston (45). During a 3-year period, 176 procedures were performed on SVG stenoses. The acute success rates were 88% for conventional PTCA (50/57), 94% for DCA (33/35), and 99% for Palmaz-Schatz stenting (83/84). There were no major complications (death, Q-wave MI, or emergent CABG) after either DCA or stenting. Angiographic follow-up was obtained for 78% (50/64) of the eligible patients. The rate of restenosis, defined as ≥50% stenosis, was 28% (5/18) for DCA, compared with 25% (8/32) for stenting.

The preliminary results of CAVEAT II, a randomized trial of PTCA versus DCA for the treatment of de novo vein graft stenoses, were presented at the 1993 Scientific Session of the American Heart Association. Three hundred five patients were enrolled at 56 centers in North America and Europe. The mean age of the grafts, the location of the target lesions, and the lesion morphology were similar for the two groups (Table 25.2). Predilation was necessary in 15% of the DCA procedures, and 22% required adjunctive PTCA after DCA, compared with a 4% rate of DCA in the patients randomized to PTCA. DCA was associated with higher rates of distal embolization, abrupt closure, and non–Q-wave MI (Tables 25.3 and 25.4). The QCA angiographic analysis revealed both a larger acute gain for DCA (1.46 mm) than for PTCA (1.12 mm) and a greater late loss (0.62 mm versus 0.52 mm), resulting in a net gain of 0.68 mm for DCA compared with 0.52 mm for PTCA. The 6-

Table 25.2.
CAVEAT II Graft Data

	DCA (n = 149)	PTCA (n = 156)
Graft age (yrs)	9.6	9.9
Lesion location		
Aortic anastomosis	14%	8%
Body	81%	92%
Distal anastomosis	5%	4%
Lesion morphology		
Eccentric	71.8%	70.5%
Irregular contour	29.5%	26.9%
Thrombus present	15.4%	18.0%

Table 25.3.
CAVEAT II Procedural Data

	DCA (%)	PTCA (%)
Thrombolytics	7	7
Complications		
Distal embolus	12	4
Dissection	13	19
Occlusion	3	2
Perforation	0.7	0
Visual success (<50% stenosis)	98.6	97.4
Final % stenosis	10	20

Table 25.4.
CAVEAT II Acute Clinical Data

	DCA n (%)	PTCA n (%)
Death	3 (2.0)	3 (1.9)
MI	24 (16.1)	17 (10.9)
Q-wave	2 (1.3)	3 (1.9)
CABG	1 (0.67)	2 (1.3)
Abrupt closure	7 (4.7)	4 (2.6)
Composite clinical Endpoints (death, MI, CABG, acute closure)	30 (20.1)	19 (12.2)

Table 25.5.
CAVEAT II Clinical Data Follow-up

	DCA (n = 149)	PTCA (n = 156)
Restenosis by QCA	45.5%	50.0%
MI	28 (18.8)	25 (16.0)
Q-wave	4 (2.7)	6 (3.8)
Repeat intervention	36 (24.2)	54 (34.6)
Death	8 (5.4)	12 (7.7)
Composite	60 (40.3)	78 (50.0)

month restenosis rates were not significantly different, 45.5% for DCA versus 50.0% for PTCA, but repeat intervention was more common in the PTCA group (Table 25.5).

Transluminal Extraction Atherectomy (TEC) (Figure 25.4)

Although DCA is an effective treatment for focal SVG lesions, the device may cause distal embolization if employed to treat diffusely diseased or degenerated SVGs. The TEC catheter has been advocated as a suitable device for use in SVGs because of its ability to aspirate clot and atheromatous material. Safian et al. (46) reported their experience with TEC in 146 consecutive patients with 158 SVG lesions. The average age of the grafts was 8.3 years, and the lesion morphology was characterized as focal or tubular in 83% of lesions and diffuse in 17%. Although the TEC device was successfully advanced through 144 lesions (91%), the minimal lumen diameter increased only from 0.9 ±

0.5 mm before TEC to 1.5 ± 0.7 mm after TEC, reflecting the relative undersizing of the TEC cutter compared with the reference diameter of the vein grafts (3.8 ± 0.9 mm). Therefore adjunctive PTCA was used after TEC in 144 lesions: to achieve a larger lumen in 115, to salvage technical failures in 14, and to manage no-reflow or abrupt closure after TEC in 15. The mean diameter stenosis was 75% ± 14% before TEC, 58% ± 20% after TEC, and 36% ± 22% after adjunctive PTCA.

The following angiographic complications occurred after TEC and before adjunctive PTCA: distal embolization in 18 (11.3%), severe dissection causing abrupt closure in eight (5%), and no-reflow in seven (4.4%). After adjunctive PTCA an angiographic complication persisted in 16% of cases: 10 no-reflow, five distal embolization, and one abrupt closure. There were three in-hospital deaths (2.0%), three Q-wave MIs (2.0%), four non–Q-wave MIs (2.7%), and four hemorrhagic strokes (2.7%). Vascular injury necessitated blood transfusion in seven patients (4.7%) and surgical repair in two patients (1.4%). Angiographic follow-up data were obtained in 105 of 132 eligible lesions (80%). The minimal lumen diameter measured by quantitative angiography was 1.3 ± 1.0 mm. Defined as a diameter stenosis >50%, restenosis occured in 72 of 105 lesions (69%), including total occlusion of the original target lesion in 30 (29%). The authors' have modified their technique in the presence of angiographic thrombus to emphasize use of large cutters and very slow cutter advancement to facilitate aspiration. Nonetheless, the high rates of angiographic

complications and restenosis are sobering, justifying the authors' conclusion that ". . . the application of TEC atherectomy to diffusely diseased and severely degenerated vein grafts should be used cautiously and only after repeat bypass surgery has been strongly considered."

The clinical significance of distal embolization was discussed in a report of 86 SVG lesions treated with TEC at the Washington Hospital Center (47). There were 11 instances of distal embolization, two after passage of the guidewire, two immediately after TEC, and seven after adjunct PTCA was used to treated a suboptimal result after TEC. In patients with distal embolization the mean

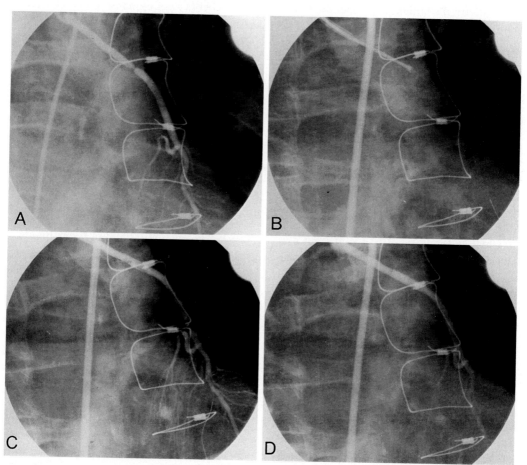

Figure 25.4. **A.** Angiogram of an LAD SVG before TEC. **B.** TEC was performed using a 7.5 Fr device. **C.** Adjunctive PTCA resulted in dissection of the SVG. **D.** Final angiogram after placement of a Palmaz-Schatz biliary stent.

age of the SVGs was 8.4 years, which was not significantly different from the mean age of the SVGs without distal embolization, 7.7 years. The presence of SVG thrombus before TEC was more common in patients with distal embolization than in those without distal embolization (82% versus 40%). Distal embolization was associated with higher rates of both minor and major complications. In patients with distal embolization, five of the 11 had major complications, with three deaths and two nonfatal Q-wave myocardial infarctions, and the remaining six patients had non–Q-wave myocardial infarctions. Patients without distal embolization had a major complication rate of 1.9% (1/54) and non–Q-wave MI occurred in 11% (6/54). Based on these observations, the authors have modified their approach to adjunct PTCA after TEC. Adjunct PTCA is performed immediately after TEC only to treat a residual stenosis >60% or a major angiographic complication. Otherwise, treatment of the residual stenosis with PTCA or a stent is delayed until anticoagulation with warfarin has been maintained for 1 to 4 weeks.

EXCIMER LASER CORONARY ANGIOPLASTY (ELCA) OF VENOUS BYPASS GRAFTS

As noted above, restenosis rates are very high after either PTCA or DCA of stenoses of the proximal anastomosis of SVGs. Recent data suggest that ELCA may be a suitable alternative treatment for such lesions (48, 49). The Percutaneous Excimer Laser Coronary Angioplasty Registry included a total of 495 patients who underwent treatment with ELCA for 545 SVG stenoses (49). Ostial lesions (n = 65) tended to have higher clinical success (95%) and lower complications (0%) than lesions in the body of the SVG. A multicenter registry of 200 patients included 59 cases of aorto-ostial SVG stenoses treated with ELCA (48). After ELCA and adjunctive PTCA, a final diameter stenosis ≤50% was achieved in 54 cases (91.5%). The following procedural complications were observed:

seven non–Q-MIs, 1 Q-wave MI, four embolizations, two extensive dissections, one perforation, and no deaths. Restenosis, defined as >50% diameter stenosis, was documented in 35% of SVGs, although angiographic follow-up was obtained in only 20 cases. Nevertheless, the data suggest that ELCA may be an option for treatment of aorto-ostial SVG stenoses.

ACUTE MI IN PATIENTS WITH PREVIOUS CABG

Patients with previous CABG constituted 12% of the total population of 614 patients who underwent PTCA as the primary treatment for acute MI at the Mid America Heart Institute (50). Acute MI in patients with previous CABG is often caused by SVG thrombosis. Kahn et al. (50) identified the infarct artery as an SVG in 48 patients (67%) and a native coronary artery in 24 patients (33%) in their series of 72 patients with acute MI and previous CABG. Similar data were reported by Grines et al. (51) who reviewed 50 cases of acute MI >1 year after CABG who underwent either angiography (n = 46) or autopsy (n = 4) within 1 week of the acute MI. The infarct artery was identified as an SVG in 38 patients (76%), a native artery in eight patients (16%), and indeterminate in four patients (8%).

There are limited data regarding intravenous thrombolytic therapy for acute MI in patients with previous CABG because these patients have been excluded from many of the thrombolytic trials. Grines et al. (51) reported that only two of eight grafts were successfully reperfused after intravenous thrombolytic therapy, while graft patency was restored by intragraft infusion of a thrombolytic drug in eight of the 10 grafts. Kahn et al. (50) employed primary PTCA as the initial therapeutic strategy for treatment of acute MI in patients with previous CABG. PTCA was successful in 41 of 48 (85%) grafts. Patency was documented in 25 of 27 vein grafts that were restudied before hospital discharge. The two reocclusions were asymptomatic. Thus pre-

Table 25.6.
Recommendations for Percutaneous Intervention in SVG Disease

PTCA—stenosis of distal anastomosis or stenosis in younger SVG
Stent—discrete stenosis of SVG body or aorto-ostial stenosis
DCA—discrete, bulky, complex, or eccentric stenosis of SVG body
ELCA—aorto-ostial stenosis
TEC—discrete stenosis of body with associated thrombus
Thrombolysis—extensive thrombosis
CABG—diffusely diseased or degenerated SVG

liminary data support an invasive approach to the management of acute MI in patients with previous CABG, with emergency angiography to identify the infarct artery, and PTCA if appropriate.

TREATMENT ALGORITHM FOR DISEASED VEIN GRAFTS

Based on the information reviewed in this chapter, we recommend the following approach for the treatment of diseased SVGs (Table 25.6). The operator should always consider the option of preserving the native circulation by dilating the native, grafted artery before performing an intervention in an SVG. PTCA should provide high initial success and long-term patency rates for stenoses of the distal anastomosis, especially those that occur within the first postoperative year. Stents are emerging as the treatment of choice for discrete stenoses involving the body of SVGs, with high success rates and acceptable complication and restenosis rates. There is no ideal approach to the treatment of aorto-ostial lesions, although the excimer laser and possibly stenting may be tried in patients who are considered to be poor candidates for reoperation. Directional atherectomy may be optimal for smooth, eccentric, bulky lesions in SVGs that are less than 3 years old. We reserve TEC for treatment of stenoses with angiographic evidence of thrombus. Alternatively, adjunctive urokinase infusion may be attempted to reduce the risk of distal embolization. Finally, reoperation should always be considered

before attempting percutaneous revascularization. The data suggest that the natural history of SVG disease is altered little by percutaneous interventions and may be considered as end-stage disease that can only be palliated for a while. CABG should be the treatment of choice in patients with diffusely diseased or degenerated grafts who have suitable conduits and distal targets and no other contraindications to surgery. "Heroic" attempts to salvage degenerated grafts should be confined to patients who are not candidates for repeat CABG because of, for example, inadequate conduits, severe left ventricular dysfunction, or other medical conditions.

REFERENCES

1. Nwasokwa ON, Koss JH, Friedman GH, Grunwald AM, Bodenheimer MM. Bypass surgery for chronic stable angina: predictors of survival benefit and strategy for patient selection. Ann Intern Med 1991;114:1035–1049.
2. Campeau L, Lesperance J, Hermann J, Corbara F, Grondin CM, Bourassa MG. Loss of the improvement of angina between 1 and 7 years after aortocoronary bypass surgery. Circulation 1979;60:I-1–I-5.
3. Loop FD, Lytle BW, Cosgrove DM et al. Influence of the internal-mammary-artery graft on 10-year survival and other cardiac events. N Engl J Med 1986;314:1–6.
4. Cox JL, Chiasson DA, Gotlieb AI. Stranger in a strange land: the pathogenesis of saphenous vein graft stenosis with emphasis on structural and functional differences between veins and arteries. Prog Cardiovasc Dis 1991;34:45–68.
5. Vlodaver Z, Edwards JE. Pathologic analysis in fatal cases following saphenous vein coronary arterial bypass. Chest 1973;64:555–563.
6. Chesebro JH, Clements IP, Fuster V et al. A platelet-inhibitor-drug trial in coronary-artery bypass operations. N Engl J Med 1982;307:73–80.
7. Goldman S, Copeland J, Moritz T et al. Improvement in early saphenous vein graft patency after coronary artery bypass surgery with antiplatelet therapy: results of a Veterans Administration cooperation study. Circulation 1988; 77:1324–1332.
8. Chesebro JH, Fuster V, Elveback LR et al. Effect of dipyridamole and aspirin on late vein-graft patency after coronary bypass operations. N Engl J Med 1984;310:209–214.
9. Goldman S, Copeland J, Moritz T et al. Saphenous vein graft patency 1 year after coronary artery bypass surgery and effects of antiplatelet therapy. Circulation 1989; 80:1190–1197.
10. Walts AE, Fishbein MC, Matloff JM. Thrombosed, ruptured atheromatous plaques in saphenous vein coronary artery bypass grafts: ten years' experience. Am Heart J 1987; 114:718–723.

11. Kalan JM, Roberts WC. Morphologic findings in saphenous veins used as coronary arterial bypass conduits for longer than 1 year: necropsy analysis of 53 patients, 123 saphenous veins, and 1865 five-millimeter segments of veins. Am Heart J 1990;119:1164–1184.

12. The VA Coronary Artery Bypass Surgery Cooperative Study Group. Eighteen-year follow-up in the veterans affairs cooperative study of coronary artery bypass surgery for stable angina. Circulation 1992;86:121–130.

13. Campeau L, Enjalbert M, Lesperance J et al. The relation of risk factors to the development of atherosclerosis in saphenous-vein bypass grafts and the progression of disease in the native circulation. N Engl J Med 1984;311:1329–1332.

14. Blankenhorn DH, Nessim SA, Johnson RL, Sanmarco ME, Azen SP, Cashin-Hemphill L. Beneficial effects of combined colestipol-niacin therapy on coronary atherosclerosis and coronary venous bypass grafts. JAMA 1987; 257:3233–3240.

15. Cashin-Hemphill L, Mack WJ, Pogoda JM, Sanmarco ME, Azen SP, Blankenhorn DH. Beneficial effects of colestipol-niacin on coronary atherosclerosis. JAMA 1990;264:3013–3017.

16. Campos EE, Cinderella JA, Farhi ER. Long-term angiographic follow-up of normal and minimally diseased saphenous vein grafts. J Am Coll Cardiol 1993;21:1175–1180.

17. Lytle BW, Loop FD, Taylor PC et al. Vein graft disease: the clinical impact of stenoses in saphenous vein bypass grafts to coronary arteries. J Thorac Cardiovasc Surg 1992;103:831–840.

18. Douglas JS. Percutaneous intervention in patients with prior coronary bypass surgery. In: Topol EJ, ed. Textbook of interventional cardiology. 2nd ed., 1993.

19. Platko WP, Hollman J, Whitlow PL, Franco I. Percutaneous transluminal angioplasty of saphenous vein graft stenosis: long-term follow-up. J Am Coll Cardiol 1989;14:1645–1650.

20. Plokker HWT, Meester BH, Serruys, PW. The Dutch experience in percutaneous transluminal angioplasty of narrowed saphenous veins used for aortocoronary arterial bypass. Am J Cardiol 1991;67:361–366.

21. Webb JG, Myler RK, Shaw RE et al. Coronary angioplasty after coronary bypass surgery: initial results and late outcome in 422 patients. J Am Coll Cardiol 1990;16:812–820.

22. deFeyter PJ, van Suylen R, de Jaegere P, Topol EJ, Serruys PW. Balloon angioplasty for the treatment of lesions in saphenous vein bypass grafts. J Am Coll Cardiol 1993;21:1539–1549.

23. Chapekis AT, George BS, Candela RJ. Rapid thrombus dissolution by continuous infusion of urokinase through an intracoronary perfusion wire prior to and following PTCA: results in native coronaries and patent saphenous vein grafts. Catheterization and Cardiovascular Diagnosis 1991;23:89–92.

24. Saber RS, Edwards WD, Holmes DR, Vlietstra RE, Reeder GS. Balloon angioplasty of aortocoronary saphenous vein bypass grafts: a histopathologic study of six grafts from five patients, with emphasis on restenosis and embolic complications. J Am Coll Cardiol 1988;12:1501–1509.

25. Weintraub WS, Cohen CL, Curling PE et al. Results of coronary surgery after failed elective coronary angioplasty in patients with prior coronary surgery. J Am Coll Cardiol 1990;16:1341–1347.

26. Morrison DA, Crowley ST, Veerakul G, Barbiere CC, Grover F, Sacks J. Percutaneous transluminal angioplasty of saphenous vein grafts for medically refractory unstable angina. J Am Coll Cardiol 1994;23:1066–1070.

27. deFeyter PJ, Serruys P, van den Brand M, Meester H, Beatt K, Suryapranata H. Percutaneous transluminal angioplasty of a totally occluded venous bypass graft: a challenge that should be resisted. Am J Cardiol 1989;64:88–90.

28. Kahn JK, Rutherford BD, McConahay DR et al. Initial and long-term outcome of 83 patients after balloon angioplasty of totally occluded bypass grafts. J Am Coll Cardiol 1994;23:1038–1042.

29. Hartmann JR, McKeever LS, Stamato NJ et al. Recanalization of chronically occluded aortocoronary saphenous vein bypass grafts by extended infusion of urokinase: initial results and short-term clinical follow-up. J Am Coll Cardiol 1991;18:1517–1523.

30. Douglas JS. Angioplasty of saphenous vein and internal mammary artery bypass grafts. In: Topol EJ, ed. Textbook of interventional cardiology. 1990.

31. Cote G, Myler RK, Stertzer SH et al. Percutaneous transluminal angioplasty of stenotic coronary artery bypass grafts: 5 years' experience. J Am Coll Cardiol 1987;9:8–17.

32. Dorros G, Lewin RF, Mathiak LM et al. Percutaneous transluminal coronary angioplasty in patients with two or more previous coronary artery bypass grafting operations. Am J Cardiol 1988;61:1243–1247.

33. Pinkerton CA, Slack JD, Orr CM, van Tassel JW, Smith ML. Percutaneous transluminal angioplasty in patients with prior myocardial revascularization surgery. Am J Cardiol 1988;61:15G–22G.

34. Reeves F, Bonan R, Cote G et al. Long-term angiographic follow-up after angioplasty of venous coronary bypass grafts. Am Heart J 1991;122:620–627.

35. Piana RN, Moscucci M, Cohen DJ et al. Palmaz-Schatz stenting for treatment of focal vein graft stenosis: immediate results and long-term outcome. J Am Coll Cardiol 1994;23:1296–1304.

36. De Scheerder IK, Strauss BH, De Feyter PJ et al. Stenting of venous bypass grafts: a new treatment modality for patients who are poor candidates for reintervention. Am Heart J 1992;123:1046–1054.

37. Strumpf RK, Mehta SS, Ponder R, Heuser RR. Palmaz-Schatz stent implantation in stenosed saphenous vein grafts: clinical and angiographic follow-up. Am Heart J 1992;123:1329–1336.

37a. Wong SC, Popma JJ, Pichard AD et al. Comparison of clinical and angiographic outcomes after saphenous vein graft angioplasty using coronary versus "biliary" tubular slotted stents. Circulation 1995;91:339–350.

38. Zampieri P, Colombo A, Almagor Y, Maiello L, Finci L. Results of coronary stenting of ostial lesions. Am J Cardiol 1994;73:901–903.

38a. Rocha-Singh K, Morris N, Wong SC et al. Coronary stenting for treatment of ostial stenoses of native coronary arteries or aortocoronary saphenous venous grafts. Am J Cardiol 1995;75:26–29.

39. Keren G, Douek P, Oblon C, Bonner RF, Pichard AD, Leon MB. Atherosclerotic saphenous vein grafts treated with different interventional procedures assessed by intravascular ultrasound. Am Heart J 1992;124:198–206.

39a. Mudra H, Klauss V, Blasini R et al. Ultrasound guidance of Palmaz-Schatz intracoronary stenting with a combined intravascular ultrasound balloon catheter. Circulation 1994;90:1252–1261.

40. Nakamura S, Colombo A, Gaglione A et al. Intracoronary ultrasound observations during stent implantation. Circulation 1994;89:2026–2034.

40a. Wong SC, Popma J, Mintz G et al. Preliminary results from the reduced anticoagulation in saphenous vein graft stent (RAVES) Trial. Circulation 1994;90:I-124 (abstract).

40b. Gaglione A, Tiecco F, Hall P et al. High-pressure–assisted intracoronary stent implantation without subsequent anticoagulation. Circulation 1994;90:I-622 (abstract).

40c. Blengino S, Maiello L, Hall P et al. Randomized trial of coronary stent implantation without anticoagulation: aspirin vs ticlopidine. Circulation 1994;90:I-124 (abstract).

41. Cowley MJ, DiSciascio G. Directional coronary atherectomy for saphenous vein graft disease. Cathet Cardiovasc Diagn 1993;1(Suppl):10–16.

42. Kahn JK, Hartzler GO. Retrieval of vein graft suture fragments with directional coronary atherectomy: a note of caution. Am Heart J 1990;120:692–696.

43. Hinohara T, Robertson GC, Selmon MR et al. Restenosis after directional coronary atherectomy. J Am Coll Cardiol 1992;20:623–632.

44. Stephan WJ, Bates ER, Garrett K, Muller DWM. Directional coronary atherectomy of ostial stenoses. Circulation 1993;88:I-496.

45. Pomerantz RM, Kuntz RE, Carrozza JP et al. Acute and long-term outcome of narrowed saphenous venous grafts treated by endoluminal stenting and directional atherectomy. Am J Cardiol 1992;70:161–167.

46. Safian RD, Grines CL, May MA et al: Clinical and angiographic results of transluminal extraction coronary atherectomy in saphenous vein bypass grafts. Circulation 1994;89:302–312.

47. Hong MK, Popma JJ, Pichard AD et al. Clinical significance of distal embolization after transluminal extraction atherectomy in diffusely diseased saphenous vein grafts. Am Heart J 1994;127:1496–1503.

48. Eigler NL, Weinstock B, Douglas JS et al. Excimer laser coronary angioplasty of aorto-ostial stenoses. Circulation 1993;88(1):2049–2057.

49. Bittl JA, Sanborn TA, Yardley DE et al. Predictors of outcome of percutaneous excimer laser coronary angioplasty of saphenous vein bypass graft lesions. Am J Cardiol 1994;74:144–148.

50. Kahn JK, Rutherford BD, McConahay DR et al. Usefulness of angioplasty during acute myocardial infarction in patients with prior coronary artery bypass grafting. Am J Cardiol 1990;65:698–702.

51. Grines CL, Booth DC, Nissen SE et al. Mechanism of acute myocardial infarction in patients with prior coronary artery bypass grafting and therapeutic implications. Am J Cardiol 1990;65:1292–1296.

EDITORIAL SUMMARY

The treatment of vein graft disease remains problematic for several reasons including the following: (a) the underlying pathophysiology, particularly of older vein grafts (in older vein grafts, the atheromatous material is particularly friable leading to an increased incidence of embolization); (b) the presence of multivessel disease; (c) the fact that the patient has already undergone CABG makes repeat urgent CABG surgery more difficult if an acute complication arises; and (d) restenosis.

The specific approach depends on consideration of these factors. Matching the specific device to the specific lesion is important for optimizing outcome. The lesions should be categorized as (a) discrete (realizing that pathologically old vein grafts rarely have isolated discrete lesions) or diffuse, and (b) by their location—ostial, shaft, or distal anastomosis. Other considerations include the size of the vein graft and the distal bed.

For discrete lesions, conventional PTCA, directional atherectomy, and stents can all result in good initial success rates. Directional atherectomy gives larger initial minimal luminal diameter than PTCA, particularly in ostial lesions; this does not translate into statistically significant differences in restenosis. Stents also give larger initial minimal luminal diameter. Preliminary data suggest that restenosis rates may be decreased. There is currently a randomized trial comparing PTCA and stents for vein graft disease.

For diffuse disease, TEC has been used in addition to laser and long balloon dilation. In this setting of diffuse disease, distal embolization rates are definitely increased. There is increasing interest in one specific stent configuration (Wallstent). These self-expanding stents are long enough to cross long segments of diseased vein grafts and may improve results.

Lesion location also plays an important role. Ostial lesions dilate poorly. Alternative techniques have been studied, most prominently eccentric laser, directional atherectomy, and stenting. Although these techniques give better initial results, restenosis rates remain substantially increased. For shaft lesions, device selection depends on lesion length, vide supra. Finally, anastomotic lesions are the most favorable. Discrete lesions in this location are very well treated with conventional PTCA with low restenosis rates.

26. Complete Versus Incomplete Revascularization

A. Complete Versus Incomplete Revascularization After PTCA

MARTIAL G. BOURASSA

Percutaneous transluminal coronary angioplasty (PTCA) is performed more and more frequently in patients seeking care for severe manifestations of multivessel coronary artery disease (CAD) (1). The majority of these patients previously underwent coronary artery bypass grafting (CABG). In patients in whom complete revascularization is planned and has a reasonable likelihood of success following PTCA, this procedure can be a less invasive and less costly alternative to CABG. However, complete revascularization is not possible or not planned in many of these patients, and therefore the value of this common PTCA strategy deserves further scrutiny.

DEFINITION OF COMPLETE REVASCULARIZATION

In previous reports (2) multivessel CAD is usually defined as 50% or greater luminal diameter stenosis in two or three major coronary territories, that is, areas of myocardium supplied by vessels with a diameter of 1.5 mm or greater. In a given patient with multivessel CAD, complete revascularization is achieved if all significant lesions are reduced to less than 50% luminal diameter stenosis following PTCA.

INCIDENCE OF INCOMPLETE REVASCULARIZATION

The proportion of patients undergoing PTCA for the treatment of multivessel CAD in North America in the 1990s varies widely according to the experience and preference of clinicians, angioplasty operators, and cardiac surgeons in different institutions. However, it can be estimated that patients with double or triple vessel CAD represent over one-half of the patients currently undergoing PTCA in major cardiovascular centers (1). In more than half of these patients, complete revascularization is not intended nor achieved after PTCA (2). This approach is quite different from that which has guided the practice of CABG where complete revascularization has traditionally been viewed as an important objective to achieve optimal early and late results (3–5).

The most important factor influencing the degree of revascularization after PTCA is whether partial revascularization is planned prior to the procedure.

In the 1985–1986 NHLBI PTCA Registry (6–7), the angioplasty operator was asked prior to the procedure to describe his treatment plan for each significant lesion as one of the following: PTCA amenable and intend to dilate, PTCA amenable but do not intend to dilate, and not PTCA amenable. After the procedure he described the outcome in terms of which intended lesions were attempted and which among them were successfully dilated.

This led to a classification of the patients into five subgroups (Fig. 26A.1):

1. Patients in whom not all lesions were amenable to PTCA.
2. Patients in whom all lesions were amenable but PTCA was not intended for all of them.

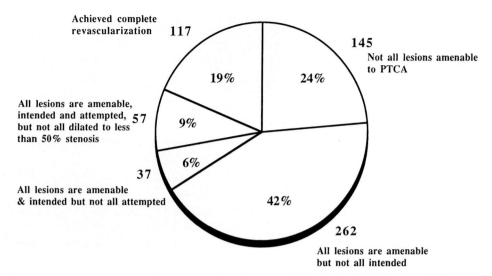

Figure 26A.1. Operator strategy and reasons for incomplete revascularization for the total group of 618 patients with multivessel coronary artery disease in the 1985–1986 NHLBI PTCA Registry. (Reprinted with permission from Bourassa MG, Holubkov R, Yeh W, Detre KM. Am J Cardiol 1992;70:174–178.)

3. Patients in whom all lesions were amenable and intended but not all were actually attempted.
4. Patients in whom all lesions were amenable, intended, and attempted but not all were dilated to less than 50% stenosis.
5. Patients in whom complete revascularization was achieved.

Complete correction was not intended in two-thirds of these patients; it was not possible in 24%, and although it was theoretically possible, the angioplasty operator did not plan to achieve complete revascularization in 42%. Thus complete correction was planned in only one-third of the patients with multivessel CAD in the registry. It was achieved in 19%, whereas in 6% some lesions were not attempted, and in 9% some lesions could not be dilated successfully. Overall, in more than 80% of the patients in whom complete revascularization was not achieved, it had not been planned in the first place.

In other recent reports (2) the incidence of complete revascularization in patients with multivessel CAD undergoing PTCA was higher, ranging from 32 to 58%. However, even among the different clinical sites participating in the NHLBI PTCA registry, there was a wide variability in operator strategy and

outcome. The frequency with which complete revascularization was intended ranged from 8 to 61%, and the frequency with which it was achieved ranged from 0 to 38% (7).

Overall, in the NHLBI PTCA registry, complete revascularization was achieved in 67% of the patients in whom it was planned and attempted. These rates were comparable for patients with double- and triple-vessel CAD (68% and 62%, respectively) (7).

Thus the incidence of complete revascularization in patients with multivessel CAD varies widely depending on patient selection and more importantly on whether it is planned. It is usually not planned in a large proportion of patients, and when it is planned and attempted, it is achieved in most patients irrespective of whether they have double- or triple-vessel CAD.

CLINICAL AND ANGIOGRAPHIC FACTORS INFLUENCING COMPLETE REVASCULARIZATION

Patients with multivessel CAD and incomplete revascularization following PTCA have significantly worse baseline clinical characteristics than those in whom complete re-

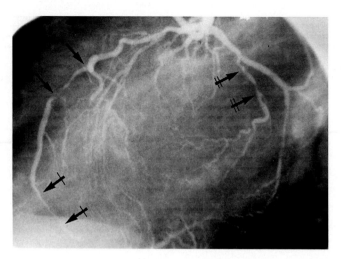

Figure 26A.2. Cineangiogram of a patient with multivessel coronary artery disease in whom coronary anatomy was judged not to be technically suitable for PTCA because of excessive length of the stenosis of the mid left anterior descending artery (→); diffuse disease of the distal left anterior descending artery (→); excessive length of the narrowing of the second marginal branch of the left circumflex artery (→); and chronic right coronary artery occlusion with collaterals from the left anterior descending artery system to the distal right coronary artery.

vascularization is achieved (8, 9). In general, they are older, they are more often female and they have more unstable angina, left ventricular dysfunction, triple-vessel CAD, and urgent/emergent PTCA. However, these unfavorable clinical characteristics are seen primarily in patients in whom complete revascularization is not intended. Particularly, unstable angina, triple-vessel CAD, and urgent/emergent revascularization are strong predictors, in multivariate analysis, of whether incomplete revascularization is planned before PTCA (9). Patients with recent myocardial infarction were excluded from this analysis. However, we know that incomplete revascularization is almost routinely planned in these patients prior to PTCA. Thus it is most often in these higher-risk patients with multivessel CAD that incomplete revascularization is planned prior to the procedure.

Among the angiographic factors, chronic total occlusions and adverse stenosis morphology are usually the major reasons why patients with multivessel CAD are judged not to be amenable to complete revascularization prior to PTCA.

In the NHLBI PTCA Registry, only 63% of total occlusions were considered amenable to PTCA and only 54% of those attempted were successfully dilated (7).

In the Bypass Angioplasty Revascularization Investigation (BARI), the three major angiographic factors (not mutually exclusive) why patients with multivessel CAD were not technically suitable for PTCA were chronic total occlusions, diffuse CAD, and excessive lesion length (10) (Fig. 26A.2). Total occlusions were present in 68% of the patients, diffuse CAD in 32%, and excessive lesion length in 26%. Excessive calcification and excessive angulation each accounted for 5% of the exclusions and excessive tortuosity for 3%.

Stenosis severity, on the other hand, is a major factor influencing whether PTCA is intended in patients with multivessel CAD (7). Among the lesions suitable for PTCA in the NHLBI PTCA registry, the procedure was planned for only 38% of 50 to 69% stenoses, compared with 80% of 70 to 89% narrowings, and over 85% of 90 to 99% narrowings. Overall, 93% of all stenoses in which the operator intended to perform PTCA were actually attempted. As expected, successful dilatation was inversely related to the initial severity of the stenosis: 94% for 50 to 69% narrowings, 86% for 70 to 89% narrowings, and 79% for 90 to 99% narrowings.

Lesion location is also a significant factor influencing whether PTCA is intended (7). PTCA is most frequently planned for lesions of the right coronary artery (80% of the lesions), compared with 70% for the left anterior descending artery and 65% for the left circumflex artery.

Thus complete revascularization is not planned in many patients with multivessel CAD undergoing PTCA because it is precluded by the presence of chronic total occlusions, diffuse CAD, or excessive lesion length. It is also often not planned, although it would be possible, in patients with less than severe (50 to 69%) coronary narrowings, presumably because of the risk of abrupt closure or severe restenosis in these lesions of borderline clinical significance.

PROGNOSIS OF INCOMPLETE REVASCULARIZATION

Several recent studies have described the early outcome of PTCA in patients with multivessel CAD (1, 2). These reports show that, although the risk of the procedure is significantly higher than in patients with single vessel CAD, PTCA can be achieved with a high initial success rate and a relatively low incidence of major complications in patients with multivessel CAD. In the 1985–1986 NHLBI PTCA Registry, over 90% of attempted lesions were successfully dilated, and the major in-hospital events included death, 1.6%; myocardial infarction, 5.5%; and emergency CABG, 4.4% (11). When patients with incomplete revascularization were compared with those with complete correction, there was no significant difference in procedure-related mortality and incidence of myocardial infarction between the two groups. However, emergency CABG was significantly more frequent in patients without than in patients with complete revascularization.

After adjustment for major differences in baseline characteristics, patients in whom complete revascularization was not planned prior to the procedure did not have more in-hospital events than those in whom it was planned and achieved (unpublished data). However, patients in whom complete revascularization was planned but not achieved had a significantly higher incidence of in-hospital complications. This was particularly true, of course, in the subgroup of patients in whom complete revascularization was planned but not attempted because of procedural complications.

This provides a strong argument for deliberately choosing not to attempt complete revascularization prior to PTCA in higher-risk patients with multivessel CAD.

The most important issue then is the long-term outcome of patients in whom complete revascularization is not intended prior to PTCA. Is it comparable or significantly worse than that of patients in whom complete correction is intended, attempted, and achieved?

The currently available midterm data comparing complete versus incomplete revascularization after PTCA in patients with multivessel CAD are controversial (2). Some reports suggest that there is no difference in outcome, whereas others show a significantly higher incidence of events in patients with incomplete revascularization from 1 to several years after the procedure.

In the 1985–1986 NHLBI PTCA Registry, the 5-year follow-up events after PTCA in patients with multivessel CAD included deaths, 10.4%; late myocardial infarctions, 8.6%; recurrent angina, 16.2%; repeat PTCA, 26.4%; and CABG, 21.8% (11). Of these only recurrent angina and CABG were significantly more frequent in patients without than in those with complete revascularization. After adjustment for the prognostic influence of several major baseline characteristics, incomplete revascularization remained a major correlate of increased late CABG after PTCA. This was true in patients in whom complete correction was not intended prior to PTCA, as well as in those in whom it was planned but not achieved (11). However, patients in whom complete revascularization was intended but not attempted had a higher frequency of all events at 5 years.

Although these reports suggest that incomplete revascularization, when it is planned prior to PTCA, may be an acceptable alternative to more complete correction following CABG, they do not allow us to reach any definitive conclusions. All of these studies are retrospective, based on highly selected subsets of patients, and they all suffer from a severe lack of power. Only prospective, controlled studies will provide the appropriate answers. Fortunately, at least five large-scale randomized clinical trials are currently in progress (12). They will not provide all the answers, and additional studies will be needed to answer more specific questions, for example, is single-vessel PTCA acceptable in patients with unstable angina and multivessel CAD? Nevertheless, studies such as BARI, which only requires optimal, not necessarily complete, revascularization, will be very helpful (10).

SUMMARY

Incomplete revascularization is often part of the PTCA strategy and can usually be predicted prior to the procedure in patients with multivessel CAD. When complete revascularization is planned in these patients, it is usually achieved. Patients with incomplete revascularization are typically older, female, and suffering from unstable angina, recent myocardial infarction, severe left ventricular dysfunction, or triple-vessel CAD or requiring urgent/emergent PTCA. Angiographically, complete correction is often not possible because of chronic total occlusions or adverse stenosis morphology (diffuse or distal CAD, excessive lesion length, etc.) or simply not planned in the presence of less than severe (50 to 69%) coronary narrowings. Incomplete revascularization, particularly when it is planned prior to PTCA, is associated with a higher incidence of CABG but not of death, myocardial infarction, or repeat PTCA early and late after the intervention. However, these results will have to be confirmed by long-term, prospective, controlled studies.

REFERENCES

1. Detre K, Holubkov R, Kelsey S, Cowley M, Kent K, Williams D, Myler R et al. Percutaneous transluminal coronary angioplasty in 1985–1986 and 1977–1981. The National Heart, Lung, and Blood Institute Registry. N Engl J Med 1988;318:265–270.
2. De Feyter PJ. PTCA in patients with stable angina pectoris and multivessel disease: Is incomplete revascularization acceptable? Clin Cardiol 1992;15:317–322.
3. Tyras DH, Barner HB, Kaiser GC, Codd JE, Laks H, Pennington DG, William VL. Long-term results of myocardial revascularization. Am J Cardiol 1979;44:1290–1296.
4. Cukingnam RA, Carey JS, Wittig JH, Brown BG. Influence of complete coronary revascularization on relief of angina. J Thorac Cardiovasc Surg 1980;79:188–193.
5. Jones EL, Craver JM, Guyton RA, Bone DK, Hatcher CR Jr, Riechward N. Importance of complete revascularization in performance of the coronary bypass operation. Am J Cardiol 1983;51:7–12.
6. Bourassa MG, Holubkov R, Detre KM, Wilson J. Complete revascularization in patients with multivessel coronary disease: an uncommon outcome. J Am Coll Cardiol 1991;17:113A.
7. Bourassa MG, Holubkov R, Yeh W, Detre KM. Strategy of complete revascularization in patients with multivessel coronary artery disease (A report from the 1985–1986 NHLBI PTCA Registry). Am J Cardiol 1992;70:174–178.
8. Reeder GS, Holmes DR, Detre K, Costigan T, Kelsey SF. Degree of revascularization in patients with multivessel coronary disease: a report from the National Heart, Lung, and Blood Institute Percutaneous Transluminal Coronary Angioplasty Registry. Circulation 1988;77:638–644.
9. Bourassa MG, Yeh W, Holubkov R, Detre KM. Incomplete revascularization (ICR) after multivessel PTCA. J Am Coll Cardiol 1992;19:139A.
10. Bourassa MG, Roubin GS, Detre KM, Sopko G, Krone RJ, Attabuto MJ, Bjerregaad P et al. Bypass Angioplasty Revascularization Investigation (BARI): patient screening, selection and recruitment. Am J Cardiol (in press).
11. Bourassa MG, Yeh W, Holubkov R, Detre KM. Long-term prognosis of complete revascularization after multivessel PTCA. Circulation 1992;86:I-54.
12. BARI, CABRI, EAST, GABI, and RITA. Coronary angioplasty on trial. Lancet 1990;335:1315–1316 editorial.

B. Complete Versus Incomplete Revascularization

DAVID P. FAXON

Coronary angioplasty is the most frequently performed revascularization procedure in the United States, now approaching nearly 350,000 cases per year (1). Its growth is in part the result of increased operator experience and improved relevant technology, which has permitted the use of angioplasty in multivessel coronary disease. Angioplasty in the setting of multivessel disease frequently results in incomplete revascularization either through failure of the procedure or, more commonly, as a result of a strategy of dilating the clinically important lesions and leaving others behind. This strategy of culprit lesion angioplasty has resulted in a larger number of patients who now undergo the procedure, but the long-term benefits and risks of this strategy remain unclear.

BACKGROUND

In the early days of coronary bypass surgery, incomplete revascularization was not infrequent. Surgical studies comparing the long-term outcome of complete revascularization with that of incomplete revascularization demonstrated a less favorable long-term outcome, with a higher mortality and less relief of symptoms (2–4). In addition, early graft closure is associated with a poorer long-term outcome. Based on these studies, the current surgical strategy has been to revascularize all major coronary territories. However, extrapolation of the results of bypass surgery to coronary angioplasty is probably not justified. First of all, bypass surgery is defined as being complete when all large epicardial vessels have been bypassed. However, the actual success of the bypass is not assessed by angiography, and a small percentage of bypass grafts are known to occlude early. Also, the early studies looking at the completeness of revascularization did not factor in the importance of the coronary stenosis, its location, nor the magnitude of the ischemic territory. Since the risk of the procedure is not significantly influenced bypassing a larger number of vessels, there is no reason not to completely revascularize a patient surgically. Finally, the prior surgical studies comparing complete revascularization with incomplete revascularization were not randomized, and frequently patients who had incomplete revasculariza-

tion had diffusely diseased or nonbypassable vessels, placing them in a high-risk subgroup of patients who are likely to fare less well. To date, no randomized comparison of bypass patients has been conducted to truly demonstrate that incomplete revascularization results in a less favorable outcome.

The other problem with prior surgical studies, as well as angioplasty studies, is the definition of incomplete revascularization. While most authors suggest that it should be defined as the presence of a significant residual stenosis of more than 50% in an artery of greater than 1.5 mm in diameter, some studies have used a 70% cutoff, the successful dilation of all attempted stenoses but not all lesions, the successful dilation of all proximal stenoses, or dilation of all vessels serving a significant amount of residual myocardium. In fact, there are at least 17 definitions of adequate revascularization in the literature, yet in only one study, that by Cowley and colleagues, has the predictive value of these definitions been tested (5).

There are a number of potential advantages to incomplete revascularization. First, incomplete revascularization can treat a culprit lesion that may be principally responsible for the patient's anginal symptoms. The concept of culprit angioplasty was first introduced by Wohlgelernter and colleagues (6). They described the efficacy of single-vessel percutaneous transluminal coronary angioplasty (PTCA) in 27 patients with unstable angina. In three-quarters of the patients a culprit lesion could be identified either by distribution of the electrocardiogram (ECG) changes or the anatomic features of the lesion. All were successfully treated by angioplasty. The follow-up showed an excellent long-term outcome. Unfortunately, this concept of culprit lesion angioplasty has been expanded by some to apply not only to unstable angina, but to all patients undergoing angioplasty. In addition, while a culprit lesion was adequately identified in Wohlgelernter's study in three-quarters of the patients, in a larger series of patients with unstable angina studied by Ambrose, a culprit lesion could be identified in only 58% of patients (7). In the Bypass Angioplasty Revascularization Intervention (BARI) Trial, only 21% of lesions were identified as being culprit, using angiographic criteria (KM Detre, personal communication). Nevertheless, if a culprit lesion can be identified in a patient with unstable angina, it seems reasonable to use the approach of incomplete revascularization, since treatment of this particular lesion may result in improvement of symptoms without the necessity to treat all lesions. The second principal advantage of treating only a single or several important lesions is that it is technically easier to perform the angioplasty and, presumably, this approach results in a lower risk of complications and a lower risk of subsequent restenosis. Finally, the number of patients who would be candidates for angioplasty, given a strategy of incomplete revascularization, is much larger than if complete revascularization needed to be obtained in all patients (9).

The disadvantages of incomplete revascularization include inadequate relief of symptoms, a less favorable long-term mortality and complication rate, and the need for subsequent bypass surgery because of unacceptable symptoms. As mentioned above, the inability to accurately identify a culprit lesion makes it difficult to be sure that important ischemic territories are treated with angioplasty. It is clear from the review of numerous studies reporting the incidence of incomplete revascularization that the vast majority of patients with multivessel disease undergoing angioplasty have incomplete revascularization, ranging from 40 to 80% of patients (9–10). A recent report by Bourassa and colleagues from the National Heart, Lung, and Blood Institute Percutaneous Transluminal Coronary Angioplasty (NHLBI PTCA) Registry indicated that the incidence of incomplete revascularization may be even higher (9).

Studies looking at the long-term outcome of a strategy of incomplete revascularization have been mixed (Table 26B.1). While five studies have shown no difference in outcome with complete revascularization (6, 11–14), seven studies have shown significant and important differences (5, 15–20). By and

Table 26B.1.
Completeness of Revascularization and Outcome After PTCA

Author (Ref.)	R	n	FU (y)	Death	MI	% CABG	PTCA	No Sx
Faxon (11)	C	72	1	3	7	15	30	76
	IR	67		6	13	18	19	67
Reeder (12)	C	127	2	3	7	33	20	69
	IR	159		5	9.4	35	8	67
Thomas (13)	C	19	1	0	0	5	11	63
	IR	73		0	1	1	12	63
Deligonul (15)	C	118	2	5	2.5	7	14	80
	IR	225		5.4	3.5	16	13	78
Vandormel (17)	C	35	$\frac{1}{2}$	0	3	3	3	63
	IR	31		0	0	16	16	63
Mabin (18)	C	31	1	0	3	13	6	87
	IR	35		0	3	23	6	63
O'Keefe (20)	C	445	4.5	11		24		67
	IR	201		12		34		67
Bourassa (9)	C	173	1	1.2	5.2	5.8	23	79
	IR	565		3.4	8.3	15	17	75
Cowley (5)	C	91	3	Event-free survival				92
	IR	248		Event-free survival				74

R, Revascularization; C, complete revascularization; IR, incomplete revascularization; n, number; FU (y), follow-up in years; MI, myocardial infarction; CABG, coronary artery bypass surgery; PTCA, percutaneous transluminal coronary angioplasty; No Sx, asymptomatic at follow-up.

large, the clinical trials have not demonstrated a significant increase in overall mortality. The study by Bourassa and colleagues showed a higher incidence of complications for patients who had incomplete revascularization because of a complication during the procedure (9, 19). However, in those in whom incomplete revascularization was planned, there was no difference in acute or long-term mortality after adjusting for baseline characteristics. The study did show differences in event-free rates during the 6-year follow-up period, with nearly twice the events in the incomplete revascularization group compared with the complete (19). This was principally because of a need for either repeat bypass surgery or angioplasty. Not unexpectedly, the completely revascularized patients had a higher incidence of repeat PTCA, while the incomplete revascularized group had a higher incidence of bypass surgery. Another study by O'Keefe, which included 646 patients with multivessel disease, also showed a less favorable outcome with incomplete revascularization (20). Most of the reported series do demonstrate a higher incidence of recurrent angina and the need for bypass surgery in incomplete revascularized patients. A recent study by Cowley and colleagues evaluated 370 patients followed for 27 months after angioplasty (5). The 3-year, event-free survival for the entire group was 76.5%.

Complete revascularization was strongly and negatively associated with long-term cardiac events. Using a Cox proportional hazard regression analysis, better left ventricular ejection fraction, lower Canadian Cardiovascular Society anginal class, less severe complex disease, and complete revascularization were associated with better event-free survival. Interestingly enough, when incomplete revascularization was defined as no stenosis of greater than 60% in large vessels, an improved prediction occurred. Other studies have also emphasized that the degree of incomplete revascularization is most impor-

tant. In a study from our center (11) we showed that if adequate revascularization was realized, defined as revascularization of all stenoses (>50%) in vessels of greater than 1.5 mm in diameter and serving viable territory, then no difference was found when compared with completely revascularized patients. However, when lesions were left in bypassable vessels that served viable territory, the outcome was much poorer, principally because of the need for repeat bypass surgery. The location of the lesion is also important, and this has not been clearly defined in previous studies. In a study from the NHLBI PTCA Registry, a favorable 1-year outcome, defined as no clinical events and minimal or no angina, was highly predicted by the absence of a significant proximal stenosis of more than 50%. The importance of proximal versus distal disease is probably a surrogate for the size of the ischemic myocardium. As pointed out in the study by Cowley (5), other factors such as LV function, age, and comorbidity need to be taken into consideration in determining long-term outcome and therefore the appropriateness of incomplete revascularization in any individual patient.

PRACTICAL APPROACH

Deciding Whether To Perform Incomplete Revascularization

The first important issue that needs to be decided in approaching a patient in whom incomplete revascularization is contemplated is whether a culprit lesion can be accurately identified. Angiographic criteria have been reported by Ambrose and colleagues (7), as well as others, and lesion characteristics such as wall irregularities and intraluminal filling defects consistent with thrombi, as well as extremely high-grade lesions with delayed flow, have all been used to identify the culprit lesions by angiography. In the study by Ambrose, however, only 58% of patients with unstable angina had so-called type 2 eccentric morphology, while 65% of patients with nonacute myocardial infarction (MI) had a similar morphology (7). Interestingly, 17% of the unstable angina patients had a abnormal morphology in some other vessel, suggesting that multiple lesions may be the culprit in some patients.

Clinically, however, the use of electrocardiographic changes in a territory subtended by a high-grade coronary stenosis is often used to identify the culprit lesion. The thallium exercise test has also been suggested by Breisblatt and colleagues as a reasonable way of identifying the most ischemic territory (21), but it clearly is not a tool that can identify all ischemic territories, since it is a measure of relative perfusion of one area versus another. All of us have seen patients in whom there is one major defect and then, following revascularization of that territory, a repeat exercise test shows new ischemic territories in other distributions. This suggests that these areas were always ischemic, but were masked by the very positive defect in one area. The other problem with exercise testing or ECG changes in the setting of multivessel coronary disease is that global ischemia may be seen, making identification of a culprit lesion very difficult.

As previously mentioned, the culprit lesion was identified in only 21% of patients undergoing angioplasty in the BARI Trial (8), indicating the difficulty in truly identifying a culprit lesion. In the setting of unstable angina, I believe it is appropriate to try to identify a culprit lesion and to be sure that angioplasty will be able to treat this particular lesion or lesions. As indicated from the Ambrose study, it is much more likely to identify a culprit lesion in the setting of unstable angina or subendocardial myocardial infarction (SEMI). If intravascular ultrasound and/or angioscopy are used, a culprit lesion can be identified with a high degree of success. I primarily use the angiographic appearance of the lesion and electrocardiographic changes to determine a culprit lesion and rely on thallium scanning to a much lesser degree in this clinical setting. In patients with stable, multivessel, coronary disease in whom all significant coronary territories need to be identified, then noninvasive testings may be much more important and helpful. The thallium exercise test, single photon emission computer tomography (SPECT) scanning, and even positron emission tomography (PET) scanning are useful ways of determining both the presence of ischemic myocardium and, perhaps equally important, the viability of the myocardium. In settings where large vessels serve apparent infarct territories but there is suspicion that ischemia may occur in that area, a resting PET scan using ammonium and deoxyglucose can be extremely helpful in understanding the viability of the potentially ischemic territory. Reinjection of thallium is also an alternative means of identifying viability, if PET scanning is not readily available.

Finally, the importance of the territory served by the vessel is also an important consideration in my practice in determining the need for complete or incomplete revascularization. Cowley's study pointed this out, as did our own study on incomplete revascularization (5, 10). If the vessel in question serves a small territory, for example, 10% or less of the myocardium, then I am much less inclined to worry about it as a significant factor in long-term outcome. The only studies that help validate this approach are some preliminary studies using PET scanning where the ischemic territory has been quantified and long-term outcome has been obtained. In these studies, less than a 10% area of ischemic myocardium does not seem to be important for the long-term outcome. The larger the area at jeopardy, the greater importance it has and the greater the need for revascularization. When 50% of the contour of the left ventricular outline on ventriculography is jeopardized by a significant stenosis, then angioplasty needs to be done on that critical stenosis; if angioplasty cannot be done, then I would be unwilling to perform angioplasty in that setting.

Table 26B.2.
Decision Analysis in Incomplete Revascularization

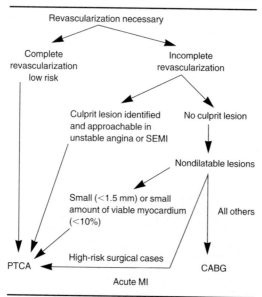

Therefore my algorithm (Table 26B.2) for deciding whether angioplasty should be done includes the determination of whether complete revascularization or incomplete revascularization can be accomplished by carefully evaluating the morphology and location of the stenoses in vessels of greater than 1.5 mm in diameter. I always favor complete revascularization if possible. I pay particular attention to the lesion location, favoring a proximal location as compared with a distal location. If complete revascularization can be obtained with reasonable safety, then angioplasty should be considered. If the patient cannot be completely revascularized, but the stenoses that are left behind are not functionally important because they either served infarcted territory or are too small to be bypassed, then I would refer that patient for angioplasty as well. In unstable angina I would insist that the culprit lesion, regardless of its size, be treated successfully by angioplasty. Finally, incomplete revascularization seems a reasonable option, as long as a majority of the ischemic territory can be adequately treated and no more than 10% of the myocardium at jeopardy is left behind. If this cannot be obtained, then the patient should be referred for surgical treatment. Clearly, there are some caveats that need to be considered that may change these general guidelines. If the patient is extremely elderly or has numerous other medical problems that would make surgical treatment impossible or of extremely high risk, then it may be reasonable to consider incomplete revascularization, even though there may not be complete relief of symptoms. In addition, incomplete revascularization is clearly the correct strategy in the patient who is in the midst of an acute myocardial infarction, where complete revascularization may be obtained at a later date or where the patient could be referred for bypass surgery if necessary. It may also be reasonable to consider a staged procedure in unstable angina, when multiple, high-grade lesions need to be dilated and the risk of the procedure is high for each of the lesions to be treated. There is some potential disadvantage to this strategy in that symptomatic relief may not be obtained and it may place the patient at higher risk than a strategy of dilation of all lesions at the same setting.

The Strategy of Dilation in the Setting of Incomplete Revascularization

As previously mentioned, identification of a culprit lesion is important and it should be the first lesion that is attempted. If successful dilation of the major lesion is accomplished without significant complications, my strategy would then be to continue to dilate all significant lesions thereafter in order of their importance. I define importance by the proximal location of the stenosis, the viability of the myocardium that it is serving, and the size of viable myocardium. As stated before, if the patient is at high risk for complications and palliation is the strategy, only the proximal lesions serving large areas of viable myocardium should be attempted during one procedure.

The difficulty with incomplete revascular-

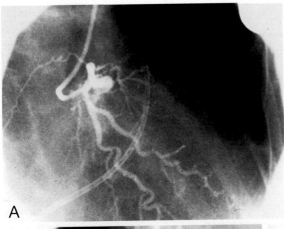

A

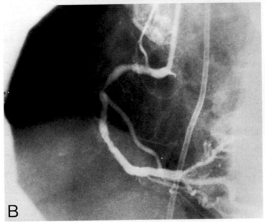

B

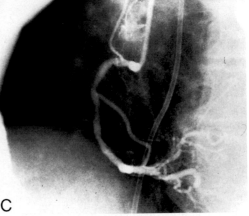

C

Figure 26B.1. This 54-year-old woman had prior anterior MI 3 years earlier and a recent episode of unstable angina. Cardiac catheterization showed two-vessel disease with severe hypokinesia of the anterior wall on ventriculography. The RCA lesion was dilated successfully, but the patient continued to have symptoms because of the totally occluded LAD. Following bypass surgery the patient became asymptomatic.

ization is that the tools we use to define important ischemic territories are relatively inadequate and there are a number of cases where the patient continues to have symptoms despite our best judgement that incomplete revascularization is reasonable. One such case, shown in Figure 26B.1, is that of a 54-year-old woman who had a myocardial infarction 3 years earlier, had a symptom-free period, but then began to develop recurrent angina that progressed to unstable angina. She was found to have a total occlusion of the left anterior descending (LAD) that was visible from collaterals from the left side. The anterior wall was severely hypokinetic and a high-grade lesion in the midright coronary artery (RCA) was also present. We reasoned that her RCA was her culprit lesion, since she

had a previous anterior myocardial infarction and was symptom-free following it. We felt that treatment of the RCA would satisfactorily take care of her anginal symptoms without the need to treat her totally occluded LAD. Angioplasty was successfully accomplished; however, the patient continued to have pain immediately following the procedure and 3 months later underwent bypass surgery of the LAD with relief of her symptoms. At the time we felt that the anterior wall was primarily infarcted and that, if there were viable myocardium, it was a small territory. However, in retrospect it appeared that the LAD was also important. In this setting a more careful evaluation of the viability of the anterior wall should have been done prior to revascularization.

In another example of a patient with incomplete revascularization, a similar situation occurred (Fig. 26B.2). This 65-year-old man had a history of a prior anterior MI 5 years earlier and had gradually developed worsening angina over a 3-year period. Despite medical therapy, he remained class 3. On catheterization he was found to have a diffusely diseased LAD, a high-grade stenosis in the circumflex just after a large, obtuse, marginal branch, and a significant lesion in the mid-RCA. The left ventricular angiogram

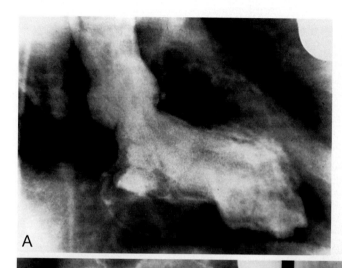

Figure 26B.2. This 65-year-old man had a prior MI 5 years earlier without symptoms until angina occurred and increased over 3 years. Cardiac catheterization showed three-vessel disease and an aneurysm of the anterior wall. PTCA of the RCA and circumflex resulted in complete cessation of symptoms.

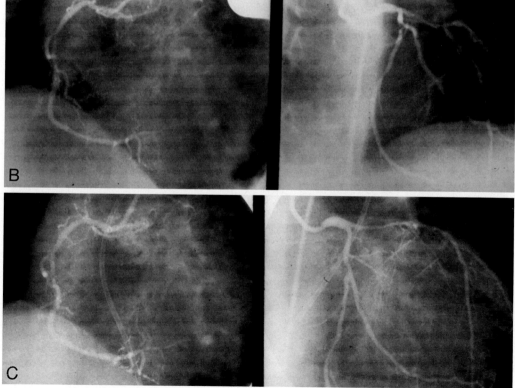

showed an anterior aneurysm, but good wall motion in the lateral wall and the inferior wall. We again reasoned that the LAD served the prior infarct territory and that the ischemic territories were the circumflex and the RCA. We therefore did angioplasty of the circumflex and the RCA without complications, and in this patient complete relief of symptoms occurred with a negative exercise test and a good long-term follow-up.

Another patient illustrates the difficulty in determining the culprit lesion (Fig. 26B.3). This 58-year-old man presented with a 6-week history of increasing angina with several

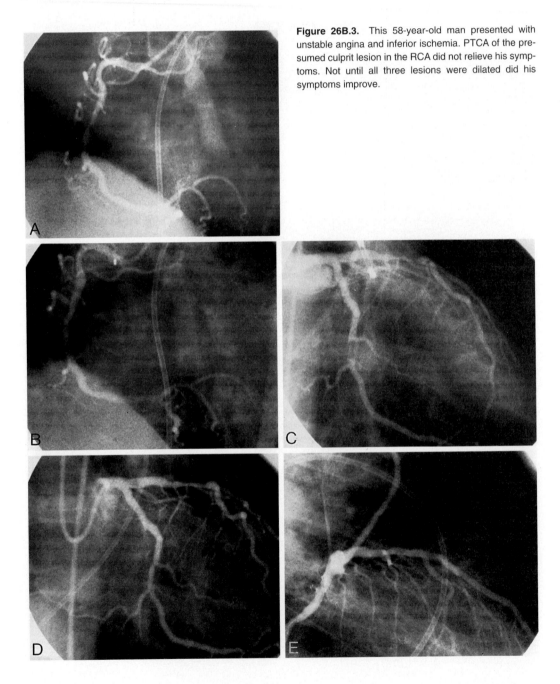

Figure 26B.3. This 58-year-old man presented with unstable angina and inferior ischemia. PTCA of the presumed culprit lesion in the RCA did not relieve his symptoms. Not until all three lesions were dilated did his symptoms improve.

episodes of rest pain. On admission to the coronary care unit he demonstrated inferior ischemia and subsequently underwent cardiac catheterization, which showed a significant lesion in the mid-RCA, a significant lesion in the distal circumflex, and a 50% stenosis in the mid-LAD. On the basis of inferior ST-segment changes with chest pain and the high-grade nature of the RCA lesion serving a large amount of myocardium, the RCA lesion was successfully dilated and the patient was taken back to the coronary care unit. Over the next 2 days the patient continued to have recurrent chest pain with minimal ECG changes. He was taken back to the cardiac catheterization laboratory where the RCA remained widely patent, but because of the previous, inferior ST-segment changes, the circumflex was now felt to also be a culprit lesion and was dilated with a successful result. The patient was returned to the coronary care unit, but continued to have recurrent episodes of mild angina over the next several days. He again returned to the cardiac catheterization laboratory where both the right and circumflex arteries remained widely patent and the LAD was successfully dilated. Following dilation of all three vessels and complete revascularization, the patient remained asymptomatic and was discharged from the hospital. This final case illustrates the difficulty in identifying a culprit lesion and, in this particular situation, suggests that all three lesions were of clinical importance in the patient's presenting symptoms. No functional test would have significantly aided in defining the territory, and perhaps the strategy of complete revascularization should have been attempted at the time of the initial angioplasty.

SUMMARY

Incomplete revascularization is very common in multivessel angioplasty. If performed in appropriately selected patients, it can result in an excellent long-term outcome with less risk and less restenosis. This strategy is not reasonable, however, when large areas of viable myocardium are left behind,

since clinical studies and experience indicate that the outcome is much less favorable. The results of the current, large, multicenter trials comparing PTCA with bypass surgery should help better define those in whom incomplete revascularization is an acceptable strategy.

REFERENCES

1. Graves EJ. National hospital discharge survey: annual summary 1991. National Center for Health Statistics 1993, DHHS publication (PHS);44:1775–1793.
2. Cukingnan RA, Carey JS, Wittig JH, Brown BG. Influence of complete coronary revascularization on relief of angina. J Thorac Cardiovasc Surg 1980;79:188–193.
3. Lawrie GM, Morris GC, Silvers A et al. The influence of residual disease after coronary bypass on the 5-year survival rate of 1274 men with coronary artery disease. Circulation 1982;66:717–723.
4. Gould BL, Clayton PD, Jensen RL, Liddle HV. Association between early graft patency and late outcome for patients undergoing artery bypass graft surgery. Circulation 1984;69:569–576.
5. Cowley MJ, Vandermael M, Topol EJ et al. Is traditionally defined complete revascularization needed for patients with multivessel disease treated by elective coronary angioplasty? J Am Coll Cardiol 1993;22:1289–1297.
6. Wohlgelernter D, Cleman M, Highman HA, Zaret BL. Percutaneous transluminal coronary angioplasty of the "culprit lesion" for management of unstable angina pectoris in patients with multivessel coronary artery disease. Am J Cardiol 1986;58:400–464.
7. Ambrose JA, Hjemdahl-Monsen CE, Borrico S, Gorlin R, Fuster V. Angiographic demonstration of a common link between unstable angina pectoris and non–Q-wave acute myocardial infarction. Am J Cardiol 1988;61:244–247.
8. Deleted in proofs.
9. Bourassa MG, Holubkov R, Wanlin Y, Detre KM, and the co-investigators of the NHLBI PTCA. Strategy of complete revascularization in patients with multivessel coronary artery disease (a report from the 1985–1986 NHLBI PTCA Registry). Am J Cardiol 1992;70:174–178.
10. DeFeyter PJ. PTCA in patients with stable angina pectoris and multivessel disease: Is incomplete revascularization acceptable? Clin Cardiol 1992;15:317–322.
11. Faxon DP, Ghalili K, Jacobs AK et al. The degree of revascularization and outcome after multivessel coronary angioplasty. Am Heart J 1992;123:854–859.
12. Reeder GS, Holmes DR, Detre K, Costigan T, Kelsey SF. Degree of revascularization in patients with multivessel coronary disease: a report from the National Heart, Lung, and Blood Institute Percutaneous Transluminal Coronary Angioplasty Registry. Circulation 1988;77:638–644.
13. Thomas ES, Most AS, Williams DO. Coronary angioplasty for patients with multivessel coronary artery disease: follow-up clinical status. Am Heart J 1988;115:8–13.
14. Bell MR, Bailey KR, Reeder GS, Lapeyre AC, Holmes DR. Percutaneous tranluminal angioplasty in patients with mul-

tivessel coronary disease: how important is complete revascularization for cardiac event-free survival? J Am Coll Cardiol 1990;16:553–562.

15. Deligonul U, Vandormael MG, Kern MJ, Zelman R, Galan K, Chaitman BR. Coronary angioplasty: a therapeutic option for symptomatic patients with two- and three-vessel coronary disease. J Am Coll Cardiol 1988;11:1173–1179.

16. Shaw RE, Anwar A, Myler RK et al. Incomplete revascularization and complex lesion morphology: relationship to early and late results in multivessel coronary angioplasty. J Invest Cardiol 1990;2:93–101.

17. Vandormael MG, Chaitman BR, Ischinger T et al. Immediate and short-term benefit of multilesion coronary angioplasty: influence of degree of revascularization. Am Coll Cardiol 1985;6:982–994.

18. Mabin TA, Holmes DR, Smith HC et al. Follow-up clinical results in patients undergoing percutaneous transluminal coronary angioplasty. Circulation 1985;71:754–760.

19. O'Keefe JH, Rutherford BD, McConahay DR et al. Multivessel coronary angioplasty from 1980 to 1989: procedural results and long-term outcome. J Am Coll Cardiol 1990; 16:1097–1102.

20. Bourassa MG, Yeh W, Detre KM. Five-year event rates after multivessel PTCA when complete revascularization is not possible or not intended. Presented at the American College of Cardiology 43rd Annual Scientific Session. J Am Coll Cardiol 1993;22:223A (abstract).

21. Breisblatt WM, Barnes JV, Weiland F, Spaccavento LJ. Incomplete revascularization in multivessel percutaneous transluminal coronary angioplasty: the role for stress thallium-201 imaging. J Am Coll Cardiol 1998;11:1183–1190.

C. Completeness of Revascularization and Multivessel Disease Dilation

DAVID R. HOLMES JR. and MALCOLM R. BELL

The issues of completeness of revascularization and multivessel disease dilation are intertwined and have assumed increasing importance as the frequency of multivessel dilation has increased. Complete myocardial revascularization was initially a surgical concept and was applied to surgical series. Although the definition of complete revascularization was variable in these series, there was general consensus that achievement of complete revascularization was associated with improved long-term survival and freedom from symptoms, including late myocardial infarction. With further follow-up, because of graft attrition, these differences may decline. There are other confounding variables, including the status of left ventricular function, the presence and severity of regional wall motion abnormalities in the distribution of the vessels to be treated, and the effect of diffuse distal disease (Table 26C.1).

These same considerations are extremely important for the practice of interventional

Table 26C.1.
Multivessel Disease: Interventional Cardiology Considerations

Assessment
- Coronary anatomy
- Clinical setting
- Left ventricular function
- Degree, extent and location of ischemia

Coronary anatomy
- Match coronary anatomy with clinical and functional assessment to identify significant lesions.
- Determine if all significant lesions can be dilated.
- Match technology available with specific lesion.
- Assess risk of each lesion.
- Plan sequence—most importantly, functional lesion first (exception being chronic total occlusion supplying target lesion), then subsequent lesions. Complete revascularization goal.
- Consider bailout options.
- If significant lesions cannot be treated, consider other options.
- Stage procedures if target lesion treatment results in suboptimal result.

Clinical setting
- Acute ischemic syndromes: optimize antithrombotic, anticoagulant drugs—IIb/IIIa receptor antibodies when available
- Culprit lesion dilation

Left ventricular function
- The more abnormal the left ventricular function, the greater the importance of complete revascularization. If complete revascularization cannot be achieved with catheter-based therapy in severe three-vessel disease and left ventricular dysfunction, consider surgical options.
- Abnormal left ventricular function may affect response to PTCA. If artery to be treated supplies most of the remaining viable myocardium, consider placement of partial cardiopulmonary bypass system or intraaortic balloon pump.

Degree, extent, and location of ischemia
- Ischemic territories should be matched with coronary anatomy. Severe ischemia in multiple regions mandates complete revascularization.

cardiology. The issue is further complicated by three additional problems.

1. *Chronic occlusion.* There is an abundance of data on dilation for chronic occlusions. Success rates even in highly selected series are substantially lower than seen with subtotal stenoses and average approximately 70%. Specific features have been identified that are associated with improved success rates, including short duration, short length of occlusion, and lack of bridging collaterals at the site. In these patients an inability to pass the occlusion with a guidewire is the limiting step, although in 5 to 10% of patients a wire can be used to cross the occlusion but a balloon cannot be passed. In this setting laser angioplasty or rotational atherectomy may be very helpful. The presence of an undilatable chronic occlusion is one of the most frequent reasons for inability to achieve complete revascularization.

   At the present time, newer technology is being focused on alternative means to approach these chronic total occlusions. The optimal approach would be to create a small pilot channel through the occlusion that would then facilitate placement of either a balloon or a debulking technology. A laser wire, 0.018 inch, is currently being tested in a randomized trial. This wire is delivered through a conventional PTCA balloon up to the occlusion. Then, using biplane fluoroscopy for guidance, the wire is used to lase a small pilot channel. Whether this approach will allow greater success rates remains to be determined.

2. *The incremental risk of dilating each additional lesion.* Dilation may result in unpredictable outcome. Dissections are common. While they usually do not result in adverse outcome, in 4 to 7% of lesions, abrupt or threatened closure may occur. This results in substantial increased morbidity and even mortality. Although higher-risk lesions can be identified using angiographic criteria, dilation of even ideal lesions can result in a suboptimal outcome. In a patient with multivessel disease the operator may limit the number of vessels dilated, in part because of this incremental risk, and just concentrate on those lesions felt to be the most severe. In several recent series the most frequent reason for failure to achieve complete revascularization was a decision to not dilate lesions, even though they could have been dilated. This decision is in part based on the incremental risk associated with each lesion dilated. Other considerations include the amount of contrast required if multiple lesions are to be treated, patient comfort if the procedure has been very long, scheduling concerns, and difficulty in identifying the culprit lesion. In some situations not all lesions may be amenable to conventional dilation, a fact that should be apparent to the operator prior to the procedure. In such cases there should be consideration of alternative methods of percutaneous intervention or consideration of surgical revascularization if more appropriate.

   A complicating factor in assessment of the risk of dilating additional lesions is the potential series of subsequent events that may result from a complication; if acute closure of the second lesion being dilated results in hypotension, then the first lesion dilated may also close and result in worsening hemodynamics. If significant hypotension occurs after dilation of a second lesion, the operator should be prepared to recheck the initially dilated lesion.

   Subacute closure or worsening of the initial lesion treated can be also be suspected based on collateral patterns. In a patient with a dilatable chronic occlusion of the right coronary artery and severe proximal left anterior descending stenosis with visible collaterals from the distal left anterior descending feeding the right coronary artery, the right coronary artery would be dilated first. After right coronary artery dilation, the left anterior descending would be approached. After dilation of the left anterior descending, if collaterals are still seen to fill the distal right coronary artery, the right coronary artery should again be injected to see if the result is suboptimal.

3. *Restenosis.* Although there is an increasing amount of information available on the pathophysiology and mechanisms of restenosis, much remains unknown. Specific lesion morphology may affect restenosis. In general, the greater the number of lesions dilated, the greater the chance one or more will have restenosis that may be symptomatic. However, it is important to realize that the risk of restenosis per patient is not double or triple with two- or three-vessel dilation compared with single-vessel dilation.

These issues are perhaps the most important areas affecting dilation practice in patients with multivessel disease, in addition to the variables previously mentioned that affect both the practice of dilation and surgery alike, including diffuse disease, left ventricular function, and prior infarction in the region of the vessel to be treated.

In published series of patients undergoing PTCA for multivessel disease, the frequency with which complete revascularization can be achieved and the importance of this on long-term follow-up have been studied. In multiple series the completeness of revascularization has varied, being higher in patients with two-vessel disease than three-vessel disease. With two-vessel disease, up to 50% of patients have been completely revascularized, while with three-vessel disease, the frequency has been approximately 25 to 30%. In the recent NHLBI PTCA Registry, complete revascularization was achieved in 19% of patients. As previously mentioned, in 42% of patients all of the lesions were amenable to PTCA, but all were not intended to be dilated.

The concept of culprit lesion dilation or functionally adequate revascularization has assumed increasing importance. There are specific lesion characteristics felt to be associated with unstable lesions, including the presence of coronary arterial thrombus and irregular lumen borders. Successful PTCA in some of these patients will result in excellent symptomatic improvement. Identification of the culprit lesion in the setting of severe three-vessel disease, however, remains difficult. Recently the concept of functionally adequate revascularization has been discussed. This has been defined as successful dilation of all stenoses ≥70% in vessels that are larger than 1.5 mm in diameter, that could be bypassed, and that serve viable myocardium. Inclusion of the viable myocardium is the important addition to this definition and requires careful predilation evaluation using nuclear perfusion testing or studying wall motion with angiographic or echocardiographic techniques.

The long-term follow-up of patients with complete and incomplete revascularization has also been studied. It is complex and depends on several factors, including the length of follow-up, the baseline characteristics of the patients, and the coronary anatomy. In patients with predominantly two-vessel disease and well-preserved left ventricular function, during short or intermediate follow-up, complete revascularization may not be required. In patients with severe three-vessel disease and abnormal left ventricular function, achievement of complete revascularization is very important. In the NHLBI PTCA Registry, when differences in left ventricular function and degree of coronary artery disease were taken into consideration, intermediate-term outcome did not differ between complete and incompletely revascularized patients. In other series, particularly with abnormal left ventricular function, complete revascularization has been very important

and a major determinant of improved outcome. In a matched case control series with abnormal left ventricular function and multivessel disease, the most important determinant of long-term outcome was achievement of complete revascularization, whether by surgery or PTCA. In general, the more severe the angina, the more extensive the coronary artery disease and ischemic burden, and the more abnormal the left ventricular function, the more important complete revascularization becomes.

The relationship between survival, severity of disease, and revascularization has been evaluated in the Duke Database Registry for 9263 patients with symptomatic coronary artery disease undergoing cardiac catheterization between 1984 and 1990. This was a nonrandomized study, and the specific treatment was chosen by the individual physician and patient for clinical, nonprotocol reasons. In this group, of the 9263 patients, 2788 (30%) were treated with PTCA, while 3422 (37%) underwent initial coronary bypass graft surgery. The patients were then followed, and the primary endpoint of mortality was studied. The extent of coronary artery disease had a major impact on survival. For single-vessel disease, there were no survival advantages at 5 years of revascularization compared with medical therapy. For three-vessel disease, surgery provided a consistent advantage over medical therapy and appeared superior to PTCA. For some patients with two-vessel disease, PTCA had an advantage over coronary bypass graft surgery. In these analyses the issue of crossover is of great importance—this is difficult to categorize. Crossover may be considered a "failure" of one treatment limb or may be considered appropriate or even the optimal treatment of a patient over time as clinical conditions change.

Given these issues, the approach to dilation in patients with multivessel disease involves consideration of the specific clinical pattern problem, the coronary anatomy, and the left ventricular function, as well as of the comorbid conditions.

SPECIFIC CLINICAL PATTERNS AND LEFT VENTRICULAR FUNCTION

In patients with unstable angina, the angiogram should be carefully reviewed to identify a possible culprit lesion. Although it is not always possible to identify such a lesion, it helps to guide dilation when present. This is easiest in a patient with single-vessel disease with a very severe stenosis. In patients with moderate stenoses in a number of different vessels and one single severe stenosis with, for example, coronary arterial thrombus, it is also relatively straightforward. In patients with severe multivessel disease and what is felt to be a culprit lesion, it is important to address the other lesions as well, particularly if abnormal left ventricular function is present. Additional dilation can be performed either at the time of initial dilation if this is uncomplicated; alternatively, it can be performed later before hospital discharge.

CORONARY ANATOMY

The strategy of dilation in these patients involves consideration of the specific lesion characteristics. In general, the lesion felt to be responsible for the clinical symptoms should be approached first with the optimal technology for the specific lesion. If only the culprit lesion can be approached and dilated, particularly if it is in a small vessel, and if other severe lesions that cannot be dilated will remain, consideration should be given to an alternative means for revascularization.

Exceptions to beginning with the culprit lesion are occasionally made. The most frequent exception occurs when there is a chronic occlusion that supplies collaterals to the distribution of the culprit lesion. There is no real scientific data to support this approach, but theoretically it does make sense to provide a source of collaterals should acute closure occur. With the more widespread use of intracoronary stents, this approach may be required less often, as higher-risk lesions can be treated with a safety net. The results of dilating the most severe or culprit lesion must be assessed before approaching other lesions.

If there is any concern about the dilated lesion, it is best to stage the procedure. This depends, however, on the clinical setting. In patients being treated for acute myocardial infarction, only the infarct-related artery should be treated. In these patients, PTCA of other lesions can be performeed prior to hospital dismissal. Other considerations in the decision on whether to stage a procedure include the amount of contrast used, the duration of the procedure, and patient comfort. Staging can be performed the next day while the sheath is still in place. Alternatively, it can be performed at a later time after sheath removal. This does require repeat arterial puncture, however.

The treatment of moderate stenoses remains problematic. The early experience with dilation documented that the risk of dilation of moderate stenosis was similar to that of more severe, functionally important stenoses and that restenosis occurred with similar frequency. Given the fact that these were only moderate stenoses, not severe and not resulting in functionally important hypoperfusion, in general the recommendation was made to avoid PTCA.

Since that time, the means available for assessment of lesions have changed. Currently, intravascular ultrasound is more commonly used to define anatomy and intravascular Doppler studies to interrogate the lesions and to study some measure of functional significance. With the use of these tests in conjunction with angiography, if a lesion does not appear to be functionally significant, then dilation is not usually performed even though the lesion would be amenable to treatment. Alternatively, if the procedure is to be changed, nuclear stress testing can be performed, for example, adenosine or dipyridamole thallium or sestamibi imaging, prior to the second procedure in cases where there is debate about the functional significance of a moderate lesion. Such lesions, if they manifest evidence of myocardial ischemia, can then be dilated, particularly if three-vessel disease is present with abnormal left ventricular function or if extensive ischemia is present. If a lesion of borderline significance is present, is in a large vessel, and supplies viable myocardium, then PTCA is often performed to improve the completeness of revascularization.

SUGGESTED READINGS

Bell MR, Bailey KR, Reeder GS, Lapeyre AC III, Holmes DR Jr. Percutaneous transluminal angioplasty in patients with multivessel coronary disease: How important is complete revascularization for cardiac event-free survival? J Am Coll Cardiol 1990;16(3):553–562.

Bell MR, Gersh BJ, Schaff HV et al. Effect of completeness of revascularization on long-term outcome of patients with three-vessel disease undergoing coronary artery bypass surgery: a report from the Coronary Artery Surgery (CASS) Study. Circulation 1992;86:446–457.

Berger PB, Holmes DR Jr. Dilation strategies in patients with multivessel disease. In: Faxon DP, ed. Practical angioplasty. New York; Raven Press, 1993.

Bourassa MG, Holubkov R, Yeh W et al. Strategy of complete revascularization in patients with multivessel coronary artery disease (a report from the 1985–1986 NHLBI PTCA Registry). Am J Cardiol 1992;70:174.

de Feyter PJ, Serruys PW, Arnold A et al. Coronary angioplasty of the unstable angina–related vessel in patients with multivessel disease. Eur Heart J 1986;7(6):460–467.

Ellis SG, Cowley MJ, DiSciascio G et al. Determinants of 2-year outcome after coronary angioplasty in patients with multivessel disease on the basis of comprehensive pre-procedural evaluation. Implications for patient selection. The Multivessel Angioplasty Prognosis Study Group. Circulation 1991;83:1905.

Faxon DP, Ghalilli K, Jacobs AK. The degree of revascularization and outcome after multivessel coronary angioplasty. Am Heart J 1992;123:854.

Holmes DR Jr, Detre KM, Williams DO et al. Long-term outcome of patients with depressed left ventricular function undergoing percutaneous transluminal coronary angioplasty: The NHLBI PTCA Registry. Circulation 1993; 87:21–29.

Holmes DR Jr, Holubkov R, Vlietstra RE et al. Comparison of complications during percutaneous transluminal coronary angioplasty from 1977 to 1981 and from 1985 to 1986: the National Heart, Lung, and Blood Institute Percutaneous Transluminal Coronary Angioplasty Registry. J Am Coll Cardiol 1988;12:1149–1155.

Kussmaul WGI, Krol J, Laskey WK et al. One-year follow-up results of "culprit" versus multivessel coronary angioplasty trial. Am J Cardiol 1993;71:1431–1433.

Myler RK, Topol EJ, Shaw RE et al. Multiple vessel coronary angioplasty: classification, results, and patterns of restenosis in 494 consecutive patients. Cathet Cardiovasc Diagn 1987;13:1.

Reeder GS, Holmes DR Jr, Detre K et al. Degree of revascularization in patients with multivessel coronary disease: a report from the National Heart, Lung, and Blood Institute Percutaneous Transluminal Coronary Angioplasty Registry. Circulation 1988;77:638–644.

Stevens T, Kahn JK, McCallister BD et al. Safety and efficacy of percutaneous transluminal coronary angioplasty in patients with left ventricular dysfunction. Am J Cardiol 1991; 68:313.

Wohlgelernter D, Cleman M, Highman HA, Zaret BL. Percutaneous transluminal coronary angioplasty of the "culprit lesion" for management of unstable angina pectoris in patients with multivessel coronary artery disease. Am J Cardiol 1986;58(6):460–464.

EDITORIAL SUMMARY

The concept of completeness of revascularization is extremely important for interventional cardiology. There has been conflicting information on its effect on long-term outcome following PTCA. Initially, the concept of complete revascularization was evaluated in the surgical arena, and there it was found that patients who received a conduit to each diseased major arterial distribution segment had better outcomes than patients who were incompletely revascularized. There have been multiple dilation series that have assessed this. In general, patients with incomplete revascularization have worse outcomes; it must be kept in mind that these patients usually have more adverse baseline characteristics with a higher incidence of prior infarction, more severe coronary artery disease, and an increased frequency of chronic total occlusion. Their long-term follow-up may be equally affected by their more adverse baseline characteristics, as well as the status of revascularization.

Achievement of complete revascularization is inversely related to the number of vessels diseased—as the number increases, the ability to achieve complete revascularization decreases. The two major reasons for failure to achieve complete revascularization are the presence of a chronic total occlusion that is felt to be not dilatable or the presence of a lesion that, while significant, is not felt to be responsible for ischemia and therefore is not electively dilated. Attempts to identify new technology (e.g., laser crossing guidewires that can increase success rates with chronic total occlusion) should have a great impact on the frequency with which complete revascularization can be achieved.

The concept of functional complete revascularization has been proposed and evaluated and has substantial merit. This takes into account the size of the vessel and the status of the left ventricle it supplies and is based on the premise that dilation of a vessel supplying a completely scarred, akinetic region of myocardium will not improve outcome. Instead, attempts should be made to identify ischemia-producing stenoses, and concentrate on these. An important additional concept is the degree of left ventricular dysfunction and the total amount of ischemic myocardium. In general, the greater the degree of ischemic burden, the more important complete revascularization becomes. If multiple viable areas of left ventricular myocardium are supplied by vessels that cannot be treated with a percutaneous technique, then alternative strategies (e.g., coronary bypass surgery) should be considered.

27. Left Ventricular Dysfunction

A. Percutaneous Revascularization of the Patient with Poor Left Ventricular Function

FAYAZ A. SHAWL

Severe coronary artery disease in patients with markedly depressed left ventricular function is associated with a poor prognosis (1). Coronary artery bypass graft surgery has been the mainstay of treatment in such patients in the past, but is associated with significant morbidity and mortality (2, 3). Coronary angioplasty has been offered as an alternative to coronary artery bypass surgery in these patients. The results of PTCA in patients with left ventricular ejection fraction (LVEF) between 35% and 40% have been reported and show a procedural success of >80% and a mortality of 2.7 to 5% (4, 5). These reports also suggest that coronary angioplasty is usually well tolerated in patients with moderately depressed ejection fraction, but coronary occlusion caused by balloon inflation or abrupt closure in patients with more severely depressed ejection fraction may result in hemodynamic collapse. Additionally, these patients may not survive the delay required to institute emergency bypass surgery.

Percutaneous cardiopulmonary bypass support (PCPS) provides complete systemic hemodynamic support independent of intrinsic cardiac function and has been employed prophylactically in high-risk patients prior to angioplasty or emergently following abrupt closure (6–9). A recent report (10) by the National Registry of Elective Supported Angioplasty indicated patients with a left ventricular ejection fraction of 20% or lower had significantly less hospital mortality when prophylactic support was employed compared with standby support. Complications are mostly related to the cannula insertion site and can be minimized by use of current techniques (11). The discussion that follows details the author's experience with the technique, the basic principles, and patient management during percutaneously established cardiopulmonary bypass support in patients with poor left ventricular function undergoing coronary intervention.

TECHNIQUE OF ELECTIVE PERCUTANEOUS CARDIOPULMONARY BYPASS SUPPORT

Patients are prepped and draped in the catheterization laboratory in the usual sterile manner, exposing both groins. All items necessary for the percutaneous cannula insertion are available in a compact percutaneous insertion kit (C.R. Bard, Billerica, MA). Using the Seldinger technique, a 7 Fr pigtail catheter is introduced into the right femoral artery to perform iliofemoral angiography, initially visualizing the left side and then, if necessary, the right side. The tip of the pigtail is positioned just above the bifurcation of the aorta, and 16 cc of contrast agent is power-injected at the rate of 8 cc/second. Prior to angiography a needle (the same as used for percutaneous vascular access) is placed along the groin crease to establish the relationship of the skin crease to the bifurcation of the femoral system and to use as a guide for arterial entry (Fig. 27A.1).

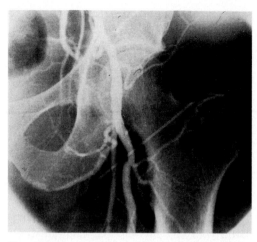

Figure 27A.1. Left iliofemoral cineangiogram performed prior to cannulation to assess the adequacy for cannula placement. The skin crease is marked with a radiopaque needle placed on the surface of the skin before angiography.

If the left iliofemoral system indicates a suitable anatomy, a Swan-Ganz catheter is placed in the right femoral vein and advanced to the pulmonary artery for the monitoring of hemodynamic parameters prior to, during, and after the procedure. If the anatomy of the left iliofemoral system is unsuitable for bypass cannulas, angiography is performed on the right side using the same technique. If the left iliofemoral system reveals acceptable anatomy for the insertion of a bypass cannula, the pigtail catheter is exchanged over a standard 0.038-inch guidewire with a standard 8 Fr angioplasty sheath that is introduced in the right femoral artery. Access to the left femoral artery and vein is obtained using a standard, single-wall needle, and 7 Fr sheaths are left in place. The knowledge of the iliofemoral anatomy, together with its relationship to the skin crease (needle marker), the common femoral artery, or the femoral artery below the bifurcation (if of adequate caliber) of the profunda and the superficial femoral artery is critical. Care is taken to ensure that the actual arterial puncture site is below the inguinal ligament to facilitate subsequent external clamp placement for hemostasis.

Patients are then heparinized with 225 units of heparin (as a single bolus) per kg body weight to obtain an activated clotting time of 400 seconds or greater, which is checked after 10 or 15 minutes. The percutaneous insertion kit containing the 18 Fr cannulas is opened next. Then the 0.038-inch flexible guidewire is introduced through the arterial sheath. Keeping this 0.038-inch flexible guidewire in place, the arterial sheath is removed and a long, 8 Fr dilator is introduced. The tip of this long dilator usually lies above the bifurcation of the descending aorta. The 0.038-inch flexible guidewire is removed and replaced with the stiff 0.038-inch guidewire with a flexible tip. Holding the stiff guidewire in place, the long, 8 Fr dilator is removed and the vessel is then dilated with a 12 Fr and then a 14 Fr dilator. Before the 14 Fr dilator is removed, a 1 to 2 mm skin incision is made at the entry site using a No. 11 blade to accommodate the bypass cannulas. The 14 Fr dilator is removed, and an 18 Fr cannula is advanced over the stiff guidewire using a rotary motion, taking care to advance both dilator and cannula assembly as a single unit so that the cannula does not buckle. This is best accomplished by having an assistant hold the proximal end of the cannula dilator unit firmly together. After the introduction of the 18 Fr arterial cannula, the guidewire and the dilator are removed and the tube is closed quickly using the available Robert's clamp.

Employing a similar approach, an 18 Fr multihole venous cannula is advanced until the tip is positioned just above the junction of the inferior vena cava and right atrium. During advancement of the venous cannula, the soft tip of the guidewire is positioned in the superior vena cava (Fig. 27A.2). It takes less than 5 minutes to cannulate a patient for PCPS using the author's technique after venous and arterial access is obtained. While cannulation is being performed, a perfusionist primes the disposable perfusion circuit.

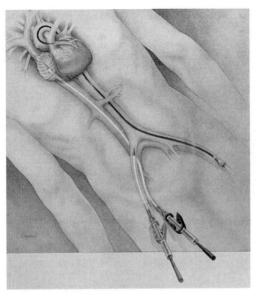

Figure 27A.2. Schematic representation of the appropriate position of the arterial and venous cannulas. Note placement of the tip of the venous cannula just above the junction of the inferior vena cava and right atrium. The arterial cannula is advanced until the hub is flush with the skin. Also note that a right femoral approach is shown in the diagram, whereas the left femoral approach is more commonly used in elective cases, with the PTCA performed from the contralateral side.

PORTABLE CARDIOPULMONARY BYPASS SUPPORT SYSTEM

The portable cardiopulmonary bypass support system (Bard CPS ReAct System, C.R. Bard, Inc., Billerica, MA) is a battery-operated, portable system on a hospital cart with a disposable CPS circuit that includes a centrifugal, nonocclusive pump; a propylene, hollow-fiber–membrane oxygenator; clamps; connectors; and a heat exchanger (Fig. 27A.3). The perfusion circuit is primed by a perfusionist using 1300 cc of Normosol. It takes less than 10 minutes to set up and prime this system.

PATIENT SELECTION FOR SUPPORTED ANGIOPLASTY

The basic indication for supported angioplasty is a severely symptomatic patient in whom the risk of unsupported percutaneous transluminal coronary angioplasty (PTCA) or

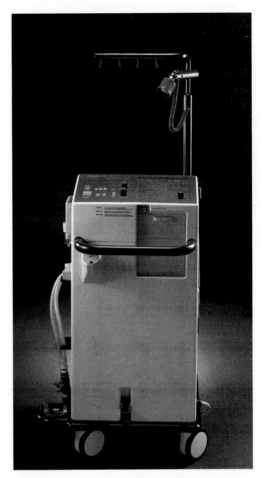

Figure 27A.3. Portable cardiopulmonary bypass support system (Bard CPS ReAct System, C.R. Bard, Inc., Billerica, MA).

coronary artery bypass graft surgery is extremely high but in whom there is an appropriate lesion or lesions. High operative risk can be based on severe left ventricle dysfunction, multiple previous bypass surgeries, advanced age, or associated medical illnesses present. The risk of PTCA is also extremely high in such patients, particularly those in whom the only remaining patent vessel is to be dilated. At times it is impossible to determine which mode of therapy is preferable in such patients. If patients are considered inoperable, emergency bypass surgery in the event of PTCA complication may be of no benefit. In cases truly deemed

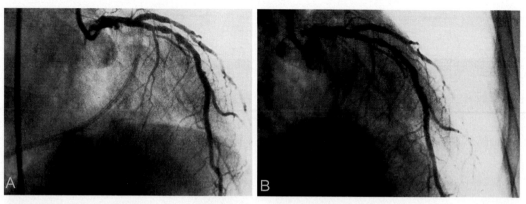

Figure 27A.4. **A.** A 67-year-old man with unstable angina caused by critical mid anterior descending artery stenosis, who also had a totally occluded left circumflex and right coronary artery. **B.** After successful coronary angioplasty, the repeat coronary angiogram shows an excellent angiographic result.

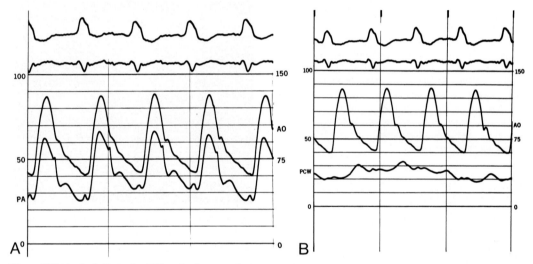

Figure 27A.5. **A & B.** Aortic *(AO)* and pulmonary *(PA)* pressures prior to bypass. Note reduction in AO, PA, and PCW **(C & D)** pressures. During balloon inflation on bypass, the patient had no chest pain. Note there was no increase in PCW, but a reduction in pulse pressure was present **(E)** without much change in the diastolic AO pressure. *PCW,* Pulmonary capillary wedge pressure.

inoperable, the patient, his or her family, the referring cardiologist, and the surgeons have all agreed that no emergency coronary bypass surgery would be undertaken even if the need arises. Contraindications to supported angioplasty include situations where dilation of the target vessel is not technically feasible or where the lesion is considered at high risk for abrupt closure (particularly if the patient is not a candidate for coronary bypass graft surgery). Additional contraindications are the presence of severe ilio-

femoral disease or a history of bleeding diathesis. When coronary artery bypass surgery is not an option under any circumstances, angioplasty should be undertaken only if an ideal lesion is present.

SAMPLE CASE HISTORY

A 67-year-old man was admitted with an acute inferior myocardial infarction and congestive heart failure. The patient had a prior history of liver disease and alcoholic cardiomyopathy, with multiple prior admissions

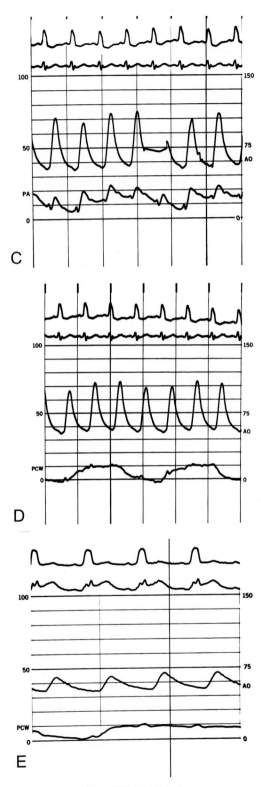

Figure 27A.5.C, D, & E.

for congestive heart failure. He had resection of one lobe of his lung for carcinoma and had chronic obstructive lung disease caused by a long history of heavy cigarette abuse. Because of postinfarction angina, he underwent cardiac catheterization, which revealed moderately severe pulmonary hypertension, elevated left ventricular end-diastolic pressure, and severe diffuse global hypokinesis, with a left ventricular ejection fraction of 15%. Coronary angiography revealed proximal total occlusions of the right coronary and left circumflex and a critical narrowing in the midleft anterior descending (LAD) coronary artery (Fig. 27A.4*A*).

Coronary bypass surgery, while technically feasible, was felt to be very high risk. Therefore the decision was made to do supported angioplasty.

Hemodynamics prior to PCPS revealed a systemic blood pressure of 128/60 mm Hg (Fig. 27A.5*A*), and a pulmonary capillary wedge pressure (PCW) of 25 mm Hg (Fig. 27A.5*B*). PCPS was instituted and gradually increased to 3.0 L/minute with a decrease in the systemic and PA pressures to 105/58 mm Hg and 8 mm Hg, respectively (Fig. 27A.5*C* and *D*). PTCA of the midLAD was then performed successfully using a prolonged balloon inflation of 5 minutes. The patient had no chest pain during the inflation and there was no increase in the PCW (Fig. 27A.5*E*) because the patient was on PCPS.

During balloon inflation there was a decrease in pulse pressure caused by transient, segmental, left ventricular dysfunction without any change in the aortic diastolic pressure. Following balloon deflation, pulse pressure immediately returned to its baseline value. A repeat angiogram revealed an excellent result (Fig. 27A.4*B*).

INITIATION OF CARDIOPULMONARY BYPASS SUPPORT

Baseline hemodynamic measurements, which include arterial, pulmonary artery, and pulmonary capillary wedge pressures, are obtained prior to the insertion of bypass cannulas. The arterial cannula is backbled by opening the Robert's clamp prior to disconnection to the primed perfusion circuit. Next, venous and arterial cannulas are attached to the CPS perfusion circuit, making sure that there are no air bubbles, particularly on the arterial side. Before the initiation of any flow, it is important to keep venous lines closed to the atmosphere. The patients are kept well hydrated before starting cardiopulmonary bypass support. If pulmonary artery diastolic or pulmonary capillary wedge pressure is <8 mm Hg, rapid volume infusion through the pump is given prior to full institution of bypass flow.

During elective supported angioplasty, cardiopulmonary bypass support is started using 2 L/minute flow with increments of 0.5 L/minute if pulmonary artery diastolic pressure is >5 mm Hg or >50% of the baseline or if chest pain or electrocardiographic changes occur with an increase in the filling pressures after less than 2 minutes of balloon inflation. At times a "chattering" of the venous line occurs during an attempt to increase the flow rate with the reduction in blood flow, as reflected on the blood flowmeter. This is an indication of intimal collapse of the vena cava around the venous cannula, which can be resolved by reducing the speed of the blood pump, adding volume, and then increasing pump speed until a corresponding increase of blood flow cannot be demonstrated.

Significant hypotension, defined as a mean pressure of <60 mm Hg (a lower blood pressure can be tolerated if the patient is awake and responding to verbal commands), can be corrected in most cases by volume infusion through the pump. In certain circumstances, particularly if the systemic vascular resistance is low, Neosynephrine infusion may be necessary. Activated clotting time is measured every 15 minutes and is maintained at or about 400 seconds. Arterial blood gas and mixed venous oxygen saturations are determined periodically in all patients.

PTCA TECHNIQUE

Patients who undergo elective, supported angioplasty are premedicated with aspirin 325 mg daily prior to the procedure, when feasible. An infusion of low molecular-weight dextran is started 3 to 4 hours prior to the procedure at a rate of 50 cc/hour, unless the patient is in congestive cardiac failure. PTCA is then performed from the contralateral femoral artery in the standard fashion after the establishment of cardiopulmonary bypass support. PTCA of the culprit vessel is initially performed and, if successful, additional vessels are also attempted. If patients are receiving intravenous nitroglycerin or heparin prior to PTCA, it is continued. The heparin infusion, however, is discontinued after receiving the standard bolus of heparin at the time of cannulation of CPS.

TERMINATION OF CARDIOPULMONARY BYPASS SUPPORT

After the completion of PTCA, cardiopulmonary bypass support is gradually weaned over a period of 5 to 15 minutes and the cannulas are clamped. Every effort is made to ensure excellent angiographic results following PTCA. If there is any doubt regarding the results following PTCA, repeat angiography should be performed 15 to 20 minutes later, prior to the termination of cardiopulmonary bypass support. Patients should be observed in the catheterization laboratory for an additional 15 to 30 minutes prior to transport to the coronary care unit. During weaning from bypass support, the bypass flow is reduced by about 0.5 L/minute. Volume is infused as necessary to increase the left ventricular filling pressure, estimated by the pulmonary capillary wedge pressure or the pulmonary diastolic pressure, to at least 8 to 10 mm Hg or to the prebypass level, whichever is less. In some patients, particularly those with severe left ventricular dysfunction or recent myocardial infarction, inotropic agents (dopamine and dobutrex) may be necessary to wean the patient from bypass. In the rare instance where an intraaortic balloon pump is needed, it is placed via the contralateral femoral artery.

The patient is then transported to the coronary care unit on a stretcher. Weaning and subsequent termination of PCPS can be done in the coronary care unit if the patient has not been weaned within about 30 minutes in the catheterization laboratory (which seldom happens). The stretcher commonly used consists of a flat metal surface with an adjustable headrest. A mattress with an egg-carton supplement and a pillow with the head elevated approximately 15° is used for patient comfort. A Cell Saver is used to autotransfuse the blood remaining in the bypass perfusion circuit. After autotransfusion is completed, the activated clotting time is checked on the coronary care unit.

REMOVAL OF BYPASS CANNULAS

Bypass cannulas are removed when the activated clotting time falls below 240 seconds. It takes 4 to 8 hours after the last dose of heparin to achieve this level of activating clotting time. After the cannulas are removed, manual compression for hemostasis is performed for 15 to 20 minutes. During this period of manual compression, an assessment of the appropriate point of clamp compression is made. To assess the status of the pedal pulse, pressure is slightly relaxed without allowing bleeding after 15 to 20 minutes of local compression. This allows an estimate of the degree of clamp pressure necessary for subsequent clamp compression. Mechanical clamp compression is then achieved using a new, modified disk (Comfort Disc, Instromedix, Hillsboro, OR) and applying a locked compression clamp (Compressar, Instromedix, Hillsboro, OR) (Fig. 27A.6). Clamp compression is adjusted so that the pedal pulses remain palpable or there is good capillary filling. After 90 minutes of compression and if there is no bleeding, the clamp is gradually released 2 mm every 20 minutes.

When the partial thromboplastin time

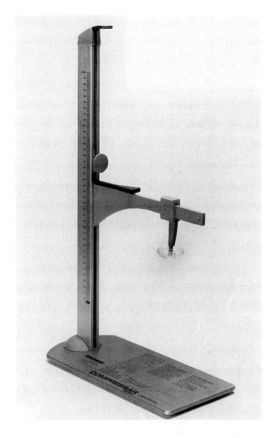

Figure 27A.6. Compression clamp with a self-locking mechanism and disk in place.

declines to <70 seconds or the activating clotting time declines to <180 seconds, low-dose heparin 600 to 800 units/hour infusion is begun and is continued until the patient is fully ambulatory. The angioplasty sheath and the Swan-Ganz catheter are removed the following day. Most patients are discharged at ≥72 hours after the procedure.

OBSERVATION ON CARDIOPULMONARY BYPASS SUPPORT DURING SUPPORTED ANGIOPLASTY

Once cardiopulmonary bypass support is instituted and the flow is increased, patients usually complain of generalized warmth, and in some cases, nausea. Administration of 5 mg compazine given intravenously prior to the initiation of cardiopulmonary bypass support can substantially reduced the incidence of nausea. Another way to significantly reduce nausea is by starting the flow at 0.5 L/minute and increasing by 0.5 L/minute every 30 seconds until a flow rate of 2 L/minute is achieved. With the current use of 18 Fr cannulas, a flow of up to 5 L/minute can be achieved if the patient is well hydrated prior to the procedure.

With the initiation of cardiopulmonary bypass support, there is a rapid fall (over a few minutes) in the filling pressures, manifested by reduction in the pulmonary capillary wedge pressure. There is also a reduction in the systolic arterial blood pressure, with a slight increase in diastolic pressure, the latter feature known to be present with nonpulsatile flow. Echocardiography performed during cardiopulmonary bypass support demonstrates a reduction in the left atrial and left ventricular dimensions. These observations, together with reduction of the preload and afterload, suggest that CPS reduces myocardial oxygen demand, which may be responsible, in part, for the absence of angina during balloon inflation in most patients undergoing supported angioplasty. Nonetheless, segmental wall motion irregularities and reduced pulse pressure are present during balloon inflation, indicating ischemia distal to the occlusion. Patients may experience numbness and tingling in the left leg when PCPS cannulas are inserted; in such cases sedation in the form of intravenous morphine may be necessary. Intravenous nitroglycerin or sublingual nifedipine may be helpful in some cases to counteract any spasm, particularly when iliofemoral angiography has revealed a good-caliber vessel prior to cannulation. Also, in patients with good-caliber iliofemoral vessels, such complaints may disappear spontaneously.

In some patients, significant hypotension, defined as a mean blood pressure of 60 mm Hg, occurs during bypass or when increasing the flow rate. This is more common and pronounced in patients who are volume depleted or have low filling pressures in the setting of a dilated, poorly functioning, left ventricle. Therefore it is imperative to have adequate filling pressures prior to the institution of bypass flow. Urinary output increases after the institution of PCPS. Therefore inserting a Foley catheter prior to the procedure is necessary. In most patients in whom PCPS is terminated in the catheterization laboratory, volume infusion of 150 to 1000 cc is necessary prior to the termination of PCPS. Recently, 25% albumin 50 to 75 cc has been given prior to the start of the procedure through the pump, which has resulted in a dramatic decrease in the volume requirement during the procedure.

OBSERVATIONS AFTER THE TERMINATION OF BYPASS SUPPORT

It is recommended that PCPS not be extended beyond 6 hours. However, in the author's experience (9) clinically significant microcirculatory compromise has not been noted even with prolonged bypass times up to 8 hours. If there is difficulty in weaning the patient from PCPS, then insertion of an intraaortic balloon pump (IABP) from the contralateral groin and additional inotropic support have been quite useful in such cases. The IABP is inserted in the laboratory and then the weaning of PCPS is undertaken in the coronary care unit. Some patients may complain of numbness and a tingling sensation in the leg when cannulas are still in place while waiting for the activated clotting time to fall below 240 seconds in the coronary care unit. Such patients may require sedation, as well as vasodilators (IV nitroglycerin or sublingual nifedipine). Interestingly, these complaints are usually transient and disappear in an hour or so, particularly when angiography in such patients has revealed a good-caliber iliofemoral system. Observation is safe so long as there is good capillary filling. The total clamp compression time necessary for hemostasis using the current method is less than 3 hours with a maximum compression for 90 minutes followed by a subsequent gradual release over the next 90 to 120 minutes.

DISCUSSION

The development of percutaneous cardiopulmonary bypass support provides an additional technique to support patients undergoing high-risk coronary angioplasty in the catheterization laboratory. Our initial results do suggest that supported angioplasty can be successful in patients with poor left ventricular function (11) with an acceptable morbidity and mortality (12). Local complications resulting from cannula insertion have been virtually eliminated using the current removal technique (13). The hemodynamic stability achieved during supported angioplasty not only permits PTCA to be performed in such high-risk patients, but also reduces the operator's anxiety about arrhythmias and hemodynamic instability. Also, in the event of abrupt closure (9) during supported angioplasty, emergency surgical revascularization, repeat dilatation, or even stent placement can be performed safely. Multicenter experience (10) suggests that patients with an ejection fraction of 20% or lower clearly benefit from prophylactic support. With experience, cardiopulmonary bypass support can be initiated in the standby situation promptly in almost all cases. The ability to initiate support in the standby circumstance reduces the need for emergency bypass surgery, as well as procedural mortality. The use of bypass support during cardiac emergencies is most successful when initiated within 25 minutes (14).

The IABP is the only other device readily available for use in the catheterization laboratory capable of supporting certain high-risk patients (15, 16). Indeed, in some patients this may provide adequate support. However, in patients who cease to have an effective cardiac rhythm, the intraaortic balloon pump is ineffective (17, 18). Also, the circulatory support provided is limited, and patients with severe hemodynamic compromise (evidence of hypoperfusion unresponsive to IABP sup-

port and inotropic agents) will not benefit (19). However, IABP placed prophylactically prior to catheter intervention may be beneficial in patients with moderately severe left ventricular dysfunction (LVEF >20%), with unstable angina, or with a recent myocardial infarction, especially when prolonged balloon inflations may be anticipated.

The experience to date suggests that patients with poor left ventricular function (LVEF ≤20%) are suitable candidates for PCPS-supported angioplasty with acceptable morbidity and mortality, improvement in anginal status and left ventricular function, and good long-term survival (20, 21). In our series of 103 high-risk patients with left ventricular ejection fractions ≤25% (mean 20.4 ± 3.8%), we reported a clinical success rate of 94% with an in-hospital mortality rate of 5.8%. On long-term follow-up (39 ± 18 months) 76% of the patients were functionally improved and had an increase in their ejection fraction from a baseline of 20.4% to 29.3% postprocedure.

A recent report by the National Registry of Elective Supported Angioplasty compared the use of prophylactic cardiopulmonary support with standby support (10). Both the prophylactic and the standby groups were comparable with respect to important baseline characteristics, except that the left ventricular ejection fraction was lower in the prophylactic group (Table 27A.1). A subgroup analysis showed that patients with a left ventricular ejection fraction ≤20% receiving prophylactic support had significantly lower procedural mortality (Table 27A.2) than did those in the standby group. Although procedural mortality was lower in the prophylactic group (4.8% versus 18.8%), femoral complications were significantly higher than that of the standby group (12.6% versus 6.1%). Also, the need for blood transfusion was higher in the prophylactic group (39% versus 11%). However, with meticulous aftercare using the author's technique (13), the local complications have been reduced to <2%. These data, however,

Table 27A.1.
Baseline Characteristics and Procedural Outcome of 569 Patients With Prophylactic or Standby Cardiopulmonary Support

	Prophylactic CPS[a] (n = 389)	Standby CPS[a] (n = 180)
Age >75 years	54 (13.9)	32 (17.8)
Female	88 (22.6)	56 (31.1)
LVEF (mean)	27.5%	36.7%[b]
LVEF ≤20%	126 (32.4)	32 (17.8)[c]
Procedural success	345 (88.7)	152 (84.4)
Mortality	25 (6.4)	11 (6.1)
Femoral complications	49 (12.6)	11 (6.1)[c]
Lesions dilated per patient	1.75	1.65
Unprotected left main dilated	36 (9.3)	10 (5.6)
Only patent vessel dilated	119 (30.6)	37 (20.6)

[a]Unless otherwise indicated, data is expressed as number (%) of patients.

[b]P <.01.

[c]P <.05.

CPS, Cardiopulmonary support; LVEF, left ventricular ejection fraction.

Table 27A.2.
Outcome in the Subgroup of 158 Patients With a Left Ventricular Ejection Fraction ≤20%

	Prophylactic CPS[a] (n = 126)	Standby CPS[a] (n = 32)
Procedural success	112 (90.5)	26 (81.2)
Major complications		
Death	6 (4.8)	6 (18.8)[b]

[a]Data expressed as number (%) of patients.

[b]P <.05.

suggest that patients with extremely depressed left ventricular function will benefit most from prophylactic rather than from standby support.

ACKNOWLEDGMENTS

The excellent contribution in the preparation of this manuscript by my research assistant Kathryn Dougherty is greatly appreciated as is the secretarial support provided by Karen Ellis.

REFERENCES

1. Serota H, Ubeydullah D, Woo-Hyeong L, Aquirre F, Kern MJ, Taussig SA, Vandormael MG. Predictors of cardiac survival after percutaneous transluminal coronary angioplasty in patients with severe left ventricular dysfunction. Am J Cardiol 1991;2:367–372.

2. Bounous EP, Mark DB, Pollock BG, Hlatky MA, Harrel FE Jr, Lee KL, Rankin JS et al. Surgical survival benefits for coronary disease patients with left ventricular dysfunction. Circulation 1988;78:I155–I157.

3. Alderman EL, Fisher LD, Litwin P et al. Results of coronary artery surgery in patients with poor left ventricular function (CASS). Circulation 1983;68:785–795.

4. Dorros G, Lewin RF, Mathiak L. Percutaneous transluminal coronary angioplasty in patients with severe left ventricular dysfunction (LVEF ≤35%). Cathet Cardiovasc Diagn 1989; 17:62 (abstract).

5. Kohli RS, DiSciascio G, Cowley MJ, Nath A, Goudreau E, Vetrovec GW. Coronary angioplasty in patients with depressed left ventricular function. J Am Coll Cardiol 1990; 16:807–811.

6. Shawl FA, Domanski MJ, Punja S, Hernandez TJ. Percutaneous cardiopulmonary bypass support in high-risk patients undergoing percutaneous transluminal coronary angioplasty. J Am Coll Cardiol 1989;64:1258–1263.

7. Vogel RA, Shawl F, Tommaso C, O'Neill W, Overlie P et al. Initial report of the National Registry of Elective Cardiopulmonary Bypass–Supported Coronary Angioplasty. J Am Coll Cardiol 1990;15:23–29.

8. Shawl FA, Domanski MJ, Hernandez TJ et al. Emergency percutaneous cardiopulmonary bypass support with cardiogenic shock from acute myocardial infarction. Am J Cardiol 1989;64:967–970.

9. Shawl FA, Domanski MJ, Wish MH, Davis M, Punja S, Hernandez TJ. Percutaneous cardiopulmonary bypass support in patients with cardiac arrest in the catheterization laboratory. Cathet Cardiovasc Diagn 1990;19:8–12.

10. Teirstein PS Vogel RA, Dorros G, Stertzer SH et al. Prophylactic versus standby cardiopulmonary support for high-risk percutaneous transluminal coronary angioplasty. J Am Coll Cardiol 1993;21:590–596.

11. Shawl FA, Bajaj S, Domanski MJ, Hoff S. Percutaneous cardiopulmonary bypass–supported coronary angioplasty in severely depressed left ventricular function. J Am Coll Cardiol 1993;21(2):140A.

12. Shawl FA, Domanski MJ, Wish M, Punja S, Hernandez TJ. Cardiopulmonary bypass–supported PTCA: experience in 75 high-risk patients. Circulation 1989;80(4):II-271.

13. Shawl FA, Domanski MJ, Wish MH, Davis M. Percutaneous cardiopulmonary bypass support in the catheterization laboratory: technique and complications. Am Heart J 1990; 120:195–203.

14. Shawl FA, Dougherty KG, Hoff SB, Ellis KO. Percutaneous cardiopulmonary bypass during cardiac arrest: factors influencing survival. Circulation 1993;88(Suppl 4):I226.

15. Kahn JK, McConahay DR, Rutherford BD et al. Supported "high risk" coronary angioplasty using intra-aortic balloon pump counterpulsation. J Am Coll Cardiol 1990;15:41A (abstract).

16. Hartzler GO, Rutherford BD, McConahay DR et al. High-risk percutaneous transluminal coronary angioplasty. Am J Cardiol 1988;81:33G–37G.

17. Alcan KE, Stertzer SH, Wallash E, DePasquale NP, Bruno MS. The role of intra-aortic balloon counterpulsation in patients undergoing percutaneous transluminal coronary angioplasty. Am Heart J 1983;105:527–530.

18. Phillips SJ. Percutaneous cardiopulmonary bypass and

innovations in clinical counterpulsation. Crit Care Clin 1986;2:297–318.

19. Myler RK, Stertzer SH. Left ventricular support during high-risk coronary angioplasty: an argument for the use of cardiopulmonary support. J Invas Cardiol 1990;2:155–156.

20. Shawl FA, Dougherty KG, Hoff SB, Ellis KO. Treatment option for inoperable or high-risk patients with left main coronary artery disease (LMCAD). Circulation 1993;88:I-297 (abstract).

21. Shawl FA, Bajaj S, Domanski MJ, Hoff S. Percutaneous cardiopulmonary bypass–supported coronary angioplasty in severely depressed left ventricular function. J Am Coll Cardiol 1993;21(Suppl 2):140A.

B. Hemodynamic Support and Revascularization of the Patient With Very Poor Left Ventricular Function

JOEL K. KAHN and GEOFFREY O. HARTZLER

Percutaneous interventions in patients with very poor left ventricular (LV) function may pose many challenges to the cardiovascular interventionalist. A careful consideration of patient preparation, equipment selection, and hemodynamic support in each case is necessary to maximize the likelihood of an uncomplicated and successful procedure. In this chapter we will review our approach to intervention in these patients and the potential complications that must be avoided.

PATIENT CHARACTERISTICS

Traditionally, patients have been identified as high risk for major ischemic complications related to poor LV function using an assessment of the LV ejection fraction (EF). In our own series of 845 elective percutaneous transluminal coronary angioplasty (PTCA) procedures in patients with poor LV function, the procedural mortality was 4% in patients having an EF $\leq 40\%$ compared with 1% in patients having an EF $>40\%$ (1). Furthermore, among patients with an EF $\leq 40\%$, there was a trend, albeit lacking statistical

significance, toward a higher procedural mortality the lower the EF. Clearly, a careful assessment of both global and regional LV function should be made prior to the performance of any interventional procedure.

Ellis et al. has suggested a jeopardy score as an alternative to the EF as a marker of increased risk for procedural mortality caused by LV dysfunction (2). The jeopardy score was a summation of the number of coronary segments that would potentially become ischemic if acute vessel closure occurred. In an analysis of 8052 elective PTCA procedures at Emory University, procedural mortality correlated better with the jeopardy score than with the EF (2).

It is intuitive that both the EF and the number of viable myocardial regions being treated are factors that must be considering in planning a dilation and support strategy. Other clinical factors should also be contemplated before the procedure begins. Patients with very poor LV function often are older, have more diffuse coronary artery and peripheral vascular disease, and more frequently have diabetes mellitus and renal insufficiency (1). A peripheral vascular examination should be carefully performed and documented in anticipation of the possible need for large-bore arterial support devices.

To minimize intraprocedural risks, patients with very poor LV function should be carefully assessed. Pulmonary congestion may require admission to the hospital for diuresis prior to the procedure. Electrolytes should be checked and normalized if possible. If patients are taking beta-blockers, careful withdrawal of these agents should be considered to maximize the responsiveness to catecholamine agents if needed during the procedure. In patients with significant renal dysfunction, low-dose dopamine, mannitol, and diuretic therapy may be used during the periprocedural period to minimize renal tubular injury.

A final clinical consideration before the procedure commences is the potential need for emergency surgical revascularization.

Certain patients with very poor LV function are offered PTCA as palliation and are unacceptable candidates for emergency CABG because of poor target arteries or comorbid illnesses. This should be carefully discussed ahead of the procedure with the patient and family and documented on the chart. A surgical opinion corroborating this palliative approach is probably wise from a medicolegal standpoint. In other cases it is often wise to have formal cardiac surgical review before the case begins to alert the surgical staff to a potentially high-risk situation should instability or poor results develop during percutaneous intervention.

TECHNICAL CONSIDERATIONS

We generally place 8 Fr or larger arterial sheaths and guides in these higher risk cases to minimize the chances that the procedure will be prolonged or fail because of the inadequate guide support or contrast visualization that may result from the use of smaller guides. Furthermore, many of these patients have complex anatomies that may require new interventional devices necessitating sheaths as large as 11 Fr. It is far better to have the appropriate sheath and guide in place ahead of time than to try to accomplish difficult guide exchanges in the middle of the procedure. It is not our routine to place femoral venous sheaths in stable patients with poor LV function, but if pulmonary congestion or hypotension is present, a venous sheath and a balloon-tipped pulmonary catheter may prove helpful to monitor the patient during the procedure and guide therapy should pulmonary edema or hypotension worsen.

As discussed below, some patients with very poor LV function are candidates for hemodynamic support devices during coronary intervention. If support is being considered, we will perform iliac angiography of the side contralateral to our guiding catheter access to evaluate whether there is sufficient arterial size and patency to permit ready access to the central arterial circulation. If it

is anticipated that the intervention will be poorly tolerated, we will usually place an intraaortic balloon pump before intervention (see below).

We will routinely select low-osmolar contrast agents in patients with very poor LV function. We are cautious about the use of calcium channel blockers during procedures in patients with very poor LV function and avoid them entirely in patients with low arterial pressures. We also modify our dosing of Dextran-40 if this is administered during the procedure because of the volume expanding effects of this drug; in patients with very poor ventricles we may omit it entirely, and in others only 100 to 200 cc will be infused compared with our usual administration of 500 cc.

The dilation strategy planned before the procedure differs little from routine interventions. Whenever possible, consideration is given to recanalizing chronically occluded arteries at the beginning of the procedure before subtotal stenoses are approached. This may open collateral routes of coronary flow to stenotic vessels and improve the hemodynamic stability during these inflations. The decision to attempt chronic total occlusion PTCA in patients with very poor LV function may be complex. Careful consideration of the recognized morphologic features favorable for successful PTCA, such as a tapered stump, short segment of occlusion, absence of bridging collaterals, and no major side branches, plays a role. A consideration of the additional time and contrast requirements that may develop by initially attempting PTCA of a chronic total occlusion before other stenotic areas must be judged for each patient. We do strive whenever possible, however, to achieve complete revascularization of all major arteries in a single setting.

Positioning of the guide catheter throughout the case is extremely important during interventions in patients with very poor LV function. To prevent cumulative and repetitive ischemia, ventricularization should be avoided except for a few seconds if it is necessary to deliver the balloon catheter to the stenosis. We are meticulous in backing the guide catheter out of the ostium at all times during the procedure except to deliver the device and to perform contrast injections. With active control of the guide-catheter position, we rarely resort to guide catheters with side holes. We feel that the decreased coronary artery visualization with side-hold guide catheters often leads to increased contrast media utilization, which must be avoided in patients with poor LV function.

Balloon selection requires more thoughtful consideration in patients with very poor LV function. Standard, low-profile balloon catheters are selected most commonly. Autoperfusion balloon catheters may be considered, however, as primary dilation catheters if the coronary anatomy is proximal, nontortuous, and not longer than 20 to 25 mm. The delivery of 40 to 60 cc/minute of coronary flow may be adequate for successful PTCA in even the most impaired ventricles. The trade-off, however, of the higher-profile balloon and catheter shaft must be contemplated. Very complex stenoses or chronic total occlusions may be poor targets for the primary use of autoperfusion balloons because of the anticipated difficulties in delivering the balloon to the lesion. A lower-profile balloon catheter with greater crossing potential may be a better choice in these lesions even without the coronary perfusion. Similarly, a small-diameter proximal artery with diffuse narrowing may be a poor choice for the primary use of an autoperfusion balloon catheter because of the possibility of creating ischemia proximal to the balloon material by compromise of a small left main coronary or the side branches by the higher-profile catheter shaft. In our experience the recent improvements in catheter performance of the latest generation of autoperfusion balloon catheters (Flow-Track, Advanced Cardiovascular Systems, Santa Clara, CA) has improved the catheter performance and permitted dilation of more distal anatomy. Overall, in straightforward anatomy,

a perfusion balloon will likely improve the tolerance of the procedure.

We monitor the volume of contrast administered during the procedure and attempt to limit the dose as much as possible without compromising our judgments. If the creatinine is normal, we have seen few problems with using as much as 400 to 500 ml of contrast media (3).

HEMODYNAMIC SUPPORT

One of the most challenging decisions facing the interventionalist before embarking on a procedure in a patient with very poor LV function is whether hemodynamic support is needed to avoid pulmonary edema, prevent hypotension, or permit longer coronary manipulation as may be required if a nonballoon device is selected. There are several clinical scenarios that have been suggested as sufficiently high risk to consider the prophylactic placement of a support device before intervention. The criteria that we have suggested are listed in Table 27B.1 (4). Alternative criteria have been suggested by the National Registry of Elective Cardiopulmonary Bypass and include (a) the presence of severe unstable angina, (b) an LVEF <25%, or (c) intervening on an artery supplying more than half of the viable myocardium (5).

We believe that the problem with almost any list of criteria for elective hemodynamic support is that we have found it nearly impossible to predict which patients will develop hypotension or other life-threatening prob-

Table 27B.1.

Recommended Guidelines for Patient Selection for Consideration of Prophylactic Placement of Hemodynamic Support Prior to Coronary Intervention[a]

1. Severe left ventricular dysfunction (ejection fraction <30%)
2. Unprotected left main coronary intervention
3. Intervention of single remaining conduit to viable myocardium
4. Arterial hypotension during multivessel intervention

[a]Adapted from Kahn JK, Rutherford BD, McConahay DR et al. J Am Coll Cardiol 1990;15:1151–1155.

lems during electively scheduled coronary interventions. Patients with very poor LV function will on occasion tolerate inflations in critical vessels for several minutes or longer without obvious explanation. Collaterals from unappreciated sources, such as conus branches of an occluded right coronary artery to a proximal anterior descending artery or intramyocardial collaterals, may account for the stability in these patients. For this reason, in most cases of patients with a very poor EF, we have elected not to place hemodynamic support ahead of time. Instead, if the initial arterial pressure is over 100 mm Hg, we will usually proceed with the procedure and assess the blood pressure and clinical response carefully in the first few seconds of arterial manipulation. If the treatment is well tolerated, the procedure will be continued and the patient will be monitored carefully for slowly progressive, hemodynamic deterioration requiring support. If short balloon inflations or positioning on nonballoon devices results in dramatic changes in the blood pressure or rhythm, a support device will be placed early in the procedure. Finally, if a patient with poor LV function presents to the laboratory with an arterial blood pressure under 100 mm Hg, we will usually place a balloon-tipped pulmonary artery flotation catheter to assess whether the hypotension results from hypovolemia. If this is the case, small fluid boluses will be administered until either the blood pressure increases or the filling pressures are optimized. If the patient is not hypovolemic or the arterial pressure does not respond adequately to fluid boluses, we will usually place a support device before any coronary manipulation is started.

INTRAAORTIC BALLOON PUMP SUPPORT

Of the various methods of hemodynamic support available, we select, when necessary, intraaortic balloon pump counterpulsation. There are rare circumstances, of course, when intraaortic balloon pump counterpulsation cannot provide meaningful cir-

culatory support such as full cardiac arrest and disorganized cardiac rhythms. These, however, are very rare circumstances to be performing coronary interventions, arising at most a few times a year even in the busiest of interventional centers. In such circumstances femoral-femoral percutaneous cardiopulmonary support, if available, may offer an advantage.

There are two ways in which we use intraaortic balloon pump support. The balloon pump is most commonly placed at the initiation of the procedure or early during coronary manipulation. In these cases the contralateral femoral artery is prepared and bilateral sheaths are placed. The balloon pump catheter is positioned, and 1:1 counterpulsation is continued throughout coronary manipulation. The balloon pump often needs to be placed on standby during guide-catheter exchanges to permit atraumatic advancement of the guide catheter to the central aorta.

The second situation where a balloon pump is used is at the end of the coronary intervention. In these cases the coronary manipulation is tolerated without support, but the balloon pump is inserted at the end of the case in the hope that benefits will accrue after the procedure. The common setting for this approach is in infarct intervention involving the anterior wall or in the setting of infarct patients with multivessel coronary artery disease and significantly depressed LV function. In these settings it has been suggested that intraaortic balloon pump counterpulsation may lower reocclusion and early restenosis rates (6). Another setting where we have placed intraaortic balloon pumps at the end of coronary procedures is in patients treated electively with multivessel intervention with marginal blood pressures at the end of the procedure. It is our feeling that the augmented diastolic pressure may maintain superior coronary perfusion and patency during the 24 to 48 hours after the procedure and reduce the likelihood of out-of-laboratory acute arterial occlusion. Furthermore, postprocedural pulmonary edema may be reduced with the maintenance of counterpulsation for up to 48 hours. When the intraaortic balloon pump is placed at the end of the procedure, the contralateral femoral artery does not need to be accessed. The existing femoral arterial sheath can be removed over a guidewire with firm pressure at the puncture site, and the intraaortic balloon pump catheter can be advanced through the existing puncture tract. We have used the sheathless 9.5 Fr balloon pump catheters with guide success in this setting as the catheter easily traverses through the subcutaneous tissues after predilation with the 8 Fr sheath.

We have had less success using the sheathless balloon pump insertion method when the balloon pump is inserted primarily, perhaps because the stepped dilator does not provide adequate tissue separation. We usually select 50-cc intraaortic balloon pumps in medium- or large-framed individuals, usually men, with the more standard 40-cc balloon being reserved for small-framed patients.

We have previously reported our results with prophylactic placement of intraaortic balloon pump catheters in high-risk coronary interventions (4). Over a 30-month period during which we performed 3408 coronary interventions, we electively placed an intraaortic balloon pump catheter in 28 patients (0.9%). The most common indication for prophylactic placement was severe LV dysfunction (EF ≤30%), but others included a single remaining vessel providing circulation to the heart, and left main disease. We performed multivessel angioplasty in 21 of the patients and dilated a total of 94 narrowings. Lesion success to a diameter stenosis of <40% was achieved in 90 lesions (96%). Profound procedural hypotension developed in 11 patients despite intraaortic balloon pump support, but in all cases the augmented diastolic pressure remained above 90 mm Hg. There were no procedural deaths or myocardial infarctions. Peripheral vascular complications developed in three patients requiring embolectomy in

two and repair of a pseudoaneurysm in the third. We concluded that intraaortic balloon pump support in patients with high-risk features undergoing elective coronary interventions was effective and usually uncomplicated. At least two other experienced interventional centers have reported similar findings with the prophylactic placement of intraaortic balloon pumps for high-risk coronary intervention (7, 8). For these reasons, it remains our support device of choice.

CLINICAL RESULTS

We have analyzed in detail our experience with coronary angioplasty in patients with poor LV function through 1990 (1). Up to that time, 8962 elective coronary angioplasties had been performed and entered into a prospective computer database. In 845 procedures the LVEF was ≤40%, and in the remaining 8117 procedures the LVEF was >40%. When we compared the clinical characteristics of the two groups, the patients with poor LV function were generally older, were more likely to have had a prior myocardial infarction and coronary artery bypass surgery, were more often diabetic, had more advanced angina pectoris, and were more likely to have three-vessel coronary artery disease (Table 27B.2).

Of the 845 patients with poor LV function,

Table 27B.2.

Clinical and Angiographic Baseline Characteristics of Patients With Left Ventricular Ejection Fractions (LVEF) ≤40% Compared With >40% Treated With Coronary Angioplasty[a]

	LVEF <40%	LVEF >40%	P Value
Number	845	8117	
Mean age (year)	63	60	<.01
Prior infarction	713 (84%)	3490 (45%)	<.001
Prior bypass	333 (39%)	1736 (21%)	<.001
Diabetes mellitus	208 (25%)	1108 (14%)	<.001
Class IV angina	405 (48%)	3175 (41%)	<.001
Three-vessel disease	526 (62%)	2646 (33%)	<.001

[a]Adapted from Stevens T, Kahn JK, McCallister BD et al. Am J Cardiol 1991;68:313–319 with permission.

angioplasty was successful in 93% of 2211 lesions compared with 95% in patients with better LV function ($P = .007$). An intraaortic balloon pump was used in 113 procedures (13%), prophylactically in 76 and emergently in the rest. Intraaortic balloon pumps were most frequently used in patients with an LVEF <20%. Complete revascularization was achieved in 249 procedures (29%).

A major procedural complication occurred in 6% of the patients with poor LV function. Procedural death complicated the procedure in 35 patients (4%). Urgent bypass surgery was performed in 18 patients (2%), and a nonfatal infarction occurred in 15 patients (2%). The yearly procedural death rate was <3% from 1987 to 1989. The most frequent cause of procedural death was acute vessel closure, but other causes included contrast nephropathy and congestive heart failure.

Because many of the patients with poor LV function in our series may have been considered for bypass surgery at other institutions, we calculated the predicted operative mortality for coronary bypass grafting for the 100 most recent patients using the Coronary Artery Surgery Study formula. The predicted operative mortality was 10.3% compared with an observed mortality with angioplasty of 3% ($P = .08$).

We reported the follow-up of 99% of the hospital survivors for a mean of 33 months following hospital discharge (1). The 1- and 4-year actuarial survival rates were 87% and 69%, respectively. Cox multivariate analysis identified age >70 years, the number of diseased vessels, and class IV angina as independently related to long-term mortality (1).

ANGIOPLASTY OR BYPASS SURGERY IN POOR LV FUNCTION?

A randomized comparison of the safety and outcome of patients treated with coronary intervention or bypass grafting is not available at the time of this writing. In the interim, we performed a retrospective comparison of safety and long-term efficacy of angioplasty

and bypass surgery in patients with multivessel disease and impaired LV function (9). One hundred consecutive patients who underwent coronary artery bypass surgery were matched with a concurrent cohort of 100 patients who underwent coronary angioplasty from 1985 to 1988. All patients had an LVEF <40% and two- or three-vessel disease. Angina was more severe in the surgical group, but the groups otherwise were well matched. Angioplasty was able to achieve complete revascularization in only 37% of patients compared with 82% in the surgical group ($P < .001$).

Early results favored angioplasty with a shorter hospital stay (4 versus 13 days, $P < .001$) and a somewhat lower hospital mortality (3% versus 5%, $P = $ NS). Stroke occurred significantly more often in the bypass group (7% versus 0%). During 5-year follow-up, superior relief from disabling angina was observed in the surgical group (99% versus 89%, $P = .01$) and a trend toward improved survival was identified (76% versus 67%, $P = .09$).

SUMMARY

The technical approach to coronary intervention in patients with very poor LV function that we have outlined has resulted in a steady lowering of the procedural mortality over the past decade. This remains a high-risk patient group, however, both for in-hospital complications and for later adverse events. In no other subgroup of coronary intervention is it as important to weigh the advantages and disadvantages for surgical or percutaneous coronary revascularization for each patient. In patients without significant comorbidities and in whom complete revascularization cannot be achieved with coronary intervention, surgical therapy generally should be selected. In patients in whom comparable revascularization can be anticipated with either surgical or percutaneous interventions, the lower, predicted, procedural mortality with angioplasty generally is preferred provided close follow-up can be maintained following the procedure. In patients with significant comorbidities greatly increasing the risks of surgical therapy, coronary interventions can be selected as palliative therapy, even if unable to achieve complete

revascularization. The results of ongoing randomized trials will help clarify the optimal therapy for
selected patients with poor LV function.

REFERENCES

1. Stevens T, Kahn JK, McCallister BD et al. Safety and efficacy of percutaneous transluminal coronary angioplasty in patients with left ventricular dysfunction. Am J Cardiol 1991;68:313–319.
2. Ellis SG, Myler RK, King SB et al. Causes and correlates of death after unsupported coronary angioplasty: implications for use of angioplasty and advanced support techniques in high-risk settings. Am J Cardiol 1991;68:1447–1451.
3. Kahn JK, Rutherford BD, McConahay DR et al. High-dose contrast media administration during complex coronary angioplasty. Am Heart J 1990;120:533–536.
4. Kahn JK, Rutherford BD, McConahay DR et al. Supported "high-risk" coronary angioplasty using intraaortic balloon pump counterpulsation. J Am Coll Cardiol 1990;15:1151–1155.
5. Vogel RA, Shawl F, Tommaso C et al. Initial report of the National Registry of Elective Cardiopulmonary Bypass Supported Coronary Angioplasty. J Am Coll Cardiol 1990;15:23–29.
6. Ishihara M, Sato H, Tateishi H, Uchida T, Dote K. Intraaortic balloon pumping as the postangioplasty strategy in acute myocardial infarction. Am Heart J 1991;122:385–389.
7. Anwar A, Mooney MR, Stertzer SH et al. Intraaortic balloon counterpulsation support for elective coronary angioplasty in the setting of poor left ventricular function: a two-center experience. J Invasive Cardiol 1990;2:175–180.
8. Voudris V, Marco J, Morice MC et al. "High-risk" percutaneous transluminal coronary angioplasty with preventive intraaortic balloon counterpulsation. Cathet Cardiovasc Diagn 1990;19:160–164.
9. O'Keefe JH, Allan JJ, McCallister BD et al. Angioplasty versus bypass surgery for multivessel coronary artery disease with left ventricular ejection fraction ≤40%. Am J Cardiol 1993;71:897–901.

C. Periprocedural Strategies in the Patient with Very Poor Left Ventricular Function

ALICE K. JACOBS

Since the advent of percutaneous coronary
revascularization with coronary angioplasty,
enormous technologic advances have allowed expansion of the technique to higher-
risk patients with more complex coronary
anatomy and comorbid disease. Patients in
whom the risk of an adverse outcome was previously considered prohibitive are now being
considered candidates for the procedure.
Certainly, in patients with coronary artery
disease, one of the most important prognostic
clinical factors that adversely affects both
acute and long-term outcome is left ventricular dysfunction (1). It has been well documented that surgical revascularization in
such patients with multivessel disease and
stable or unstable angina improves survival
(2–4). However, although the role of percutaneous revascularization in the setting of reduced left ventricular function is less clearly
defined, the use of coronary angioplasty in
these patients is increasing (5, 6). Most studies report a similar procedural outcome in patients undergoing coronary angioplasty with
both normal and reduced left ventricular
function, although long-term survival is reduced in patients with depressed left ventricular function. Specifically, in patients with
left ventricular dysfunction (mean left ventricular ejection fraction 39%) undergoing
percutaneous transluminal coronary angioplasty within the NHLBI PTCA Registry,
there was no difference in in-hospital rate of
death or nonfatal infarction in comparison
with patients with preserved left ventricular
function. However, during long-term follow-
up, left ventricular dysfunction was associated with a significantly higher mortality rate
even after adjustment for variables such as
older age, diabetes mellitus, congestive heart
failure, multivessel disease, and clinical success of the procedure (7).

Recently, in an effort to safely perform percutaneous revascularization in patients with
depressed left ventricular function who are
deemed to be at high risk for an adverse outcome, both systemic and regional support
techniques have been gaining more widespread use (Table 27C.1). The goals of these
modalities are to support the systemic circulation and/or to provide oxygenated blood to
the ischemic myocardium. In our laboratory
the intraaortic balloon and the antegrade and

Table 27C.1.
Myocardial Support Techniques

Systemic support
  Intraaortic balloon counterpulsation
  Cardiopulmonary bypass
  Partial left heart bypass
  Hemopump
Regional support
  Antegrade perfusion
    Passive hemoperfusion
    Active hemoperfusion
    Fluosol
  Retrograde perfusion
    Coronary sinus retroperfusion
    Pressure-controlled intermittent coronary sinus occlusion
    Coronary sinus retrograde cardioplegia

Table 27C.2.
Preprocedural Approach to the High-Risk Patient

1. Risk assessment
2. Cardiac surgical consultation
3. Detailed discussion with patient and family
4. Assessment of ability to use support modalities
5. Preprocedural technical strategy

retrograde regional support techniques are used most often. Other than the indirect benefit from improvement in left ventricular function, the perfusion balloon catheters and synchronized retroperfusion do not provide direct peripheral circulatory support as do percutaneous bypass systems or the Hemopump and do not improve the peripheral hemodynamic profile as does the intraaortic balloon.

APPROACH TO THE PATIENT

Management Prior to the Procedure

The preprocedural approach to the patient is of critical importance, and our overall strategy is outlined in Table 27C.2.

DECISION MAKING AND RISK MANAGEMENT

The decision to perform percutaneous revascularization in patients with very poor left ventricular function is based on multiple factors and determined by the overall risk of

the procedure. Conceptually, we divide this risk assessment into high-risk patients and high-risk lesions. Patient factors contributing to the risk of an adverse outcome include, importantly, the degree of left ventricular dysfunction, female gender, advanced age, and the presence of diabetes mellitus, as well as other comorbid illness (8). Lesion characteristics associated with abrupt closure have been well described and based on morphologic features such as angulation, tortuosity, eccentricity, thrombus, and lesion length (9).

In addition to consideration of patient and lesion factors that increase the risk of the procedure, we attempt to assess the risk of hemodynamic compromise. In a retrospective review of 28 clinical and angiographic variables in a group of consecutive patients undergoing coronary angioplasty at our institution, multivariate analysis identified multivessel disease, diffuse disease, myocardium at risk, and the degree of target lesion stenosis as independent predictors of hemodynamic compromise (decrease in systolic blood pressure by >20 mm Hg to <90 mm Hg during balloon inflation) (Table 27C.3). Using this analysis, a 13-point weighted scoring system was created based on the regression coefficients of the variables (Table 27C.4). This scoring system was then prospectively applied to another group of consecutive patients undergoing coronary angioplasty. In using a

Table 27C.3.
Multivariate Analysis of Predictors of Hemodynamic Compromise[a]

Angiographic Characteristics	Unit	Odds Ratio	P Value	Confidence Interval
Multivessel disease	0, +	4.3	.03	1.1–16.1
Diffuse disease	0, +	4.1	.05	1.0–16.9
Myocardium at risk	10%	1.7	.03	1.1–2.7
Pre-PTCA stenosis	10%	0.6	.05	0.3–1.0

[a]Reprinted with permission from Bergelson et al. Am J Cardiol 1992; 70:1540–1545.

PTCA, Percutaneous transluminal coronary angioplasty.

Table 27C.4.
Scoring System[a]

Angiographic Characteristic	Score
Myocardium at risk (%)	
6–14	−2
15–23	−1
24–32	0
33–41	1
42–50	2
51–59	3
60–68	4
Multivessel disease	3
Pre-PTCA stenosis (%)	
50–57	3
58–65	2
66–73	1
74–81	0
82–89	−1
90–97	−2
98–100	−3
Diffuse disease	3

[a]Reprinted with permission from Bergelson et al. Am J Cardiol 1992; 70:1540–1545.

PTCA, Percutaneous transluminal coronary angioplasty.

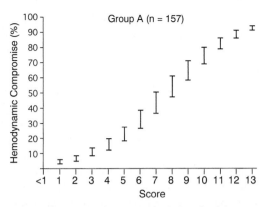

Figure 27C.1. Relation of Boston University risk score to the incidence of hemodynamic compromise during percutaneous intervention (see also Tables 27C.1 and 27C.2). (From Bergelson BA et al. Am J Cardiol 1992; 70:1540–1545.)

risk score of ≥4 to define high risk for hemodynamic compromise, this scoring system had a sensitivity of 92% and a specificity of 92% (Fig. 27C.1) (10). Currently, the risk score influences our decision to use prophylactic or standby support modalities.

Finally, the assessment of overall risk of the procedure is greatly influenced by the patient's candidacy for coronary bypass surgery and for systemic support techniques. In the setting of very poor left ventricular function and abrupt vessel closure unresponsive to the usual repeat dilation strategies, the ability to support the systemic circulation (and regional myocardium, if possible) and safely transport the patient to the operating room for emergency coronary bypass surgery is a major factor in our decision to perform the procedure. Except in unusual cases, if the patient is not considered to be a surgical candidate under any circumstance and if severe peripheral vascular disease precludes the use of the intraaortic balloon, we would not consider the patient to be eligible for percutaneous revascularization in the setting of

a high-risk lesion profile, particularly if the risk of hemodynamic compromise was also increased.

SURGICAL CONSULTATION

In the patient with very poor left ventricular function, prior to proceeding with percutaneous revascularization, formal cardiac surgical consultation is obtained. The patient is evaluated by our thoracic surgical colleagues, and the suitability of the patient for coronary bypass surgery either on an elective or in an emergency situation is discussed. Occasionally, when the patient is deemed to be a candidate for surgery on an elective basis but not on an emergency basis (i.e., in the setting of multiple previous cardiac surgical procedures), the optimal revascularization strategy is reassessed. More often, in these high-risk patients the surgeon agrees to an on-line assessment at the time of the failed or complicated procedure. If the patient is experiencing ongoing ischemia but is hemodynamically stable and supported by systemic and regional modalities, emergency surgical revascularization will be provided. Alternatively, if there is only minimal ongoing ischemia or, in contrast, severe hemodynamic compromise and instability, the patient will not be considered a candidate for emergency coronary bypass surgery.

DISCUSSION WITH THE PATIENT AND FAMILY

Prior to proceeding with any percutaneous revascularization procedure and, in particular, in the patient deemed to be at high risk because of reduced left ventricular function, the options for treatment and the risks of the procedure are discussed in detail with the patient and family. The likelihood of a major or minor complication is explained in terms that can be understood. In these high-risk circumstances and especially in the setting where surgical backup is refused, we agree to perform the procedure only with the support and understanding of both the patient and family and in consultation with the referring physician.

ASSESSMENT OF THE ABILITY TO USE SUPPORT MODALITIES

In the patient with reduced left ventricular function, it is mandatory that preprocedural evaluation include an assessment of the likelihood of successful placement of both systemic and regional support devices. A history and physical exam focusing on peripheral vascular disease or other pathology (i.e., aortic insufficiency) precluding intraaortic balloon placement are performed. A detailed cineangiographic review is undertaken, noting lesion location and morphologic characteristics, which determine the ability to maintain antegrade (or retrograde) perfusion. As noted previously, in the patient in whom hemodynamic compromise during percutaneous revascularization is likely, candidacy for support technology strongly influences the decision to perform the procedure.

PREPROCEDURAL STRATEGY

Prior to the procedure, careful assessment of the dilation and device strategy is undertaken during a review of the cineangiogram. Therefore in this setting of increased risk and severely reduced left ventricular function, we

rarely perform "on-line" revascularization unless absolutely necessitated by limited vascular access sites. When studying the diagnostic angiogram, careful consideration is given to the relationship between the diagnostic catheter and coronary orifice and to the takeoff of the proximal coronary artery from the ascending aorta. In addition, the size and shape of the aorta, the amount of backup support needed, the length of the left main trunk, and the location of the coronary ostium are important considerations in choosing the appropriate devices and the guiding and balloon catheters. In the setting of multivessel disease, the order of the target lesions approached is carefully considered. Most often, the lesion deemed to be the "culprit" is approached first. However, in certain circumstances revascularization of another lesion prior to the "culprit" lesion may provide collateral flow and thereby reduce the risk of the procedure. In the patient with severely reduced left ventricular function, we strongly consider a staged procedure, and we would not attempt to instrument a second lesion if there is evidence of a dissection, thrombus, or a suboptimal result in the first lesion.

Management in the Interventional Laboratory

PERIPHERAL ANGIOGRAPHY

In all high-risk patients with reduced ventricular function and, in particular, in those patients at increased risk for hemodynamic compromise, we initially prep both femoral access sites. One femoral artery is instrumented with a pigtail catheter, and peripheral angiography of the aortoiliac and common femoral arteries is obtained either via hand injection of approximately 20 cc of contrast or by a Medrad power injector. Review of the angiography aids in the decision to use one femoral site for the procedure and the other for the purpose of providing systemic support using large catheters such as the intraaortic balloon. In these patients we routinely instrument the contralateral femoral artery with a 5

Fr sheath to ensure rapid deployment of support devices if necessary.

PROPHYLACTIC VERSUS STANDBY SUPPORT

In general, in the patient who arrives in the laboratory in stable condition without evidence of active or ongoing ischemia, the systemic (intraaortic balloon) and regional (perfusion balloon and/or reperfusion) catheters are placed in a standby ready mode. However, as noted above, the majority of patients undergo contralateral femoral artery sheath insertion, and selected patients in whom synchronized retroperfusion is an attractive strategy undergo right internal jugular vein cannulation with a 9 Fr sheath. However, the following situations are notable exceptions to this practice during which prophylactic support techniques are instituted:

1. Acute ischemia refractory to intravenous medical therapy.
2. Hemodynamic instability (Fig. 27C.2).
3. Stable but marginal hemodynamic profile with relative hypotension (systolic blood pressure ≤90 mm Hg) and

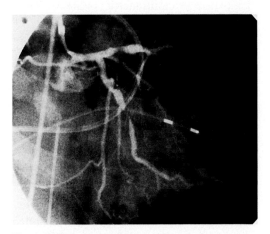

Figure 27C.2. Cineangiogram of the left coronary artery (right anterior oblique projection with caudal angulation) in a patient in cardiogenic shock. The intraaortic balloon *(left)* was inserted prior to angiography. The left anterior descending artery (infarct artery) has delayed filling (thought to represent "no-reflow"), but is without a significant stenosis. The left circumflex obtuse marginal artery has a significant stenosis that was thought to be contributing to the hemodynamic instability. The patient underwent successful angioplasty of the obtuse marginal artery lesion using a perfusion balloon catheter.

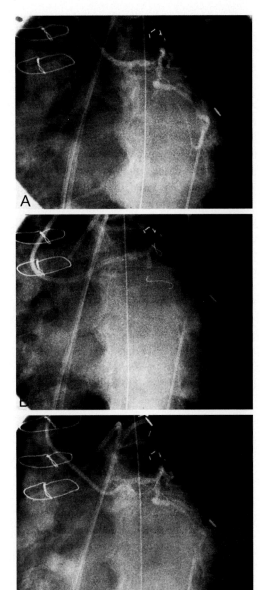

Figure 27C.3. **A.** Cineangiogram of the left coronary artery (shallow left anterior oblique projection) illustrating a significant left main stenosis in an elderly patient with prior bypass surgery (patent graft to left anterior descending artery) who was no longer considered an operative candidate and in whom unstable angina was refractory to maximal medical management. Because of ongoing ischemia, the intraaortic balloon *(right)* was inserted prior to angiography. **B.** Balloon inflation in the left main coronary artery using a "kissing" balloon strategy and requiring the use of a left Amplatz guide for support. **C.** Follow-up cineangiogram illustrating an insignificant residual stenosis in the left main coronary artery.

elevated filling pressure (pulmonary artery diastolic pressure ≥25 mm Hg).

4. Severely reduced left ventricular function (left ventricular ejection fraction ≤20%).

5. Instrumentation of an artery supplying the only viable myocardium (in the setting of poor left ventricular function) (Fig. 27C.3).

6. Demonstrated hemodynamic compromise during previous revascularization of the same target lesion.

HEMODYNAMIC MONITORING

During interventional procedures, all patients with poor left ventricular function undergo continuous hemodynamic monitoring with a pacing catheter positioned in the pulmonary artery. Importantly, prior to instrumenting the coronary artery, arterial blood pressure, filling pressures, and heart rate are optimized with intravenous therapy, including, where appropriate, administration of fluids, nitroglycerin, pressor agents, and Lopressor.

Management Postprocedure

In the vast majority of patients undergoing percutaneous revascularization in this high-risk setting, heparin is continued until the following day when sheaths (and the intraaortic balloon) are removed. If the angiographic results reveal evidence of a dissection or residual thrombus, the sheaths are removed on half-dose heparin and full-dose heparin is resumed 2 hours following sheath removal and continued for a prolonged period (24 to 72 hours). Patients in whom abrupt closure would result in hemodynamic compromise or collapse are observed in the interventional unit an additional 24 to 48 hours following sheath removal, preferably until heparin has been discontinued.

CHOOSING A SUPPORT TECHNIQUE

Systemic Support

INTRAAORTIC BALLOON COUNTERPULSATION

Physiology. By far the most widely used systemic (or global myocardial) support modality is intraaortic balloon counterpulsation. Enthusiasm for use of this device is based on its availability and ease of implementation. There are multiple hemodynamic effects of intraaortic balloon counterpulsation, which are based, in part, on the pathophysiologic state of the patient (11). Myocardial ischemia is reliably relieved by a combination of an increase in coronary perfusion pressure and a reduction in myocardial workload. Balloon inflation during diastole increases coronary flow to all regions, and rapid deflation at end-diastole is associated with a reduction in system afterload; stroke volume and cardiac output are thereby improved.

Practical Considerations. Percutaneous placement of the intraaortic balloon and the use of smaller-diameter catheters and sheaths have greatly improved the ease of insertion and expanded the use of the technique to smaller patients with moderate peripheral vascular disease. In our laboratory, in the setting of peripheral vascular disease and/or a small (short) patient, we have recently been using pediatric intraaortic balloons. These smaller catheters (8 Fr, 30.5-inch-long) and balloons (30 cc) have been effective in providing the expected hemodynamic effects without compromising the peripheral arterial circulation. Of note, when the intraaortic balloon is deployed, the balloon pump is turned off when angioplasty or atherectomy catheters are introduced or withdrawn (over a wire) through the descending thoracic aorta. Otherwise, the balloon actively pumps during the procedure.

Despite the beneficial hemodynamic features of intraaortic balloon counterpulsation, its use is limited to patients with a stable ventricular rhythm, and its ability to provide circulatory support is modest, with a maximum increase in cardiac output between 10% and 40%. In addition, the intraaortic balloon does not provide regional myocardial protection during coronary balloon inflation or after abrupt closure (although it may provide some theoretical benefit because of improved collateral flow from increased coronary perfusion pressure). Therefore, in addition to intraaortic balloon counterpulsation, we routinely provide myocardial support via antegrade or retrograde perfusion during periods of prolonged ischemia.

Despite the lack of controlled clinical trials demonstrating the efficacy of intraaortic balloon counterpulsation, extensive single-center and anecdotal experience has been accumulated (12, 13). The vast majority of these reports (as well as our own experience) suggest that this modality is effective in providing clinical and hemodynamic stability during percutaneous revascularization, particularly in the setting of reduced left ventricular function. In addition, intraaortic balloon counterpulsation may provide a valuable bridge to emergency cardiac surgery. Recently, use of the intraaortic balloon to treat recurrent acute closure of the target lesion has been described (14).

Regional Myocardial Support

ANTEGRADE PERFUSION

The possibility of maintaining coronary flow distal to coronary balloon occlusion during angioplasty was first evaluated by Gruentzig and colleagues, but since brief coronary occlusions were well tolerated, these observations did not undergo widespread clinical evaluation (15). More recently, there has been enormous interest in distal coronary perfusion, based on the increased number of high-risk patients in whom coronary angioplasty is being performed, as well as on the tendency to perform more prolonged balloon inflations in the setting of a coronary artery dissection. Therefore use of perfusion balloon catheters (autoperfusion or passive hemoperfusion) has dramatically increased, and their popularity is based on simplicity and ease of use.

Physiology. In the majority of patients undergoing percutaneous revascularization, coronary occlusion time is limited by angina,

electrical instability, or hemodynamic compromise and, in patients with reduced left ventricular function, perhaps by hemodynamic collapse. This ischemic response depends on the presence of collateral flow, the preprocedure coronary stenosis and the size and viability of the regional myocardial territory. If the coronary occlusion time is brief, restoration of oxygenated blood flow rapidly reverses the manifestations of ischemia. In fact, numerous experimental and clinical studies have demonstrated the efficacy of antegrade perfusion in reducing the ischemic response to coronary occlusion (16–18).

The aortic pressure serves as the driving force in passive perfusion systems, where a lumen with side holes before and after the balloon serves as a conduit for distal perfusion. Flow rates are linearly proportional to proximal artery perfusion pressure. Hemoperfusion is dependent on catheter length, lumen diameter, and blood viscosity.

Practical Considerations. In the patient with severely reduced left ventricular function, preservation of arterial blood flow during coronary angioplasty may be essential, and often we use a perfusion balloon catheter as our primary strategy. Once the balloon is properly positioned, we maximize distal flow by removing the wire, withdrawing the guide from the coronary ostium, and limiting inflation pressures to avoid encroaching the central lumen. Distal flow is limited by relative hypotension, tandem lesions, and side branch occlusion. However, by maintaining distal flow, these perfusion balloon catheters may be particularly useful during dilation of the more proximal lesion during a multilesion procedure in the same vessel. Patient comfort with less angina is an added benefit of this approach. In procedures complicated by coronary dissection and/or abrupt closure in which repeat dilation is unsuccessful, the catheter serves as a "bail-out" device and a bridge to emergency coronary bypass surgery (19, 20).

RETROGRADE PERFUSION

Of all the support modalities, the retrograde perfusion techniques in general, and specifically synchronized coronary sinus retroperfusion, have undergone the most extensive experimental and preclinical evaluation (21–24). The efficacy of these techniques is based on the unique microcirculation of the heart with its extensive venovenous and arteriovenous anastomoses (25). When used during coronary angioplasty, several studies have shown that synchronized retroperfusion reduces but does not abolish the ischemic response to coronary balloon occlusion as determined by angina, electrocardiographic changes, and left ventricular regional wall motion (26–28).

Physiology.   During synchronized retroperfusion, arterial blood is pumped via the coronary sinus during diastole, and normal venous drainage occurs during systole. This sequence avoids myocardial edema, which occurs when venous drainage is impaired. Inflation of a balloon catheter positioned in the coronary sinus allows arterial blood to be pumped toward the ischemic myocardium without reflux into the right atrium. Retrograde delivery of flow tracers and enhanced glucose metabolism in the risk region during synchronized retroperfusion have been documented by positron emission tomography (29). Efficacy in reducing myocardial ischemia is based on direct delivery of arterial blood to the myocardium, but enhanced myocardial washout may occur as well (30).

Practical Considerations.   Coronary sinus catheterization is most successful from the right internal jugular vein and requires fluoroscopic guidance and pressure monitoring. Placement of the catheter into the great cardiac vein is facilitated with a wire once the catheter enters the coronary sinus, and we usually use contrast media to visualize the anatomy. After a short learning curve, successful cannulation of the great cardiac vein

is achieved in approximately 90% of patients within 5 minutes.

The retroperfusion system consists of a coronary sinus catheter (8.5 Fr triple lumen with a 10-mm-diameter balloon at the tip), an arterial cannula (single-lumen 7 or 8 Fr catheter with distal end and side holes), a synchronized pneumatic pump for blood triggered on the R wave of the electrocardiogram, and an electropneumatic balloon inflation mechanism. The arterial cannula connects to the pumping console; arterial blood is delivered to the distal port of the coronary sinus catheter during balloon inflation, which occurs during diastole. The pumping console functions to maintain selective flow rates, to provide balloon inflation with a fixed volume of gas and synchronization with each pump stroke, and to monitor coronary sinus pressure from the distal port of the catheter. Maximum flow rates of 250 cc/minute can be delivered, but flow rates are set to prevent exceeding a coronary sinus systolic pressure of 60 mm Hg.

We usually reserve coronary sinus retroperfusion for patients undergoing high-risk procedures in the left anterior descending artery in whom severe peripheral vascular disease precludes systemic support modalities. In these patients the pump and catheters are in a standby ready mode, but we do perform internal jugular venous cannulation with a 9 Fr sheath prior to the procedure (and with administration of heparin). For ongoing ischemia or an angiographic result necessitating prolonged coronary balloon inflation, we institute synchronized retroperfusion on-line.

The advantages to retrograde perfusion during percutaneous revascularization are numerous and are outlined in Table 27C.5. This technique is effective in maintaining circulation to side branches otherwise compromised by coronary lesions or angioplasty balloon catheters. It is particularly useful when antegrade access to the artery is lost and can serve as a bridge to the operating room where the coronary sinus catheter can be used to

Table 27C.5.
Advantages of Retrograde Perfusion

1. Avoids manipulation of arterial system
2. Venous system is rarely diseased
3. Maintains access to ischemic microvasculature even when antegrade access to artery is lost
4. Serves as bridge to operating room
5. Coronary sinus pressure monitoring provides a continuous recording of left ventricular end-diastolic pressure (32).

rapidly institute coronary sinus retrograde cardioplegia.

However, synchronized retroperfusion is limited by the lack of efficacy in all patients (and the ability to predict which patients will benefit). In addition, experience with this technique is limited to disease in the left anterior descending artery, although positioning the catheter in the proximal coronary sinus should theoretically provide similar efficacy in all myocardial regions. This hypothesis is supported by the fact that retrograde coronary sinus cardioplegia performed during cardiac surgery has not been shown to provide inadequate protection of the right ventricle or the inferior and posterior walls of the left ventricle (31).

SUMMARY

Currently, the efficacy of global and regional myocardial support modalities has allowed the expansion of percutaneous revascularization procedures to patients with complex disease and very poor left ventricular function in whom the risk of death would have previously been considered prohibitive. After thoughtful consideration of which support techniques are indicated, detailed discussion with the patient, family, and thoracic surgeons and careful preprocedural planning of the technical strategy, percutaneous revascularization can usually be performed safely and with a high rate of success. Therefore the most difficult question we face is not whether the procedure *can* be performed but whether it *should* be performed, based on the procedural risk and anticipated long-term outcome.

REFERENCES

1. Detre K, Holubkov R, Kelsey S et al. One-year follow-up results of the 1985–1986 National Heart, Lung, and Blood Institute's Percutaneous Transluminal Coronary Angioplasty Registry. Circulation 1989;80:421–428.

2. Alderman EL, Fisher LD, Litwin P et al. Results of coronary artery surgery in patients with poor left ventricular function (CASS). Circulation 1983;68:785–795.

3. Pigott JD, Kouchoukos NT, Oberman A, Cutter GR. Late results of surgical and medical therapy for patients with coronary artery disease and depressed left ventricular function. J Am Coll Cardiol 1985;5:1036–1045.

4. Bournous EP, Mark DB, Pollock BG et al. Surgical survival benefits for coronary disease patients with left ventricular dysfunction. Circulation 1988;78(Suppl 1):I-151–I-157.

5. Stevens T, Kahn JK, McCallister BD et al. Safety and efficacy of percutaneous transluminal coronary angioplasty in patients with left ventricular dysfunction. Am J Cardiol 1991;68:313–319.

6. Kohli RS, DiSciascio G, Cowley MJ, Nath M, Goudreau E, Vetrovec GW. Coronary angioplasty in patients with severe left ventricular dysfunction. J Am Coll Cardiol 1990;16:807–811.

7. Holmes DR, Detre KM, William DO et al. Long-term outcome of patients with depressed left ventricular function undergoing percutaneous transluminal coronary angioplasty. Circulation 1993;87:21–29.

8. Holmes DR, Holubkov R, Vlietstra RE et al. Comparison of complications during percutaneous transluminal coronary angioplasty from 1977 to 1981 and from 1985 to 1986: the National Heart, Lung, and Blood Institute Percutaneous Transluminal Coronary Angioplasty Registry. J Am Coll Cardiol 1988;12:1149–1155.

9. Ellis SG, Roubin GS, King SB III et al. Angiographic and clinical predictors of acute closure after native vessel coronary angioplasty. Circulation 1988;77:372–379.

10. Bergelson BA, Jacobs AK, Cupples LA et al. Prediction of risk for hemodynamic compromise during coronary angioplasty. Am J Cardiol 1992;70:1540–1545.

11. Weber KT, Janicki JS. Intra-aortic balloon counterpulsation: a review of physiological principles, clinical results, and device safety. Ann Thorac Surg 1974;17:602–636.

12. Kahn JK, Rutherford BD, McConahay DR, Johnson WL, Giorgi LV, Hartzler GO. Supported "high-risk" coronary angioplasty using intraaortic balloon pump counterpulsation. J Am Coll Cardiol 1990;15:1151–1155.

13. Anwar A, Mooney MR, Stertzer SH et al. Intra-aortic balloon counterpulsation support for elective coronary angioplasty in the setting of poor left ventricular function: a two-center experience. J Invasive Cardiol 1990;2:175–180.

14. Suneja R, Hodgson JM. Use of intraaortic balloon counterpulsation for treatment of recurrent acute closure after coronary angioplasty. Am Heart J 1993;125:530–532.

15. Anderson HV, Leimgruber PP, Roubin GS, Nelson DL, Gruentzig AR. Distal coronary artery perfusion during percutaneous transluminal coronary angioplasty. Am Heart J 1985;110:720–726.

16. Cambell CA, Rezkalla S, Kloner RA, Turi ZG. The autoperfusion balloon angioplasty catheter limits myocardial ischemia and necrosis during prolonged balloon inflation. J Am Coll Cardiol 1989;14:1045–1050.

17. Quigley PJ, Hinohara T, Phillips HR et al. Myocardial protection during coronary angioplasty with an autoperfusion balloon catheter in humans. Circulation 1988;78:1128–1134.

18. Leitschuh ML, Mills RM, LaRosa D, Jacobs AK, Ruocco NA, Faxon DP. Outcome after major dissection during coronary angioplasty using the perfusion balloon catheter. Am J Cardiol 1991;67:1056–1060.

19. Sundram P, Harvey JR, Johnson RG, Schwartz MJ, Baim DS. Benefit of the perfusion catheter for emergency coronary artery grafting after failed percutaneous transluminal coronary angioplasty. Am J Cardiol 1989;63:282–285.

20. Tomaki H, Simpson JB, Philips HR, Stack RS. Transluminal intracoronary reperfusion catheter: a device to maintain coronary perfusion between failed coronary angioplasty and emergency coronary bypass surgery. J Am Coll Cardiol 1988;11:977–982.

21. Mohl W, Glogar D, Mayr H et al. Reduction of infarct size induced by intermittent coronary sinus occlusion. Am J Cardiol 1984;53:923–928.

22. Jacobs AK, Faxon DP, Coats WD, Vogel RM, Ryan TJ. Coronary sinus occlusion: effect on ischemic left ventricular dysfunction and reactive hyperemia. Am Heart J 1991;121:442–449.

23. Drury JK, Yamazaki S, Fishbein MC, Meerbaum S, Corday E. Synchronized diastolic coronary venous retroperfusion: results of a preclinical safety and efficacy study. J Am Coll Cardiol 1985;2:328–335.

24. Yamazaki S, Drury JK, Meerbaum S, Corday E. Synchronized coronary venous retroperfusion: prompt improvement of left ventricular function in experimental myocardial ischemia. J Am Coll Cardiol 1985;5:655–663.

25. Wearn JT. The role of the thebesian vessels in the circulation of the heart. J Exp Med 1928;47:293.

26. Kar S, Drury JK, Hajduczki I et al. Synchronized coronary venous retroperfusion for support and salvage of ischemic myocardium during elective and failed angioplasty. J Am Coll Cardiol 1991;18:271–282.

27. Nanto S, Nishida K, Hirayama A et al. Supported angioplasty with synchronized retroperfusion in high-risk patients with left main trunk or near left main trunk obstruction. Am Heart J 1993;125:301–309.

28. Incorvati RL, Tauberg SG, Pecora MJ et al. Clinical applications of coronary sinus retroperfusion during high-risk percutaneous transluminal coronary angioplasty. J Am Coll Cardiol 1993;22:127–134.

29. O'Byrne GT, Nienaber CA, Miyazaki A et al. Positron emission tomography demonstrates that coronary sinus retroperfusion can restore regional myocardial perfusion and preserve metabolism. J Am Cardiol 1991;18:257–270.

30. Chang BL, Drury KJ, Meerbaum S, Fishbein MC, Whiting JS, Corday E. Enhanced myocardial washout and retrograde blood delivery with synchronized retroperfusion during acute myocardial ischemia. J Am Coll Cardiol 1987;9:1091–1098.

31. Menasche P, Piwnica A. Cardioplegia by way of the coronary sinus for valvular and coronary surgery. J Am Coll Cardiol 1991;18:628–636.

32. Faxon DP, Jacobs AK, Kellett MA, McSweeney SM, Coats WD, Ryan TJ. Coronary sinus occlusion pressure and its relation to intracardiac pressure. Am J Cardiol 1985;56:457–460.

D. Supported Percutaneous Intervention: The Duke Experience

E. MAGNUS OHMAN, JOHN WILSON, HARRY R. PHILLIPS III, and RICHARD S. STACK

Percutaneous interventions in patients with left ventricular dysfunction and multivessel disease are frequently called "high-risk" interventions. Although few clinicians agree on the exact criteria for defining "high-risk" patients, most physicians and surgeons would agree that patients with an ejection fraction $<25\%$, clinical evidence of congestive heart failure, multivessel disease, and interventions on vessels supplying $>50\%$ of the viable myocardium represent the broad spectrum of this group. The role of percutaneous revascularization in patients with poor left ventricular function is dependent on the use and selection of various left ventricular support devices. Relatively few interventional operators individually perform a high volume of these procedures. However, some hospitals and operators have built a large experience with these procedures over the last few years. This chapter will review the experience with these procedures over the last few years. This chapter will review the experience at our institution coupled with the published information on percutaneous interventions in "high-risk" patients with particular reference to left ventricular support devices. In addition, a percutaneous revascularization approach will be put in perspective with other treatment strategies such as continued medical management and coronary artery bypass grafting.

PROGNOSIS WITH MEDICAL AND CABG THERAPY

The prognosis of patients with ischemic heart disease is very strongly correlated to the age of the patient, type of clinical presentation, presence of congestive heart failure, and findings from cardiac catheterization. Of this constellation of clinical and anatomic variables, left ventricular function is the most important variable for predicting short- and long-term mortality. It has been estimated that approximately 2% of the adult population in the United States may be suffering from congestive heart failure and that the prevalence may be as high as 4.5% in individuals between 65 and 74 years of age (1). In the Framingham study the overall 5-year mortality rate was 75% in patients with the clinical diagnosis of congestive heart failure (2). The etiology of heart failure in this cohort of 652 patients was coronary artery disease in 54%, and the mortality rate was not affected by the cause of heart failure. In a study at Duke University Medical center of 571 medically treated patients who had an exercise ejection fraction <30% and three-vessel coronary artery disease, there was a 50% mortality rate during a 3-year follow-up period (3). Patients with an exercise ejection fraction >30% and with three-vessel coronary artery disease had a 20% 5-year mortality rate.

The location of significant lesions within the coronary anatomy has been found to be important prognostically. In particular, the left anterior coronary artery has been found to supply a proportionally greater part of the myocardium than the remaining coronary arteries. For this reason the degree of multivessel coronary artery disease has been further refined by applying a jeopardy score to specific lesions, where the presence of a lesion in the proximal left anterior descending artery provides further prognostic information (4). This scoring system is shown in Figure 27D.1. By applying a point score of 2 for each significant lesion and an additional 2 points for each vessel distal to that

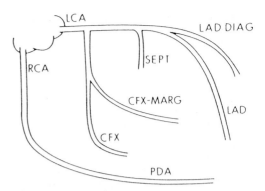

Figure 27D.1. Diagram of coronary artery tree demonstrating the six segments counted in the jeopardy score. *CFX*, Left circumflex coronary artery; *CFX-MARG*, major marginal branch of the left circumflex coronary artery; *LAD*, left anterior descending artery; *LAD DIAG*, major diagonal branch of the left anterior descending artery; *LCA*, left main coronary artery; *PDA*, posterior descending coronary artery; *RCA*, right coronary artery; *SEPT*, major septal perforating artery.

lesion, a total of score of 12 can be achieved. Thus a significant lesion in the proximal left anterior descending (before the first septal branch) will be ascribed a point score of 6. A proximal lesion in the circumflex artery would be given a score of 4, and a lesion in the proximal right coronary artery would have a score of 2. The 3-year survival in patients with two- and three-vessel coronary artery disease was 87% and 77%, respectively. Using the jeopardy score of 6 or 12, the corresponding survival was 89% and 63%, respectively. The jeopardy score was also found to add additional prognostic information to the degree of left ventricular function (4).

The clinical markers of ischemia provide an independent contribution to event-free survival (5). These clinical markers that provide prognostic information include a history of unstable or progressive angina and ST-T–wave changes on the electrocardiogram. A patient with three-vessel coronary artery disease and an ejection fraction <50% without unstable angina or ECG changes has a 76% infarction-free survival at 2 years. A patient with similar anatomic findings but with unsta-

Table 27D.1.
Review of the Literature of CABG for Patients With Severely Reduced Ejection Fraction (EF)[a]

First Author (Ref.)	No. of Patients	Years	EF	30-Day Mortality	Late Mortality
Vlietstra (98)	10	1966–72	<0.25		60% (2 yr)
Manley (99)	183	1968–71	Mean 0.22	16.0%	43% (5 yr)
Yatteau (100)	24	1968–72	<0.25	42.0%	50% (2 yr)
Oldham (101)	11	1969–72	≤0.25	55.0%	
Zubiate (102)	140	1969–72	<0.20	22.0%	41% (6 yr)
Faulkner (103)	46	1969–75	Mean 0.21	4.0%	17% (2 yr)
Mitchel (104)	9		<0.20	0.0%	11% (1 yr)
Fox (105)	7	1971–74	<0.20	0.0%	14%
Jones (106)	41	1973–77	<0.20	2.5%	10% (1 yr)
Alderman (8)	82	1975–79	≤0.25	8.0%	37% (5 yr)
Mochtar (107)	62	1975–83	Mean 0.25	4.8%	30% (5 yr)
Zubiate (108)	93	1976–81	<0.20	5.0%	50% (5 yr)
Hochberg (109)	51	1976–82	0.20–0.24	12.0%	42% (3 yr)
Hochberg (109)	41	1976–82	<0.20	37.0%	85% (3 yr)
Sanchez (110)	23	1982–89	Mean 0.28	9.0%	24% (2 yr)
Kron (111)	39	1983–88	<0.20	2.6%	17% (3 yr)
Blakeman (112)	20	1984–88	Mean 0.18	15.0%	30% (1 yr)
Christakis (113)	487	1982–90	<0.20	9.8%	

[a]Modified from Milano CA, White WD, Smith LR et al. Ann Thorac Surg 1993;56:487–493 with permission.

ble angina and ECG changes has a 56% infarction-free survival.

The described prognostic information from medically treated patients should serve as a framework for decisions regarding percutaneous interventions and surgical revascularization. Several published series have noted a considerable in-hospital mortality in patients with severely reduced left ventricular function undergoing CABG. A recent review of the literature (Table 27D.1) has shown that the 30-day mortality rate has improved steadily since the late 1960s. In a series of 118 patients from Duke University with an ejection fraction <25%, the operative mortality (30 days) was 11% (6). One- and 5-year survival was 77% and 58%, respectively. There were five variables that predicted a higher risk of mortality: the presence of other vascular disease (P <.005), female gender (P <.005), history of hypertension (P <.005), elevated left ventricular end-diastolic pressure (P <.005), and depressed cardiac index (P <.05). Inherent to any observational series of interventions in patients with severely reduced left ventricular function is the selection bias that these series rep-

resent. The improvement in survival may result from both improved surgical techniques and improved selection of patients, with the more recent series having included patients more likely to survive. In the coronary artery surgery study (CASS) only 20% of patients enrolled had an ejection fraction between 35% and 50% (7). After 7 years of follow-up the survival in patients randomized to CABG was 84% compared with 70% for the medical group (P = .01). More importantly, in the 651 excluded patients with an ejection fraction <35% a multivariate analysis documented a survival benefit with surgical revascularization (P <.05)(8). Surgical benefit was most apparent in patients with an ejection fraction of <26% who had a 63% 5-year survival when treated with CABG compared with 43% when treated medically. A 15-year retrospective analysis of 5809 patients treated at Duke University found similar survival benefit with surgical revascularization in patients with depressed left ventricular function (9). Although the survival benefit with CABG appeared the greatest in patients with more extensive coronary artery disease and acute clinical presentation, the relative survival benefit with CABG in patients with varying degrees of depressed left ventricular function appeared constant when other baseline characteristics were taken into account (10). The long-term survival difference is particularly noteworthy when considering that almost 50% of saphenous vein grafts are occluded at 10 years after the operation (11). In addition, failure to use internal mammary grafting has been found to be associated with a higher likelihood for death caused by heart failure during follow-up after CABG (12).

These observations in patients with left ventricular failure treated with CABG suggest that the degree of left ventricular dysfunction is related to the clinical and angiographic extent of coronary artery disease and that, when revascularization is achieved, left ventricular function will improve in proportion to the degree of revascularization achieved. This coupled with the importance of complete revascularization during CABG (13) suggests that when percutaneous interventions are considered in patients with left ventricular dysfunction, complete revascularization should be the goal whenever possible.

PERCUTANEOUS INTERVENTIONS IN HIGH-RISK SUBSETS

A useful comparison can be made between ischemia developing during percutaneous interventions in high-risk patients and the pathophysiology of cardiogenic shock. Although actual cellular necrosis is not part of the initial insult during angioplasty, ischemic left ventricular dysfunction can become catastrophic, and the dramatic downward spiral seen in cardiogenic shock may ensue in this high-risk population as well. Once hypotension results, coronary perfusion pressure may be inadequate to allow blood flow to the ischemic myocardium and further left ventricular dysfunction occurs. Various definitions have been used to describe patients at high risk for percutaneous interventions. In the past, high-risk characteristics included advanced age,

multivessel disease, multiple lesions to be dilated, prior coronary artery bypass grafting, poor left ventricular function, and left main stenosis as the target lesion (14). Today, the majority of the patients considered at high risk have significantly depressed left ventricular function and/or lesion(s) in vessels supplying a substantial amount of myocardium. The common thread in all these definitions is that the patient would not be expected to tolerate a device occlusion or abrupt closure of the vessel during or following the procedure.

It remains difficult to accurately predict which patient will be hemodynamically intolerant of balloon or device occlusion, develop abrupt closure, or die. When considering whether to perform high-risk interventions it is useful to consider the procedural risk as a combination of the risk of abrupt closure (see Chapter 36B) and the risk of mortality. The latter variable is predominantly a reflection of the risk of abrupt closure or other ischemic events such as myocardial infarction. In an overview from the literature of 25,000 patients undergoing angioplasty, the overall mortality rate was only 0.7% (15). The patient characteristics independently correlated with a higher in-hospital mortality were cardiogenic shock or heart failure, older age, and female gender. Cardiac catheterization variables that correlated with mortality were depressed left ventricular function and multivessel coronary artery disease. The most important post-PTCA characteristic that has been found to be related with higher in-hospital mortality is abrupt closure, which had an incidence of approximately 7% when data on nearly 9,000 patients were combined (15). Unstable angina and multivessel coronary artery disease were independent predictors of abrupt closure, as were certain lesion characteristics as described elsewhere in this book (see Chapter 36B). Ellis and colleagues (16) have built on the experience of the coronary jeopardy score developed by Califf and colleagues (4), which was previously described (see above). In Ellis' observations a score of

>3 (of a maximum of 6) would be applied if >50% of viable myocardium were dilated. A jeopardy score >2.5 was associated with an in-hospital mortality of over 10%. An ejection fraction of less than 25% was associated with a 4% mortality, and this characteristic did not contribute independently to in-hospital mortality. Similarly, Bergelson and colleagues found that preprocedural ejection fraction did not predict hemodynamic collapse (defined as a fall of 20 mm Hg with a systolic blood pressure <90 mm Hg) in 157 patients undergoing angioplasty (17). In their observations the four variables predicting hemodynamic collapse were multivessel disease, diffuse disease, myocardium at risk, and pre-PTCA stenosis.

Although percutaneous interventions are now more frequently performed in patients with left ventricular dysfunction, there is relatively little information available on the procedural or long-term outcomes in this patient population. Holmes and colleagues reviewed the experience from the NHLBI PTCA Registry in 244 patients with an ejection fraction <45% compared with 1802 patients with normal left ventricular function (18). Patients with depressed left ventricular function had a lower frequency of successful dilations of all lesions attempted (76% versus 84%, P <.01). In-hospital complications were similar in both depressed and normal left ventricular function groups, respectively: death 0.8% versus 0.7%, nonfatal myocardial infarction 4.9% versus 4.5%, and emergency CABG 4.5% versus 3.2%. During a 4-year follow-up period, 87% remained alive and 77% had not had a myocardial infarction or CABG. However, in the small subgroup of 11 patients who had an ejection fraction <25% the long-term survival was only 45%. Similar findings have been observed in two studies examining patients with an ejection fraction of <35% having PTCA (19, 20). In a report of 845 patients with an ejection fraction <40%, who were undergoing elective PTCA by one group of operators, the angiographic success

was lower (93% versus 95%, P <.01) when compared with 8117 patients with normal left ventricular function having PTCA during the same 10-year period (21). The procedural mortality was also increased (4% versus 1%, P <.001). Survival at 1 year and 4 years in patients with left ventricular dysfunction treated with angioplasty was 87% and 69%, respectively. Predictors of long-term mortality were multivessel disease, age >70 years, unstable angina, and incomplete revascularization. In a follow-up study 100 patients from the above-described PTCA cohort were matched and compared with 100 patients with an ejection fraction <40% who had CABG (22). The early results favored PTCA with a shorter hospitalization (4 versus 13 days, P <.001), fewer strokes (0% versus 7%), and similar in-hospital mortality (3% versus 5%) compared with CABG. However, during five-year follow-up, patients treated with CABG had less disabling angina (1% versus 11%, P = .01) and a trend toward improved survival (76% versus 67%, P = .09).

Current randomized clinical trials comparing PTCA with CABG are going to be fundamental in exploring the merits of CABG versus percutaneous interventions. The bypass angioplasty revascularization investigation (BARI) trial will have only a few patients with an ejection fraction less than 25% and/or congestive heart failure making worthwhile comparisons difficult (Edwin Alderman, personal communication). These results will be available in 1995 but will not include a large experience with the use of support devices during high-risk percutaneous interventions. A randomized clinical trial comparing PTCA, CABG, and medical therapy is currently being conducted, which should provide very important information on optimal treatment strategies for patients with severe left ventricular dysfunction (Mitchell Krucoff, personal communication).

Risk stratification for planned percutaneous intervention should include an estimate of long-term outcome with alternative

Table 27D.2.
Support Strategies

Coronary (local) support
    Anterograde local support
        Auto perfusion
            Bailout balloon
            Perfusion balloon
            Temporary stent
        Distal coronary hemoperfusion
        Perfluorocarbon coronary perfusion
    Retrograde local support
        Synchronized coronary sinus retroperfusion
Systemic support
    Intraaortic balloon counterpulsation (IABP)
    Cardiopulmonary support (CPS)
    Hemopump
    Partial left heart bypass

Table 27D.3.
Intraaortic Balloon Counterpulsation

Advantages
    Displacement not catastrophic
    Pulsatile flow
    FDA approved
    Ability to place in >90%
    Full heparinization not required
    Perfusion technician unnecessary
    Long-term use (weeks)
    May augment coronary perfusion
    Percutaneous
    Small size (10.5 Fr to 9.5 Fr)
    Rapid insertion
Disadvantages
    Synchronization with rhythm necessary
    Dependent on LV function
    May not augment coronary perfusion with critical stenoses
    Complications in 9 to 43%
    Relatively modest hemodynamic effects
    May cause hemolysis/thrombocytopenia
    Contraindicated with aortic insufficiency

approaches such as medical therapy and CABG. Once the decision has been made to proceed with percutaneous intervention, the procedural risk and associated complications need to be evaluated with the knowledge of the various support techniques available to reduce in-hospital complications and mortality. Contemporary methods and devices that support the heart and patient during interventions are listed in Table 27D.2. The methods of "local" coronary support include those of anterograde support (auto perfusion balloons (23, 24), distal coronary hemoperfusion (25, 26), perfluorocarbon perfusion (27, 28), and retrograde support via the coronary sinus (29–31). Since these methods are presented in depth elsewhere in this text, we will focus in this chapter on systemic support techniques and applications. These include intraaortic balloon pump counterpulsation, percutaneous cardiopulmonary support, the Hemopump, and partial left heart bypass.

INTRAAORTIC BALLOON COUNTERPULSATION

Intraaortic balloon counterpulsation (IABP) has become widely accepted since its development in the early 1960s (32) and introduction into clinical practice in 1968 (33). Between 75,000 and 80,000 intraaortic balloon pumps are inserted each year just in the United States (34). Although the hemody-

namic effects of the pump are modest, its main advantages over other support devices are its ease of insertion and widespread availability. Patients in whom IABP is to be used, however, must have a stable rhythm and some basal cardiac output. While complications occur in 9% to 43% of patients in whom it is inserted (34–36), they are generally limited to limb ischemia, vascular damage requiring repair, and embolic phenomena.

The intraaortic balloon pump is placed in the descending aorta percutaneously through the femoral artery. By inflating during diastole and deflating during systole, it reduces left ventricular afterload and myocardial oxygen consumption; it also may augment diastolic coronary perfusion. The overall hemodynamic effects include a decrease in both peak systolic and end-diastolic pressures with a large increase in overall diastolic pressure and a slight increase or no change in mean aortic pressure. Pulmonary capillary wedge pressure and left ventricular end-diastolic pressure decrease by 10 to 20%, while cardiac output increases 10 to 40% (34). Table 27D.3 lists the major advantages and disadvantages of aortic counterpulsation.

Several investigators have examined the

ability of the IABP to augment diastolic perfusion of the coronary arteries. In an early study of seven patients with refractory unstable angina and critical proximal LAD stenoses, Fuchs and colleagues demonstrated a good correlation between changes in coronary sinus blood flow and IABP-augmented aortic mean diastolic pressure, but they could not determine how much of this flow was related to collateral circulation (37). Six patients studied by Williams and coworkers had anginal pain relief while the IABP was inserted, but the investigators were not able to demonstrate an increase in regional coronary blood flow and felt that the most likely mechanism was reduced myocardial oxygen consumption secondary to systolic unloading of the ventricle (38). Three recent studies examined IABP augmentation of coronary flow after PTCA. MacDonald and colleagues failed to show significant augmentation of coronary perfusion pressure by IABP distal to a stenosis, but their measurements were made through the central lumen of the PTCA balloon catheter, which may impede usual blood flow (39). Using a 3 Fr coronary Doppler catheter, Ishihara and colleagues showed an increase in peak coronary flow but no change in mean coronary flow, which they suggested may reduce reocclusion after PTCA, a clinical finding that other investigators have demonstrated (40). Kern and co-

workers, using a 0.018-inch, Doppler-tipped angioplasty guidewire, showed an increase in both mean and peak coronary blood flow velocity after PTCA, which was further increased by IABP (41). Importantly, there was no significant augmentation before the critical stenoses were dilated. While unloading of the ventricle may reduce ischemia somewhat, PTCA is essential to maximize the effects of the IABP. In summary, these results may help explain the beneficial effects of IABP in preventing reocclusion after successful reperfusion (42–44) and in improving survival of patients with cardiogenic shock treated with IABP plus revascularization as compared with IABP alone (45).

Although the use of intraaortic balloon pumping to support high-risk angioplasty has yet to be studied with a randomized trial, four small retrospective studies show reasonable success with IABP (Table 27D.4) (29, 46–48). The two earlier studies (29, 47) predated the availability of perfusion balloon catheters, which may further improve high-risk angioplasty in conjunction with IABP.

Patients who have had unsuccessful PTCA and patients who have had abrupt closure following PTCA may benefit from IABP for hemodynamic support (49, 50). One study of this use of IABP included 777 patients undergoing PTCA and 2068 patients undergoing CABG (50). Among patients who developed

Table 27D.4.
IABP Before High-Risk PTCA In-Hospital Follow-Up

Author (Ref.)	n	Mean F/U (Months)	Lesion Success	IABP Complications (%)	Events (%)			
					Death	MI	CABG	Repeat Intervention
Alcan (1983) (47)	9	NA	9/9	33	11	NA	11	NA
					0	NA	NA	NA
Szatmary (1988) (29)	16	22	27/30	0	6	0	0	0
					13	0	6	6
Voudris (1990) (48)	27	13.1	39/39	4	0	0	0	0
					7	0	4	22
Kahn (1990) (46)	28	NA	90/94	11	7	0	0	NA
					NA	NA	NA	NA

IABP, Intraaortic balloon counterpulsation; PTCA, percutaneous transluminal coronary angioplasty; F/U, follow-up; MI, myocardial infarction; CABG, coronary artery bypass graft; NA, not applicable.

ST-T changes and chest pain after PTCA, all 12 who did not have intraaortic balloon pumping developed Q-waves after CABG as opposed to only two of eight in whom IABP support was used prior to surgery. Three other studies showed hemodynamic stabilization and some resolution of EKG changes with IABP (47, 49). It is important to note that intraaortic balloon counterpulsation has very little, if any, role in patients with cardiac arrest in the absence of cardiac output or an intrinsic rhythm (51).

Intraaortic balloon counterpulsation can allow for a longer balloon inflation by ventricular unloading and can serve as a useful bridge in patients with failed angioplasty or complications requiring urgent CABG. The precise role of IABP is unclear in high-risk patients with stable hemodynamics undergoing angioplasty. Patients who have demonstrated instability with balloon inflation in the same lesion would be suitable for IABP support. In addition, ventricular unloading may benefit patients with poor left ventricular function. A reasonable option in many situations is to gain arterial access with a small diameter sheath in the opposite groin prior to any intervention so that the balloon pump can be readily inserted if the patient becomes unstable. Prophylactic IABP use after a successful intervention may decrease the incidence of abrupt closure with an acceptably low complication rate.

Aortic Counterpulsation Catheter Insertion

In experienced hands the IABP can be inserted percutaneously in less than 5 minutes and is the fastest support technique that can be instituted in the catheterization laboratory or other acute care facility. The IABP is best inserted percutaneously through the femoral artery using the Seldinger technique. Other access sites, including the left axillary or subclavian arteries, usually require the assistance of a vascular surgeon. Sheathless insertion is preferable in smaller patients or those with peripheral vascular disease because it reduces the access hole from 10.5 Fr to 9.5 Fr and reduces the limitation of flow in the iliac artery. Using this technique may reduce the incidence of limb ischemia without increasing the risk of hemorrhagic complications (52). In obese patients it is preferable to use the standard approach with a 10.5 Fr sheath with the IABP catheter to avoid kinking of the catheter through the long subcutaneous path.

Aortic Counterpulsation Complications

Major complications of IABP are rare and are generally related to the acuity of the patient's condition during the insertion. Recent series have demonstrated complication rates following elective insertion of 0% to 11% (35, 46, 53). In patients with cardiogenic shock or other emergencies, however, the complication rate is considerably higher, varying from 4% to 36% (54). This may reflect the fact that patients requiring emergency insertions also have more risk factors that predispose to complications, including female gender, diabetes, mellitus, or peripheral vascular disease.

Limb ischemia and vascular trauma or laceration with hemorrhage are the most common major complications of IABP. Rarer complications include aortic dissection, platelet destruction, emboli to renal or peripheral arteries, and balloon rupture with gas embolus. Nonvascular complications tend to occur in <1% of cases. Patients who have IABP inserted for >5 days are at increased risk of local or systemic infection (55).

Role of Aortic Counterpulsation in Myocardial Infarction

The TAMI group demonstrated that patients who had an intraaortic balloon pump inserted had less reocclusion following successful reperfusion than patients who did not (42). Ishihara and colleagues demonstrated similar findings in patients undergoing primary angioplasty for acute myocardial infarction (40). A randomized trial was performed in 182 patients with acute MI requiring mechanical reperfusion to test the hypothesis that IABP reduces the risk of reocclusion without undue vascular or hemorrhagic complications (44). Patients were randomized to 48 hours of IABP and IV heparin (96 patients) or heparin alone (86 patients). The group receiving IABP/heparin had a higher patency rate and fewer recurrent ischemic events than the control group with very few complications. Among 106 patients undergoing primary PTCA, there was no difference in vascular complications or major bleeding between the IABP group and the control group (56). Overall, prophylactic IABP support after successful reperfusion resulted in less recurrent ischemia, less need for repeat intervention, and a lower reocclusion rate. Following successful rescue PTCA, 36 patients treated with IABP for 24 hours had a significantly lower reocclusion rate, better LV function, and a trend toward a decrease in mortality compared with 20 patients not treated with IABP (57). While this study addressed only patients with acute MI, IABP-augmented diastolic coronary flow after intervention may help to prevent reocclusion in other groups of patients as well. The high-risk PTCA group who might not tolerate abrupt closure may be such a group, but further studies are needed to support this claim.

CARDIOPULMONARY SUPPORT

The cardiopulmonary support (CPS) device uses the percutaneous femoral vein to femoral artery cardiopulmonary bypass to support patients with cardiac decompensation. It was initially developed for emergent or elective open heart surgery but has become widely used over the past few years. Today, it is also used in patients with cardiogenic shock, cardiac arrest, massive pulmonary embolism, hypothermia, and drug overdose and in high-risk patients undergoing elective angioplasty.

The CPS system includes a centrifugal pump, a flow probe, a heat exchanger, and a hollow fiber membrane oxygenator, all connected in closed series with a long femoral vein/right atrial cannula on one end and a femoral artery cannula on the other. Originally, the CPS was placed via femoral cutdown, but it is now routinely inserted percutaneously via 18 Fr or 20 Fr cannulas in the femoral artery and femoral vein. Because it does not rely on gravity but actively pumps blood from the right atrium by the centrifugal pump, the device is able to generate cardiac output between 4 (18 Fr) and 6 (20 Fr) liters per minute.

To reduce vascular complications a contrast injection is performed first to establish that there is adequate patency of the femoral artery. Then the arterial cannula is inserted because of the difficulty of adequately controlling bleeding while dilating the vessel if the venous cannula has already been placed. Next, the venous cannula is placed in the right atrium fluoroscopically over a stiff guidewire. Lastly, the cannulas are attached to the tubing connected to the centrifugal pump, oxygenation, and heater. CPS requires experienced operators, and trained personnel. Besides the cardiologist, a perfusionist and a cardiac anesthesiologist should be present for the initiation and maintenance of CPS.

Complications of the procedure occur frequently, including vascular complications and bleeding. Because there is also a risk of air embolism, special steps must be taken to ensure that unnecessary intravenous lines are clamped during CPS and that necessary lines have all the air removed from the IV solution bag. Central lines such as Swan-Ganz catheters should not be opened to air under any circumstances because the negative pressure on the venous side can draw in large amounts of air. Obese patients create a special problem because the relatively short arterial catheter can have its side holes close to the entrance into the femoral artery in such patients, and even slight withdrawal of the cannula can cause massive subcutaneous bleeding if the side holes are outside the femoral artery. Close attention must therefore be paid to

Table 27D.5.
Cardiopulmonary Support

Advantages
  FDA approved
  Synchronization with rhythm unnecessary
  Provides full circulatory support
  Independent of LV function
  Decreases myocardial energy consumption
  Percutaneous access
Disadvantages
  No LV decompression
  Large size (18 to 20 Fr)
  Short-term use (<24 to 48 hours)
  Full-dose heparin
  Displacement from groin catastrophic
  Perfusion technician/cardiac anesthesiologist necessary
  Fails to augment myocardial perfusion beyond stenoses
  Can cause thrombocytopenia/hemolysis
  High complication rate
  Nonpulsatile flow

suturing the cannulas in place and preventing dislodgment when the patient must be moved. The major advantages and disadvantages of cardiopulmonary support are represented in Table 27D.5.

Different patient care settings require different size CPS cannulas. Larger cannulas (20 Fr) are able to generate flow of up to 6 liters per minute, the appropriate rate for CPS in patients with cardiac arrest or cardiogenic shock. In hemodynamically stable patients undergoing supported angioplasty, the smaller 18 Fr size may be used, as the flow rates necessary to provide support may be less and complications may be reduced by the smaller size. The weight and height of the patient should always be taken into consideration.

After the patient has been weaned from CPS, the cannulas can be removed, either manually with prolonged pressure application or surgically. Surgical closure may reduce vascular complications and it allows for uninterrupted heparinization of the patient, but it may preclude repeat percutaneous access through that groin. Therefore we prefer prolonged clamping of the groin, resorting to surgical closure only in those patients who cannot be taken off anticoagulation or who fail

clamping. Extreme obesity may preclude percutaneous removal.

Hemodynamically, the nonpulsatile pumping of blood results in systolic unloading of the ventricle and a dramatic reduction in right atrial and pulmonary artery pressures from preload reduction. In addition, the pulse pressure narrows as flow rates are increased, and mean arterial pressure may decline as well. CPS is able to maintain perfusion to vital organs even in the setting of electromechanical dissociation, ventricular fibrillation, or asystole. The main disadvantage in these particular situations is that CPS provides no left ventricular decompression (blood still enters passively from the pulmonary circulation), so if the heart becomes enlarged, decompression may have to be done manually with a pigtail catheter in the ventricle.

The exact effect of CPS on myocardial function remains to be conclusively evaluated. Pavlides and colleagues [58] assessed global and regional myocardial function by echocardiography in 20 patients undergoing PTCA with cardiopulmonary support. Wall stress (afterload) was significantly decreased with the initiation of CPS. Global left ventricular function was unchanged when the patients were on CPS, but did decrease with balloon inflation. Interestingly, regional wall motion deteriorated in areas supplied by arteries with greater than or equal to 50% stenosis just by going on CPS, and a further decrease was seen with balloon inflation. Thus, while many patients will have little or no chest pain or EKG changes on CPS with balloon inflation, CPS may not prevent ischemia in the myocardium supplied by the target vessel or by other vessels with significant stenoses. In addition, CPS does not offer any myocardial protective effect beyond a lesion if abrupt closure occurs.

Cardiopulmonary support was first applied in a portable fashion in 1966 [59], although the majority of the experience has been in the last few years. Several studies have reported its use in patients suffering from cardiac arrest or cardiogenic shock, and these are presented in Table 27D.6 (59–68). Although the numbers in the studies are small, in-hospital mortality in this group after cardiopulmonary support (and in some circumstances revascularization) is high, running between 20% and 88%. Most of the studies show mortality rates of 70% or higher. Obviously, this group of patients would be expected to do poorly without CPS, so it is very difficult to know what role it has in this population. The outcome certainly tends to be better if the arrest happens in a setting in which CPS can be initiated almost immediately (i.e., cardiac catheterization laboratory) (69) and if revascularization is an option.

By the late 1980s cardiopulmonary support was being used for high-risk patients undergoing angioplasty. The currently available data are presented in Table 27D.7 (70–76). The largest series to date is that of the National Registry of Elected Supported Angioplasty (76, 77). The initial series of 105 patients included in the 1988 National Registry was reported in 1990 (76). The suggested criteria for entry were patients with severe or unstable angina and at least one likely dilatable coronary artery stenosis, left ventricular ejection fraction less than 25%, and/or a target vessel supplying more than half of the viable myocardium. Twenty-nine percent of the patients had dilation of their only patent coronary vessel, and 19% of patients were deemed to have inoperable disease. While the angioplasty success rate was 95%, major complications occurred in 39% of patients and overall in-hospital mortality was 8%. It became evident during the 1988 experience that patients may benefit by having cardiopulmonary support available but not necessarily instituted during high-risk angioplasty (the so-called standby support). The 1989 National Registry, which was reported in 1992 (77), included 258 patients who had prophylactic CPS and 98 patients who underwent their high-risk angioplasty with standby support only. Although there was some difference in baseline ejection fraction between the two groups, procedural success was similar, as was the rate of emergency CABG and death. However, major complications occurred in 41% of the patients who underwent

Table 27D.6.
Outcome of Cardiopulmonary Support for Cardiac Arrest or Cardiogenic Shock

Author (Ref.)	n	Successful Weaning (%)	% In-Hospital Mortality
Kennedy (1966) (59)	8	NR	88
Mattox (1977) (68)	43	67	60
Phillips (1989) (65, 66)	20	NR	70
Shawl (1989) (60, 67)	10	NR	20
Overlie (1990) (61)	35	43	77
Reedy (1990) (63)	38	69	76
Sugimoto (1991) (62)	8	NR	75
Rees (1992) (64)	9	44	56

NR, Not recorded.

Table 27D.7.
Outcome in High-Risk PTCA Utilizing Prophylactic Cardiopulmonary Support

Author (Ref.)	n	EF Mean	Lesion Success/ Attempt %	Major Complications[a] %	Emergency CABG %	Abrupt Closure %	In-Hospital Deaths %
Vogel (1988) (71)	9	26	11/12	11	0	0	11
Tommaso (1989) (70)	10	25	12/13	40	0	0	10
Taub (1989) (74)	7	32	10/10	86	0	0	14
Freedman (1989) (73)	4	30	9/9	0	0	0	0
Shawl (1989) (72)	51	NR	115/117	?	0	4	6
1988 National Registry (1990) (76)	105	32	173/182	39	4	7	8
Ott (1990) (75)	5	24	12/12	40	0	0	0

[a]Death, myocardial infarction, abrupt closure, CABG, or repeat PTCA.

EF, Ejection fraction; *CABG*, coronary artery bypass graft; *NR*, not recorded.

Table 27D.8.
Prophylactic Versus Standby Cardiopulmonary Support

Author (Ref.)		n	EF%	Procedural Success (%)	Major Complications[a] (%)	Emergency CABG (%)	Death (%)
Tommaso (1989) (78)	Prophylactic	14	26	86	14	0	14
	Standby	9	25	100	0	0	0
Herz (1990) (79)	"Standby"[b]	56	NR	95	2	5	0
1989 National Registry	Prophylactic	258	28	89	41	2	6
(1992) (77)	Standby	98	34	88	12	2	6

[a]Death, myocardial infarction, abrupt closure, CABG, or repeat PTCA.

[b]Compared their series with the 1988 National Registry (76).

EF, Ejection fraction; *CABG,* coronary artery bypass graft; *NR,* not recorded.

their procedure with CPS and in only 12% of patients who did not. Two other studies have examined prophylactic versus standby cardiopulmonary support and are presented in Table 27D.8 (78, 79). Herz and colleagues reported a series of patients with high-risk features that would have qualified for CPS in the National Registry, although none of their patients actually underwent prophylactic CPS (79). They compared their results with the 1988 National Registry and found similar rates of procedural success without the extent of major complications. Unfortunately, there has been no randomized prospective study evaluating the outcome of standby versus prophylactic cardiopulmonary support. The findings of the 1989 National Registry underscore our inability to determine who is at greatest risk and in need of supported angioplasty. Because of the high complication rates and lack of indisputable benefit in patients considered high risk for coronary intervention, the ACC/AHA Task Force has suggested that individual use of CPS as a prophylactic measure remains to be clarified by further clinical investigation. In our experience CPS is the support strategy of choice in patients with an ejection fraction of <20% and where the target artery supplies >50% of viable myocardium. Its use in this setting is supported by published data from the National Registry of CPS, where patients with these characteristics had a higher mortality when CPS was *not* used.

THE HEMOPUMP

The Hemopump (Johnson & Johnson, Skilman, NJ) is an investigational device developed as an alternative to other ventricular assist devices. Its main advantage is that it is intraarterial and semipercutaneous and can be inserted relatively easily. The Hemopump is a catheter-mounted axial flow pump with an Archimedes spiral vein screw that rotates at 15,000 to 27,000 RPM (80). It is made of silicone rubber reinforced by a coil spring and has a beveled tip that is placed in the left ventricle. The pump portion of the assembly is 20 cm long and 7 mm in diameter so that the pump end is 21 Fr in size and the shaft is 11 Fr as it traverses the femoral artery. The screw is located in the cannula in the arch of the aorta and is powered by a driveshaft connected to an electromagnetic motor outside the body. The Hemopump delivers 0.5 to 3.5 L/minute of nonpulsatile flow and does not need to be synchronized with the cardiac cycle or rhythm (81). The device decompresses the left ventricle by pumping blood from the left ventricle into the descending aorta.

Several studies have described the hemodynamic effects of the Hemopump. Merhige and colleagues demonstrated that in the absence of ischemia, the Hemopump reduced left ventricular end-diastolic pressure in dogs and resulted in systolic unloading of the ventricle while maintaining mean aortic pressure (82). The same effects were noted in the presence of ischemia with an increase in regional myocardial perfusion with the Hemopump turned on. Shiiya and coworkers confirmed these findings in six open-chest dogs and also showed a reduced O_2 demand and improved blood flow: O_2 demand ratio in the nonoccluded coronaries (83). These hemodynamic effects also appear to be superior to those of intraaortic balloon pumping in dogs (84). One study of four patients with cardiogenic shock after acute myocardial infarction showed the Hemopump increased the cardiac index by 120% and the mean arterial pressure by 48% and reduced the pulmonary capillary wedge pressure by 37% (85).

A few of the major advantages of the Hemopump are that it does not require synchronization with rhythm, it operates independently of left ventricular function, and it has a myocardial protective effect and offers decompression for the left ventricle. In approximately 15 to 20% of patients, however, the Hemopump cannot be inserted because of size limitations. Smaller devices (14 Fr) currently under investigation may allow the Hemopump to be applied to a wider range of patients. The tradeoff is that the smaller devices may cause more hemolysis (86) and provide less flow. Additional advantages and disadvantages of the Hemopump are listed in Table 27D.9. The Hemopump was initially used for postpericardiotomy shock or allograft failure and allowed weaning from cardiopulmonary bypass (87–89). It has also been used with some limited success in patients with cardiogenic shock following myocardial infarction (80, 88, 90, 91). The device appears most beneficial in patients with cardiogenic shock or when used as a bridge in patients awaiting heart transplantation or revascularization. It does not appear to have a well-defined role in patients with cardiomyopathy.

Most studies of the Hemopump to date have contained small numbers of patients with a wide range of causes of their cardiac decompensation. The largest clinical trial thus far was a multicenter trial of 123 patients

Table 27D.9.
Hemopump

Advantages
  Decompresses the ventricle
  Decreases myocardial energy consumption
  Augments coronary perfusion
  Perfusion technician unnecessary
  Full heparinization not required
  No significant hemolysis or complement activation
  No synchronization with rhythm necessary
  Works independently of LV function
  May be used up to 14 days
Disadvantages
  Requires arterial cutdown
  Dependent on LV filling
  Limited by size (21 Fr)
  Inability to place device in 20%
  Smaller devices may cause more hemolysis
  Investigational
  Ventricular arrhythmias
  Displacement from LV could be catastrophic
  Nonpulsative flow

with cardiogenic shock (either postmyocardial infarction or postcardiotomy). Of the 53 patients in whom published data are available (92, 93), the Hemopump was successfully inserted in 41 (77%). The 30-day survival of the Hemopump group was 32%, and the survival of those who could not have the device inserted for technical reasons was 17%. While this trial showed a trend toward improved survival with the Hemopump, it was not randomized and preliminary results in all 123 patients found no statistically significant difference in survival between the two groups (34). Loisance and coworkers reported on nine patients with ischemia unresponsive to medical therapy who were at high risk to undergo either surgery or PTCA (94, 95). The high-risk surgical characteristics included age >75 years in two patients, ejection fraction less than 20% in six patients, and no adequate bypass conduit in five patients. The high-risk PTCA characteristics included uncontrolled ischemia in seven patients, ejection fraction less than 20% in six patients, and a target lesion located in the last remaining patent vessel perfusing a major mass of myocardium, with three patients having a lesion located in an unprotected left main coronary artery. Six of the nine patients had the pump implanted, with results that included an increase in cardiac index by 25% and a decrease in pulmonary capillary wedge pressure by 19%. All six underwent PTCA without "significant" complications, although three had ventricular tachycardia and one had high-degree AV block. Five of the six patients remained symptom free at follow-up 5 to 15 months later, and the remaining patient underwent elective surgical revascularization for persistent angina. Three patients were not able to receive the Hemopump: two had small iliac vessels, and one had aortoiliac disease. One of these three patients died during angioplasty and a second patient died 2 weeks later of uncontrolled myocardial ischemia; the third patient underwent coronary artery bypass grafting.

There are no other published studies of the Hemopump as a supportive device for high-risk angioplasty. It is therefore unclear whether it will emerge as a viable option with more widespread applicability. Its precise role in supported angioplasty will need to be defined in the future.

PARTIAL LEFT HEART BYPASS SUPPORT

Partial left heart bypass is another potential means of supporting patients during high-risk angioplasty. This method is performed percutaneously using a transseptal approach with large-bore catheters placed in the left atrium and femoral artery (14 to 20 Fr). The advantage of this system is that it does not require an oxygenator because blood is pumped from the oxygenated left atrium to the femoral artery. Its disadvantages are its limited use and the large catheters required for the roller pump to effectively increase the cardiac output (96, 97). Further clinical investigation is needed to clarify the exact role of this device in supporting critically ill patients.

SUMMARY

Performing revascularization in patients with left ventricular dysfunction, multivessel disease, and an unstable clinical presentation is a considerable challenge. In general, our belief is that revascularization should be attempted, since the prognosis with continued medical management in all published series has been worse when compared with an aggressive revascularization approach. If all significant lesions can be approached with percutaneous intervention with an estimated lesion success greater than 90%, a percutaneous approach may be taken with or without support devices. If lesion success is deemed to be low, then CABG may be the preferred therapy. In a few selected patients with comorbid disease or prior CABG, a percutaneous approach may also be considered as preferential. The decision regarding which revascularization strategy to use should include discussions with the cardiothoracic surgeons, and the availability of surgical backup should also be considered prior to the procedure. Once a percutaneous approach has been chosen, the need for percutaneous support devices should be explored.

The decision to use support devices to assist high-risk percutaneous interventions is complex. The appropriate selection should be based on patient characteristics, whether complete or culprit lesion strategy is applied, the area in jeopardy for reduced blood supply, the procedure's ischemic duration, and the patient's clinical status. Thus the selection of support strategy will be different when a discrete (suitable for perfusion balloon angioplasty) culprit lesion in the mid-LAD coronary artery in a patient with an ejection fraction of 20% and stable angina is considered compared with multiple lesions in the mid-LAD, other target lesions in the LCX and the RCA, an ejection fraction of 20%, and unstable angina. In the former scenario the combination of perfusion balloon angioplasty and IABP support may be adequate. In the latter the prophylactic use of percutaneous CPS may be considered as a better alternative. Ultimately, every case needs to be considered with all the risk factors for procedural mortality, risk of abrupt closure, and technical issues reviewed. For elective procedures, the laboratory experience with CPS should also be considered. In general, for patients with an ejection fraction of >20% the IABP is the support device of choice. For patients with an ejection fraction of <20% IABP with CPS standby or prophylactic CPS should be considered. The decision between these two strategies will depend on the amount of myocardium in jeopardy and the degree of clinical heart failure. Patients with a large area of jeopardy and heart failure should have CPS-supported percutaneous interventions.

Patients requiring hemodynamic support during acute myocardial infarction should have IABP started as soon as possible during the acute cardiac catheterization procedure. Observational data have suggested that the combination of acute angioplasty and IABP use improves in-hospital mortality (45) and can improve sustained coronary artery patency (42). In our experience the use of CPS should be limited to patients who are undergoing emergency CABG, where IABP cannot fully sustain the patient because of life-threatening arrhythmias. All patients who have sustained cardiac arrest in the cardiac catheterization laboratory should have CPS started as soon as possible. Observational data have noted that if CPS can be started within 10 minutes of cardiac arrest this can be a lifesaving procedure (69).

Along with percutaneous interventions, the use of support devices by interventional cardiologists has risen over the last decade. The ultimate challenge has been applying this technology to the "right" patient and thereby making percutaneous revascularization a safer procedure. In the future less invasive procedures will combine the physiologic benefits of aortic counterpulsation with the considerable peripheral support of CPS. The challenge for the future will be how such an approach should be developed and more importantly in which patients it should be applied.

REFERENCES

1. Schocken DD, Arrieta MI, Leaverton PE, Ross EA. Prevalence and mortality rate of congestive heart failure in the United States. J Am Coll Cardiol 1992;20:301–306.
2. Kalon KLH, Anderson KM, Kannel WB, Grossman W, Kevy D. Survival after the onset of congestive heart failure in Framingham heart study subjects. Circulation 1993; 88:107–115.
3. Lee KL, Pryor DB, Pieper KS et al. Prognostic value of radionuclide angiography in medically treated patients with coronary artery disease. A comparison with clinical and catheterization variables. Circulation 1990;82:1705–1717.
4. Califf RM, Phillips HR, Hindman MC et al. Prognostic value of a coronary artery jeopardy score. J Am Coll Cardiol 1985;5:1055–1063.
5. Califf RM, Mark DB, Harrell FE Jr et al. Importance of clinical measures of ischemia in the prognosis of patients with documented coronary artery disease. J Am Coll Cardiol 1988;11:20–26.
6. Milano CA, White WD, Smith LR et al. Coronary artery bypass in patients with severely depressed ventricular function. Ann Thorac Surg 1993;56:487–493.
7. Passamani E, Davis KB, Gillespie MJ, Killip T, and the CASS principal investigators and their associates. A randomized trial of coronary artery bypass surgery: survival of patients with a low ejection fraction. N Engl J Med 1985;312:1665–1671.
8. Alderman EL, Fisher LD, Litwin P et al. Results of coronary artery surgery in patients with poor left ventricular function (CASS). Circulation 1983;68:785–795.
9. Califf RM, Harrell FE Jr, Lee KL et al. The evolution of medical and surgical therapy for coronary artery disease. A 15-year perspective. JAMA 1989;261:2077–2086.
10. Bounous EP, Mark DB, Pollock BG et al. Surgical survival benefits for coronary disease patients with left ventricular dysfunction. Circulation 1988;78:I-151–I-157.
11. FitzGibbon GM, Leach AJ, Kafka HP, Keon WJ. Coronary bypass graft fate: long-term angiographic study. J Am Coll Cardiol 1991;17:1075–1080.
12. O'Connor GT, Morton JR, Diehl MJ et al. Differences between men and women in hospital mortality associated with coronary artery bypass graft surgery. Circulation 1993;88:2104–2110.
13. Bell MR, Gersh BJ, Schaff HV et al. Effect of completeness of revascularization on long-term outcome of patients with three-vessel disease undergoing coronary artery bypass surgery: a report from the Coronary Artery Surgery Study (CASS) Registry. Circulation 1992; 86:446–457.
14. Hartzler GO, Rutherford BD, McConahay DR, Johnson WJ, Giorgi LV. "High-risk" percutaneous transluminal coronary angioplasty. Am J Cardiol 1988;61:33G–37G.
15. Phillips HR, Califf RM. An approach to percutaneous revascularization in patients with stable coronary ischemia. In: Roubin GS, Califf RM, O'Neill WW, Phillips HR, Stack RS, eds. Interventional cardiovascular medicine: principles and practice. New York: Churchill Livingstone, 1994.
16. Ellis SG, Myler RK, King SB III et al. Causes and correlates of death after unsupported coronary angioplasty: implications for use of angioplasty and advanced support techniques in high-risk settings. Am J Cardiol 1991; 68:1447–1451.
17. Bergelson BA, Jacobs AK, Cupples LA et al. Prediction of risk for hemodynamic compromise during percutaneous transluminal coronary angioplasty. Am J Cardiol 1992; 70:1540–1545.
18. Holmes DR Jr, Detre KM, Williams DO et al. Long-term outcome of patients with depressed left ventricular function undergoing percutaneous transluminal coronary angioplasty: the NHLBI PTCA Registry. Circulation 1993; 87:21–29.
19. Kohli RS, Disciascio G, Cowley MJ, Nath A, Goudreau E, Vetrovec GW. Coronary angioplasty in patients with severe left ventricular dysfunction. J Am Coll Cardiol 1990;16:807–811.

20. Serota H, Deligonul U, Lee WH et al. Predictors of cardiac survival after percutaneous transluminal coronary angioplasty in patients with severe left ventricular dysfunction. Am J Cardiol 1991;67:367–372.

21. Stevens T, Kahn JK, McCallister BD et al. Safety and efficacy of percutaneous transluminal coronary angioplasty in patients with left ventricular dysfunction. Am J Cardiol 1991;68:313–319.

22. O'Keefe JH Jr, Allan JJ, McCallister BD et al. Angioplasty versus bypass surgery for multivessel coronary artery disease with left ventricular ejection fraction ≤40%. Am J Cardiol 1993;71:897–901.

23. Quigley PJ, Kereiakes DJ, Abbottsmith CW et al. Prolonged autoperfusion angioplasty: immediate clinical outcome and angiographic follow-up. J Am Coll Cardiol 1989;13:155A (abstract).

24. Hinohara T, Simpson JB, Phillips HR et al. Transluminal catheter reperfusion: a new technique to reestablish blood flow after coronary occlusion during percutaneous transluminal coronary angioplasty. Am J Cardiol 1986; 57:684–686.

25. Snyder R, Wijay B, Angelini P. Percutaneous transluminal coronary angioplasty with hemoperfusion. ASAIO Trans 1991;37:M367–M368.

26. Lehmann KG, Atwood JE, Snyder EL, Ellison RL. Autologous blood perfusion for myocardial protection during coronary angioplasty: a feasibility study. Circulation 1987; 76:312–323.

27. Tokioka H, Miyazaki A, Fung P et al. Effects of intracoronary infusion of arterial blood or Fluosol-DA 20% on regional myocardial metabolism and function during brief coronary artery occlusion. Circulation 1987;75:473–481.

28. Christensen CW, Reeves WC, Lassar TA, Schmidt DH. Inadequate subendocardial oxygen delivery during perflurocarbon perfusion in a canine model of ischemia. Am Heart J 1988;115:30–37.

29. Szatmary LJ, Marco J, Fajadet J, Caster L. The combined use of diastolic counterpulsation and coronary dilation in unstable angina due to multivessel disease under unstable hemodynamic conditions. Int J Cardiol 1988; 19:59–66.

30. Gore JM, Weiner BH, Benotti JR et al. Preliminary experience with synchronized coronary sinus retroperfusion in humans. Circulation 1986;74:381–388.

31. Nanto S, Nishida K, Hirayama A et al. Supported angioplasty with synchronized retroperfusion in high-risk patients with left main trunk or near left main trunk obstruction. Am Heart J 1993;125:301–309.

32. Moulopoulos SD, Topaz S, Kolff WL. Diastolic balloon pumping (with carbon dioxide) in the aorta—a mechanical assistance to the failing circulation. Am Heart J 1962; 63:669–675.

33. Kantrowitz A, Tjonneland S, Freed PS, Phillips SJ, Butner AN, Sherman JL. Initial clinical experience with intraaortic balloon pumping in cardiogenic shock. JAMA 1968; 203:135.

34. Goldenberg IF. Nonpharmacologic management of cardiac arrest and cardiogenic shock. Chest 1992;102(Suppl 2):596S–616S.

35. McCabe JC, Abel RM, Subramanian VA, Gay WA. Complications of intra-aortic balloon insertion and counterpulsation. Circulation 1977;57:769–773.

36. Scheidt S, Wilner G, Mueller H et al. Intra-aortic balloon counterpulsation in cardiogenic shock. N Engl J Med 1973;288:979–984.

37. Fuchs RM, Brin KP, Brinker JA, Guzman PA, Heuser RR, Yin FCP. Augmentation of regional coronary blood flow by intra-aortic balloon counterpulsation in patients with unstable angina. Circulation 1983;68:117–123.

38. Williams DL, Korr KS, Gerwirtz H, Most AS. The effect of intra-aortic balloon counterpulsation on regional myocardial blood flow and oxygen consumption in the presence of coronary artery stenosis in patients with unstable angina. Circulation 1982;66:593–597.

39. MacDonald RG, Hill JA, Feldman RL. Failure of intraaortic balloon counterpulsation to augment distal coronary perfusion pressure during percutaneous transluminal coronary angioplasty. Am J Cardiol 1987;59:359–361.

40. Ishihara M, Sato H, Tateishi H, Kawagoe T, Muraoka Y, Yoshimura M. Effects of intraaortic balloon pumping on coronary hemodynamics after coronary angioplasty in patients with acute myocardial infarction. Am Heart J 1992;124:1133–1138.

41. Kern MJ, Aguirre F, Bach R, Donohue T, Siegal R, Segal J. Augmentation of coronary blood flow by intra-aortic balloon pumping in patients after coronary angioplasty. Circulation 1993;87:500–511.

42. Ohman EM, Califf RM, George BS et al. The use of intraaortic balloon pumping as an adjunct to reperfusion therapy in acute myocardial infarction. The Thrombolysis and Angioplasty in Myocardial Infarction (TAMI) Study Group. Am Heart J 1991;121:895–901.

43. Campeau L, Lesperance J, Bourassa MG. Natural history of saphenous vein aortocoronary bypass grafts. Mod Concepts Cardiovasc Dis 1984;53:59–63.

44. Ohman EM, George BS, White CJ et al. The use of aortic counterpulsation to improve sustained coronary artery patency during acute myocardial infarction: results of a randomized trial. Circulation 1994;90:792–799.

45. Bengtson JR, Kaplan AJ, Pieper KS et al. Prognosis in cardiogenic shock after acute myocardial infarction in the interventional era. J Am Coll Cardiol 1992;20:1482–1489.

46. Kahn JK, Rutherford BD, McConahay DR, Johnson WL, Giorgi LV, Hartzler GO. Supported "high-risk" coronary angioplasty using intraaortic balloon pump counterpulsation. J Am Coll Cardiol 1990;15:1151–1155.

47. Alcan KE, Stertzer SH, Wallsh E, DePasquale NP, Bruno MS. The role of intra-aortic balloon counterpulsation in patients undergoing percutaneous transluminal coronary angioplasty. Am Heart J 1983;105:527–530.

48. Voudris V, Marco J, Morice MC, Fajadet J, Royer T. "High-risk" percutaneous transluminal coronary angioplasty with preventive intraaortic balloon counterpulsation. Cathet Cardiovasc Diagn 1990;19:160–164.

49. Margolis JR. The role of the percutaneous intra-aortic balloon in emergency situations following percutaneous transluminal coronary angioplasty. Transluminal coronary

angioplasty and intracoronary thrombolysis. Coronary heart disease IV. Berlin: Springer-Verlag, 1982.

50. Jones EL, Murphy DA, Craver JM. Comparison of coronary artery bypass surgery and percutaneous transluminal coronary angioplasty including surgery for failed angioplasty. Am Heart J 1984;107:830–835.

51. Lincott AM, Popma JJ, Ellis SG, Vogel RA, Topol EJ. Percutaneous support devices for high-risk or complicated coronary angioplasty. J Am Coll Cardiol 1991; 17:758–769.

52. Nash IS, Lorell BH, Fishman RF, Baim DS, Donahue C, Diver DJ. A new technique for sheathless percutaneous intraaortic balloon catheter insertion. Cathet Cardiovasc Diagn 1991;23:57–60.

53. Alcan KE, Stertzer SH, Wallsh E, Bruno MS, DePasquale NP. Current status of intra-aortic balloon counterpulsation in critical care cardiology. Crit Care Med 1984; 12:489–495.

54. Scheidt S. Preservation of ischemic myocardium with intraaortic balloon pumping: modern therapeutic intervention or *primum non nocere*. Circulation 1978;58:211–214.

55. Lazar JM, Ziady GM, Dummer SJ, Thompson M, Ruffuer RJ. Outcome and complications of prolonged intraaortic balloon counterpulsation in cardiac patients. Am J Cardiol 1992;69:955–958.

56. Ohman EM, George BS, White CJ et al. Reocclusion of the infarct-related artery after primary or rescue angioplasty: effect of aortic counterpulsation. Circulation 1993;88(Suppl I):I-107.

57. Ishihara M, Sato H, Tateishi H et al. Intraaortic balloon pumping following rescue coronary angioplasty after failed thrombolysis. Circulation 1993;88(Suppl I):I-107.

58. Pavlides GS, Hauser AM, Stack RK et al. Effect of peripheral cardiopulmonary bypass on left ventricular size, afterload and myocardial function during elective supported coronary angioplasty. J Am Coll Cardiol 1991; 18:499–505.

59. Kennedy JH. The role of assisted circulation in cardiac resuscitation. JAMA 1966;197:615–618.

60. Shawl FA, Domanski MJ, Hernandez TJ, Punja S. Emergency percutaneous cardiopulmonary bypass support in cardiogenic shock from acute myocardial infarction. Am J Cardiol 1989;64:967–970.

61. Overtie PA. Emergency use of portable cardiopulmonary bypass. Cathet Cardiovasc Diagn 1990;20:27–31.

62. Sugimoto JT, Baird E, Bruner C. Percutaneous cardiopulmonary support in cardiac arrest. ASAIO Trans 1991; 37:M282–M283.

63. Reedy JE, Swartz MT, Raitnel SC, Szukalski EA, Pennington DG. Mechanical cardiopulmonary support for refractory cardiogenic shock. Heart Lung 1990; 19:514–525.

64. Rees MR, Browne T, Sivanantnay VM et al. Cardiac resuscitation with percutaneous cardiopulmonary support. Lancet 1992;340:513–514.

65. Phillips SJ, Ballentine B, Slonine D et al. Percutaneous initiation of cardiopulmonary bypass. Ann Thorac Surg 1983;36:223–225.

66. Phillips SJ, Zeff RH, Kongtahworn C et al. Percutaneous cardiopulmonary bypass: application and indication for use. Ann Thorac Surg 1989;47:121–123.

67. Shawl FA, Domanski MJ, Wish M, Punja S, Hernandez TJ. Emergency percutaneous cardiopulmonary support in cardiogenic shock: long term follow-up. Circulation 1989;80(Suppl II):II-258 (abstract).

68. Mattox KL, Beall AC. Application of portable cardiopulmonary bypass to emergency instrumentation. Med Instrum 1977;11:347–349.

69. Overtie PA, Reichman RT, Smith SC et al. Emergency use of portable cardiopulmonary bypass in patients with cardiac arrest. J Am Coll Cardiol 1989;13:160A.

70. Tommaso CL, Gundry SR, Zoda AR, Stafford JL, Johnson RA, Vogel RA. Supported angioplasty: initial experience with high-risk patients. J Am Coll Cardiol 1989;13:159A (abstract).

71. Vogel RA. The Maryland experience: angioplasty and valvuloplasty using percutaneous cardiopulmonary support. Am J Cardiol 1988;62:11k–14k.

72. Shawl FA, Domanski MJ, Punja S, Hernandez TJ. Percutaneous cardiopulmonary bypass support in high-risk patients undergoing percutaneous transluminal coronary angioplasty. Am J Cardiol 1989;64:1258–1263.

73. Freedman RJ, Wrenn RC, Godley ML, Knoepp JD, Smith C, LaCroix C. Complex multiple percutaneous transluminal coronary angioplasties with vortex oxygenator cardiopulmonary support in the community hospital setting. Cathet Cardiovasc Diagn 1989;17:237–242.

74. Taub JO, L'Hommedieu BD, Raithel SC et al. Extracorporeal membrane oxygenation for percutaneous coronary angioplasty in high-risk patients. ASAIO Trans 1989;35:664–666.

75. Ott RA, Mills TC, Tobis JM, Allen BJ, Dwyer ML. ECMO-assisted angioplasty for cardiomyopathy patients with unstable angina. ASAIO Trans 1990;36:M483–M485.

76. Vogel RA, Shawl F, Tommaso C et al. Initial report of the National Registry of Elective Cardiopulmonary Bypass Supported Coronary Angioplasty. J Am Coll Cardiol 1990,15:23–29.

77. Tierstein PS. Cardiopulmonary support. Am J Cardiol 1992;69:19F–21F.

78. Tommaso CL, Vogel RA. Supported vs. standby supported angioplasty. Circulation 1989;80(Suppl II):II-272.

79. Herz I, Fried G, Feld H et al. High-risk PTCA without cardiopulmonary support. Circulation 1990;82(Suppl III):III-654.

80. Lincott AM, Popma JJ, Bates ER et al. Successful coronary angioplasty in two patients with cardiogenic shock using the Numbus Hemopump support device. Am Heart J 1990;120:970–972.

81. Wamples RK, Mose JC, Frazier OH, Olsen DB. In vivo evaluation of a peripheral vascular access axial flow blood pump. ASAIO Trans 1988;34:450–454.

82. Merhige ME, Smalling RW, Cassidy D et al. Effect of the Hemopump left ventricular assist device on regional myocardial perfusion and function: reduction of ischemia during coronary occlusion. Circulation 1989;80(Suppl III):III-158–III-166.

83. Shiiya N, Zelinsky R, Delevze PM, Loisance DY. Effects of Hemopump support on left ventricular unloading and coronary blood flow. ASAIO Trans 1991;37:M361–M362.

84. Smalling RW, Cassidy DB, Merhige M et al. Improved hemodynamic and left ventricular unloading during acute ischemia using the Hemopump left ventricular assist device compared to intraaortic balloon counterpulsation. J Am Coll Cardiol 1989;13:160A (abstract).

85. Smalling RW, Sweeney MJ, Cassidy DB et al. Hemodynamics in cardiogenic shock after acute myocardial infarction with the Hemopump assist device. Circulation 1989;80(Suppl II):II-624 (abstract).

86. Mooney MR, Mooney JF, Van Tassel RA et al. The Nimbus Hemopump: a new left ventricular assist device that combines myocardial protective with circulatory support. J Invasive Cardiol 1990;2:169–173.

87. Frazier OH, Wamples RK, Duncan JM et al. First human use of the Hemopump, a catheter-mounted ventricular assist device. J Am Coll Cardiol 1989;13:121A (abstract).

88. Frazier OH, Nalcatan T, Duncan JM, Parnis SM, Fuqua JM. Clinical experience with the Hemopump. ASAIO Trans 1989;35:604–606.

89. Burnett CM, Vega JD, Radovancevic B et al. Improved survival after Hemopump insertion in patients experiencing post cardiotomy cardiogenic shock during cardiopulmonary bypass. ASAIO Trans 1990;36:M626–M629.

90. Deeb GM, Bolling SF, Nicklas J et al. Clinical experience with the Nimbus pump. ASAIO Trans 1990;36:M632–M636.

91. Phillips SJ, Barker L, Balentine B et al. Hemopump support for the failing heart. ASAIO Trans 1990;36:M629–M632.

92. Wampler RK, Frazier OH, Lansing AM et al. Treatment of cardiogenic shock with the Hemopump left ventricular assist device. Ann Thorac Surg 1991;52:506–513.

93. Wampler RK, Johnson DV, Rutan PM, Riehle RA. Multicenter clinical study of the Hemopump in the treatment of cardiogenic shock. Circulation 1989;80(Suppl II):II-670 (abstract).

94. Loisance D, Deboise-Rande JL, Deleuze P, Okude J, Rosenval O, Geschwind H. Prophylactic intraventricular pumping in high-risk coronary angioplasty. Lancet 1990; 335:438–440.

95. Loisance D, Deleuze P, Dubois-Rande JL et al. Hemopump ventricular support for patients undergoing high-risk coronary angioplasty. ASAIO Trans 1990;36:M623–M626.

96. Glassman E, Chinitz L, Levite H, Slater J, Winer H. Partial left heart bypass support during high-risk angioplasty. Circulation 1989;80(Suppl II):II-272 (abstract).

97. Babic VV, Brojicic S, Kjurisic Z, Vucinic M. Percutaneous left atrial-aorta bypass with a roller pump. Circulation 1989;80(Suppl II):II-272 (abstract).

98. Vlietstra RE, Assad-Morell JL, Frye RL et al. Survival predictors in coronary artery disease: medical and surgical comparisons. Mayo Clin Proc 1977;52:85–90.

99. Manley JC, King JF, Zeft HJ, Johnson WD. The "bad" left ventricle: results of coronary surgery and effect on late survival. J Thoracic Cardiovasc Surg 1976;72:841–848.

100. Yatteau RF, Peter RH, Behar VS, Bartel AG, Rosati RA, Kong Y. Ischemic cardiomyopathy: the myopathy of coronary artery disease—natural history and results of medical versus surgical treatment. Am J Cardiol 1974; 34:520–525.

101. Oldham HN, Kong Y, Bartel AG et al. Risk factors in coronary artery bypass surgery. Arch Surg 1972;105:918–923.

102. Zubiate P, Kay JH, Dunne EF. Myocardial revascularization for patients with an ejection fraction of 0.2 or less: 12 years' results. West J Med 1984;140:745–749.

103. Faulkner SL, Stoney WS, Alford WC et al. Ischemic cardiomyopathy: medical versus surgical treatment. J Thorac Cardiovasc Surg 1977;74:77–82.

104. Mitchel BF, Alivizatos PA, Adam M, Geisler GF, Thiele JP, Lambert CJ. Myocardial revascularization in patients with poor ventricular function. J Thorac Cardiovasc Surg 1975;69:52–62.

105. Fox HE, May IA, Ecker RR. Long-term functional results of surgery for coronary artery disease in patients with poor ventricular function. J Thorac Cardiovasc Surg 1975;70:1064–1072.

106. Jones EL, Craver JM, Kaplan JA et al. Criteria for operability and reduction of surgical mortality in patients with severe left ventricular ischemia and dysfunction. Ann Thorac Surg 1978;25:413–424.

107. Mochtar B, Meeter-Laird K, Brower RW, Verbaan N, Haalebos MMP, Box E. Aorto-coronary bypass surgery in 62 patients with severe left ventricular dysfunction—a follow-up study. Thorac Cardiovasc Surg 1985;33:30–33.

108. Zubiate P, Kay JH, Mendez AM. Myocardial revascularization for the patient with drastic impairment of function of the left ventricle. J Thorac Cardiovasc Surg 1977; 73:84–86.

109. Hochberg MS, Parsonnet V, Gielchinsky I, Hussain SM. Coronary artery bypass grafting in patients with ejection fractions below forty percent: early and late results in 466 patients. J Thorac Cardiovasc Surg 1983;86:519–527.

110. Sanchez JA, Smith CR, Drusin RE, Reison DS, Malm JR, Rose EA. High-risk reparative surgery—a neglected alternative to heart transplantation. Circulation 1990;82:IV-302–IV-305.

111. Kron IL, Flanagan TL, Blackbourne LH, Schroeder RA, Nolan SP. Coronary revascularization rather than cardiac transplantation for chronic ischemic cardiomyopathy. Ann Surg 1989;210:348–354.

112. Blakeman BM, Pifarre R, Sullivan H, Costanzo-Nordin MR, Zucker MJ. High-risk heart surgery in the heart transplant candidate. J Heart Transplant 1990;9:468–472.

113. Christakis GT, Weisel RD, Fremes SE et al. Coronary artery bypass grafting in patients with poor ventricular function. J Thorac Cardiovasc Surg 1992;103:1083–1092.

28. Multivessel Disease

DANIEL B. MARK and JAMES G. JOLLIS

Coronary artery disease (CAD) is a chronic disorder that many patients must endure for decades. The course of the disease for an individual patient is typically characterized by long periods of clinical stability punctuated by acute exacerbations, often taking the form of unstable angina or acute myocardial infarction. Management of the patient with multivessel coronary artery disease requires an understanding of the natural history of CAD along with the potential short- and long-term effects of the different treatment options available. Multivessel CAD may either be diagnosed at cardiac catheterization or suspected from the result of a noninvasive stress test. For this chapter we will assume that the patient has already undergone cardiac catheterization and that the clinician is now faced with the problem of deciding which treatment option to pursue. The major management options in this setting involve choices of medications and coronary revascularization techniques. Other portions of this text deal in detail with the technical aspects of revascularization. In this chapter we will briefly review the key concepts involved in the prognostic stratification of the patient with multivessel disease. We will then show how the prognosis of the patient relates to treatment selection.

PROGNOSIS IN THE MEDICALLY TREATED PATIENT

CAD Risk Continuum

It is important to understand that multivessel coronary artery disease is not a homogeneous anatomic or prognostic entity but rather a spectrum of disease severity that includes very low risk to very high risk individuals (1). The efficient estimation of the patient's short- and long-term risks of adverse cardiac events (especially death and myocardial infarction) is the principal foundation on which treatment decisions are made. It is conceptually helpful in thinking about the risks of coronary disease to view the patient's prognosis as the sum of the risks attributable to the patient's current disease state and the risks that the patient's disease will progress to a higher- or lower-risk state.

The risks associated with the patient's current disease state can be understood with reference to four major types of prognostic measures (Table 28.1). The strongest individual prognostic indicator in coronary disease is the extent of left ventricular damage present. Typically, the ejection fraction is the variable most often used to summarize the state of the left ventricular function (2). However, because it is a ratio (stroke volume over left ventricular end-diastolic volume), compensatory responses to left ventricular damage that serve to maintain cardiac output (e.g., Frank Starling mechanism) may make the ejection fraction an optimistic measure of true left ventricular contractile abilities (3). More recent studies have therefore focused directly on ventricular volumes as indicators of myocardial systolic dysfunction and decompensation (4). Even the observation at left ventricular angiography of a dilated left ventricle (an informal ventricular volume assessment) indicates a higher-risk state for any given ejection fraction value than that same ejection fraction with a nondilated ventricle. Cardiomegaly on the plain chest radiograph is

Table 28.1.
Major Prognostic Factors in Coronary Disease Relating to Current Risk State[a]

Left ventricular function/damage
    History of prior MI
    CHF symptoms
    Cardiomegaly on chest radiography
    Ejection fraction
    Regional LV wall-motion abnormalities
    LV diastolic function
    LV end-systolic and end-diastolic volumes
    Mitral regurgitation
    Atrial fibrillation
    Conduction disturbances on ECG
Coronary disease severity
    Anatomic extent of CAD
    Transient ischemia
    Collateral vessels
Ongoing coronary plaque event
    Symptom course (unstable, progressive, stable)
    Transient ischemia
    Hematologic milieu
Electrical instability
    Ventricular arrhythmias
    Late potentials
    Decreased heart rate variability

[a]From Mark DB. In: Roubin GS et al, eds. Interventional cardiovascular medicine: principles and practice. New York: Churchill Livingstone, 1994.

MI, Myocardial infarction; CHF, congestive heart failure; I.V., left ventricular; ECG, electrocardiography; CAD, coronary artery disease.

a similar measure that has been shown repeatedly to have independent prognostic value (5–7). Another such measure is the presence and severity of congestive heart failure symptoms (6, 8). For any given ejection fraction value, symptomatic heart failure indicates a patient at substantially higher risk than a similar patient without congestive heart failure symptoms (9).

Ischemic mitral regurgitation is now recognized as an important and often underdiagnosed problem in multivessel coronary disease patients (6, 10, 11). Overall, about 20% of CAD patients presenting for diagnostic cardiac catheterization have some degree of mitral regurgitation and 3% have severe regurgitation. Pathophysiologically, there are three major forms of this disorder, each with somewhat different prognostic implications. The most common form is papillary muscle dysfunction, which is typically initiated by an inferior or posterior wall myocardial infarction involving the posterior descending artery and the posteromedial papillary muscle. Mitral regurgitation resulting from papillary muscle dysfunction may be associated with a good long-term prognosis if it is caused by a culprit lesion in the arterial supply to the papillary muscle that can be revascularized and if the overall state of the left ventricle is good. The second type of mitral regurgitation seen in ischemic heart disease is that resulting from global left ventricular dilation with secondary disruption of the function of the mitral valve apparatus. Dilation of the left ventricle caused by ischemic damage will move the papillary muscles out of proper alignment with resulting incomplete systolic coaptation of the mitral leaflets and varying degrees of regurgitation. In addition, longstanding left ventricular dilation may result in secondary dilation of the mitral annulus, also disrupting proper valvular function. This form of mitral regurgitation is associated with a poor prognosis, largely because of the severity of underlying left ventricular dysfunction. The final and least common type of ischemic mitral regurgitation is papillary muscle rupture, which typically occurs as a consequence of acute myocardial infarction and is seen in less than 1% of such patients. The picture here is one of abrupt hemodynamic deterioration with acute pulmonary edema and a rapid downhill course unless the disorder is promptly recognized and aggressively treated. In studies in the Duke Database for Cardiovascular Diseases, we have found that mitral regurgitation of any degree is a significant adverse prognostic factor, and severe regurgitation is a major independent determinant of survival in coronary disease (11–13). Because mitral regurgitation provides a form of afterload reduction to the left ventricle, the combination of a significantly depressed left ventricular ejection fraction and moderate or severe mitral regurgitation is a worrisome combination, since it indicates that the true systolic performance of the ventricle is probably significantly worse than the ejection fraction would suggest.

There is an ongoing debate about whether ventricular arrhythmias and late potentials are merely markers of a significantly damaged myocardium or are actually independent indicators of a separate dimension of risk for the patient with coronary disease (14). A similar debate exists about the prognostic significance of atrial arrhythmias and interventricular conduction defects. Atrial fibrillation is an uncommon arrhythmia in coronary disease, with an estimated prevalence of 0.6% in the Coronary Artery Surgery Study (CASS) registry (15). The CASS investigators reported that atrial fibrillation in coronary disease correlated particularly with the presence of ischemic mitral regurgitation and with symptomatic heart failure. Even after accounting for these factors, however, atrial fibrillation was associated with approximately a doubling of the patient's risk of dying compared with sinus rhythm. Similar observations have been made about interventricular conduction disturbances, particularly left bundle branch block or incomplete conduction defects that did not meet full criteria for left bundle branch block (16).

After left ventricular function, the most important prognostic characteristics of the coronary disease patient relate to the anatomic extent and severity of coronary atherosclerosis. Traditionally, the extent of disease is measured as "the number of diseased vessels." In this system the coronary tree is divided into three distributions, the left anterior descending (including diagonal branches), the left circumflex (including marginal branches), and the posterior descending artery. If a 70% (visual assessment) or greater diameter stenosis is present in any large segment of the distribution, it is considered "diseased." Conceptually, the number of diseased vessels is intended to convey a sense of the magnitude of jeopardy faced by the corresponding three major segments of the left ventricle. While this classification is very widely used, it is in-

sufficiently informative for either clinical decision making or for prognostic studies. For example, a patient with a 75% distal right coronary lesion and a 75% second circumflex marginal lesion has two-vessel disease as does a patient with a 99% proximal left anterior descending lesion and a proximal 99% right coronary lesion (assuming right dominance), but they clearly have significantly different prognoses and may require different therapeutic strategies.

Over the last two decades, many investigators have tried to improve on the "number-of-diseased-vessels" classification system. Although some innovations may provide a more informative and prognostically rich classification, no such effort to date has met with general clinical acceptance. The one system that has achieved some use in research studies is the coronary artery jeopardy score derived by Johnson and colleagues at the Massachusetts General Hospital and validated independently by Califf and coworkers at Duke (17). The score divides a stereotypic coronary tree into six major segments and assigns two points to each segment with a 70% or greater stenosis. The score values thus range from 0 (no significant CAD) to 12 (significant left main and right coronary artery disease) and stratify prognosis significantly better than a simple, number-of-diseased-vessels classification. However, the score has several important limitations that are characteristic of most attempts in this area. First, all lesions of 70% or greater are treated as prognostically equivalent without actually taking into account the true amount of myocardium at risk or the varying risk associated with different degrees of "significant" coronary stenosis. Second, the score does not take into account the presence of serial lesions or collateral vessels, and the variable branching pattern of the coronary tree in different patients cannot be accounted for. Third, the score does not take into account morphologic and pathophysiologic characteristics of the atherosclerotic plaques, such as the presence of attached thrombus. Finally, the viability of myocardium downstream from each lesion is not considered in assessing whether that lesion truly "jeopardizes" myocardium.

New approaches in this area involve taking advantage of powerful new computerized coronary tree programs and processing much more detailed information than the typical clinician is capable of assimilating.

Recently, our group proposed an intermediate strategy that took advantage of more detailed information available from the typical clinician interpretation of the coronary angiogram, but did not require quantitative analysis of the coronary tree or microcomputer processing to create the score (1, 18, 19). The new Duke index (Table 28.2), which is hierarchical and assigns each patient to the worst category applicable to them, takes into account prognostically important information about lesion severity (e.g., a 95% lesion represents a higher risk than a 75% stenosis) and location (e.g., a proximal lesion represents a higher risk than a nonproximal lesion, especially in the left anterior descending artery). To keep this system relatively simple, categories with similar prog-

noses were collapsed together to reduce the total number of categories in the final index. Prognostic weights have been assigned using Cox regression analyses and a linear transformation so that the score ranges from 0 (no CAD) to 100 (≥95% left main disease). Early experience with this new index suggests that it may help to identify important anatomic subsets of patients with multivessel disease who derive particular benefit from PTCA or from CABG that were not evident using the overall number-of-diseased-vessels classification (20).

Recent work in quantitative coronary angiography has challenged the primacy of the long-accepted, visually determined, "significant" coronary stenosis (21). While the percent diameter stenosis assessed by quantitative coronary angiography is undoubtedly both more accurate and more consistent than the visual determination, it is as yet unclear that use of these measurements improves clinical decision making or prognostic risk stratification. Recently, investigators in the Angioplasty Compared to Medicine study found that visual stenosis measurements actually correlated better with exercise capacity on the treadmill than did stenosis measurements with quantitative angiography or handheld calipers (22).

The occurence of transient ischemia provides another marker of the severity of coronary artery disease. Although many investigators refer to this phenomenon as "silent ischemia," the use of this term emphasizes an artificial dichotomy among ischemic episodes that is probably no longer relevant. The original reason for making such a distinction was based on the hypothesis of Cohn that silent ischemia reflected a "defective anginal warning system" that would place patients who manifested this phenomenon at a particularly increased risk of adverse prognostic events relative to their symptomatic counterparts (23). For the most part, the defective anginal warning system theory has not been borne out by the evidence. It is now well established

Table 28.2.
Duke Prognostic CAD Index

Extent of CAD	Prognostic Weight (0–100)
No CAD ≥50%	0
1 VD 50–74%	19
>1 VD 50–74%	23
1 VD, 75%	23
1 VD, ≥95%	32
2 VD	37
2 VD, both ≥95%	42
1 VD, ≥95% proximal LAD	48
2 VD, 95% LAD	48
2 VD, ≥95% proximal LAD	56
3 VD	56
3 VD, ≥95% in at least one	63
3 VD, proximal LAD	67
3 VD, ≥95% proximal LAD	74
Left main 75%	82
Left main ≥95%	100

1 VD, One-vessel disease; *2 VD*, two-vessel disease; *3 VD*, three-vessel disease; *LAD*, left anterior descending; *CAD*, coronary artery disease.

that many CAD patients have a majority of their ischemic events without symptoms (24, 25). Growing evidence now suggests that ischemia occurs on a continuum and that the frequency and extent of transient ischemic episodes (both symptomatic and silent) correlates strongly with the severity of underlying coronary disease. What remains unsettled is the extent to which transient ischemia provides independent prognostic information about the patient's disease beyond that available from an examination of the coronary arteriogram. It is possible, and many clinicians believe, that transient ischemia during exercise testing or ambulatory monitoring helps to differentiate otherwise similar appearing coronary lesions with differing "functional" importance.

The third major group of prognostic variables related to risks of the current disease state in CAD consists of indicators of whether a recent coronary plaque event has occurred. Current thinking, supported by a growing body of pathologic, angioscopic, and ultrasound data, is that atherosclerotic plaque rupture is the initiating event for most of the adverse clinical consequences of coronary disease (26–28). Coronary plaque rupture appears to occur most commonly in high-risk plaques, which are those with a cholesterol-rich core and a thin, fibrous cap (28, 29). Rupture appears to take place most often at the shoulder of the plaque in an area where the cap of the plaque is particularly thin. The proximate cause is still a matter of active investigation and is believed related to transient hemodynamic changes, as well as to changes in the composition of the plaque itself (30). The extent of disruption of the plaque cap caused by rupture varies considerably. In less severe cases there is minimal associated thrombus formation; the plaque may enlarge during the healing process, but otherwise such cases are usually asymptomatic. At the other end of the spectrum, severe disruption of the plaque cap may lead to a large, obstructive coronary thrombus and

acute myocardial infarction. Interestingly, while most of the focus in the treatment of coronary disease has been on plaques judged to be "significant" by coronary angiography (i.e., at least 75% stenosis), these are not the plaques that are now believed to be the highest risk for rupture and associated thrombosis. The "insignificant" plaques that are noted with varying frequency on coronary angiography and that are not suitable for treatment with either PTCA or CABG are now believed to be the principal source of risk for many coronary disease patients.

Clinically, the principal marker of an unstable coronary plaque is a change in the patient's symptom pattern, typically manifesting as a sudden increase in the frequency, severity, or ease with which ischemic attacks are provoked. In a detailed evaluation of the prognostic information available from the patient's routine anginal history, we found that the presence of increasingly progressive symptoms over the preceding 6 weeks and a greater frequency of symptoms were both strong predictors of prognosis, even when information on left ventricular ejection fraction and coronary disease severity from cardiac catheterization was taken into account (31). Conversely, a stable symptom pattern suggests the absence of a recent plaque event of clinical consequence, although there are clearly some situations in which a crescendo pattern of ischemia develops without the patient's awareness of symptoms.

Despite the substantial limitation of symptom status as a measure of disease activity, as yet there is not a more efficient objective method for identifying CAD patients experiencing a significant plaque event. Neither exercise testing nor ambulatory monitoring is practical for screening for plaque events, as they cannot be repeated frequently enough to provide an adequate surveillance. It is quite clear from recent work (and our own experience bears this out) that plaque events can develop and progress quite rapidly, so that it is possible for a patient to have a negative adequate exercise study and shortly after to develop a large anterior myocardial infarction.

The fourth major domain of CAD risk relates to the electrical stability (or lack thereof) of the myocardium. A large number of studies have evaluated the relationship between various forms of ventricular arrhythmias and prognosis in coronary disease. In general, the findings from these studies are that malignant ventricular arrhythmias (e.g., sustained ventricular tachycardia, ventricular fibrillation) are significant adverse prognostic markers except when they occur in the earliest phase (e.g., first 48 hours) of acute myocardial infarction. The significance of lesser degrees of ventricular arrhythmias, such as frequent premature ventricular contractions or nonsustained ventricular tachycardia, remains more controversial. There are two points of view represented in the current literature. One suggests that these lesser ventricular arrhythmias are markers for myocardial electrical instability. The other point of view is that such arrhythmias are a consequence of left ventricular dysfunction and scarring and do not convey independent prognostic information. This debate has been complicated by the recent report from the Cardiac Arrhythmia Suppression Trial (CAST) showing that antiarrhythmic drugs that were quite effective in suppressing ventricular arrhythmias actually increased mortality in a cohort of post-MI patients (32). In contrast, beta blockers and coronary bypass surgery, two therapies whose primary impact is on ischemia rather than on arrhythmias, have both been reported to diminish sudden cardiac death (33, 34). Thus it remains unsettled at present whether any therapies whose principal effects are to suppress ventricular arrhythmias can improve survival in coronary disease. Ongoing randomized trials with implantable defibrillators (which effectively treat rather than suppress malignant arrhythmias) should provide important additional information in this area.

In recent years, interest had increased in the use of measurement of late potentials on the signal-averaged ECG to identify patients at risk for sudden cardiac death. Late potentials are believed to indicate the electrophysiologic substrate for reentrant ventricular tachycardia, and numerous studies have reported that late potentials are powerful adverse prognostic findings that are independent of the results of ambulatory monitoring for ventricular arrhythmias and left ventricular ejection fraction (35). The clinical utility of this measure continues to be debated. Investigations into heart rate variability have yielded another marker for high risk that is of uncertain pathophysiologic or therapeutic significance (36, 37). Heart rate variability is presumed to reflect the net effects of the parasympathetic and sympathetic nervous systems, both of which have been shown to be important in affecting the threshold for ventricular fibrillation. Neither late potentials nor heart rate variability have yet been accepted as part of the standard risk assessment for coronary artery disease.

Along with the above measures of risk from the current disease state, prognosis in coronary disease depends importantly on the probability that the disease process will move to a higher- or lower-risk state. For the most part, we now believe that shifts in risk state are related to changes in coronary plaques as described earlier. Since detection of plaque events is still very indirect and imprecise, our understanding of their pathophysiology remains poor. It is believed that high-risk atherosclerotic plaques, that is, those plaques that have a large liquid cholesterol core and a thin, fibrous cap (as discussed above), cycle through phases of particular vulnerability to rupture because of factors that are incompletely defined. A vulnerable, high-risk plaque is one in which a plaque event can be initiated by normal physiologic stresses on the circulatory system. In the setting of a vulnerable plaque, a fortuitous triggering event (such as a surge in blood pressure that might be caused by a sudden change in physical activity or emotional state) might then initiate an active plaque event (38). At present, the best we can do to identify the major risks of progression of disease is to target those factors that predict the occurrence of the disease, namely, the standard cardiovascular risk factors such as smoking, diabetes, hypertension, and hypercholesterolemia.

EFFECTS OF MEDICAL THERAPY ON PROGNOSIS

As fundamental as the question is, surprisingly little of the literature on the prognosis of CAD deals with the issue of whether medical therapy itself affects the natural history of the disease. Most prognostic studies of CAD have passively assumed that medical therapy does not affect outcome and that all forms of medical therapy perform equivalently in this regard. It is now clear, however, that these are pragmatic rather than scientific decisions. Given the profusion of individual therapeutic agents available for treatment of CAD and the lack of consensus about the optimal medical regimen for any given type of patient, analysis of the effects of medical therapy can become prohibitively complex outside the realm of a carefully controlled, randomized trial. The complexity of the problem notwithstanding, there is now strong evidence that many agents do in fact affect survival in CAD.

Some of the most convincing evidence available to date about the benefits of medical therapy in CAD relate to aspirin (39). Since platelets are one of the principal participants in the thrombotic consequences of a coronary plaque event, platelet inhibition is now viewed as a key therapeutic strategy in controlling the acute manifestations of the disease. Evidence about the survival benefits of aspirin come from several, large-scale trials (39, 40). In the asymptomatic population (subjects with preclinical CAD) the evidence is still inconclusive, although aspirin has been shown to reduce the risk of a first nonfatal MI by 33%. In chronic stable angina the Physician's Health Study reported an 87%

statistically significant reduction in the risk of a first nonfatal MI and a 49% nonstatistically significant reduction in mortality (41). In unstable angina, aspirin has been shown in four randomized trials to improve prognosis relative to placebo, producing reductions in mortality and MI rates of around 50% (40). In acute MI the ISIS II trial showed that low-dose aspirin given immediately reduced the 30-day mortality by a magnitude equivalent to and additive with that of thrombolytic therapy. At least eight separate trials have evaluated the role of aspirin after acute MI. While individually these trials have arrived at conflicting conclusions, when pooled they suggest a 10 to 15% reduction in long-term mortality and a 20 to 30% reduction in reinfarction rates (39).

Beta-adrenergic blocking agents are another class of pharmacologic agents for which there is strong evidence of prognostic benefit in CAD. Most of the data available so far, however, relate to the acute MI and post-MI phases of the disease. There are no data supporting the use of prophylactic beta-blockers in asymptomatic subjects, and there are no adequate controlled data about the survival effects of beta-blockers in stable angina. Three double-blind randomized trials have compared beta-blockers to placebo in unstable angina (40). A meta-analysis of the available trials indicates a 13% reduction in the risk of progression of acute MI (42). However, no clear effect on mortality has yet been demonstrated. In acute MI patients not receiving thrombolytic therapy, beta-blockers lower mortality by approximately 15% when given acutely (43). They also lower mortality by around 20% and reduce the risk of reinfarction by approximately 25% when started in the predischarge phase and continued for the first several years after MI. Whether beta-blockers also provide prognostic benefits in patients who are given reperfusion therapy is at present less clear-cut. The mechanism of benefit of beta-blockers in preventing cardiac death is uncertain, may be multifactorial, and is believed to be a class effect rather than the property of one or more of the individual agents in this class of drugs.

Nitrates are the oldest class of pharmacologic agents used for treatment of ischemic heart disease. There are no controlled trials that have tested the prognostic effects of these drugs on asymptomatic subjects or on patients with stable angina. There are also no randomized, placebo-controlled trials in unstable angina dealing with effects on cardiac events. Approximately 900 patients have been randomized in seven trials of intravenous nitroglycerin in acute myocardial infarction during the prethrombolytic era (44). In aggregate, these data suggest a 49% reduction in mortality associated with early nitrate therapy. Recently, the GISSI 3 (transdermal glyceryl trinitrates) and the ISIS 4 (isosorbide mononitrate) trials showed that routine nitrate use for 6 weeks after acute MI in a population receiving thrombolytic therapy does not produce clinically relevant benefit (45). In addition, the long-term prognostic effects of nitrates after MI remains undefined, although one retrospective study has suggested benefit. The potential mechanism of prognostic benefit with nitrates is assumed to relate to their hemodynamic effects (decreased preload and afterload) or their direct dilating effects on epicardial coronary vessels and collateral vessels. In addition, an antiplatelet effect of nitrates has recently been suggested (46).

Calcium channel blocking agents represent the newest class of antianginal drugs. The prognostic effects of these medications remains controversial (47). Five trials of nifedipine in acute MI have all shown better survival in the placebo-treated patients. One large trial of diltiazem in acute MI showed no overall mortality effect but an increased mortality in patients with impaired left ventricular function and a decreased mortality in the subgroup of patients with well-preserved left ventricular function (48). Two trials of verapamil in acute MI have reported beneficial

trends for the treatment group. Diltiazem has also been shown to reduce early nonfatal reinfarction in patients with non–Q-wave MI (49). However, in three separate randomized trials involving about 900 patients with unstable angina, nifedipine did not affect the risk of death or nonfatal myocardial infarction. Calcium blockers have vasodilatory properties that make them potent antianginal agents, and they also reduce cardiac preload and afterload. In addition, some work has suggested that these drugs may inhibit the progression of atherosclerosis. However, the potential for adverse prognostic effects, particularly in patients with left ventricular dysfunction, is disturbing and remains incompletely defined at present. Therefore many have advised using these drugs as second or third line agents in CAD patients (40).

Angiotensin-converting enzyme (ACE) inhibitor use has substantially increased over the last few years following the demonstration in several clinical trials of an improved survival for patients with left ventricular dysfunction (50–53). Two recent trials have also suggested that these agents may produce a reduction in nonfatal MI, although the mechanism for this effect has yet to be defined (50).

In summary, there is much evidence that medical therapy importantly affects the prognosis of CAD, although not necessarily always in a beneficial fashion. In addition, it seems reasonable to assume that medical therapy has improved over the past 20 years in its efficacy, although few direct empirical data are available to support this contention. The relationship between the prognostic effects of medical therapy and the angiographic extent of CAD has gone largely unexplored.

EFFECTS OF REVASCULARIZATION THERAPY ON CAD PROGNOSIS

Much of our understanding of the prognostic effects of coronary revascularization come from the earlier work comparing coronary bypass surgery with medical therapy (12, 54).

Investigations by our group and others using statistical models have shown that coronary bypass surgery acts specifically to reduce long-term mortality risk attributable to coronary disease by an amount proportional to the extent of the coronary disease present. In other words, an effective coronary bypass surgery procedure substantially mitigates or even neutralizes the risk of dying attributable to the coronary disease present. Bypass surgery, however, does not alter the risk from noncoronary prognostic factors, such as older age or low ejection fraction. It also does not prevent the subsequent occurrence of myocardial infarction (55). What coronary bypass surgery does do is to make any subsequent myocardial infarction likely to be significantly smaller than it otherwise would have been and consequently more survivable for the patient (56).

The prognostic benefits of coronary bypass surgery can be summarized in terms of its relative effect (e.g., a 50% reduction in the risk of dying relative to medical therapy) or its absolute effect (e.g., an increase in the 5-year survival rate from 75 to 90%) or both. The relative scale tells us about the magnitude of efficacy of the procedure. Thus bypass surgery in a patient with critical left main disease produces a substantially greater relative reduction in mortality risk than does a procedure performed on a patient with two-vessel disease, even though both patients may have a significant improvement in their life expectancy from the procedure. On the other hand, the absolute difference in survival rates with surgery versus medicine provides information reflecting both the relative efficacy of the procedure and the degree of risk associated with continued conservative (i.e., medical) therapy. Thus a group of patients with three-vessel disease who are 55 years old and have good left ventricular function and no major comorbidity will have the same relative benefit from bypass surgery as a group of patients with the same exact coronary anatomy who are all 75 years old and have an

ejection fraction of 35%, but the latter group will have a substantially greater absolute increment in their survival from the procedure. In other words, while bypass surgery does not work any better in high-risk patients, the relative benefits of the procedure are magnified by the noncoronary factors that increase the patient's medical risk of cardiovascular death. The largest survival benefits of bypass surgery in absolute terms are thus observed in patients with the most severe CAD and the highest absolute medical risk.

The prognostic effects of coronary angioplasty and other percutaneous intervention relative to medicine and bypass surgery are still controversial and remain incompletely defined. To address this question, we examined our experience with over 9000 patients with symptomatic CAD treated with medicine, coronary angioplasty, or coronary bypass surgery at Duke Medical Center over a 7-year period (18). Our major findings can be summarized as follows (Figs. 28.1–28.7). In patients with the most severe coronary disease (i.e., three-vessel disease, and two-vessel disease with a 95% proximal left anterior descending lesion), bypass surgery significantly improved survival relative to both medical therapy and angioplasty. In intermediate levels of CAD (i.e., other forms of two-vessel disease), revascularization appeared to offer a modest survival benefit with coronary angioplasty having a slight advantage over bypass surgery because of its lower procedural mortality rate. In single-vessel disease patients, revascularization did not offer any prognostic advantage up to 5 years over initial medical therapy.

Some of the results of the major angioplasty/bypass surgery randomized trials in multivessel CAD have been reported, although the results of the largest, the BARI trial, will not be available until the fall of 1995 (57–60). To date these studies have found an equivalent cardiac event rate (death or infarction) with the two revascularization strategies, while coronary angioplasty pa-

1 Vessel Disease

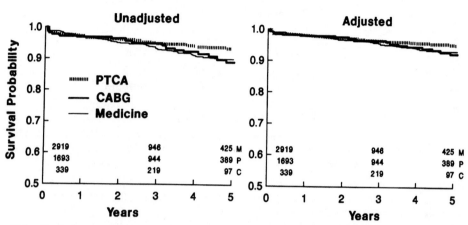

Figure 28.1. Survival curves for one-vessel disease showing unadjusted *(left)* and adjusted *(right)* comparisons of the three treatment groups to demonstrate absolute survival differences. *X* axis shows follow-up time out to 5 years. *Y* axis shows cardiovascular survival probability from 1.0 to 0.5. Numbers at the bottom of the plots show number of patients in each treatment group remaining to be followed at 0, 3, and 5 years of follow-up. PTCA indicates percutaneous transluminal coronary angioplasty *(P)*; CABG, coronary artery bypass graft survey *(C)*; and M, medically treated. (From Mark DB et al. Circulation 1994;89(5):2015–2025 with permission.)

2 Vessel Disease

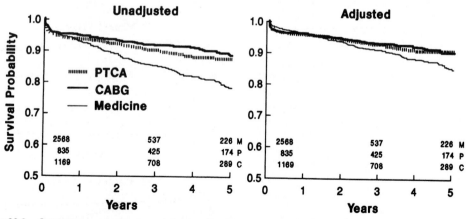

Figure 28.2. Survival curves for two-vessel disease. See Figure 28.1 for orientation. PTCA indicates percutaneous transluminal coronary angioplasty *(P)*; CABG, coronary artery bypass graft surgery *(C)*; and M, medically treated. (From Mark DB et al. Circulation 1994;89(5):2015–2025 with permission.)

3 Vessel Disease

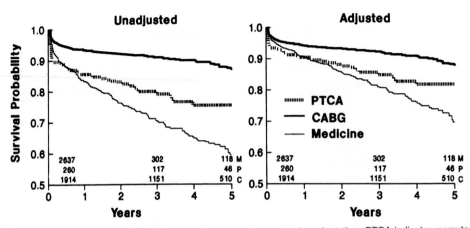

Figure 28.3. Survival curves for three-vessel disease. See Figure 28.1 for orientation. PTCA indicates percutaneous transluminal coronary angioplasty *(P)*; CABG, coronary artery bypass graft surgery *(C)*; and M, medically treated. (From Mark DB et al. Circulation 1994;89(5):2015–2025 with permission.)

Figure 28.4. Adjusted survival curves for one-, two-, and three-vessel disease, excluding patients with acute myocardial infarction within 2 weeks. Patterns seen in Figures 28.1 through 28.3 are clearly preserved in the nonacute myocardial infarction portion of the study population. *PTCA,* Percutaneous transluminal coronary angioplasty; *CABG,* coronary artery bypass graft surgery; *Med,* medically treated. (From Mark DB et al. Circulation 1994; 89(5):2015–2025 with permission.)

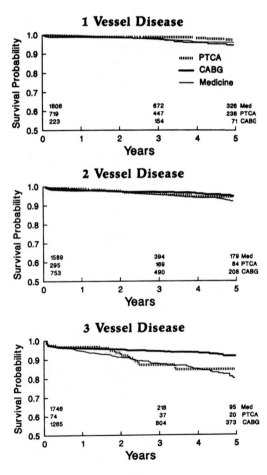

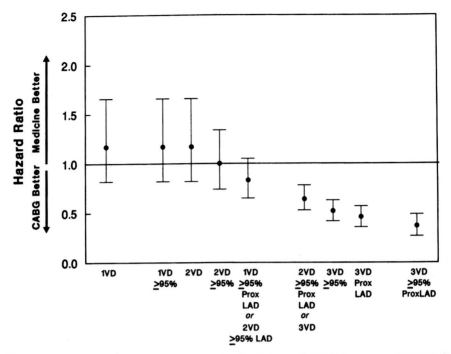

Figure 28.5. Hazard (mortality) ratios for coronary artery bypass graft surgery (CABG) versus medicine calculated from the Cox regression model to evaluate relative survival differences. Points indicate hazard ratios for each level of the coronary artery disease index; bars indicate 99% confidence intervals. Horizontal line at ratio of 1.0 indicates point of prognostic equivalence between treatments. Hazard ratios below the line favor CABG, those above the line favor medicine. *VD,* Vessel disease; *Prox LAD,* proximal left anterior descending coronary artery. (From Mark DB et al. Circulation 1994;89(5):2015–2025 with permission.)

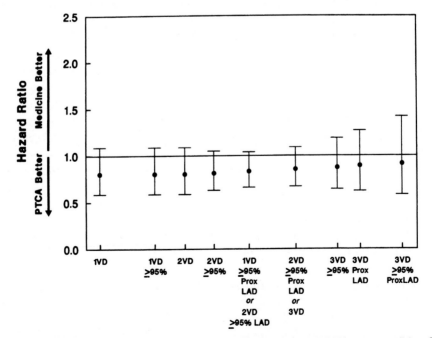

Figure 28.6. Hazard ratios for percutaneous transluminal coronary angioplasty (PTCA) versus medicine. See Figure 28.5 for orientation. Points below 1.0 favor PTCA. *VD,* vessel disease; *Prox LAD,* proximal left anterior descending coronary artery. (From Mark DB et al. Circulation 1994;89(5):2015–2025 with permission.)

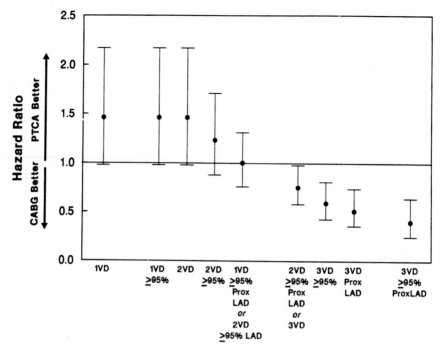

Figure 28.7. Hazard ratios for coronary artery bypass graft surgery (CABG) versus percutaneous transluminal coronary angioplasty (PTCA). See Figure 28.5 for orientation. Points below 1.0 favor CABG. *VD*, Vessel disease; *Prox LAD*, proximal left anterior descending coronary artery. (From Mark DB et al. Circulation 1994;89(5):2015–2025 with permission.)

tients have had more angina in follow-up and substantially more repeat revascularization procedures. Given the relatively small size of all of these studies, it will be important to supplement the individual study analyses with a pooled analysis of all the available trials when the data can be made available.

OVERVIEW OF THERAPEUTIC APPROACH TO THE PATIENT WITH MULTIVESSEL CAD

Despite the enormous number of revascularization procedures done in the United States each year, there is surprisingly still no consensus about their appropriate use. There are six main factors that we take into account when assessing treatment options for multivessel disease patients: (a) their overall risk of cardiac events with continued medical therapy, considering the factors described earlier in this chapter; (b) the projected prognostic benefits of revascularization as described in the last section of this chapter; (c) the severity of ischemic symptoms and associated impair-

ment of functional status; (d) the technical feasibility of PTCA and of CABG; (e) the presence and extent of major comorbidity; and (f) the patient's preferences. The first two considerations generally dictate that for significant left main disease or high-risk multivessel disease (e.g., with a proximal high-grade left anterior descending stenosis and depressed left ventricular function, or an acute coronary syndrome) bypass surgery remains the preferred option. Limitations in physical activities and functional status caused by ischemic symptoms are another indication for revascularization. Coronary angioplasty demonstrated a modest advantage over medical therapy in improving exercise performance and symptom relief in single-vessel disease in the ACME trial (61). For multivessel disease patients, both angioplasty and surgery improve functional status relative to medicine (62). In addition, recent results from the EAST trial suggest that bypass surgery is associated with somewhat better symptom relief in such patients than angioplasty (63). Whether an individual patient is having enough ischemic symptoms to make revascularization the preferred approach depends both on the initial success of medical therapy in controlling such symptoms and the willingness of that patient to accept the procedural risks of revascularization to achieve better symptom control and a higher functional status.

A number of anatomic considerations guide selection of coronary revascularization techniques. Morphologic lesion characteristics that favor percutaneous interventions include short length, lack of calcification, location in a straight segment, and lack of associated thrombus. Characteristics that make percutaneous intervention less likely to be successful include tortuous vessels, long-standing total occlusions, and eccentric or ostial plaques. Significant left main lesions (e.g., $\geq 50\%$ diameter stenosis) generally preclude percutaneous intervention in the left coronary system unless the system is "protected" by a previously placed bypass graft. The availability of and experience with newer-generation percutaneous techniques such as directional and rotational atherectomy, laser, and coronary stents has broadened the range and complexity of lesions that may be successfully approached. The presence of anatomic characteristics unfavorable to percutaneous intervention will often lead us to recommend bypass surgery in patients for whom revascularization is deemed desirable.

Anatomic and morphologic considerations may also weigh against selection of bypass surgery as the preferred therapeutic option. Diffuse distal-vessel disease or small vessel diameter may preclude satisfactory placement of grafts. Lack of adequate bypass conduit because of previous vein stripping, bypass surgery, or subclavian artery disease (limiting internal mammary artery flow) may also limit the therapeutic choices. Similarly, previous inflammatory pericardial processes

or severely impaired left ventricular function are factors that may weigh against selection of bypass surgery. The availability of and experience with newer surgical techniques such as use of the gastroepiploic artery may broaden the range of complex patients that can be considered for surgery.

Major comorbidity such as advanced chronic obstructive lung disease or dialysis-dependent renal failure substantially alters the risk:benefit ratio for invasive therapies. Unfortunately, these patients often present with high-risk multivessel disease and thus pose the dilemma of having the most to gain from invasive therapy but also the highest risk of major complications and a prolonged postprocedural recovery. The literature in this area is still inadequate to define when, in these patients, the risks associated with their comorbidity exceed the projected benefits of revascularization. Thus each clinician tends to approach such patients with a level of aggressiveness dictated by their recent experience with other similar patients (e.g., "the last patient like this I did an angioplasty on did great" or ". . . spent months in the Intensive Care Unit after the procedure"). Clearly, more work is needed in this area to put therapeutic decision making on a firmer footing.

We listed patient preferences last in the factors we consider in making treatment recommendations for our patients, not because they are least important but because it is least clear how best to assess and incorporate them. Some patients come to the hospital expressing strong preferences for a particular therapy or strong aversions to a particular therapy, often based on experiences of family members, friends, or colleagues at work. Such opinions may reflect an inadequate information base rather than carefully reasoned preferences. Of course, deciding whether to undergo a high-risk angioplasty or bypass operation is not like deciding which automobile or television to buy. Consumers usually have a much better understanding of what such purchases will provide in the way of benefits. In addition, consumers do not usually face an overt risk of immediate death or major comorbidity from their nonmedical purchasing decisions.

In contrast, selecting medical therapy or one of several revascularization options is usually done without a full understanding of the choices or their downstream consequences and does involve some immediate personal risk of death or disability. We are currently investigating better ways of incorporating individual patient preferences into the therapeutic decision-making process as part of the Ischemic Heart Disease Patient Outcome Research Team (PORT) project. One such method involves the use of an interactive video disk that presents an individualized risk profile and a thorough description of treatment options to the patient. Work in this project has shown that patients vary greatly in the degree to which they are bothered by anginal symptoms and diminished functional capacity. They also vary greatly in their willingness to accept short-term risks in exchange for long-term gains. Over the next 5 years, we anticipate that bedside tools will become readily available to help better educate the patient on treatment options and to allow therapeutic decisions to better reflect the preferences of the patient along with the objective risk:benefit considerations.

REFERENCES

1. Mark DB. Assessment of prognosis in patients with coronary artery disease. In: Roubin GS, Califf RM, O'Neill WW, Phillips HR III, Stack RS, eds. Interventional cardiovascular medicine: principles and practice. New York: Churchill Livingstone, 1994.
2. Pryor DB, Bruce RA, Chaitman BR, Fisher L, Gajewski J, Hammermeister KE, Pauker SG, Stokes J III. Task force I: determination of prognosis in patients with ischemic heart disease. J Am Coll Cardiol 1989;14(4);1016–1025.
3. Konstam MA, Kronenberg MW, Udelson JE, Kinan D, Metherall J, Dolan N, Edens T et al. Effectiveness of preload reserve as a determinant of clinical status in patients with left ventricular systolic dysfunction. Am J Cardiol 1992;69:1591–1595.
4. Eng C. Enlargement of the heart. Heart Failure 1991; 15–24.
5. Harrell FE Jr, Lee KL, Califf RM, Pryor DB, Rosati RA. Regression modeling strategies for improved prognostic prediction. Stat Med 1984;3:143–152.
6. Harris PJ, Harrell FE Jr, Lee KL, Behar VS, Rosati RA. Survival in medically treated coronary artery disease. Circulation 1979;60:1259–1269.
7. Hammermeister KE, DeRouen TA, Dodge HT. Variables predictive of survival in patients with coronary disease: selection by univariate and multivariate analyses from the clinical, electrocardiographic, exercise, arteriographic, and quantitative angiographic evaluations. Circulation 1979; 59:421–430.
8. Bounous EP Jr, Mark DB, Pollock BG, Hlatky MA, Harrell FE Jr, Rankin JS, Wechsler AS et al. Surgical survival benefits for coronary disease patients with left ventricular dysfunction. Circulation 1988;78(Suppl I):I151–I157.
9. Clements IP, Brown ML, Zinsmeister AR, Gibbons RJ. Influence of left ventricular diastolic filling on symptoms and survival in patients with decreased left ventricular systolic function. Am J Cardiol 1991;67:1245–1250.
10. Tcheng JE, Jackman JD, Nelson CL, Gardner LH, Smith LR, Rankin JS, Califf RM et al. Outcome of patients sustaining acute ischemic mitral regurgitation during myocardial infarction. Ann Intern Med 1992;117:18–24.
11. Hickey MS, Smith LR, Muhlbaier LH, Harrell FE Jr, Reves JG, Hinohara T, Califf RM et al. Current prognosis of ischemic mitral regurgitation: implications for future management. Circulation 1988;78(Suppl I):I51–I59.
12. Califf RM, Harrell FE Jr, Lee KL, Rankin JS, Hlatky MA, Mark DB, Jones RH et al. The evolution of medical and surgical therapy for coronary artery disease: a 15-year perspective. JAMA 1989;261:2077–2086.
13. Rankin JS, Livesey SA, Smith LR, Sheikh KH, Van Trigt P, de Bruijn NP, Califf RM et al. Trends in the surgical treatment of ischemic mitral regurgitation: effects of mitral valve repair on hospital mortality. Semin Thorac Cadiovas Surg 1989;1:149–163.
14. Califf RM, McKinnis RA, Burks J, Lee KL, Harrell FE Jr, Behar VS, Pryor DB et al. Prognostic implications of ventricular arrhythmias during 24-hour ambulatory monitoring in patients undergoing cardiac catheterization for coronary artery disease. Am J Cardiol 1982;50:23–31.
15. Cameron A, Schwartz MJ, Kronmal RA, Kosinski AS. Prevalence and significance of atrial fibrillation in coronary artery disease (CASS Registry). Am J Cardiol 1988; 61:714–717.
16. Bateman TM, Weiss MH, Czer LSC, Conklin CM, Kass RM, Stewart ME, Matloff JM et al. Fascicular conduction disturbances and ischemic heart disease: adverse prognosis despite coronary revascularization. J Am Coll Cardiol 1985;5:632–639.
17. Califf RM, Phillips HR, Hindman MC, Mark DB, Lee KL, Behar VS, Johnson RA et al. Prognostic value of a coronary artery jeopardy score. J Am Coll Cardiol 1985; 5:1055–1063.
18. Mark DB, Nelson CL, Califf RM, Harrell FE Jr, Lee KL, Jones RH, Fortin DF et al. The continuing evolution of therapy for coronary artery disease: initial results from the era of coronary angioplasty. Circulation 1994;89(5):2015–2025.
19. Smith LR, Harrell FE Jr, Rankin JS, Califf RM, Pryor DB,

Muhlbaier LH, Lee KL et al. Determinants of early versus late cardiac death in patients undergoing coronary artery bypass graft surgery. Circulation 1991;84(Suppl III):245–253.

20. Mark DB, Nelson CL, Harrell FE Jr, Fortin D, Pryor DB, Jones RH, Stack RS et al. Improved survival benefits with coronary angioplasty and coronary bypass surgery: assessment using a new coronary prognostic index. Circulation 1992;86:I-536 (abstract).

21. Uren NG, Melin JA, De Bruyne B, Wijns W, Baudhuin T, Camici PG. Relation between myocardial blood flow and the severity of coronary-artery stenosis. N Engl J Med 1994;330:1782–1788.

22. Folland Ed, Vogel RA, Hartigan P, Bates ER, Beauman GJ, Fortin T, Boucher C et al., and the Veterans Affairs ACME investigators. Relation between coronary artery stenosis assessed by visual, caliper, and computer methods and exercise capacity in patients with single-vessel coronary artery disease. Circulation 1994;89:2005–2014.

23. Cohn PF. Silent myocardial ischemia in patients with a defective anginal warning system. Am J Cardiol 1980; 45:697–702.

24. Rocco MB, Nabel EG, Campbell S, Goldman L, Barry J, Mead K, Selwyn AP. Prognostic importance of myocardial ischemia detected by ambulatory monitoring in patients with stable coronary artery disease. Circulation 1988; 78:877–884.

25. Pepine CJ. Is silent ischemia a treatable risk factor in patients with angina pectoris? Circulation 1990;82:II-135–II-142.

26. Davies MJ, Thomas AC. Plaque fissuring: the cause of acute myocardial infarction, sudden ischemic death, and crescendo angina. Br Heart J 1985;53:363–373.

27. Davies MJ, Thomas A. Thrombosis and acute coronary-artery lesions in sudden cardiac ischemic death. N Engl J Med 1984;310(18):1137–1140.

28. Falk E. Morphologic features of unstable atherothrombotic plaques underlying acute coronary syndromes. Am J Cardiol 1989;63:114E–120E.

29. Fernandez-Ortiz A, Badimon JJ, Falk E, Fuster V, Meyer B, Mailhac A, Weng D et al. Characterization of the relative thrombogenicity of atherosclerotic plaque components: implications for consequences of plaque rupture. J Am Coll Cardiol 1994;23(7):1562–1569.

30. Rasheed Q, Nair R, Sheehan H, Hodgson JM. Correlation of intracoronary ultrasound plaque characteristics in atherosclerotic coronary artery disease patients with clinical variables. Am J Cardiol 1994;73:753–758.

31. Califf RM, Mark DB, Harrell FE Jr, Hlatky MA, Lee KL, Rosati RA, Pryor DB. Importance of clinical measures of ischemia in the prognosis of patients with documented coronary artery disease. J Am Coll Cardiol 1988; 11:20–26.

32. Echt DS, Liebson PR, Mitchell LB, Peters RW, Obias-Manno D, Barker AH, Arensberg D et al., and the CAST investigators. Mortality and morbidity in patients receiving encainide, flecainide, or placebo. The Cardiac Arrhythmia Suppression Trial. N Engl J Med 1991;324(12):781–788.

33. Holmes DR, Davis KB, Mock MB, Fisher LD, Gersh BJ, Killip T III, Pettinger M, participants in the Coronary Artery Surgery Study. The effect of medical and surgical treatment on subsequent sudden cardiac death in patients with coronary artery disease: a report from the coronary artery surgery study. Circulation 1986;73:1254–1263.

34. Furberg CD, Hawkins CM, Lichstein E. Effect of propranolol in postinfarction patients with mechanical or electrical complications. Circulation 1984;69:761–765.

35. Steinberg JS, Regan A, Sciacca RR, Bigger JT, Fleiss JL. Predicting arrhythmic events after acute myocardial infarction using the signal-averaged electrocardiogram. Am J Cardiol 1992;69:13–21.

36. Kleiger RE, Miller JP, Bigger JT, Moss AJ. Decreased heart rate variability and its association with increased mortality after acute myocardial infarction. Am J Cardiol 1987;59:256–262.

37. Bigger JT Jr, Fleiss JL, Steinman RC, Rolnitzky LM, Kleiger RE, Rottman JN. Correlations among time and frequency domain measures of heart period variability two weeks after acute myocardial infarction. Am J Cardiol 1992;69:891–898.

38. Muller JE, Abela GS, Nesto RW, Tofler GH. Triggers, acute risk factors and vulnerable plaques: the lexicon of a new frontier. J Am Coll Cardiol 1994;23(3):809–813.

39. Antiplatelet Trialist's Collaboration. Collaborative overview of randomized trials of antiplatelet therapy. I. Prevention of death, myocardial infarction, and stroke by prolonged antiplatelet therapy in various categories of patients. Br Med J 1994;308:81–106.

40. Braunwald E, Mark DB, Jones RH, Cheitlin MD, Fuster V, McCauley K, Edwards C et al. Unstable angina: diagnosis and management. AHCPR Monograph No. 94-0682, 1994.

41. Steering Committee of the Physicians' Health Study Research Group. Final report on the aspirin component of the ongoing physicians' health study. N Engl J Med 1989;321:129–135.

42. Yusuf S, Wittes J, Friedman L. Overview of results of randomized clinical trials in heart disease. II. Unstable angina, heart failure, primary prevention with aspirin, and risk factor modification. JAMA 1988;260:2259–2263.

43. Yusuf S, Wittes J, Friedman L. Overview of results of randomized clinical trials in heart disease. I. Treatments following myocardial infarction. JAMA 1988;260:2088–2093.

44. Yusuf S, MacMahon S, Collins R, Peto R. Effect of intravenous nitrates on mortality in acute myocardial infarction; an overview of the randomised trials. Lancet 1988;1:1088–1092.

45. Gruppo Italiano per lo Studio della Sopravvivenza nell'Infarto Miocardico. GISSI-3: effects of lisinopril and transdermal glyceryl trinitrate singly and together on 6-week mortality and ventricular function after acute myocardial infarction. Lancet 1994;343:1115–1122.

46. Diodati J, Theroux P, Latour JG, Lacoste L, Lam JYT, Waters D. Effects of nitroglycerin at therapeutic doses on platelet aggregation in unstable angina pectoris and acute myocardial infarction. Am J Cardiol 1990;66:683–688.

47. Held PH, Yusuf S, Furberg CD. Calcium channel blockers in acute myocardial infarction and unstable angina: an overview. Br Med J 1989;299:1187–1192.

48. The Multicenter Diltiazem Postinfarction Trial Research Group. The effect of diltiazem on mortality and reinfarction after myocardial infarction. N Engl J Med 1988; 319:385–392.

49. Gibson RS, Boden WE, Theroux P, Strauss HD, Pratt CM, Gheorghiado M, Capone RJ et al. The Diltiazem Reinfarction Study Group. Diltiazem and reinfarction in patients with non–Q-wave myocardial infarction. N Engl J Med 1986; 315:423–429.

50. Yusuf S, Pepine CJ, Garces C, Pouleur H, Salem D, Kostis J, Benedict C et al. Effect of enalapril on myocardial infarction and unstable angina in patients with low ejection fractions. Lancet 1992;340:1173–1178.

51. The SOLVD Investigators. Effect of enalapril on survival in patients with reduced left ventricular ejection fractions and congestive heart failure. N Engl J Med 1991;325:293–302.

52. Kjekshus J, Swedberg K, Snapinn S. Effects of enalapril on long-term mortality in severe congestive heart failure. Am J Cardiol 1992;69:103–117.

53. Pfeffer MA, Braunwald E, Moye LA, Basta L, Brown EJ, Cuddy TE, Davis BR et al. for the SAVE Investigators. Effect of captopril on mortality and morbidity in patients with left ventricular dysfunction after myocardial infarction. Results of the survival and ventricular enlargement trial. N Engl J Med 1992;327:669–677.

54. Yusuf S, Zucker D, Peduzzi P, Fisher LD, Takaro T, Kennedy JW, Davis K et al. Effect of coronary artery bypass graft surgery on survival: overview of 10-year results from randomised trials by the Coronary Artery Bypass Graft Surgery Trialists Collaboration. Lancet 1994; 344:563–570.

55. Davis KB, Alderman EL, Kosinski AS, Passamani E, Kennedy JW. Early mortality of acute myocardial infarction in patients with and without prior coronary revascularization surgery. Circulation 1992;85:2100–2109.

56. Wiseman A, Waters DD, Walling A, Pelletier GB, Roy D, Theroux P. Long-term prognosis after myocardial infarction in patients with previous coronary artery bypass surgery. J Am Coll Cardiol 1988;12:873–880.

57. RITA trial participants. Coronary angioplasty versus coronary artery bypass surgery: the Randomised Intervention Treatment of Angina (RITA) trial. Lancet 1993; 341:573–580.

58. King SB III, Lembo NJ, Weintraub WS, Kosinski AS, Barnhart HX, Kutner MH, Alazraki NP et al. for the EAST investigators. A randomized trial comparing coronary angioplasty with coronary bypass surgery: the Emory Angioplasty Versus Surgery Trial. N Engl J Med 1994; 331:1044–1050.

59. Hamm CW, Reimers J, Rupprecht HJ, Ischinger T. Angioplasty vs bypass-surgery in patients with multivessel disease: re-interventions and complications during 6 months follow-up. J Am Coll Cardiol 1993;21:72A (abstract).

60. The BARI investigators. Protocol for the Bypass Angioplasty Revascularization Investigation. Circulation 1991; 84(6)(Suppl V):V-1–V-27.

61. Parisi AF, Folland ED, Hartigan P. A comparison of angioplasty with medical therapy in the treatment of single-vessel coronary artery disease. N Engl J Med 1992; 326:10–16.

62. Mark DB, Nelson C, Delong E, Fortin D, Pryor DB, Stack RS, Jones RH et al. Comparison of quality of life outcomes following coronary angioplasty, coronary bypass surgery and medicine. J Am Coll Cardiol 1993;21(2):216A (abstract).

63. Weintraub W. Preliminary economic and quality of life outcomes from the Emory Angioplasty Surgery Trial (EAST). Presented at the American Heart Association Annual Scientific Sessions, November 1993.

29. Proximal Left Anterior Descending Vessel Disease

A. The Role of PTCA

DOUGLAS M. BURTT and
ALFRED F. PARISI

Other than left main coronary stenosis, perhaps the most compelling anatomic finding at coronary angiography is disease of the proximal left anterior descending (LAD) coronary artery. Because the percentage of left ventricular myocardium dependent on supply from the LAD is so high (on average, 42% of the left ventricular mass) (1), patency of this vessel is most crucial. An average patient suffering anterior myocardial infarction is left with an impaired ejection fraction of 35% and is more likely to suffer from heart failure, lethal ventricular arrhythmias, and peripheral embolization than a counterpart with occlusion of the right coronary artery (RCA) or circumflex. For this reason, isolated significant disease of the proximal LAD (greater than 70% stenosis) most often will mandate intervention. Our premise is that coronary angioplasty (PTCA) remains the most practicable method for intervention in the majority of such patients, although, for some, atherectomy and even surgery are reasonable alternatives. We wish to address briefly the rationale for PTCA in proximal LAD disease, discuss the ways in which patients may present with proximal LAD disease that in our estimation mandate catheterization, and then focus on the anatomic and other factors that help us to make a decision for or against PTCA.

NATURAL HISTORY OF MEDICALLY TREATED PROXIMAL LAD DISEASE

Accurate data on the natural history of medically treated patients with proximal LAD disease is virtually impossible to obtain because of selection bias. Nonrandomized studies such as the Duke University database analysis by Califf et al. (2) and the Mid-Atlantic Heart and Vascular Institute database review by Klein et al. (3) suggest that 3- and 5-year mortality is higher in patients with proximal LAD disease than in those with nonproximal LAD disease and that this is particularly true for patients with decreased left ventricular function. In addition, Klein's study suggests that the severity of a proximal LAD stenosis correlates directly with prognosis, with the highest mortality seen in the cohort with 90% or greater stenosis, an intermediate mortality seen in those with 70 to 89% stenosis, and the lowest mortality seen in those with less than 70% proximal LAD stenosis (Fig. 29A.1).

With these data in mind, our general approach has been to perform cardiac catheterization according to the guidelines presented herein, and if greater than 70% stenosis is present in the proximal LAD, to proceed with interventional therapy as discussed below.

CHOICE OF INTERVENTIONAL THERAPY— RATIONALE FOR PTCA

The choice of treatment for patients with significant proximal LAD disease and normal left ventricular function continues to be somewhat controversial for several reasons. First, no surgical study (Coronary Artery Surgery Study (4), VA Cooperative (5) or European cooperative (6)) has definitively shown surgical revascularization to improve survival or to reduce the risk of myocardial infarction in single-vessel coronary artery disease. Secondly, some data (7) have suggested that surgical revascularization with an internal mam-

Figure 29A.1. Influence of severity of proximal LAD narrowings on survival (Kaplan-Meier analysis). Taken from database analysis of 866 patients with significant CAD for whom medical therapy was chosen by their physicians. Stenosis number grades refer to percent luminal narrowing. The divergence of the curves is highly significant ($P <.0001$). (Adapted with permission from Klein LW et al. Am J Cardiol 1986;58:42–46.)

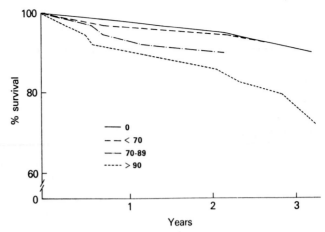

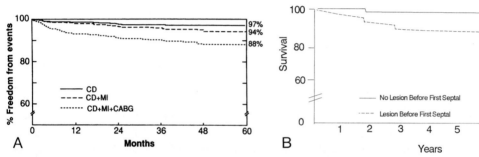

Figure 29A.2. **A.** Five-year Kaplan-Meier actuarial freedom from cardiac death (CD), myocardial infarction (MI), and coronary bypass surgery (CABG) in 537 consecutive patients undergoing elective PTCA of the proximal LAD. (Adapted with permission from Frierson JH et al. J Am Coll Cardiol 1992;19:745–751. **B.** Seven-year Kaplan-Meier survival curves from 224 consecutive, medically treated patients with isolated, significant LAD stenosis, comparing them according to the status of the proximal segment ($P = .01$). Five-year cardiac survival for patients with proximal LAD stenosis was 90%. (Adapted with permission from Califf RM et al. Circulation 1983;67:283–289.)

mary graft demonstrates some superiority to PTCA in isolated LAD disease.

An enlightening study of PTCA for proximal LAD disease was presented in a review of 537 consecutive patients at the Cleveland Clinic by Frierson et al. (8) in 1992. The majority of these patients (77%) had isolated proximal LAD disease, and all underwent single-vessel LAD PTCA. Patients were followed for a mean of 44 months with a 99.8% follow-up rate. In addition, routine follow-up angiography was performed in 76% of patients.

The Cleveland Clinic patients underwent successful PTCA 96.1% of the time with complication rates as follows: myocardial infarction in 2.2%, in-hospital bypass surgery in

3%, and death in 0.4%. While follow-up angiography demonstrated restenosis (defined as ≥50% stenosis at the PTCA site) in 39.6% of patients, only 19% developed clinical restenosis requiring reintervention. Of most interest was the long-term follow-up data, which demonstrated a 5-year cardiac survival rate of 97% and a freedom from myocardial infarction or cardiac death rate of 94% (Fig. 29A.2*A*). These figures can be compared with previous natural history studies of patients with proximal LAD disease, such as the Duke Registry study (with a 90% 5-year cardiac survival rate, Fig. 29A.2*B*) and the study by Klein et al. demonstrating a 93% *3-year* survival rate, suggesting superior survival in patients with isolated significant proximal

LAD disease treated with PTCA compared with medical therapy.

The prime importance of Frierson's study, however, is the demonstration that, even in patients with ostial LAD lesions (9), the risks of PTCA have significantly fallen over the past decade, while procedural success rates have increased. With the advent of bailout devices for acute LAD occlusion in the laboratory, such as prolonged inflations with the perfusion balloon, directional atherectomy for intimal flap removal, and intracoronary stent placement, and with more careful monitoring of the activated clotting time (ACT) resulting in far less periprocedural thrombus formation, the rate of acute closure and the risk of emergency surgery have fallen even lower in the last 3 years. With all these factors taken together, the use of angioplasty as the initial procedure of choice in most patients with proximal LAD disease seems reasonable.

PTCA VERSUS CORONARY ARTERY BYPASS GRAFTING

A study by Kramer et al. (7) published in 1989 received substantial attention because of its conclusion that single-vessel coronary artery bypass grafting (CABG) may be superior to PTCA for isolated LAD disease. This retrospective review of 781 patients with isolated LAD disease treated with either PTCA or CABG between 1980 and 1984 at the Cleveland Clinic looked at endpoints of death and "event-free survival" after 5 years of follow-up. Their conclusions that CABG offers "better long-term benefit" and "superior long-term results" compared with PTCA do not seem justified after a careful examination of their data. Firstly, by including the very first PTCA patients angioplastied at the Cleveland Clinic (*one* patient in 1980, *12* patients in 1981), the authors looked at a skewed PTCA population with "novice" angioplasty physicians who were, by definition, on their learning curve. In contrast, the surgical patients underwent remarkably complication-free surgery, with *no* operative deaths and only *one* perioperative myocardial infarction (0.3%). These remarkably low numbers do not accurately reflect the broader experience with CABG, even in single-vessel coronary artery disease.

Secondly, their analysis of the data unfavorably compares the five-year mortality after PTCA (4.7%) with that after CABG (2.0%). A closer review of their data shows that nine of 13 deaths in the PTCA group were noncardiac (eight from malignancy) and that the 5-year *cardiac* mortality after PTCA and CABG were identical at 1.4%. In addition, the number of late myocardial infarctions at 5 years was identical for the two groups (8 of 368 CABG patients, and 8 of 413 PTCA patients). Finally, angina functional classification in follow-up patients who did not require reintervention was superior in the PTCA patients compared with the CABG patients with 7.8% of CABG patients having class II to IV angina, while only 2.5% of PTCA patients remained in these functional classes.

FUNCTIONAL IMPROVEMENT FOLLOWING LAD PTCA

The Angioplasty Compared to Medicine (ACME) (10) study compared angioplasty as the sole intended therapy with medical therapy in patients with single-vessel coronary artery disease. Six months after randomization the PTCA patients had superior angina relief, used less antianginal medication, and had better treadmill performance at higher double products than their medically assigned counterparts.

Of the 212 patients with single-vessel disease in this trial, 69 had lesions in the proximal (first half of the) LAD while the remaining 143 had lesions either in the distal LAD or in one of the remaining arteries. The proximal LAD patients treated by PTCA improved their treadmill performance by 2.2 minutes, as did the PTCA-treated patients who did not have proximal LAD disease. Patients treated medically also improved their total exercise

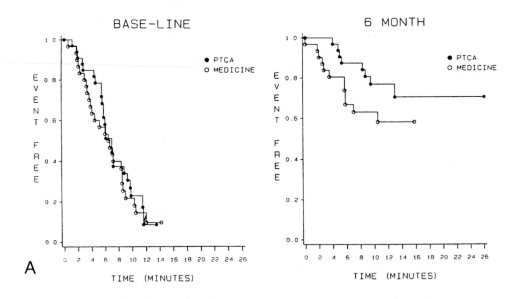

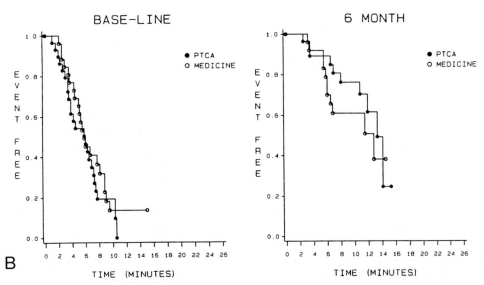

Figure 29A.3. Duration of angina-free exercise in the ACME Trial. The proportion of patients who were free of angina on the treadmill is plotted on the vertical axis, and the length of time to the onset of angina on the horizontal axis. Data were censored at the patients' total exercise time if they did not have angina during the test. The left panels show the specified treatment groups at baseline, and the right panels show the same groups 6 months after randomization. LAD patients who had PTCA fared better than their medically treated counterparts at 6 months. (Reproduced with permission from AF Parisi, MD, ACME Investigator.)

Table 29A.1.
Outcomes in ACME Patients Subgrouped by Lesion Location at 6-Month Follow-up (n = 200)

	Prox RCA/LCx		Prox LAD		Distal	
	Med	PTCA	Med	PTCA	Med	PTCA
ETT						
No. Patients	26	29	31	33	43	38
Δ Total exercise duration (minutes)	0.1	2.0	0.5	1.7	0.8	2.3
Δ Double product (× 10³)	−4.1	3.1	−5.0	1.7	−0.5	0.8
Δ Onset angina (minutes)	0.9	3.1	−1.5	1.2	1.3	1.2
% Angina-ETT	42	34	39	24	33	24
CABGs	0	0	0	4	0	3
Clinical						
% Angina free	46	61	42	56	49	72
% Beta-blocker	62	29	58	25	44	36
% Ca blocker	81	32	90	34	73	42
% Nitrates	62	25	68	22	67	28

ACME, Angioplasty Compared to Medical Therapy Trial; *Prox*, proximal; *RCA*, right coronary artery; *LCx*, left circumflex; *LAD*, left anterior descending; *PTCA*, percutaneous transluminal coronary angioplasty; *ETT*, exercise tolerance test; *CABGs*, coronary artery bypass grafts; *Ca*, calcium.

duration on the treadmill, but only by 0.5 minutes ($P < .01$). Of particular interest, however, is the performance of the proximal LAD–treated subgroup relative to the other subgroups in terms of angina-free time on the treadmill (Fig. 29A.3) and change in double product as compared with the baseline (Table 29A.1). These data suggest that patients with proximal LAD disease, when treated by PTCA, may gain more functional benefit at higher levels of myocardial oxygen demand. By comparison, their medically treated counterparts with proximal LAD lesions had the greatest fall in maximal achieved double product consistent with both earlier angina and greater use of concomitant medical therapy (Table 29A.1). In addition, the medically treated subgroup with proximal LAD disease had the lowest angina-free rate of any subgroup at 6-month follow-up. The improvement in symptoms and exercise performance has been shown to be persistent at later follow-up.

CLINICAL PRESENTATION

With the above data in mind, there are a number of clinical scenarios that can lead to the decision for cardiac catheterization and, thereafter, to coronary intervention. A crucial point in the decision process therefore is *when* to proceed with cardiac catheterization, since the finding of significant proximal LAD stenosis will often mandate intervention. We would usually recommend catheterization in the following clinical situations.

Silent Ischemia

Perhaps the most common circumstance that brings an asymptomatic patient to our attention for catheterization is the finding of a strongly positive exercise or dipyridamole-thallium test while screening the patient prior to vascular surgery. We have tended to follow the guidelines of Eagle (11), Boucher (12), and their colleagues, initially stratifying patients based on clinical variables associated with increased perioperative risk. (Clinical variables include Q waves on EKG, age >70 years, history of angina, history of ventricular ectopic activity requiring treatment, and history of medically treated diabetes mellitus.) These guidelines also include recommending coronary angiography for all patients with positive exercise-thallium tests occurring at a low workload (less than 6 minutes of the standard Bruce protocol) or at a low rate-pressure product (less than 15,000) or in those with scans showing multiple territories of redistribution, increased lung uptake, or cavity dilation. Dipyridamole-thallium scans with large or multiple areas of redistribution, increased lung uptake (greater than 60% of myocardium), or cavity dilation also mandate catheterization. We have, in general, extended these guidelines to include patients with a moderate area of redistribution in the anterior and apical regions consistent with proximal LAD disease.

An exception to the above guidelines would be the asymptomatic patient who has *none* of the high-risk clinical variables described by Eagle and in whom the perioperative event rate has been shown to be very low (3.1%) (Fig. 29A.4). Such patients can reasonably be managed without preoperative catheterization, since the combined morbidity of catheterization and interventional therapy may well outweigh the risks of cautious surgery under close scrutiny by an informed anesthesiologist and surgical team.

Another setting in which asymptomatic patients are discovered is that of the "routine screening" stress test in patients with multiple coronary risk factors or patients whose profession may mandate "routine" testing, such as airline pilots or high-level corporate executives (as part of the "executive physical"). While we ordinarily do not order screening stress tests as a part of our routine, such patients are often referred for evaluation after abnormal testing, and our approach to catheterization has been similar to those being screened prior to vascular surgery, as outlined above. In particular, emphasis is given to the duration of exercise on the treadmill in an effort to avoid "routine catheterization" in patients who can reach high levels of exercise (greater than stage III of the Bruce protocol) or reach high rate-pressure products (greater than 25,000) without symptoms. These patients are generally placed on medical therapy and followed with periodic stress testing, unless any of the above-mentioned thallium indicators of severe coronary artery disease are present, or unless catheterization is mandated by their employer or (in the case of airline pilots) by the FAA.

Stable Angina Pectoris

Patients with stable angina pectoris are recommended for PTCA for three major reasons: persistent exertional angina despite medical therapy with limitation of lifestyle, angina occurring with minimal activity, and stable angina with a "high-risk" ETT. There are clearly some patients who have had stable exertional symptoms for months or years and who, despite all efforts with medical therapy, continue to have symptoms that restrict their lifestyle and diminish their sense of well-being. Some patients cannot tolerate optimal doses of medication because of side-effects, including mental sluggishness, asthma, intolerable gastrointestinal irritation, or sexual

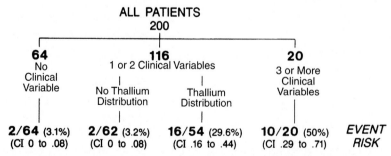

Figure 29A.4. Algorithm for using clinical variables and results of dipyridamole-thallium imaging to stratify cardiac risk as applied to a group of 200 patients. "Event" refers to postoperative cardiac ischemic events, including unstable angina, ischemic pulmonary edema, myocardial infarction, or cardiac death. Clinical variables are Q wave on electrocardiogram, age >70 years, history of angina, history of ventricular ectopic activity requiring treatment, and diabetes mellitus requiring treatment. (Adapted with permission from Eagle KA et al. Ann Intern Med 1989;110:859–866.)

dysfunction, and for this reason wish to explore the option of PTCA with an eye toward reducing their medication requirements.

Those patients with stable angina who, despite medication, continue to have "high-risk" ETT results, with greater than 2 mm of ST-segment depression within the first two stages of the Bruce protocol or with strongly positive thallium scans as outlined above, are also reasonable candidates for PTCA.

Unstable Angina Pectoris

Perhaps the majority of patients referred for PTCA at our institution are referred for therapy of unstable angina. For simplification we have used the classification of unstable angina introduced by Hultgren (13) in which patients with new onset angina that stabilizes or with stable angina that becomes more frequent or prolonged are labeled "type I" and in which patients with prolonged angina occurring at rest often associated with ST-changes or with systemic signs of ischemia (diaphoresis, dyspnea, etc.) are labeled "type II" unstable angina.

Our practice, which is relatively "conservative," has been to manage type I patients expectantly, with increased doses of medical therapy, and if they remain stable for 48 hours, to proceed with symptom-limited exercise testing, usually with thallium imaging. We base the need for catheterization primarily on the stress test results in these patients.

Alternatively, the patients who present with type II unstable angina are referred directly for catheterization, usually after 24 hours of stabilization on intravenous nitrates and heparin, with the expectation that further intervention will likely be necessary. The subgroup of patients we are most concerned with are those who initially manifest ST segment deviation on presentation, followed by deep, symmetrical T-wave inversion across the precordial leads, which has been shown to be most often associated with high-grade proximal LAD stenosis (14).

Acute Myocardial Infarction

Finally, those patients presenting with acute anterior myocardial infarction often manifest one of the following scenarios, which mandate intervention with catheterization and PTCA:

1. Patients who present early into the course of anterior myocardial infarction and in whom thrombolytic therapy is strongly contraindicated should be taken directly to the catheterization laboratory with the expectation of emergent PTCA, or, if anatomy dictates, emergency CABG. Some investigators (15) would take the stand that all patients with acute anterior myocardial infarction presenting within 4 hours of pain onset should be taken to the catheterization laboratory for primary PTCA to be performed if feasible, although the majority of patients presenting in this time frame do not present to an institution with an immediately available laboratory. Our policy has been to institute thrombolytic therapy in almost all acute myocardial infarction patients, with the exception of those with impending or full-blown cardiogenic shock or those who begin to infarct while in the hospital, when there is a laboratory available within 30 minutes.

2. Patients who have already received thrombolytic therapy who continue to have ongoing chest pain for greater than 2 hours after treatment, patients who develop recurrent "waxing and waning" ischemic pain within 24 hours after thrombolytics, or patients who, despite thrombolytic therapy, are verging on or entering into cardiogenic shock (16) are all brought to the laboratory with the expectation of intervention.

3. Patients with post–myocardial infarction angina, more than 24 hours from presentation, especially if ST changes are present (17), are all candidates for urgent intervention.

4. Patients who appear to have had successful thrombolytic therapy, who remain pain-free, but go on to have abnormal thallium exercise testing, with a significant area of redistribution on either 4-hour or (if we continue to suspect viability despite the 4-hour scan) on 24-hour delayed imaging, are all taken to the laboratory with the expectation of intervention.

It should be pointed out that there has been a recent resurgence of interest in the use of immediate PTCA in the setting of acute myocardial infarction, particularly with anterior infarcts presenting early, since the publication of the Primary Angioplasty in Myocardial Infarction Study Group (PAMI) data by Grines et al. (15). This study randomized 395 patients presenting within 12 hours of the onset of acute myocardial infarction either to receive heparin, aspirin, and intravenous t-PA or to receive heparin, aspirin, and immediate PTCA. The study demonstrated a higher success rate for opening infarct-related vessels than had previously been reported (97%), pointing out that improvements in guidewire technology and in balloon trackability and pushability have impacted favorably on the performance of PTCA in acutely ill patients. In addition, no patient in the PTCA group required emergency CABG. The results demonstrated a significant reduction in mortality in those patients treated with immediate PTCA who were "not low risk," defined as having anterior myocardial infarction, age greater than 70, or heart rate greater than 100/minute on presentation (although the mortality results were not statistically significant for the study group as a whole). In addition, immediate PTCA reduced the combined occurrence of reinfarction or death both in the hospital and at 6-month follow-up, and the incidence of intracranial bleeding with t-PA (2.0% in this study) was eliminated by the use of immediate PTCA without thrombolytic therapy.

This study brings out an important point that our group has discovered anecdotally, which is that, in acute infarct patients undergoing PTCA, adequate anticoagulation with high doses of heparin is essential for success. We concur with the dosage regimen outlined in the PAMI study, using a total heparin bolus of between 15,000 and 20,000 units, scrupulously maintaining the ACT around 350 seconds. In addition, we have tended to use prolonged balloon inflations at relatively low atmospheres as the preferred initial inflation strategy. An initial 5-minute inflation at 4 to 6 atm, with an ACT greater than 350, often produces remarkably good results. Heparin is usually continued overnight, discontinued for 2 to 3 hours to allow sheath removal in the morning, and then resumed without a bolus 1 to 2 hours later, maintaining a partial thromboplastin time of 60 to 80 for 48 more hours.

Utilizing this regimen, the acute success rate has been quite high, and the incidence of acute symptomatic reclosure has been less than 1% at our institution.

ANGIOGRAPHIC FINDINGS

Once the decision has been made for cardiac catheterization, the next step in the decision-making tree involves the interpretation of the angiographic findings. Assuming that a proximal LAD stenosis has been found, what steps enter into the decision for or against PTCA?

Percent Angiographic Stenosis

At one end of the spectrum are lesions that are clearly less than 50% in severity and for which there is general agreement that medical therapy is the most reasonable option. Of more concern are those lesions that appear angiographically to fall within the 50 to 70% range, which on some views appear no more than 50% and on other views appear closer to 70% in severity. With these "borderline" lesions we have taken the approach advanced by Kalff et al. (18) who demonstrated a very good correlation between presence of exercise-induced, anteroapical thallium perfusion defects and the presence of a significant gradient across the stenosis. In short, if thallium has demonstrated significant ischemia in the appropriate location, then our approach is to dilate the "borderline" proximal LAD stenosis, but if there is little or no thallium-proven ischemia, then we would opt not to dilate but to follow medically. Our observation has also been that patients with 70% lesions in the proximal LAD are more likely to be symptomatic than those with similar lesions in other locations, perhaps because of the extent of myocardium supplied.

When a "70% stenosis" is discussed, it is always interesting to observe the way in which different observers reach their respective determinations of lesion severity. Depending on one's bias, some individual observers seem always to be "overreading" lesion severity, while others appear to be chronic optimists. Our group has been under-impressed with the usefulness of various computer-assisted algorithms to aid in the determination of lesion severity, such as the angiographic densitometric methods and edge-detection algorithms used to facilitate computation of percent diametric and percent geometric stenosis. The numbers obtained are not highly reproducible, and depending on how one chooses the "region of interest," the numbers can be made to vary accordingly. We tend to use the old-fashioned hand-caliper and "eyeball" methods, coupled with a major emphasis on the clinical presentation and the noninvasive data. Interestingly, data from the ACME trial, which used visual, hand-held caliper, and computer-assisted edge-detection algorithms, have shown no definitive advantage to the last two methods (19).

Lesion Morphology

Once the decision has been made that the lesion is of sufficient severity to dilate, the next question is how to approach the lesion based on the morphology. We will examine several morphologic scenarios and give our approach to each.

TOTAL OCCLUSIONS

In the setting of acute proximal LAD occlusion with evolving myocardial infarction, we would always attempt to dilate the lesion with a conventional over-the-wire balloon, unless there were either a ≥70% left main stenosis or there were severe, operable three-vessel coronary artery disease. In the case of more chronic total occlusions, we would always attempt to dilate if the lesion was likely less than 3 months old, if there were a reasonable "stump" visualized in which to maneuver the guidewire, and if there were no visualized "bridging collaterals."

Technically, we would begin with a flexible guidewire, usually working in a steeply angulated right anterior oblique (RAO) cranial view (80° RAO, 40° to 50° cranial), begin-

ning by trying to cross the lesion with a rotational movement of the wire through the occlusion. If the wire alone did not cross easily, and if the "stump" of the occlusion were clearly seen, we would advance the over-the-wire balloon to within 0.5 centimeter of the occlusion and then try to rotate the wire across the lesion. It is highly important to keep the balloon tip directed at the stump in a coaxial manner, or else the wire may become subintimal. Finally, if the lesion could not be crossed in this manner, different varieties of guidewire could be used to replace the initial, flexible wire. We would usually exchange first for a stiffer wire, and then, if the lesion still could not be crossed, exchange for a finer, 0.010-inch wire, which occasionally finds a channel that has been opened up by the larger wire, but could not be traversed by the larger-diameter wire.

Following successful crossing of the total occlusion, we would opt to use relatively prolonged, low-atmosphere inflations (Fig. 29A.5) and would generally continue intravenous heparin at least overnight.

LONG LESIONS

With the advent of several newer techniques, longer lesions have been approached with a high degree of success, utilizing long conventional balloons, excimer laser, rotational atherectomy, and intracoronary stents. Prior to approaching longer lesions, it is most reasonable to discuss the risks of restenosis and of acute closure with the patient and the referring physician. With lesions greater than 10 mm in length, the restenosis rate approaches 50% regardless of the method used for dilation. Of interest, however, is that the length of the restenotic segment is often significantly less than that of the original lesion (Fig. 29A.6), and a second dilation may be associated with a lower rate of restenosis (20). In addition to a higher rate of restenosis, longer lesions are associated with a higher risk of acute closure. Several abstracts have advocated the use of intracoro-

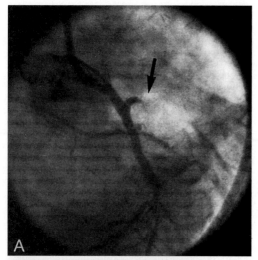

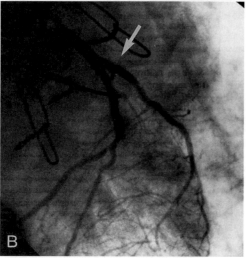

Figure 29A.5. A. Angiogram demonstrating a total proximal LAD occlusion *(arrow)* just beyond the left main coronary artery. The patient had recently undergone bypass surgery, but the distal internal mammary anastomosis was technically unsatisfactory and not amenable to PTCA. To relieve severe unstable angina, PTCA of the occluded native LAD was performed. **B.** Angiographic result following several prolonged inflations of an over-the-wire balloon in the proximal LAD *(arrow),* resulting in freedom from angina at 6-month follow-up.

discrete lesions, and several deaths have been reported during attempted dilation of long lesions, particularly during the "learning curve" of operator experience with rotational atherectomy. Finally, excimer laser has been advocated as a "debulking" strategy to be used in long lesions and then followed by dilation using a long balloon.

Our approach has been to avoid balloon dilation of heavily calcified lesions greater than 1 cm in length and to refer patients for internal mammary artery grafting, particularly if the distal vessel is relatively free from disease. An emerging alternative to bypass in some of these patients is rotational atherectomy, although the restenosis rate after Rotablator therapy of long lesions will need to be scrutinized in large clinical trials.

In noncalcified or minimally calcified vessels, we have used long balloons as the primary approach and have tried to avoid oversizing the balloon to prevent large intimal dissections. After the initial inflations, if more prolonged inflations are required because of recoil or a small intimal flap, the long balloon can be exchanged for a 3-cm perfusion balloon to allow for longer inflation times. If a large dissection occurs, with compromise of the lumen or reduction of distal flow, our approach has been to leave a perfusion balloon across the lesion, place an intraaortic balloon if ischemia is present, and then either deploy an intracoronary bailout stent or send the patient for emergency CABG.

This overall approach to long, complex lesions has been very successful in many cases and has been particularly useful in patients with severely compromised distal flow pre-PTCA in whom it was not clear whether the distal vessel was of sufficient size to permit CABG.

SERIAL AND BIFURCATION LESIONS

Serial lesions in the proximal (or proximal and mid) LAD usually respond well to conventional PTCA, as long as each separate lesion is appropriate for dilation. In general,

nary stents to "bail out" failed PTCA in long lesions (21). Other centers have been advocating the use of rotational atherectomy devices, particularly the Rotablator, for dilation of long, calcified stenoses (22). Again, the risks of acute closure are higher than for

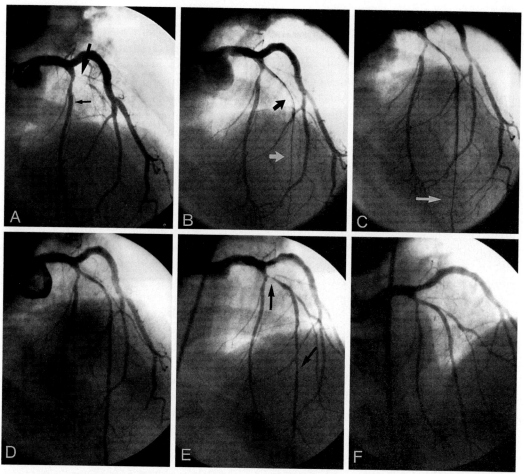

Figure 29A.6. **A.** Angiogram demonstrating a subtotal occlusion of the LAD *(large arrow)* at the takeoff of the first septal perforator *(small arrow)*. Because of very faint distal flow, the caliber of the mid and distal vessel could not be well visualized and suitability of the vessel for CABG was questionable. **B.** After initial dilation of the LAD at the site of subtotal occlusion, significant disease could be seen in the midportion of the vessel *(arrows)*. **C.** After dilation of the midportion of the LAD, significant disease could be visualized in the distal vessel as well *(arrow)*. **D.** Following dilation of all segments of the vessel, a satisfactory result was achieved with good flow all the way to the apex. Because of the length of the dilated segments, however, restenosis was anticipated. **E.** Angiography performed 4 months after initial PTCA for evaluation of abnormal thallium testing demonstrated discrete areas of restenosis at the initial site of dilation and in the midportion of the vessel *(arrows)*. **F.** After reangioplasty a satisfactory result was achieved, and follow-up exercise-thallium testing 4 months later was normal.

we try to dilate each lesion separately, beginning with the most proximal lesion and moving distally. We tend to place a final inflation on the proximal lesion "on the way out" to ensure that the lesion has not been disturbed by the shaft of the balloon catheter during distal dilations. The additional risk of restenosis in serial lesions is not additive as one might intuitively expect, but rises from approxi-

mately 20 to 30% (clinical) restenosis for single proximal LAD lesions to 35 to 40% for multiple lesions (23).

Bifurcation lesions involving a large first diagonal branch can present several potential difficulties. If the diagonal is a relatively large vessel and is involved in the LAD lesion, the vessel is usually protected with a second guidewire. It may be difficult to engage the takeoff of the diagonal with the guidewire, particularly if it arises just beyond the bulk of the lesion. A relatively acute angle can be formed at the tip of the flexible guidewire, usually about 60°, to facilitate wiring the diagonal. Sometimes a mild secondary bend, slightly more proximal to the tip, can be useful.

We have tended to use a system of two fixed-wire devices for most bifurcation lesions because of the ease of delivery and the increased visualization with two fixed-wire devices in place. These are both introduced through the central lumen of a single Tuohy-Borst adapter rather than through a Y-connection, again to facilitate steerability and balloon placement (24).

Our experience with dilating bifurcation lesions using "kissing balloons" has been that one of the two branches usually remains slightly underdilated. We usually begin with inflations in the LAD proper, until a satisfactory result has been achieved. If the diagonal lesion appears 70% or less, it is usually left alone, depending on the vessel's size. If it is highly stenotic, then inflations are performed in the diagonal proper, aiming for less than 50% residual, but not aiming for a "perfect result," since more inflations in the diagonal often result in shifting of plaque back into the LAD proper. If alternating inflations in the LAD and diagonal do not provide satisfactory results, then "kissing balloon" inflations are performed in both vessels simultaneously, again concentrating on a minimal residual in the LAD proper, with good flow into the diagonal (Fig. 29A.7).

More recently, we have begun using directional coronary atherectomy (DCA) to treat bifurcation lesions, particularly when vessel caliber is ≥3.0 mm and the takeoff angle of the side branch is ≤75°. If plaque can be successfully removed from the bifurcation site, the overall appearance of both vessels following the procedure may be improved compared to conventional PTCA.

ECCENTRIC LESIONS

With the advent of directional coronary atherectomy (DCA), noncalcified eccentric lesions in the proximal LAD, particularly in the most proximal portion of large, straight vessels, are now being approached more frequently with DCA with excellent angiographic results. Although the "ideal" lesion for DCA is not often present, DCA is probably the procedure of choice for highly eccentric proximal LAD lesions if the following criteria are met: no visualized calcium in the lesion, no acute bend in the vessel at or just beyond the lesion, no disease in the ostium of the left main (since there is poor control of the guiding catheter tip), and vessel caliber is 3.0 mm or greater.

It should be noted that, in addition to the usefulness of DCA for eccentric lesions, DCA has been used successfully both as a treatment for "balloon-resistant" lesions that have not successfully dilated with conventional balloon maneuvers (such as the use of high-inflation pressures or "upsizing" the balloon by 0.5 mm) and as a "bailout" procedure for patients receiving conventional PTCA who developed local intimal flaps that could not be successfully "tacked up" with recurrent or prolonged balloon inflations (25).

SUMMARY

The finding of isolated, significant proximal LAD stenosis at cardiac catheterization most often will mandate an interventional approach to the patient. Guidelines for the decision to proceed with catheterization and for an interventional strategy to approach various lesions have been presented and are outlined in summary flow-diagrams (Figs. 29A.8 and 29A.9).

Improvements in conventional balloon angioplasty, as well as new approaches with directional and rotational atherectomy, excimer laser, and intracoronary stenting, allow a nonsurgical approach in the majority of these patients, with a low procedural morbidity and mortality. Follow-up studies have documented very low 5-year mortality after successful LAD PTCA, comparing

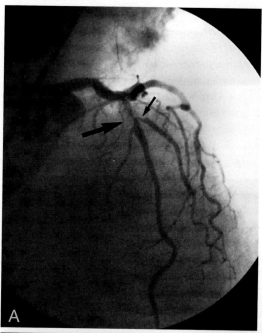

Figure 29A.7. **A.** Angiography demonstrating a proximal LAD stenosis *(large arrow)* involving the origin of the first diagonal branch *(small arrow).* **B.** After alternating inflations of balloons placed in the LAD and diagonal, a simultaneous "kissing" balloon inflation was performed (with a monorail balloon in the LAD and a fixed-wire device in the diagonal). Both balloons were advanced through the central lumen of a Tuohy-Borst adapter. **C.** Appearance of the bifurcation following "kissing balloon PTCA." A small intimal tear is seen in the proximal aspect of the diagonal branch.

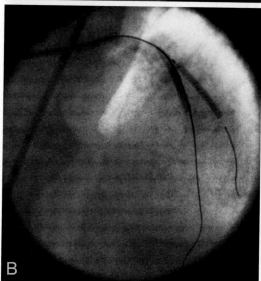

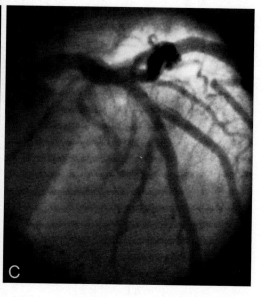

favorably with previous studies of medically treated patients. A recent randomized, controlled study in single-vessel disease has documented significant improvement in levels of angina and in treadmill performance for PTCA patients compared with their medically treated counterparts, and the differences are most apparent in patients with proximal LAD lesions. Presently, we would advise that all patients with proximal, isolated LAD disease producing significant symptoms or ischemia be seriously considered for revascularization using interventional catheterization techniques as the best method to palliate their coronary disease.

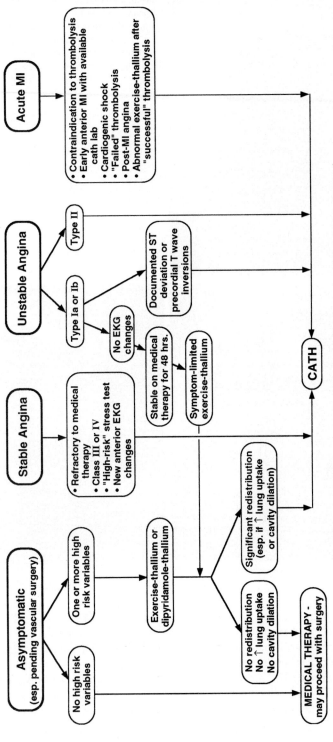

Figure 29A.8. Guidelines for the decision to proceed with cardiac catheterization (see text).

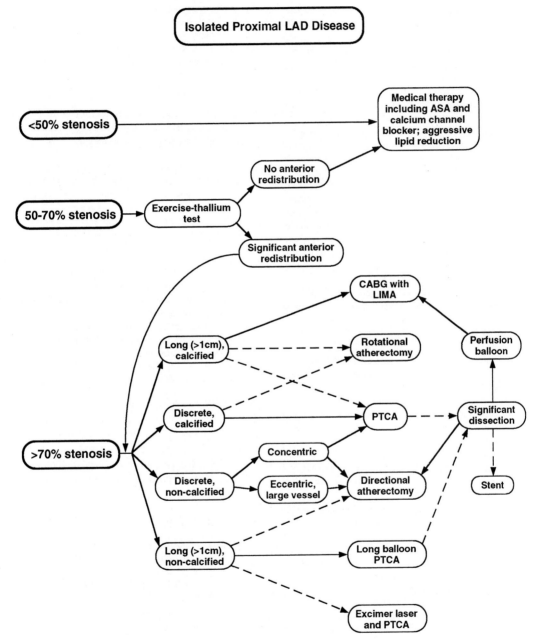

Figure 29A.9.   An interventional strategy to approach proximal LAD disease (see text).

REFERENCES

1. Verani MS, Mahmarian JJ, Pratt CM, Boyce TM. The variable extent of jeopardized myocardium in patients with single-vessel coronary artery disease: quantification by thallium-201 single photon emission computer tomography. J Am Coll Cardiol 1991;17:355–362.

2. Califf RM, Tomabechi Y, Lee KL et al. Outcome in one-vessel coronary artery disease. Circulation 1983;67:283–290.

3. Klein LW, Weintraub WS, Agarwal JB et al. Prognostic significance of severe narrowing of the proximal portion of the left anterior descending coronary artery. Am J Cardiol 1986;58:42–46.

4. Mock MB, Ringqvist I, Fisher LD et al. Survival of medically treated patients in the Coronary Artery Surgery Study (CASS) registry. Circulation 1982;66:562–568.

5. Murphy ML, Hultgren HN, Detre K, Thomsen J, Takaro T. Treatment of chronic stable angina: a preliminary report of the survival data of the randomized Veterans Administration Cooperative Study. N Engl J Med 1977;297:621–627.

6. European Coronary Artery Bypass Surgery Study Group. Prospective randomized study of coronary artery bypass surgery in stable angina pectoris. Lancet 1980;2:491–495.

7. Kramer JR, Proudfit WL, Loop FD et al. Late follow-up of 781 patients undergoing percutaneous transluminal coronary angioplasty or coronary bypass grafting for an isolated obstruction in the left anterior descending coronary artery. Am Heart J 1989;118:1144–1153.

8. Frierson JH, Dimas AP, Whitlow PL et al. Angioplasty of the proximal left anterior descending coronary artery: initial success and long-term follow-up. Am J Cardiol 1992;19:745–751.

9. Brown R, Kochar G, Maniet AR, Banka VS. Effects of coronary angioplasty using progressive dilation on ostial stenosis of the left anterior descending artery. Am J Cardiol 1993;71:245–247.

10. Parisi AF, Folland ED, Hartigan P. A comparison of angioplasty with medical therapy in the treatment of single vessel coronary artery disease. N Engl J Med 1992;326:10–16.

11. Eagle KA, Coley CM, Newell JB et al. Combining clinical and thallium data optimizes preoperative assessment of cardiac risk before major vascular surgery. Ann Intern Med 1989;110:859–866.

12. Boucher CA, Brewster DC, Darling RC, Okada RD, Strauss HW, Pohost GM. Determination of cardiac risk by dipyridamole-thallium imaging before peripheral vascular surgery. N Engl J Med 1985;312:389–394.

13. Hultgren HH, Giacomini JC, Miller C. Treatment of unstable angina. JAMA 1985;253:2555–2557.

14. Zwaan C, Bar FW, Janssen JHA et al. Angiographic and clinical characteristics of patients with unstable angina showing an ECG pattern indicating critical narrowing of the proximal LAD coronary artery. Am Heart J 1989;117:657–665.

15. Grines CL, Browne KF, Marco J et al. A comparison of immediate angioplasty with thrombolytic therapy for acute myocardial infarction. N Engl J Med 1993;328:673–679.

16. Lee L, Bates ER, Pitt B, Walton JA, Laufer N, O'Neill WW. Percutaneous transluminal coronary angioplasty improves survival in acute myocardial infarction complicated by cardiogenic shock. Circulation 1988;78:1345–1351.

17. Schuster EH, Bulkley BH. Early post-infarction angina. Ischemia at a distance and ischemia in the infarct zone. N Engl J Med 1981;305:1101–1105.

18. Kalff V, Kelly MJ, Soward A et al. Assessment of hemodynamic significance of isolated stenoses of the left anterior descending coronary artery using thallium-201 myocardial scintigraphy. Am J Cardiol 1985;55:342–346.

19. Folland ED, Vogel RA, Hartigan P et al. Relation between coronary artery stenosis assessed by visual, caliper, and computer methods and exercise capacity in patients with single-vessel coronary artery disease. Circulation 1994;89:2005–2014.

20. Zidar JP, Jackman JD, Tenaglia AN et al. Late outcome for PTCA of long coronary lesions using long angioplasty balloon catheters. Circulation 1992;86(Suppl 1):2036a (abstract).

21. Cannon AD, Hearn JA, Bilodeau L et al. Long balloon angioplasty and adjuvant stenting for long type B and C lesions. Circulation 1992;86:(Suppl 1):2035a (abstract).

22. Fajadet J, Doucet S, Cailllard J, Cassagneau B, Robert G, Marco J. Coronary rotational ablation in complex lesions: clinical, angiographic and procedural predictors of success and complications. Circulation 1992;86:(Suppl 1):2034a (abstract).

23. Pooled data, including NHLBI PTCA Registry data.

24. Korr KS, Burtt DM. "Intimate" double balloon coronary angioplasty with a single Y connector. Cathet Cardiovasc Diagn 1991;24:321–322.

25. Hofling B, Gonschior P, Simpson L, Bauriedel G, Nerlich A. Efficacy of directional coronary atherectomy in cases unsuitable for percutaneous transluminal coronary angioplasty (PTCA) and after unsuccessful PTCA. Am Heart J 1992;124:341–348.

ACKNOWLEDGMENT

The authors of this chapter would like to acknowledge the expert secretarial assistance of Ms. Teresa Silva and Mrs. Suzanne Bailey, as well as the technical expertise of Dr. Steven Herman in the preparation of this manuscript.

B. The Role of Bypass Surgery

JEAN-JACQUES GOY, ERIC EECKHOUT, MICHEL HURNI, BERNARD BURNAND, PATRICK RUCHAT, FRANK STUMPE, PIERRE VOGT, JEAN-CHRISTOPHE STAUFFER, NADIA DEBBAS, LUKAS KAPPENBERGER, and HOSSEIN SADEGHI

BACKGROUND

The management of patients with proximal left anterior descending coronary artery stenosis is of critical importance and remains controversial. Surgeons often advocate a surgical approach. On the other hand cardiologists define an isolated proximal LAD stenosis as one of the best indications for coronary angioplasty. The survival rate of patients with multivessel coronary artery disease and proximal LAD lesion is 92% at 5 years and 75% at 10 years after cardiac surgery (1). When the left internal mammary artery is used, the in-hospital mortality (<30 days) is very low (<2%) and the relief of angina excellent with 92% of the patients free of symptoms at 5 years (2). In a similar group of patients with proximal LAD stenosis and multiple-vessel disease, medical treatment carries a significantly worse prognosis with a survival rate of 83% and 64% at 5 and 10 years, respectively, as shown by the European Coronary Surgery study (1). Thus the benefit of surgery over medical therapy in the specific group of patients with proximal LAD stenosis and multiple-vessel disease is widely accepted.

However, coronary angioplasty has to be considered as a possible option for coronary revascularization. Angioplasty is usually performed in patients with single-vessel disease and offers a slight benefit over medical therapy at 6 months in terms of exercise tolerance and relief of angina as demonstrated by Parisi et al. (3). However, they studied a heterogeneous group of patients with a single coronary artery stenosis of any vessel. The number of patients with LAD stenosis is unknown, and their conclusion might be slightly different for the particular group of patients with proximal LAD stenosis. No prospective study addresses the specific question of the exact role of angioplasty in this group of patients. Based on retrospective data, the survival rate after angioplasty for single coronary stenosis compares favorably with surgery in a heterogeneous group of patients (4). Another retrospective evaluation of a group of proximal LAD stenosis treated with angioplasty shows the 5-year actuarial freedom from cardiac death to be 97% and from death and myocardial infarction to be 94%. Adding surgical or

percutaneous revascularization to cardiac death and myocardial infarction, the proportion of patients free from events decreases to 71% (5). The initial success rate of angioplasty is high (>95%), but 25 to 30% of the patients experience a recurrence of symptoms caused by a restenosis within the first 6 months after the initial intervention, making additional investigations, angiography, and angioplasty necessary and increasing therefore the final cost and the morbidity. Although the in-hospital outcome is similar in patients treated with surgery or angioplasty, the length of the in-hospital stay and the cost and morbidity of the procedure are lower for the latter. These advantages are counterbalanced by the need for further reintervention to achieve a good clinical result, penalizing patients treated with angioplasty. Finally, the quality of the revascularization seems equally good with the two strategies, but no prospective trial has tested this hypothesis.

A previous report based on a retrospective analysis of 781 patients with isolated proximal obstruction of the LAD treated with surgery (venous graft or left internal mammary artery graft) or angioplasty suggested a better long-term result after surgery (the analyzed endpoints being death, myocardial infarction, and additional revascularization) (6). This study does not provide information on the patients' functional status postprocedure. Moreover, this was a retrospective analysis of a heterogeneous group of patients with different types of grafts and various degrees of left ventricular function. Several ongoing studies are comparing surgery and angioplasty in patients with ischemic heart disease (7–10). In most of them, except for the RITA trial (8), patients with single coronary stenosis are excluded. In the RITA trial the results of the subgroup of patients with proximal LAD lesion have not yet been reported. The major problem with the aforementioned trials is that they represent a "melting pot" of many different coronary situations (various ejection fractions, proximal or distal stenosis, one or more stenoses on a vessel, various sizes of vessel, presence of collaterals, etc.), making extrapolation of their conclusions to any individual patient difficult.

PATIENTS AND METHOD

We designed a prospective, randomized trial comparing surgery using left internal mammary artery graft and angioplasty in a group of patients with isolated proximal LAD stenosis and normal left ventricular ejection fraction. Documented clinical or silent ischemia was an inclusion criteria. Previous Q-wave myocardial infarction, unstable angina pectoris, or left ventricular ejection fraction below 0.50 were exclusion criteria.

Study design made provision for clinical and functional assessments at 6 months, 1, 2, 3, 4, and 5 years after treatment. Clinical parameters prospectively collected were cardiac death, myocardial infarction (Q and non-Q wave), repeat revascularization, angina functional class, exercise tolerance, clinical need for reangiography, and postprocedural antianginal drug regimen. Functional status was estimated by means of the functional class and the stress test. Two variables were used, the double product at peak exercise and the duration of the exercise before the occurrence of ST depression >1 mm, angina, dyspnea, or fatigue.

Randomization to surgery or angioplasty was done according to the Zelen method (11) and after a consensual decision by the cardiologist and the surgeon to minimize crossover from the surgical group to the angioplasty group. In a 4-year period 5119 patients underwent coronary angiography in our institution. Single coronary stenosis was documented in 1786 patients, and in 142 of them an isolated proximal LAD stenosis with normal left ventricular function was present. Finally, 134 patients accepted to be randomized and entered the trial: 68 were assigned to angioplasty and 66 surgery. Most patients were very symptomatic with CCS (Canadian cardiovascular classification) class III or IV and were on optimal medical therapy. The risks

factors were equally distributed between the two groups (Table 29B.1). The angiographic characteristics of the stenosis, assessed by quantitative coronary angiographic analysis, were similar in the two groups. The groups were matched for number of ostial lesions, as well as by lesion type A, B, or C (Table 29B.2).

Table 29B.1.
Clinical Characteristics of the Study Population at Time of Randomization

Characteristic		CABG (n = 66)	PTCA (n = 68)
Sex[a]	Male	53 (80%)	55 (80%)
Age[b] (yr)		55 ± 10	58 ± 11
Angina (Canadian Cardiovascular Society)			
	Class I	0	1
	Class II	9	5
	Class III	30	33
	Class IV	22	21
	Unstable	5	8
Medication			
	β-Blockers	40	48
	Calcium antagonists	54	57
	Nitrates	59	62
	Molsidomine	4	3
Risk factors			
	Current smoker	34	40
	Diabetes	8	8
	Family history	32	34
	Hypertension	27	31
	Hyperlipidemia	34	38

[a]Percentages shown are percentages of each study group.

[b]Plus-minus values are means ± SD.

Table 29B.2.
Angiographic Characteristics of the Study Population at Time of Randomization

Characteristic		CABG (n = 66)	PTCA (n = 68)
Preprocedure minimal luminal diameter (mm)[a]		0.60 ± 0.28	0.66 ± 0.23
Post-PTCA minimal luminal diameter (mm)[a]		—	2.10 ± 0.34
Preprocedure percentage stenosis[a]		79 ± 8	71 ± 6
Post-PTCA percentage stenosis[a]		—	25 ± 6
Lesion type[b]			
	Type A	30 (46%)	40 (59%)
	Type B	20 (30%)	20 (29%)
	Type C	16 (24%)	8 (12%)

[a]Plus-minus values are means ± SD.

[b]Percentages shown are percentages of each study group.

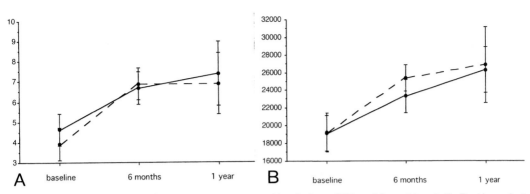

Figure 29B.1. A. Exercise duration at stress test expressed in minutes ± 95% confidence interval. **B.** Double product at stress test ± 95% confidence interval.

Functional parameters were also matched (Fig. 29B.1). Statistics were performed using the intention-to-treat analysis.

RESULTS

Standard percutaneous and surgical revascularization procedures were used. Only experienced operators having performed over 500 angioplasties or 350 grafting procedures were allowed to treat the patients included in the present trial. All the 68 patients randomized to the angioplasty group were treated with angioplasty. Of the 66 patients randomized to surgery, five refused surgery and were treated with angioplasty, one patient developed unstable angina while awaiting surgery and underwent angioplasty because of the unavailability of the surgical team, and one patient experienced a myocardial infarction awaiting his operation. Thus 59 patients were grafted.

The procedural outcome was uneventful in 98% of the patients in the surgical group (one patient developed a non–Q-wave perioperative myocardial infarction). In the angioplasty group 97% had an uneventful outcome (two patients had an acute closure during the procedure and underwent emergency bypass surgery). At a mean follow-up time of 24 ± 12 months (range 6 to 55), the overall rate of cardiac death and myocardial infarction (including in-hospital events) was not different in the two groups (Table 29B.3).

Table 29B.3.
Ranking Scale of the Primary Endpoints at a Mean Follow-Up Period of 2 Years

Endpoint	CABG (n = 66)	PTCA (n = 68)	P Value (Fisher's Test)
Cardiac death	1	0	.049
Myocardial infarction			
Q-wave	1	2	
Non–Q-wave	1	6	
Total	2	8	.09
Cardiac death and myocardial infarction	3	8	.21
Revascularization			
CABG	0	9	
PTCA	2	8	
Total	2	17	.0009
None of the above	61	43	.0001

Repeat revascularization was significantly more frequent in the angioplasty group. This was mainly because of restenosis, which occurred in 22 patients (32%). The outcome of the two groups is presented in Figures 29B.2 and 29B.3. The higher incidence of events after angioplasty is related mainly to restenosis. With the Kaplan-Meier method the estimated proportion of patients with no adverse event is 0.86 in the surgical group versus 0.43 in the angioplasty group ($P < .01$) (Fig. 29B.4). The calculated relative risk for further revascularization in patients treated by angioplasty was 8.3 (95% confidence interval: 4.7 to 12) compared with patients treated by surgery. Respectively, the risk for any major adverse cardiac event was 4.4 (3.0

Figure 29B.2. Outcome of the patients treated by surgery.

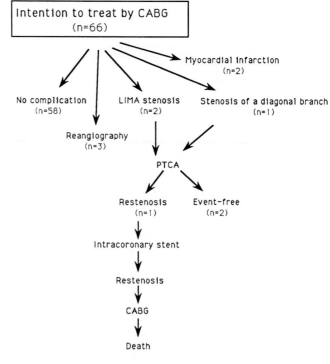

Intention to treat by CABG
(n=66)

Myocardial infarction
(n=2)

No complication
(n=58)

LIMA stenosis
(n=2)

Stenosis of a diagonal branch
(n=1)

Reangiography
(n=3)

PTCA

Restenosis
(n=1)

Event-free
(n=2)

Intracoronary stent

Restenosis

CABG

Death

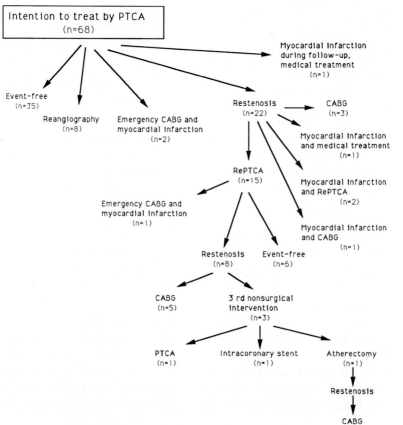

Intention to treat by PTCA
(n=68)

Myocardial infarction
during follow-up,
medical treatment
(n=1)

Event-free
(n=35)

Reangiography
(n=8)

Emergency CABG and
myocardial infarction
(n=2)

Restenosis
(n=22)

CABG
(n=3)

Myocardial infarction
and medical treatment
(n=1)

RePTCA
(n=15)

Myocardial infarction
and RePTCA
(n=2)

Emergency CABG and
myocardial infarction
(n=1)

Myocardial infarction
and CABG
(n=1)

Restenosis
(n=8)

Event-free
(n=6)

CABG
(n=5)

3 rd nonsurgical
intervention
(n=3)

PTCA
(n=1)

Intracoronary stent
(n=1)

Atherectomy
(n=1)

Restenosis

CABG

Figure 29B.3. Outcome of the patients treated by angioplasty.

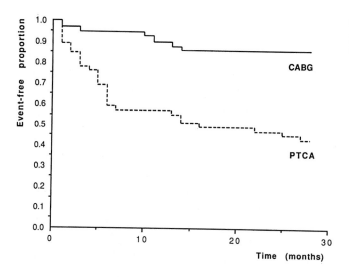

Figure 29B.4. Kaplan-Meier estimated proportions without adverse event at 30 months.

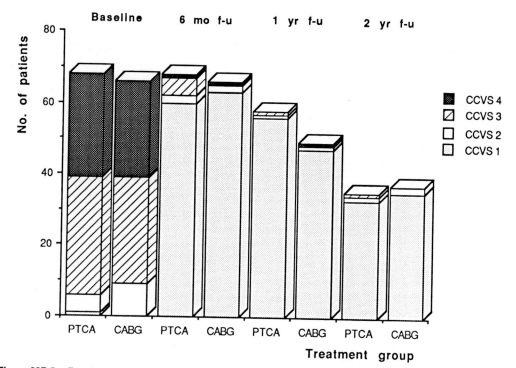

Figure 29B.5. Functional class at baseline and during follow-up (F/U) expressed by means of the Canadian cardiovascular classification (CCVS).

to 6.3). Angina functional class (Fig. 29B.5) and stress test results (Fig. 29B.1) were not different in the two groups at follow-up; indeed, at 2 years 77% of the patients in the angioplasty group were asymptomatic compared with 82% in the surgical group. There was a significant and durable increase in the exercise capacity and exercise duration after both treatments. However, patients treated with angioplasty were taking more antianginal drugs than those treated with surgery as shown in Table 29B.4.

Table 29B.4.
Drug Regimen at 2-Year Follow-Up

Drug	CABG[a] (n = 66)	PTCA[a] (n = 68)	P Value Chi-Square Test
None	3	1	
Aspirin	54	14	
Aspirin and 1 antianginal drug	36	51	<.01
Aspirin and 2 antianginal drugs	7	29	
Aspirin and 3 antianginal drugs	0	5	

[a]Values shown are percentages of each study group.

DISCUSSION

Patients with single coronary artery disease have a very good long-term prognosis when treated medically (4). When symptoms persist, angioplasty can be performed and has been shown to have some benefit over medical therapy in this group of patients (3). Surgery is considered only when medical therapy fails, when angioplasty is not feasible, or if multiple restenosis occurs. However, these cases are very rare, especially when the vessel concerned is the right coronary artery or the circumflex coronary artery, as long-term benefit of surgery is limited by the long-term patency of the venous graft. It is often stated that surgery should be postponed as long as possible in patients with ischemic heart disease mainly because of the high occlusion rate of venous grafts after 10 years. To compare angioplasty and surgery in patients with single right or circumflex coronary artery stenosis would have been unethical. The prognostic importance of a proximal LAD lesion and the excellent long-term patency of a left internal mammary graft (90 to 95% at 10 to 15 years) justify a surgical approach to such lesions even in single-vessel disease. This supported the rationale and ethics behind the present trial, which, in fact, clearly shows that surgery remains a very good therapeutic option for patients with proximal LAD stenosis.

In our study both left internal mammary artery grafting and angioplasty improved the clinical status of symptomatic patients with isolated proximal left anterior descending artery stenosis and normal left ventricular function. The higher rate of events with angioplasty is because of the need for repeat revascularization, mainly related to restenosis. For angioplasty to result in the same relief of angina as surgery, more intensive antianginal treatment and successful reintervention are necessary. In view of these results, both surgery and angioplasty are possible treatments for an isolated proximal LAD stenosis. Indication for angioplasty in the treatment of single LAD stenosis should be considered in the light of these results. After surgery some patients will develop other lesions of the right or circumflex artery; in those, angioplasty can certainly be used. Moreover, adequate control of risk factors can probably slow the progression of the atherosclerotic process. The possible need for future reintervention should not influence the choice of treatment when proximal LAD stenosis is documented.

Clearly, the final choice between surgery and angioplasty should be based on the angiographic aspect of the lesion, the estimated rate of complications, and a careful discussion with the patient who must be fully informed of both the advantages and possible complications of each treatment option. Physicians should consider surgery and angioplasty as complementary therapeutic options in patients with ischemic heart disease and isolated proximal LAD stenosis, knowing that for some patients surgery is the best choice and for others angioplasty is better. However, two major trials, comparing elective stenting and conventional balloon angioplasty for de novo stenoses in native vessels, have shown a significant reduction in the restenosis rate and of clinical events following stenting (12, 13). Therefore a more liberal and optimal use of stents may improve the long-term efficacy of transcatheter coronary therapeutics and partially modify the present conclusions. To answer this question, randomized trials comparing elective stenting with surgery in patients with isolated proximal LAD stenosis are mandatory.

SUMMARY

Isolated proximal LAD stenosis and normal left ventricular function comprise a particular subset of coronary disease. When an aggressive approach is required, angioplasty and surgery can both be safely recommended. Surgery has a place in the treatment of these lesions but only if the left internal mammary artery is used.

REFERENCES

1. Varnauskas E, and the European Coronary Surgery Study Group. Twelve-year follow-up of survival in the randomized European Coronary Surgery Study. N Engl J Med 1988; 319:332–337.
2. Sergeant P, Lesaffre E, Flameng W, Suy R. Internal mammary artery: methods of use and their effect on survival. Eur J Cardiothorac Surg 1990;4:72–78.
3. Parisi AF, Folland ED, Hartigan P. A comparison of angioplasty with medical therapy in the treatment of single-vessel coronary artery disease. N Engl J Med 1992; 326:10–16.
4. Akins CW, Block PC, Palacios IF, Gold HK, Carroll DL, Grunkemeier GL. Comparison of coronary artery bypass grafting and percutaneous transluminal coronary angioplasty as initial treatment strategies. Ann Thorac Surg 1989;47:507–516.
5. Frierson JH, Dimas AP, Whitlow PL et al. Angioplasty of the proximal left anterior descending coronary artery: initial success and long-term follow-up. J Am Coll Cardiol 1992;19:745–751.
6. Kramer JR, Proudfit WL, Loop FD et al. Late follow-up of 781 patients undergoing percutaneous transluminal coronary angioplasty or coronary artery bypass grafting for an isolated obstruction in the left anterior descending coronary artery. Am Heart J 1989;118:1144–1153.
7. BARI, CABRI, EAST, GABI and RITA: coronary angioplasty on trial. Lancet 1990;335:1315–1316 (editorial).
8. RITA participants. Coronary angioplasty versus coronary artery bypass surgery: the Randomized Intervention Treatment of Angina (RITA) trial. Lancet 1993;341:573–580.
9. King SB III, Lembo NJ, Weintraub WS et al. A randomized trial comparing coronary angioplasty with coronary bypass surgery. New Engl J Med 1994;331:1044–1050.
10. Hamm CW, Reimers J, Ischinger T et al. A randomized study of coronary angioplasty compared with bypass surgery in patients with symptomatic multivessel coronary disease. N Engl J Med 1994;331:1037–1043.
11. Zelen M. A new design for randomized clinical trials. N Engl J Med 1979;300:1242–1245.
12. Serruys PW, de Jaegere P, Kiemeneij F et al. A comparison of balloon-expandable-stent implantation with balloon angioplasty in patients with coronary artery disease. N Engl J Med 1994;331:489–495.
13. Fischman DL, Leon MB, Baim DS et al. A randomized comparison of coronary stent placement and balloon angioplasty in the treatment of coronary artery disease. N Engl J Med 1994;331:496–501.

C. Optimal Management of the Patient with Single-Vessel Proximal Left Anterior Descending Stenosis

STEPHEN G. ELLIS

BACKGROUND

Because of the feared consequences of its occlusion, narrowing of the proximal left anterior descending (LAD) coronary artery has been called "the widow-maker" lesion (1). Indeed, occlusion at this site typically results in ischemia to 50% of the left ventricular myocardium (2) and, if not quickly relieved, is often fatal.

In the early 1980s several studies found a 10 to 18% 3-year mortality for patients with single-vessel disease at this location when they were treated medically, although often only nitrates (but not beta-blockers or aspirin) were utilized (3, 4).

The demonstrated excellent long-term patency of internal mammary arteries (IMA) (5), which are often utilized for stenoses at this site, suggested that IMA grafting might be the preferred treatment for this high-risk patient group. The relatively small number of these patients enrolled in the three randomized trials of the 1970s (6–8) and the changes in both medical and surgical care since that time make firm recommendations difficult to justify, but most physicians today feel that patients with proximal LAD disease require revascularization.

Balloon angioplasty has been performed to this site since 1977. However, the risk of ischemic complications and restenosis are both higher with treatment at this site compared with that of other sites, especially if the ostium of the LAD is involved (9, 10). Until recently, however, there had never been randomized trials or convincing database studies on which to base decisions regarding the preferred form of revascularization.

CONTEMPORARY TRIALS OF PTCA VERSUS MEDICAL THERAPY

In the only randomized trial of balloon angioplasty versus medical therapy, the ACME investigators (11) randomized 64 patients with proximal LAD involvement to either therapy. With only a 6-month follow-up reported, the PTCA group seemed to have improved exercise tolerance (+1.2 versus −1.5 min to angina on a standard exercise test) but a somewhat greater need for bypass surgery (12% versus 0%). No mortality difference was noted.

CONTEMPORARY TRIALS OF CABG VERSUS PTCA

Two recently reported randomized trials have for the first time given more definitive data on which to base decision making in this area. From the SALAD trial Goy and colleagues report the results in 134 patients of randomization between internal mammary artery grafting and PTCA (12). At 2 years the surgery patients were doing better, with an 86% versus 43% event-free survival (P <.01), 3% versus 12% myocardial infarction (P = .05), and less severe angina (Table 29C.1). In a three-way trial also including randomization to medical therapy (and also involving disease in the mid LAD), Hueb and colleagues (13) found similar results after a 2-year follow-up. Death, infarction, or late revascularization was reported in only 2% of patients who had undergone surgery using an internal mammary artery, while 27% of PTCA patients and 12% of medically treated patients had adverse events. Thus, with the possible exception that early IMA surgery may make latter surgery more difficult, such surgery

Table 29C.1.
Incidence of Complications During Follow-Up

Complication	CABG (n = 66)	PTCA (n = 68)
Cardiac death	1	0
Noncardiac death	0	3
Myocardial infarction	2	8
Revascularization		
CABG	1	13
PTCA	3	10
Reangiography	6	30
Restenosis	—	22
Graft stenosis	2	—
Stenosis of an untreated vessel	1	0
No adverse endpoint	58	35

Reprinted with permission from Goy J-J et al. A comparison of coronary angioplasty with left internal mammary artery grafting in the treatment of isolated proximal left anterior descending artery stenosis. Lancet 1994 (in press).

clearly seems to be preferred over other traditional therapies.

THE ROLE OF NEW DEVICES AND NEW DILATION STRATEGIES

Several new device techniques, notably directional coronary atherectomy (DCA) and stent implantation, have been touted as advances in treatment for proximal LAD disease compared with standard balloon angioplasty.

In the CAVEAT I trial 1004 patients with de novo stenoses <12 mm in length in arteries ≥3.0 mm in diameter (visually) were randomized to either standard PTCA or DCA (14). Boehrer recently reported the results of the study for ostial and also proximal LAD disease (15). For the 487 patients with proximal (but nonostial) lesions, DCA had a higher initial success rate (91% versus 78%, P = .0003) and lower restenosis (50% versus 66%, P = .01), no difference in death or urgent bypass surgery, but a higher incidence of Q-wave and non–Q-wave infarctions (8% versus 3%, P = .02). For the 73 patients with ostial disease there was no difference between DCA and PTCA for success (87% versus 87%), restenosis (48% versus 46%), or complications. Of note, it is suspected that there may have been an investigator bias to exclude patients from the study if they were "ideal" for DCA (short and highly eccentric lesions), and post-DCA PTCA was discouraged; hence results may have been slightly substandard compared with those using current techniques. Thus a subsequent study, *Balloon versus Optimal Atherectomy Trial* (BOAT) has been initiated. Enthusiasm for a dramatic difference between the results of CAVEAT and BOAT should be tempered by the realization that even in the best quartile of procedural result within CAVEAT I ($<27\%$ stenosis by quantitative angiography (or about $<15\%$ by "eyeball"), the restenosis rate was 40% (16). Hence the restenosis rates, which drive most of the late events with percutaneous treatment and make it look inferior to IMA surgery, remain quite high.

Coronary stent placement to prevent restenosis has recently been tested in two trials, STRESS (17, 18) and BENESTENT (19), both of which focused on de novo, short lesions in arteries normally ≥3.0 mm in diameter. A breakout of the proximal LAD results is available from the BENESTENT trial, which found in the 168 patients randomized in this subgroup that restenosis was reduced in these patients to the same degree as in the other patients (Fig. 29C.1). This technique will be even more promising if short- and long-term anticoagulation can be minimized in patients with excellent initial angiographic and intravascular ultrasound results, as first suggested by Columbo and colleagues (20). Still, there may be some concern about subacute thrombosis at this site in particular, with possible backward propagation into the left main trunk.

There has also been recent interest in prolonged balloon inflations with perfusion balloons to perhaps improve on the results of PTCA. For example, Cribier recently reported (21) the results of a randomized trial of long ≥12 min) versus shorter (≤3 min) balloon inflation in 278 lesions. Long inflation led to a higher procedural success rate (91% versus 78%, $P<.01$), less frequent severe dissections (10% versus 27%, $P<.01$), but no difference in the restenosis rate (47% versus 43%). A similar result was found by Ohman and colleagues (22). Thus, while improved initial results may be obtained with this technique, restenosis does not appear to be decreased.

SUMMARY

Despite high initial success rates, all percutaneous approaches to revascularization of the proximal LAD have high ($>40\%$) restenosis rates, with the exception of placement of Palmaz-Schatz stents. While individualization to each patient's situation is required, it is the author's opinion that if the LAD will not safely accommodate a Palmaz-Schatz stent or the patient is a poor candidate for surgery, that IMA bypass is the approach most likely to lead to long-term event-free survival. There will, of course, be patients who prefer to avoid surgery and take their chances with restenosis. In this situation, DCA or prolonged inflation PTCA is probably best for most proximal lesions, although Rotablator or laser may have an appropriate role for initially debulking ostial or calcified lesions prior to further definitive treatment with DCA or PTCA. Hopefully, site-specific therapy to prevent restenosis will someday allow patients long-term results similar to that seen after IMA surgery, but without having the long recuperation required with surgery.

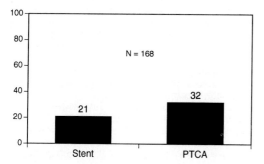

Figure 29C.1. Restenosis after stenting versus PTCA in proximal LAD lesions (BENESTENT).

REFERENCES

1. Schuster EH, Griffith LS, Bulkley BH. Preponderance of acute proximal left anterior descending coronary arterial lesions in fatal myocardial infarction: a clinicopathologic study. Am J Cardiol 1981;47:1189–1196.

2. Kalfbleisch H, Horst W. Quantitative study on the size of coronary artery supplying areas postmortem. Am Heart J 1977;94:183–192.

3. Klein LW, Weintraub WS, Agarwal JB, Schneider RM, Seelaus PA, Katz RI, Helfant RH. Prognostic significance of severe narrowing of the proximal portion of the left anterior descending coronary artery. Am J Cardiol 1986;58:42–46.

4. Califf RM, Tomabechi Y, Lee KL, Phillips H, Pryor DB, Harrell FE, Harris PJ et al. Outcome in one-vessel coronary artery disease. Circulation 1983;67:283–289.

5. Loop FD, Lytle BW, Cosgrove DM, Stewart RW, Goormastic M, Williams GW, Golding LAR et al. Influence of the internal-mammary-artery graft on 10-year survival and other cardiac events. N Engl J Med 1986;314:1–6.

6. VA Coronary Artery Bypass Surgery Cooperative Study Group. Eighteen-year follow-up in the Veterans Affairs cooperative study of coronary artery bypass surgery for stable angina. Circulation 1992;86:121–130.

7. Coronary Artery Surgery Study Group. Coronary Artery Surgery Study (CASS): a randomized trial of coronary artery bypass surgery: survival data. Circulation 1983; 68:939–950.

8. European Coronary Surgery Study Group. Long-term results of prospective randomised study of coronary artery bypass surgery in stable angina pectoris. Lancet 1982; 1173–1180.

9. Topol EJ, Ellis SG, Fishman J, Leimgruber P, Myler RK, Stertzer SH, O'Neill WW et al. Multicenter study of percutaneous transluminal angioplasty for right coronary artery ostial stenosis. J Am Coll Cardiol 1987;9:1214–1218.

10. Hirschfeld JW, Schwartz JS, Jugo R, MacDonald RG, Goldberg S, Savage MP, Bass TA et al. and the M-Heart investigators. Restenosis after coronary angioplasty: a multivariate statistical model to relate lesion and procedure variables to restenosis. J Am Coll Cardiol 1991;1 8:647–656.

11. Parisi AF, Folland ED, Hartigan P and Veterans Affairs ACME investigators. A comparison of angioplasty with medical therapy in the treatment of single-vessel coronary artery disease. N Engl J Med 1992;326:10–16.

12. Goy JJ, Eeckhout E, Vogt P, Stauffer JC, Hurni M, Ruchat P, Stumpe F et al. Surgery versus angioplasty for proximal left anterior descending (LAD) coronary artery stenosis (SALAD). A prospective randomized trial. J Am Cardiol 1994;23:268A (abstract).

13. Hueb WA, Arie S, Almeida Oliveira S, Bellotti G, Jatene A, Pileggi F. Randomized trial of surgery, angioplasty or medical therapy for single-vessel proximal left anterior de-

EDITORIAL SUMMARY

The clinical outcome of patients with significant proximal left anterior descending coronary artery disease has been felt to be characterized by increased event rates of angina, myocardial infarction, and cardiac mortality. Accordingly, clinicians have had hesitation about treating these patients medically. This arterial segment has been able to be approached since the early days of PTCA even with the early equipment available because it is usually a straight segment without significant proximal tortuosity. Therefore, since the early days of PTCA, patients with proximal left anterior descending lesions were felt to be excellent candidates for treatment. PTCA was felt to be such an important treatment modality for these patients that early attempts at designing a randomized trial of PTCA versus coronary bypass surgery were not felt achievable because either patients or their physicians would have already decided what their best treatment option should entail. Recently, however, the first randomized trial of left internal mammary artery versus PTCA for left anterior descending disease has been reported. As has been true with other randomized studies of PTCA versus coronary bypass surgery, the initial and intermediate outcome using mortality and myocardial infarction were similar; the patients randomized to PTCA needed more repeat procedures.

The issues of treatment of the proximal left anterior descending include (a) potential for hemodynamic compromise if acute closure occurs; (b) potential for left main coronary artery involvement if a significant dissection of the left anterior descending occurs with retrograde propagation; (c) involvement of major diagonal branches arising in the vicinity of the left anterior stenosis; and (d) restenosis.

The outcome of acute closure depends on the amount of myocardium at risk, which, for proximal left anterior descending lesions, is substantial. Once it has occurred, stents may be very effective and have been shown to decrease infarction rates and the need for urgent coronary bypass surgery. For ostial lesions, the stents are not ideal because they would overlap the left main coronary artery. Also, depending on the type of stent, it can trap large side branches, either the diagonal or the circumflex, making it impossible to ever dilate lesions in these side branches. It must be remembered that even if the stent fails to "normalize" the arterial segment with acute closure, it can be used as a bridge to surgery so that surgery can be performed under more elective conditions, allowing the surgeon more opportunity to use internal mammary arteries as the conduits.

It is optimal to avoid acute or threatened closure rather than treat it after the fact. For this reason, new devices are often used. Large bulky lesions in the proximal left anterior descending are often ideal for directional coronary atherectomy or primary stenting. Directional laser or Rotablator are usually used in smaller vessels with more diffuse disease or ostial stenoses.

The final issue to be considered is restenosis, which has been found to be increased in proximal left anterior descending lesions—particularly more ostial locations. Three randomized trials have shown that use of newer devices can decrease restenosis: CAVEAT I found decreased restenosis rates in patients with proximal left anterior descending stenoses, particularly if the final angiographic result was optimal with residual stenosis <20%, while STRESS and BENESTENT found that the use of the JJIS coronary stent was associated with decreased restenosis rates. The results of these trials are often used in choosing the therapeutic strategy for patients with proximal left anterior descending disease.

scending artery stenosis. Results of long-term follow-up. J Am Coll Cardiol 1994;23:268A (abstract).

14. Topol EJ, Leya F, Pinkerton CA, Whitlow PL, Hofling B, Simonton CA, Masden RR et al. and for the CAVEAT Study Group. A comparison of directional atherectomy with coronary angioplasty in patients with coronary artery disease. N Engl J Med 1993;329:221–227.

15. Boehrer JD, Ellis SG, Keeler GP, Debowey D, Califf RM, Topol EJ for the CAVEAT investigators. Differential benefit of directional atherectomy over angioplasty for left anterior descending in proximal, non-ostial lesions: results from CAVEAT. J Am Coll Cardiol 1994;23:386A (abstract).

16. Ellis SG, Umans VA, Whitlow PL, Pinkerton CA, Keeler GP, Kuntz RE on behalf of the CAVEAT investigators. Angiographic restenosis in CAVEAT is determined by the acute result (not the device used to obtain it). Circulation 1993;88:I-495.

17. Fischman D, Savage M, Leon M, Schatz R, Baim D, Penn I, Detre K et al. for the STRESS investigators. Acute and late angiographic results of the STent REStenosis Study (STRESS). J Am Coll Cardiol 1994;23:60A (abstract).

18. Leon MB, Fischman D, Schatz RA, Baim DS, Penn I, Nobuyoshi M, Colombo A et al. for the STRESS investigators. Analysis of early and late clinical events from the STent REStenosis Study (STRESS). J Am Coll Cardiol 1994;23:60A (abstract).

19. de Jaegere P, Macaya C, Fiemeneij F, Rutsch W, de Bruyne B, Emanuelsson H, Legrand V et al. on behalf of the Benestent Study Group. Critical evaluation of the immediate angiographic results after stent implantation in the first 260 patients randomized in the Benestent study. Circulation 1993;88:I-640.

20. Colombo A, Hall P, Almagor Y, Maiello L, Gaglione S, Nakamura S, Borrione M et al. Results of intravascular ultrasound guided coronary stenting without subsequent anticoagulation. J Am Coll Cardiol 1994;23:335A (abstract).

21. Cribier A, Eltchaninoff H, Chan C, Koning R, Jolly N, Baala B, Khotari M et al. Comparative effects of long (>12 min) versus standard (≤3 min) sequential balloon inflations in PTCA. Preliminary results of a prospective randomized study: immediate results and restenosis rate. J Am Coll Cardiol 1994;23:58A (abstract).

22. Ohman EM, Marquis J-F, Ricci DR, Brown RIG, Knudtson ML, Kereiakes DJ, Samaha JK et al. for the Perfusion Balloon Catheter Study Group. A randomized comparison of the effects of gradual prolonged versus standard primary balloon inflation on early and late outcome. Results of a multicenter clinical trial. Circulation 1994;89:1118–1125.

EDITORIAL SUMMARY

Treatment	Comments
Internal mammary artery bypass	Best long-term results. Avoid if due to young age, diffuse disease, or other reasons; bypass is likely to be needed soon or more than once more.
Stenting	Use of Palmaz-Schatz stent with focal stenosis in a >3 mm diameter vessel is the best percutaneous treatment. Use caution or avoid, however, with ostial location, thrombus present, or poor run-off. Has not been tested directly versus IMA surgery and may provide results that are nearly comparable.
Directional atherectomy	Probably the next best percutaneous choice when technically feasible.
Saphenous vein bypass	Decidedly inferior to use of the IMA. Still may be a better choice than percutaneous treatment when these approaches are high risk.
Balloon angioplasty	Should be used only when stenting and DCA are not possible and the patient wishes to avoid bypass surgery.
Rotablator	A reasonable pretreatment for stenting or DCA in a heavily calcified vessel. May be reasonably used as a stand-alone treatment or with balloon angioplasty only when an excellent angiographic result is obtained (e.g., ≤15% diameter stenosis by QCA or ≤0% diameter stenosis visually) or when stenting and DCA are not possible.
Laser (Excimer or Holmium)	Unproven. Probably of no advantage.
TEC	Unproven. Probably of no advantage.
Medical therapy	On the basis of considerable randomized and registry data, this form of therapy is difficult to justify unless both surgery and percutaneous treatments are high risk or unless the patient has limited life expectancy.

30. Retained Components

DAVID R. HOLMES JR. and KIRK N. GARRATT

The problem of retained components in the vascular system following percutaneous revascularization is extremely uncommon. Fortunately, there are no large series of reported experience with retained components. Nonetheless, advances in technology and skill level encourage operators to approach increasingly difficult cases and employ increasingly complex equipment, which may increase the chances of misadventure. Conventional angioplasty equipment has been refined to such a high level of quality that fracturing of these components or trapping of equipment in vascular spaces is exceedingly rare. Newer technologies, though, are less well refined and may incorporate mechanisms that increase the chances of loss of equipment in the coronary system. Some atherectomy devices, for instance, are capable of sheering through guidewires, and implantable devices such as stents may be lost from a deployment catheter system during attempts at placement.

GUIDEWIRES

In the past the most common foreign body was part of a guidewire (Fig. 30.1). Coronary angioplasty guidewires are generally constructed of a stainless steel alloy that is strong enough to resist kinking during manipulation and that allows torque transmission from the proximal end to the distal end. The distal tip of the guidewire is generally constructed of a forming ribbon that allows the operator to form or shape the tip of the wire. The forming ribbon is usually surrounded by a safety coil that wraps around the forming ribbon and adheres it to the steel alloy core of the wire (1).

Fracture of the wire tip may occur if the wire tip becomes fixed at its most distal end in a hard occlusion or intramurally within the vessel wall and if excessive turning is applied to the proximal end of the guidewire. Although advances in guidewire technology make tip fracture less likely today, it is still possible to embed the tip of the wire in atheroma or the vessel wall, particularly when attempting to cross a chronic total occlusion. In this setting vigorous turning of the wire should be avoided as separation may still occur. Separation can be recognized when attempts at withdrawing the wire result in wire stretching without any movement of the tip itself. The frequency with which guidewires fracture and are retained in the coronary system is difficult to determine accurately, because such complications are rarely reported. In one series of 5400 consecutive patients, complications related to retention of guidewire material in the coronary circulation were reported in eight (0.15%) patients (2). Retention of guidewire fragments is a serious matter and has led to acute epicardial coronary occlusion (3, 4). In one reported case the guidewire tip was inadvertently passed completely through the coronary vascular wall and was lodged in the pericardial space (5). When the guidewire was retracted, the tip fractured and was left free in the pericardial space.

The forming ribbon at the tip of the guidewire is the most likely portion to come free. As described, this ribbon is wrapped by a retaining coil. When the ribbon comes free, the steel wrapping gradually uncoils as the guidewire is retracted. Occasionally this "safety line" is strong enough to tug the fractured wire tip out

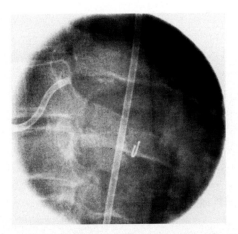

Figure 30.1. Right anterior oblique view of the left coronary artery. A tip of a fixed wire dilation has been displaced and retained within the distal circumflex.

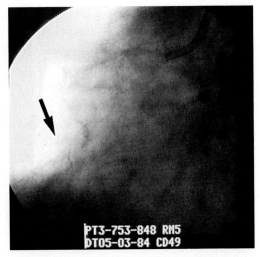

Figure 30.2. Left anterior oblique view of the right coronary artery. The guidewire had fractured within the right coronary artery; however, a loop protrudes into the ascending aorta. The guidewire is rather radiolucent and hard to visualize.

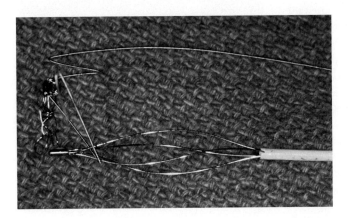

Figure 30.3. A Dotter retrieval catheter can be used to remove foreign bodies (e.g., stents or guidewires) from the aorta. In this case it has been used to extract a stent that failed to deploy.

of the coronary, but often the safety wire fractures as well. The uncoiled safety wire may extend well out of the coronary artery and into the guide catheter, however, providing the opportunity for retrieval of the retained fragment. Unfortunately, this very thin steel wire is radiolucent (Fig. 30.2). Grasping of this safety wire, even if done blindly, forms the basis for succccessful percutaneous removal of retained guidewire fragments.

The approach to a retained guidewire depends on the position of the guidewire, the length of the guidewire retained, and the arterial segment involved. The major concern is that of thrombosis of the affected segment. If the fragment is short and distal in a small side branch, nothing may be required as the risk of removing it may be greater than the risk of leaving it behind. In other circumstances, with a proximal segment in a large vessel or a proximal loop in the aorta (Fig. 30.2), attempts at removal are mandated.

Several approaches can be used (2, 4, 6–8). If a loop is protruding into the aorta, it may be snared with a Dotter retrieval catheter (Fig. 30.3) or even a bioptome, although the

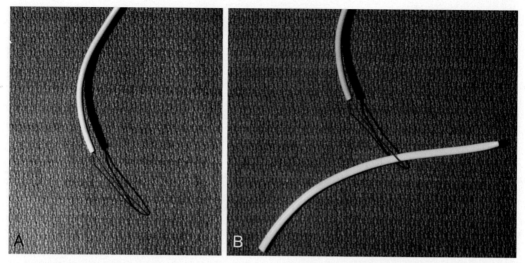

Figure 30.4. **A.** A simple loop snare can also be used. **B.** This can snare retained catheters or wire.

latter could result in cutting the wire. In addition, a variety of loop snares are available (Fig. 30.4). The wire must be firmly grasped so that it is not lost in the systemic circulation during withdrawal.

If the wire is completely within the coronary artery, a loop snare can still be used. Unfortunately, some retrieval devices are not long enough to reach the coronary ostium through a conventional guide catheter. Alternatively, another catheter can be positioned next to the fragment and rotated to trap the loop; balloon catheters, diagnostic coronary catheters, and even pigtail catheters have been successfully used for this purpose.

Wire fractures can also occur with newer rotational therapeutic devices. With directional atherectomy, if the guidewire is trapped in a side branch distal to the lesion to be treated, rotation of the cutter may fracture the tip. Similarly, with rotational atherectomy, if the brake is not used properly, the wire can rotate at very rapid speeds and again, if fixed, can fracture.

RETAINED BALLOON CATHETER COMPONENTS

In general, the integrity of current balloon catheters makes disruption or fragmentation

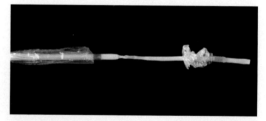

Figure 30.5. Rupture of balloon during inflation can make withdrawal difficult and can result in dislodgment of part of the catheter.

of any element in the catheter extremely unlikely. Even angioplasty balloons that rupture under high pressure are so designed to tear linearly, rather than fragment into small pieces. This greatly facilitates removal of the damaged catheter without concern over retained fragments. There have been occasional reports of balloon catheter components being lost in the coronary or systemic circulation from older balloon catheter designs (Fig. 30.5).

CORONARY STENTS

A more common group of retained components or devices will be intracoronary stents. This complication can be expected to increase, given the U.S. Food and Drug Administration approval of stents for treatment of acute or threatened closure and prevention of restenosis. Stents can be delivered without problem in properly selected patients. However, use of optimal guide catheters and guidewires is essential for proper placement. Without optimizing equipment, delivery failure may occur. This may result in a stent that is delivered proximal to the intended target lesion. This will be more of a problem with bare-wire stents without delivery sheaths but occur with the latter. Failure of stent delivery will be further complicated by the fact that the indication for placement will often be abrupt or threatened closure with ongoing patient ischemia. The wire coil stents, which are probably more likely to be at risk, are extremely fragile, constructed out of metallic strands as thin as 0.007 inch. Some stents are made of stainless steel, which is very difficult to visualize. This further compounds the problem since proper placement of the stent may be difficult to confirm angiographically. Premature deployment may occur in several locations at different times during the procedure (Table 30.1).

Passage Through the Hemostatic Adapter and Guiding Catheter

Unless the Tuohy Borst hemostatic adapter is sufficiently open, the stent can be displaced on initial entry into the guiding catheter. If the guiding catheter is too small for the stent size selected, this can also result in the stent being stripped from the delivery balloon. An uncommon problem may occur if side holes have been placed in the catheter with a hole punch or if the catheter tip has kinked; in

Table 30.1.
Factors That May Be Associated With Premature Stent Deployment

Passage through Tuohy Borst or guiding catheter
Entry into the coronary or vein graft ostium with bare wire stent
Proximal to lesion
Withdrawal of the stent sheath proximal to the lesion and
   advancement of the bare stent

either case the irregularity that results on the inner lumen of the guiding catheter can strip the stent off the delivery balloon. For radiolucent stents (e.g., the Cook Flex-Stent) this mishap may only be recognized as loss of the characteristic indentation of the stent on the balloon. For this reason it is important to carefully examine the delivery balloon when it reaches the distal end of the guide catheter in the ascending aorta before the balloon exits the distal tip of the guiding catheter. Recognition of stent loss from the delivery balloon, onto the proximal part of the balloon catheter, before the delivery balloon is exited from the guide catheter may greatly reduce the chance of further mishap related to the stent. If the stent has been stripped off the balloon and is in the guide but this is not recognized by the operator, the delivery balloon may be advanced into place and inflated. Absence of the stent at this time may be recognized by a change in the characteristic pattern of balloon expansion when the balloon is inflated. Typically, the deployment balloon will expand from the ends symmetrically toward the center of the balloon. When the stent is stripped, however, the balloon inflates relatively symmetrically over its entire length. Under some circumstances, this may be the only clue that the stent has been lost from the delivery balloon. Of course, stripping of a radiopaque stent is much more readily identified.

Entry Into the Coronary Artery or Vein Graft Ostium

Meticulous attention must be paid to the alignment of the guiding catheter. If an acute angle is present between the guiding catheter tip and the vessel ostium, the rather bulky delivery balloon may be unable to be passed smoothly into the vessel. The stent delivery balloon may exit the guide catheter but be unable to negotiate the turn into the ostium, resulting in dislodgment of the guide catheter position. At this point, the stent delivery balloon may be fully out of the guiding catheter, may be only partially engaged into the coronary ostium, or under some circumstances may be completely outside of the coronary or vein graft system. Firm guide support catheters and heavy-bodied guidewires help to prevent this situation, but this may occur even when optimal equipment is used. Clearly, disease at the vessel ostium may further contribute to this problem. Since the distal tip of most guiding catheters is angulated, retraction of the delivery balloon and stent to pull the stent back into the guiding catheter generally requires that the stent negotiate some angle to reenter the guiding catheter tip. This usually results in damage to the stent as it catches the end of the guide catheter. Under the worst of circumstances, the stent may catch in the guide catheter tip and be completely stripped off the delivery balloon as the balloon catheter is withdrawn into the guide catheter. This leaves the stent free of the delivery balloon, generally outside of the coronary system, and held in place only by the coronary guidewire.

Proximal to the Lesion

The final location of premature deployment is proximal to the lesion but within the coronary artery. This may occur when the proximal vessel is too tortuous or is diffusely diseased. Passage of the stent delivery balloon into the vessel may bring the stent into the proximal portion of the vessel, but it may not be possi-

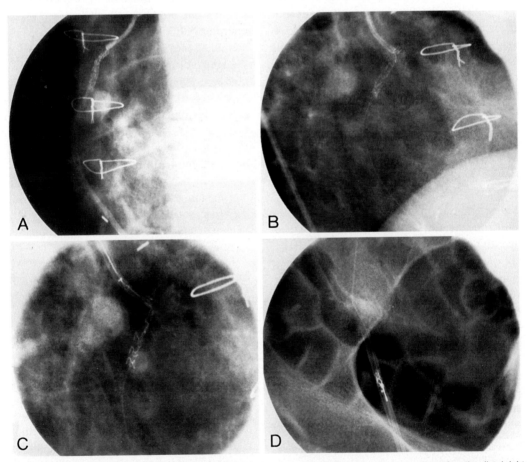

Figure 30.6. **A.** A bare metal coil stent has been implanted in an ostial lesion in a saphenous vein graft to the distal right coronary artery. Full deployment was not possible. **B** and **C.** The stent was grasped and slowly withdrawn into the guiding catheter. **D.** The stent was then removed through the femoral arterial sheath.

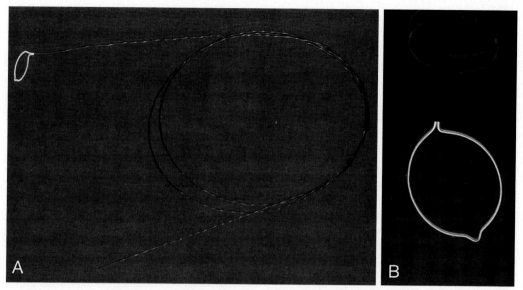

Figure 30.7. An Amplatz loop snare can also be used to remove stents.

ble to reach the target lesion. Withdrawal of the stent delivery balloon can cause the stent to be stripped away from the balloon, as the stent may catch on luminal irregularities of the proximal vessel. This seems to be a particular problem in heavily calcified vessels. Under such circumstances, the best option may be to inflate the deployment balloon and deliver the stent in a more proximal location than would be ideal.

Although bare wire coil stents are more apt to be damaged than "sheathed" stents, the latter can be deployed in the wrong location. During sheath withdrawal the entire stent catheter may be moved proximal to the lesion. Attempts at advancing the stent under these circumstances may strip the sheath.

Retrieval Techniques

Although these conditions can usually be avoided, there are cases in which the stent is deployed prematurely. The approach to this "retained component" varies depending on where the stent is located, whether it is damaged or partially inflated, and whether the guidewire remains through the stent into the distal vessel.

If the guidewire remains through the stent, the most important principle is to retain the guidewire position (Fig. 30.6). Perhaps the easiest approach, particularly if the stent is in the proximal coronary artery or in the ascending aorta, is to place a 1.5-mm or even 2.0-mm conventional balloon through the noninflated stent. The balloon is then inflated and withdrawn, trapping the stent between the balloon and the guiding catheter. The guiding catheter and balloon can then be withdrawn as a unit while leaving the guidewire positioned through the lesion. Alternatively, the stent can be snared with a loop (Fig. 30.7) or with a bioptome if it is in the ostium of the coronary artery and then withdrawn.

A variety of snares or grasping devices can also be used within the coronary artery itself. The majority of these are relatively bulky, but can be delivered through a sheath. If the stent is partly inflated within the vessel, it can still be extracted although arterial damage may occur. Alternatively, if retraction looks difficult, it may be more reasonable to dilate and implant the stent where it is, provided that it does not prevent access to an important side branch. Another stent can then be placed in the arterial segment originally intended for stenting. Prior to that, care should be taken to rectify any problems that led to the initial premature deployment.

SUMMARY

Retained components remain an uncommon problem for the interventional cardiologist. This situation can usually be avoided by meticulous attention to details, but may still occur. Assessment of the problem requires optimal radiographic equipment. High-definition fluoroscopy is needed to visualize retained components, particularly the stainless steel stents. Assessment of the three-dimensional relationship between the coronary arterial structures and the foreign body is essential to select the optimal retrieval system. Efforts should be made to ensure access to the distal coronary arterial bed and to allow for atraumatic removal if possible. If safe removal is not possible, the stent may be deployed, provided it does not compromise an important side branch. Alternatively, in rare cases, surgical removal may be required.

REFERENCES

1. Kaufmann UP, Meier B. Guidewires. In: Vlietstra RE, Holmes DR Jr, eds. Coronary balloon angioplasty. Cambridge, MA: Blackwell Scientific, 1993.

2. Hartzler GO, Rutherford BD, McConahay DR. Retained percutaneous transluminal coronary angioplasty equipment and their management. Am J Cardiol 1987;60:1260–1264.

3. Kaltai M, Barteak I, Beiro V. Guidewire snap causing left main coronary occlusion during coronary angioplasty. Cathet Cardiovasc Diagn 1986;12:324–326.

4. Arce-Gonzalez JM, Schartz L, Ganassin L et al. Complications associated with the guidewire in percutaneous coronary angioplasty. J Am Coll Cardiol 1987;10:218–221.

5. Khonsari S, Livermore J, Mahrer P et al. Fracture and dislodgment of floppy guidewire during percutaneous transluminal coronary angioplasty. Am J Cardiol 1986;58:855–856.

6. Steele PM, Holmes DR Jr, Mankin HT, Schaff HV. Intravascular retrieval of broken guidewire from the ascending aorta after percutaneous transluminal coronary angioplasty. Cathet Cardiovasc Diagn 1985;11:623–628.

7. Foster-Smith KW, Garratt KN, Higano ST, Holmes DR Jr. Retrieval techniques for managing flexible intracoronary stent misplacement. Cathet Cardiovasc Diagn 1993; 30:63–68.

8. Krone RJ. Successful percutaneous removal of retained broken coronary angioplasty guidewire segment. Cathet Cardiovasc Diagn 1986;12:409–410.

31. Management of the Vascular Sheath Following PTCA

HARRY H. GIBBS and TIMOTHY A. SANBORN

The introduction of the Seldinger technique of percutaneous arterial catheterization provided rapid and easy access to the coronary circulation and expedited the dramatic development of interventional cardiac catheterization (1). The placement of a vascular sheath in the femoral artery facilitated catheter exchanges, but had no major impact on procedural techniques or complications. With the introduction of coronary angioplasty by Gruentzig in 1977 (2), however, placement of a vascular sheath became necessary since the need for periprocedural anticoagulation with heparin prevented immediate catheter removal because of the inability to achieve hemostasis. To minimize the incidence of peripheral vascular complications of PTCA, patients at risk of vascular complications should be identified and meticulous care exercised with the arterial access procedure, with the timing of sheath removal, and with the hemostasis procedure (3).

VASCULAR RISK ASSESSMENT

There are several factors that identify those patients at risk of developing peripheral vascular complications. These risk factors should be sought prior to PTCA and meticulous care taken with both the arterial access and hemostasis procedures to minimize complications. Female gender, advanced age, a history of congestive heart failure, peripheral vascular disease, a smaller body surface area, or a cardiac intervention (e.g., PTCA, valvuloplasty, atherectomy, stent placement) rather than a diagnostic cardiac catheterization all predict a greater risk of vascular complication (4, 5). In patients undergoing PTCA, anticoagulation or thrombolytic therapy and the use of a larger sheath also are associated with more complications (4, 6). A number of epidemiologic factors that are associated with the development of atherosclerotic vascular disease are not, however, associated with an increased risk of peripheral vascular complications. These include diabetes, hyperlipidemia, cigarette smoking, hypertension, family history of heart disease, and cerebrovascular disease (5). In the subset of patients undergoing IABP placement, however, diabetes has been reported to significantly increase the risk of vascular complications (7). PTCA has a reported incidence of vascular complication requiring surgery of 0.9 to 1.5% and a risk of bleeding requiring transfusion of up to 6.6% (4, 6, 8). Identification of high-risk patients may help reduce the occurrence of these complications.

ARTERIAL ACCESS PROCEDURE

Arterial puncture and sheath placement should only be performed in the common femoral artery (CFA). Inadvertent puncture of the superficial femoral artery (SFA) may result in subsequent pseudoaneurysm or arteriovenous fistula formation (9). There are several reasons why puncture of the SFA rather than the common femoral artery (CFA) increases the incidence of pseudoaneurysm formation: (a) the CFA overlies the femoral head, which provides bony support for better vessel compression following sheath removal; (b) the

SFA has a smaller diameter than the CFA, increasing the size of the puncture relative to the vessel circumference; and (c) the CFA has additional support from the femoral sheath in which it lies with the common femoral vein. Arteriovenous fistula formation is associated with simultaneous puncture of the artery and vein, the risk of which is greater with puncture of the SFA as it lies over the femoral vein, whereas the CFA has a relative paucity of overlying venous side branches. Localization of the skin puncture site to a position directly above the inferior border of the femoral head will result in successful puncture of the CFA in 95% of cases when the needle is angled between 30° and 45° to the skin (9). The skin puncture site is easily identified by positioning the needle tip over the inferior border of the femoral head under fluoroscopic control. The inguinal skin crease should be avoided as an anatomic marker since its relation to the CFA is quite variable, particularly in the obese patient when it is displaced inferiorly by pannus.

HEMOSTASIS METHOD

Hemostasis following sheath removal has traditionally been achieved by direct compression over the arterial puncture site to allow thrombus formation. This may be performed manually or by the use of mechanical devices. During manual compression, digital pressure is exerted to partially occlude the femoral artery for a period of about 20 minutes after which time pressure is slowly released and hemostasis assessed. A number of mechanical devices have also been used to apply pressure to the femoral puncture site. The commonest device in clinical practice is the mechanical clamp, which consists of a C arm attached to a flat base. The base is positioned under the patient's hip; the C arm, with a small, plastic disk at its end, is lowered onto the skin over the puncture site; and sufficient pressure is applied to prevent bleeding, while maintaining a palpable distal pulse. Once applied, the device remains in position and

frees the operator to perform other duties. This device has been shown to reduce hemostasis time and hematoma formation when compared with manual compression (10).

A pneumatic compression device has recently been described (11). This device consists of an inflatable, transparent bubble that is attached to an arch made of hard plastic. The bubble is positioned over the femoral arterial puncture site and secured there by means of the plastic arch and a belt under the patient's hips. As the catheter is removed from the femoral artery, the bubble is inflated to a high pressure to temporarily occlude the vessel. Since the bubble is transparent, it is possible to see when bleeding has stopped. After brief total occlusion of the femoral artery, pressure within the bubble is lowered to allow palpation of the pedal pulses but without bleeding from the puncture site. Pressure is then applied until hemostasis is achieved. Preliminary data have shown this device to be safe and effective in achieving hemostasis; however, the time to achieve hemostasis and the incidence of bleeding and hematomas was not significantly different from manual compression (11). Whether this device can reduce patient discomfort or postprocedure care remains to be determined.

It is common for a pressure dressing to be applied to the groin site following femoral arterial puncture. This practice, however, has not been shown to reduce the incidence of local complications. Pressure dressings that use adhesive tape have a high incidence of allergic skin reactions, which limit their usefulness (12).

NEW HEMOSTATIC TECHNIQUES

Extravascular Collagen Hemostatic Device

A collagen vascular hemostatic device (Vasoseal, Datascope, Oakland, NJ) has recently been reported to be effective in achieving hemostasis following femoral arterial catheterization with a significantly reduced groin compression time (13–16). The hemostasis procedure involves positioning a short, 11.5

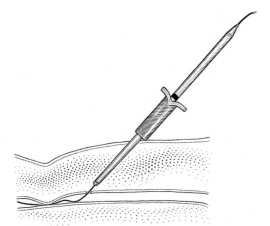

Figure 31.1. The 11.5 Fr dilator and sheath system is advanced over a guidewire to the surface of the femoral artery.

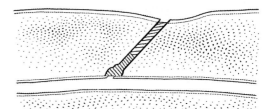

Figure 31.3. Hemostasis is completed following a short period of manual compression.

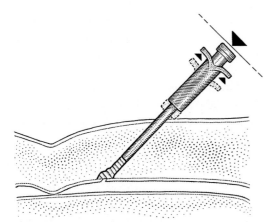

Figure 31.2. During complete manual arterial compression, the guidewire and dilator are removed and collagen is advanced through the sheath into the tract from the femoral artery to the skin.

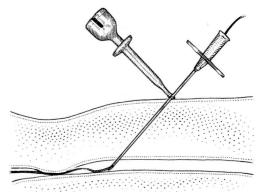

Figure 31.4. At the time of initial arterial puncture, a clamp is attached to the needle to measure the skin-to-artery distance. Using a needle depth indicator, the skin-to-artery distance is used to determine the desired vascular hemostatic device kit size.

Fr sheath on the adventitial surface of the femoral artery and instilling absorbable bovine collagen in the tract from the femoral artery to the skin surface (Figs. 31.1 and 31.2). Complete manual compression of the femoral artery is then performed for 1 minute after which light pressure is maintained for a variable time, usually between 2 and 5 minutes, until hemostasis is achieved (Fig. 31.3). Intraarterial instillation of collagen is avoided by measuring the distance from the skin to the femoral arterial puncture site at the time of

sheath placement to determine the length of collagen required for the hemostasis procedure (Fig. 31.4). In addition, the delivery sheath is at least 2.5 Fr sizes larger than the arterial sheath used for the interventional procedure, which aids in preventing the collagen from entering the artery. Currently, the hemostatic device is restricted to use with sheaths of ≤9 Fr to avoid inadvertent intraarterial collagen injection and possible arterial thrombosis. Clinical trials have demonstrated this device to be safe and effective in achieving hemostasis following PTCA, as well as diagnostic catheterization (14–16). Arterial compression times and the time to ambulation are reduced. In the largest series to date, 466 patients undergoing diagnostic catheterization and PTCA both on and off heparin were randomized to hemostasis by Vasoseal or conventional arterial compression (14). In the 134 control patients having manual or mechanical arterial compression, hemostasis time was 35.5 ± 27.1 minutes. In the group of 71 Vasoseal patients undergoing PTCA in whom heparin was discontinued 4 hours prior to the hemostasis procedure, compression time to achieve hemostasis was 4.6 ± 4.1 minutes. In the 85 PTCA patients in whom Vasoseal was used during full anticoagulation with heparin, 7.4 ± 11.4 minutes of compression time was required for hemostasis. These reductions in hemostasis times were highly statistically significant. In a second study 145 patients were randomized either to immediate sheath removal on full anticoagulation using Vasoseal (81 pts) or to standard sheath removal by arterial compression the morning following PTCA after discontinuation of heparin (64 patients) (15). Vasoseal patients were fully anticoagulated (mean ACT 338 ± 50 seconds) at the time of sheath removal and remained on full anticoagulation overnight, as did the control patients. The times to ambulation following the PTCA procedure were 15.1 ± 10.3 and 33.7 ± 10.4 hours for the Vasoseal and control groups, respectively, which was highly statistically significant.

Hemostatic Puncture-Closuring Device With Intraluminal Anchor

Another device that attaches a plug of collagen to the adventitial surface of the femoral artery with an intraluminal anchor by way of a positioning suture is also currently under investigation. To date there are no reports of long-term follow-up after the use of this device (17).

TIMING OF SHEATH REMOVAL

There is little data to support a firm recommendation for the most appropriate timing of vascular sheath removal. Clinical practice and the angiographic result of PTCA dictate the timing of sheath removal rather than the results of randomized trials (18). Following uncomplicated PTCA, sheath removal may be performed 3 to 4 hours after the initial heparin bolus. Bleeding complications may be more frequent following prolonged anticoagulation. In patients with a suboptimal PTCA result who have an arterial dissection, an angiographic appearance suggestive of thrombus at the dilation site, or other procedural predictors of abrupt closure, the usual clinical practice has been to continue intravenous heparin for 12 to 24 hours and, if clinically stable, to then discontinue heparin and remove the sheath 4 hours later. This approach allows maintenance of full anticoagulation and rapid access to the coronary circulation in the event of abrupt closure. New hemostatic devices that allow sheath removal during full anticoagulation have been discussed above. Monitoring the level of anticoagulation by the activated clotting time (ACT) aids in the timing of sheath removal. The ACT provides a rapid assessment of heparin effect and may be performed serially until it falls below the therapeutic range. An ACT of less than 200 indicates a low level of anticoagulation that should allow effective hemostasis by arterial compression. Sheath removal during anticoagulation increases the incidence of pseudoaneurysm formation, and measurement of the ACT may reduce this complication, although there are no published data to this effect (6).

CARE OF THE PATIENT WITH AN INDWELLING SHEATH

Patients with a sheath remaining in situ in the femoral artery should remain supine and be observed closely for the development of vascular complications. The commonest complications are bleeding and hematoma formation at the arterial puncture site. This is often only mild oozing associated with overanticoagulation. This problem may usually be controlled by a reduction or temporary discontinuation of the heparin infusion and by light digital pressure over the arterial puncture site. More severe bleeding, however, may be controlled by changing the vascular sheath to one of a larger size (e.g., replace a 7 Fr sheath with an 8 Fr sheath). If these methods fail and significant blood loss continues, then the sheath may need to be removed as anemia or hypotension may produce myocardial ischemia and abrupt closure. In this instance arterial compression may be required for a number of hours until the anticoagulation effect of heparin has reversed. Mechanical compression devices such as the C arm clamp or the pneumatic compression device greatly relieve operator fatigue during these prolonged hemostasis procedures. Alternatively, a collagen vascular hemostasis device may be used to achieve arterial hemostasis even during full anticoagulation. A new, flexible, vascular sheath has been developed that allows the patient to sit up to $60°$ with the sheath in place (19). Patient discomfort, as assessed by the need for analgesia, is less using the flexible sheath. Hemostasis times and vascular complication rates were not different in the small group of patients in whom the use of this sheath has been reported.

REFERENCES

1. Seldinger SI. Catheter placement of the needle in percutaneous angiography: a new technique. Acta Radiol 1953; 39:368.
2. Gruentzig AR, Senning A, Seigenthaler WE. Nonoperative dilatation of coronary artery stenosis: percutaneous coronary angioplasty. N Engl J Med 1979;301:61.
3. Gibbs H, Sanborn T. Peripheral vascular complications of diagnostic and interventional cardiac catheterization. Cardiovasc Intervent 1992;2:10.
4. Oweida SW, Roubin GS, Smith RB, Salam AA. Postcatheterization vascular complications associated with percutaneous transluminal coronary angioplasty. J Vasc Surg 1990;12:310.
5. McCann RL, Schwartz LB, Pieper KS. Vascular complications of cardiac catheterization. J Vasc Surg 1991;14:375.
6. Muller DW, Shamir KJ, Ellis SG, Topol EJ. Peripheral vascular complications after conventional and complex percutaneous coronary interventional procedures. Am J Cardiol 1992;69:63.
7. Kantrowitz A, Wasfie T, Freed P et al. Intraaortic balloon pumping 1967 through 1982: analysis of complications in 733 patients. Am J Cardiol 1986;57:976.
8. Grines CL, Glazier S, Bakalyar D et al. Predictors of bleeding complications following coronary angioplasty. Circulation 1991;84:II-591.
9. Kim D, Orron DE, Skillman JJ et al. Role of superficial femoral artery puncture in the development of pseudoaneurysm and arteriovenous fistula complicating percutaneous transfemoral cardiac catheterization. Cathet Cardiovasc Diagn 1992;25:91.
10. Semler HJ. Transfemoral catheterization: mechanical versus manual control of bleeding. Radiology 1985;154:234.
11. Nordrehaug J, Chronos N, Foran J et al. Randomized evaluation of a new inflatable femoral artery compression device after cardiac angiography. Circulation 1992;86:I-382.
12. Eisenberg RL, Mani RL. Pressure dressings and postangiographic care of the femoral puncture site. Radiology 1977;122:677.
13. Merino A, Faulkner C, Corvalan A, Sanborn TA. Percutaneous vascular hemostatic device for interventional procedures. Cathet Cardiovasc Diagn 1992;26:319.
14. Sanborn T, Brinker J, Kosinski E et al. Reduced compression time using a vascular hemostatic device after diagnostic angiography and angioplasty: a multicenter randomized trial. Circulation 1992;86:I-372.
15. Gibbs H, Molloy T, Shaftel P, Barra L, Sanborn T. Reduced hemostasis time and early ambulation following percutaneous transluminal coronary angioplasty using a collagen vascular hemostatic device. Presented at the Cardiac Society of Australia and New Zealand Annual Scientific Meeting, 1993.
16. Gibbs J, Slade A, Nordrehaug J et al. The use of a collagen plug for femoral arterial haemostasis following cardiac catheterization: single institution experience. Eur Heart J 1992;13(Suppl):428.
17. Kensey KR, Evans DG, McGill LD, Nash JC. In vivo feasibility testing of a bioresorbable hemostatic puncture closing device. J Am Coll Cardiol 1991;17:263A.
18. Popma J, Dehmer G. Care of the patient after coronary angioplasty. Ann Intern Med 1989;110:547.

32. Acute Myocardial Infarction

A. Acute Myocardial Infarction

JOEL K. KAHN and WILLIAM W. O'NEILL

The use of coronary interventions in the treatment of acute myocardial infarction (MI) has been advocated for over a decade, but the pendulum of enthusiasm for this approach has swung widely during this period. We have remained dedicated to this approach because of the inherent advantages that we appreciated in the management of patients with acute MI in the catheterization laboratory (Table 32A.1). The controversy has been resolved with the completion of the Primary Angioplasty Myocardial Infarction (PAMI) I trial (1), which documented a lower frequency of nonfatal reinfarction and death in patients with acute MI treated with direct angioplasty compared with intravenous tissue plasminogen activator (Table 32A.2). A striking reduction in recurrent ischemia and stroke was also observed in the angioplasty-treated patients. It is appropriate therefore to consider coronary interventions as the optimal approach to acute MI and thrombolytic therapy as a second-line treatment for patients where coronary intervention is not readily available. The purpose of this chapter is to familiarize coronary interventionalists with our protocol for treating patients with acute MI at William Beaumont Hospital.

PRE–CATHETERIZATION LABORATORY PHASE

Patients presenting to the emergency room at William Beaumont Hospital with a suspected acute myocardial infarction are managed by a multidisciplinary team as a true medical emergency similar to a major trauma case. A triage nurse at the entrance directs the patient to a dedicated chest pain emergency room, where a specialized nursing staff with experience in coronary care unit or catheterization laboratory nursing quickly obtains a brief history, vital signs, and a 12-lead electrocardiogram. An emergency room physician is assigned to the area to facilitate the evaluation and early therapy of ischemic syndromes, but a staff interventional cardiologist, assigned by a formal call schedule, is available routinely within 15 minutes. In obvious cases of acute MI, pharmacologic therapies (see below) are begun while the catheterization laboratory is readied. In unclear cases, a state-of-the-art echocardiographic recorder dedicated to the chest pain center is used to assess left ventricular wall motion. The chest pain center nurses have been formally instructed in the use of the echocardiogram. All patients with inferior wall myocardial infarction on initial electrocardiography and all patients with chest pain and normal 12-lead electrocardiography have right-sided precordial electrocardiograms recorded (2). Patients with initially normal or nondiagnostic tracings will have the electrocardiogram repeated as often as every 30 minutes if symptoms continue to assess for evolving signs of ischemia.

Emergency room therapy is begun rapidly and involves multiple pharmacologic agents to ameliorate myocardial ischemia and pretreat patients for possible coronary intervention. All patients receive 325 mg of soluble aspirin that is chewed. Patients are bolused intravenously with 10,000 units of heparin, and an infusion is begun. Intravenous nitroglycerin is infused if the systolic blood pressure is >100 mm Hg. This medication is used in very low doses in patients with electro-

Table 32A.1.

Potential Advantages of Direct Angioplasty for the Treatment of Acute Myocardial Infarction

1. Contraindications limited to absent vascular access and severe contrast allergy (<1% of patients)
2. Rapid confirmation of diagnosis with coronary arteriography
3. Rapid appreciation of prognosis by assessment of left ventricular function and coronary anatomy
4. Recanalization rates over 90% in native coronary arteries
5. Recanalization rates over 80% in saphenous vein grafts
6. Final residual lumen typically <40%
7. Rapid access to life-sustaining treatments (temporary pacemaker, intraaortic balloon pump, intubation ventilation) if needed
8. Extremely low rate of complicating stroke
9. Low rates of in-hospital reinfarction
10. Potential for early discharge in low-risk patient

Table 32A.2.

A Comparison of Immediate Angioplasty Versus Intravenous Thrombolytic Therapy (t-PA) in the Primary Angioplasty Myocardial Infarction I Study[a]

	Angioplasty	t-PA
Patient number	195	200
Success	97%	—
Reinfarction	5 (2.6%)	13 (6.5%)
Death	5 (2.6%)	13 (6.5%)
Stroke	0	7 (3.5%)
Recurrent ischemia	10 (5.1%)	47 (23.5%)
Six-week ejection fraction	53%	53%
Six-month reinfarction or death	16 (8.5%)	32 (16.8%)

[a]Adapted from Grines CL, Browne KF, Marco J et al. N Engl J Med 1993; 328:673–679.

cardiographic, clinical, or echocardiographic evidence of right ventricular infarction because of the hypotension that may be precipitated. Patients with tachycardia (rate >100 beats/minute) who are free of rales, wheezing, or advanced heart block receive intravenous beta-blockers, typically metoprolol 5 mg administered three times over 15 minutes. Finally, after a preprinted informed consent is obtained that lists the possibility of angioplasty, atherectomy, intravessel thrombolytics, intraaortic balloon pumping, and emergency bypass surgery, liberal dosing of morphine sulfate is prescribed to achieve sedation and chest pain relief. We have been omitting intravenous lidocaine except in patients with frequent multiform premature ventricular contractions or salvos of nonsustained ventricular tachycardia.

In the past a major question existed as to whether pretreatment with intravenous thrombolytic agents should occur when coronary intervention is anticipated. To clarify this important question, we performed a randomized trial of infarct angioplasty with and without adjunctive thrombolytic therapy using intravenous streptokinase (3). Overall, we found that thrombolytic therapy was harmful. Angioplasty was not facilitated, ventricular function was equally preserved, and long-term patency was not augmented by

adjunctive streptokinase. Intravenous streptokinase was associated with more frequent local and systemic bleeding, a greater need for emergency bypass surgery, and a longer length of stay with higher hospital costs. For these reasons we would strongly advocate withholding thrombolytic agents when infarct angioplasty is planned. We feel that intravenous thrombolytic agents should be administered only when a protracted length of time (>120 minutes) is anticipated prior to initiation of intervention. One of the major advantages of infarct angioplasty is the fact that this therapy is highly successful without the added risk of stroke associated with thrombolytic therapy.

CATHETERIZATION LABORATORY

Our goal is to have patients on the catheterization laboratory table within 30 minutes of presenting to the emergency department. In the laboratory, electrocardiographic monitors are attached, oxygen is continued, and intravenous lines are sorted and organized. We use radiolucent precordial electrodes to permit monitoring of 12-lead electrocardiograms in the laboratory. Both inguinal regions are shaved and prepared with iodine solution. The patient is quickly draped and the injector and manifold are loaded with low-ionic contrast media. We routinely obtain arterial and venous access with 8 Fr sheaths. The venous sheath permits the reliable administration of medications and allows ready placement of a transvenous pacemaker or pulmonary artery catheter when needed. The pulmonary artery catheter is especially useful in patients with signs of right ventricular infarction to aid in management of volume administration. However, we do not routinely place these catheters in uncomplicated cases. In patients with low blood pressures, arterial access with a Doppler needle (Smart Needle, Peripheral Systems Group, Santa Clara, CA) may aid in cannulation.

During this early catheterization period, attention must also be focused on the status of the patient. If needed, stabilization of the patient's hemodynamics with fluids, vasopressors, or inotropes should be begun. We have routinely used intravenous dextran to provide added antiplatelet therapy. Transcutaneous oxygen monitoring should be attached and supplementation provided as needed. If necessary, it is preferable to electively intubate patients with pulmonary edema and respiratory difficulties before the angioplasty as compared with dealing with obtunded patients requiring emergency intubation later. Patients with frank cardiogenic shock will usually benefit from the percutaneous placement of an intraaortic balloon pump before the angioplasty is begun. Throughout this early period, liberal sedation with benzodiazepines and opiates are administered to reduce the anxiety of the patient.

We perform contrast ventriculography as the initial procedure in almost all patients with suspected acute MI. The only exception is in patients with profound cardiogenic shock with hypotension and respiratory distress. This study can be performed with as little as 25 to 30 cc of contrast and provides invaluable information. End-diastolic pressures can be measured, left ventricular systolic performance can be judged, regional wall motion abnormalities can be identified confirming the presence of ongoing and prior ventricular damage, the presence and sever-

ity of mitral regurgitation can be estimated, true and false aneurysms of the left ventricle can be identified, and intracardiac clot may be observed. We have recently studied a patient with an evolving inferior wall MI who unexpectedly demonstrated a contained rupture of the inferior wall on routine contrast ventriculography. This was not observed on the echocardiogram performed in the emergency department, and it led to immediate referral of the patient for bypass surgery and successful repair of the rupture.

We generally select a 7 Fr diagnostic catheter to inject the suspected noninfarct artery. Adequate views are obtained for complete diagnosis. An 8 Fr guiding catheter is then used to select the suspected infarct artery. Although it may be tempting to use 7 Fr guide catheters to avoid the additional arterial stretch, firm guide support may be required in infarct intervention and we rely on the 8 Fr systems. Angiograms are obtained in multiple views to completely document the coronary anatomy. In about 15% of cases, the force of the injections alone will recanalize an artery totally occluded with fresh thrombus. More commonly, contrast will stain the site of recent occlusion, but will not restore flow. In patients with prior bypass surgery, surgical reports are generally not available and saphenous and mammary grafts are sought with appropriate catheters. Freshly occluded saphenous vein bypass grafts typically have a meniscus appearance with thrombus that stains with contrast. In up to 10% of patients with prior bypass surgery presenting with acute MI, however, it may be impossible to ascertain the infarct vessel because of occlusion of both the native and graft vessels.

An individualized strategy for revascularization must be determined for each patient at this point in the procedure. In the PAMI I trial 90% of patients with acute MI studied with emergency angiography had coronary anatomy appropriate for intervention (1). Certain patients, however, may require alternative approaches. The presence of a severe narrowing of the left main coronary artery is generally a reason for referral for emergency bypass surgery rather than transcatheter revascularization. Rarely, we have revascularized a freshly occluded right coronary artery in the setting of left main narrowing with subsequent referral for elective bypass surgery several days later. We also consider patients for emergency coronary bypass surgery who have critical multivessel disease with a coronary lesion in the infarct vessel that is poorly suited for intervention because of tortuosity, excessive length, or extreme calcification. In the PAMI I trial nine of 195 patients (5%) were referred for emergency bypass surgery (1). In all of these cases the outcome was successful. Occasionally, by the time of emergency angiography, the infarct vessel will have reperfused, perhaps as a result of the actions of intravenous heparin and aspirin. If an artery less than 70% narrowed is present with TIMI grade III flow, we will not perform an intervention and medical therapy will be pursued. In the PAMI I study eight of 195 patients (4%) met these criteria (1). Rarely, the infarct vessel cannot be identified because of multiple occluded arteries. This is slightly more common in patients with prior bypass surgery as mentioned. In these patients medical therapy may be selected if ischemia has resolved or if ongoing, careful probing with an angioplasty guidewire of the most likely infarct vessel is attempted.

When a commitment to intervention is determined, a second bolus of 10,000 units of heparin is usually administered. Activated thrombin times are measured frequently throughout the procedure and are kept over 350 seconds. We usually select an 0.014-inch compatible balloon catheter sized to match the infarct vessel proximal to the site of narrowing or occlusion. We generally do not predilate with an undersized balloon, and we do not use perfusion balloons since the trade-off in crossing profile has not proven advantageous. A soft-tip guidewire is chosen and carefully shaped based on the anatomy to be navigated. Recently we have selected longer balloon catheters (30 to 40 mm) routinely for infarct angioplasty and have found them useful for balloon positioning without the "watermelon-seed" effect. The guidewire is directed to the site of occlusion. If a tapered stump provides a clue to the path of the true lumen, it is followed. Otherwise, the stump is gently probed, and when an area permitting slight penetration of the guidewire is identified, it is pursued. Most commonly, a soft guidewire can be manipulated through the occlusion without tremendous force. Occasionally, the balloon catheter and guide will need to be advanced to provide increased support for the balloon. It is uncommon to have to bring the balloon catheter all the way down to the occlusion to facilitate crossing of the guidewire, but when gently probing of the wire is met repeatedly by buckling, this may be necessary. In less than 5% of acute infarcts a stiffer guidewire of either an intermediate or a standard construction may be required to pierce a firm occlusion. This is most likely to occur when symptom duration is longer than 6 hours. Generally, we have found that the earlier the patient is treated, the softer and easier the thrombus is to cross. Great care should be taken not to create a dissection plane, which may complicate all further attempts at recanalization. In only a small number of cases will it be difficult or impossible to cross a total occlusion presumed to be causing an MI. Even recently occluded saphenous vein grafts usually yield to deliberate and careful attempts to wire the true lumen (4). Repeated failure should prompt a consideration of whether the vessel being instrumented might be a chronic total occlusion erroneously judged to be the site of recent thrombosis. In unusual cases of complete failure to cross infarct vessels with the guidewire, efforts at recanalization may have to be abandoned. Alternatively, an infusion catheter can be left at the occluded vessel stump, and urokinase can be infused for several hours or overnight in an attempt to salvage the effort.

Once crossed with a guidewire, many occluded infarct vessels will demonstrate restored antegrade flow. Reperfusion arrhythmias and hypotension should be carefully monitored for, particularly when the infarct vessel is the right coronary artery (5). The balloon catheter is then advanced to the lesion. We have found repeatedly that low-pressure inflations (2 to 4 atm) for prolonged periods (60 to 180 seconds) will result in full balloon expansion. If the operator is willing to give lower-pressure inflations a chance, it is the rare infarct vessel that requires greater than 8 atm for complete dilation. We generally inflate two to three times with a goal of achieving the smallest possible residual stenosis with brisk antegrade flow. Not uncommonly, restoration of flow following angioplasty leads to dilation of the distal vessel requiring an exchange for a larger balloon.

Problems can be encountered that require special maneuvers. Intense spasm of the infarct vessel after the first few dilations is relatively common and probably relates to the release of potent vasoconstrictors from platelets and endothelium (6). Time is the greatest ally in restoration of true arterial dimensions, but if the pressure is >100 mm Hg systolic, intracoronary nitroglycerin can be administered to accelerate the phenomenon. Refractory spasm is uncommon but may require brief, low-pressure balloon inflations to terminate.

Dissection can result from guidewire trauma or oversizing of balloons. If flow is TIMI grade III with a large residual lumen, the dissection can be observed for several minutes; if stable, the patient can be left with intravenous heparin infusing, or if more threatening, dissections can be handled in the usual manner. We have used perfusion balloon catheters to repair intimal dissections during infarct angioplasty with good results. Alternatively, we have resorted to salvage directional atherectomy during infarct angioplasty if the dissection does not involve an extraluminal cap implying severe transmural injury. In these cases we have felt that the risk of perforation with directional atherectomy is too high.

Residual thrombus is a challenging problem that complicates less than 25% of infarct interventions. Most commonly, visible thrombus will respond to prolonged balloon inflations with generous-sized balloon catheters. If extensive thrombus is present, the activated thrombin time should be rechecked and further boluses of heparin administered. The next step is to consider intravessel urokinase (250,000 to 500,000 units) administer over 10 to 20 minutes. This may increase the bleeding complications and therefore should be considered carefully. The usefulness of urokinase as an adjunct in infarct intervention has been demonstrated by Morishita et al. who reported that, in infarct vessels demonstrating persistent thrombus after balloon inflation, urokinase improved the angiographic appearance and reduced the rate of restenosis for arteries restudied at 1 month (7). We have also placed intracoronary infusion catheters at the site of narrowing in rare cases of refractory thrombus for local infusions of urokinase for several hours or overnight. In cases of recent thrombosis of saphenous vein grafts, thrombus refractory to balloon dispersion may occur. In cases selected for straight graft anatomy without diffuse friable disease we have advanced multipurpose guiding catheters up to the sight of thrombosis and have applied steady suction to aspirate the debris out of the graft (8). Constant suction must be applied until the guiding catheter completely exits the body to avoid embolization of the thrombus to other arterial circulations.

We have also resorted to using the transluminal extraction catheter (TEC) (Interventional Technologies Inc.) in cases of refractory thrombus, vein graft thrombosis, or salvage of thrombolytic failures during evolving acute MI. This device has a cutting surface that rotates at 800 to 1200 rpm, excising debris. An aspiration port provides constant irrigation and removal of shavings into a vacuum bottle. In data submitted to the Food and Drug Administration, the TEC device has been useful for treatment of intracoronary thrombus. In this investigation 92 patients were treated with a 100% angiographic success and a 96% clinical success. To further explore the role of this device in the management of high-risk acute-infarct patients, a two-center 70-patient trial has recently been completed (9). Although early results appear promising, further studies in larger numbers of patients will be needed before the role of TEC in the therapy of acute MI is resolved.

We have observed embolism of thrombotic fragments to the distal circulation in a small number of cases of infarct intervention. Large fragments can usually be disrupted with agitation of the guidewire. Alternatively, the balloon catheter can be used to inflate and disrupt the debris at low pressures. Greater burdens of distal debris may be precipitated, especially during intervention in occluded vein grafts, and may result in a no-reflow phenomenon. We have recently had some success with large doses of intravessel nitroglycerin (>500 μg) or small doses of intravessel verapamil (0.1 mg) if hypotension and heart block are not present.

Hypotension and bradycardia related to the Bezold-Jarisch reflex can be anticipated with recanalization of totally occluded proximal right coronary arteries (5). Volume replacement may be helpful, particularly if a pulmonary artery catheter has been placed confirming right ventricular involvement. This problem is usually short-lived and responds promptly to intravenous atropine and small boluses of short-acting vasopressors such as metaraminol or neosynephrine. In more refractory cases we have resorted to intraaortic balloon pump counterpulsation for stabilization. Hypotension during any infarct intervention should prompt placement of a pulmonary artery catheter for determination of the pulmonary capillary wedge pressure. If volume replacement, pressors, and intraaortic balloon pumping do not correct the blood pressure, we have resorted in rare cases to using percutaneous cardiopulmonary bypass.

Ventricular tachycardia can complicate infarct intervention. It is usually responsive to standard antiarrhythmic therapy. During right coronary artery reperfusion, however, it may be particularly resistant to standard drug therapy. Intravenous magnesium can be tried but has not been uniformly effective in our experience. We have seen unusual cases where every time the infarct artery is reperfused with balloon deflation, ventricular tachycardia develops and responds only to repeat inflation of the balloon catheter. Intraaortic counterpulsation has stabilized some patients, but others seem very responsive to the administration of 1 to 2 mg of intravenous propanolol. This unusual electrical storm of ventricular tachycardia can take hours to stabilize.

POSTPROCEDURAL CARE

Once a stable luminal result is achieved, the patient's overall status is assessed before transfer from the catheterization laboratory. If hemodynamic instability or pulmonary congestion has occurred, a pulmonary artery catheter is often floated for continuous monitoring in the coronary care unit. If the infarct involved the proximal left anterior descending artery and threatened a large portion of the anterior wall, an intraaortic balloon pump is often inserted at the end of the case through the preexisting arterial access site. This approach has been reported to result in a lower rate of abrupt reclosure and improved ventricular recovery (10), although preliminary data from the randomized PAMI II trial did not find a conclusive benefit with intraaortic balloon pump placement. At this point we feel that an IABP should be placed for hemodynamic instability, but not necessarily routinely for all patients with large infarcts.

In the intensive care unit, intravenous nitroglycerin is infused, usually for 48 hours and then weaned. Intravenous heparin is infused continuously to achieve an activated clotting time of 160 to 200 seconds. Approximately 24 hours after the infarct intervention, if the patient is stable, the heparin will be reduced to between 200 and 500 units/hour; the lower the rate the larger the arterial and venous sheath. The sheaths are removed when the activated clotting time is less than 160 seconds. Two to 4 hours later, while the patient remains at strict bed rest with a sandbag on the groin, the heparin infusion is increased to approximately 1000 units/hour and clotting times are measured and adjusted. In uncomplicated cases heparin is continued intravenously for 2 to 3 days and is then tapered off. Preliminary data from PAMI II suggest that in low-risk patients (age <70, inferior infarction, no hemodynamic compromise or recurrent ischemia) the ICU phase may be eliminated and that patients can be safely discharged on day 3 to 4 (with a 7 day mortality of <2%). In cases complicated by heavy thrombus, saphenous vein graft intervention, suboptimal results, or anteroapical injury, heparin is continued until orally administered warfarin achieves an appropriate degree of anticoagulation. Intra-aortic balloon pumps are generally removed 48 hours after infarct intervention if hemodynamic stability has been observed.

Previously, the mainstay of therapy at discharge following infarct intervention has consisted of aspirin and a calcium channel antagonist, usually diltiazem. This regimen was employed in the PAMI I trial and a cumulative incidence or death or recurrent reinfarction of 8.5% was observed at 6-month follow-up (1). It has recently been suggested by O'Keefe and coworkers at the Mid America Heart Institute that oral beta-blocker therapy at discharge following coronary infarct intervention is associated with a survival advantage compared with calcium antagonist therapy (11). Therefore it would seem proper to discharge patients following infarct interventions on medical programs similar to those of most other infarct patients.

SUMMARY

As we have demonstrated in the PAMI I trial and recently corroborated in the study by Zijlstra and coworkers (12), direct infarct angioplasty is a highly attractive alternative to intravenous thrombolytic therapy for acute infarction. Angioplasty therapy provides a long-term survival advantage, results in shorter and less complicated hospital stays, and lowers the risk of stroke. While angioplasty is clearly more effective, logistic constraints and lack of technical expertise with this therapy may limit its application. In the future it is possible that local centers of excellence for the treatment of infarction may evolve as trauma centers have evolved. This may aid in expanding applicability of this therapy. Interventionalists embarking on infarct angioplasty must be prepared to coordinate the emergency care of extremely ill patients. It must be remembered that infarct angioplasty may be the most challenging of all coronary interventions to safely and successfully complete. A large experience with elective angioplasty is mandatory prior to undertaking this therapy. We are convinced that the information that acute intervention provides when appropriately applied, the extremely high rate of recanalization achieved, and the ability to provide immediate hemodynamic support or emergency bypass surgery, if needed, for high-risk cases make emergency intervention the optimal method of managing acute myocardial infarction.

REFERENCES

1. Grines CL, Browne KF, Marco J et al. A comparison of immediate angioplasty with thrombolytic therapy for acute myocardial infarction. N Engl J Med 1993;328:673–679.
2. Kahn JK, Bernstein M, Bengtson JR. Isolated right ventricular myocardial infarction. Ann Intern Med 1993; 118:708–712.
3. O'Neill WW, Weintraub R, Grines CI et al. A prospective, placebo-controlled, randomized trial of intravenous streptokinase and angioplasty versus lone angioplasty therapy of acute myocardial infarction. Circulation 1992;86:1710–1717.
4. Kahn JK, Rutherford BD, McConahay DR et al. Usefulness of angioplasty for acute myocardial infarction in patients with prior bypass grafting. Am J Cardiol 1990;65:698–702.
5. Kahn JK, Rutherford BD, McConahay DR et al. Catheterization lab events during direct infarct angioplasty: a contemporary analysis. Circulation 1990;82:1910–1915.
6. Kahn JK, Hartzler GO. Evidence for dynamic coronary vasoconstriction in the early minutes of acute myocardial infarction. Am Heart J 1991;121:188–190.
7. Morishita H, Hattori R, Aoyama T. The intracoronary administration of urokinase following direct PTCA for acute myocardial infarction reduces early restenosis. Am Heart J 1992;123:1153–1156.

8. Kahn JK, Hartzler GO. Percutaneous thrombus aspiration in acute myocardial infarction. Cathet Cardiovasc Diagn 1990;20:54–57.

9. Larkin TJ, Grines CL, Safian RD et al. A prospective pilot study of transluminal extraction atherectomy in acute myocardial infarction. Circulation (abstract).

10. Ishihara M, Sato H, Tateishi H, Uchida T, Dote K. Intraaortic balloon pumping as the postangioplasty strategy in acute myocardial infarction. Am Heart J 1991;122:385–389.

11. Sayed-Taha K, Krikorian R, Bresnahan DR et al. Beta-blockers with direct infarct angioplasty: liability or useful adjunct? J Am Coll Cardiol 1993;21:77A (abstract).

12. Zijlstra F, de Boer MJ, Hoorntje JCA et al. A comparison of immediate coronary angioplasty with intravenous streptokinase in acute myocardial infarction. N Engl J Med 1993;328:680–684.

Table 32B.1.
Coronary Intervention for Acute Myocardial Infarction

Primary therapy
Thrombolytic contraindication
Chest pain in absence of ST elevation
Shock
Recurrent myocardial ischemia postthrombolysis
Failure of thrombolysis (rescue PTCA)

B. Intervention in Acute Myocardial Infarction

GUY S. REEDER

Acute myocardial infarction, virtually always the result of thrombotic coronary artery occlusion, has become a major indication for mechanical coronary intervention. To the experienced interventionalist, it is perhaps somewhat ironic that in most cases the technical aspects of this procedure are often more simple, faster, and straightforward than other more "complex" lesions often tackled electively and yet perhaps yield the most gratifying results, both to the operator and to the patient.

INDICATIONS

Indications for acute coronary intervention in myocardial infarction are shown in Table 32B.1. Used as primary therapy for Q-wave infarction, angioplasty results in higher patency rates than any thrombolytic regimen and in equal or better clinical outcomes as demonstrated by the results of three recently published randomized trials comparing acute angioplasty and thrombolytic therapy (1–4). Details of these trials have been discussed elsewhere in this textbook. While patency rates in excess of 90% can be expected with experienced operators, the timely application of this strategy is limited to approximately 15 to 20% of the population. Primary angioplasty is best limited to patients who develop infarction in-hospital or close to catheterization facilities where intervention can be performed within 30 to 45 minutes of patient presentation. Otherwise, thrombolytic therapy should remain the mainstay of treatment for Q-wave infarction.

Thrombolytic contraindications are another important indication for acute coronary intervention. The most devastating complication of thrombolytic therapy is hemorrhagic stroke; risk factors include age >75 years, systolic hypertension >175 mm Hg, and low body weight, as well as prior history of stroke or intracranial neoplasm. In such cases direct angioplasty (with essentially no risk of hemorrhagic stroke) is preferable.

Another important subgroup includes patients who present with chest pain in absence of electrocardiographic ST-segment elevation, as such cases are not generally considered for thrombolytic therapy. (One exception is the patient presenting with ischemic chest pain and ST-segment depression in leads V1 through V3, which may represent posterior wall transmural infarction. Such patients may be thrombolytic candidates.) However, most other patients will usually undergo rapid medical stabilization followed by urgent angiography and angioplasty of appropriate lesions. New enzymatic serum tests such as rapid CK assay, CK isoforms, and troponin-T may allow very early identification of patients with myocardial infarction as opposed to those with prolonged angina or noncardiac pain.

Patients presenting with cardiogenic shock have an extremely high mortality, and noncontrolled trials suggest that this may be significantly reduced with successful angioplasty (5, 6). Therefore urgent angioplasty should be considered in all patients with cardiogenic shock, including those with hemodynamic derangement caused by right ventricular infarction.

Recurrent myocardial ischemia following thrombolytic therapy is a well-accepted indication for angiography and angioplasty as demonstrated by multiple randomized trials (7–11). In the absence of demonstrable ischemia, routine or adjunctive angioplasty is of no benefit and imparts a higher risk of morbidity. Finally, failed thrombolytic therapy has been an accepted indication for so-called rescue angioplasty. Observational data (12) would suggest that rescue angioplasty is successful slightly less often than primary angioplasty and is associated with relatively low mortality in successful cases but high mortality in patients in whom the artery cannot be reopened.

The only randomized trial to investigate this issue was RESCUE (13) (Randomized Comparisons of Rescue Angioplasty with Conservative Management of Patients with Early Failure of Thrombolysis for Acute Anterior Myocardial Infarction). One hundred fifty-one patients with first anterior wall infarction treated with a thrombolytic agent and who angiographically demonstrated occluded infarct vessel within 8 hours of symptom onset were randomized to RESCUE angioplasty or conservative therapy with aspirin, heparin, and coronary vasodilators. The angioplasty success rate was 92%. The combined endpoint of death plus severe congestive heart failure at 30 days was less common in the angioplasty arm than control (6 versus 17%, $P = .05$). Similarly, exercise but not resting ejection fraction also reached statistical significance ($43 \pm 15\%$ versus $38 \pm 13\%, P = .04$).

Logistic problems with the application of rescue angioplasty relate to the difficulty of bedside diagnosis of failed thrombolysis, prompt availability of angioplasty, and a substantially increased risk of morbidity in patients with right coronary occlusion.

In the EPIC trial (14) (Evaluation of 7E3 for the Prevention of Ischemic Complications) 2099 high-risk patients undergoing angioplasty were randomized to 7E3 or placebo and received standard ancillary angioplasty medical treatment. Following a bolus and 12-hour infusion of 7E3, the 30-day composite endpoint of death, myocardial infarction, bypass, or repeat intervention, including stent, was reduced by 35% versus control. Bleeding was increased with twice as many transfusions required in the treatment group and was predominantly related to the groin puncture site and gastrointestinal tract. At 6-month follow-up (15) treated patients had a 23% reduction in major ischemic events or elective revascularization.

CONTRAINDICATIONS

Contraindications to angioplasty for myocardial infarction are shown in Table 32B.2. Numerous randomized studies have demonstrated that routine angioplasty performed very early, during hospitalization, or late following hospitalization (16) for acute infarction in the absence of exercise-induced or spontaneous myocardial ischemia provides no benefit and produces a small increase in patient morbidity. Thus routine angioplasty in the absence of demonstrable ischemia cannot be routinely advised. The second major contraindication is the situation in which thrombolytic therapy can be applied much more quickly than angioplasty. This example may

Table 32B.2.
Coronary Intervention for Acute Myocardial Infarction

Successful thrombolysis without evidence of ischemia
Thrombolytic therapy can be given with much less delay

Table 32B.3.
Procedural Factors

Clinical
  Pain relief
  Hemodynamic stabilization
  Adjunctive therapies
Angiographic
  Prior knowledge of coronary anatomy; bypass graft location, anomalies
  Lesions and vessel characteristics
  Flush occlusion versus stub
  Thrombus
  Graft versus native vessel

relate to the rural hospital where transport of the patient to an angioplasty center might take 1 to 2 hours. Unless thrombolytic contraindications are present, this patient should receive immediate thrombolysis rather than transport for primary angioplasty.

The bulk of data regarding the use of coronary intervention for acute infarction has centered on the patient with Q-wave myocardial infarction. No randomized trials have investigated the role of angioplasty in non–Q-wave infarction. At our institution, most of these patients find their way to early catheterization following medical stabilization, and angioplasty of the culprit vessel is frequently performed.

PROCEDURAL FACTORS

Some of the clinical and angiographic factors useful in guiding the interventional approach are listed in Table 32B.3. From the clinical standpoint, the importance of adequate pain relief and hemodynamic stabilization, including the use of intraaortic balloon pumping or even percutaneous cardiopulmonary support, cannot be overemphasized. The generally accepted adjunctive therapies commonly used for patients undergoing thrombolysis are also appropriate for those undergoing primary angioplasty. These include aspirin and full heparinization with monitoring of the activated clotting time (ACT) with a target of approximately 400 seconds. Nitrates and beta-blockade are also mainstays of treatment.

Angiographic factors play an important role in planning the strategy of revascularization. Any prior knowledge of the coronary anatomy is useful, especially in the presence of prior bypass grafting or if coronary anomalies are known. In patients with acute infarction, we generally use 7 Fr catheters to perform diagnostic angiography because of the almost certain likelihood for subsequent rapid intervention. In patients presenting with unstable symptoms following thrombolysis, 5 or 6 Fr diagnostic catheters are preferable initially since they reduce the risk of groin hematoma and because approximately 15 to 30% of these patients will have multivessel disease or substantially impaired left ventricular function or will otherwise be candidates for surgical revascularization.

Important anatomic characteristics include the location of the coronary or graft ostium and the proximal tortuosity of the vessel. In general, Judkin's guides are suitable for almost all patients with native lesions, as guide support is not a major issue with most acute occlusions. The single most important lesion characteristic is the ability to angiographically identify the stub of the occluded vessel. Most of the time this is possible with the use of angulated views; when no stub is apparent, the operator should consider the possibility of an anomaly such as a separate ostium of the occluded vessel. Aortic flush injections, aortic root angiography, or even transesophageal echocardiography may be useful in identifying an anomalous origin. In the presence of a flush occlusion, it may be necessary to blindly probe with the guidewire, but the success rate is relatively low in this situation.

In contradistinction to chronic total occlusion (where lesion factors such as concentric tapering of the vessel stub, absence of side branches or bridging collaterals, and ability to obtain strong guide support are all necessary for success), with acute occlusions the ability to identify a vessel stub is usually sufficient to ensure initial vessel reopening. Similarly, the selection of a balloon and guidewire are probably not critically important because of the soft nature of fresh thrombus. In general, we favor a soft to medium wire, usually 0.014 inch in diameter with just enough distal bend to allow it to traverse the proximal artery and enter the occluded segment. Gentle advancement and probing of the occlusion with slow wire rotation and a moderate degree of patience will almost always allow the occlusion to be crossed, and then as much wire as possible should be advanced into the distal vessel to prevent inadvertent loss of position during advancement of the balloon. While a low-profile balloon is of theoretical advantage, for these soft lesions probably any of the newer, over-the-wire, prewrapped balloons will be adequate, and inflated balloon size should approximate the size of the nonoccluded proximal segment.

Determining the length of the occlusion can be useful for balloon selection; sometimes there will be faint antegrade opacification of the vessel, which usually indicates a short segment of occlusion. On other occasions retrograde collateralization from the contralateral artery will allow some estimation of occlusion length. Rarely 30- to 40-mm balloon length will be required. The amount of intraarterial thrombus is inversely related to procedural success and tends to be increased in proximal right coronary occlusions, especially in vein graft occlusions. When thrombus is very proximal, such as in the left main or proximal right coronary, there is a risk of systemic embolization with balloon inflation since thrombus can be displaced into the aortic root. In the presence of substantial amounts of thrombus, an intracoronary infusion of urokinase, given by infusion pump both through the guiding catheter and the balloon catheter positioned within or proximal to the thrombus, has sometimes been useful for decreasing thrombus burden.

PROBLEMS (TABLE 32B.4)

Difficulties in dealing with excessive intracoronary thrombus have been outlined above. Thrombus no doubt predisposes to reclosure

Table 32B.4.
Problems of Dilation During Acute Infarction

Excessive thrombus
Repeated reclosure
Unable to cross lesion
Acute dissection
Unable to dilate
Reflex hypotension

of the dilated segment, which for the experienced interventionalist is probably the most common problem with primary angioplasty for infarction. While not extensively described in the literature, repeated reclosure occurs in approximately 15% of cases. Besides ensuring the adequacy of heparin anticoagulation, multiple repeated balloon inflations, especially prolonged inflation of an autoperfusion catheter, have helped solve this problem considerably. When repeated reclosure seems to be related to recoil rather than a thrombotic mechanism, the use of an intracoronary stent can be considered, though in this setting the risk of stent thrombosis is higher. Additional mechanisms to reduce the occurrence of rethrombosis include the use of hirudin, an antithrombin derived from the European leech, and/or monoclonal antibodies designed to block the 2B3A platelet receptor.

Inability to cross the occlusion usually mandates a trial of different guidewires of various stiffness and distal bend. Review of the preprocedure angiogram, especially with regard to possible abrupt angulation of the vessel at the site of occlusion or the presence of a small, poorly seen branch vessel in which the wire tip may inadvertently lodge, may be useful. Angulated views and biplane injections can help ensure that the wire is positioned in the appropriate position. The smaller and stiffer wires may have a propensity to track subintimally, producing unrecognized dissection. The use of an 0.0018-inch wire of softer, intermediate stiffness or a blunt-tipped wire (Magnum wire) may be useful to avoid dissection. Large dissections are best treated with acute stenting if they are obstructive. Inadequate guide support is an uncommon problem with acute occlusions, but occasionally the guiding catheter must be replaced with a more aggressive variety such as the Amplatz or Voda designs. Inability to dilate the lesion is rare in acute occlusions and would indicate the use of a high-pressure balloon.

Severe reflex hypotension is a significant problem in procedures involving occluded right coronary arteries (17). The typical scenario is one where the patient has an ongoing inferior wall infarct, but is relatively stable from a hemodynamic standpoint up to the first balloon deflation. With reperfusion of the right coronary artery, profound systemic hypotension and bradycardia rapidly ensue. This problem is commonly resistant to atropine, fluids, and dopamine and may require small amount of epinephrine (25 to 50 μg boluses) for resolution. The Bezold-Jarisch reflex is responsible for this problem, and the interventionalist must anticipate the possible need for aggressive management should it occur.

ROLE OF NEWER INTERVENTIONS (TABLE 32B.5)

The use of intracoronary stenting has been alluded to above. Stent placement should be avoided in arteries with a large amount of residual intracoronary thrombus unless refractory, repeated vessel reclosure has occurred. Additionally, patients must be candidates for long-term anticoagulation with coumadin. Directional atherectomy, as well as extraction atherectomy, has been insufficiently tested in acute infarction to draw any firm conclusions regarding its benefit. While directional atherectomy can certainly remove thrombus material from the artery, there are no data to suggest an advantage over angioplasty in this setting. The transluminal extraction catheter (TEC device) has theoretical appeal

in this situation, and at least one trial investigating its use in infarction is currently under way. None of the currently available laser coronary angioplasty systems have been adequately tested in patients with acute infarction. At the present time there is no indication for laser over angioplasty in this setting. There is continuing interest in ultrasound guidewire thrombolysis. While in vitro experiments have demonstrated the feasibility of thrombus dispersal using ultrasound energy, methodologic problems with attenuation of ultrasound energy at bend points of the guidewire have precluded the practical application of this technology to the coronary anatomy.

In conclusion, human coronary interventions, predominantly balloon angioplasty, will continue to play an important role in therapy for acute myocardial infarction. The major limitation for more widespread use of direct angioplasty for infarction is the timely access to this treatment for patients not close to an angioplasty center. The elective use of angioplasty following thrombolytic therapy should be preceded by demonstration of ischemia. The techniques employed for opening totally occluded vessels are straightforward and, in many cases, less complex than for other lesions such as bifurcation stenoses or chronic total occlusions. The major impediment to success is the presence of large amounts of intracoronary thrombus and repeated vessel reclosure for which the newer antithrombotic agents offer great hope. Whether the newer interventional devices will make a major impact in this application remains to be seen.

Table 32B.5.
Role of Newer Interventions

Stenting
Atherectomy
Laser
Ultrasound thrombolysis

REFERENCES

1. Grines CL, Browne KF, Marco J et al. A comparison of immediate angioplasty with thrombolytic treatment of myocardial infarction. Circulation 1992;86:1400–1406.
2. Zijlstra F, deBoer MJ, Hoorntje JCA et al. A comparison of immediate coronary angioplasty with intravenous streptokinase in acute myocardial infarction. N Engl J Med 1993;328:680–684.
3. Gibbons RJ, Holmes DR Jr, Reeder GS et al. Immediate angioplasty compared with the administration of a thrombolytic agent followed by conservative treatment for myocardial infarction. N Engl J Med 1993;328:685–691.

4. Lange RA, Hillis LD. Immediate angioplasty for acute myocardial infarction. N Engl J Med 1993;328:726-728.

5. Goldberg RJ, Gore JM, Alpert JS et al. Cardiogenic shock after acute myocardial infarction: incidence and mortality from a community-wide perspective, 1975 to 1988. N Eng J Med 1991;325:1117–1122.

6. Lee L, Bates ER, Pitt B et al. Percutaneous transluminal coronary angioplasty improves survival in acute myocardial infarction complicated by cardiogenic shock. Circulation 1988;78:1345–1351.

7. Topol EJ, Califf RM, George BS et al. A randomized trial of immediate versus delayed elective angioplasty after intravenous tissue plasminogen activator in acute myocardial infarction. N Engl J Med 1987;317:581–588.

8. Simoons ML, Arnold AER, Betriu A et al. Thrombolysis with tissue plasminogen activator in acute myocardial infarction: no additional benefit from immediate percutaneous coronary angioplasty. Lancet 1988;1:197–203.

9. The TIMI Study Group. Comparison of invasive and conservative strategies after treatment with intravenous tissue plasminogen activator in acute myocardial infarction: results of the thrombolysis in myocardial infarction (TIMI) trial, phase II. Circulation 1992;85:1254–1264.

10. Topol EJ, Califf RM, George BS et al. Coronary arterial thrombolysis with combined infusion of recombinant tissue–type plasminogen activator and urokinase in patients with acute myocardial infarction. Circulation 1988; 77:1100–1107.

11. DeBono DP, Pocock SJ, for the SWIFT Investigators Group. The SWIFT study of intervention versus conservative management after anistreplase thrombolysis. Circulation 1989;80(Suppl 2):II-418 (abstract).

12. Ellis SG, O'Neill WW, Bates ER et al. Implications for patient triage from survival and left ventricular functional recovery analyses in 500 patients treated with coronary angioplasty for acute myocardial infarction. J Am Coll Cardiol 1989;13:1251–1259.

13. Ellis SG, da Silva ER, Heyndrickx G et al for the RESCUE investigators. Randomized comparison of Rescue angioplasty with conservative management of patients with early failure of thrombolysis for acute anterior myocardial infarction. Circulation 1994;90:2280–2284.

14. The EPIC investigators. Use of a monoclonal antibody directed against the platelet glycoprotein IIb/IIIa receptor in high-risk coronary angioplasty. N Engl J Med 1994; 330:956–961.

15. Topol EJ, Califf RM, Weisman HF, Ellis SG, Cheng JE, Worley S, Ivanhoe R et al. on behalf of the EPIC investigators. Randomised trial of coronary intervention with antibody against platelet IIb/IIIa integrin for reduction of clinical restenosis: results at six months. Lancet 1994; 343:881–886.

16. Ellis SG, Mooney Mr, George BS et al. Randomized trial of late elective angioplasty versus conservative management for patients with residual stenoses after thrombolytic treatment of myocardial infarction. Circulation 1992;86:1400–1406.

17. Gacioch GM, Topol EJ. Sudden paradoxic clinical deterio-
ration during angioplasty of the occluded right coronary artery in acute myocardial infarction. J Am Coll Cardiol 1989;14:1202–1209.

EDITORIAL SUMMARY

The treatment of acute myocardial infarction has evolved rapidly over the last decade. New studies continue to be performed and evaluated, which will further our understanding of the problem and help identify optimal treatment strategies.

PTCA will play an expanding role even though it has been rigorously tested far less frequently or scientifically than thrombolytic therapy. A number of important principles have become more well understood.

1. The goal of reperfusion therapy is prompt restoration of TIMI-3 blood flow to the infarct-related coronary artery. TIMI-2 flow results in outcomes similar to TIMI-1 or 0 flow, which are distinctly less favorable than outcomes seen with TIMI-3 flow. Accelerated rtPA is associated with improved outcome because it results in higher reperfusion rates and more frequent TIMI-3 flow than does streptokinase.

2. Direct angioplasty results in significantly higher early reperfusion rates (>90%) than thrombolytic therapy, even accelerated rtPA. In addition, in the overwhelming majority of patients undergoing direct PTCA, TIMI-3 flow results in full reperfusion.

3. Direct angioplasty can be used in a wider group of patients with acute myocardial infarction. Even though there is heightened awareness of the benefits of thrombolytic therapy, <50% of patients with acute myocardial infarction receive thrombolytic therapy for one of several reasons. PTCA can be technically applied in the overwhelming majority of patients as there are few exclusion criteria.

4. In low-risk patients, direct PTCA and thrombolytic therapy will result in similar outcomes. In higher risk patients— those with large anterior infarctions, prior infarctions, and hemodynamic instability—PTCA results in improved outcome defined as decreased mortality and decreased recurrent ischemia as compared with thrombolytic therapy and should be strongly considered if personnel and facilities are available. Thrombolytic therapy should not be withheld if the patient cannot undergo immediate direct PTCA. For patients with cardiogenic shock, direct angioplasty appears to be even more important and results in improved outcome.

5. Following failed thrombolytic therapy, PTCA should still be attempted if possible, although in this setting success rates are decreased and complication rates are increased. Following successful thrombolytic therapy, on the other hand, PTCA should still be delayed as was documented in the early reperfusion trials of TAMI, TIMI, and the European Cooperative Study Group.

6. New adjunctive medications hold great promise in optimizing outcome. Of particular note are the IIb/IIIa receptor blocking drugs, which may decrease recurrent ischemia and improve outcome.

33. Internal Mammary Artery Stenoses

MALCOLM R. BELL

BACKGROUND: USE OF THE INTERNAL MAMMARY ARTERY FOR CORONARY SURGICAL REVASCULARIZATION

The remarkable ability of the internal mammary artery (IMA) to remain patent for long periods was first demonstrated in patients who had undergone the Vineberg operation. However, implantation of the left IMA into the left anterior descending coronary artery was not performed until the late 1960s, but in view of the relative ease and success of using the saphenous vein to provide bypass conduits to the coronary arteries, its use remain limited. However, the usefulness and importance of using the IMA as a bypass graft were highlighted by Loop and his coworkers at the Cleveland Clinic in 1986 (1). In their landmark paper there was convincing evidence that the IMA graft reduced the risk of late myocardial infarction and decreased the risk of late cardiac events and need for a cardiac reoperation. Most importantly, the 10-year survival was superior in patients who had a mammary artery graft placed in their left anterior descending coronary artery versus those in whom only saphenous veins were used. Since then the IMA graft has become the graft of choice for patients undergoing coronary artery bypass surgery whenever it is technically feasible. Although the most common implementation of mammary artery grafting is the use of the left IMA (LIMA) to bypass obstructions of the left anterior descending coronary artery, bilateral and sequential IMA grafts have also been employed.

The explanation for improved patency rates of IMA grafts compared with saphenous vein grafts may lie in the apparent resistance to atherosclerosis of the IMA. Detailed autopsy studies confirm that the incidence of atherosclerosis in the IMA is extremely low, even in the presence of significant coronary artery disease (2, 3). Accelerated atherosclerosis does not appear to occur in IMA grafts, whereas it is common in saphenous vein grafts (4). There is also preliminary evidence that there may be differences in endothelial receptor expressions in the IMA compared with other vascular beds. Despite the apparent "resistance" of the IMA to atherosclerosis, postsurgical graft stenoses or occlusions may occur. However, it appears that the development of graft obstructions may be related, in many cases, to technical factors at the time of surgery, such as "rough" handling of the artery during its mobilization or difficulties in securing the anastomosis. Therefore, whether the excellent patency rates will be reproduced in the majority of other centers remains to be seen. Meanwhile, as the utilization of IMAs as coronary conduits increases, it can be anticipated that interventional cardiologists will be faced with a growing number of mammary artery obstructions in need of dilation.

OUTCOME OF PERCUTANEOUS TRANSLUMINAL ANGIOPLASTY OF IMA GRAFT STENOSES

To date the total number of published reports of patients undergoing percutaneous transluminal coronary angioplasty (PTCA) for IMA graft stenoses is small, but as can be seen from Table 33.1, the overall success rate appears to be at least 90% in these selected

Table 33.1.
Summary of Reports of Use of Angioplasty for Internal Mammary Artery Graft Stenoses

| Author | Number of Patients | Location of Stenosis | | | Angiographic Success (%) |
		IMA	Anastomosis	Native Vessel	
Dorros et al (7)	8	—	6	1	88
Cote et al (6)	5	—	5	—	100
Pinkerton et al (8)	9	—	7	4	91
Shimshack et al (10)	45	12	20	25	95
Bell et al (5)	11	—	7	4	91
Popma et al (9)	20	—	12	8	83

IMA, Internal mammary artery.

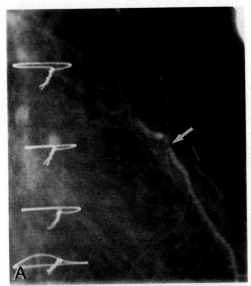

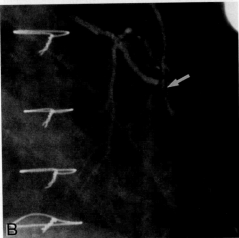

series (5–10). Most of the reported IMA PTCA procedures have involved dilation at the distal anastomotic site (Fig. 33.1) with a smaller number of dilations in the distal native vessel (Fig. 33.2), whereby the IMA was used as a conduit for the balloon catheter and wire. In our experience it has been unusual to find a stenosis within the body of the graft that requires dilation.

TECHNICAL APPROACH

Preprocedural Preparation

When faced with a potential IMA PTCA procedure, three fundamental questions should be addressed during the initial assessment and planning of the technical approach:

1. In situations in which the stenosis is within the native vessel, can this be approached from the proximal native vessel (if patent) rather than through the IMA conduit?
2. Should arterial access be obtained through the femoral or ipsilateral brachial artery?
3. How tortuous is the IMA?

These are very important questions to address since IMA angioplasty can be technically very challenging and often presents unique obstacles to the cardiologist.

PTCA VIA THE NATIVE VESSEL

Native coronary vessel stenoses that are distal to the IMA graft anastomosis can poten-

Figure 33.1. Angiographic example of an anastomotic stenosis in an internal mammary artery graft to the distal left anterior descending coronary artery before **(A)** and after **(B)** successful angioplasty. The site of stenosis is indicated by the arrow. Both images were obtained in the right anterior oblique projection.

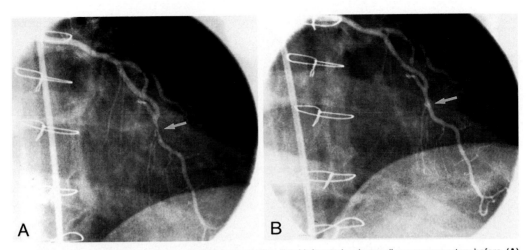

Figure 33.2.   Angiographic example of a stenosis in the native distal left anterior descending coronary artery before **(A)** and after **(B)** successful angioplasty. In this case the internal mammary artery graft was used as a conduit for the balloon catheter. The site of stenosis is indicated by the arrow. Both images were obtained in the right anterior oblique projection.

tially be dilated without passage through the IMA graft. This approach may be preferable if the native vessel has remained patent. Any stenosis proximal to the graft insertion site should be assessed for suitability of dilation—occasionally, this may not be necessary if the obstruction is not considered to be significant. The distal lesion should preferably be crossed with the wire prior to dilating the proximal lesion. Once the proximal lesion has been successfully dilated, the balloon can be advanced across the distal stenoses—this may entail the use of a smaller balloon catheter than the one used for the proximal lesion. This approach avoids the need to negotiate the IMA, thus avoiding the risk of potential trauma to the IMA or other technical difficulties.

TORTUOSITY OF THE IMA

If the IMA is to be negotiated, one of the more challenging features will be the presence of extreme tortuosity. Tortuous IMAs are not uncommon and will generally require very patient and skillful manipulation of the catheter system to reach the graft anastomosis (Figs. 33.3 and 33.4). Extreme tortuosity adds length to the total route, and the operator will need to take this into account when selecting equipment to avoid being frustrated when it becomes apparent that the catheter appears to be "too short" and is unable to reach its intended target (vide infra).

ARTERIAL ACCESS SITE

Choice of arterial access site will clearly be individualized and will be based on a number of factors. PTCA performed during the same setting as diagnostic angiography can generally be attempted using the existing arterial access if the engagement of the IMA has been successful. PTCA involving the IMA can usually be successfully performed using the femoral approach (5, 8, 9), but others have advocated the ipsilateral brachial approach as an alternative (7). Many catheterization laboratories are not well suited to using the left brachial approach because of placement of video monitors and other equipment, and under these circumstances a femoral approach may be less cumbersome. However, the brachial approach to the IMA is relatively straightforward and should be considered whenever there is anticipated difficulty with use of the femoral approach. This is particularly relevant when the right IMA is the target vessel since its engagement from the aorta is often very difficult. Since we often continue

Figure 33.3. In this right anterior oblique projection image, significant tortuosity of the proximal segment of the internal mammary artery is evident. The severe bends to the vessel are indicated by the arrows. In such a case one would anticipate significant technical difficulties in negotiating the entire vessel and at the same time would be faced with the potential problem of inability to reach a distal target because of loss of effective "catheter system length" within the tortuous vessel.

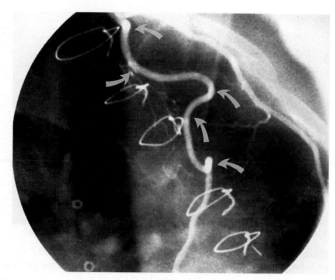

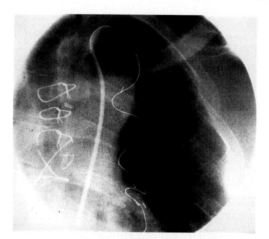

Figure 33.4. Fluoroscopic view of an angioplasty guidewire demonstrating significant tortuosity throughout the length of the left internal mammary artery. Despite this, successful dilation of a native left anterior descending coronary artery stenosis was accomplished.

Choice and Use of Equipment

CONTRAST MEDIA

To minimize patient discomfort, we always use nonionic contrast during diagnostic and interventional procedures involving the IMA. This lessens the pain and discomfort that many patients experience during angiography of this vessel. Ionic, but low-osmolar contrast media are also helpful in this regard.

GUIDE CATHETERS

We generally use 7 or 8 Fr guiding catheters that have a "LIMA" curve at the end of the catheter and use these from either the arm or the leg. Other guide catheters that are occasionally used include a right Judkins and right bypass catheter. The curve of the LIMA catheter is such that the catheter tip is more coaxial with the takeoff of the vessel, thereby reducing the risk of trauma. The use of soft-tip catheters is advocated. The catheter is advanced over a guidewire when using the arm approach; once the guidewire has been removed, intubation of the IMA is usually accomplished without difficulty. When the femoral approach is employed, access to the subclavian artery is usually obtained by first positioning a right Judkins diagnostic catheter within this vessel and then exchanging

the administration of heparin for at least the first few hours after PTCA, we always employ a cut-down technique for isolating the brachial artery, rather than puncture the artery percutaneously, so the catheter can be removed at the conclusion of the procedure and the arteriotomy closed. Finally, the brachial approach may be preferable to the femoral approach if there is extreme tortuosity of the IMA since shorter guide catheters can be used (vide infra).

this for the LIMA catheter over a long exchange wire. The LIMA catheter is placed in the left (or right) subclavian artery and slowly withdrawn using small contrast test injections to identify the origin of the IMA vessel. Gentle counterclockwise rotation on the left side and clockwise rotation on the right will usually help position the catheter correctly. Then with careful manipulation of the tip of the LIMA catheter, the ostium of the IMA is intubated. The operator needs to be particularly vigilant for pressure damping and awkward guide engagement to minimize the risk of ostial vessel dissection. Although we generally do not use guidewires to intubate the ostium, other operators have advocated their use (8); their use may facilitate successful guide catheter placement into an IMA that has an unusual site of origin (e.g., brachiocephalic artery) or an unusual takeoff angle. The IMA appears to be susceptible to dissection (11), and therefore great care should be taken with the tip of the guide catheter whenever it is moved in or out of the IMA. The acute takeoff angle of the IMA from the subclavian artery or the finding of a small caliber IMA in some patients can present problems with satisfactory guide catheter engagement. When catheter damping is a persistent problem, we will generally use a 7 Fr catheter or smaller size; 6 Fr catheters or catheters with side holes are very helpful.

GUIDEWIRES

When over-the-wire systems are employed, regular guidewires can be used in most cases such as the 0.014- to 0.018-inch Hi-Torque Floppy (Advanced Cardiovascular Systems, Inc., Temecula, CA) or Hy-Per Flex (USCI Division, C.R. Bard, Inc., Billerica, MA). If there is a lot of tortuosity, then use of larger diameter wires such as 0.018 inch, which provide more steerability, should be considered. Other wires such as the Reflex wire (Cordis Corporation, Miami, FL), which consists of a single wire core, may also be useful in difficult cases by virtue of its being very "push-

able," thereby avoiding prolapse of the proximal wire around multiple bends.

BALLOON CATHETERS

In the absence of extreme tortuosity, balloon-on-wire systems can be very useful for PTCA of distal lesions in the native vessel or anastomotic stenoses. Because of the overall low profile of these catheters, visualization is usually excellent and positioning across tight lesions is usually easily accomplished. The other advantage of these angioplasty systems is the added length that some have compared with many over-the-wire systems. They can therefore be useful when the usable length of the entire system becomes important. Thus the Probe catheter (USCI Division, C.R. Bard, Billerica, MA), which has a usable shaft length of 145 cm, is 10 cm longer than most conventional balloon catheter systems.

In terms of over-the-wire systems, we have no strong preference for any one type of PTCA catheter—most modern PTCA catheters are low profile and will perform satisfactorily. However, selecting a catheter that is very "pushable" with a favorable crossing profile will be important when there is a lot of proximal tortuosity; careful selection of such a system is required particularly when the lesion to be crossed appears to be severely narrowed.

An important cautionary note is necessary concerning withdrawal of the PTCA balloon catheter. Whenever this is done, there is the potential for the guide catheter to be pulled further into the proximal vessel. If the operator is not vigilant, the guide catheter can be dragged deeply into the IMA. This may lead to significant catheter-induced dissection of the vessel and bring the procedure to a quick conclusion. As emphasized earlier, the IMA is very susceptible to catheter trauma, and to avoid this mechanism of trauma the operator needs to watch the tip of the guide catheter very carefully for any forward motion. It is safer to withdraw the guide catheter simultaneously with the balloon catheter. This is particularly important when the IMA is very tortuous since there will be a considerable amount of "drag" or friction along the entire system as it is withdrawn.

Catheter System Length. As discussed above, situations in which the IMA is extremely tortuous and long may result in the catheter system in use being too short to reach the target lesion. For example, when using a "standard" operating system of a 100-cm guide catheter and a 135-cm-long balloon catheter shaft, the usable portion of the balloon catheter amounts to only 35 cm. The effective length will actually be a few centimeters less because the balloon itself needs to be advanced across the lesion, and there is also the "dead space" within the "Y" adaptor to consider. Therefore any stenosis that is 30 cm (approximately) or more distal to the tip of the guide catheter cannot be reached by such a system.

The major limiting factor is the length of the guide catheter itself; using a shorter catheter (e.g., 80 cm) adds another 20 cm to the usable length, but these catheters are not widely available. There is only a limited choice of short guide catheters, and on occasion we have shortened longer catheters ourselves to overcome such obstacles. Shorter catheters are ideally suited to the brachial approach, but can be used from the leg in the absence of significant aortoilial tortuosity or if the patient is not too tall. Although most conventional systems have a usable shaft length of 135 to 137 cm, at least one manufacturer has available a 145-cm-long system (The Mystic, Schneider (USA) Inc., Minneapolis, MN), although this does include the balloon length itself. Therefore the majority of distal lesions should be reachable when these options are considered. Such strategies should be determined ahead of time to avoid the frustration of having crossed a lesion with a guidewire and then discovering that the catheter is too short. At this point the operator will be faced with the options of a guide catheter exchange or removing the entire system.

MANAGEMENT OF COMPLICATIONS

Most reported series of PTCA involving IMAs report a low incidence of complications and include coronary spasm, dissection, and abrupt closure (5–10). Acute myocardial infarction and need for emergency bypass surgery may result from persistent abrupt closure. These complications are not unique to IMA PTCA and are generally approached in the same manner as conventional PTCA. However, the options for rescue intervention are more limited with this type of PTCA. Generally, the "tacking up" of a significant dissection following conventional PTCA involves the use of an autoperfusion balloon as an initial step. This can also be attempted when one is faced with a dissection following IMA PTCA, but if there is any significant tortuosity of the IMA, one can expect considerable difficulty in successfully advancing such a system. The support offered by the guide catheter will probably be extremely limited; a 0.018-inch guidewire may provide additional support over which to advance the system. Should this strategy fail or prolonged balloon inflations fail to restore adequate antegrade flow, no other viable options are currently available. We have yet to require placement of an intracoronary stent in this situation; this could be a very challenging maneuver, particularly if the IMA was very tortuous. The loss of a stent within a tortuous IMA or embolization of the stent while attempting to retrieve a "stray" stent—particularly in view of the proximity of the cerebral circulation—could lead to potentially disastrous consequences of such a technical misadventure.

REFERENCES

1. Loop FD, Lytle BW, Cosgrove DM et al. Influence of the internal-mammary-artery graft on 10-year survival and other cardiac events. N Engl J Med 1986;314:1–6.
2. Kay HR, Korns ME, Flemma RJ et al. Atherosclerosis of the internal mammary artery. Ann Thorac Surg 1976; 21:504–507.
3. Sims FH. A comparison of coronary and internal mammary arteries and implications of the results in the etiology of arteriosclerosis. Am Heart J 1983;105:560–566.

4. Shelton ME, Forman MB, Virmani R et al. A comparison of morphologic and angiographic findings in long-term internal mammary artery and saphenous vein bypass grafts. J Am Coll Cardiol 1988;11:297–307.

5. Bell MR, Holmes DR Jr, Vlietstra RE et al. Percutaneous transluminal angioplasty of left internal mammary artery grafts: two years' experience with a femoral approach. Br Heart J 1989;61:417–420.

6. Cote G, Myler RK, Stertzer SH et al. Percutaneous transluminal angioplasty of stenotic coronary artery bypass grafts: 5 years' experience. J Am Coll Cardiol 1987;9:8–17.

7. Dorros G, Lewin RF. The brachial artery method to transluminal internal mammary artery angioplasty. Cathet Cardiovasc Diagn 1986;12:341–346.

8. Pinkerton CA, Slack JD, Orr CM et al. Percutaneous transluminal angioplasty involving internal mammary artery bypass grafts: a femoral approach. Cathet Cardiovasc Diagn 1987;13:414–418.

9. Popma JJ, Cooke RH, Leon MB et al. Immediate procedural and long-term clinical results of internal mammary artery angioplasty. Am J Cardiol 1992;69:1237–1239.

10. Shimshak TM, Giorgi LV, Johnson WL et al. Application of percutaneous transluminal coronary angioplasty to the internal mammary artery graft. J Am Coll Cardiol 1988; 12:1205–1214.

11. Farooqi S, Jain AC, O'Keefe M. Catheter-induced left internal mammary artery bypass graft dissection. Cathet Cardiovasc Diagn 1985;11:597–601.

34. The Brachial Approach

A. Transbrachial, Transaxillary, and Transradial Angioplasty

KIRK N. GARRATT and DAVID R. HOLMES JR.

RATIONALE

Most coronary interventional procedures performed today make use of the transfemoral approach. Since open arteriotomy and repair are not required, the procedure can be performed rapidly. Manual compression is usually satisfactory to secure hemostasis, and since this task can often be delegated to an assistant, the operator is then free to apply his or her time to other tasks. The procedure is associated with a high degree of safety, with only rare infectious complications. Although local ecchymoses and hematomas occur with some frequency, serious vascular complications are not common. As Grossman has pointed out (1), multiple catheterization procedures at the same site are possible, whereas use of an access site requiring open arteriotomy is usually associated with so much local scar formation that the procedure cannot be repeated more than two or three times with safety.

Despite these considerations, use of the brachial approach has many advantages. The long tradition of cardiac catheterization procedures began with the isolation and cannulation of a brachial vessel when Warner Forssmann inserted a catheter into his own left brachial vein (2). In the past, diagnostic angiographers were thoroughly trained in the transbrachial approach, which was the standard of coronary catheterization for many years. With increasing use of the transfemoral approach, many operators have seen their skills in the transbrachial approach dull with disuse, and some young operators may receive limited training in the technique. At one time most coronary catheters were designed for use from the brachial access site, so there was a greater selection of catheters for transbrachial angiography. The popularity of the transfemoral approach has led to the proliferation of catheters designed to be advanced retrogradely from the femoral artery.

Nonetheless, there are many reasons to consider use of the brachial arterial access site for coronary intervention. Circumstances under which a transfemoral approach is impractical include severe ileofemoral atherosclerotic disease, occlusion of the distal aorta or femoral arteries, and severe aortic coarctation (Table 34A.1). Although percutaneous puncture of ileofemoral bypass grafts has been described, many operators are reluctant to perform this out of concern for continued bleeding after removal of the catheters and the risk of a potentially devastating infection. Although catheters can frequently be passed safely through abdominal aortic aneurysms, aneurysms associated with abundant thrombus should not be approached. Shaggy atheroma, particularly in the thoracic aorta, may also pose a significant hazard for retrograde passage of large interventional catheters from the femoral artery. The transbrachial approach represents the shortest practical route for accessing coronary arteries or saphenous vein graft ostia, which may be a consideration in treatment of very distal lesions, particularly those involving lesions in the terminal target vessel of a long sequential vein graft.

By far, the Sones catheter (USCI Division of Bard, Billerica, MA) was the mainstay for transbrachial diagnostic coronary angiography for many years. This catheter, available in 7, 7.5, and 8 Fr, is 80 cm long with an angled, tapering tip (Fig. 34.A.1) and was the first catheter to reliably achieve selective coronary artery intubation. Today, a greater variety of catheter iterations, including several preformed brachial shapes, make selective coronary intubation achievable even under circumstances in which the Sones catheter is inadequate. During the early years of coronary intervention, guide catheters were bulky and clumsy. The smallest available angioplasty guide catheters were 9 Fr and were not very well suited for passage through the brachial artery of many patients. Guide catheters have become much more refined; new polymeric formulations have allowed thinner catheter walls to be used without impairing the handling characteristics of the guide. As a consequence, 5 and 6 Fr guide catheters are currently available that are well suited for transbrachial balloon angioplasty (3, 4). These very small guide catheters have

internal dimensions sufficient to accommodate many over-the-wire angioplasty balloon systems, since the profile of the balloon catheters has also been greatly reduced recently. Recognizing the interest in ultrasmall guide catheters, several major guide catheter manufacturers now produce a complete line of very small guides, with some companies exploring guide catheter equipment as small as 4 Fr in outer diameter. The availability of this equipment may enhance coronary intervention using the transbrachial approach, as well as the transfemoral approach.

A substantial advantage of transbrachial balloon angioplasty is the ability to perform coronary intervention in the setting of full anticoagulation. A transfemoral approach is impractical in this setting, since complete hemostasis can rarely be fully assured with manual pressure alone and direct repair of the femoral artery requires the participation of a vascular surgeon. However, the ability to visually assess the arteriotomy at the close of a transbrachial procedure permits the operator to be certain that adequate hemostasis has been achieved at the end of the case.

ANATOMY

Most catheterization laboratories are configured to allow the operator to approach the patient from the right. As a consequence, the right brachial artery is usually preferred over the left brachial artery. The brachial artery is the terminal branch of the axillary artery, which is the terminal branch of the subclavian artery, which arises off the brachiocephalic trunk (innominate artery) (Fig.

Table 34A.1.
Patients in Whom Transbrachial Angioplasty is Preferred Over Transfemoral Angioplasty

- Obliterative atherosclerosis of iliac arteries, femoral arteries, or distal aorta
- Extreme aortoiliac tortuosity
- Skeletal abnormalities limiting hip extension or ability to lay flat
- Anticoagulated state
- Recent administration of thrombolytic drug
- Abdominal aortic aneurysm with friable thrombus
- Abdominal aortic or descending thoracic aortic stable dissection
- Aortic coarctation
- Internal mammary (thoracic) artery angioplasty
- Very distal lesions, particularly within or beyond sequential vein grafts

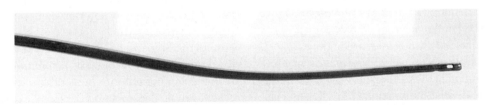

Figure 34A.1. Sones catheter. The tapering tip with slight angulation and side holes made this catheter the first to be suitable for selective coronary intubation.

Figure 34A.2. Overview of the chest, shoulder, and upper extremity arterial anatomy. See text for discussion.

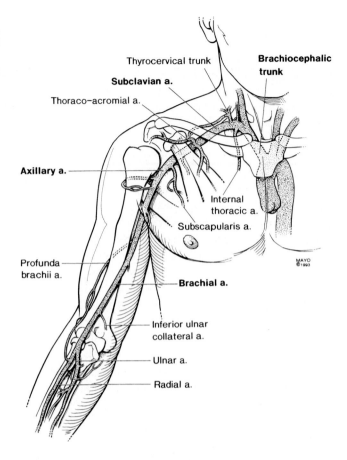

34A.2). The brachial artery, vein, and median nerve form a neurovascular bundle that extends from the teres major insertion site to the olecranon fossa. This neurovascular bundle travels along the medial aspect of the brachialis and biceps muscles and courses beneath the bicipital aponeurosis as it enters the olecranon fossa. The brachial artery bifurcates into the radial and ulnar arteries; this usually occurs just distal to the olecranon fossa. To avoid entering the bifurcation point or one of the smaller distal arterial branches, the brachial artery should be entered above the level of the olecranon fossa. This is easily identified as the flexor crease of the elbow. At this level, the brachial artery lies in close apposition to the median nerve and the terminal branch of the brachial vein. The inferior ulnar collateral artery (supratrochlear artery) arises from the medial aspect of the brachial

artery at a variable distance above the olecranon fossa. The superior ulnar collateral artery arises even more proximally, generally well beyond the area of exposure during a brachial arteriotomy procedure.

Proximal to the teres major muscle is the axillary artery. As one passes retrogradely from the brachial into the axillary artery, several branches are encountered. The most distal branches of the axillary artery include the subscapular artery, which courses posteriorly and medially to supply the subscapularis musculature, and the anterior humeral circumflex artery, which passes posteriorly around the humeral head. This branch wraps the humerus and frequently communicates with the smaller anterior humeral circumflex artery, which also arises off the distal axillary artery. In the mid portion of the axillary artery, the lateral thoracic artery arises and passes inferomedially along the pectoralis minor, ultimately coursing along the lateral thoracic wall. Proximal to the pectoralis minor muscle, the thoracoacromial artery arises and passes anteriorly into the pectoralis major.

Passing retrograde through the axillary artery, the subclavian artery is entered proximal the level of the first rib. The subclavian artery extends from the common carotid artery to the first rib. In this vascular segment, the internal thoracic (internal mammary) artery arises, which typically passes inferiorly and anteriorly within the thoracic cavity along the lateral sternal edge. Anterior and superior to the internal thoracic artery is the thyrocervical trunk, which gives rise to the suprascapular artery, the transverse cervical artery, and the thyroglossal artery. Posterior and a bit proximal to this trunk is the vertebral artery. Between the subclavian artery and the aortic arch is the brachiocephalic trunk (innominate artery). The only other branch of the brachiocephalic trunk is the common carotid artery.

The path of the venous system mirrors that of the arterial system. Viewed from distal to proximal, the brachial vein joins the basilic vein in the shoulder girdle to form the axillary vein. The cephalic vein joins the axillary vein between the first and second rib. Proximal to the first rib, the axillary vein becomes the subclavian vein. At this point the external and anterior jugular veins usually anastomose with the subclavian vein. Proximal to this, the subclavian vein joins with the internal jugular vein to form the short, right brachiocephalic (right innominate) vein, which joins with the longer, left brachiocephalic (left innominate) vein to form the superior vena cava.

EQUIPMENT AND TECHNIQUE

Arteriotomy

Transbrachial angioplasty may be performed by either the open arteriotomy (cut-down) or percutaneous technique. To perform an open arteriotomy, the right arm is secured to an arm board that extends the right arm out from the body at an angle of about 70° relative to the vertical axis of the body. Pads and towels should be placed beneath the arm for comfort and to maintain the desired orientation of the arm. A circulating nurse or assistant holds the arm up while disinfecting solution is scrubbed over the antecubital fossa, around to the posterior aspect of the elbow, and distal and proximal from the olecranon fossa over the volar surface for a distance of at least 6 inches. Once the skin has been disinfected, the arm is rested back on the padded arm board. I prefer to secure the hand to the arm board using tape, with the palm upward. This prevents the normal pronator drift that occurs as the patient relaxes. After draping the area, the medial and lateral epicondyles of the distal humerus are palpated and the flexor crease of the elbow identified. The skin is infiltrated with 2% lidocaine along a line running parallel to the flexor crease and about 1 cm superior (proximal) to it. The brachial artery is palpated to find its course, and deep infiltration of anesthetic is performed. The skin is then incised along the anesthetic line using a number 15 scalpel blade (Fig. 34A.3). An incision no less than 2 cm in length should be made.

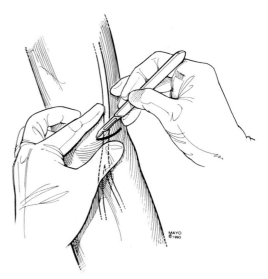

Figure 34A.3. A skin incision is made about 1 cm superior to and parallel with the olecranon flexor crease. The incision should be at least 2 cm in length.

Sharp dissection may be used through the superficial fasciae, but thereafter blunt dissection only is used (Fig. 34A.4). Once the deep fasciae has been opened, the bicipital aponeurosis is identified. Dissecting away the fat and adventitial layers, the medial aspect of the bicipital aponeurosis is usually easily defined. The brachial artery generally lies just beneath this aponeurosis. Fingertip palpation can be very helpful in locating the brachial artery at this point (Fig. 34A.5). Using blunt retractors, the aponeurosis is pulled laterally, and further blunt dissection is made to expose the neurovascular bundle. The bundle is opened with blunt dissection and the brachial artery isolated.

Care must be taken at this point to avoid trauma to branch vessels. As mentioned, the brachial artery generally bifurcates below the level of the olecranon fossa, but high brachial bifurcations may occur. Also, the inferior ulnar collateral artery, which can arise near the level of the olecranon fossa, may cause significant bleeding if lacerated. When the artery is isolated and cleaned of adventitia, umbilical tape or rubber straps are passed around the vessel (Fig. 34A.6) and brought to the surface of the skin (Fig. 34A.7). The vessel may now be entered.

Either a transverse or longitudinal incision may be made into the artery. The latter has a lower risk of accidental complete transection of the brachial artery. Curved forceps used to grasp the artery can limit the incision

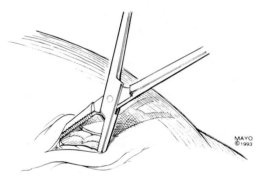

Figure 34A.4.   After sharp dissection is used to open the skin and superficial fasciae, all further dissection is conducted bluntly, using forceps to spread tissue.

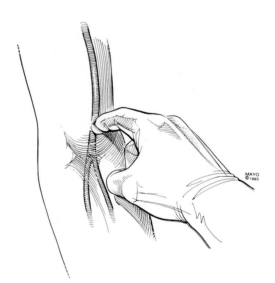

Figure 34A.5.   Inserting a fingertip to palpate for an arterial impulse can be very helpful in guiding the dissection to the brachial artery.

Figure 34A.6.   Once the brachial artery is located and cleaned of periadventitial tissue, a curved forceps is passed behind the vessel. Umbilical straps are grasped with the forceps and pulled around the vessel.

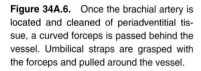

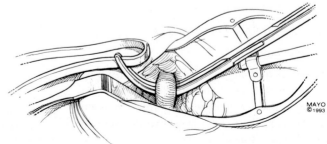

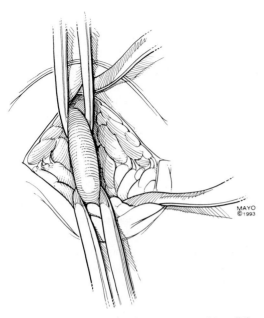

Figure 34A.7. The umbilical straps are used to pull the brachial artery to the skin surface.

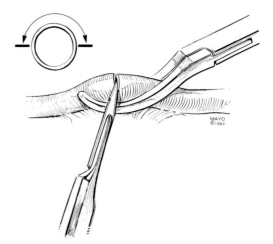

Figure 34A.8. The brachial artery is incised. If a transverse incision is used, curved forceps placed longitudinally around the artery can limit the depth of the incision. The incision must not involve an arc of greater than 180° *(insert)*; larger incisions put the artery at risk of complete transection.

depth when making a transverse incision (Fig. 34A.8). Tension is applied with the umbilical straps to prevent excessive bleeding. The incision is made with a number 11 scalpel blade. Once an arteriotomy is made, a curved blunt-tipped syringe is introduced into the distal artery and a solution containing heparin 50 to 100 units/cc is injected. Installation of this heparin solution is continued until a burning sensation is appreciated in the hand. At that time the syringe is removed and tension is applied with the distal umbilical strap while a 0.035-inch soft-tipped guidewire is passed retrogradely into the proximal segment of the brachial artery. Over this wire an appropriately sized vascular hemostatic sheath is placed. Tension on both umbilical straps may be reduced at this time. The sheath is flushed with heparinized saline and secured in place (Fig. 34A.9) with a suture or clamp. (Under some conditions, a high systolic blood pressure or pulse pressure can propel the vascular sheath out of the brachial artery.) Angioplasty may be conducted through the vascular sheath.

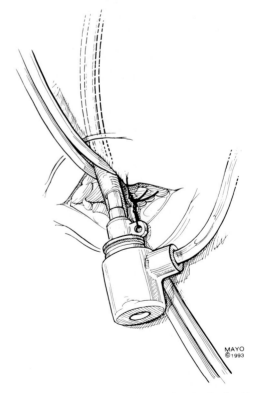

Figure 34A.9. The hemostatic vascular sheath should be anchored in place with a clamp or suture to prevent accidental removal.

Following the end of the procedure, the vascular sheath is aspirated and then removed while tension is again applied with umbilical straps. Vascular clamps may be placed proximal and distal to the arteriotomy site to stabilize the segment for repair. These must be applied using the minimum pressure required for hemostasis to avoid unnecessary crush injury to the artery. The brachial arterial segment is allowed to forcefully bleed for 1 or 2 seconds by first releasing the distal umbilical strap and then the proximal umbilical strap. If the return of blood is not forceful, a Fogerty catheter is advanced into the vascu-

lar segment, the balloon inflated to low pressure, and the catheter retracted to remove any in situ thrombus. Since this maneuver causes extensive endothelial denudation, it should not be routinely performed unless blood return is not adequate. The arteriotomy site is then closed with 6.0 proline suture. We prefer to place anchoring sutures at the corners of the incision (Fig. 34A.10) and then close the remainder of the wound while maintaining slight tension on these lateral anchoring lines (Fig. 34A.11). Sutures should be evenly spaced; five sutures usually are sufficient (Fig. 34A.12). Even after meticulous suture placement, a small amount of oozing is not uncommon. This usually responds to a few minutes of digital compression with a fingertip. Local use of Gelfoam or similar hemostatic material may also be helpful in some circumstances. The skin is then sutured closed.

During isolation of the brachial artery, great care must be taken to identify and avoid injury to the median nerve. This glistening white structure can often have a superficial appearance similar to the artery, particularly in the setting of brachial arterial atherosclerosis. The pulsatile character of the brachial artery usually makes identification simple. However, if doubt exists, puncture of the structure with a 23-gauge needle should per-

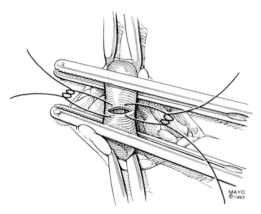

Figure 34A.10. When closing the arteriotomy site, anchoring sutures should be placed first at the corners of the incision.

Figure 34A.11. Placing traction on the corner-adhering sutures brings the wound edges into opposition. This simplifies proper placement of additional sutures.

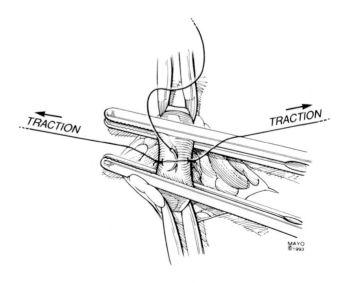

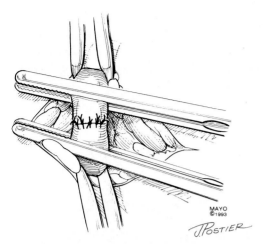

Figure 34A.12. Five evenly spaced stitches will usually close the arteriotomy satisfactorily.

mit aspiration of blood if the artery has been properly identified. Occasionally, the median nerve will fan out as a network over the surface of the brachial artery. Transient or permanent median nerve injury can be produced by passage through this neural network. If the nerve cannot be gently retracted away from the artery, an alternative arterial access route should be used.

The large brachial vein may be used for right heart catheterization or installation of fluids and drugs. The vein can be isolated and cannulated in a manner similar to the brachial artery, although it must be handled gently because of its thin structure.

Some operators prefer to perform a cutdown procedure to isolate the brachial artery, then puncture the artery with a thin-wall, 18-gauge needle, and insert a guidewire through it. The vascular sheath can usually be easily passed into the artery (Fig. 34A.13) and will generally produce a small arteriotomy wound. The advantage of this approach is that the arteriotomy site, if formed cleanly, is quickly and easily repaired. Unfortunately, arterial tearing may occur with attempts to insert the vascular sheath. Extensive, irregular tears are difficult to close and may require the assistance of a vascular surgeon to repair.

The percutaneous approach to the brachial

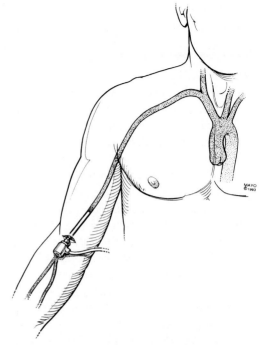

Figure 34A.13. Whether placed through an open arteriotomy, by needle puncture or an isolated artery, or percutaneously, the vascular hemostatic sheath should be positioned above the bifurcation of the ulnar and radial arteries.

artery is similar to the transfemoral percutaneous approach (5–8). The area of maximal pulsation of the brachial artery is identified by palpation and is usually found $1\frac{1}{2}$ cm above the flexor crease of the elbow. An area immediately over the point of maximal pulsation is slowly infiltrated with 2% lidocaine, and a skin nick is made with a number 11 scalpel. Blunt dissection is made until the superficial fasciae has been penetrated. A thin-wall, 18-gauge needle is advanced into the brachial artery, and a 0.035-inch, soft-tip introducing guidewire is advanced into the proximal segment of the brachial artery. An appropriately sized hemostatic vascular sheath is advanced over the guidewire, aspirated, and flushed. The sheath must remain in place until anticoagulant therapy has been discontinued, which is a liability with respect to interventional procedures. However, short-term, indwelling brachial sheaths, particularly if small caliber, do not seem to pose undue risk of thrombosis.

Guide Catheter Selection

Since the brachial artery is typically a smaller vessel than the femoral artery, some operators are reluctant to use an 8 Fr sheath routinely for transbrachial angioplasty. Since guide manufacturers now produce 6 and 7 Fr guide catheters with nearly every available tip configuration and excellent handling characteristics, they are generally preferred.

The diagnostic "grandfather" of coronary catheters is the Sones catheter. As previously described, this tapering-tip catheter can be manipulated from the brachial root into both the left and right coronary arteries. However, the inner diameter of most diagnostic catheters, the Sones included, are too small to easily accommodate many balloon catheters. Patterned after the Sones design, Simon Stertzer developed the brachial Stertzer guide (USCI, Division of Bard, Billerica, MA) for performing balloon dilation. The overall catheter design was similar to the Sones, although the angulation of the primary curve was altered slightly. The tapering tip remained; this was thought to minimize trauma to the coronary ostium, particularly since this guide catheter could be easily and inadvertently inserted deeply into the coronary artery. Although used for many years, declining demand has resulted in discontinuation of the Stertzer guide catheter production.

The Judkins left and right guide catheters are the most common guide catheters used during transfemoral angioplasty. These common catheter shapes are manufactured by every major catheter company in Europe and North America. Judkins catheters can be used during transbrachial angioplasty (9). The catheter tends to follow its usual course around the aortic knob best when the approach is from the left brachial artery. When the right brachial access site is used, the arch of the aorta no longer deflects the distal portion of the guide catheter. As a consequence,

the Judkins catheters tend to appear somewhat overbent (Fig. 34A.14). Undersizing by one catheter size (e.g., from a Judkins L4 to a Judkins L3.5) will usually compensate for

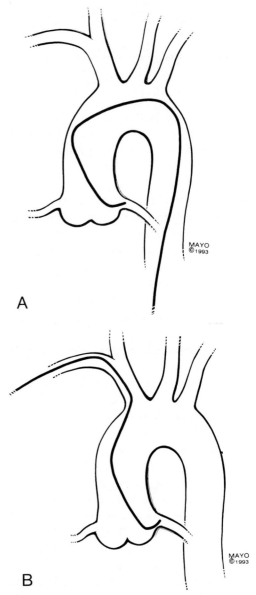

Figure 34A.14. A. Judkins guide catheters are designed to fit the shape of the aortic arch when passed retrogradely from the femoral artery. **B.** Use of these guides from the brachial artery changes the relationship between the aorta and the catheter, causing the catheter tip to seem overbent. Downsizing by one size (e.g., JL4 to JL3.5) usually corrects the fit.

this change. The Judkins right catheters usually fit well, although they occasionally will fail to reach the right coronary ostium sufficiently to firmly engage the vessel.

The Amplatz design catheters (multiple manufacturers) will generally perform as well from the transbrachial as from the transfemoral approach when attempting to engage the left coronary ostium. Depending on vascular tortuosity, the handling characteristics of the Amplatz (and any other guides, for that matter) will be variable. The Amplatz right guide catheters will occasionally fail to seat into the right coronary ostium when advanced from the right brachial artery, but the Amplatz left guide catheters usually seat in the right coronary without difficulty.

The brachial preformed catheters (multiple manufacturers) are essentially modifications of the Amplatz design. The primary curve is the same, but the distal tip has been lengthened. The secondary curve is somewhat flattened relative to Amplatz catheters. This guide catheter generally can be deflected off the aortic cusps into the coronary ostia without too much difficulty, and the added length of the catheter tip beyond the primary curve aids engagement. Because of the relative ease of handling and the firm support offered by this guide, it is my first choice for most brachial angioplasties.

Most other guide catheters have been employed from the transbrachial approach, but the efficacy of these guide catheters will be dependent on the individual anatomy involved. Angioplasty of lesions within an internal mammary artery graft represent a special concern (10–12). The internal mammary artery is frequently better approached by the transbrachial than the transfemoral route, but the guide catheter employed for this must possess a relatively sharp distal angulation because of the sharp angle of departure of the internal mammary artery off the subclavian artery. Several guide catheters are suitable for this, including the usual internal mammary artery guide catheter. A line of

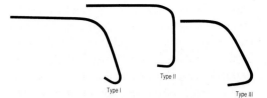

Figure 34A.15. The Dorros brachial guide catheters designed for angioplasty of internal mammary artery lesions. A variety of shapes permit successful intubation of almost any internal mammary artery ostium.

guide catheters specifically designed for this purpose were designed by Gerald Dorros (10), and this family of catheters bears his name (USCI Division of Bard). Three distinct internal mammary guide catheters constitute the family, with angulations varying substantially between the three members (Fig. 34A.15). With this group of guide catheters, nearly any internal mammary artery should be approachable, and the guides offer a good level of support for angioplasty. They are currently available only in 8 Fr, although newer 6 Fr guides have been successfully used (13, 14). For a more complete discussion of guide catheters, see reference No. 3.

An advantage of the transbrachial approach is the ability to shorten the distance from the access site to the coronary lesion. As mentioned, this can be of importance when a very distal lesion is to be approached, such as a lesion at the distal anastomosis of a long sequential vein graft. Although some guide catheters are available in 80- and 90-cm lengths for transbrachial use, many guide catheter configurations are still available only in the 100- to 110-cm length range. As a consequence, it may occasionally be necessary to modify the length of the guide catheter to complete the procedure. This can be done by cutting the guide catheter with a fresh number 15 scalpel blade and attaching a hub to the cut end. In the past, we have machined replaceable hubs for use in our laboratory, but plastic hubs suitable for use with 6, 7, and 8 Fr catheters are now commercially available from Cook, Inc. (Bloomington, IN). Since the middle layer of most guide catheters consists of a woven steel or kevlar braid, the catheter may be somewhat difficult to cut. Care must be taken not to flatten or crush the catheter unduly during the shortening process, as this may impede easy passage of the balloon angioplasty equipment.

Balloon Catheters

The only special concern regarding balloon catheter selection for transbrachial angioplasty is the need to use equipment compatible with small guide catheters. A variety of over-the-wire balloon catheters with excellent push, track, and cross capabilities, having outer diameters as small as 2.7 Fr, are available and are suitable for use with 6 Fr and 7 Fr guide catheters. These small balloon catheters not only fit through the guides but also generally allow satisfactory opacification of the vessel during contrast injections. Balloon catheters designed to work with 0.010-inch guidewires (ACS, Temecula, CA) offer a lower profile because of a reduction in the obligate lumen size for the guidewire. Fixed-wire balloon catheters are available with outer diameters that are virtually the size of a guidewire. These catheters can be easily advanced through 6 Fr guide catheters, and satisfactory opacification during contrast injection is generally the rule. Prior to the availability of 6 Fr guide catheters, we employed 6 Fr diagnostic catheters for the performance of balloon angioplasty using fixed-wire balloon catheters. The inner diameter of these diagnostic catheters was sufficient to permit advancement of the balloon catheter into place, but opacification was problematic. Also, the inflated balloon usually was difficult to withdraw back into the diagnostic catheter. Six Fr guide catheters have obviated the need for this.

Patient Preparation and Selection

Before the brachial site is used, an Allen's test should be performed to ensure patency of both of the terminal branches of the brachial artery. This may be important in the event of a thrombotic complication, since it is possible that only one distal branch may become completely occluded. Furthermore, it may be possible to clear one distal branch but not the other using a Fogerty balloon catheter. Adjunctive thrombolytic drugs and balloon angioplasty of the arm vasculature have been useful in resolving complications related to use of the brachial artery site (15–18). The traditional means of managing occlusive complications of the brachial artery is vein patch angioplasty, which is associated with a very high success rate. More extensive arterial resections or bypass procedures are rarely needed (19).

Balloon angioplasty is an appropriate therapy for patients who fail to recanalize following the administration of lytic drugs. To test the efficacy of the brachial approach to emergency cardiac catheterization (with or without balloon angioplasty) following thrombolytic therapy, the Thrombolysis and Angioplasty in Myocardial Infarction (TIMI) study group reviewed their experience with 202 patients who underwent transbrachial catheterization after thrombolysis. The results were compared to 502 patients who underwent transfemoral catheterization (20). The time interval from lytic therapy to coronary angiography was not different between the groups, and the technical success with acute PTCA was slightly greater using the brachial approach (89% versus 78%). The frequency of death, vascular reocclusion, need for emergency bypass surgery, and significant vascular bleeding, and the need for vascular repair were similar between the two groups. The investigators conclude that the transbrachial approach is associated with a risk and efficacy profile equal to that of the transfemoral approach for coronary intervention following thrombolytic therapy.

Postangioplasty Management

Most operators prefer to withdraw the vascular sheath at the earliest possible time. Significant intimal dissection, intravascular haziness, or frank filling abnormalities suggesting intraluminal thrombus are optimally treated with a period of postprocedural heparin infusion. Because the consequence of distal thrombosis in the upper extremity can be devastating, most operators elect to withdraw the sheath and close the arteriotomy site under direct visualization and then proceed with anticoagulant therapy. However, if the risk of an abrupt closure is perceived to be high, then a period of observation with the vascular sheath in place may be indicated; this may facilitate rapid access to the coronary system should recurrent ischemia develop. If distal pulses are intact, then the sheath may be left in place, provided high-dose anticoagulant therapy is used. When the anticoagulant therapy is to end or the desired period of observation has passed, the sheath can be removed and the arteriotomy site closed, or in the case of a percutaneous sheath placement, manual compression applied to achieve hemostasis. While indwelling, the side arm of the sheath should be attached to a pressurized fluid delivery system that infuses heparinized saline through the guide catheter at a slow rate.

Noncoronary Angioplasty

The transbrachial approach may also facilitate balloon angioplasty of noncoronary vascular structures. A syndrome of coronary-subclavian artery steal has been described among patients with internal mammary artery bypass grafts and subclavian arterial stenoses. In this circumstance, use of the arms may provoke angina. A transbrachial approach to the subclavian artery to facilitate angioplasty of that vessel is a useful alternative to carotid subclavian bypass surgery and may involve a lower complication rate than surgery with equally good results (21–23). There is a risk of cerebral embolization with this procedure; the presence of antegrade vertebral blood flow may identify patients at highest risk of cerebral embolization (24). The transbrachial approach has also been utilized to effect dila-

tion and thrombolytic treatment of lesions in the distal aorta (25), and even in the lower extremities (26), and under circumstances in which a transfemoral approach was impractical.

Saphenous vein grafts involved with abundant thrombus may be best treated with an infusion of lytic agents prior to balloon dilation. This is not commonly performed from the brachial artery because of concerns regarding the risks of an indwelling brachial sheath during ongoing lytic therapy. Successful prolonged transbrachial urokinase infusion has been described, however (27).

Outpatient Angioplasty and the Transbrachial Approach

With the rapid changes occurring in the delivery of medical care in the United States, a greater emphasis is being placed on cost-effective medical treatments. Coronary angiography and balloon dilation necessitate a brief hospital stay, but means of shortening that interval further are being explored. A potential benefit of transbrachial angioplasty is the ability to perform vascular interventional procedures and secure optimal hemostasis afterwards. As a result early hospital discharge may be possible. Outpatient noncoronary angioplasty has been successful using both the transfemoral and transbrachial approaches (28). There is limited experience with outpatient coronary angioplasty, but results reported from William Beaumont Hospital suggest that this is also feasible (29). Since antiplatelet, and frequently anticoagulant, therapies are commonly used after coronary intervention, primary closure of the arteriotomy site may be superior to manual compression of a percutaneous puncture wound for outpatient coronary procedures.

COMPLICATIONS AND LIMITATIONS

The most important complications related to transbrachial angioplasty involve vascular, neurologic, or cerebrovascular accidents (Table 34A.2). Limited ability to apply newer

Table 34A.2.
Principal Complications and Limitations Related to Transbrachial Angioplasty

Vascular complications
   Brachial lacerations
   Inability to repair arteriotomy
   Upper extremity arterial thrombosis
   Postclosure bleeding
Neurologic complications
   Median nerve mechanical trauma
   Ischemic neurologic trauma
Cerebrovascular complications
   Embolic cerebrovascular accident
   Thrombotic cerebrovascular accident
Limited ability to apply new interventional technologies
   Atherectomy devices
   Stents
   Vascular lasers

technologies that can minimize or overcome some complicating events may also be considered a liability of transbrachial angioplasty.

Vascular Complications

The four principal vascular complications seen with transbrachial angioplasty are tears or lacerations of the brachial artery during the procedure, an inability to properly close the arteriotomy and achieve hemostasis, thrombosis in the vessel (usually distal to the arteriotomy), and late bleeding complications. Arterial spasm occurring near the arteriotomy site is a less common complication and is easily handled with use of systemic vasodilators such as nitrates and calcium antagonists. Local installation of 2% lidocaine around the artery is also very effective in overcoming focal brachial arterial spasm.

Serious tears and lacerations of the brachial artery may occur as a consequence of overly aggressive dissection to free the artery. Although the artery itself is rarely injured with blunt dissection, avulsion of a side branch can occur relatively easily. If this is a significant side branch (such as the inferior ulnar collateral artery), then bleeding can be substantial. This complication is generally manageable with local compression and time, although the length of the procedure may be significantly prolonged and the surgical field obscured as a consequence of the bleeding episode. Occasionally, a ligature must be placed to contain the bleeding. More serious injuries may occur with a poorly placed arteriotomy. This is particularly true if transverse (rather than longitudinal) incisions are used (see Fig. 34A.3). An excessive transverse incision may result in bleeding around the hemostatic sheath. A wide transverse incision also weakens the integrity of the artery to a greater degree than a more limited incision. An incision that extends through one-half or more of the circumference of the vessel may present the risk of complete arterial transection when an attempt is made to pass the sheath into the arteriotomy site (see Fig. 34A.8). With this disastrous complication, the bleeding stump of the brachial artery may vanish from the surgical field as it is retracted proximally by the tension of tissues within the brachioradialis groove. This constitutes a surgical emergency. Direct pressure should be placed along the bicipital groove well above the incision site to contain bleeding until a vascular surgeon has arrived. Placing a tourniquet onto the upper extremity can also be useful in limiting blood loss.

Occasionally wounds are difficult to close, either because of an irregular arteriotomy configuration or the presence of significant atherosclerotic disease in the region of the arteriotomy. Also, if the arteriotomy is closed in an improper fashion, significant "dog ears" may form at the corners of the arteriotomy. Under these circumstances, hemostasis may be difficult to achieve. Some small amount of oozing is common after suturing closed the arteriotomy, but this generally responds well to a few moments of digital pressure. Local application of Gelfoam may also be helpful with minor oozing. More substantial bleeding should be controlled with placement of sutures where appropriate, and the assistance of a vascular surgeon should be recruited if necessary. In our laboratory a case of excessive bleeding was encountered when suture material attached to a cutting needle was used to close an arteriotomy; the tracks left by the cutting needles resulted in significant oozing that required the assistance of a vascular surgeon to control. Passing suture material through the posterior wall of the brachial artery when trying to repair an anterior wall arteriotomy must be avoided; this may result in excessive bleeding or thrombosis.

Focal thrombosis is usually manageable with a Fogerty catheter in conjunction with systemic anticoagulant and antiplatelet therapy. Local installation of thrombolytic drugs can be considered if Fogerty embolectomy is insufficient, although even low doses of fibrinolytic agents may present a risk of bleeding at the arteriotomy site. Systemic fibrinolytic therapy is contraindicated, since late bleeding may occur even after excellent hemostasis has been achieved.

Late bleeding may occur as a consequence of insufficient hemostasis at the close of the procedure or excessive patient movement causing disruption of the hemostatic plug. Strict upper extremity immobilization will minimize the risk of this complication. It is our practice to keep the upper extremity immobilized for 6 hours after documentation of complete reversal of the effect of anticoagulant drugs. Since the upper extremity cannot hide a large volume of blood as easily as the pelvis, bleeding is usually evident soon after it occurs. This is fortunate, since a tense hematoma within the neurovascular sheath around the brachial artery may result in compression of the median nerve. Late bleeding is initially managed with local pressure. Because of the risk of ischemic or pressure injury to the neurologic structures, evaluation by a vascular surgeon is indicated. Under some circumstances, the wound must be reopened to relieve the pressure within the neurovascular sheath.

Generally, complication rates of transbrachial arteriography and angioplasty have compared favorably with the transfemoral approach (Table 34A.3). Surgeons at the St. John Hospital and Medical Center in Detroit, Michigan, recently reported complications related to transbrachial and transfemoral catheterization procedures over a 3-year period at their institution (30). At their hospital a large proportion of diagnostic catheterizations are performed via the brachial artery (3137 versus 4055 via the femoral artery). In addition, balloon angioplasty was also performed via the brachial artery in some patients (32 via the brachial artery versus 1573 via the femoral artery). The authors note that the frequency of complications was greater with brachial artery catheterization, and balloon dilatation was associated with a higher complication rate than diagnostic studies. However, the chief brachial artery complication reported was arterial thrombosis, which was easily diagnosed and treated.

Table 34A.3.

Complications of Transbrachial Versus Transfemoral Cardiac Catheterization and Angioplasty

Author (Ref)	Year	Transbrachial No. Complications/Total (%)	Transfemoral No. Complications/Total (%)	P Value
Babu (31)	1989	60/10,500[a] (0.57)	14/850[a] (1.65)	.0002
George (20)[b]	1990	20/202[a] (1)	15/502[a] (2.99)	.0001
Khoury (30)	1992	62/3169 (1.96)	33/5628 (0.59)	.0001
Total of above studies		142/13,871 (1.02)	62/6980 (0.89)	.348

[a]Complications requiring surgical intervention.

[b]Patients received thrombolytic therapy before catheterization.

The difference in complication rates was significant for each study, but the combined data did not demonstrate any significant difference in complication rates with transbrachial compared with transfemoral catheterization.

By comparison, complications associated with the transfemoral approach were generally more complicated, were more difficult to identify, and were associated with significant morbidity. Also, brachial arterial complications were almost always diagnosed by physical exam alone (97% of cases), whereas additional studies such as Doppler flow imaging or angiography were needed in 70% of femoral arterial complications to make the diagnosis.

In the largest available series on complications after brachial procedures, surgeons from the New York Medical Center in Valhalla, New York, reported in 1989 on arterial complications among more than 16,000 patients undergoing catheterization procedures (31). The brachial artery was used for vascular access in 10,500 patients, and the femoral artery was used in 850 patients. They note that hand ischemia was the most frequent complication in the former group and bleeding the most common complication in the latter group. Surgical intervention was required more frequently in the brachial artery group (0.57%) than in the femoral artery group (0.23%); however, complications among the femoral artery group were more serious and associated with greater morbidity. They also note that delayed intervention was associated with a high morbidity despite satisfactory surgical intervention.

Neurologic Injury

The principal neurologic structure threatened by transbrachial angioplasty is the median nerve. Mechanisms of injury include sharp or blunt injury to the nerve during the arteriotomy procedure, injury related to prolonged and excessive traction on the nerve, ischemic injury, and compression injury. The variable relationship of the median nerve to the brachial artery can result in inadvertent injury to the nerve during attempts to isolate the brachial artery. The nerve may have an appearance similar to the artery, and in the setting of significant upper extremity atherosclerosis or prior brachial artery cut-down

procedures, the pulsatile nature of the artery may be difficult to fully appreciate. Attempts to pass a guidewire or even a hemostatic sheath into the median nerve can obviously have disastrous consequences. Use of a fine-gauge needle in an attempt to aspirate blood from the structure under question should help clarify whether the median nerve or brachial artery has been located. Spreading tissues with forceps during blunt dissection can risk injury to the median nerve, particularly if tissues are spread in a transverse manner over the surface of the nerve. For this reason, some operators feel that tissue should be spread only in a longitudinal manner relative to the path of the median nerve and brachial artery. In patients with well-developed upper extremity musculature, vigorous retraction of muscle and tendon may be necessary to identify the artery. Care should be taken not to apply excessive retraction pressure on the median nerve. Crush injury to the nerve can occur and may result in permanent disability.

The most devastating neurologic injury is ischemic neurologic paralysis of the upper extremity, which results in a dysfunctional arm. Not only is the function of the arm lost, but muscular contractures result in the formation of a "claw hand" deformity (Volkmann's contracture). Although classically associated with excessively tight casts, which cause ischemic injury to all of the major upper extremity nerve beds, a large, untreated brachial arterial bleed could compress the ventral nerves of the upper limb (median and ulnar nerves), and extensive posterior edema or tissue displacement could also threaten the dorsal nerve network (radial nerve) of the upper extremity. Fortunately, this dreaded complication occurs only when a major complication is left untreated for a prolonged period and therefore is completely avoidable. The potential for these serious complications makes involvement of a vascular surgeon mandatory at the earliest sign of a serious complication.

Cerebrovascular Events

As guide catheters are advanced from the brachial approach, their path is a relatively straight one up to the subclavian artery, where the catheters turn to enter the ascending aorta. Manipulations of guide catheters may cause a certain stress on the vascular segment extending from the origin of the innominate artery to the axillary artery; both the common carotid and vertebral arteries arise from within that vascular segment. As a consequence, guide manipulation poses the potential risk of dislodging atheromatous or thrombotic materials and causing an embolic event into the cranial circulation. Fortunately, clinical cerebrovascular events are uncommon using this approach. It is likely that the vascular segment from the innominate to the axillary artery is less likely to be burdened with shaggy atheromatous disease than is the aortic knob, which is the equivalent vascular segment that endures the risk of guide manipulations during the transfemoral approach. Lethal episodes of systemic cholesterol emboli have resulted from aggressive guide manipulations against the thoracic aorta in the presence of severe atheromatous disease. The presence of such disease in the proximal upper extremity vasculature will probably be unknown to the operator in most circumstances. If shaggy or thrombotic disease is known to exist in the innominate artery, subclavian artery, or axillary artery, or if the origins of the vertebral or common carotid arteries are known to be highly diseased, then an alternative vascular approach should be considered.

NEW DEVICES AND THE TRANSBRACHIAL APPROACH

Balloon angioplasty via the transbrachial approach is facilitated by the small size of the balloon catheters available. However, new interventional devices are generally much larger. As a consequence, large guide catheter systems must be used.

Directional coronary atherectomy was the first new intracoronary device approved. The coronary directional atherectomy catheters are available in 5, 6, and 7 Fr sizes. However, because of the relatively long, rigid housing and the low-pressure balloon that is attached to the housing, a minimum 10 Fr guide catheter is necessary to conduct directional coronary atherectomy. Successful transbrachial directional coronary atherectomy has been performed (32). However, the large guide catheter required would not be appropriate for use in patients with small brachial arteries or extensive brachial atherosclerosis. It should be noted that the large guide catheters are typically available in fewer iterations, tend to be less easily managed, and may present special difficulties for transbrachial coronary intervention.

The transluminal extraction endarterectomy catheter and the Rotablator catheter have both been recently approved by the Food and Drug Administration (FDA) for general use. The Rotablator device consists of a diamond chip–impregnated burr that rotates at high speeds over a guidewire. Burr sizes vary between 1.25 and 3.5 mm for coronary use; a 9 or 10 Fr guide catheter is required. A transluminal extraction endarterectomy catheter (TEC) consists of a flexible rotating torque tube with a set of stainless steel blades attached to a conical head that rotates at 750 rpm. This system is also advanced over a guidewire. Unlike the Rotablator device, which allows pulverized fragments to drift away into the distal vasculature, the TEC catheter uses a vacuum apparatus to aspirate formed debris. This catheter requires the use of 10 or 11 Fr guide catheters. Although successful coronary treatment with the Rotablator using the transbrachial approach has been described (33), experience with the TEC device from the brachial artery is more limited. As with directional coronary atherectomy, guide iterations and handling characteristics may be limiting factors.

Coronary lasers also represent an alternative to conventional balloon angioplasty.

The most widely used laser is the excimer laser, which uses ablating light energy at 308 nanometers generated by a xenon chloride–excited dimer laser source. Laser fibers range from 1.3 to 2.2 mm in diameter. Although the 1.3 fiber may be passed through an 8 Fr guide catheter, the larger fibers do not pass easily through 8 Fr guides, and require 9 Fr systems. The major limitation to transbrachial laser therapy is guide handling and ostial fit. When treating proximal lesions with the laser device, an excellent coaxial alignment with the vessel is mandatory to avoid dissection formation and the potential for vessel perforation.

The FDA recently approved the Cook FlexStent (Cook, Inc.) for general use. This is the first intracoronary stent device to be released. At least three other stents, the Schatz-Palmaz stent (Johnson and Johnson, Warren, NJ), the Wiktor stent (Medtronic, Minneapolis, MN), and the Wallstent (Schneider-Shiley, Minneapolis, MN), are involved in widespread clinical trials in North America and Europe, and several other stent designs are involved in more limited clinical trials. All permanent coronary stents currently under study require a minimum of 1 or 2 months of poststent anticoagulant and antiplatelet therapy to prevent subacute thrombosis. Since the risk of thrombosis begins the moment the stent is placed, removal of the sheath becomes problematic, because anticoagulant therapy must be interrupted to complete the task. Recently, Rosenschein and Ellis (34) described successful multivessel balloon dilation with intracoronary stent placement using a large-lumen, 7 Fr guide catheter from the left brachial artery. The point is made that warfarin therapy may begin before the procedure, which may substantially shorten the hospital stay and reduce stent-related expenses. Cardiologists at the Clinique Pasteur in Dakota Medical Center, University of North Dakota School of Medicine in Fargo, North Dakota, described successful intracoronary stent placement using a

7 Fr catheter from the left brachial approach. They also note the benefit of continued anticoagulant therapy through the stenting procedure (35). Recently, transradial stenting has been introduced and is being studied. It allows easy compression and rapid full ambulation. The palmar arch must be intact in this approach in case radial artery occlusion occurs.

Although no special concerns are evident with respect to placing stents from the brachial artery, retrieval of misplaced or displaced stents from the transbrachial approach is untested, and thus uncertainty exists regarding stent retrievability. It is our practice to withdraw stents that have been displaced from their deployment balloons around the aortic arch to below the level of the renal arteries whenever possible, before attempting to trap the stent and remove it (36). This would not be possible using the transbrachial approach, and consequently any stent mishap may have an increased risk of cerebral or renal embolization.

The Johnson and Johnson Schatz-Palmaz biliary/peripheral vascular stents have been used in saphenous vein grafts (37, 38). The stent is now packaged in a smaller (7.5 Fr) stent delivery sheath system, which does not require predilation of the lesion prior to stent placement. The smaller delivery system is designed for a transbrachial approach (39). The utilization of this system for coronary or vein graft stent placement is untested.

Columbo and associates at Centro Cuore Columbus, in Milano, Italy, reported last year on their initial 100 Johnson and Johnson Schatz-Palmaz stent placement experiences. The transbrachial approach was used in 17 patients. No specific problems were associated with this approach (40).

Severe calcific aortic stenosis in patients who are nonoperative candidates may still be treated with percutaneous transluminal balloon valvuloplasty. These balloon catheters are large and require 9 or 10 Fr guide catheters. Nonetheless, valvuloplasty may be successfully accomplished via the transbrachial approach. Because of the poor long-term results of aortic valvuloplasty, the procedure is being performed less frequently than in the past (41).

Intravascular ultrasound and angioscopy are new intracoronary imaging modalities being used at an increasing number of investigative centers. These devices require a minimum 8 Fr guide catheter size; their use should not be impacted by a transbrachial approach, provided appropriate guide catheter alignment and support are available.

TRANSAXILLARY, TRANSRADIAL, AND OTHER POTENTIAL VASCULAR ROUTES FOR CORONARY ANGIOPLASTY

On occasion, a patient with such severe atherosclerosis obliterans presents with coronary disease that neither the femoral nor brachial arterial access routes are feasible. This can occur when there is obliterative atherosclerosis within the distal aorta or both iliac arteries and within both upper extremity vascular networks. If the upper extremity obstruction occurs distal to the level of the teres major muscle, then the transaxillary approach may be used (42). To accomplish this, the patient is positioned with the right upper extremity extended away from the body at an angle of 90° or more relative to the long axis of the body. The axilla is draped and prepped in a sterile fashion, and the axillary artery is identified by palpation. The point of maximal impulse is usually evident near the lateral aspect of the pectoralis major muscle. If a small guide catheter (7 Fr or less) is to be used, the skin may be infiltrated with 2% lidocaine, a skin nick made with a number 11 blade through the superficial fasciae, and the deep fasciae perforated using blunt dissection. A percutaneous approach may then be used to enter the vessel and place an appropriately sized vascular sheath. If larger vascular sheaths are to be used, the assistance of a vascular surgeon should be recruited to expose the vessel. The complex neurovascular anatomy of the region prohibits the interventionalist with limited experience in this anatomic area from undertaking the dissection without the assistance of a vascular surgeon. As previously mentioned, a transradial approach has also been used with initial excellent success.

Largely as a means to minimize bleeding complications associated with full anticoagulation and stents, Kiemeneij and Marco have developed the transradial approach for coronary access (41a). Patients are chosen who are unlikely to require a pacemaker or to become hemodynamically unstable. After assuring ulnar artery patency by means of an Allen's test, the radial artery is punctured at the level of the styloid process after local anesthesia and using the Seldinger technique. A wrist board placing the wrist in modest dorsiflexion is useful. A short, 6 Fr sheath is then inserted over an appropriately sized flexible wire. The fascia is often dense and predilation with an introducer is helpful. Arterial spasm with considerable pain is common, and intraarterial nitroglycerin may be helpful. The guiding catheter is then advanced over a wire in the same fashion as with a brachial approach to the coronary ostium and the procedure performed. As "passive" guide support with 6 Fr catheters is sometimes inadequate, deep coronary intubation (usually by advancing the guiding catheter over the wire and balloon) is frequently necessary. This must be done with caution, and requires the use of soft guide catheters (e.g., Pink Power, Schneider, Inc.). After the dilation of stent placement is complete, the sheath is removed and manual pressure is applied. Even with full anticoagulation, hemostasis is usually obtained within 20 minutes. The wrist board should be left in place to stabilize the area for several hours. Patients may be ambulatory within a few minutes after hemostasis has been assured. Ulnar artery occlusion is reported in about 5%, but symptomatic occlusion is extremely uncommon.

It must be remembered that even with large-lumen, 6 Fr guiding catheters, stents with delivery sheaths, for example, JJIS, cannot be used because of their size. For these stents, larger guiding catheters are required, which may prevent a radial approach.

The eventual role that this approach will play is uncertain. Stenting without anticoagulation after IVUS guidance or with postdeployment, high-pressure dilation may relegate a radial approach to a small niche.

Vascular radiologists routinely use a translumbar aortic puncture to access the aorta when the distal aorta or iliac arteries are occluded with atheromatous disease. Small (5 Fr) catheters are typically used for this, although larger catheters may be placed. Several logistic problems make this approach impractical for coronary arteriography or angioplasty. First, the patient must be positioned on his or her side, which makes coronary imaging difficult. Second, manipulation of the guide catheter using this access route is difficult. Third, since these patients frequently have extensive four-extremity atherosclerosis, their true central blood pressure is often unknown until the puncture is made. Bleeding complications related to translumbar aortic puncture in normotensive patients are infrequent, but the risk can rise to 25% in patients with severe systemic hypertension. Clearly, manual pressure cannot be applied nor can an open repair procedure be easily performed, so hemostasis is problematic. For these reasons, this approach is rarely considered.

Vascular radiologists and cardiologists with an interest in peripheral vascular disease have become increasingly deft at reestablishing patency in occluded iliac and femoral arteries and in the distal aorta. Thus an approach to the patient with bilateral lower extremity occlusions may be an initial transfemoral recanalization procedure to regain access to the aorta. When a long, occluded segment is present, the approach is often complicated by passage of the probing catheter into the subintimal space. Although

the dissection that occurs as a consequence of this is rarely associated with any significant clinical consequence, gaining entry into the subintimal space usually prevents successful recanalization through to the distal aorta.

The subclavian artery remains a theoretical possibility, but because of difficulty with hemostasis following the procedure, this artery is rarely considered. When faced with a patient with bilateral axillary occlusions, bilateral iliac occlusions, and a distal aortic occlusion that could not be recanalized using a transfemoral approach, we performed diagnostic angiography using a transcarotid approach. It should be remembered that the first cardiac catheterization was performed by Claude Bernard in 1844, when the right ventricle of a horse was entered via the jugular vein, and the left ventricle was entered retrogradely via the carotid artery (39). For human application the carotid artery was isolated by a vascular surgeon and then punctured using an 18-gauge needle. Five Fr diagnostic catheters were then advanced into the vessel. This was performed under continuous electroencephalographic monitoring. Although the procedure was successful and uncomplicated, this approach is clearly associated with high risk and is not recommended for diagnostic or therapeutic procedures.

Digital subtraction angiography can be used to identify appropriate vascular access routes in patients with extensive atherosclerosis obliterans. Using this technique, a venous injection of a radiolabeled tracer is made, and scans are made over the right and left shoulder girdles and over the abdomen and pelvis. Using subtraction techniques, the venous phase can be removed, and the arterial structures can be analyzed. Although the technique lacks the fine definition of arteriography, it is generally possible to determine whether a vessel is patent or occluded.

SUMMARY

Advances in guide catheter and balloon catheter technologies have permitted the "downsizing" of angioplasty systems. This has made transbrachial angioplasty more attractive than in the past, when 8 or 9 Fr vascular sheaths were necessary. Although untested, it is expected that smaller vascular sheaths will translate into fewer vascular complications. The success of transbrachial angioplasty is determined by the same factors that determine success with transfemoral angioplasty. Most complications occur with a frequency similar to those of transfemoral angioplasty, although theoretical considerations suggest that the transbrachial approach may be preferred for some interventions. The most serious complications related to vascular and neurologic injury can be minimized or avoided by exercising care to avoid trauma to the median nerve during isolation of the brachial artery and by prompt attention to vascular complications with the close collaboration of a vascular surgeon.

REFERENCES

1. Grossman W. Cardiac catheterization: historical perspective and present practice. In: Grossman W, ed. Cardiac catheterization and angiography. 3rd ed., Philadelphia: Lee & Febiger, 1986.
2. Forssmann W. Die Sondierung Des Rechten Herzens. Klin Wochenschr 1929;8:2085.
3. Garratt KN, Menke KK. Angioplasty guiding equipment. In: Vliestra RE, Holmes DR Jr, eds., Coronary balloon angioplasty. Cambridge, MA; Blackwell Scientific, 1993.
4. Kern MJ, Talley JD, Deligonul U, Serota H, Aguirre F et al. Preliminary experience with 5 and 6 French diagnostic guiding catheters for coronary angioplasty. Cathet Cardiovasc Diagn 1991;22:60–63.
5. Maouad J, Hebert JL, Guermonprez JL. Percutaneous brachial approach for transluminal coronary angioplasty. Cathet Cardiovasc Diagn 1989;18:118–120.
6. Kamada RO, Fergusson DJ, Itagaki RK. Percutaneous entry of the brachial artery for transluminal coronary angioplasty. Cathet Cardiovasc Diagn 1988;15:132–133.
7. Deligonul U, Gabliani G, Kern MJ, Vandormael M. Percutaneous brachial catheterization: the hidden hazard of high brachial artery bifurcation. Cathet Cardiovasc Diagn 1988;14:44–45.
8. Korr KS, Januski V. Percutaneous brachial coronary angioplasty utilizing a standard de arm sheath introducer system. Cathet Cardiovasc Diagn 1989;18:121–124.
9. Spaccavento LJ, Breisblatt WM. Use of femoral artery guiding catheters via the left brachial artery for transluminal coronary angioplasty. Cathet Cardiovasc Diagn 1990; 20:182–184.
10. Dorros G, Lewin RF. The brachial artery method to transluminal internal mammary artery angioplasty. Cathet Cardiovasc Diagn 1986;12:341–346.
11. Salinger M, Drummer E, Furey K, Bott Silverman C, Franco

I. Percutaneous angioplasty of internal mammary artery graft stenosis using the brachial approach: a case report. Cathet Cardiovasc Diagn 1986;12:261–265.
12. Singh S. Coronary angioplasty of internal mammary artery graft. Am J Med 1987;82:361–362.
13. Brown RI, Galligan L, Penn IM, Weinstein L. Right internal mammary artery graft angioplasty through a right brachial artery approach using a new custom guide catheter: a case report. Cathet Cardiovasc Diagn 1992;25:42–45.
14. Ueno K, Kotoo Y, Arai M, Matsubara T, Watanabe S, Ito H, Hirakawa S. Coronary angioplasty using an over-the-wire balloon catheter through a new 6 French guiding catheter. Cathet Cardiovasc Diagn 1992;26:61–68.
15. Dorros G, Lewin RF. Percutaneous transluminal angioplasty of a brachial artery occlusion after cardiac catheterization. Am J Cardiol 1987;59:163.
16. Mouad J, Guermonprez JL. Percutaneous femoral transluminal angioplasty of a right brachial artery occluded after Sones coronary angiography. Cathet Cardiovasc Diagn 1988;14:165–168.
17. Widlus DM, Venbrux AC, Benati JF, Mitchell SE et al. Fibrinolytic therapy for upper extremity arterial occlusions. Radiology 1990;175:393–399.
18. Angelini P, Bush HS. Brachial artery injury as a complication of cardiac catheterization: percutaneous transluminal angioplasty and streptokinase as a treatment alternative. Cathet Cardiovasc Diagn 1988;15:243–246.
19. Mann JW, Davidson JT. Vein patch angioplasty for brachial arterial occlusion after cardiac catheterization. Am Surg 1990;56:520–522.
20. George BS, Candela RJ, Topol EJ, Stack RS et al. Brachial approach to emergency cardiac catheterization during thrombolytic therapy for acute myocardial infarction. TAMI study group. Cathet Cardiovasc Diagn 1990;20:221–226.
21. Dorros G, Lewin RF, Jamnadas P, Mathiak LM. Peripheral transluminal angioplasty of the subclavian and innominate arteries utilizing the brachial approach: acute outcome and follow-up. Cathet Cardiovasc Diagn 1990;19:71–76.
22. Shapira S, Braun SD, Puram B, Patel G, Rotman H. Percutaneous transluminal angioplasty of proximal subclavian artery stenosis after left internal mammary to left anterior descending artery bypass surgery. J Am Coll Cardiol 1991;18:1120–1123.
23. Selby JB Jr, Matsumoto AH, Tegtmeyer CJ, Hartwell GD et al. Balloon angioplasty above the aortic arch: immediate and long-term results. Am J Roentgenol 1992; 160:631–635.
24. Sharma S, Kaul U, Rajani M. Identifying high-risk patients for percutaneous transluminal angioplasty of subclavian and innominate arteries. Acta Radiol 1991;32:381–385.
25. Iyer SS, Hall P, Dorros G. Brachial approach to management of an abdominal aortic occlusion with prolonged lysis and subsequent angioplasty. Cathet Cardiovasc Diagn 1991;23:290–293.
26. Dacie JE, Daniell SJ. The value of percutaneous transluminal angioplasty of the profunda femoris artery in threatened limb loss and intermittent claudication. Clin Radiol 1991; 44:311–316.

27. Doorey AJ, Rosenbloom MA, Zolnick MR. Successful angioplasty of a chronically occluded saphenous vein graft using a prolonged urokinase infusion from the brachial route. Cathet Cardiovasc Diagn 1991;23:127–129.

28. Rogers WF, Kraft MA. Outpatient angioplasty. Radiology 1990;174:753–755.

29. Cragg DR, Friedman HZ, Almany SL, Glazier SM, O'Neill WW. Interim safety analysis of the Beaumont Outpatient Angioplasty Trial. J Am Coll Cardiol 1991;17:30A (abstract).

30. Khoury M, Batra S, Berg R, Rama K, Kozul V. Influence of arterial access sites and interventional procedures on vascular complications after cardiac catheterizations. Am J Surg 1992;164:205–209.

31. Babu SC, Piccorelli GO, Shah PM, Stein JH, Clauss RH. Incidence and results of arterial complications among 16,350 patients undergoing cardiac catheterization. J Vasc Surg 1989;10:113–116.

32. Michelson B, Schwengel RH, English P, Patrick C, Herpel K, Ziskind AA. Successful use of the right brachial approach to perform directional atherectomy of the left coronary artery. Cathet Cardiovasc Diagn 1993;(Suppl 1):45–47.

33. Rosenblum J, Stertzer SH, Schechtmann NS, Hidalgo B et al. Brachial rotational atherectomy. Cathet Cardiovasc Diagn 1991;24:32–36.

34. Rosenschein U, Ellis SG. Preprocedure warfarinization and brachial approach for elective coronary stent placement—a possible strategy to decrease cost and duration of hospitalization. Cathet Cardiovasc Diagn 1992;25:290–292.

35. Jenny DB, Robert GP, Fajadet JC, Cassagneau BG, Marco J. Intracoronary stent implantation: new approach using a monorail system and new large-lumen 7F catheters from the brachial route. Cathet Cardiovasc Diagn 1992;25:297–299.

36. Foster-Smith KW, Garratt KN, Higano ST, Holmes DR Jr. Retrie Valsalva techniques for managing flexible intracoronary stent misplacement. Cathet Cardiovasc Diagn 1993;30:63–68.

37. White CJ, Ramee SR, Collins TJ, Escobar A, for Main STATUS POST. Placement of "biliary" stents in saphenous vein coronary bypass grafts. Cathet Cardiovasc Diagn 1993;30:91–95.

38. Friedrich SP, Davis SF, Kuntz RE, Carrozza JP Jr, Baim DS. Investigational use of the Palmaz-Schatz biliary stent in large saphenous vein grafts. Am J Cardiol 1993;71:439–41.

39. Dorros G, Mathiak L. Direct deployment of the iliofemoral balloon expandable Palmaz stent utilizing a small (7.5 French) arterial puncture. Cathet Cardiovasc Diagn 1993;28:80–82.

40. Colombo A, Maiello L, Almagor Y, Thomas J, Zerboni S et al. Coronary stenting: single institution experience with the initial 100 cases using the Palmaz-Schatz stent. Cathet Cardiovasc Diagn 1992;26:171–176.

41. Cribier A, Savin T, Berland J, Rocha P et al. Percutaneous transluminal balloon valvuloplasty of adult aortic stenosis: report of 92 cases. J Am Coll Cardiol 1987;9:381–386.

41a. Kiemeneij F, Laarman GJ, de Melker E. Percutaneous radial artery entry for coronary angioplasty. European Heart J 1993;14:288 (abstract).

42. McIvor J, Rhymer JC. Two hundred forty-five transaxillary arteriograms in arteriopathic patients: success rate and complications. Clin Radiol 1992;45:390–394.

43. Cornand A. Cardiac catheterization. Development of the technique, its contributions to experimental medicine, and its initial application in man. Acta Med Scand Suppl 1975;579:1–32.

B. The Brachial Approach to Coronary Intervention

SIMON H. STERTZER

HISTORICAL PERSPECTIVES

The art and science of coronary angiography emerged fully in 1958 when F. Mason Sones perfected the selective brachial method (1). Sones' seminal contribution not only opened the floodgate to a clearer understanding of the morphologic correlates of clinical coronary atherosclerosis, but helped to accelerate the development of coronary revascularization surgery as well. Selective coronary angiography ultimately ushered in the present era of interventional cardiology that began in 1977. Indeed, the femoral approach to selective coronary angiography was perfected some 4 years after Sones' contribution by the dedicated radiographer Melvin Judkins (2). All interventionalists working today owe their subspecialty's infrastructure to these historic achievements.

In 1978 Myler and Stertzer began percutaneous transluminal coronary angioplasty in the United States following the monumental effort of Andreas Gruentzig in Zurich in 1977. Shortly thereafter, Stertzer, Dorros, and Kaltenbach paved the way for coronary angioplasty to be adapted to the brachial approach, utilizing the principles of the original Sones technique (3). The author developed the first safe and effective multipurpose guiding catheter tool for the conduct of upper extremity

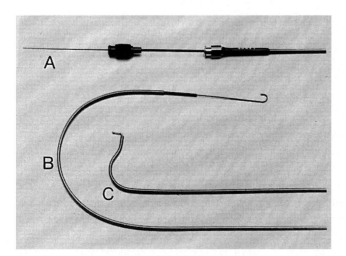

Figure 34B.1. **A.** Proximal hub of guiding catheter with introducer and guidewire. **B.** Straight tip of brachial guiding catheter (Stertzer), showing introducer and J wire. **C.** Bent-tip brachial guide with forming stylet in place.

balloon angioplasty (4). This so-called Stertzer guide is still in use (USCI-BARD, Billerica, MA) and has been the mainstay conduit of brachial angioplasty (Fig. 34B.1). Dorros, Stertzer, George, DeLaFuente, Kaltenbach, Kober, and their associates have collectively exceeded 12,000 brachial balloon angioplasty procedures since 1978.

After 1985 the rapid improvement in femoral guiding catheters, coupled with the astonishing advances in balloon and guidewire technology, led to a gradual decrease in the use of brachial angioplasty, as well as to an unmistakable attenuation of its instruction in domestic training programs. Although the surgical cut-down method remains extremely reliable and attended by very low complication rates, its art has somewhat disappeared from catheterization laboratory teaching programs. Moreover, not only is the surgical handling of the brachial artery meticulously demanding, but the angiographic catheter manipulations from the upper extremity require at least 18 to 24 months of intensive training for unequivocal expertise.

Nonetheless, the inclusion of a discussion of this method remains appropriate since some interventions are still easier, safer, and occasionally addressable only via the brachial approach.

BRACHIAL ARTERY ACCESS

The access to the right or left brachial artery may be from either the percutaneous or the direct cut-down method. The cut-down is traditional, requires definite surgical skill, and is the subject of this section. The percutaneous method, while feasible, is accomplished by a modified Seldinger technique and involves the placement of a sheath in the vessel. Generally, preformed Judkins, Amplatz, or multipurpose guides are placed into a 7 or 8 Fr sheath, and diagnostic or therapeutic interventions are then carried out in fashion similar to the retrograde femoral approach (5). Despite communications reporting the safety and efficacy of percutaneous brachial angioplasty, it is a method clearly associated with greater difficulty in gaining access to smaller vessels, and repeatedly engenders more spasm secondary to the sheath's presence in the vessel. Diagnostic and therapeutic interventions are now possible percutaneously with 6 Fr and even 5 Fr sheaths, but are quite limited in scope compared with the versatility of 8 Fr and larger guiding catheter interventions. In addition, the percutaneous brachial approach is definitely attended by more hemorrhagic complications in the postprocedural period, since hemostasis is affected by compression rather than by direct suturing of an arteriotomy. This is particularly problematic in patients who require prolonged post-procedural anticoagulation. Indeed, in the author's view, it is probably safer to have a vascular surgeon assist an operator who is unfamiliar with direct cut-down than to have a percutaneous brachial artery puncture performed on an infrequent basis. Moreover, as stated by George (6), it is better to refer the patient to an experienced brachial operator than to attempt a rare upper-extremity procedure.

Although much has been written about the brachial cut-down (6, 7), some descriptive facts are still worth retaining. Firstly, it is clear that the brachial cut-down can be performed repeatedly in the same vessel (usually the right brachial artery), provided normal or near-normal brachial and radial pulses return after each procedure. Indeed, even one repeat procedure may be ill-advised in a patient whose first procedure was complicated by brachial obstruction and surgical reconstruction after pulse loss, whereas four or five interventions may be completely feasible if the prior intervention returned both the radial and brachial pulses to normal.

In general, second and succeeding cut-downs are performed by making skin incisions about 1 cm above the previous cut-down site. However, if multiple incisions are made more and more cephalad, the artery tends to lie more deeply in muscle and follows more closely the median nerve. Although this is not an insurmountable technical problem, deep proximal cut-downs can sometimes be avoided if the brachial artery (a) is undiminished by prior procedures and (b) is easily palpable below the most distal incision site. In those cases where the brachial artery is still fully palpable superficially below the most distal incision site, a cut-down can be performed with relative ease and a catheter introduced retrograde past the healed arteriotomy sites.

First-time incisions for brachial artery cut-

down are still performed in the antecubital space where the vessel is felt most prominently, usually just above the arm crease. The incision length is generally about 15 mm, but varies directly with the depth of the brachial artery. The incision is retracted with a self-retaining ophthalmic or pediatric retractor, and the brachial artery is isolated with umbilical or elastic tapes. Most angiographers still employ a horizontal skin incision with a vertical arteriotomy.

The standard Stertzer guide may be used for retrograde diagnostic angiography, as well as for coronary angioplasty. If the Stertzer guide is used, it is introduced after the arteriotomy by first introducing its inner sheath and then passing a 0.032 or 0.035-inch J guidewire up to the subclavian artery (Fig. 34B.1). The nontapered guide is then eased through the arteriotomy using the inner introducer (Fig. 34B.2).

As the J guidewire is advanced through the innominate artery on the right (or the left subclavian on the left), the introducer catheter is withdrawn into the guiding catheter.

After the 0.035-inch wire reaches the sinus of Valsalva, both the introducer and the wire are then removed and the guiding cath-

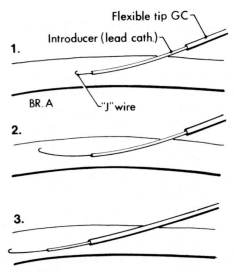

Figure 34B.2. Brachial artery cut-down. *GC,* Guiding catheter; *BR.A,* brachial artery.

eter attached to the rotating adaptor in the standard fashion. At the time of the arteriotomy, 4000 units of heparin (diluted in 10 cc of saline) are introduced into the distal brachial circulation just before the guiding catheter is introduced. The remainder of the heparin required for an angioplasty procedure (6000 to 11,000 units) is given as soon as the guiding catheter arrives at the sinus of Valsalva. An activated clotting time is checked and followed (every 30 minutes) throughout the procedure and is regularly maintained above 300 seconds.

At the termination of the procedure, the vertical arteriotomy is repaired with 6-0 monofilament nylon interrupted sutures. Although much discussion still centers about arteriotomy opening and closing patterns, the safest method still appears to be vertical arteriotomy and vertical interrupted closure. These statements are made as guidelines to those unfamiliar with the method, recognizing that the pursestring and other closures that experienced hands have used over the years yield excellent results as well.

Finally, the surgical care of the brachial wound is critical for complication-free results. If the radial pulse is absent after the procedure, the arteriotomy site is immediately reexplored by the operator. If thrombus or antegrade flap is identified, it is corrected immediately. If full flow is not restored in the hemodynamics laboratory, a vascular surgeon should be asked to see the patient. Occasionally, a diminished pulse can be caused by spasm alone. Should complications result in more than 1% of the cases, the operative technique should be reevaluated.

The skin closures are effected with sutures of 4-0 Dermalon or similar monofilament nylon, and the wound is kept dry until suture removal at 1 week. Patients may obviously remain fully anticoagulated after brachial cut-down and repair, provided that (a) the arteriotomy has been neatly and completely sealed surgically at the end of the procedure, and (b) a firm, wide, but nonocclusive (arte-rial) pressure dressing of elastic bandage is utilized for several hours, or overnight, after the procedure. This dressing must be watched closely in heparinized patients so that oozing is prevented from creating subcutaneous intrafascial hematomas. Care must be taken to avoid hand ischemia or severe venous congestion, since the only way to prevent oozing in heparinized patients is to encircle the arm dressing completely with the elastic bandage.

BRACHIAL GUIDE MANIPULATION FOR ROUTINE PTCA

As stated above, the Stertzer guide with its 3-inch flexible tip is not only still a standard guide for low-profile balloon percutaneous transluminal coronary angioplasty, but it may also be used for diagnostic angiography since its longer tip makes it easier to access the coronary orifice than the standard Sones diagnostic catheter. However, the guiding catheter is 8.3 Fr as opposed to the standard Sones 8 Fr, thus requiring a minimally longer arteriotomy (about 1 mm) for the introduction and for the repair of the brachial artery.

When the brachial guide is advanced into the sinus of Valsalva, a gentle loop is made in the left coronary sinus. The simplest projection for learning brachial guide manipulation is the right anterior oblique projection for the left coronary artery (Fig. 34B.3).

Figure 34B.4A shows a brachial catheter directly intubating the left main coronary artery in a discrete type A lesion of the left anterior descending coronary artery. The left anterior descending coronary artery can frequently be selectively entered by rotating the Sones diagnostic or Stertzer guiding catheter clockwise in the left main coronary artery. In Figure 34B.4B the brachial guide is in the classical J form in a gentle loop in the left sinus of Valsalva with the tip engaging in the left main coronary artery in the right anterior oblique position. In Figure 34B.4C, postangioplasty, the guide slack has been removed from the semi-power position in Figure

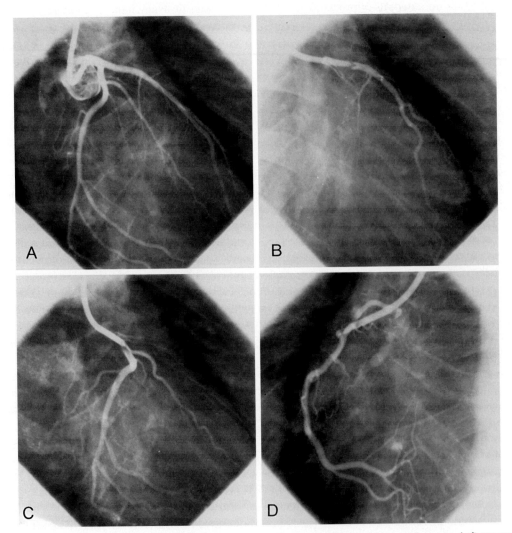

Figure 34B.3.   A. The Stertzer guiding catheter in formation of an appropriate loop in a smaller aorta. Left coronary artery is seen in RAO projection. **B.** Selective intubation of the LAD seen in **A,** in the RAO projection. **C.** Selective intubation of the left circumflex artery in the RAO projection. **D,** Right coronary artery, selective intubation LAO view of Figure 34B.13, *A* and *B.*

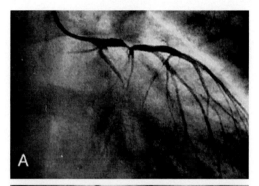

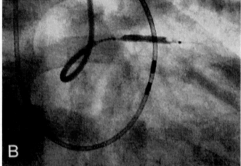

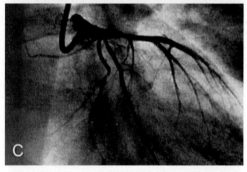

Figure 34B.4. **A.** Left anterior descending coronary artery stenosis prior to dilation. **B.** Brachial guiding catheter with standard dilation catheter inflated. **C.** Left anterior descending coronary artery after angioplasty; right anterior oblique position.

34B.4*B* to a smaller loop diagnostic configuration.

In summary, introduction of the brachial guiding catheter into the left coronary artery is thus accomplished by first maneuvering it into a J shape in the left main coronary artery and then rotating it counterclockwise from this loop, in the left coronary sinus in the RAO projection (Fig. 34B.3*A*). This manipulation will direct the tip of the catheter poste-

riorly, where it can be seen to engage the left coronary orifice. Power backup is usually achieved by levering the guiding catheter in its J shape into the left main coronary artery, backing its loop against the opposite wall, and then increasing the guiding shaft pressure by pushing at the brachial incision site.

Subselective engagement into the left anterior descending is sometimes achievable as stated above, by lifting the loop of the J and turning the main stem–engaged guiding catheter clockwise into the left anterior descending itself (see Fig. 34B.3*B*). For selective intubation of the left circumflex, the loop may be turned counterclockwise (Fig. 34B.3*C*), but more reliably, a bent-tip Stertzer guide is the key to subselective intubation of the circumflex vessel (Fig. 34B.1*C*).

Examples of subselective intubation of the left anterior descending and circumflex arteries (required for backup support during balloon angioplasty) are also seen in Figures 34B.5 and 34B.6.

In Figure 34B.7*A* note how the upwardly directed brachial guiding catheter approaches a long segment of disease in the origin of the left anterior descending coronary artery. Yet, in 34B.7*B* observe how the balloon equipment redirects the guide tip. Finally, although in 34B.7*C* the end result is satisfactory, it is more likely that high-speed rotational atherectomy would be used primarily to debulk an original lesion of this type today.

The right coronary artery is perhaps the best target vessel for balloon angioplasty via the brachial approach. Indeed, anterior takeoffs creating noncoaxial guide positions, and "shepherd's crook" curves in the right coronary artery occasionally render balloon angioplasty extremely difficult in this vessel. Most of those guiding catheter problems associated with the groin approach are readily avoided by a brachial approach. In the past few years, however, the advent of the Arani double loop and the so-called hockey-stick guides have clearly joined with the lower pro-

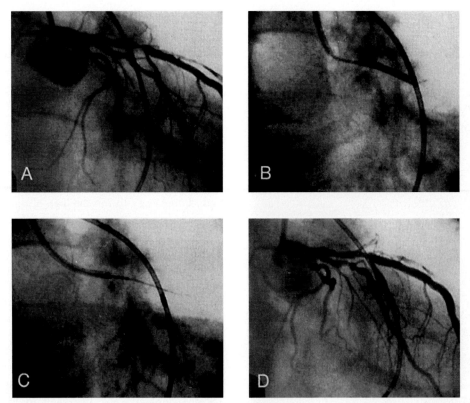

Figure 34B.5. **A.** Stenosis in the mid anterior descending artery just beyond pacing catheter. **B.** Superselective guide entry up to the lesion with balloon force-through. **C.** Guiding catheter retracted during balloon inflation. **D.** Result of angioplasty is seen directly under pacing catheter.

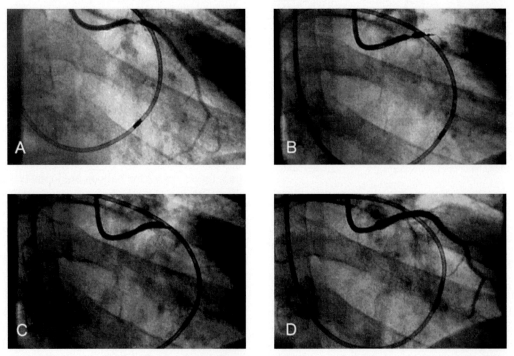

Figure 34B.6. **A.** High-grade, isolated circumflex lesion, superselectively photographed with the guiding catheter directly at the lesion. **B.** Balloon forced through with proximal portion of dilation catheter still within guide. **C.** Full balloon inflation. **D.** Result of angioplasty.

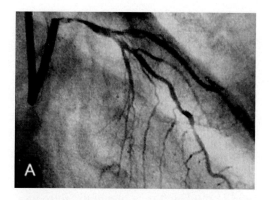

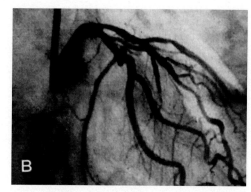

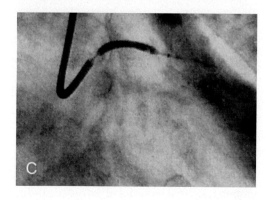

Figure 34B.7. **A.** Long segment, high-grade stenosis of anterior descending artery filmed through guiding catheter, selectively injecting anterior descending ramus. **B.** Balloon inflation—right anterior oblique view. **C.** Reconstitution of anterior descending artery.

file, more pushable balloons to decrease the necessity for utilizing the upper extremity approach. Nonetheless, some angioplasty procedures remain extremely difficult, if not impossible, to complete in the right coronary artery from the femoral approach. In Figure 34B.8 a severe "shepherd's crook" resulted in PTCA failure from the groin in an experienced center. The ascending portion of the hairpin curve is not dissected, but merely represents streaming of contrast in a single 35-mm frame. The guiding catheter here is functioning as a diagnostic catheter. In Figure 34B.8B the 3-inch, medium-curve brachial guiding catheter is advanced into a power position at the apex of the "shepherd's crook," permitting backup for the passage of a high-torque floppy wire and 3.5-mm balloon catheter beyond and into the lesion, respectively. In Figure 34B.8C the post-PTCA frame shows the patency of the final successful result.

In another "failure-to-cross" right coronary femoral case (Fig. 34B.9A) a total occlusion of the right coronary artery is seen. In Figure 34B.9B deep penetration of the brachial guiding catheter permits enough backup to force the 3.0-mm angioplasty balloon across the lesion. In Figure 34B.9C the total occlusion has been opened via the brachial approach, and a bifurcation lesion of the posterior descending and posterolateral branch has been identified. The upper extremity approach now permitted a second "kissing wire" and balloon to complete the bifurcation angioplasty successfully as seen in Figure 34B.9D.

The more classic type A lesion (Fig. 34B.10A) was approached via the right brachial artery in a patient with iliac vessels too tortuous for any femoral access. In Figure 34B.10B the 3.5-mm balloon is inflated, and in Figure 34B.10C the post-PTCA result is

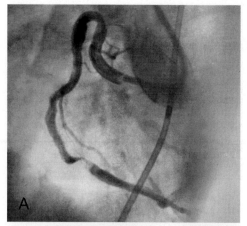

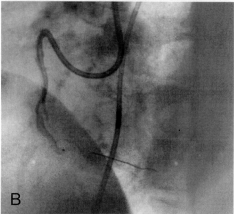

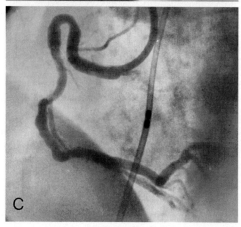

Figure 34B.8. A. "Shepherd's crook" right coronary artery with high-grade lesion at 7 o'clock, photographed via brachial guide 8 Fr. Pacing catheter in pulmonary artery. **B.** Power position of 3-inch medium brachial guide in power position of shepherd's crook. High-torque floppy II wire distal to 3.5-mm balloon catheter *(dot at 7 o'clock).* Balloon centered in lesion. **C.** Post-PTCA angiogram via brachial guide.

shown. Deep penetration into the right coronary artery is usually effected by turning the catheter in Figure 34B.10*B* in the clockwise direction.

The brachial approach to coronary intervention includes a full capability to deal with coronary bypass grafts, as well as with native circulation disease. Both saphenous vein grafts and internal mammary arteries are readily accessed via the arm approach. Indeed, the mammary arteries are often only readily intubated by a brachially introduced guiding catheter in cases where groin access is tortuous or impossible. Brachial guide access to the IMA orifice is frequently done from the ipsilateral extremity by first intubating the LIMA or RIMA with an appropriate diagnostic catheter and then introducing the brachial guide carefully over an exchange wire.

NEW-DEVICE UPPER EXTREMITY INTERVENTIONS

In addition to the 90-cm Stertzer guiding catheter, several varieties of extruded guiding catheters are technically capable of being introduced into the brachial artery. The so-called Castillo (modified Amplatz) guiding catheters are usable conduits for balloon angioplasty in some vein grafts of the left circumflex arteries that require special backup powers not provided by the woven-Dacron USCI brachial guide. In addition, new-device interventions by the brachial approach, such as stent delivery, high-speed rotational ablation, and even directional atherectomy, are all feasible using the upper extremity pathway when the groin is inaccessible for standard operations.

The brachial cut-down is still usually performed via the right brachial artery for new-device intervention. The arteriotomy incision for stent guide introduction (usually 8 Fr) is identical to that performed in balloon PTCA.

However, high-speed rotational atherectomy, directional atherectomy, and balloon valvuloplasty require a modified approach because of the requirement for 9 Fr, 10 Fr, and

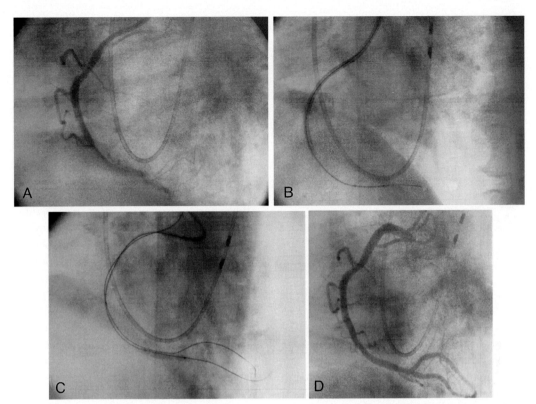

Figure 34B.9. **A.** Total occlusion RCA at crux of heart. **B.** Deep penetration of brachial guide into RCA permitting 3.0-mm balloon to cross lesion. **C.** Total occlusion opened with bifurcation lesion identified ("kissing-balloon," double-arm guide technique). **D.** Post-PTCA result.

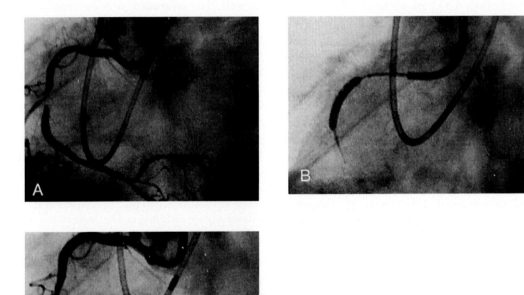

Figure 34B.10. **A.** Type A lesion in LAO projection seen via right brachial approach. **B.** Fixed-wire balloon inflated in RCA via a brachial guide. **C.** Postangioplasty control injection, RAO view. Pacing catheter in pulmonary artery.

Table 34B.1.
Modification of Brachial Artery Management for
>8.3 Fr Guiding Catheters

1. Horizontal skin incision up to 9 Fr guides. Vertical skin incision perhaps usually more cephalad than standard Sones incision for greater than 9 Fr guides. (Arteriotomy incision may be carried up or down with Potts' scissors to accommodate the larger device.)
2. Longitudinal arteriotomy incision mandatory.
3. The 6-0 monofilament nylon closure may be continuous suture rather than interrupted because of the length of the arteriotomy.
4. Utilize brachial arteries that appear to be at least 4 mm in diameter (e.g., older patients, more proximal arterial incisions).

11 Fr guiding catheters on occasions. Indeed, double-balloon aortic valvuloplasty has routinely been carried out by Dorros and the author using one balloon from the groin, one balloon from the brachial artery, or both balloon valvuloplasty catheters (up to 15 mm in diameter) from the right and left brachial arteries simultaneously (8). Table 34B.1 depicts the technique modifications used for these more extensive arteriotomies where greater than 8.3 Fr guides are used.

If the caveats of Table 34B.1 are followed, spasm, bleeding, or pulse loss are no more frequent than in arteriotomies done for standard balloon angioplasty with the 8.3 Fr guiding catheter.

In Figure 34B.11A a calcified right coronary artery lesion is seen in the left anterior oblique position in the patient with a high right coronary take-off and no femoral access. Figure 34B.11B shows the diagnostic study with an Amplatz catheter in the right anterior oblique projection demonstrating the anterior position of the right coronary origin. In Figure 34B.11C one of the Rotablator (Heart Technology Inc., Bellevue, WA) burrs is seen passing into the right coronary lesion via a 9 Fr guiding catheter introduced from the right brachial artery. Figure 34B.11, D and E show the LAO and RAO views, respectively, after high-speed rotational ablation. In Figure 34B.11C note the platinum tip of the 0.009-inch Heart Technology wire in the distal right

coronary artery as the guide for the Rotablator burr.

Directional atherectomy, as noted above, is also feasible via the upper extremity approach, provided the brachial artery is large enough for the appropriate guiding catheter introduction. In Figure 34B.12 there is a thrombotic total occlusion of the left anterior descending coronary artery in a patient 3 days after anterior myocardial infarction. Because of the presence of clinical ischemia and the passage of 72 hours since failed thrombolysis, the Simpson Atherocath (DVI, Mountain View, CA) is introduced into the total left anterior descending obstruction via a brachially introduced DVI guide (Fig. 34B.12B). The thrombus and atherosclerotic plaque have been extracted by the device, and patency with TIMI 3 flow has been restored to the left anterior descending coronary artery (Fig. 34B.12C).

The upper extremity approach to vascular intervention is extended to the treatment of peripheral vascular and renal artery disease as well. The treatment of acute myocardial infarction is also eminently feasible utilizing this approach. Indeed, the upper extremity route of intervention continues to adapt to new devices and remains a useful adjunct for the modern interventional cardiologist or radiographer.

SUMMARY

Future directions in coronary intervention may continue to rely on brachial approaches for certain subsets. Currently, even radial artery percutaneous stent introduction via 6 Fr catheters is being extensively investigated in The Netherlands and in France.

Deep but safe power positions remain feasible using the woven-Dacron brachial guides. This is of particular help in patients with ostial lesions when there is concern that a femoral approach may result in guide catheter trauma (Fig. 34B.13, A and B). Finally, it should also be observed that full left ventriculography may be carried out by hand injection using the 8.3 Fr brachial guide (Fig. 34B.13C).

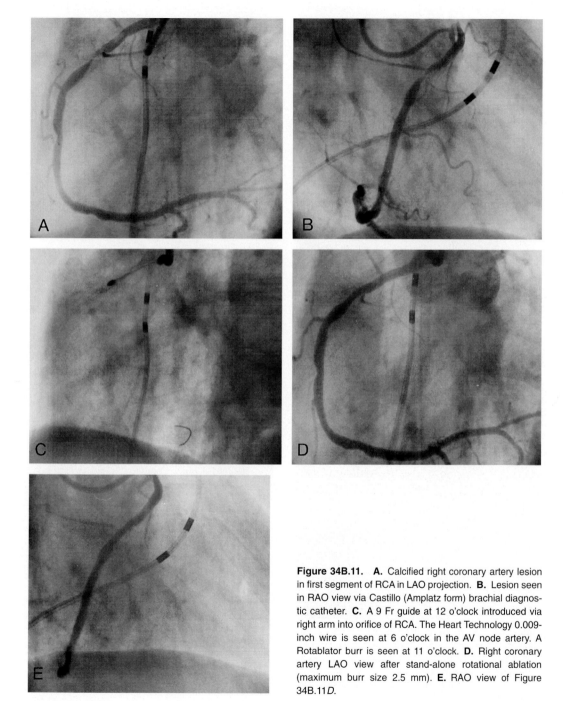

Figure 34B.11. **A.** Calcified right coronary artery lesion in first segment of RCA in LAO projection. **B.** Lesion seen in RAO view via Castillo (Amplatz form) brachial diagnostic catheter. **C.** A 9 Fr guide at 12 o'clock introduced via right arm into orifice of RCA. The Heart Technology 0.009-inch wire is seen at 6 o'clock in the AV node artery. A Rotablator burr is seen at 11 o'clock. **D.** Right coronary artery LAO view after stand-alone rotational ablation (maximum burr size 2.5 mm). **E.** RAO view of Figure 34B.11*D*.

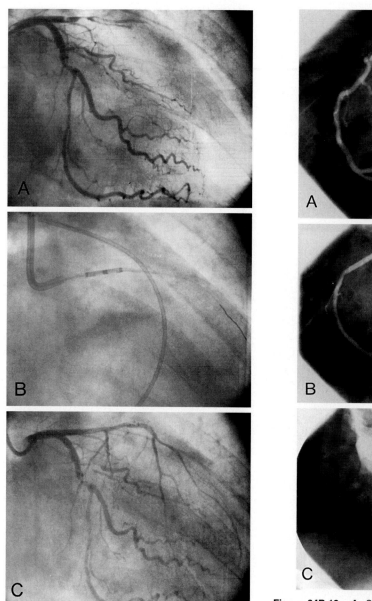

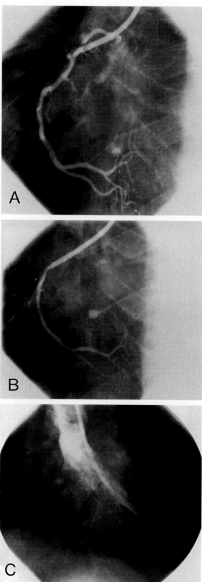

Figure 34B.12. **A.** Thrombotic occlusion LAD, RAO view. **B.** Atherocath EX 6 Fr being advanced into LAD over high-torque floppy II 0.014-inch guidewire into occlusion. Brachial guide is a left DVI 9 Fr. **C.** After standalone directional atherectomy, RAO view via Sones diagnostic catheter.

Figure 34B.13. **A.** Selective angiography of the RCA. LAO using Stertzer brachial guide in firm diagnostic position (see Fig. 34B.3D). **B.** Same RCA as in **A** with deep penetration power position. LAO projection. **C.** Left ventriculogram, end systole, RAO projection, hand injection via Stertzer brachial guide.

REFERENCES

1. Sones FM, Shirey EK. Cine coronary arteriography. Mod Conc Cardiovasc Dis 1962;31:735.
2. Judkins MP. Selective coronary arteriography: a percutaneous transfemoral technique. Radiology 1967;89:815–824.
3. Dorros G, Stertzer S, Kaltenbach M, Bruno MS. The brachial artery approach to (percutaneous) transluminal coronary angioplasty. Circulation 1980;62(Suppl III):III-161 (abstract).
4. Stertzer SH. Brachial approach to transluminal coronary angioplasty. In: Angioplasty. New York: McGraw-Hill, 1986.
5. Maouad J, Hebert JL, Guermonprez JL. Percutaneous brachial approach for transluminal coronary angioplasty. Cathet Cardiovasc Diagn 1989;18:118–120.
6. George BS, Stertzer S. Brachial technique to intervention. In: Topol EJ, ed. Textbook of interventional cardiology. Philadelphia: WB Saunders, 1990.
7. Jang DJ. Angioplasty. New York: McGraw-Hill, 1986.
8. Dorros G, Lewin RF, Stertzer SH, King JF, Waller BF, Myler RK, Mathiak L et al. Percutaneous transluminal aortic valvuloplasty—the acute outcome and follow-up of 149 patients who underwent the double balloon technique. Eur Heart J 1990;11:429–440.

35. Approach to Elastic Recoil

ROBERT D. SAFIAN

Prior to Food and Drug Administration (FDA) approval of the Simpson Directional Coronary Atherocath (DCA, Devices for Vascular Intervention, Mountain View, CA) in 1989, the only percutaneous device approved for use in human coronary arteries was the balloon angioplasty catheter. Since that time, several other devices have been approved by the FDA, including the transluminal extraction catheter (TEC, Interventional Technologies, San Diego, CA), the high-speed mechanical rotational atherectomy device (Rotablator [MRA], Heart Technologies, Bellevue, WA), excimer lasers (ELCA, Advanced Interventional Systems, Irvine, CA), and intracoronary stents (Cook, Indianapolis, IN, and Johnson and Johnson Interventional Systems, Warren, NJ). Within the next few years, other percutaneous devices, including thermal angioplasty devices, biodegradable stents, and temporary stents may gain FDA approval and be available for widespread use in human coronary arteries. All of these devices have been developed with the hope of addressing the various limitations of balloon angioplasty (PTCA). The purpose of this chapter is to describe the treatment approach, using balloons and other devices, to the problem of elastic recoil.

DEFINITION OF ELASTIC RECOIL

Elastic recoil occurs to some extent after PTCA in virtually all lesions. This fact was recognized in early studies of PTCA, which reported residual stenoses of 25 to 35% despite full balloon inflation (1). Despite improvements in operator experience and angioplasty equipment, contemporary studies continue to report similar residual stenoses after PTCA (2). In fact, stretching of the arterial wall with subsequent elastic recoil appears to be more common than "remodeling" the arterial wall by cracking the arterial wall with controlled dissection (3). Since a residual stenosis of 25 to 35% is generally considered "acceptable" for PTCA, "significant" elastic recoil is usually associated with residual stenoses $\geq 50\%$ after full balloon inflation.

Certain lesion characteristics (e.g., ostial location, calcification, thrombus, severe angulation, total occlusion, eccentricity, and ulceration) are readily apparent by angiography before intervention. In contrast, although some lesion characteristics (eccentricity) *may* be associated with elastic recoil (4), most cases of significant elastic recoil are not predictable and become apparent only after PTCA. The post hoc recognition of elastic recoil is therefore similar to the post hoc recognition of dissection or abrupt closure, and treatment strategies are generally based on the fact that the lesion has already been dilated by conventional angioplasty techniques. For purposes of this discussion, it is important to distinguish true elastic recoil (that is, suboptimal luminal enlargement despite full balloon expansion) from failure to dilate a rigid lesion (that is, suboptimal luminal enlargement caused by failure to fully expand the inflated balloon).

ASSESSMENT OF ELASTIC RECOIL

From a practical standpoint, most operators estimate the extent of elastic recoil in the catheterization laboratory, based on apparent full expansion of the inflated balloon and visual estimation of the residual diameter stenosis. However, Hermans and colleagues have described more precise methods for estimating elastic recoil using computerized quantitative angiographic analysis to measure the minimal inflated balloon diameter (MBD), the residual luminal diameter after intervention (RLD), and the normal reference diameter (REF) (5). Elastic recoil was calculated by the following formula:

$$Elastic\ recoil = MBD - RLD/REF$$

Using densitometric and edge-detection techniques, elastic recoil accounted for an immediate loss of luminal diameter equivalent to 21 to 34% of the reference diameter, which is similar to the 25 to 35% residual stenosis commonly reported after PTCA.

The extent of elastic recoil after intervention with stents, atherectomy devices, and lasers has also been studied. Kuntz and associates reported virtual elimination of elastic recoil after stent implantation in native vessels and vein grafts (6). In the same study the extent of elastic recoil was 6% for directional atherectomy and 15% for laser balloon angioplasty. Safian and coworkers used measurements of device efficiency to estimate the extent of elastic recoil after TEC atherectomy, MRA, and excimer laser angioplasty (7). In their study device efficiency was defined as the ratio of the residual luminal diameter (RLD) to the diameter (D) of the largest device used (RLD/D), and elastic recoil was estimated by the following equation:

$$Elastic\ recoil = [1 - RLD/D] \times 100$$

Their data suggest that the efficiency of luminal enlargement was 73% for TEC, 92% for MRA, 85% for ELCA, and 71% for PTCA, corresponding to elastic recoil of 27% for TEC, 8% for MRA, 15% for ELCA, and 29% for PTCA. Unfortunately, there are no data to evaluate the extent of elastic recoil for these devices for specific lesion subsets. Furthermore, it is important to understand that adjunctive PTCA is required in 70 to 90% of lesions treated with TEC, MRA, and ELCA. The data reported by Safian et al. reflect the

extent of elastic recoil immediately after devices (before adjunctive PTCA). The impact on elastic recoil of pretreating lesions with these devices before subsequent PTCA is also under investigation. Preliminary studies from our institution suggest that PTCA after MRA (14% elastic recoil) and after DCA (22% elastic recoil) had significantly less recoil than PTCA alone (32% elastic recoil), or PTCA after TEC (31% elastic recoil) or after ELCA (31% elastic recoil) (8).

POTENTIAL TREATMENT STRATEGIES FOR ELASTIC RECOIL

In general, there are several potential treatment strategies to manage elastic recoil. The simplest initial approach is to perform repeat balloon inflations using a balloon:artery ratio of approximately 1.0. In some cases, a long (40-mm) balloon may be useful to completely cover the "shoulders" of the lesion and prevent dissection at the interface between plaque and normal vessel wall. If necessary, prolonged balloon inflations (10 to 30 minutes) can be performed with a perfusion balloon catheter. Although repeat PTCA may improve immediate luminal dimensions and achieve acceptable angiographic results, I am always concerned that these prolonged balloon inflations will not sufficiently "remodel" the vessel, and that within a few minutes to hours (once the patient has left the catheterization laboratory) recoil will recur. This is especially likely if the final residual stenosis is still 40 to 50%.

A second approach is to slightly oversize the balloon, using a balloon:artery ratio of 1.1 to 1.3. This can be accomplished by using compliant balloons inflated repeatedly above nominal inflation pressure, or by using noncompliant balloons which are 0.25 to 0.5 mm larger than the normal reference diameter, inflated to nominal inflation pressure. In my experience, this technique has been more effective than simply using prolonged balloon inflations, but the improvement in luminal dimensions may be achieved at the expense of

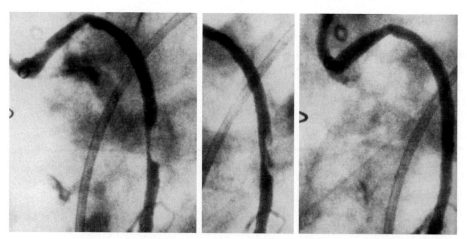

Figure 35.1. Eccentric stenosis in the body of a saphenous vein graft to the left anterior descending coronary artery *(left panel)*. Although PTCA resulted in no appreciable change in luminal diameter because of elastic recoil *(middle panel)*, there was no significant residual stenosis after implantation of a single Palmaz-Schatz stent *(right panel)*.

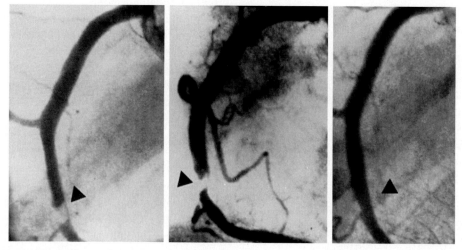

Figure 35.2. Eccentric stenosis in the right coronary artery *(left panel)*, which remained unchanged after conventional PTCA because of elastic recoil *(middle panel)*. After DCA there was no significant residual stenosis *(right panel)*. (Courtesy of Dr. Gregory Robertson and Devices for Vascular Intervention, Inc.)

an increased incidence of dissection leading to abrupt closure (9). In addition, recent studies suggest that the diameters of compliant balloons are unpredictable after multiple inflations, whereas the diameters of noncompliant balloons seem to be more predictable. Finally, Rensing et al. suggested that use of oversized balloons may not result in larger luminal dimensions since more stretch leads to more elastic recoil (10).

A third approach to elastic recoil is the intracoronary stent, which may offer the best solution to elastic recoil via its metal "scaffolding effects" (Fig. 35.1). Although self-expanding and certain balloon-expandable stents virtually eliminate elastic recoil (6, 11), some balloon-expandable stents may occasionally be compressed by vessel recoil, mandating the need for multiple overlapping stents. In addition, stents may require vigorous anticoagulation regimens to prevent stent thrombosis, sometimes require in-hospital admission for 6 to 7 days, may be associated with vascular and other bleeding complications, and are less useful in smaller (<3 mm) vessels. Although temporary stents are theoretically attractive because the need for long hospitalizations and chronic anticoagulation can be avoided, their utility for elastic recoil is uncertain for the same reasons as perfusion balloon angioplasty.

Directional coronary atherectomy (DCA) is a fourth approach to elastic recoil that may have significant value (12). Since eccentric lesions are often associated with elastic recoil caused by "stretching" the normal vascular wall, DCA can be used effectively to excise eccentric plaque (Fig. 35.2). DCA may also be useful in aortoostial and origin lesions, which are commonly associated with elastic recoil. However, although tissue excision may increase vascular compliance and facilitate luminal enlargement, DCA has limited utility in vessels <2.5 mm in diameter and in lesions associated with significant calcification.

Finally, the role of other atherectomy and laser devices for treatment of elastic recoil is unknown. Success of the Rotablator for these lesions is highly dependent on the nature of these lesions. Because of the principle of differential cutting, the Rotablator is much more effective at treating inelastic tissue associated with rigid and/or heavily calcified lesions, but is of much less value in the run-of-the-mill elastic lesion, not associated with calcification. The transluminal extraction catheter (TEC) does not appear to have any value for management of elastic recoil per se, and its use in native coronary arteries is frequently complicated by dissection and by a high incidence of restenosis. The real value of excimer lasers for treating elastic recoil is unknown, but they may also be useful for elastic recoil associated with plaque rigidity and calcification (Fig. 35.3). The directional laser may be useful for elastic recoil associated with eccentric lesions in smaller vessels.

In the future, thermal angioplasty devices may prove useful for treatment of elastic recoil. These devices have potentially broad appeal because of their ease of use, similarity to

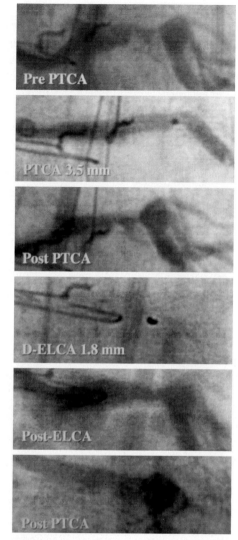

Figure 35.3. Highly eccentric and irregular stenosis in the distal left main coronary artery *(top panel)*. This lesion could not be treated with DCA because of inability to negotiate the right angle bend in the left circumflex coronary artery. Despite full balloon inflation using a 40-mm-long balloon *(2nd panel)*, there was no improvement in luminal diameter after PTCA because of marked elastic recoil *(3rd panel)*. Excimer laser angioplasty was performed with a 1.8-mm directional laser fiber *(4th panel)*, leaving a moderate residual stenosis *(5th panel)*, which was then redilated with the original balloon resulting in marked improvement in luminal diameter and minimal residual stenosis *(6th panel)*.

and compatibility with conventional balloon angioplasty systems, availability in a wide range of balloon diameters, and lack of need for special medications or prolonged hospitalization. Although laser balloon angioplasty (LBA) appeared to be quite effective at decreasing immediate elastic recoil in a randomized study compared with conventional PTCA, late (6-month) arterial dimensions were similar and there were no differences in restenosis rates (13). However, because of marketing concerns, further development of this device was terminated by the manufacturer. Physiologic low-stress angioplasty (PLOSA, Boston Scientific, Watertown, MA) is another thermal angioplasty system that relies on radiofrequency energy (rather than a laser source) to deliver heat to the arterial wall, and preliminary studies also suggest an early reduction in elastic recoil. Finally, thermal perfusion balloon angioplasty may offer additional promise for treatment of elastic recoil.

TREATMENT ALGORITHM FOR ELASTIC RECOIL

Unfortunately, there have not been any studies comparing the various treatment strategies for elastic recoil. However, the following strategies have worked effectively in a very busy interventional practice consisting of tertiary referrals from other interventional cardiologists:

If significant elastic recoil (residual stenosis ≥50%) occurs immediately following PTCA in a vessel ≥2.7 mm in diameter, I would strongly encourage directional atherectomy as the next therapeutic option, provided extensive dissection and/or heavy calcification are absent. Elastic recoil associated with mild or moderate focal dissection is readily treated by directional atherectomy. For relatively uncomplicated elastic recoil, I prefer DCA to stenting, to avoid prolonged hospitalization and the potential complications of stent thrombosis and bleeding. However, *if elastic recoil is also associated with significant dissection,* stenting would be my first choice of therapy, and I would discourage DCA because of the risk of coronary perforation.

If elastic recoil is associated with heavy vessel calcification, I would recommend Rotablator atherectomy to debulk the lesion, followed by either conventional PTCA or directional atherectomy. *If recoil is associated with significant dissection and vessel calcification,* I would recommend stenting. However, stenting should be avoided in situations where the original balloon cannot be fully inflated in the lesion, since it may then be impossible to deploy and fully expand the stent.

If significant elastic recoil occurs in a vessel <2.7 mm in diameter, DCA and stenting may not be practical solutions. If prolonged balloon inflations or slight oversizing with a noncompliant balloon are ineffective, I would recommend the Rotablator, particularly for calcified vessels, followed by conventional PTCA if necessary to achieve definitive luminal enlargement. For eccentric or long (≥20 mm) lesions, excimer laser angioplasty may be useful, followed by PTCA if necessary. If elastic recoil is associated with severe dissection, the best initial therapy is repeat PTCA, with a long (40 mm) balloon or perfusion balloon catheter.

A technical tip that may be useful concerns the exchange of guiding catheters. Occasionally, it may become necessary to exchange guiding catheters to adequately manage an elastic lesion, and it may be desirable to leave a guidewire in place to avoid recrossing the lesion. The most common circumstance is when conventional PTCA is performed using 6 to 8 Fr guiding catheters and the decision is made to insert a stent through a 9 Fr guide or perform DCA through a 10 Fr guide. Although several techniques can be used successfully, the technique I have found to be most useful and reliable is as follows:

Exchange the guidewire for a 0.018-inch, 300-cm-long Platinum-Plus guidewire (Meditech, Mansfield, MA), which is extremely stiff and durable. The 3-cm floppy tip should be placed in the distal vessel, and the original guiding catheter and sheath can then be removed. A new vascular sheath and guiding catheter can then be positioned over the Platinum-Plus guidewire, and stents can be delivered on a compatible balloon. If DCA is indicated, the 0.018-inch Platinum-Plus guidewire should be exchanged for an appropriate 0.014-inch guidewire.

SUMMARY

Elastic recoil is perhaps one of the most frequent and frustrating dilemmas faced by interventional cardiologists. However, the availability of stents, atherectomy devices, and lasers may simplify the management of elastic recoil by improving luminal dimensions and reducing the incidence of complications.

REFERENCES

1. Kent KM, Bentivoglio LG, Block PC et al. Percutaneous transluminal coronary angioplasty: report from the Registry of the National Heart, Lung and Blood Institute. Am J Cardiol 1982;49:2011.
2. Rensing BJ, Hermans WRM, Vos J et al. Angiographic risk factors of luminal narrowing after coronary balloon angioplasty using balloon measurements to reflect stretch and elastic recoil at the dilatation site. Am J Cardiol 1992; 69:584.
3. Jain A, Demer LL, Raizner AE, Hartley CJ, Lewis JM, Roberts R. In vivo assessment of vascular dilatation during percutaneous transluminal coronary angioplasty. Am J Cardiol 1987;60:988.
4. Rensing BJ, Hermans WR, Strauss BH, Serruys PW. Regional differences in elastic recoil after percutaneous transluminal coronary angioplasty: a quantitative angiographic study. J Am Coll Cardiol 1991;17:34B.
5. Hermans WRM, Rensing BJ, Strauss BH, Serruys PW. Methodological problems related to the quantitative assessment of stretch, elastic recoil, and balloon-artery ratio. Cathet Cardiovasc Diagn 1992;25:174.
6. Kuntz RE, Safian RD, Levine MJ et al. Novel approach to the analysis of restenosis after the use of three new coronary devices. J Am Coll Cardiol 1992;19:1493.
7. Safian RD, Freed M, Lichtenberg A et al. Are residual stenoses after excimer laser angioplasty and coronary atherectomy due to inefficient or small devices: comparison to balloon angioplasty. J Am Coll Cardiol 1993; 22:1628.
8. Safian RD, Fishman RF, Freed M. "Facilitated angioplasty": Does it occur? Circulation 1992;86(Suppl I):I-734 (abstract).
9. Roubin GS, Douglas JS Jr, King SB III et al. Influence of balloon size on initial success, acute complications, and restenosis after percutaneous transluminal coronary angioplasty. A prospective randomized study. Circulation 1988;78:557.
10. Rensing BJ, Hermans WRM, Beatt KJ et al. Quantitative angiographic assessment of elastic recoil after percutaneous transluminal coronary angioplasty. Am J Cardiol 1990;66:1039.
11. Haude M, Erbel R, Hassan I, Meyer J. Quantitative analysis of elastic recoil after balloon angioplasty and after intracoronary implantation of balloon-expandable Palmaz-Schatz stents. J Am Coll Cardiol 1993;21:26.
12. Hofling B, Gonschior P, Simpson L, Bauriedel G, Nerlich A. Efficacy of directional coronary atherectomy in cases unsuitable for percutaneous transluminal coronary angioplasty (PTCA) and after unsuccessful PTCA. Am Heart J 1992;124:341.
13. Spears JR, Reyes VP, Plokker HWT et al. Laser balloon angioplasty: coronary angiographic follow-up of a multicenter trial. J Am Coll Cardiol 1990;15:26A (abstract).

36. Treatment of Closure After Coronary Intervention

A. Approach to Acute and Threatened Closure

KUMAR SRIDHAR and SHELDON GOLDBERG

Acute or threatened closure is the most common serious immediate complication of percutaneous transluminal coronary angioplasty (PTCA). Its occurrence is associated with major clinical sequelae, including acute myocardial infarction (35 to 50%), emergency coronary bypass surgery (30 to 70%), and death (5%) (1). Therefore it is important to develop a practical, efficacious approach in treating patients who develop this complication.

OVERVIEW

Acute closure is defined as a worsening stenosis with TIMI grade 0 to 2 distal flow in a previously patent vessel during or after coronary angioplasty. Threatened acute closure is defined as an angiographic appearance during or after coronary angioplasty thought to be at increased risk for development of acute closure. This includes the appearance of a dissection or a new thrombus despite persistent TIMI grade 3 flow (2).

Acute or threatened closure complicates 2 to 10% of PTCA procedures (3–5). With the increasingly widespread application of balloon angioplasty to patients with multivessel disease and LV dysfunction, this complication takes on ever-increasing importance.

Certain patient- and lesion-related variables are predictive of an increased risk of acute closure. Clinical factors include female gender, unstable angina, and acute myocardial infarction. Baseline angiographic preprocedural characteristics include lesions on bend points $>45°$, branch point stenoses, calcification, eccentricity and complexity, and significant distal disease. Other factors associated with acute closure include the presence of thrombus, multivessel disease, and lesion length >2 luminal diameters (4). Analysis of the preprocedural angiogram will help target those lesions at risk. Being attentive to lesion and patient variables can give the interventionalist an estimate of the risk of acute closure. Once determined, important preparation can be used to help avoid or treat the complication. Furthermore, anticipation of the problem may lead to use of agents such as platelet glycoprotein receptor antibodies (20) to prevent acute complications or to technical strategies in the catheterization suite that can effectively overcome this complication of balloon angioplasty. The addition of chimeric monoclonal fragment (REOPRO) treatment has been shown to reduce cardiac complications by 35% in high-risk cases (20).

The mechanism of acute or threatened closure involves several interactions, including elastic recoil, intimal dissection, and thrombosis. Certain angiographic features herald a higher risk of acute complications. These include dissection, residual stenosis greater than 35%, and persistent translesional gradient (4). The most important predictor of acute complication is the intraprocedural appearance of an intimal dissection. Several series have shown that patients who develop intraprocedural dissection have a higher risk of acute closure. In one study intraprocedural dissection occurred in 29% of elective angioplasty cases. When intimal dissection occurred, there was a 10.5% chance of major cardiac complications. This contrasted with a 1.6% of incidence of major complications when a tear was not present. This represented a 6.5-fold increase in the risk of major complications (6, 7). Once a dissection has occurred, certain factors increase the risk of late ischemic complications. These include angiographic features such as dissection length, significant residual stenosis, and the presence of extraluminal contrast (8).

TREATMENT OF ACUTE CLOSURE

When acute or threatened closure occurs, several options are available to the interventionalist. In the past, repeat inflations of standard balloon catheters were used, but these were often unsuccessful because inflation duration was limited by ischemia. At present, four major catheter interventions are feasible. These include the use of perfusion balloon catheters (PBC), intracoronary stenting, directional atherectomy, and intracoronary thrombolysis.

Perfusion Balloon Catheters

Perfusion balloon catheters are usually the first line of defense in acute or threatened closure. These devices are designed with side holes prior and distal to the balloon to allow passive perfusion of blood to the jeopardized myocardium. The adequacy of perfusion and control of ischemia depend on the central aortic pressure; flow rates vary from 30 to 60 cc per minute. Perfusion balloon catheters have the advantage of easy deployment and the benefit of obtaining long inflation times. Theoretically, the longer the inflation time, the greater the chance of "tacking up" the dissection. Studies involving the use of perfusion balloon catheters in failed PTCA patients have shown variable benefits. Longer inflation times led to decreased residual diameter

stenoses and higher angiographic success, as well as fewer Q-wave myocardial infarctions (9, 10). In our experience prolonged inflations of 10 minutes or more have led to acute successful results in approximately 50% of cases (Fig. 36A.1).

Perfusion balloon catheters have certain important drawbacks. They are of limited value in patients with systemic hypotension since they rely on the patient's intrinsic central pressure to maintain coronary perfusion pressure. They may be less efficacious in long spiral dissections as the balloon may not cover these adequately. Longer balloon length perfusion catheters have made inroads in this area. In addition, these devices may be difficult to use in tortuous anatomy or heavily calcified noncompliant vessels. The balloon catheter itself has a limited inflation pressure that allows distal perfusion; the distal catheter tip may be also cause trauma to the distal vasculature. Finally, side-branch ischemia may occur if the balloon catheter covers this area. Perfusion balloon catheters are less likely to prove beneficial in dissections that are long or spiral, involve major side branches, or are associated with hemodynamic compromise of the patient. Randomized trials of immediate coronary stenting versus perfusion balloon therapy in failed angioplasty have recently been reported. The trial of angioplasty and stents in Canada (TASCII) recently randomized 43 failed angioplasty patients to prolonged perfusion balloon therapy versus primary stent placement. Failed angioplasty was defined as residual stenosis greater than 50% with either (a) persistent ischemia associated with a major dissection or (b) reduction in TIMI flow. Of 22 patients randomized to primary perfusion balloon therapy only 10 were successfully resolved. In contrast, 19 of 21 (90%) of primary stent patients were successfully treated. Eleven of the 12 perfusion balloon failures were crossed over to stent therapy of which 83% were successfully managed. Coronary bypass surgery was required in only four patients in the series. Clinical

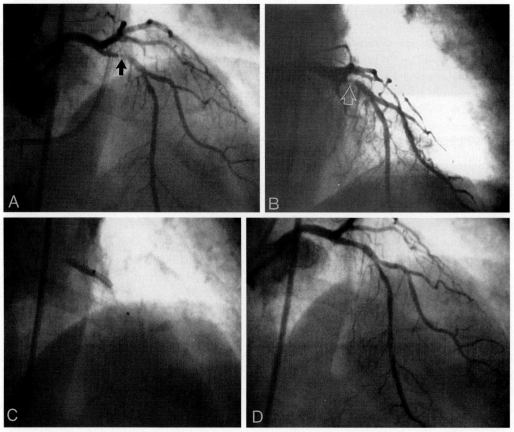

Figure 36A.1. Use of perfusion balloon catheter. A 73-year-old white female with CCS class IV angina refractory to medical management. Anterior ECG changes were present with symptoms. **A.** Baseline left coronary angiogram in the RAO projection indicating a stenosis *(arrow)* in the mid left anterior descending artery. The lesion was at higher risk because of the acute ischemic syndrome. **B.** After balloon angioplasty, threatened closure occurred because of recoil *(arrow)*. **C.** A 3.0-mm perfusion balloon catheter in place spanning the lesion for 30 minutes. **D.** Final RAO projection angiogram after PBC inflation illustrating resolution of threatened closure.

follow-up at 6 weeks indicated no difference between the two groups with respect to angina frequency and mean exercise time. This small study suggests that primary stent placement may be more effective angiographically but the combined strategy is equally effective in avoiding bypass surgery (19).

Use of a perfusion balloon catheter requires greater guiding catheter support than standard balloon angioplasty because of the higher profile of the catheter. The perfusion balloon catheter should be placed initially with the guidewire distal to the dissection. Balloon markers should be placed to span the

dissection length or at the point where the interventionalist believes the initial disruption occurred. To achieve greater perfusion, the guidewire may be removed; the guide catheter may need to be gently eased out of coronary ostium to allow for enhanced passive perfusion. Once properly positioned, a small injection of contrast can document the adequacy of distal coronary flow.

Coronary Stenting

Although initially conceived as a treatment for restenosis, coronary stents are ideally suited to deal with certain components of acute or threatened closure. Elastic recoil is prevented by the radial strength of stents. Quantitative analysis performed after standard balloon angioplasty and after stent implantation has demonstrated reduced elastic recoil with stents as compared with standard PTCA (11).

The problem of intimal dissection is successfully treated by the stents because of the "scaffolding effect." Quantitative coronary analysis of the Palmaz-Schatz stent deployed in postangioplasty dissections revealed a 94% improvement in dissection grade with 87% of complex and simple dissections completely resolved (12). However, coronary stents, because of their metallic composition, are associated with the problem of subacute thrombosis, which complicates 5 to 16% of stent implantations.

Coronary stenting has significantly altered the interventionalist's approach to acute closure. These devices may substantially reduce the rate of emergency coronary bypass surgery from angioplasty complications (2). However, the procedure demands significant technical expertise and operator experience, especially in the acute setting. This procedure also demands rigorous postprocedure evaluation and aftercare to prevent late complications.

The most widely investigated stents include the flexible Gianturco-Roubin stent (Cook) and the articulated, rigid Palmaz-Schatz stent (Johnson and Johnson).

GIANTURCO-ROUBIN STENT

The Gianturco-Roubin stent was recently approved by the FDA for use in bailout situations. It has a single-strand, surgical-grade stainless steel structure woven into a cylindrical, interdigitating loop configuration; the stent is mounted on a compliant balloon. This device has the advantage of relatively easy delivery because of its flexibility and easy preparation. The hoop strength reduces shortening, and its expanded length of 20 mm allows for coverage of most dissections with a single device. Disadvantages include the desirability for 0.18-inch, extrasupport wire and 9 Fr catheter systems for large-vessel stent deployment. The stent is relatively radiolucent and often difficult to visualize. Because of its fine structure, it can be traumatized during placement. The stent cannot be overexpanded because of its "clam shell" design and so it must be appropriately sized at the start. Incomplete dissection coverage may occur as a result of extravasation of dissection material between the loops (Fig. 36A.2).

Clinical evaluation of the Gianturco-Roubin stent in failed PTCA patients has not involved randomized trials. Case control series patients matched for closure type and acute versus threatened closure indicated improved TIMI flow grade and residual stenosis with the use of the Gianturco-Roubin stent; but no improvement in death or myocardial infarction rates. Q-wave infarction was particularly a problem in patients who underwent delayed stenting because of closure outside of the cardiac catheterization laboratory.

Unfortunately, angiographic improvement did not translate as well into clinical improvement. Most of this was attributed to the delay in stent implantation (2). In a recent series of 518 consecutive patients with acute or threatened closure, the Gianturco-Roubin stent was successful in resolving the problem in 95%. In approximately 5% of patients the coronary stents could not be deployed because of technical problems. Disrupted vessels treated with these stents showed an improvement in residual stenosis from 65% diameter narrowing prior to stenting to 15% after stenting. Myocardial infarction occurred in 5% of the patients and emergency coronary artery bypass grafting was required in 7% of cases. The mortality rate was 2.2%. Vascular complications and subacute thrombosis were the major problems associated with this device. Eighteen percent of patients had bleeding complications requiring transfusion, usually for entry site problems, and subacute thrombosis occurred in 8.7% of patients. Interest-

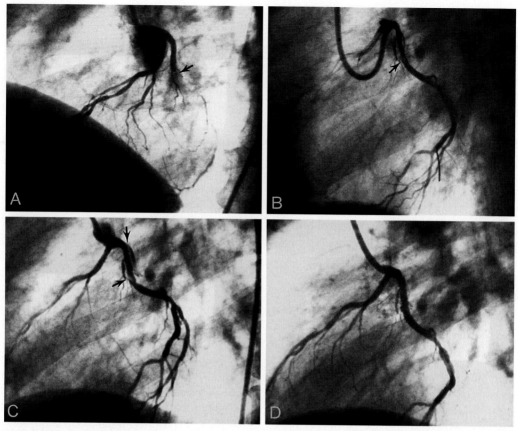

Figure 36A.2.   Use of Gianturco-Roubin coronary stent. A 47-year-old white male with a recent inferoposterior myocardial infarction and postinfarction angina. **A.** Baseline LAO projection of a subtotally occluded dominant circumflex *(arrow)*. **B.** Following balloon angioplasty, an intimal flap was present *(arrow)*. **C.** Subsequently, the patient developed chest pain with ECG changes. LAO projection angiography reveals a spiral dissection with significant luminal encroachment *(arrows)*. **D.** Final angiography, after Gianturco-Roubin coronary stenting, reveals minor luminal irregularities with resolution of the dissection.

ingly, multiple stent implantation was not associated with a higher rate of subacute thrombosis (13).

PALMAZ-SCHATZ STENT

The Palmaz Schatz stent is an articulated slot of stainless steel mesh. Two 7-mm segments are connected by a 1-mm central bridging strut. The articulation allows some degree of flexibility. The device is 15 mm in unexpanded length. The stent delivery system uses a sheath to cover the stent to avoid embolization or proximal deployment. Because of the high profile nature of the system, large-lumen 8 Fr guide catheters are required along with adequate guide support to aid in visualization and deployment.

A recent retrospective series of patients was reported in which Palmaz-Schatz stents were implanted for failed PTCA, including suboptimal PTCA results, threatened closure, and acute closure. Initial deployment success was achieved in 98% of the patients with only four of 56 patients having significant clinical complications (Fig. 36A.3). However, by 30 days, 16% of these patients developed subacute thrombosis with associated complications. A major predictor of subacute thrombosis was angiographically visible thrombus after coronary stenting (14).

We favor the use of the coronary stent in patients with relatively discrete dissections without significant thrombotic burden in vessels ≥3 mm in diameter. Importantly, patients with bleeding diatheses cannot undergo this procedure because of the intense anticoagulation regimen required including aspirin, heparin, warfarin and dextran. Regimens that omit warfarin may permit treatment of these patients. To optimize the results of coronary artery stenting, certain important principles should be followed. Patients at high risk of acute closure who may be candidates for coronary stents should be pretreated with intravenous dextran, in addition to the usual pre-PTCA medications. In addition, the operator should make sure that appropriate backup support is provided by the guide catheter chosen. We favor the 9 Fr guides for the Gianturco-Roubin stents and large-lumen 8 Fr guides for the Palmaz-Schatz stents. Every effort should be made to optimize the backup support available. This may involve the use of Amplatz, hockey-stick, or multipurpose catheter shapes, depending on the anatomic situation.

Next, to ensure smooth tracking of the devices, we recommend the use of extrasupport guidewires, which provide a firmer rail on which the stent can track. The 0.014-inch, extrasupport device for the Palmaz-Schatz stent and the 0.018-inch extrasupport wire for the Gianturco-Roubin stent are recommended. Newly developed guidewires that combine the properties of a firm rail and floppy wire steerability have also shown promise. Once the decision is made to use intracoronary stenting, the operator must determine the length of dissection that needs to be covered. Multiple projections may be

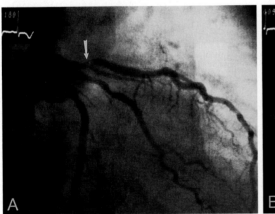

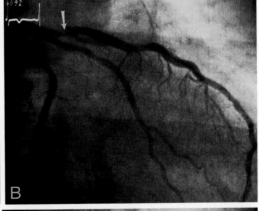

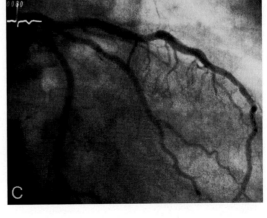

Figure 36A.3. Use of Palmaz-Schatz coronary stent. A 54-year-old male with unstable angina. **A.** Baseline RAO projection angiogram illustrating an eccentric proximal LAD stenosis *(arrow)*. **B.** After balloon angioplasty, the proximal LAD has a hazy angiographic appearance with associated dissection *(arrow)* suggesting threatened closure. **C.** After Palmaz-Schatz stent implantation, the lesion has been stabilized with resolution of the initial dissection.

required to assure complete visualization of the entire disrupted segment. During intracoronary stenting, the entire length of the dissection needs to be covered by the stent(s). This is critical since areas of uncovered disruption lead to increased rates of subacute thrombosis. We also recommend using a continuous series of stents as opposed to leaving gaps of uncovered vessel between disrupted segments. If thrombus appears during coronary stenting, intracoronary urokinase administration is advised.

After the required number of stents are deployed, the interventionalist must ascertain the following: (a) Is the dissection completely covered (distal or proximal ends)? If the dissection is not completely spanned, especially the distal end, then coronary bypass surgery should be considered. (b) Are the stent struts fully expanded? Full expansion of stent struts is often difficult to determine by coronary angiography. We usually use a noncompliant balloon inflated to high pressure after stent delivery to fully expand the struts and assure stent-vessel contact. Intracoronary ultrasound improves the evaluation of stent expansion. (c) Is there evidence of intraluminal residual dissection or residual thrombus? If intraluminal residual thrombus is present, then the administration of intracoronary urokinase is recommended. Intraluminal residual dissection can sometimes be treated with reinflation of a perfusion balloon catheter within the stented segment; however, if the dissection is persistent, coronary surgery should be considered. (d) Is there inflow or outflow obstruction (stenosis >50%, immediately adjacent to the stented segment)? Inflow or outflow obstruction may predispose to subacute thrombosis. This can be treated with low-pressure inflation of a compliant balloon.

Subacute thrombosis is a major concern related to coronary stenting in the failed PTCA setting, occurring in 5 to 20% of patients (13–15). The trend in recent years has been toward a higher degree of anticoagulation postprocedure. While vigorous anticoagulation may help lessen the incidence of subacute thrombosis, it may result in higher rates of bleeding complications. In some series the rates of bleeding and vascular complications have been as high as 16 to 20% (2, 13).

Directional Atherectomy

This technique has been reported in small series of patients with acute closure or with suboptimal PTCA results. These studies have shown improvement in the angiographic appearance of lesions complicated by acute closure and unresolved with standard treatment (16).

Practically, directional atherectomy has limited usefulness. Both sheaths and guiding catheters must be upsized to accommodate the device. The device itself is cumbersome and requires significant operator expertise. Distal lesions and tortuous segments are difficult to approach, and there is a risk of coronary perforation with aggressive cutting. Directional atherectomy can only be used in situations where the luminal flap is localized and can be contained within the length of the catheter housing. We recommend its use in only selective situations.

Intracoronary Thrombolysis

Intracoronary thrombus formation before or during angioplasty frequently heralds a later adverse event and is notoriously difficult to treat. If thrombus is present prior to angioplasty, we recommend a 48- to 72-hour course of intravenous heparin to reduce the total thrombus burden prior to coronary intervention. If thrombus is still present at the time of intervention, then adjunctive treatment with intracoronary urokinase is also recommended.

Intracoronary thrombolytics should be administered in patients who develop angiographically visible defects during angioplasty or in situations where acute or threatened closure is caused by significant thrombus formation. Although there are no randomized trials using these agents, the outcome is so poor if left untreated that this course of action seems prudent. A small series of patients treated with urokinase for acute closure caused by thrombus suggested an improvement in acute angiographic success (TIMI 3 flow and <50% residual stenosis). The mean dosage of urokinase administered was approximately 400,000 units with the median dosage being 250,000 units. Since systematic lytic states are less common with a dose below 500,000 units, we recommend consideration of the risks if surgical intervention will be required before proceeding with further urokinase. Subsequent follow-up studies have suggested poor short-term patency despite strict anticoagulation regimens (17, 18). Improved antiplatelet agents and thrombin inhibitors may be necessary if this problem is to be dealt with successfully.

SUMMARY

Acute or threatened closure represents the most serious complication the interventionalist will face in the cardiac catheterization lab. Major treatment options include perfusion balloon catheters, coronary stents, directional atherectomy, and intracoronary thrombolytics. Perfusion balloon catheters are widely available, and we recommend them as first-line treatment. Prolonged inflations (15 to 20 minutes) may be necessary to seal underlying dissections. Perfusion balloon catheters can be expected to improve approximately half of the acute or threatened events. Stenting should be reserved for those patients who have larger vessels with unresolved dissections and reduced TIMI flow. Stents are effective in treating acute closure, but are at increased risk for delayed closure caused by subacute thrombosis. A combination of perfusion balloon catheters and coronary stenting can be expected to resolve the majority of acute or threatened closures. Intracoronary thrombolytics should be used in any patients with extensive clot burden or angiographically visible filling defects complicating PTCA.

Coronary bypass surgery, although often the last option, is still a viable treatment for acute closure, especially if interventional approaches are not successful in improving flow to TIMI grade 3.

It is our feeling that if a patient does not have normal flow along with minimal thrombus burden, as well as a completely covered and stable dissection, these patients should be treated with bypass surgery.

Acute closure at present remains a difficult problem. Further development such as coated stents, refined mechanical devices, and new pharmacologic agents may improve future outcomes.

REFERENCES

1. Freed M, Grines C, eds., Manual of interventional cardiology. Physician's Press Michigan, 1992.
2. Lincoff AM, Topaz EJ et al. Intracoronary stenting compared with conventional therapy for abrupt vessel closure complicating coronary angioplasty: a matched case control study. J Am Coll Cardiol 1992;21:866–875.
3. Detre KM, Holmes DR et al. Incidence and consequences of periprocedural occlusion. Circulation 1990;82:739–750.
4. Ellis SG, Roubin GS, King SB III et al. Angiographic and clinical predictors of acute closure after native vessel coronary angioplasty. Circulation 1988;77:372–379.
5. Lincoff AM, Popma JJ, Ellis SG et al. Abrupt vessel closure complicating coronary angioplasty: clinical, angiographic and therapeutic profile. J Am Coll Cardiol 1992; 19:926–935.
6. Waller BF, Orr CM et al. Coronary balloon angioplasty dissections: "The good, the bad and the ugly." J Am Coll Cardiol 1992;20:701–706 editorial.
7. Bredlau C, Roubin CS et al. In-hospital morbidity and mortality in patients undergoing elective coronary angioplasty. Circulation 1985;72:1044–1052.
8. Black AJR, Namay DL et al. Tear or dissection after coronary angioplasty: morphologic correlates of an ischemic complication. Circulation 1989;79:1035–1042.
9. Leitschuh ML, Mills RM Jr et al. Outcomes after major dissection during coronary angioplasty using the perfusion balloon catheter. Am J Cardiol 1991;G7:1056–1060.
10. Jackman D Jr., Zider JP et al. Outcome after prolonged balloon inflation of >20 minutes for initially unsuccessful percutaneous transluminal coronary angioplasty. Am J Cardiol 1992;69:1417.
11. Haude M, Erbel R et al. Quantitative analysis of elastic recoil after balloon angioplasty and after intracoronary implantation of balloon-expandable Palmaz-Schatz stent. J Am Coll Cardiol 1993;21:26–34.
12. Fischman D, Savage MP et al. Effect of intracoronary stenting on intimal dissection after balloon angioplasty: review of quantitative and qualitative coronary analysis. J Am Coll Cardiol 1991;18:1445–1451.
13. George BS, Voorhees WD III, Roubin GS et al. Multicenter investigation of coronary stenting to treat acute or threatened closure after percutaneous transluminal coronary angioplasty: clinical and angiographic outcomes. J Am Coll Cardiol 1993;22:135–143.
14. Herrmann HC, Buchbinder M et al. Emergent use of balloon-expandable coronary stenting for failed percutane-

ous transluminal coronary angioplasty. Circulation 1992;
86:812–819.

15. Maiello L, Columbus A et al. Coronary stenting for treatment of acute or threatened closure following dissection
after coronary balloon angioplasty. Am Heart J 1993;
125:1570–1574.

16. McKeever LS, Merck JC et al. Bail-out directional atherectomy for abrupt coronary artery occlusion following conventional angioplasty. Cathet Cardiovasc Diagn 1993;
1(Suppl)31–36.

17. Gulba DC, Daniel WS et al. Role of thrombolysis and thrombin in patients with acute coronary occlusion during percutaneous transluminal coronary angioplasty. J Am Coll Cardiol 1990;16:563–568.

18. Goudreau E, DiSciascio G et al. Intracoronary urokinase as
an adjunct to percutaneous transluminal coronary angioplasty in patients with complex coronary narrowings or
angioplasty-induced complications. 1992;69:57–62.

19. Ricci DR, Buller CE et al. Coronary stent servus prolonged
perfusion balloon for failed coronary angioplasty—a randomized trial. Circulation 1994;90:I-651 (abstract).

20. The EPIC Investigators. Use of a monoclonal antibody
directed against the platelet glycoprotein IIb/IIIa receptor in
high-risk coronary angioplasty. N Engl J Med 1994;
330:956–961.

B. Prevention and Management of Abrupt Closure

ROBERT FEDERICI, ALAN TENAGLIA,
WILLIAM HILLEGASS, ROBERT
HARRINGTON, PAUL A. GURBEL,
and E. MAGNUS OHMAN

Abrupt closure of a dilated coronary segment during or after percutaneous interventions has plagued the interventional cardiologist since the inception of coronary angioplasty. Despite considerable improvement in angioplasty techniques, use of new devices, and understanding of the importance of anticoagulation and antiplatelet therapy, the incidence of abrupt closure has remained steady at approximately 7% over the last decade. Although restenosis is by far the most common problem following percutaneous coronary intervention, abrupt closure leads to the vast majority of the in-hospital morbidity and mortality associated with percutaneous pro-

cedures. Furthermore, the "cost" of abrupt closure in hospital charges and duration of hospitalization after either stent placement or coronary artery bypass grafting (CABG) is considerable. The severe and sometimes unexpected way in which periprocedural occlusion occurs has provoked much interest in this area of interventional cardiology. In this chapter we will outline the clinical characteristics, management, and prevention of abrupt closure as a practical approach to harnessing this vexing problem. We will also outline the future research needs in the area of abrupt closure.

PATHOPHYSIOLOGY OF ABRUPT CLOSURE

An understanding of the mechanism and pathophysiology of percutaneous coronary interventions is important to elucidate the mechanisms of abrupt closure. Dissection, thrombosis, and spasm are the main processes responsible for closure of a coronary segment. Unfortunately, plaque fracture, which in a limited form gives rise to a successful coronary intervention, is in a more extensive form the predominant feature of abrupt closure (1, 2). Animal and human cadaveric models, as well as necropsy specimens, have elucidated the process of balloon injury. When cadaveric coronary arteries are balloon injured, splitting of the intima and media, plaque fracture, and overstretching of the muscle fibers occur (3–5). The atherosclerotic plaque tends to be relatively incompressible and does not contribute greatly to luminal opening. Animal models have similarly shown that balloon injury causes plaque fracture, intimal and medial splitting, and stretching of the arterial segment. In addition, there is desquamation of the intima at the angioplasty site and rapid deposition of platelets and fibrin (3, 6, 7). Autopsy data from patients who recently underwent angioplasty corroborate the data from animal and postmortem PTCA observations (1, 2, 8–12). The pathologic specimens show tears in the intima and media in almost all of the patients.

Plaque disruption and thrombus were also found. Dissecting hematomas, larger dissections, and thrombus were more frequently found in patients who died because of abrupt closure compared with patients who died because of abrupt closure compared with patients who died of causes unrelated to the angioplasty procedure (2, 10).

Imaging during coronary angioplasty reinforces the proposed mechanisms of balloon injury (12–17). More recently, intravascular ultrasound and angioscopy have been helpful in validating the mechanisms of angioplasty and abrupt closure as hypothesized from pathologic observations. Intracoronary ultrasound demonstrates that dissection and plaque rupture are responsible for approximately 80% of the luminal enlargement. Vessel stretch contributes significantly less to a successful lumen enlargement (16). Angioscopy, the only technique to directly visualize coronary arteries in vivo, demonstrates obstructive dissection flaps and thrombus in patients who have suffered abrupt closure (18, 19).

Spasm has been implicated in the pathogenesis of abrupt closure (20). Altered vasomotor function of the arterial segments is present following angioplasty (21), possibly resulting from mechanical stretch of the artery or endothelial denudation (19). After balloon injury, spasm probably contributes to the occurrence of abrupt closure only to a small degree. In contrast, spasm is a major mechanistic culprit of abrupt closure following laser angioplasty and other thermal angioplasty procedures (22).

Intimal and medial tearing, plaque fracture, desquamation of the endothelium, platelet and fibrin deposition, and arterial stretching are all involved in the pathophysiology of balloon injury. Abrupt closure develops when mechanical obstruction (dissection), thrombus formation, and/or spasm cause obliteration or near-obliteration of the vessel lumen. From these pathologic observations, with some indirect corroboration of different imaging modalities, a process that does not lead to abrupt closure appears to be characterized by a small-to-modest injury that, because of flow characteristics, causes little hemostatic "repair" response with thrombus formation. On the other hand, severe flow limitations caused by either major dissection or spasm lead to reduced or turbulent flow favoring local thrombus formation leading to abrupt closure.

INCIDENCE AND CONSEQUENCES OF ABRUPT CLOSURE

Abrupt closure complicates between 2 and 14% of angioplasty procedures. This rate varies depending on the definition used and the patient population studied (23–33). Interestingly, the incidence of abrupt closure has not changed significantly since the early angioplasty experience, despite more careful attention to anticoagulation and aspirin use. One reason for this may be that coronary interventions are being performed on patients with more complex anatomy and on patients who are generally sicker (28). The overall incidence of periprocedural occlusion was approximately 7% when data on 11,133 patients were reviewed, as shown in Table 36B.1 (23, 25–27, 29, 34). More than two-thirds of these patients occluded in the angioplasty laboratory. Patients who suffer abrupt closure after leaving the laboratory will most likely reocclude within the first 24 hours (25, 30). However, some patients, especially those who undergo stent implantation, can occlude up to 7 to 10 days after the procedure (35).

The importance of abrupt closure is underscored by its association with adverse outcomes and ischemic complications following the procedure. Among patients who have an angioplasty procedure and do not suffer periprocedural occlusion, the risk of having a myocardial infarction, requiring coronary bypass grafting, and dying is 3%, 2%, and less than 1%, respectively (27). Conversely, among patients who have abrupt closure, approximately 40% will have a myocardial

Table 36B.1.
Incidence of Abrupt Closure

Study (Ref.)	Year	No. of Patients	Total (%)	Abrupt Closure	
				In Laboratory (%)	Out of Laboratory (%)
NHLBI (27)	1985–1986	1801	6.8	4.9	1.9
Beth Israel (29)	1981–1986	1160	4.7	3.8	0.9
Michigan (26)	1988–1990	1319	8.3	6.8	1.5
Duke (23)	1986–1989	658	8.2	4.5	3.7
Thorax center (25)	1986–1988	1423	7.3	5.6	1.7
Emory (34)	1982–1986	4772	4.4	2.3	2.1
Total		11,133	6.6	4.7	2.0
		95% CI	6.1–7.1%	4.3–5.1%	1.7–2.3%

Table 36B.2.
Complications After Abrupt Closure

Study (Ref.)	Year	No. of Patients	In-hospital Events		
			Death (%)	MI (%)	CABG (%)
Emory (34)	1982–1986	140	2	54	55
NHLBI (27)	1985–1986	122	5	40	35
Beth Israel (29)	1981–1986	54	2	35	33
Michigan[a] (26)	1988–1990	109	8	20	20
Thorax center (25)	1986–1988	104	6	36	30
Total		529	5	37	35
		95% CI	3.1–6.7%	33–41%	31–39%

[a]DCA and STENTS available.

Table 36B.3.
Predictors of Abrupt Closure or Ischemic Complications

Study (Ref.)	Clinical Hx	Angiographic	Postprocedural
Tenaglia et al (23)	—	Total occlusion	—
		Branch point	
		Lesion length	
		Thrombus	
		RCA	
Ellis et al (24)	—	Total occlusion	—
		Angulation	
		High-grade lesion	
		Tortuosity	
deFeyter et al (25)	Unstable angina	Complex lesions	—
	Multivessel disease	Thrombus	
Ellis et al (34)	Multivessel disease	Branch point	Post-PTCA stenosis
	Female gender	Angulation	Dissection
		Other stenosis in same vessel	
		Lesion length	
		Thrombus	
Bredlaw et al (32)	Female gender	Calcification	Dissection
	Multivessel disease	Lesion length	
		Eccentricity	
Detre et al (27)	3-vessel disease	Diffuse morphology	Dissection
	Unstable angina	Thrombus	
	High risk for surgery	Collateral flow	

infarction, 35% will require bypass surgery, and 4% will die, as shown in Table 36B.2 (25–27, 29, 34).

The ability to predict which patients will ultimately develop abrupt closure would be of great clinical utility. Improving patient selection and modifying techniques in high-risk patients could then minimize the procedural risks. Many studies have been published to evaluate predictive factors of abrupt reclosure (23–25, 27, 29–32, 34, 36–40). Because the ability to predict an infrequent event depends on the prevalence of the characteristic in the population and the size of the study cohort, there is some discordance between the studies (23). However, a common theme is becoming evident.

The predictors of abrupt closure or periprocedural complications can be broken into three groups; clinical characteristics, angiographic results, and postprocedural results. The presence of multivessel coronary artery disease, unstable angina, and female gender all convey an increased risk of periprocedural complications, as shown in Table 36B.3 (23–25, 27, 32, 34). Although these variables increase the risk for abrupt closure, the effect

is only modest. For example, in the NHLBI PTCA Registry (27) the incidence of abrupt closure was statistically significantly associated with the presence of unstable angina (9.9% versus 6.1%; $P <.05$) and the presence of three-vessel coronary artery disease (9.8% versus 6.0%; $P <.05$). Among all 14 different baseline clinical characteristics, the rate of abrupt closure was above 6% if the characteristic was absent; in the majority of variables assessed, the incidence was also below 10% when it was present. These findings suggest that the incidence of abrupt closure is more closely related to angiographic or procedural factors rather than the clinical scenario.

The angiographic features of coronary lesions are probably the most important characteristics predictive of acute success and complication rates. The AHA/ACC task force classification of lesion morphology has simplified the task of determining which patients possess inherently greater risk during the angioplasty procedure (41). This classification system assigned risk groups depending on lesion morphology and is shown in Table 36B.4. If a lesion meets the criteria for type A

Table 36B.4.
ACC/AHA Classification of Type A, B, and C Lesions: Lesion-Specific Characteristics[a]

Type A Lesions (high success, 85%; low risk)	
Discrete (<10 mm length)	Little or no calcification
Concentric	Less than totally occlusive
Readily accessible	Not ostial in location
Nonangulated segment, <45 degrees	No major branch involvement
Smooth contour	Absence of thrombus

Type B Lesions (moderate success, 60 to 85%; moderate risk)	
Tubular (10 to 20 mm length)	Moderate to heavy calcification
Eccentric	Total occlusion <3 months old
Moderate tortuosity of proximal segment	Ostial in location
Moderately angulated segment, >45 and <90 degrees	Bifurcation lesions requiring double guidewires
Irregular contour	Some thrombus present

Type C Lesions (low success, <60%; high risk)	
Diffuse (>2 cm length)	Total occlusion >3 months old
Excessive tortuosity of proximal segment	Inability to protect major side branches
Extremely angulated segments >90 degrees	Degenerated vein grafts with friable lesions

[a]Modified from Ryan TJ et al. Circulation 1988;78:486–502.

morphology, the system predicts high success (greater than 85%) and low risk for adverse events. Type B lesions have moderate success (60 to 85%) and carry a moderate risk. Type C lesions are thought to have low success (less than 60%) and high risk (41). This classification system, which was initially devised by a panel of experts, was improved by Ellis and colleagues after extensive review of angioplasty outcomes in large databases. Based on this review a subclassification of type B lesions into B1 and B2 was devised, where B1 lesions were those that had only one B feature and B2 lesions had more than one B feature (24). The ability of this updated classification system to risk-stratify patients based on the morphology of lesions has been validated by clinical studies. Pivotal research by Ellis and colleagues has provided a framework for predicting complication rates using the AHA/ACC classification. They have observed an increasing incidence of complication rates with more complex lesion morphology; type A 3%, type B1 6%, type B2 9%, and type C lesions 18% (23, 24). Although this classification is useful because of its simplicity, it is also apparent that the morphology classification is heterogeneous, with diverse morphologies being grouped together.

To explore the relationship between lesion morphology and complication rates by evaluating the morphology individually versus comparing a type A to a type C lesion, Tenaglia and coworkers examined 779 lesions in 658 patients (23). They confirmed the increasing risk of abrupt closure with more complex lesion morphology: type A—4.6%, type B1—7.0%, type B2—9.6%, and type C—13.4%. Their observations confirmed the heterogeneity of the classification to predict the rate of abrupt closure. For example, in patients with type B1 characteristics (39% of lesions dilated), 25% of the lesions had an individual risk of abrupt closure <4.5%, and 25% of the lesions had a risk >8.1%. In this cohort the multivariate predictors of abrupt closure

were: total occlusion ($P = .0003$, prevalence 7%); branch point ($P = .0007$, prevalence 10%); lesion length ($P = .01$, >10 mm prevalence 21%); thrombus score ($P = .02$, prevalence 12%); and right coronary artery ($P = .03$, prevalence 36%). Based on the relationship of these characteristics a patient-specific scoring system could be devised using a formula [Score = (5 × lesion length) + (6 × thrombus score) + (13 × branch location) + (6 × right coronary) + (40 × total occlusion)]. Thus an 8-mm lesion (lesion length score 1) at a branch point (location #1) with hazy appearance (thrombus score 1) would have a score of 24 with an estimated risk of abrupt closure of 25%. A lesion without any of the five lesion morphologies described in the formula would have an estimated risk of abrupt closure of <3% (score = 0). With the knowledge of the scoring system, the AHA/ACC classification added no significant prognostic value to the risk of abrupt closure (23).

Other studies have observed that the length of the stenosis, presence of thrombus, angulation at the site of stenosis, branch stenoses, total occlusions, diffuseness of coronary artery disease, tortuosity of the vessel, eccentricity of the lesion, severity of the stenosis, presence of collaterals, and presence of calcification have all been associated with an increased risk of abrupt closure and periprocedural complications as shown in Table 36B.3 (23–25, 27, 32, 34). The preinterventional framework for evaluation of a patient undergoing percutaneous intervention should incorporate the clinical history and, more importantly, a careful review of the angiogram. If the risk of abrupt closure is estimated to be high, the procedure should be modified to apply a different interventional strategy or to adjust the pretreatment or periprocedural anticoagulation, as will be discussed later.

The presence of an arterial dissection is highly associated with the development of abrupt closure (27, 32, 34, 39, 40). A patient with a dissected artery following angioplasty has a six-to tenfold increased risk of abrupt closure compared with a patient with no angiographic evidence of dissection (32, 39). Dissection is the strongest predictor of adverse outcome and ischemic complications. Since dissections complicate approximately 35% of all angioplasty procedures, it is important to identify the types of dissections that are most associated with adverse outcomes. Approximately, 90% of all dissected arteries will leave the catheterization laboratory without any flow limitation in the dilated segment; of these, about 7% will develop abrupt closure (39). Dissections with a high residual stenosis, longer dissections (>9 mm), the presence of extraluminal contrast or intraluminal filling defects, and lesions that have acutely closed in the laboratory all have a higher risk of subsequent abrupt closure, myocardial infarction, emergency CABG, and repeat PTCA. Identification and classification of a dissection can identify patients who may need further interventions and/or closer observation after coronary intervention (32, 39, 40).

Abrupt closure predisposes patients to adverse clinical outcomes, which translates into longer hospitalizations and higher costs. These patients require more repeat coronary interventions, including CABG and PTCA. They also suffer more myocardial infarctions, require more intensive care, and have longer hospital stays than patients who do not have abrupt closure (28, 42). The NHLBI registry reports an average increased length of stay of 8 days in patients who have abrupt closure (28). The CAVEAT data confirm this increased length of stay and show that the cost to the institution more than doubles from $9344 for an uncomplicated percutaneous intervention (angioplasty or atherectomy) to $24,501 in patients with abrupt closure (42). While long-term follow-up is relatively limited in patients who are successfully treated by repeat percutaneous coronary intervention for abrupt closure, these patients have been reported to have higher rates of death, CABG, and myocardial infarctions when followed for a year after the event (27, 33). Interestingly, the restenosis rates in patients who have successful intervention for the management of abrupt closure are similar to patients without abrupt closure (27, 33). However, this may represent a withdrawal bias since patients with abrupt closure have worse clinical outcomes during follow-up (43). Clearly, any therapy that can reduce the rate of abrupt closure may reduce both morbidity and health care system expenditures.

INCIDENCE OF ABRUPT CLOSURE WITH THE USE OF ADVANCED PERCUTANEOUS DEVICES

Directional coronary atherectomy (DCA), intracoronary stenting, excimer laser angioplasty, high-speed rotational atherectomy (Rotablator), transluminal extraction catheters (TEC), and perfusion balloon catheters have all been developed to improve standard balloon angioplasty techniques. Although it has been postulated that the rates of abrupt closure would decrease (44), the new devices do not appear to reduce abrupt closure (22, 45–50).

Some limitations exist in comparing the new technology with balloon angioplasty. A learning curve exists with any new device, and this may lead to some increase in complications initially that will eventually decrease with greater experience (35, 51). Also, very few direct randomized comparisons with enough statistical power to discern a difference in periprocedural abrupt closure rates have been performed.

Directional coronary atherectomy is the best studied of the new technologies. Reported abrupt closure rates vary between 4 and 8% (45, 51–54), and most abrupt closure events occur in the catheterization laboratory. The modified ACC/AHA morphology criteria have been used to predict rates of success and complications with DCA (51). Type A, B1, and B2 lesions have success rates of 93%, 88%, and 75%, respectively. The corresponding complication rates are 3%, 6%, and 13% (51). Some angiographic predictors of adverse outcome with balloon angioplasty correlate with increased complications when DCA is employed. Predictors of increased complications are angulated lesions, proximal tortuosity, severe stenosis, calcification, thrombus, and long lesions (51–53). Increased operator experience and restenotic lesions were factors that decreased the risk of abrupt closure. Also, saphenous vein graft (SVG) lesions have a trend toward lower abrupt closure rates than native coronary arteries (1.6% versus 4.4%, $P = .08$) (51, 52), with rates of death, CABG, and myocardial infarction comparable with those of angioplasty in observational studies (51–53). Two randomized trials comparing DCA with balloon angioplasty have been reported. In the CCAT trial 274 patients were randomized to directional coronary atherectomy or balloon angioplasty in the proximal left artery descending artery. No significant difference in the rates of abrupt closure was detected (DCA 4.3% versus PTCA 5.1%) (54). However, CAVEAT, the largest trial directly comparing the two technologies, showed a higher rate of abrupt closure in the DCA group (7%) compared with 3% in the PTCA group (45).

The excimer laser has been found to be of particular use in long lesions, ostial lesions, and total occlusions. The abrupt closure rates vary between 1.3 and 30% (22, 55). An initial report observed an abrupt closure rate of 30% in patients within 20 minutes of laser angioplasty. Most of the closure occurred between 5 and 12 minutes and was preceded by severe spasm. The abrupt closure was reversed in this study with nitroglycerin and PTCA with a 96% success rate compared with a 41% success rate for abrupt closure induced by balloon injury (22). The implication is that mechanisms for abrupt closure following laser angioplasty may predominantly be spasm. The excimer laser registry reports a periprocedural occlusion rate of 5.4% (55). Interestingly, clinical success in laser therapy is not related to lesion morphology. Type A, B1, B2, and C lesions all had a success rate of approximately 87% (55). Also, no specific lesion morphology predisposes the patient to abrupt closure (22, 55), although bifurcation lesions do predict a higher perforation rate (55). Excimer laser has the unique property of obtaining higher technical success in traditionally difficult lesions without an increase in complications. It may be the device of choice for preventing abrupt closure in total occlusions, a theory that requires confirmation in a randomized clinical trial.

Intracoronary stents should eliminate two potential mechanisms of abrupt closure: spasm and dissection. Presumably the stent would have a tremendous impact on the incidence of abrupt closure. With the slotted-tube Palmaz-Schatz stent, abrupt closure within the first 24 hours after stent implantation is extremely rare (35, 46, 56). Unfortunately, later subacute thrombosis or abrupt closure becomes a greater problem. The majority of subacute thrombotic occlusions with the Palmaz-Schatz stent occur between days 3 and 9 following stent implantation (46). Adequacy of anticoagulation is a major determinant in the continued patency of the stent (35, 48). Acute/subacute closure rates for the Palmaz-Schatz stent vary between 2.8 and 10% (35, 46, 47, 56). Poor flow in the vessel, preexisting luminal thrombus, small native vessels, multiple stents, type C lesions, unstable angina, incomplete covering by the stent of the dissection, and placement for bailout indications all increase the likelihood of subacute closure (46, 48). Two randomized trials directly comparing the Palmaz-Schatz stent with balloon angioplasty are under way. The Benestent preliminary data shows no difference in abrupt/subacute closure rates between conventional balloon angioplasty and intracoronary stenting: stent 3.5% and PTCA 2.7% (47). The flexible-coil Gianturco-Roubin stent has been primarily used and studied as a bailout device in the event of acute or threatened closure. Abrupt closure (less than 24 hours) has been reported with this stent, but again the majority of thrombotic occlusion occurs at 3 to 5 days postimplantation (48, 57). The acute/subacute closure rate for the Gianturco-Roubin stent is 7.6 to 11.7% (48, 57). Although stents differ in design and amount of metal, there are no comparative data to assess which design may be superior in either preventing or reducing the rate of abrupt closure. The use of a particular stent as treatment or prevention of abrupt closure should therefore be guided by the individual operator and hospital experience.

The consequences of periprocedural occlusion after stent implantation are just as devastating as those following balloon angioplasty. Myocardial infarction rates as high as 70% have been reported (46, 48). Because the major mechanism of closure in stents is thrombosis, treatment of abrupt closure in a stent accordingly uses different strategies. Local delivery of thrombolytic therapy has been used successfully (46). In addition, special attention should be paid to evaluating the outflow from the stent to ensure that there is no major restriction of flow distal to the stent, which may predispose to stent thrombosis and should be dealt with by further balloon angioplasty. Acute/subacute closure with the current stents remains a major source of morbidity and mortality; however, future improvements in stent design and periprocedural anticoagulation regimens may decrease these events.

Rotational atherectomy with the Rotablator and the transluminal extraction catheter (TEC) have been recently approved by the FDA for use in the United States. The Rotablator is particularly useful in calcified lesions and ostial and bifurcation stenoses (49, 58, 59). TEC atherectomy is used primarily in degenerated, diffusely diseased saphenous vein grafts (60). The rates of abrupt closure for these techniques is between 5 and 11% (49, 58–60). As these devices are rarely used without adjunctive balloon angioplasty, it is hard to discern the effect of the device versus the accompanying balloon angioplasty on the rate of abrupt closure after leaving the catheterization laboratory.

The perfusion balloon catheter (PBC) allows gradual prolonged inflations, which should translate into less vessel trauma compared with standard short balloon inflations (61). This hypothesis was tested in a randomized clinical trial in which 478 patients were allocated to either a gradual 15-minute dilation or four standard 1-minute dilations (50). The angiographic success rate was higher in patients assigned to the prolonged dilations (95% versus 89%, $P = .016$). Importantly, the rate of major dissections was reduced by the primary prolonged dilation strategy (3% versus 9%, $P = .003$). Because the perfusion balloon was used in both arms of the study the overall rate of abrupt closure was very low (in-laboratory, 1%; in-hospital, 2%). The use of the perfusion balloon as a primary device may reduce the rate of major dissection and therefore the rate of abrupt closure. This may be a particularly important strategy in patients with more complex lesion morphology, where prolonged dilations have been found to be a particularly useful inflation strategy to improve angiographic appearance (62).

PERIPROCEDURAL THERAPIES TO PREVENT ABRUPT CLOSURE

To prevent abrupt closure careful attention must be paid to periprocedural medications. Early clinical experience documented the need for adequate antithrombotic therapy with aspirin and heparin. As the incidence of abrupt closure has remained constant over the years, a more refined approach has been developed with both existing agents and newer agents currently under investigation.

Antiplatelet therapy is essential for the safe performance of angioplasty. Schwartz and colleagues prospectively demonstrated the importance of aspirin and dipyridamole use during the angioplasty procedure. Patients treated with aspirin had a significant reduction in Q-wave myocardial infarctions compared with those given placebo (6.9% versus 1.6%) (63). Barnathan and colleagues confirmed the need for aspirin in patients undergoing angioplasty. Patients who were not pretreated with aspirin and/or dipyridamole had a significantly higher rate of abrupt closure (10.7% versus 1.8%) and emergency CABG (9.9% versus 2.7%) (64). More recently, Lembo and colleagues demonstrated that dipyridamole confers no additional benefit to aspirin alone in reducing the frequency of ischemic complications (65). Aspirin provides significant benefits in patients undergoing angioplasty, and unless an absolute contraindication exists, aspirin should be used routinely. For patients who are allergic to aspirin, ticlopidine may be used (66). Because of the pharmacokinetics of this agent, therapy should be started >24 hours prior to the procedure.

Systemic anticoagulation with intravenous heparin therapy is standard management during the angioplasty procedure. A heparin dose to achieve an activated clotting time (ACT) of greater than 300 seconds has become the standard level of anticoagulation in North America. This level of anticoagulation was derived from observations in patients placed on extracorporeal circulation during coronary artery bypass surgery (67). The optimal level of ACT during the procedure remains controversial. The matter is further complicated by the fact that ACT levels measured by the Hemochron and the Hemotech devices do not provide similar results over the broad ranges that are used during percutaneous interventions (68). Observation from Duke University on 1290 consecutive patients undergoing angioplasty have documented an inverse relationship ($P = .02$) between ACT levels (Hemochron device) and the risk of abrupt closure as shown in Figure 36B.1 (69). Patients with abrupt closure had significantly lower ACT during balloon inflation compared with control patients (346 ± 67 versus 388 ± 81, $P < .002$). On the other hand, high levels

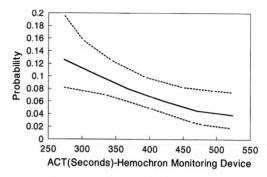

Figure 36B.1. Relationship between probability of abrupt closure (with 95% confidence intervals) and activated clotting time (ACT) during procedure as measured by the Hemachron device. (Reproduced with permission from Narins CR et al. J Am Coll Cardiol 1994;23:470A.)

of ACT achieved by high doses of heparin administration have been found to be an independent predictor ($P = .004$) of bleeding complications (70). In this study of 438 patients the best trade-off between ischemic complications and bleeding complications using risk-benefit analysis suggested the "optimal ACT" (by Hemochron device) during the procedure to be in the range of 425 to 525 seconds. These findings suggest that for each patient a trade-off decision can be made. A higher level of ACT (>400 seconds) is desirable for those patients who pose a high risk for abrupt closure. For patients with a low risk of abrupt closure, a lower level (300 to 400 seconds) may be appropriate. As empiric dosing of heparin provides a suboptimal level of anticoagulation in a substantial majority of patients (71), the ACT level should be monitored throughout the procedure. Additional heparin should be given to maintain the level above the chosen threshold to reduce the risk of abrupt closure.

Preprocedural heparinization is not thought to be required in most patients who undergo angioplasty. However, in patients with unstable angina, preprocedural heparinization has been shown to decrease the rate of abrupt closure. Thrombotic vessel occlusion was significantly higher (8.3% versus 1.5%) in patients with unstable angina who did not

Table 36B.5.
Intracoronary Thrombus and Risk of Abrupt Closure After PTCA

Study (Ref.)	Year	No. of Patients	Patients With Thrombus (%)	Abrupt Closure	
				With Thrombus (%)	Without Thrombus (%)
Sugrue et al (106)	1986	297	15 (5)	73	8
Ellis et al (24)	1988	451	48 (11)	14	9
Detre et al (27)	1990	1801	205 (11)	10	4
Lincoff et al (26)	1992	1309	—	23	—
Tenaglia et al (23)	1994	658	79 (12)	44	—
Ferguson et al (107)	1993	591	90 (12)	78	—
Total		5107	437 (10)	32	7

receive 24 hours of heparin prior to the procedure (72). The patients who were pretreated with heparin also had a higher procedural success rate (72). The need for postprocedural heparinization must also be individualized. Routine heparinization following angioplasty does not reduce ischemic complications, yet it increases the risk of bleeding complications (73,74). However, in patients with dissections induced during angioplasty, postprocedural heparinization is indicated (74–76). Unfortunately, the duration of anticoagulation required is not well defined, but patients with complex lesion morphology or dissection with a high risk for abrupt closure should receive 24 hours of intravenous heparin after the procedure.

Intracoronary thrombus has consistently been a predictor of abrupt closure (77). The presence of thrombus substantially increases the risk of abrupt closure to between 10 and 73% as shown in Table 36B.5. Eliminating thrombus may therefore be beneficial in reducing the incidence or reversing the consequences of abrupt closure. However, the use of intracoronary thrombolytic therapy either before or during angioplasty remains controversial. Results from several observational series are summarized in Table 36B.6. More recently Ambrose and colleagues performed a randomized trial of intracoronary urokinase versus placebo in 469 patients with unstable angina prior to percutaneous intervention. Consistent with previous studies,

Table 36B.6.
Intracoronary Thrombolysis for Angiographic Documented Thrombus

Study (Ref.)	No. of Patients	Agent	Angiographic Improvement (%)
Vetrovec et al (108)	13	SK	77
Mendelkorn et al (109)	9	SK	44
Rentrop et al (110)	5	SK	0
Shapiro et al (111)	18	SK	67
de Zwaan et al (112)	21	SK	52
Ambrose et al (113)	36	SK	0
Total	102	SK	40
Gotoh et al (114)	21	UK	95
Goudreau et al (115)	50	UK	80
Total	71	UK	88
DiSciascio et al (116)	7	tPa	28

SK, Streptokinase; *UK,* urokinase; *tPA,* tissue plasminogen activator.

there was an improvement in angiographic appearances. However, patients allocated to intracoronary urokinase had a higher rate of abrupt closure (11% versus 3%; $P <.05$) and ischemia (10% versus 3%; $P <.05$) (78). The lack of efficacy may have been caused by bleeding into dissections, which may increase the rate of ischemic events (79). One other potential mechanism for lack of efficacy is that local delivery may cause an increased thrombin formation (80). To explore this issue further a study has recently been completed that has evaluated intralesional tPA (20 mg) delivery through a Tracker catheter (Target Therapeutics, Inc.) over 20 minutes prior to PTCA in patients with unstable angina and

Figure 36B.2. Local delivery of therapeutic agents using the standard intracoronary route or through a delivery catheter. The intralesional delivery system has the advantage of delivering all of the agent to the culprit lesion. In addition, a possible mechanical effect of spraying the lesion may occur (Dr. Paul Gurbel, personal communication).

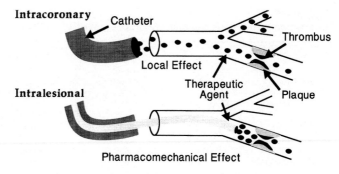

complex lesion morphology as shown in Figure 36B.2. Simultaneous to the tPA delivery into the lesion, intracoronary heparin (5000 units) is administered to inhibit the paradoxical increase in thrombin activity that accompanies fibrinolysis. Current information suggests that routine use of urokinase and possibly other thrombolytic agents is not warranted in patients with complex lesion morphology.

CLINICAL PRESENTATION AND DETECTION OF ABRUPT CLOSURE

Balloon inflations during the angioplasty procedure usually cause ischemia in the distribution of that artery. The majority of patients (80 to 90%) develop chest pain and ECG changes during balloon inflations (81, 82). The symptoms of abrupt closure can be insidious, ranging from nausea and hypotension to dramatic symptoms such as ventricular fibrillation and sudden death (25). Therefore careful postprocedural surveillance is important, particularly in high-risk patients described in Table 36B.3. In patients with abrupt closure, the majority (80 to 97%) will have chest pain (25, 30, 81–83); hypotension will occur in 15 to 20% (25, 30). Virtually any symptom that occurs with an acute myocardial infarction can be reproduced in patients with abrupt closure.

Careful attention to the 12-lead ECG during inflation and during later ischemic events is important. If an ECG is obtained during balloon inflation, that 12-lead ECG can serve as an "ischemic fingerprint" (84). If the same ischemic changes are found after the angioplasty, the diagnosis of abrupt closure can be made with virtually 100% specificity (81, 82, 84, 85). When the LAD is angioplastied, 95% of patients will have ST elevation in leads V2 and V3. Balloon occlusion of the RCA causes ST elevation in leads III and a VF about 85% of the time. When the LCx is occluded during balloon angioplasty, ST depression occurs approximately 80% of the time in V2 and V3 (82). ST elevation occurs in 77% of patients with abrupt closure by standard 12-lead ECG. ST depression occurs in 13% of patients with periprocedural occlusion. In 10% of patients with abrupt closure, no ECG changes are documented (25). If continuous 12-lead monitoring is performed on patients following a successful PTCA, 23% of patients will have transient ischemic episodes as manifested by ST elevation or depression. However, not all of these patients will develop abrupt closure. If a patient has no chest pain and no ECG changes, the incidence of major ischemic complications as manifested by infarction, CABG, or death is approximately 1%. If a patient has chest pain but no ST segment changes, the major complication rate is about 2%. ST depression without symptoms has a major complication rate of 8%. ST elevation with or without symptoms has a complication rate of approximately 60%. ST elevation in the same leads as the angioplastied artery has a major complication rate of 92% (85). It is important to note that in some cases ST elevation will precede chest pain (81, 82, 85). Limb-lead monitoring alone will identify less than half of the patients having ischemia as compared with continuous 12-lead monitoring (82, 85). For these reasons in patients identified as high risk before leaving the catheterization laboratory, the use of a 12-lead continuous monitor may prove beneficial in the early diagnosis of abrupt closure.

TREATMENTS FOR ABRUPT CLOSURE

Early treatment strategies for acute coronary occlusion involved the use of intracoronary nitroglycerin, intracoronary thrombolytic therapy, and repeat dilation with standard balloons for relatively short periods (25, 27, 29, 30). Though spasm is thought to play a role in abrupt closure, the use of nitroglycerin rarely reverses this clinical syndrome (30). Intracoronary thrombolytic therapy adds very little to the management of abrupt closure, even though thrombus formation is thought to be a significant contributor to abrupt closure (26). Repeat dilations with standard-duration balloon inflations have also shown only minimal success in reversing abrupt closure (26). In the early and mid 1980s, death occurred in approximately 5% of patients who suffered periprocedural occlusion, 35% of patients had myocardial infarctions, and emergency CABG was required in about 35% of the patients (25–27, 29, 34). Though the incidence of abrupt closure has not changed significantly since the early 1980s, the prevalence of ischemic complications has dropped substantially (57, 86–88). Initially, the treatment for abrupt closure was almost exclusively emergency CABG. Approximately 6% of the patients who underwent angioplasty required emergent coronary bypass grafting (28). With the advent of the perfusion balloon catheter and the increased use of the intraaortic balloon pump, the percentage of patients referred for emergency CABG decreased significantly to 3.5% (28). Since the widespread use of intracoronary stenting, the rate of emergency bypass grafting has decreased to approximately 2% (57). These figures need to be seen in the light of the substantially increased

complexity of lesion morphology over the last decade, as well as the new technologies that have dramatically reduced the need for emergency CABG.

Dissection is the event most strongly associated with abrupt closure and ischemic complications (32, 39). The perfusion balloon catheter and intracoronary stents have been helpful in decreasing the complication rates in patients with acute or threatened closure. The use of prolonged inflations with the perfusion balloon catheter allows the interventionist to "tack up" dissection flaps (25, 86, 87, 89–91). The perfusion balloon has been successful in reversing abrupt closure in 50 to 80% of patients in whom it has been attempted as shown in Table 36B.7 (25–27, 30). However, the optimal duration of prolonged dilation of a major dissection remains to be determined. Observation series have suggested that inflation durations of 30 minutes to 1 hour may be optimal (92), but dilations as long as 17 hours have also been found to be useful (93).

In some cases, however, prolonged dilations are not successful in achieving sustained patency of a vessel. In such patients the perfusion catheter can simply be placed without any inflation to restore blood flow down the injured vessel, which can decrease or eliminate ischemia while preparations are made for intracoronary stenting or emergency bypass grafting (90, 94). An effective combi-

Table 36B.7.
Dissection Repair Using Prolonged Perfusion Balloon Inflations

Study	No. of Patients	Average Inflation Duration (min)	Angiographic Success (%)
Smith et al (117)	28	21	57
Jackman et al (118)	40	30	80
Leitschuh et al (119)	36	18	74
Seggewiss et al (120)	63	13	81
Van Lierde et al (121)	37	29	63
de Muinck et al (122)	33	25	67
Wilson et al (92)	49	63	86
Total	286	28	73

nation of a perfusion catheter and an intraaortic balloon pump (IABP) can significantly decrease ischemia in patients who are to undergo emergency bypass grafting following a failed angioplasty (94). In patients with abrupt closure and ST elevation the perioperative myocardial infarction rate is approximately 50%. If an IABP is employed, the myocardial infarction rate drops to approximately 20% (95). Consequently, the rates of emergency CABG, myocardial infarction, and death have decreased since the introduction of the perfusion balloon catheter and the intraaortic balloon pump.

There has been limited experience with directional coronary atherectomy for treatment of major dissections. Cutting out the dissection flap has proved beneficial for periprocedural occlusion (26, 96, 97). However, operators should have considerable experience with atherectomy before this technique is attempted. In experienced hands it has been found to be particularly useful for limited eccentric dissections that partially obstruct the lumen. Perforation remains a concern with this technique. Further studies are needed to clarify the role of salvage atherectomy for acute or threatened closure.

Intracoronary stents are used effectively in patients with acute or threatened closure. The Gianturco-Roubin stent has been studied extensively as a bailout device (57, 86–89). Intracoronary stents can be successfully deployed in 95 to 97% of patients who require them for periprocedural occlusion (57, 87, 88). Case-controlled studies have compared patients treated with intracoronary stenting versus those patients treated before stenting was available. The overall success in returning patency to the vessel at risk was 97% with stenting compared with 72% using conventional techniques (87). Not surprisingly, the rates of death, myocardial infarction and emergency CABG have been reported to decrease when intracoronary stenting is employed for acute and threatened closure (57, 86–88). Patients who receive a stent for

abrupt closure have restenosis rates (39 to 46%) comparable with those of patients who were treated with redilation following abrupt closure (87, 88). Furthermore, the event-free survival during the first 6 months is equivalent at about 80% (87, 88). Hence, the benefit of using a stent and increasing the salvage rate of acute occlusion is not offset by more complications in the postdischarge period.

The perfusion balloon catheter, intracoronary stenting, and the intraaortic balloon pump have revolutionized the treatment of abrupt closure. Scott and colleagues reported that patients who were treated for abrupt closure during a period when intracoronary stents and perfusion balloons were available had a reduced incidence of periprocedural Q-wave MI from 20 to 11% compared with patients treated before these technologies were available. The rate of in-hospital CABG for patients with abrupt closure also was reduced from 39 to 30% and the mortality rate fell from 4.8 to 2.6% (86). The results of two randomized clinical trials comparing intracoronary stents versus perfusion balloon angioplasty in threatened abrupt closure are going to be formative in our understanding of the best treatment strategy for dissections and abrupt closure (Dr. Ian Penn and Dr. Patrick Serruys, personal communication). Treatment strategies for abrupt closure must be individualized for a particular patient, but appropriate use of perfusion balloon catheters, stents, and intraaortic balloon pumps significantly lower the morbidity and mortality of periprocedural occlusion.

NOVEL PHARMACOLOGIC APPROACHES IN THE PREVENTION OF ABRUPT CLOSURE

Both aspirin and heparin have limitations to their use, but are safe and inexpensive. Heparin is an indirect thrombin inhibitor that is limited by its need to combine with circulating antithrombin III, by being neutralized by circulating plasma proteins, and by its inability to inhibit clot-bound thrombin. Heparin use is further compounded by the difficulties in achieving a stable steady-state in blood. Aspirin is a very weak inhibitor of platelet function through the arachidonic acid pathway, with little effect on thrombin- or collagen-stimulated platelet aggregation. As abrupt closure results from local thrombosis in which thrombin is a pivotal enzyme regulating both hemostasis and platelet activation, an approach that encompasses both direct thrombin inhibition and platelet inhibition is being sought.

In general, the new thrombin inhibitors being evaluated as adjunctive therapies for percutaneous interventions are all direct thrombin inhibitors which can inactivate clot-bound thrombin. Agents have been developed for use as adjunctive therapies with percutaneous interventions. Hirulog, hirudin, and argatroban are direct thrombin inhibitors that are unique from heparin in that they inactivate clot-bound thrombin. These agents have been found to yield a stable dose-dependent antithrombotic effect (98–100). Hirudin, a recombinant peptide binding to both the catalytic site and the anion binding site, have been evaluated in 113 patients undergoing standard angioplasty (101). Patients randomized to hirudin had a trend toward less adverse events (death, myocardial infarction, or CABG; 1% versus 10%) and less ischemic ECG changes during continuous monitoring (4% versus 11%), which was offset by a higher incidence of dissections (35% versus 24%) and major bleeding complications (5% versus 0). No patient assigned to either hirudin or heparin suffered an abrupt closure. These initial observations with hirudin in patients having angioplasty are being evaluated in the large HELVETICA study currently under way. Hirulog, a 20-amino acid synthetic peptide binding thrombin that contains a portion of the hirudin sequence, has been examined in 291 patients undergoing elective angioplasty (102). In this dose-escalation study there appeared to be reduction in the rate of abrupt closure with a higher dose of hirulog (4% versus 11%, $P = .05$) and no

abrupt closures occurred in patients with an ACT >300 seconds. Major bleeding complications occurred in only one patient. Future randomized clinical trials will further enhance our understanding of the effect direct thrombin inhibition may have in reducing abrupt closure.

Platelets aggregate via fibrinogen binding to the platelet surface glycoprotein IIb/IIIa (GP IIb/IIIa) receptor. Blockade of this receptor results in potent platelet inhibition as it is the final pathway for platelet activation. The novel antiplatelet agents, 7E3 and integrelin, block the GP IIb/IIa receptor and inhibit platelet function to a much greater extent than aspirin with a short duration of action (103). The EPIC study was a randomized, controlled trial evaluating the efficacy of 7E3, a chimeric monoclonal antibody to the GP IIb/IIIa receptor, in a high-risk group of angioplasty patients. Though procedural success was similar in patients treated with a 7E3 bolus and infusion compared with placebo, the rate of ischemic complications was significantly decreased (8.4% versus 12.8%) (104). However, there was significant increase in major bleeding complications in patients who received the most intense GP IIb/IIIa inhibition (bolus dose + infusion) compared with placebo-treated patients (14% versus 7%). Integrelin is a synthetic cyclic heptapeptide that reversibly blocks the GP IIb/IIIa receptor. The IMPACT trial was a dose-ranging study that investigated the safety of integrelin during angioplasty (105). The integrelin-treated patients had a higher procedural success rate (97% versus 87.5%) compared with the patients treated with heparin and aspirin alone. Also, a modest reduction in ischemic complications was observed (7.9% versus 10.2%). Though minor bleeding rates were increased, there was no increase in the risk of moderate to severe bleeding. More investigation is under way to more clearly explore the benefit-to-risk ratio of these agents. The combination of potent anti-platelet agents with antithrombin therapy clearly opens new

Table 36B.8.
Proposed Management Strategy of Patients With High Risk of Abrupt Closure

High-Risk Characteristics	Potential Management		
	Preprocedure	During Procedure	Postprocedure
Patient Characteristics			
Unstable angina[a]	IV Heparin (>24 hours)	ACT >400s	⎱ IV heparin ⎰ ST-segment monitoring
Female gender[a]			
Multivessel CAD[a]		Staged procedure	
Angiographic			
Total occlusion			
Branch point			
Long lesion[a]	—	Appropriate device	⎱ IV heparin
Right coronary artery[a]		ACT >400s	⎰ ST-segment monitoring
Calcification			
Eccentricity[a]			
Complex lesion (ulcerated, hazy, etc.)	IV Heparin (>24 hours)	As above	⎱ IV heparin
Thrombus			⎰ ST-segment monitoring
Postprocedure			
Dissection	—	Stents, PBC ACT >400s	⎱ IV heparin ST-segment monitoring ⎰ IABP[b]

[a]Modify treatment strategy only if associated with other "high-risk" characteristic.

[b]Only in patients who are not candidates for CABG.

avenues to reduce the rate of abrupt closure. However, local delivery of these new potent agents may be particularly attractive to reduce the risk for hemorrhagic complications.

SUMMARY

The optimal management of patients with a high risk for abrupt closure is to prevent it. Although there is no specific strategy that can be applied to all high-risk characteristics, a general scheme based on the literature and broad-based experience is proposed in Table 36B.8. Baseline characteristics that have been associated with abrupt closure should lead to a modification to both the anticoagulation and the device used to approach the lesion. Some modification to the postprocedural management is also proposed. The angiographic lesion morphology should be approached with the appropriate device for the specific lesion being treated. Currently, there is relatively scant information to indicate that any device reduces the rate of abrupt closure. Intracoronary stenting and prolonged dilations using perfusion balloons offer some promise. The postprocedural management is limited at this point to treating or preventing major

dissections. In this regard both stents and perfusion balloons offer therapeutic options in preventing patients undergoing CABG. In patients with stable dissections careful monitoring by continuous ST-segment monitoring and prolonged heparin infusion offer some advantages.

Abrupt closure of a dilated segment remains one of the main challenges that faces the interventional cardiologist. Future application of potent targeted therapies toward the clotting cascade or platelet activation appears to offer some potential advantages that need further exploration. The future application of targeted pharmacologic therapies may be performed by local delivery to reduce any systemic effects, while pacifying the dilated coronary artery segment. These new modalities in adjunctive therapies offer some substantial hypothetical advantage to improve percutaneous intervention to become a safer procedure with minimal risk of acute ischemic complications.

REFERENCES

1. Kohchi K, Takebayashi S, Block PC, Hiroki T, Nobuyoshi M. Arterial changes after percutaneous transluminal coronary angioplasty: results at autopsy. J Am Coll Cardiol 1987;10:592–599.

2. Potkin BN, Roberts WC. Effects of percutaneous translu-minal coronary angioplasty on atherosclerotic plaques and relation of plaque composition and arterial size to out-come. Am J Cardiol 1988;62:41–50.

3. Block PC, Fallon JT, Elmer D. Experimental angioplasty: lessons from the laboratory. Am J Roentgenol 1980; 135:907–912.

4. Castaneda-Zuniga WR, Formanek A, Tadavarthy M, Vlo-daver Z, Edwards JE, Zollikofer C, Amplatz K. The mech-anism of balloon angioplasty. Diagn Radiol 1980; 135:565–571.

5. Baughman KL, Pasternak RC, Fallon JT, Block PC. Trans-luminal coronary angioplasty of postmortem human hearts. Am J Cardiol 1981;48:1044–1047.

6. Faxon DP, Weber V, Haudenschild C, Gottsman SB, McGovern WA, Ryan TJ. Acute effects of transluminal angioplasty in three experimental models of atherosclero-sis. Arteriosclerosis 1982;2:125–133.

7. O'Gara PT, Guerrero JL, Feldman B, Fallon JT, Block PC. Effect of dextran and aspirin on platelet adherence after transluminal angioplasty of normal canine coronary arter-ies. Am J Cardiol 1984;53:1695–1698.

8. Mizuno K, Kurita A, Imazeki N. Pathological findings after percutaneous transluminal coronary angioplasty. Br Heart J 1984;52:588–590.

9. Waller BF, McManus BM, Gorfinkel HJ, Kishel JC, Schmidt ECH, Kent KM, Roberts WC. Status of the major epicar-dial coronary arteries 80 to 150 days after percutaneous transluminal coronary angioplasty. Am J Cardiol 1994; 51:81–84.

10. Block PC, Myler RK, Stertzer S, Fallon JT. Morphology after transluminal angioplasty in human beings. N Engl J Med 1981;305:382–385.

11. Soward AL, Essed CE, Serruys PW. Coronary arterial find-ings after accidental death immediately after successful percutaneous transluminal coronary angioplasty. Am J Cardiol 1985;56:794–795.

12. Tobis JM, Mallery JA, Gessert J, Griffith J, Mahon D, Bessen M, Moriuchi M et al. Intravascular ultrasound cross-sectional arterial imaging before and after balloon angioplasty in vitro. Circulation 1989;80:873–882.

13. Potkin BN, Keren G, Mintz GS, Douek PC, Pichard AD, Satler LF, Kent KM et al. Arterial responses to balloon coronary angioplasty: an intravascular ultrasound study. J Am Coll Cardiol 1992;20:942–951.

14. Hodgson J McB, Reddy KG, Suneja R, Nair RN, Lesnef-sky EJ, Sheehan HM. Intracoronary ultrasound imaging: correlation of plaque morphology with angiography, clini-cal syndrome and procedural results in patients under-going coronary angioplasty. J Am Coll Cardiol 1993; 21:35–44.

15. Tenaglia AN, Buller CE, Kisslo KB, Phillips HR, Stack RS, Davidson CJ. Intracoronary ultrasound predictors of adverse outcomes after coronary artery interventions. J Am Coll Cardiol 1992;20:1385–1390.

16. Gerber T, Erbel R, Gorge G, Ge J, Rupprecht H-J, Meyer J. Classification of morphologic effects of percutaneous transluminal coronary angioplasty assessed by intravas-cular ultrasound. Am J Cardiol 1992;70:1546–1554.

17. Coy KM, Park JC, Fishbein MC, Laas T, Diamond GA, Adler L, Maurer G et al. In vitro validation of three-dimen-sional intravascular ultrasound for the evaluation of arter-ial injury after balloon angioplasty. J Am Coll Cardiol 1992;20:692–700.

18. Sassower MA, Adela GS, Koch JM, Manzo KM, Friedl SE, Vivino PG, Nesto RW. Angioscopic evaluation of periprocedural and postprocedural abrupt closure after percutaneous coronary angioplasty. Am Heart J 1993; 126:444–450.

19. Heijer Pd, Dijk Bv, Twisk SPM, Lie KI. Early stent occlusion is not always caused by thrombosis. Cathet Cardiovasc Diagn 1993;29:136–140.

20. Hollman J, Austin GE, Gruentzig AR, Douglas JS Jr, King SB III. Coronary artery spasm at the site of angioplasty in the first 2 months after successful percutaneous trans-luminal coronary angioplasty. J Am Coll Cardiol 1983; 2:1039–1045.

21. Fischell TA, Nellessen U, Johnson DE, Ginsburg R. Endothelium-dependent arterial vasoconstriction after balloon angioplasty. Circulation 1989;79:899–910.

22. Preisack MB, Athanasiadis A, Voelker W, Baumbach A, Karsch KR. Acute closure during coronary excimer laser angioplasty and conventional balloon dilatation: a com-parison of management outcome and prediction. Eur Heart J 1993;14:195–204.

23. Tenaglia AN, Fortin DF, Califf RM, Frid DJ, Nelson CL, Gardner L, Miller M et al. Individualizing the risk of angio-plasty abrupt vessel closure. J Am Coll Cardiol 1994; 24:1004.

24. Ellis SG, Vandormael MG, Cowley MJ, DiSciascio G, Deligonul U, Topol EJ, Bulle TM, and the Multivessel Angioplasty Prognosis Study Group. Coronary morpho-logic and clinical determinants of procedural outcome with angioplasty for multivessel coronary disease: implications for patient selection. Circulation 1990;82:1193–1202.

25. deFeyter PJ, Brand Mvd, Jaarman GJ, Domburg Rv, Ser-ruys PW, Suryapranata H. Acute coronary artery occlu-sion during and after percutaneous transluminal coronary angioplasty: frequency, prediction, clinical course, man-agement, and follow-up. Circulation 1991;83(3):927–936.

26. Lincoff AM, Popma JJ, Ellis SG, Hacker JA, Topol EJ. Abrupt vessel closure complicating coronary angioplasty: clinical, angiographic and therapeutic profile. J Am Coll Cardiol 1992;19:926–935.

27. Detre KM, Holmes DR, Holubkov R, Cowley MJ, Bourassa MG, Faxon DP, Dorros GR et al. Incidence and conse-quences of periprocedural occlusion: the 1985–1986 National Heart, Lung, and Blood Institute Percutaneous Transluminal Coronary Angioplasty Registry. Circulation 1990;82:739–750.

28. Holmes DR, Holubkov R, Vlietstra RE, Kelsey SF, Reeder GS, Dorros G, Williams DO et al. Comparison of compli-cations during percutaneous transluminal coronary angio-plasty from 1977 to 1981 and from 1985 to 1986: the National Heart, Lung, and Blood Institute Percutaneous Transluminal Coronary Angioplasty Registry. J Am Coll Cardiol 1988;12(5):1149–1155.

29. Sinclair IN, McCabe CH, Sipperly ME, Baim DS. Predictors, therapeutic options and long-term outcome of abrupt reclosure. Am J Cardiol 1988;61:61G–66G.

30. Simpfendorfer C, Belardi J, Bellamy G, Galan K, Franco I, Hollman J. Frequency, management and follow-up of patients with acute coronary occlusions after percutaneous transluminal coronary angiography. Am J Cardiol 1987;59:267–269.

31. Goldbaum T, DiSciascio G, Cowley MJ, Vetrovec GW. Early occlusion following successful coronary angioplasty: clinical and angiographic observations. Cathet Cardiovasc Diagn 1989;17:22–27.

32. Bredlau CE, Roubin GS, Leimbruber PP, Douglas J, King SB III, Gruentzig AR. In-hospital morbidity and mortality in patients undergoing elective coronary angioplasty. Circulation 1985;72:1044–1052.

33. Tenaglia AN, Fortin DF, Frid DJ, Gardner LH, Nelson CL, Tcheng JE, Stack RS et al. Long-term outcome following successful reopening of abrupt closure after coronary angioplasty. Am J Cardiol 1993;72:21–25.

34. Ellis SG, Roubin GS, King SB III, Douglas J, Weintraub WS, Thomas RG, Cox WR. Angiographic and clinical predictors of acute closure after native vessel coronary angioplasty. Circulation 1988;77:372–379.

35. Schatz RA, Baim DS, Leon M, Ellis SG, Goldberg S, Hirshfeld JW, Cleman MW et al. Clinical experience with the Palmaz-Schatz coronary stent: initial results of a multicenter study. Circulation 1991;83:148–161.

36. Ischinger T, Gruentzig AR, Meier B, Galan K. Coronary dissection and total coronary occlusion associated with percutaneous transluminal coronary angioplasty: significance of initial angiographic morphology of coronary stenoses. Circulation 1986;74:1371–1378.

37. Cavallini C, Giommi L, Franceschini E, Risica G, Olivari Z, Marton F, Cuzzato V. Coronary angioplasty in single-vessel complex lesions: short- and long-term outcome and factors predicting acute coronary occlusion. Am Heart J 1991;122:44–49.

38. Mabin TA, Holmes DR Jr, Smith HC, Vliestra RE, Bove AA, Reeder GS, Chesebro JH et al. Intracoronary thrombus: role in coronary occlusion complicating percutaneous transluminal coronary angioplasty. J Am Coll Cardiol 1985;5:198–202.

39. Bell M, Reeder G, Garratt K, Berger P, Bailey K, Holmes DR J. Predictors of major ischemic complications after coronary dissection following angioplasty. Am J Cardiol 1993;71:1402–1407.

40. Huber MS, Mooney JF, Madison J, Mooney M. Use of a morphologic classification to predict clinical outcome after dissection from coronary angioplasty. Am J Cardiol 1991; 68:467–471.

41. Ryan TJ, Faxon DP, Gunnar RM, Kennedy JW, King SB, Loop FD, Peterson KL et al. Guidelines for percutaneous transluminal coronary angioplasty. Circulation 1988; 78:486–502.

42. Berdan LG, Holmes DR, Davidson-Ray L, Lam LC, Talley JD, Mark DB, for the CAVEAT investigators. Economic impact of abrupt closure following percutaneous intervention: the CAVEAT experience. J Am Coll Cardiol 1994; 23:434A.

43. Nelson CL, Tcheng JE, Frid DJ, Fortin DF, Ohman EM, Califf RM, Stack RS. Incomplete angiographic follow-up results in significant underestimation of true restenosis rates after PTCA. Circulation 1990;82(Suppl III):III-312 (abstract).

44. Kuntz RE, Piana R, Pomerantz RM, Carrozza J, Fishman R, Mansour M, Safian RD et al. Changing incidence and management of abrupt closure following coronary intervention in the new device era. Cathet Cardiovasc Diagn 1992;27:183–190.

45. Topol EJ, Leya F, Pinkerton CA, Whitlow PL, Hofling B, Simonton CA, Masden RR et al. for the CAVEAT Study Group. A comparison of directional atherectomy with coronary angioplasty in patients with coronary artery disease. N Engl J Med 1993;329:221–227.

46. Haude M, Erbel R, Issa H, Straub U, Rupprecht HJ, Treese N, Meyer J. Subacute thrombotic complications after intracoronary implantation of Palmaz-Schatz stents. Am Heart J 1993;126:15–22.

47. Serruys PW, Macaya C, de Jaegere P, Kiemeneij F, Rutsch W, Heyndrickx G, Emanuelsson H et al. on behalf of the Benestent study group. Interim analysis of the Benestent-trial. Circulation 1993;88(suppl):I-594.

48. Nath FC, Muller DWM, Ellis SG, Rosenschein U, Chapekis A, Quain L, Zimmerman C et al. Thrombosis of a flexible coil coronary stent: frequency, predictors and clinical outcome. J Am Coll Cardiol 1993;21:622–627.

49. Safian RD, Niazi KA, Strzelecki M, Lichtenberg A, May MA, Juran N, Freed M et al. Detailed angiographic analysis of high-speed mechanical rotational atherectomy in human coronary arteries. Circulation 1993;88:961–968.

50. Ohman EM, Marquis J, Ricci DR, Brown RIG, Knudtson ML, Kereiakes DJ, Samaha JK et al. for the Perfusion Balloon Catheter Study Group. A randomized comparison of the effects of gradual prolonged versus standard primary balloon inflation on early and late outcome: results of a multicenter clinical trial. Circulation 1994; 89:1118–1125.

51. Ellis SG, DeCesare NB, Pinkerton CA, Whitlow P, King SB III, Ghazzal ZMB, Kereiakes DJ et al. Relation of stenosis morphology and clinical presentation to the procedural results of directional coronary atherectomy. Circulation 1991;84:644–653.

52. Popma JJ, Topol EJ, Hinohara T, Pinkerton CA, Baim DS, King SB III, Holmes J et al. for the U.S. Directional Atherectomy Investigator Group. Abrupt vessel closure after directional coronary atherectomy. J Am Coll Cardiol 1992;19:1372–1379.

53. Hinohara T, Rowe MH, Robertson GC, Selmon MR, Braden L, Leggett JH, Vetter JW et al. Effect of lesion characteristics on outcome of directional coronary atherectomy. J Am Coll Cardiol 1991;17:1112–1120.

54. Adelman AG, Cohen EA, Kimball BP, Bonan R, Ricci DR, Webb JG, Laramee L et al. A comparison of directional atherectomy with balloon angioplasty for lesions of the left anterior descending coronary artery. N Engl J Med 1993;329:228–233.

55. Bittl JA, Sanborn TA, Tcheng JE, Siegel RM, Ellis SG for the Percutaneous Excimer Laser Coronary Angioplasty Registry. Clinical success, complications and restenosis

rates with excimer laser coronary angioplasty. Am J Cardiol 1992;70:1533–1539.

56. Schatz RA, Goldberg S, Leon M, Baim D, Hirshfeld J, Cleman M, Ellis SG et al. Clinical experience with the Palmaz-Schatz coronary stent. J Am Coll Cardiol 1991;17:155B–159B.

57. Roubin GS, Cannon AD, Agrawal SK, Macander PJ, Dean LS, Baxley WA, Breland J. Intracoronary stenting for acute and threatened closure complicating percutaneous transluminal coronary angioplasty. Circulation 1992;85:916–927.

58. Teirstein PS, Warth DC, Haq N, Jenkins NS, McCowan LC, Aubanel-Reidel P, Morris N et al. High-speed rotational coronary atherectomy for patients with diffuse coronary artery disease. J Am Coll Cardiol 1991; 18:1694–1701.

59. Bertrand ME, Lablanche JM, Leroy F, Bauters C, Jaegere PD, Serruys PW, Meyer J et al. Percutaneous transluminal coronary rotary ablation with Rotablator (European experience). Am J Cardiol 1992;69:470–474.

60. Popma JJ, Leon MB, Mintz GS, Kent KM, Satler LF, Garrand TJ, Pichard AD. Results of coronary angioplasty using the transluminal extraction catheter. Am J Cardiol 1992;70:1526–1532.

61. Tenaglia AN, Quigley PJ, Kereiakes DJ, Abbottsmith CW, Phillips HR, Tcheng JE, Rendall D et al. Coronary angioplasty performed with gradual and prolonged inflation using a perfusion balloon catheter: procedural success and restenosis rate. Am Heart J 1992;124:585–589.

62. Kereiakes DJ, Knudston ML, Ohman EM, Broderick TM, Marquis J, Gurbel PA, Tcheng JE et al. for the PBC Study Group. Prolonged dilatation improves initial results during PTCA of complex coronary stenoses: results from a randomized trial. J Am Coll Cardiol 1993;21:290A.

63. Schwartz L, Bourassa MG, Lesperance J, Aldridge HE, Kazim F, Salvatori VA, Henderson M et al. Aspirin and dipyridamole in the prevention of restenosis after percutaneous transluminal coronary angioplasty. N Engl J Med 1988;318:1714–1719.

64. Barnathan ES, Schwartz S, Taylor L, Laskey WK, Kleaveland JP, Kussmaul WG, Hirshfeld JW. Aspirin and dipyridamole in the prevention of acute coronary thrombosis complicating coronary angioplasty. Circulation 1987;76:125–134.

65. Lembo NJ, Black AJR, Roubin GS, Wilenta JR, Mufson LH, Douglas J Jr, King SB III. Effect of pretreatment with aspirin versus aspirin plus dipyridamole on frequency and type of acute complications of percutaneous transluminal coronary angioplasty. Am Heart J 1990;65:422–426.

66. White CW, Chaitman B, Lassar TA, Marcus ML, Chisholm RJ, Knudson M, Morton B et al. Antiplatelet agents are effective in reducing the immediate complications of PTCA: results from the ticlopidine multicenter trial. Circulation 1987;76:IV-400.

67. Bull BS, Korpman RA, Huse WM, Briggs BD. Heparin therapy during extracorporeal circulation. J Thorac Cardiovasc Surg 1975;69:674–684.

68. Avendano A, Ferguson JJ. Comparison of hemochron and hemotec activated coagulation time target values during

percutaneous transluminal coronary angioplasty. J Am Coll Cardiol 1994;23:907–910.

69. Narins CR, Hillegass WB, Nelson CL, Harrington RA, Phillips HR, Stack RS, Califf RM. Activated clotting time predicts abrupt closure risk during angioplasty. J Am Coll Cardiol 1994;23:470A.

70. Hillegass WB, Narins CR, Brott BC, Haura EB, Phillips HR, Stack RS, Califf RM. Activated clotting time predicts bleeding complications from angioplasty. J Am Coll Cardiol 1994;23:184A.

71. Ogilby JD, Kopelman HA, Klein LW, Agarwal JB. Adequate heparinization during PTCA: assessment using activated clotting times. Cathet Cardiovasc Diagn 1989; 18(4):206–209.

72. Laskey MAL, Deutsch E, Barnathan E, Laskey WK. Influence of heparin therapy on percutaneous transluminal coronary angioplasty outcome in unstable angina pectoris. Am J Cardiol 1990;65:1425–1429.

73. Ellis SG, Roubin GS, Wilentz J, Douglas J Jr, King SB III. Effect of 18- to 24-hour heparin administration for prevention of restenosis after uncomplicated coronary angioplasty. Am Heart J 1989;117:777–782.

74. Reifart N, Schmidt A, Preusler W, Schwartz F, Storger H. Is it necessary to heparinize for 24 hours after percutaneous transluminal coronary angioplasty?. J Am Coll Cardiol 1992;19:231A.

75. McGarry TF, Gottlieb RS, Morganroth J, Zelenkofske SL, Kasparian H, Duca PR, Lester RM et al. The relationship of anticoagulation level and complications after successful percutaneous transluminal coronary angioplasty. Am Heart J 1992;123:1445–1451.

76. Gabliani G, Deligonul U, Kern MJ, Vandormael M. Acute coronary occlusion occurring after successful percutaneous transluminal coronary angioplasty: temporal relationship to discontinuation of anticoagulation. Am Heart J 1988;116:696–700.

77. Reeder GS, Bryant S, Suman V, Holmes DR Jr. Intracoronary thrombus: still a risk for PTCA failure? J Am Coll Cardiol 1994;23:184A.

78. Ambrose JA, Torre SR, Sharma SK, Israel DH, Monsen CE, Weiss M, Untereker W et al. Adjunctive thrombolytic therapy for angioplasty in ischemic rest angina: results of a double-blind randomized pilot study. J Am Coll Cardiol 1992;20:1197–1204.

79. Pavlides GS, Schreiber TL, Gangadharan V, Puchrowicz S, O'Neill WW. Safety and efficacy of urokinase during elective coronary angioplasty. Am Heart J 1991; 121:731–737.

80. Eisenberg PR, Sherman LA, Jaffe AS. Paradoxic elevation of fibrinopeptide A after streptokinase: evidence for continued thrombosis despite intense fibrinolysis. J Am Coll Cardiol 1987;10:527–529.

81. Mizutani M, Freedman SB, Barns E, Ogasawara S, Bailey BP, Bernstein L. ST monitoring for myocardial ischemia during and after coronary angioplasty. Am J Cardiol 1990;66:389–393.

82. Bush HS, Ferguson JJ III, Angelini P, Willerson JT. Twelve-lead electrocardiographic evaluation of ischemia during percutaneous transluminal coronary angioplasty and its

correlation with acute reocclusion. Am Heart J 1991; 121:1591–1599.

83. Violaris AG, Campbell S. Characteristics of transient myocardial ischaemia and acute occlusion in the immediate post-angioplasty period. Int J Cardiol 1992;34:219–221.

84. Krucoff MW, Wagner NB, Pope JE, Mortara DM, Jackson YR, Bottner RK, Wagner GS et al. The portable programmable microprocessor-driven real-time 12-lead electrocardiographic monitor: a preliminary report of a new device for the noninvasive detection of successful reperfusion or silent coronary reocclusion. Am J Cardiol 1990;65:143–148.

85. Krucoff MW, Jackson YR, Kehoe MK, Kent KM. Quantitative and qualitative ST segment monitoring during and after percutaneous transluminal coronary angioplasty. Circulation 1990;81 (Suppl IV):IV-20–IV-26.

86. Scott NA, Weintraub WS, Carlin SF, Tao X, Douglas J Jr, Lembo NJ, King SB II. Recent changes in the management and outcome of acute closure after percutaneous transluminal coronary angioplasty. Am J Cardiol 1993; 71:1159–1163.

87. Lincoff AM, Topol EJ, Chapekis AT, George BS, Candela RJ, Muller DWM, Zimmerman CA et al. Intracoronary stenting compared with conventional therapy for abrupt vessel closure complicating coronary angioplasty: a matched case-control study. J Am Coll Cardiol 1993; 21:866–875.

88. George BS, Voorhees WD III, Roubin GS, Fearnot NE, Pinkerton CA, Raizner AE, King SB et al. Multicenter investigation of coronary stenting to treat acute or threatened closure after percutaneous transluminal coronary angioplasty: clinical and angiographic outcomes. J Am Coll Cardiol 1993;22:135–143.

89. Sundram P, Harvey JR, Johnson RG, Schwartz MJ, Baim DS. Benefit of the perfusion catheter for emergency coronary artery grafting after failed percutaneous transluminal coronary angioplasty. Am J Cardiol 1989;63:282–285.

90. Ferguson TB, Hinohara T, Simpson J, Stack RS, Wechsler AS. Catheter reperfusion to allow optimal coronary bypass grafting following failed transluminal coronary angioplasty. Ann Thorac Surg 1986;42:399–405.

91. Little T. Prolonged coronary splinting in the management of acute coronary closure. Cathet Cardiovasc Diagn 1992;25:213–217.

92. Wilson JS, Ohman EM, Perez JA, Gardner LH, Nelson CL, Phillips HR, Sketch JR. Use of prolonged perfusion balloon inflations of 60 minutes as a "temporary stent" to salvage initially unsuccessful coronary interventions: acute and long-term outcome. J Am Coll Cardiol 1994;23:58A.

93. van der Linden LP, Bakx ALM, Sedney MI, Buis B, Bruschke AVG. Prolonged dilation with an autoperfusion balloon catheter for refractory acute occlusion related to percutaneous transluminal coronary angioplasty. J Am Coll Cardiol 1993;22:1016–1023.

94. Suneja R, Hodgson JM. Use of intraaortic balloon counterpulsation for treatment of recurrent acute closure after coronary angioplasty. Am Heart J 1993;125:530–532.

95. Murphy DA, Craver JM, Jones EL, Curling PE, Guyton RA, King SB III, Gruentzig AR et al. Surgical management of acute myocardial ischemia following percutaneous trans-

luminal coronary angioplasty. J Thorac Cardiovasc Surg 1984;87:332–339.

96. Topol EJ. Emerging strategies for failed percutaneous transluminal coronary angioplasty. Am J Cardiol 1989; 63:249–250.

97. Warner M, Chami Y, Johnson D, Cowley MJ. Directional coronary atherectomy for failed angioplasty due to occlusive coronary dissection. Cathet Cardiovasc Diagn 1991; 24:28–31.

98. Verstraete M, Nurmohamed M, Kienast J, Siebeck M, Silling-Engelhardt G, Buller H, Hoet B et al. on behalf of the European Hirudin in Thrombosis Group. Biologic effects of recombinant hirudin (CGP 39393) in human volunteers. J Am Coll Cardiol 1993;22:1080–1088.

99. Lidon R, Theroux P, Juneau M, Adelman B, Maraganore J. Initial experience with a direct antithrombin, hirulog, in unstable angina. Circulation 1993;88:1495–1501.

100. Clarke RJ, Mayo G, FitzGerald GA, Fitzgerald DJ. Combined administration of aspirin and a specific thrombin inhibitor in man. Circulation 1991;83:1510–1518.

101. van den Bos AA, Deckers JW, Heyndrickx GR, Laarman G, Suryapranata H, Zijlstra F, Close P et al. Safety and efficacy of recombinant hirudin (CGP 39 393) versus heparin in patients with stable angina undergoing coronary angioplasty. Circulation 1993;88:2058–2066.

102. Topol EJ, Bonan R, Jewitt D, Sigwart U, Kakkar VV, Rothman M, Bono DB et al. Use of a direct antithrombin, hirulog, in place of heparin during coronary angioplasty. Circulation 1993;87:1622–1629.

103. Bates ER, McGillem MJ, Mickelson MK, Pitt B, Mancini GBJ. A monoclonal antibody against the platelet glycoprotein IIB/IIIA receptor complex prevents platelet aggregation and thrombosis in a canine model of coronary angioplasty. Circulation 1991;84:2463–2469.

104. Tcheng JE, Topol EJ, Kleiman NS, Ellis SG, Navetta FI, Fintel DJ, Weisman HF et al. and the EPIC investigators. Improvement in clinical outcomes of coronary angioplasty by treatment with the GPIIB/IIIA inhibitor chimeric 7E3:multivariable analysis of the EPIC study. Circulation 1993;88(Suppl):I-506.

105. Mooney MR, Mooney JF, Goldenberg IF, Almquist AK, Tassel RA. Percutaneous transluminal coronary angioplasty in the setting of large intracoronary thrombi. Am J Cardiol 1990;65:427–431.

106. Sugrue DD, Holmes DR Jr, Smith HC, Reeder GS, Lane GE, Vlietstra RE, Bresnahan JF et al. Coronary artery thrombus as a risk factor for acute vessel occlusion during percutaneous transluminal coronary angioplasty: improving results. Br Heart J 1986;56(1):62–66.

107. Ferguson JJ, Bitti JA, Strony JT, Adelman B. The relationship of dissection and thrombus after PTCA to in-hospital outcome: results of a prospective multicenter study. Circulation 1993;88:I-217.

108. Vetrovec GW, Leinbach RC, Gold HK, Cowley MJ. Intracoronary thrombolysis in syndromes of unstable ischemia: angiographic and clinical results. American Heart Journal 1982;104:946–952.

109. Mandelkorn JB, Wolf NM, Singh S, Shechter JA, Kersh RI, Rodgers DM, Workman MB et al. Intracoronary thrombus in nontransmural myocardial infarction and in unstable angina pectoris. Am J Cardiol 1983;52:1–6.

110. Rentrop P, Blanke H, Karsch KR, Kaiser H, Kostering H, Leitz K. Selective intracoronary thrombolysis in acute myocardial infarction and unstable angina pectoris. Circulation 1981;63:307–317.

111. Shapiro EP, Brinker JA, Gottlieb SO, Guzman PA, Bulkley BH. Intracoronary thrombolysis 3 to 13 days after acute myocardial infarction for postinfarction angina pectoris. Am J Cardiol 1985;55:1453–1458.

112. de Zwaan C, Bar FW, Janssen JH, de Swart HB, Vermeer F, Wellens HJ. Effects of thrombolytic therapy in unstable angina: clinical and angiographic results. J Am Coll Cardiol 1988;12(2):301–309.

113. Ambrose JA, Hjemdahl-Monsen C, Borrico S, Sherman W, Cohen M, Gorlin R, Fuster V. Quantitative and qualitative effects of intracoronary streptokinase in unstable angina and non–Q-wave infarction. J Am Coll Cardiol 1987;9:1156–1165.

114. Gotoh K, Minamino T, Katoh O, Hamano Y, Fukui S, Hori M, Kusuoka H et al. The role of intracoronary thrombus in unstable angina: angiographic assessment and thrombolytic therapy during ongoing anginal attacks. Pathophysiology and Natural History 1988;77:526–534.

115. Goudreau E, Disciascio G, Vetrovec GW, Chami Y, Kohli R, Warner M, Sabri N et al. Intracoronary urokinase as an adjunct to percutaneous transluminal coronary angioplasty in patients with complex coronary narrowings or angioplasty-induced complications. Am J Cardiol 1992;69(1):57–62.

116. Disciascio G, Kohli RS, Goudreau E, Sabri N, Vetrovec GW. Intracoronary recombinant tissue-type plasminogen activator in unstable angina: a pilot angiographic study. Am Heart J 1991;122:1–6.

117. Smith JE, Quigley PJ, Tcheng JE, Bauman RP, Thomas J, Stack RS. Can prolonged perfusion balloon inflations salvage vessel patency after failed angioplasty? Circulation 1989;80(Suppl II):II-373 (abstract).

118. Jackman JD, Zidar JP, Tcheng JE, Overman AB, Phillips HR, Stack RS. Outcome after prolonged balloon inflations of greater than 20 minutes for initially unsuccessful percutaneous transluminal coronary angioplasty. Am J Cardiol 1992;69:1417–1421.

119. Leitschuh ML, Mills RM, Jacobs AK, Ruocco NA, LaRosa D, Faxon DP. Outcome after major dissection during coronary angioplasty using the perfusion balloon catheter. Am J Cardiol 1991;67:1056–1060.

120. Seggewiss H, Gleichmann U, Fassbender D, Vogt J, Mannebach H, Minami K. Therapy for acute vascular complications in percutaneous transluminal coronary angioplasty with the autoperfusion balloon catheter. Eur Heart J 1992;13:1649–1657.

121. Van Lierde J, Vrolix M, Stonis D, De Scheerder I, Stammen F, De Geest H, Piessens J. Efficacy of Stack autoperfusion catheter in acute complications of balloon angioplasty: short and intermediate-term results. Eur Heart J 1991;12:154 (abstract).

122. de Muinck E, van Dijk R, de Heijer P, Meeder J, Lie K. Prolonged autoperfusion balloon inflation for acute failure of conventional coronary angioplasty: a prospective study with retrospective controls. Eur Heart J 1991;12:155 (abstract).

EDITORIAL SUMMARY

From Dissection

Perfusion balloon angioplasty	First line therapy for dissections ≤10 to 15 mm in length. Start with a 6 to 10-minute inflation. Inflations of 20 to 60 minutes may also be helpful.
DCA	For focal and accessible PTCA-refractory dissections in which a flap protrudes into the lumen and the dissection does not appear to be deep. Guide catheter exchange will almost always have to be done—if recrossing the lesions is considered to be difficult, this approach should be only considered when stenting and CABG are considered to be poor options.
Stents	Probably best used only for refractory focal, or any long, dissection (in a patient suitable for vigorous anticoagulation). The proper use of stents remains, however, to be better defined. If the bleeding risk can be lessened, earlier stenting may be indicated. Remember to cover the entire length of the dissection and leave a good angiographic result (stenosis <10 to 20%).

From Thrombus[b]

Balloon angioplasty	Best for prompt restoration of flow when needed—but prolonged inflation probably is better at reducing recurrent obstructive thrombus.
Perfusion balloon angioplasty	May assist in restoring brisk flow.
Dispatch local delivery balloon	Delivery of 150,000 to 500,000 units urokinase ic seems to be quite efficacious.
Luminal infusion catheters	May have some role in the delivery of antithrombotic or thrombolytic agents.

[a]Anticipation and prevention are key. High-risk lesions should be treated with the lowest-risk form of therapy (including bypass surgery). Lesions that need to be treated percutaneously and are at high risk for dissection should be approached with firm ≥8 Fr guide support and a guidewire suitable for delivering a stent. Lesions at high risk for thrombotic closure should be deferred, or approached with ACT >350 seconds or advanced antiplatelet-antithrombotic pretreatment such as 7E3 or hirudin. In either instance, the possibility of needing hemodynamic support measures (IABP, PCPS) should be considered. IABP may also decrease the risk of later reclosure (as has been clearly demonstrated in the setting of acute infarction), but this is unproven.

[b]May coexist with dissection. Always ensure adequate degree of anticoagulation (ACT >350 seconds).

37. Coronary Arterial Perforation or Rupture Following Percutaneous Transluminal Coronary Angioplasty Procedure

FENG QI LIU, RAIMUND ERBEL, MICHAEL HAUDE, and JUNBO GE

Since Andreas Gruentzig et al. introduced percutaneous transluminal coronary angioplasty (PTCA) in 1977, it has gained wide acceptance and has become a very important therapeutic method for the treatment of coronary heart disease (30, 34, 52, 53). To improve the results of nonsurgical angioplasty, many new devices have been developed, including percutaneous transluminal coronary rotational angioplasty (PTCRA), directional coronary atherectomy (DCA), transluminal extraction endarterectomy catheter (TEC), and excimer laser coronary angioplasty (ELCA) (48, 63, 67, 68). Despite the high success rates, the nonsurgical coronary angioplasty is not free from complications such as acute coronary events (dissection, occlusion, spasm, embolism, and perforation) and ischemic events (myocardial infarction or prolonged angina) (11, 34, 63, 67, 68).

Coronary arterial perforation is not common. However, it can be deleterious because life-threatening events often follow, such as cardiac tamponade and acute myocardial infarction (3, 5, 11, 34, 35, 43, 64, 71). This complication calls for close observation and rapid, effective management. Although there are many studies discussing complications following angioplasty, few references exist to deal in detail with acute coronary arterial perforation. Based on our own experience, we present an intensive and comprehensive review on coronary perforation. The literature was gathered through both the Medline computer system and a hand-reference search in Medicus Index and other resources. Tables 37.1 and 37.2 show an overview of the studies reviewed.

DEFINITION

Acute coronary arterial perforation was defined as a persistent extravascular collection of contrast medium beyond the vessel wall with well-defined tears (5, 35). Bittl and associates devided perforation further into two types (5):

> Type I: It led to a major complication, for example, death, myocardial infarction, or emergency surgery.
> Type II: No clinical sequelae occurred after adjunctive balloon angioplasty.

In some studies the terms perforation and rupture were used as synonyms (3, 50, 69). To make it easier for comparison in different studies, we propose to use the term perforation alone to indicate the event when complete disruption of the arterial wall is accompanied by extravasation of contrast medium outside the vessel. In this review we mainly used "perforation." "Rupture" was used when specially necessary.

MECHANISM

Different devices and techniques played different roles in the occurrence of coronary artery perforation. Perforation might be caused by the guidewire, as well as the balloon, rotational burr, or laser (3, 41, 50, 51). All of the interventional angioplasty procedures em-

Table 37.1.
Literature Review

No.	Author (Ref).	Year	Case (n)	Method	Treatment	Death
1	Kimbiris D (43)	1982	1	PTCA	P, ECABG1	0
2	Saffitz JE (64)	1983	1	PTCA	P	1
3	Reul GJ (62)	1984	1/518 pts.	PTCA	ECABG 1	NA
4	Cowley GJ (11)	1984	3/3079 pts.	PTCA	C	0
5	Choy DSJ (10)	1984	1/5 pts.	LASER	NA	NA
6	Meng RL (51)	1985	1	PTCA	ECABG 1	0
7	Meier B (50)	1985	2/500 pts.	PTCA	C	NA
8	Pelletier LC (59)	1985	1/265 pts.	PTCA	ECABG 1	0
9	Bonzel T (6)	1986	1	PTCA	PTCA, ECABG 1	NA
10	Gonzalez-Santos JM (27)	1985	4/150 pts.	PTCA	ECABG 3	1
11	Altman F (3)	1986	1	PTCA	P	NA
12	Cherry S (9)	1987	1	PTCA	C	1
13	Jungbluth A (41)	1988	1/1000 pro.	PTCA	P	1
14	Parsonnet V (58)	1988	2/958 pro.	PTCA	ECABG 2	1
15	Abela GS (1)	1988	2/35 pts.	LASER	NA	0
16	Naunheim KS (56)	1989	3/2487 pts.	PTCA	ECABG 3	1
17	Vlietstra RE (75)	1989	1/480 pts.	DCA	NA	NA
18	Goto T (28)	1989	1/135 pts.	PTCA	NA	0
19	Sketch MH (68)	1990	3/147 pts.	TEC	ECABG 3	0
20	Iannone LA (39)	1990	1	PTCA	C	0
21	Hsn YS (37)	1990	1/750 pts.	PTCA	C	0
22	Lisanti P (47)	1990	1	PTCA	C	0
23	Margolis JR (49)	1990	<1%	ELCA	NA	NA
24	Teirstein RS (71)	1991	1/42 pts.	PTCRA	C	0
25	Bresnahan JF (8)	1991	1.1%/958 pts.	ELCA	NA	NA
26	Haase KK (32)	1991	12/1130 pts.	ELCA	ECABG 2, C 10	0
27	Sanborn TA (66)	1991	3/141 pts.	ELCA	ECABG 2, PTCA 1	0
28	Greene MA (29)	1991	1/1214 pts.	PTCA	ECABG 1	NA
29	Nassar H (54)	1991	1	PTCA	PTCA, P	0
30	van Suylen JR (73)	1991	1	PTCA, DCA	C	1
31	Parker JD (57)	1991	1	ELCA	PTCA	0
32	Holmes DR (35)	1992	32/2025 pts.	ELCA	ECABG 13, PTCA	2
33	Vetter J (74)	1992	14/1041 pts.	DCA	NA	0
34	Johnson D (40)	1992	5/463	DCA	NA	0
35	Pizzulli L (60)	1992	1/18 pts.	TEC	C	0
36	Bittl JA (5)	1992	23/764 pts.	ELCA	ECABG 8, P	0
37	Ghazzel ZMB (25)	1992	3/206 pts.	ELCA	ECABG 1, C 2	0
38	Saito S (65)	1992	1	PTCA	C	0
39	Kuntz RE (44)	1992	<0.5%/357 pts.	DCA	NA	NA
40	Eeckhaut E (18)	1993	1	PTCA	NA	NA
41	Rehders T Chr (61)	1993	1	PTCA	ECABG 1	0
42	Nilsson J (56)	1993	1	ELCA	ECABG 1	0
43	Topol EJ (72)	1993	0.2/500 pts.	PTCA	NA	NA
	Topol EJ (72)	1993	0.4/512 pts.	DCA	NA	NA
Total 43					ECABG 49	9

PTCA, Percutaneous transluminal coronary angioplasty; *TEC*, transluminal extraction endarterectomy catheter; *DCA*, directional coronary atherectomy; *ELCA*, excimer laser coronary angioplasty; *PTCRA*, percutaneous transluminal coronary rotational angioplasty; *ECABG*, emergency coronary artery bypass grafting; *pts*, patients; *pro*, procedures; *C*, conservative treatment; *NA*, not available in text of paper; *P*, pericardiocentesis or pericardial drainage.

ploy guidewires. These can penetrate the vessel wall. The perforation of an artery by a guidewire could happen when the wire is stiff-tipped or when the advancement is difficult (3, 71). Meanwhile, the guidewire technology has made great progress so that the guidewire tips are more flexible and steerable.

PTCA carries with it an inherent risk of significant complication (42). Rupture of the inner portion of the arterial wall and of atherosclerotic plaque appears to be an inevitable and also necessary event for successful PTCA (16). Regularly, subintimal and submedial dissection are found (17). Intravascular ultra-

Table 37.2.
General Data of Coronary Arterial Perforation in 17 Isolated Case Reports

Ref.	Gender	Age	Clinical Status	Involved Artery	Technique	Result	Perforation	Complication	Surgery	Other Treatment	Outcome
(3)	M	69	Angina	LAD 90%	PTCA	Good	LAD	Hemopericardium C. tamponade		Open pericardiocentesis	Good
(6)	F	51	Unstable angina	LAD 75%	PTCA	Not dilated	LAD	Hemopericardium C. tamponade	CABG	Pericardiocentesis	Good
(9)	F	82	Unstable angina	LAD 99%	PTCA	Good	LAD	LAD-RV fistula Myocardial infarction	Thoracotomy		Death
(27)	M	48	Unstable angina	LAD 80%	PTCA	Good	D	Hemopericardium C. tamponade	Ligation D		Good
(27)	M	62	Stable angina	LAD 80%	PTCA	Not dilated	D	Hemopericardium C. tamponade	CABG		Good
(27)	M	55	Unstable angina	LAD 95%	PTCA	Occlusion	D	Hypotension Hemopericardium C. tamponade	CABG		Good
(27)	F	50	Stable angina	LAD 95%	PTCA	Occlusion	D	Cardiac arrest	CABG		Death
(32)	M	56	Unstable angina	LAD 90%	ELCA	Occlusion	LAD	LAD-LV fistula			Good
(39)	F	74	Unstable angina	LAD 80%	PTCA	Good	LAD	Hemopericardium C. tamponade			Good
(41)	F	65	Unstable angina	RCA 90%	PTCA	Occlusion	RCA	Hemopericardium C. tamponade		Pericardiocentesis	Death
(43)	M	77	Unstable angina	RCA 100%	PTCA	Good	RCA	Hemopericardium C. tamponade Cardiac arrest		Pericardial drainage	Death
(50)	M	58	Unstable angina	RCA	PTCA	Good	RCA	Hemopericardium		PTCA	Good LAD
(50)	M	60	Unstable angina	LAD moderate D 100%	PTCA	Good	D	Hemopericardium		Protamine sulphate	Good D Reocclusion
(51)	M	60	Angina	LAD 99%	PTCA	Good	LAD	False aneurysm LAD-RV fistula	CABG LAD Ligation		Good
(56)	M	68	Unstable angina	RCA 95%	ELCA	Not dilated	RCA		CABG		Good
(61)	F	70	Stable angina	LAD 90%	PTCA	Good	LAD	Acute myocardial ischemia	CABG		Good
(73)	M	71	Unstable angina	RCA severe	PTCA DCA	Good	RCA	Hemopericardium C. tamponade Cardiac arrest			Good

C, Cardiac; D, diagonal branch; LAD, left anterior descending artery; RCA, right coronary artery; PTCA, percutaneous transluminal coronary angioplasty; ELCA, excimer laser coronary angioplasty; DCA, directional coronary atherectomy; LV, left ventricle; RV, right ventricle.

sound studies of coronary arteries before and after PTCA demonstrated that in concentric plaques superficial tears within the plaque occurred in 2%, deep tear in 17%, deep tear associated with subintimal or submedial dissection in 4%, and circular dissection in 31%; in eccentric plaques tearing of the plaque close to its base with dissection occurred in 29% (24). The overall rate of tearing ranges from 50 to 82% (24, 31, 76). Since the highest stress occurs at the calcified parts within a plaque, dissection frequently starts at this location (45). Risk factors include mismatch between balloon and vessel size, excessive balloon pressure, and calcified lesions. Under these situations the splitting may not be limited only to the plaque or inner part of the vessel, but may extend farther into the adventitia and result in extravasation of blood (5, 12, 62, 64). In some cases the vessel perforation occurred following rupture of a balloon (6, 64).

The second-generation angioplasty devices remove rather than displace atherosclerotic plaque for enlargement of an obstructed vessel lumen (49). The tissue ablation by the new devices is nondiscriminative. Perforation can happen with all of the mechanical or thermal techniques, since a cut can be made in any part of a vessel (2, 25). ELCA causes tissue ablation mainly through vaporization, although plaque compression and fissuring cannot be totally excluded because of a Dotter effect (25). Coronary perforation can be brought about by laser energy or mechanical effect of a catheter, for example, reflecting of the laser beam (66). DCA and TEC employ mechanical systems to enlarge narrowed lumen or to reopen an occlusion of a vessel (13, 20, 21, 44, 60, 68, 73). These approaches of angioplasty have high incidence of adventitia recovery (40, 73, 74). It was described that 23 to 30% of the specimen removed by DCA showed adventitial tissue (44, 73). Thus potential danger for perforation exists when cutting the adventitia of the vessel wall.

Besides the difference in devices, certain procedural variables are operator determined

such as the resistance of a catheter tip. Using high-frequency rotation technique (150,000 to 200,000 rpm), PTCRA works according to the principle of a microknife—hard tissue is ablated, whereas soft tissue is deflected by the diamond-coated burr. However, advancing of the burr has to be done gently; otherwise a Dotter effect could occur with dissection of the intima and media (13). Perforation could be caused particularly when the burr is pushed forward in hard segments of a vessel. The likelihood of perforation seems to be greater in occluded vessels than in partially stenosed ones because in the former case the instruments will be advanced blindly and the course of the guidewire or catheter cannot be predicted.

INCIDENCE

The reported rate of coronary artery perforation following angioplasty procedures varies greatly with different devices, as well as with different studies of the same device (Tables 37.3, 37.4, and 37.5). The conventional balloon angioplasty (PTCA) is still the most often performed procedure among all of the different techniques for nonsurgical coronary angioplasty, but its perforation rate is low. The large serial studies on PTCA documented 19 perforations out of more than 11,047 patients or procedures. The incidence of perforation in PTCA ranges from 0.1 to 2.7%. The four

Table 37.3.
Incidence of Coronary Arterial Perforation in PTCA

Reference	Method	Patient (n)	Perforation (n)	Incidence (%)
(11)	PTCA	3079	3	0.1
(56)	PTCA	2478	3	0.1
(29)	PTCA	1214	1	0.1
(41)	PTCA	1000	1	0.1
(37)	PTCA	750	1	0.1
(5)	PTCA	958	2	0.2
(62)	PTCA	518	1	0.2
(72)	PTCA	500	1	0.2
(59)	PTCA	265	1	0.4
(28)	PTCA	135	1	0.7
(27)	PTCA	150	4	2.7
Total		11047	19	

PTCA, Percutaneous transluminal coronary angioplasty.

Table 37.4.
Incidence of Coronary Arterial Perforation in ELCA

Reference	Method	Patient (n)	Perforation (n)	Incidence (%)
(49)	ELCA	255	NA	1
(32)	ELCA	1139	12	1.1
(8)	ELCA	958	NA	1.1
(25)	ELCA	206	3	1.5
(35)	ELCA	2025	32	1.6
(66)	ELCA	141	3	2.1
(5)	ELCA	764	23	3
Total		5565		

ELCA, Excimer laser coronary angioplasty.

Table 37.5.
Incidence of Coronary Arterial Perforation in DCA, TEC, and PTCRA

Reference	Method	Patient (n)	Perforation (n)	Incidence (%)
(75)	DCA	480	1	0.2
(72)	DCA	512	NA	0.4
(44)	DCA	357	NA	0.5
(40)	DCA	463	5	1.1
(74)	DCA	1041	14	1.3
(68)	TEC	147	3	2.1
(60)	TEC	18	1	5.6
(71)	PTCRA	32	1	2.4
Total		3066		

DCA, Directional coronary atherectomy; *TEC*, transluminal extraction endarterectomy catheter; *PTCRA*, percutaneous transluminal coronary rotational angioplasty.

largest reports had the same result of 0.1%, with the registry of patients from 1000 to 3079 (11, 29, 41, 56). ELCA is the second largest group in this review, showing a perforation rate of 1 to 1.1%. In two large studies with 1139 and 2025 patients the rate is 1.1 to 1.6%, respectively (32, 35). For DCA the rate is 0.2 to 1.3%. It is 2.7 to 5.6% in TEC and 2.4% in PTCRA. In comparing the different techniques, PTCA has the lowest perforation rate and ELCA the highest (almost ten times higher in ELCA than in PTCA), based on the reports with recorded patients of 500 or more.[a] For interpretation of the data, it has to be taken into account that many other studies recorded no perforation.

---

[a] References 5, 8, 11, 29, 32, 35, 37, 41, 56, 62, 72, 74.

CLINICAL FEATURES

It is of great importance to be able to recognize the clinical characteristics of acute arterial perforation. The patient's progress depends on rapid diagnosis and active treatment (27). The main clinical features are listed in Table 37.2 from isolated case reports.

Symptoms

Depending on the patient's history (i.e., angina, myocardial infarction), the location of the stenosis (large dominant vessel or side branch), the collateral supply (visible or recruitable collaterals), the balloon used (conventional balloon or perfusion), the techniques employed (PTCA, ELCA, hot-tip laser, DCA, TEC, or PTCRA), the symptoms after coronary perforation vary. Patients complained of chest pain of various severity, from dull to moderate or even severe chest pain (9, 32, 39, 50). However, in a few cases the patients felt no pain at all (51, 73). An injection of contrast medium just before further procedures (e.g., dilation of balloon, rotational cutting, or laser ablation) was considered important for avoiding enlargement of an already existing perforation.

Angiographic Charascteristics

Angiography is the most important and decisive method in the recognition of acute coronary perforation. The first angiographic sign is extravasation of contrast material outside the vessel wall (5, 35, 64). A perforation could be seen and located immediately after it took place (39, 50, 64). Then followed three different consequences (discussed mainly on case reports): (a) In most (58.8%) of the cases a free leakage of contrast medium into the pericardial space was detected by angiography (3, 27, 35). This event led frequently to cardiac tamponade (70%) (3, 27, 64) (Fig. 37.1). (b) In 18% patients' angiography demonstrated the formation of a fistula between the coronary artery and the ventricular cavity (right or left) (9, 39, 51). The cine angiograms revealed that contrast medium was

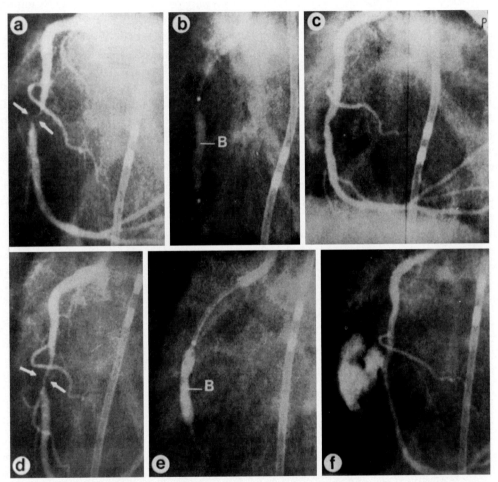

Figure 37.1. Right coronary arteriograms before (**a** and **d**), during (**b** and **e**), and after (**c** and **f**) percutaneous transluminal coronary transplasty (PTCA). **a.** A discrete severe narrowing is present *(arrows).* **b.** The stenosis was dilated by a 3-mm Gruentzig balloon *(GB)* catheter. **c.** Mild residual narrowing remained after the first PTCA procedure. **d.** The previously dilated area was again severely narrowed *(arrows)* 3 months after the first PTCA procedure. **e.** The narrowing was dilated by a 3.7-mm Gruentzig balloon *(GB)* catheter. **f.** Arteriography after PTCA showed leakage of contrast material into the epicardial tissues. The luminal diameter immediately proximal and distal to the narrowing is approximately equal to that of the pacing catheter (**d**). The diameter of the inflated balloon (**e**) is larger than that of the pacing catheter and thus exceeds the diameter of the nonstenotic arterial lumen. (From Saffitz et al. Am J Cardiol 1983;51:902–904 with permission.)

extravasated from the injured vessel into the ventricular cavity and was washed out by the ventricle rather rapidly (Fig. 37.2). (c). Subepicardial hematoma is the third development following perforation. In such cases the extravasation hematoma was limited around the broken artery and caused acute myocardial ischemia by compressing the vessel (61) (Figs. 37.3 and 37.4).

Jungbluth and colleagues reported a subacute cardiac tamponade 3.5 hours after PTCA (41). During PTCA the video recording did not show any contrast extravasation, but the coronary angiography film with high-level cine projection (CIPRO, Siemens, Erlangen) demonstrated a small fluid extravasation. The tamponade was a late development because at first it was a covered perforation that, after extension and epicardial rupture, led to pericardial effusion. Van Suylen and coworkers also described a late perforation occurring 2 days after PTCA and DCA (73). Coronary angiogram showed spiral medial dissection after PTCA and fusiform dilation after DCA.

Both of the patients with late tamponade died. Therefore, close monitoring is necessary under such situations.

Hemodynamic Effects

Coronary perforation was frequently followed by cardiac tamponade and myocardial ischemia, which could seriously influence the hemodynamics (3, 41, 64). In case reports, tamponade developed in 7 patients (41.2%), and the hemodynamics changed drastically (3, 9, 41, 61, 64). The heart rate increased, then dropped, and systolic arterial pressure fell, while the central venous pressure increased (27, 64, 73). Cardiac arrest occurred in five (29.4%) patients. Altman et al. reported an event of cardiac tamponade with a sudden hypotension of 40 mm Hg (3). The patient was treated successfully with intraaortic balloon pumping and open pericardiocentesis. Once the hemopericardium was removed and the bleeding stopped, the hemodynamic condition improved rapidly (9, 27). Rehders et al. described a case of subepicar-

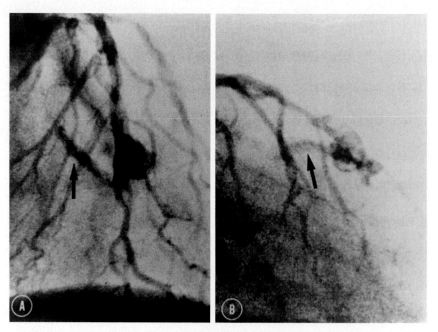

Figure 37.2. The false aneurysm and left anterior descending-right ventricle fistula *(arrows)* are seen in left **(A)** and right **(B)** anterior oblique views. (From Meng et al. J Thorac Cardiovasc Surg 1981;7:361 with permission.)

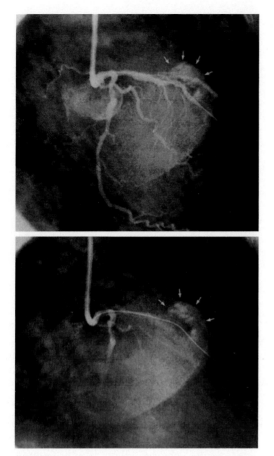

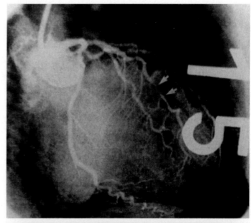

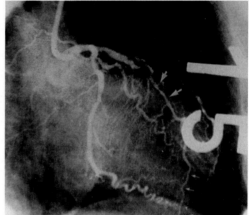

Figure 37.3. Showing the subepicardial deposit of contrast medium *(arrows)* during angiography in left anterior descending artery *(above);* after the runoff of the contrast medium the deposit can still be seen clearly *(below).* (From Rehders et al. Z Kardiol 1993;82:94–98 with permission.)

Figure 37.4. Angiograms of the left anterior descending artery (LAD) 15 minutes after the formation of the contrast deposit. The LAD was compressed in the middle third during diastole *(arrow),* and the distal LAD was seen after a delay *(above).* During systole the compression was less severe *(large arrow),* and the contrast flow was normal in the distal LAD *(small arrow).* (From Rehder et al. Z Kardiol 1993;82:94–98 with permission.)

dial hematoma (61). The patient's blood pressure dropped to 75/50 mm Hg because of acute myocardial ischemia produced by coronary compression. ECABG was performed and the patient recovered well. On the other hand, in a few benign cases (23.5%) the patients' hemodynamics remained stable when the perforation was small and not complicated by tamponade or myocardial ischemia (32, 39, 50, 51).

Echocardiographic Signs

Echocardiography, being of the most sensitive, is undoubtedly the method of choice for demonstrating pericardial fluid. It is generally believed that echocardiography can detect as little as 50 to 100 ml pericardial effusion reliably, or even 15 ml fluid (38, 70). In addition, the amount of fluid can be calculated. Also, follow-up can easily be carried out in coronary perforation. Echocardiography proved of great value in diagnosis and management of patients, especially in the presence of pericardial hemorrhage and cardiac tamponade (3, 9, 32, 37). Even localized pericardial effusion was demonstrated, representing perforation in a patient after PTCRA (22). Pericadiocentesis under echocardiographic guidance has been shown to give very promising results with a low complication rate.

Some studies observed that the right ventricular free wall and right atrial wall collapsed during diastole in tamponade. These abnormal appearances can be detected before major changes in systemic blood pressure and disappear after pericardiocentesis. Therefore, echocardiographic tamponade is a relatively early finding preceding overt clinical tamponade (38).

Electrocardiographic Signs

In acute coronary perforation electrocardiographic changes were mainly associated with myocardial ischemia (3, 9, 27, 61). Cardiac arrhythmia of any type might appear. Cherry et al. reported a case complicated with acute myocardial infarction and severe arrhythmia (9). The patient suffered severe chest pain when coronary perforation took place. The electrocardiogram showed marked anterior ST-segment elevation, which was followed by apical myocardial infarction, left bundle branch block, ventricular arrhythmia, and fatal cardiac arrest. In another patient with cardiac tamponade, initial bradycardia and subsequent artrial fibrillation were recorded (3). However, the patient did not show any signs of myocardial infarction in the electrocardiogram.

Laboratory Tests

Gonzalez-Santos et al. reported that two of four patients developed nontransmural myocardial infarction after coronary perforation. Laboratory examination showed high CK and CK-MB levels: a maximum of 1187 IU and 93 IU in one patient and 2880 IU and 180 IU in another, respectively (27).

Complications

Serious complications occurred frequently after coronary perforation. The most common ones are listed in Table 37.6 from 17 case reports. Hemopericardium was found in 10 (58.8%) patients and was the most frequent complication; of those, seven (70%) patients developed cardiac tamponade. In 17 cases the tamponade rate was 41.2%. Seven (41.2%) patients underwent emergency coronary artery bypass grafting. Cardiac arrest and cardiopulmonary resuscitation were recorded in five (29.4%) patients. Gonzaliez-Santos et al. reported four perforations, of which three had cardiac tamponade, and ECABG was performed on all four of the patients (27). Five (29.4%) patients died of whom four had tamponade. One patient died of acute myocardial infarction. Of the 151 perforations in all of the reviewed studies, nine patients died. The mortality is 6% (Table 37.1I). In four of the 17 (23.5%) cases, acute myocardial ischemia or infarction took place. Pericardiocentesis was necessary for four (23.5%) patients. Twelve of 17 patients (70.6%) suffered more than one complication. The results showed that life-threatening events took place frequently following coronary perforation.

Diagnosis

The diagnosis of acute coronary arterial perforation could be readily established

Table 37.6.

Complication of Coronary Arterial Perforation in 17 Case Reports

Complication	Case (n)	Percent (%)
Hemopericardium	10	58.8
Tamponade	7	41.2
ECABG	7	41.2
Cardiac arrest/resuscitation	5	29.4
Death	5	29.4
Acute myocardial ischemia/infarction	4	23.5
Pericardiocentesis	4	23.5
Artery-ventricular fistula	3	17.6

ECABG, Emergency coronary artery bypass grafting.

through angiography and echocardiography, together with a new chest pain, hemodynamic changes, and ECG abnormality (3, 9, 27, 35, 50, 51, 64). Usually a coronary perforation is not difficult to diagnose. However, sometimes perforation occurred not immediately after angioplasty, but a few hours or days later with a sudden manifestation (41, 51, 73). This delayed perforation carried a high risk (two deaths in three patients). It was recommended that patients with suspected deep dissection should be observed closely in the coronary intensive care unit and that emergency surgery be prepared (51). Repeat angiography was useful in diagnosis of delayed perforation. More important, however, is monitoring of the heart rate and blood pressure, as well as the right atrial and pulmonary pressures with cardiac output. An increase in right atrial pressure with constant or reduced pulmonary pressure requires echocardiography to rule out any development of pericardial effusion. It is important to know that hemorrhagic effusion may coagulate such that no echo-free space can be visualized.

Treatment

A rapid decision has to be made when coronary arterial perforation occurs, including consideration of reocclusion of the bleeding vessel, pericardiocentesis, and emergency surgery (3, 6, 27, 43, 64). In the case of perforation, rapid termination of angioplasty procedures with prompt reversal of heparinization was considered crucial in preventing cardiac tamponade (50, 71). Whether the treatment is nonsurgical or surgical depends on the clinical condition. Meier reported two patients with acute perforation who were treated conservatively and the perforation resolved spontaneously (50). However, he suggested that even in cases of no hemodynamic alteration such as these two, careful supervision and readiness for active treatment were demanded.

Balloons were used successfully in many cases for stopping the bleeding (5, 6, 9, 43, 50, 71). Erbel et al. developed the coronary perfusion catheter (CPC) to improve the ischemia tolerance of the heart (19). In their first paper they suggested the use of this catheter for treatment of coronary perforation. Subsequently, CPC was successfully used for treatment of such events.

Pericardiocentesis with subcostal or parasternal drainage was considered mandatory for treatment of pericardial hematoma or cardiac tamponade (3, 6, 27, 41, 43, 71). It was specially important when emergency surgery was not available (27).

When cardiac tamponade or myocardial ischemia or both occurred, emergency coronary artery bypass grafting was demanded to stop the bleeding, remove the pericardial hematoma, and graft a bypass to the related coronary artery (6, 27, 51, 58, 61, 62). Although the overall mortality of ECABG for failed angioplasty is high (2 to 13%), it is still worth performing if indicated by the perforation (20, 29). Since 1982 49 patients of coronary perforation underwent ECABG with four deaths.

PATHOANATOMIC FINDINGS

In 17 isolated case reports the left anterior descending artery (LAD) was involved in 12 (70.6%) patients, five of which had involvement in the diagonal branches. In five patients (29.%) the right coronary artery (RCA) was related (Table 37.2).

Saffitz et al. gave a detailed description of the pathoanatomic findings at necropsy of a perforation case (64). The epicardial adipose tissue around the RCA was hemorrhagic. There was an elliptical rupture of 0.6 cm in the long axis (Fig. 37.5). Histologic photographs showed complete rupture of the artery wall (Fig. 37.6). Other authors also reported subepicardial hemorrhagic infiltration surrounding the perforated vessel (27, 51, 61). This is a typical sign of coronary arterial perforation.

Jungbluth and colleagues provided the

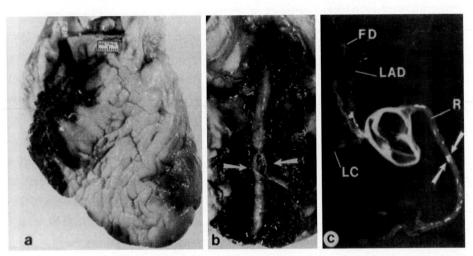

Figure 37.5. **a.** Photograph of heart showing hemorrhage in the right atrioventricular sulcus, which contains the right coronary artery. **b.** A rupture site *(arrows)* in the right coronary artery 3.5 cm from the aortic ostium. **c.** Radiograph of the major epicardial coronary arteries demonstrating focal calcific deposits. Arrows designate the site of rupture of the right *(R)* coronary artery. *FD,* First diagonal; *LAD,* left anterior descending; *LC,* left circumflex. (From Saffitz et al. Am J Cardiol 1983;51:902–904 with permission.)

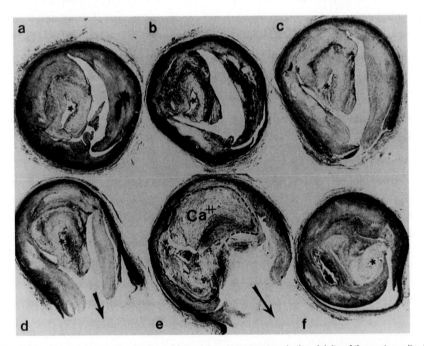

Figure 37.6. Photomicrographs of cross sections of the right coronary artery in the vicinity of the rupture site. Proximal to the rupture site **(a)** the atherosclerotic plaque is split. This split communicates with the original lumen, indicated by the asterisks. The split extends through the media **(b)** and adventitia **(c)** until through-and-through rupture *(arrows)* occurs **(d** and **e)**. Rupture occurred opposite a large calcified *(Ca++)* plaque *(outlined by dashed line)*. Distal to the rupture site **(f)**, additional splitting of the intimal plaque is seen communicating with the original lumen. (From Saffitz et al. Am J Cardiol 1983;51:902–904 with permission.)

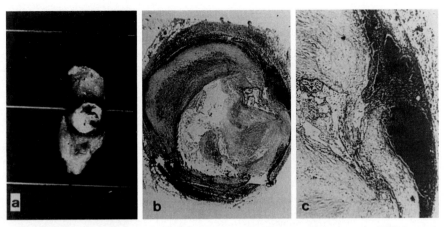

Figure 37.7.   The injured segment of right coronary artery after angioplasty. **a.** Macroscopy (× 3.75): hemorrhage in the adventitia. **b.** Histology (× 15): rupture of the intima and media, wide submedial dissection, and almost complete occlusion of the rest of the lumen by a thrombus. **c.** Part of **(b)** in the rupture site (× 50): submedial hematoma. (From Jungbluth et al. Z Kardiol 1988;77:125–129.)

autopsy report of a case with cardiac tamponade after coronary perforation (41). Pericardial hemorrhage was found. Histologic examination showed longitudinal splitting of the intima and media, as well as submedial dissection. However, disruption of the adventitia was not found (Fig. 37.7). Cardiac tamponade occurred transadventitially despite the incomplete disruption of the coronary artery. Therefore the underlying mechanism of PTCA with subintimal and submedial dissection can lead to coronary perforation, as the operator cannot predict or avoid it. New techniques, including imaging during intervention, may be useful for preventing this life-threatening event.

FOLLOW-UP

If the patient survives the acute event, the prognosis is good (27, 32, 39, 47, 50, 51). Three patients were free of symptoms during an 8 to 12-month follow-up (50, 51). Repeated angiography showed the closure of the fistula between the left anterior descending artery and the right ventricular cavity in one case at 6-month follow-up (47). Another four patients had normal exercise ECG during the 6- to 12-month follow-up.

CONCLUSION

Any type of interventional angioplasty has an intrinsic risk of acute coronary complications (11, 16, 23, 32, 74). Acute coronary arterial perforation can take place following different angioplasty procedures (5, 11, 16, 35, 51, 73). Though not common, perforation presents a great problem both to physicians and surgeons because (a) angioplasty using various techniques is performed routinely in numerous medical centers, and (b) perforation is rare but implies a high risk of death by cardiac tamponade or myocardial infarction. It is necessary for physicians to understand that nonsurgical angioplasty is not a no-risk procedure (29, 55). Caution is suggested when the following risk factors exist: a high-degree of stenosis, calcified lesion, or eccentric obstruction (Table 37.2) (64). The possibility for perforation may be reduced by avoiding a mismatch between balloon and artery or excising too deep into the adventitia (33, 64). Physicians are advised to be careful if the advance of a guidewire meets with difficulties. Repeat angiography cannot be overemphasized before proceeding with further procedures such as dilating the balloon or starting ablation with a burr or laser.

For a good prognosis, rapid diagnosis and active treatment are of utmost importance. Angiography and echocardiography are methods of choice in diagnosis and management of coronary perforation. Hemodynamics should be monitored closely. Treatment measures are control of the bleeding, evacuation of the pericardial hemorrhage, and bypass graft. Insertion of a conventional balloon or coronary perfusion balloon is satisfactory for stopping bleeding. Pericardiocentesis is essential for stabilization of hemodynamics. For some cases emergency coronary artery bypass grafting may be necessary besides the conservative treatment.

For coronary artery angioplasty, standby surgery is still necessary because of certain major complications.

REFERENCES

1. Abela GS. Laser recanalization: a basic and clinical perspective. Thorac Cardiovasc Surg 1988;36:137–141.

2. Ahn SS, Auth D, Marcus DR, Moore WS. Removal of focal atherectamous lesions by angioscopically guided high-speed rotary atherectomy. J Vasc Surg 1988;7:292.

3. Altman F, Yazdanfar S, Wertheimer J, Ghosh S, Kotler M. Cardiac tamponade following perforation of the left anterior descending coronary percutaneous transluminal coronary angioplasty: successful treatment by pericardial drainage. Am Heart J 1986;111:1196–1197.

4. Bertrand ME, Lablanehe JM, Leroy F et al. Percutaneous transluminal coronary rotary ablation with Rotablator (European experience). Am J Cardiol 1992;69:470–474.

5. Bittl JA, Sanborn TA, Tcheng JE, Siegel RM, Ellis SG, for the ELCA Registry. Clinical success, complications and restenosis rates with excimer laser coronary angioplasty. Am J Cardiol 1992;70:1533–1539.

6. Bonzel T, Kasper W, Meinertz T, Breymann T, Kameda T, Schlosser V, Just H. Koronarrupture mit Pericardtamponade waehrend PTCA: erfolgeriche Therapie. Z Kardiol 1985;74(Suppl 3):52 (abstract).

7. Bredlau CE, Raubin GS, Leimgruber PP, Douglas JS Jr, King SB III, Gruentzig AR. In-hospital morbidity and mortality in patients undergoing elective coronary angioplasty. Circulation 1985;72:1044–1052.

8. Bresnahan JF, Litvack F, Margolis J, Rothbaum D, Kenneth K, Unterecker W, Cummins F, and the ELCA investigator. Excimer laser coronary angioplasty: initial results of a multicenter investigation in 958 patients. J Am Coll Cardiol 1991;17:30A.

9. Cherry S, Vandormael M. Rupture of a coronary artery and hemorrhage into the ventricular cavity during coronary angioplasty. Am Heart J 1987;113:386–388.

10. Choy DSJ, Stertzer SH, Myler RK, Marco J, Fournial G.

Human coronary laser recanalization. Clin Cardiol 1984; 7:377–381.

11. Cowley MJ, Dorros G, Kelsey SF, van Raden M, Detre KM. Acute coronary events associated with percutaneous transluminal coronary angioplasty. Am J Cardiol 1984; 53:12c–16c.

12. Cowley MJ, Dorros SF, van Raden M, Detre KM. Emergency coronary bypass surgery after coronary angioplasty, the NHLBI PTCA registry experience. Am J Cardiol 1984; 53:22c–26c.

13. Dietz U, Erbel R, Haude M, Nixdorff U, Iversen S, Pannen P, Meyer J. Angiographische und histologische Befunde bei koconaren Hochfrequenz-Rotationsatherectomiein vitro. Z Kardiol 1989;78(Suppl):I-104.

14. Dietz U, Erbel R, Rupprecht HJ et al. High-frequency rotational angioplasty: an alternative technique for treating coronary stenosis and occlusion. Br Heart J 1993; 70:327–336.

15. Dorros G, Cowley MJ, Simpson J, Bentivoglio LG, Block PC, Bourassa M, Detre K et al. Percutaneous transluminal coronary angioplasty: report of complications from the National Heart, Lung and Blood Institute PTCA Registry. Circulation 1983;67:723–730.

16. Dueber Ch, Jungbluth A, Rumpelt HJ, Erbel R, Meyer J, Thoenes W. Morphology of the coronary arteries after combined thrombolysis and percutaneous transluminal coronary angioplasty for acute myocardial infarction. Am J Cardiol 1986;58:698–703.

17. Dueber Ch. Pathologist's findings after PTCA (the mechanism of angioplasty). In: Fleck E, Frantz E, eds. Complication in PTCA. New York: Springer-Verlag, 1990.

18. Eeckhout E, Beuret P, Lobrinus A, Genton CY, Goy JJ. Coronary artery rupture during transluminal coronary recanalization and angioplasty in a case of acute myocardial infarction and shock. Clin Cardiol 1993;16:355–356.

19. Erbel R, Class W, Busch U, v Seelen W, Brennecke R, Bloemer H, Meyer J. New balloon catheter for prolonged percutaneous transluminal coronary angioplasty and bypass flow in occluded vessels. Cathet Cardiovasc Diagn 1986;12:116–123.

20. Erbel R, O'Neill W, Auth D, Haude M, Nixdoff U, Rupprecht HJ, Dietz U et al. High-frequency rotablation of occluded coronary artery during heart catheterization. Cathet Cardiovasc Diagn 1989;17:56–58.

21. Erbel R, O'Neill W, Auth D, Haude M, Nixdoff U, Rupprecht HJ, Tschollar W et al. Hochfrequenz-Rotationsatherktomie bei koronarer Herzkrankheit. Dtsch Med Wochenschr 1989;114:487–495.

22. Erbel R, Huettemann M, Schreiner G, Darius N, Pop T, Meyer J. Ischaemietoleranz des Herzens Waerend perkutaner transluminaler Koronaangioplastie. Herz 1987; 12:302–311.

23. Erbel R, Haude M, Iversen S, Nixdoff U, Oelert H, Dietz U, Meyer J. High-frequency rotational angioplasty. In: Fleck E, Frantz E, eds. Complication in PTCA. New York: Springer-Verlag, 1990.

24. Gerber TC, Erbel R, Goerge G, Ge J, Rupprecht HJ, Meyer J. Classification of morphologic effects of percutaneous

transluminal coronary angioplasty assessed by intravascular ultrasound. Am J Cardiol 1992;70:1546–1554.

25. Ghazzal ZMB, Hearn JA, Litvack F, Goldenberg T, Kent KM, Eigler N, Douglas JS et al. Morphological predictors of acute complications after percutaneous excimer laser coronary angioplasty. Circulation 1992;86:820–827.

26. Golding LA, Loop FD, Hollman JL, Franco I, Borsh J, Stewart RW, Lutle BW. Early results of emergency surgery after coronary angioplasty. Circulation 1986;74 (Suppl 3):26–29.

27. Gonzalez-Santos JM, Vallejio JL, Pineda T, Zuazo JA. Emergency surgery after coronary disruption complicating PTCA. Report of four cases. Thorac Cardiovasc Surg 1985;33:244–247.

28. Goto T, Mitsudo K, Matsunaga K, Doi O, Nashihara Y, Awa J, Hase T. Percutaneous transluminal coronary angioplasty for treatment of acute myocardial infarction: comparison with percutaneous transluminal coronary recanalization. J Cardiol 1989;19:375–385.

29. Greene MA, Gray LA, Slater AD, Ganzel BL, Mavroudis C. Emergency aortocoronary bypass after failed angioplasty. Ann Thorac Surg 1991;51:194–199.

30. Gruentzig AR. Transluminal dilatation of coronary artery stenosis. Lancet 1978;1:263 (letter).

31. The GUIDE Trial investigators. Initial report of the "GUIDE" trial for intravascular ultrasound imaging in coronary interventions. J Am Coll Cardiol 1992;19:223A (abstract).

32. Haase KK, Baumbach A, Voelker W, Kuehlkamp V, Karsch KR. Gefaesswandperforation nach Excimer-Laser-Angioplastie. Z Kardiol 1991;80:230–233.

33. Hirohara T, Robertson GC, Simpson MR et al. Directional coronary atherectomy. J Invasive Cardiol 1990;2:217–226.

34. Holmes DR, Holubkov R, Vlietstra RE, Kelsey SF, Reeder GS, Dorros G, Williams DO, and the coinvestigators of the National Heart, Lung, and Blood Institute Percutaneous Transluminal Coronary Angioplasty Registry. Comparison of complications during percutaneous transluminal coronary angioplasty from 1977 to 1981 and from 1985 to 1986: the National Heart, Lung, and Blood Institute Percutaneous Transluminal Coronary Angioplasty Registry. J Am Coll Cardiol 1988;12:1149–1175.

35. Holmes DR, Bresnahan JF, Reeder GS, King SB III, Leon MB, Litvack F, for the ELCA Registry. Coronary perforation following excimer laser coronary angioplasty. J Am Coll Cardiol 1992;19:76A (abstract).

36. Horowitz MS, Clifford CS, Stinson EB, Harrison DC, Popp RL. Sensitivity and specificity of echocardiography diagnosis of pericardial effusion. Circulation 1974;50:239–247.

37. Hsu YS, Tamai H, Odawara K, Yamagata T, Ueda K, Tomita T, Koya M et al. Coronary arterial rupture during percutaneous transluminal coronary angioplasty: a case report. J Cardiol 1990;20:493–498.

38. Huter S, Hall R. Echocardiography. In: Julian DG, Camm AJ, Fox KM, Hall RJC, Poole-Witson PA, eds. Diseases of the heart. London: Bailliere-Tindall, 1989.

39. Iannone LA, Iannone DP. Iatrogenic left coronary artery fistula-to-left ventricule following PTCA: a previously unreported complication with nonsurgical management. Am Heart J 1990;120:1215–1217.

40. Johnson D, Hinohara T, Reberson G, Selmon M, Braden L, Simpson J. Acute complications of directional coronary atherectomy are related to the morphology of excised stenosis. J Am Coll Cardiol 1992;19:76A.

41. Jungbluth A, Dueber CH, Rumpelt HJ, Erbel R, Meyer J. Koronaarteriemorphologie nach percutaner transluminaler Koronarangioplastie (PTCA) mit Haemopericard. Z Kardiol 1988;77:125–129.

42. Kent KM, Bentivoglio LG, Block PC, Cowley MJ, Dorros G, Gosselin AF, Gruentzig A et al. Percutaneous transluminal coronary angioplasty: report from the NHLBI PTCA Registry. Am J Cardiol 1982;49:2011–2020.

43. Kimbiris D, Iskandrain AS, Goel I et al. Transluminal coronary angioplasty complicated by coronary artery perforation. Cathet Cardiovasc Diagn 1982;8:481–487.

44. Kuntz RE, Hinohara T, Safian RD, Selmon MR, Simpson JB, Baim DS. Restenosis after directional coronary atherectomy: effects of luminal diameter and deep wall excision. Circulation 1992;86:1394–1399.

45. Lee R, Loree H, Cheng G, Lieberman E, Jaramillo N, Shoen F. Computational structural analysis based on intravascular ultrasound imaging before in vitro angioplasty: prediction of plaque fracture locations. J Am Coll Cardiol 1993;21:777–782.

46. Leon MB, Hirohara T, Papma JJ et al. Strategies for coronary revascularization using different atherectomy devices: a NACI Registry report. J Am Coll Cardiol 1992; 19:92A.

47. Lisanti P, Colombo A, Pesso M. Rupture of anterior descending artery during coronary angioplasty: benign course and spontaneous repair. Description of a case. G Ital Cardiol 1990;23:236–238.

48. Litvack F, Grundfest W, Eigler N, Tsoi D, Goldenberg T, Laudenslager J, Forrester J. Percutaneous excimer laser coronary angioplasty. Lancet 1989;2:102–103 (letter).

49. Margolis JR, Litvack F, Krauthamer D, Trautwein R, Goldenberg T, Grundfest W. Coronary angioplasty with laser and high-frequency energy. Herz 1990;15:223–232.

50. Meier B. Benign coronary perforation during percutaneous transluminal coronary angioplasty. Br Heart J 1985; 54:33–35.

51. Meng RL, Harlen JL. Left anterior descending coronary artery-right ventricular fistula complicating percutaneous transluminal angioplasty. J Thorac Cardiovasc Surg 1985; 90:387–390.

52. Meyer J, Schmitz H, Erbel R, Kiesslich T, Boecker-Josephs B, Krebs W, Braun PL et al. Treatment of unstable angina pectoris with percutaneous transluminal coronary angioplasty. Cathet Cardiovasc Diagn 1981;7:361.

53. Meyer J, Erbel R, Pop T, Rupprecht HJ. Derzeitiger Stand der intrakoronaren Balloondilatation. Internist 1987; 28:736.

54. Nassar H, Hasin Y, Gotsman MS. Case report. Cardiac tamponade following coronary arterial rupture during coronary angioplasty. Cathet Cardiovasc Diagn 1991;23:177–179.

55. Nauheim KS, Fiore AC, Fagan DC, McBride LR, Barner HB, Pennington G, Willman VL et al. Emergency coronary artery bypass grafting for failed angioplasty: risk factors and outcome. Ann Thorac Surg 1989;47:816–823.

56. Nilsson J, Herzfeld I, Crip L, Aberg B, Reyden L. Immuno-histochemical analysis of a human coronary artery exposed to excimer laser angioplasty in vivo: evidence for release of fibroblast growth factor at the site of injury. Am Heart J 1993;125:908–912.

57. Parker JD, Ganz P, Selwyn AP, Bittl JA. Successful treatment of an excimer laser–associated coronary artery perforation with the Stack perfusion catheter. Cathet Cardiovasc Diagn 1991;22:118–123.

58. Parsonnet V, Fisch D, Gielkhinsky I, Hochberg M, Hussain M, Kranam R, Rothfeld L et al. Emergency operation after failed angioplasty. J Thorac Cardiovasc Surg 1988; 96:198–203.

59. Pelletier LC, Pardini A, Renkin J, David PR, Hebert Y, Bourassa MJ. Myocardial revascularization after failure of percutaneous transluminal coronary angioplasty. J Thorac Cardiovasc Surg 1985;90:265–271.

60. Pizzulli L, Koehler U, Manz M, Luederitz B. Transluminale koronary extraction Extraktionsatherektomie. Method, Akutergebniss, angiographischer und klinischer Verlauf. Z Kardiol 1992;81:133–139.

61. Rehders T, Nienaber CA. Subepikardiles Haematom (Haemorrhagia per rhexin) nach elektiver PTCA mit konsekutiver Kompressiob des distalen RIVA. Z Kardiol 1993; 82:94–98.

62. Reul GJ, Cooley DA, Hallman GL, Dunean JM, LIvesay JJ, Frazier OH, Ott DA et al. Coronary artery bypass for unsuccessful percutaneous transluminal coronary angioplasty. J Thorac Cardiovasc Surg 1984;88:685–694.

63. Ritchie JL, Hansen DD, Intlekofer MJ, Hall M, Auth CD. Rotational approaches to atherectomy and thrombectomy. Z Kardiol 1987;76:59.

64. Saffitz JE, Rose TE, Oaks JB, Roberts EC. Coronary arterial rupture during coronary angioplasty. Am J Cardiol 1983;51:902–904.

65. Saito S, Arai H, Kim K, Aoki N. Pseudoaneurysm of coronary artery following rupture of coronary artery during coronary angioplasty. Cathet Cardiovasc Diagn 1992; 26:304–307.

66. Sanborn TA, Bittl JA, Herschman RA. Percutaneous coronary excimer laser–assisted angioplasty: initial multicenter experience in 141 patients. J Am Coll Cardiol 1991; 17:169B–173B.

67. Simpson JB. Future interventional techniques. In: Califf RM, Mark DB, Wagner GS, eds. Acute coronary care in the thrombolytic era. Chicago: Year Book, 1988.

68. Sketch MH Jr, O'Nell WW, Tcheng JE, Walker C, Galichia JP, Sawchak S, Gress S et al. Early and late outcome following coronary transluminal extraction endarterectomy: a multicenter experience. Circulation 1990; 82(Suppl):III-310 (abstract).

69. Steffenino G, Meier B, Finci L, Velebit V, vo Segesser L, Faidutti B, Rutishauser W. Acute complications of elective coronary angioplasty: a review of 500 consecutive procedures. Br Heart J 1988;59:151–158.

70. Tajik AJ. Echocardiography in pericardial effusion. Am J Med 1977;63:29–40.

71. Teirstein PS, Warth DC, Haq N, Jenkins NS, MacCowan LC, Aubanel-Reidel P, Morris N et al. High-speed rotational coronary atherectomy for patients with diffuse coronary artery disease. J Am Coll Cardiol 1991;18:1694–1701.

72. Topol EJ, Leya F, Pinkerton CA, Whitlow PI, Hofling B, Simonton CA, Masden RR, for the CAVEAT study group: A comparison of directional atherectomy with coronary angioplasty in patients with coronary artery disease. N Engl J Med 1993;329:221–227.

73. van Suylen RJ, Serruys PW, Simpson JB, de Feyter PJ, Strauss BH, Zondervan PE. Delayed rupture of right coronary artery after directional atherectomy for bail-out. Am Heart J 1991;121:914–916.

74. Vetter J, Robertson G, Selmon M, Simpson J, Sheehan D, McAuley B, Branden L et al. Perforation with directional coronary atherectomy. J Am Coll Cardiol 1992;19:76A.

75. Vlietstra RE, Abbotsmith CW, Douglas JS, Hollman JL, Muller D, Safian R, Selmon MR. Complications with directional coronary atherectomy. Experience at eight centers. Circulation 1989;80(Suppl):II-582.

76. Yock PG, Fitzgerald PJ, Sudhir K. Intracoronary ultrasound scanning—clinical experience and new insights. In: Roelandt J, Gussenhoven EJ, Bom N, eds. Intravascular ultrasound. Dordrecht: Kluwer Academic, 1993.

ADJUNCTIVE THERAPIES

38. Current Antiplatelet and Antithrombotic Medications for Interventional Procedures

DAVID R. HOLMES JR. and DAVID P. FAXON

The role of anticoagulant and antithrombotic therapy during interventional cardiology procedures has been emphasized. Experimental clinical studies have shown that following vascular injury, platelets adhere and aggregate almost immediately and result in thrombosis, which, in the setting of a severe dissection or flow disturbance, can lead to abrupt closure and predispose to restenosis (1–3). The importance of this therapy has grown as the procedures have included increasing numbers of patients with acute ischemic syndromes and unstable coronary arterial lesions. In addition, the increasingly widespread use of intracoronary stents requires aggressive antiplatelet and anticoagulant therapy. New agents such as specific antithrombins (for example, Hirudin) and platelet receptor antibodies (for example, IIb/IIIa drugs) are being evaluated and will play central roles in the future once they are released. At the present time, however, three agents remain most widely used.

DEXTRAN

Dextran has been used since the inception of interventional procedures based on its mechanism of action as an antithrombotic agent. This mechanism is the result of coating and absorption on the platelet surface, which act to interfere with platelet adhesion. The pharmakinetics are such that pretreatment for at least 1 hour is necessary to have maximum antiplatelet effect (4). Experimental studies also suggest that the drug is of greater efficacy on vascular foreign bodies such as vascular grafts or stents. In one experimental angiographic study, no efficacy of dextran was demonstrated following balloon angioplasty alone (5). Given the lack of other effective antiplatelet drugs during the early years of dilation, enthusiasm for dextran was widespread. Its continued use, however, has been the subject not only of scientific study but considerable emotional debate.

The role of dextran during elective PTCA has been assessed. In a study of 152 patients undergoing elective PTCA, respectively, there was no difference in outcome in the dextran-treated patients compared with conventional agents (6). Dextran, however, was only started 30 minutes prior to the procedure so that maximal effects may not have been obtained. Another trial, also of a small number of patients, also documented no difference.

These trials led to a definite decrease in the use of dextran, particularly when some of the potential toxicity was better realized (vide infra) (7). Many interventionalists do not use dextran routinely, but reserve it for high-risk cases (for example, those with a high likelihood of dissection, the need of a bailout stent, or a large amount of clot burden) or institute dextran after a large dissection occurs. With the widespread use of stents, this trend toward a decline in the use of dextran has been reversed. All of the current stent protocols recommend dextran, although documentation of its necessity in this setting is lacking. Currently, during stenting, most protocols suggest beginning low–molecular weight dextran (40 cc) 1 to 2 hours prior to stent implantation and continuing for several hours after the procedure for a total dose of 500 to 1000 cc.

If dextran is to be administered, it must be kept in mind that untoward reactions can occur. These reactions are infrequent, are usually mild and easily treated, and include bronchospasm and urticaria. Anaphylactic reactions, however, have been reported (although are rare) and usually occur shortly after initiating therapy (7). Several strategies have been employed to prevent or ameliorate these in patients with known reactions, including pretreatment with steroids, 100 mg of Solu-Cortef or an equivalent dose, or administration of a small test dose of dextran. In some laboratories an antibody antagonist is used (PROMIT, Kabi Pharmacia, Clayton, NC). This binds to one of the two available binding sites on dextran reacting with IgG antibodies preventing the formation of large immune complexes. When given prior to dextran administration, drug reactions have been found to be ameliorated. Careful monitoring of the patient during dextran administration is still required to watch for any untoward effects. Dextran has also been associated with pulmonary hemorrhage, which can have a fatal outcome. More recently, dextran use has again decreased or stopped in an increasing number of institutions. Stents are now placed routinely without continued anticoagulation or dextran, provided that placement is optimal.

ASPIRIN

Aspirin plays a central role as a therapeutic agent in cardiovascular disease (8–12). This role is based on its inhibitory effect on platelets with irreversible inhibition of the cyclooxygenase enzymes responsible for synthesis of eicosanoids. This action irreversibly prevents generation of thromboxane A_2 and results in decreased platelet aggregation. Aspirin also acts to block synthesis of prostacyclin, which further inhibits platelet aggregation, although this latter effect occurs at higher aspirin doses. These actions are the basis for the widespread efficacy of this drug in a variety of cardiovascular disorders, including unstable angina, acute myocardial infarction, and stable coronary artery disease. The ability of aspirin to reduce platelet aggregation after angioplasty has been demonstrated experimentally, and it appears to be of greater effect than other antiplatelet agents such as Sulfinpyrazone (13,14). The addition of dipyridamole experimentally did not appear to enhance the effectiveness of aspirin.

The importance of aspirin in interventional cardiology procedures was emphasized in an early trial assessing the efficacy of aspirin and dipyridamole in prevention of restenosis. Schwartz et al. randomized 376 patients undergoing conventional PTCA either to aspirin or dipyridamole (330 mg, 75 mg) given three times daily beginning 24 hours prior to the procedure or to placebo (11). The oral dipyridamole was replaced with intravenous dipyridamole at 10 mg/hour beginning 8 hours prior to the procedure. Aspirin and dipyridamole were not associated with decreased restenosis rates (37.7% and 38.6%, drug versus placebo), but did have a dramatic effect on thromboembolic complication—13 (6.9%) of placebo patients had a periprocedural myocardial infarction compared to three of the patients (1.6%) in the group treated with aspirin and dipyridamole ($P = .01$). This effect has ·been substantiated in other prospective, as well as retrospective, trials that have documented that aspirin reduces the incidence of acute occlusion and development of procedural-related myocardial infarction. In some of these trials, aspirin was used alone; in others, it was combined with dipyridamole. Ticlopidine has also been used and shown to decrease acute complications.

At the present time all patients undergoing interventional cardiology procedures should be treated with aspirin unless it cannot be tolerated or given. Pretreatment 24 hours prior to the procedure is optimal. Because of lower absorbance, enteric-coated aspirin should be avoided if possible. Although not available in the United States, intravenous aspirin is a rapidly effective alternative to oral therapy and can be started just prior to the angioplasty procedure. Chewing an oral aspirin or use of effervescent-buffered aspirin (Alka-Seltzer) can increase absorption substantially. The exact dose and preparation are the source of debate, but should not exceed 325 mg q.d. For stent implantation, 325 mg q.d. of soluble aspirin are used in all current investigative protocols. If the patient to be treated arrives in the laboratory prior to receiving aspirin, four chewable baby aspirin are usually given to speed up absorption and effectiveness. Following the procedure, as is true with all patients with coronary artery disease, aspirin should be continued indefinitely.

Dipyridamole has often been used in combination with aspirin. This drug inhibits phosphodiesterase and also activates adenylate cyclase and increases adenosine, all of which may decrease platelet reactivity. The early use of the combination of aspirin and dipyridamole (75 mg t.i.d.) was tested and found to be effective in maintaining vein graft patency after coronary bypass graft surgery (8, 9). Subsequent reports, however, have documented that the aspirin alone is as effective as the combination of aspirin and dipyridamole. This combination remains widely used, however, when stents are placed. In this setting, the dipyridamole is started 24 to 48 hours prior to elective stenting at 75 mg t.i.d. and continued for 1 to 3 months. Whether the entire salutary effect of this regimen is related to the soluble aspirin alone has not been studied.

If aspirin cannot be used, ticlopidine is an alternative approach. This drug inhibits the first and second phase of ADP-induced platelet aggregation and is quite different than either aspirin or dipyridamole. The platelet inhibitory activity is both dose and time dependent. The onset of action after initiation of oral dosing is seen after 24 to 48 hours, with the maximum effect being attained in 3 to 5 days. Therefore patients who

are intolerant to aspirin need to be pretreated prior to interventional procedures. The usual dose is 250 mg b.i.d. Although most side effects are minor, significant hematologic abnormalities occasionally occur with neutropenia, thrombocytopenia, and even agranulocytosis. Blood counts are recommended accordingly every 2 weeks after initiation of therapy for surveillance.

HEPARIN

Heparin is the cornerstone of therapy during interventional cardiology procedures. It has a number of different effects on blood coagulation, as well as platelet action. In addition, it has multiple other properties. The major anticoagulant properties relate to its ability to catalyze the effect of antithrombin III on protein serases such as thrombin, factors XII, XI, IX, X, and tissue factor VIIa. Heparin is a heterogenous sulfonated glycosaminoglycan with variable chain lengths that result in molecular weights, ranging from 5,000 to 50,000 dalton (15). Its anticoagulant action is dependent on binding of antithrombin III, resulting in a confirmational change that allows antithrombin III to bind to certain proteinases. Not all fragments of heparin possess this anticoagulant activity.

Heparin administration is required for all interventional procedures. In the very rare patient who has a major reaction to heparin (for instance, thrombocytopenia), ancrod has been used. A number of different regimens have been described; in general, the doses of heparin have increased over the past several years. Typically, 10,000 to 15,000 units are administered intravenously. In some laboratories a 1500 U/kg dose is given as this achieves a therapeutic regimen more often than standard dosing does. However, regardless of which regimen is used, measurement of ACT is necessary given the variable effect of heparin. In some laboratories a constant infusion of 1000 U/hour are also started, while in others intermittent boluses are used often on a prespecified schedule. The effect of

Table 38.1.
Heparin Dosing

Clinical Setting	During Procedure	Target ACT	Postprocedure Heparin
Elective PTCA, excellent result	10,000–15,000	350	0–2 hr
Suboptimal result PTCA, dissection, residual thrombus	10,000–15,000	350	24–48 hr[a]
Primary angioplasty, acute infarction	10,000–15,000	350	48–72 hr[b]
Stent implanted	10,000–15,000	350	Until INR 2–3.0[c]

[a]Sheath removal after heparin stopped.

[b]Sheath removal after 24 hours, then resume heparin 6 hours later.

[c]Sheath removal same day, then resume heparin 6 hours later.

heparin is monitored in most laboratories by measurement of ACT. Two different machines are used—each has advantages and disadvantages depending on the specific measurement system used, for example, diatomaceous earth versus kaolin. In most laboratories the ACT is kept at >300 to 400 seconds. Several studies have analyzed the relationship between the ACT level and outcome of interventional procedures and have found a direct relationship emphasizing the importance of thrombus in acute closure syndromes. The optimal level of ACT is not clear, but appears to be >300 seconds. In addition to measurement of ACT alone, a variety of ACT indices have been generated, although they are not widely used. At the end of the procedure, a closing ACT should be measured and should be >300 to 350 seconds.

Following the termination of the procedure, heparin administration varies (Table 38.1). This variability is based on physician preference, specific device used, anticipated timing of sheath removal, patient factors, and angiographic features of the lesion treated. In elective conventional dilation procedures, some do not administer a heparin drip following the procedure, but instead let the ACT decrease to <150 to 160 seconds and then pull the vascular sheath. Others administer a drip a few hours and usually pull the sheath 4 hours after the procedure. In patients with a suboptimal result or residual thrombus, heparin may be continued for 24 to 48 hours at approximately 1000 U/hour to maintain the

ACT at 300 seconds or an APTT at 60 to 90 seconds. Low–molecular weight heparins are also alternatives to regular heparin. They possess three to four times greater anti-Xa activity than anti-IIa activity and have been shown to be effective in the prevention of deep vein thrombophlebitis (16). However, there has been no study as yet demonstrating superiority over regular heparin during angioplasty.

In the future there will be significant changes in the specific antithrombotic and antiplatelet medications used. Preliminary studies of both agents have demonstrated increased efficacy with reduced thrombotic complications; however, bleeding complications have increased. It is possible that specific antithrombins will take the place of heparin and IIb/IIIa receptor blockers may replace aspirin. Such specific therapy will hopefully make interventional procedures safer and better tolerated, although they will add the potential for increased bleeding.

REFERENCES

1. Wilentz JR, Sanborn TA, Haudenschild CC, Valeri CR, Ryan TJ, Faxon DP. Platelet accumulation experimental angioplasty: time course in relation to vascular injury. Circulation 1987;75:636–642.

2. Ip J, Fuster V, Israel D, Badimon L, Badimon J, Chesebro JH. The role of platelets, thrombin, and hyperplasia in restenosis after coronary angioplasty. J Am Coll Cardiol 1991:77B–88B.

3. Ring ME, Vicchione JJ, Fiore LD, Ruocco NA, Jacobs AK, Deykin D, Ryan TJ et al. Detection of intracoronary fibrin degradation after coronary balloon angioplasty. Am J Cardiol 1991;67:1330–1334.

4. Weiss HJ. The effect of clinical dextran on platelet aggregation, adhesion and ADP release in man: in vivo and in vitro studies. J Lab Clin Med 1967;69:37–46.

5. Block PC, Fallon JT, Elmer D. Experimental angioplasty: lessons from the laboratory. Am J Cardiol 1980; 135:907–918.

6. Swanson KT, Vlietstra RE, Holmes DR Jr, Smith HC, Reeder GS, Bresnahan JF, Bove AA. Efficacy of adjunctive dextran during percutaneous transluminal coronary angioplasty. Am J Cardiol 1984;54:447–448.

7. Brown RIG, Aldridge HE, Schwartz L et al. The use of dextran-40 during percutaneous transluminal coronary angioplasty: a report of three cases of anaphylactoid reactions—one near fatal. Cathet Cardiovasc Diagn 1985; 11:591–595.

8. Chesebro JH, Clements IP, Fuster V et al. A platelet-inhibitor drug trial in coronary artery bypass operations. Benefit of perioperative dipyridamole and aspirin therapy on early postoperative vein graft patency. N Engl J Med 1982;307:73–78.

9. Chesebro JH, Fuster V, Elveback LR et al. Effect of dipyridamole and aspirin on late vein graft patency after coronary bypass operation. N Engl J Med 1984; 310:209–214.

10. Patrano C. Aspirin as an antiplatelet drug. N Engl J Med 1994;330:1287–1295.

11. Schwartz L, Bourassa MG, Lesperance J et al. Aspirin and dipyridamole in the prevention of restenosis after percutaneous transluminal coronary angioplasty. N Engl J Med 1988;318:1714–1719.

12. Theroux P, Lidon RM. Anticoagulants and their use in acute ischemic syndromes. In: Topol EJ, ed. Philadelphia: *Textbook of interventional cardiology.* WB Saunders, 1994.

13. Faxon DP, Sanborn TA, Haudenschild CC, Ryan TJ. The effect of antiplatelet therapy on restenosis after experimental angioplasty. Am J Cardiol 1984;53:72C–76C.

14. Lam JVT, Chesebro JH, Steel PM, Heras M, Webster MW, Badimon L, Fuster V. Antithrombotic therapy for deep arterial injury by angioplasty. Circulation 1991;84:814–820.

15. Lane DA, Lindahl U, eds. Heparin: chemical and biological properties: clinical application. Boca Raton, FL: CRC Press, 1989.

16. Hirsh J, Levine M. Low molecular weight heparins. J Am Soc Hematol 1992;79:1–17.

39. Thrombolytic and New Antiplatelet Agents

JOSEPH F. PIETROLUNGO and ERIC J. TOPOL

Thrombolytic therapy for acute myocardial infarction (AMI) has been shown in numerous randomized trials (1–9) and a meta-analysis (10) to be unequivocally associated with an improved survival. The reduction in mortality from successful fibrinolytic administration varies because of the numerous variables, but overall is estimated to be about 30%.

This review will briefly describe the available plasminogen activators and discuss what has generally been learned about them from the large-scale trials in the treatment of AMI, offering practical suggestions for their use. In addition, the role of antithrombotic and antiplatelet agents both as adjuncts to fibrinolytic therapy and device-oriented coronary intervention is explored. Finally, a critical look at the shortcomings of our present practices and at strategies for improvement is presented.

PLASMINOGEN ACTIVATORS IN CLINICAL USE

Table 39.1 lists the plasminogen activators and some of their more salient properties. All have been studied in large trials and survival benefits demonstrated. Each could be used in the treatment of an AMI. Streptokinase, APSAC, and rt-PA are the three most commonly used agents. Urokinase is not commonly used in the United States for the treatment of AMI, although European studies have documented success with this agent (11). All have been shown to be more or less effective at saving lives in the conventional doses (7); however, debate exists over the use of adjunctive therapy, and newer dosing regimens have been trialed for rt-PA. These and other aspects of thrombolytic use are detailed throughout this review.

BENEFITS OF THROMBOLYTIC THERAPY

Mortality

Generally agreed on as the acid test for efficacy of a thrombolytic regimen (12), overall mortality reductions have been unequivocally proved with the use of all the conventional plasminogen activators to date (2, 4, 7, 13–16). The attractiveness of this endpoint is that it is easily measured and is purely objective in nature and that all other measurable variables (both positive and negative) contribute in some way to it. Currently, a large database exists consisting of 10 large randomized trials (each >1000 patients) evaluating plasminogen activator therapy in AMI. These trials represent a mix of the three commonly used fibrinolytic agents (streptokinase, APSAC, and rt-PA), varying use of aspirin and heparin and different protocols, but taken collectively, reliable recommendations on the use of thrombolytic may be made (10, 16).

Thirty-Five Day Mortality Reduction

Based on the data from the above studies, there is incontrovertible proof that when given within 12 hours of onset of symptoms, intravenous thrombolytic therapy reduces mortality following AMI. Although the search for the optimal fibrinolytic continues (see GUSTO section below), thrombolytic therapy has been shown to reliably reduce the odds of dying when given in the appropriate setting.

Table 39.1.
Comparative Features of Commonly Used Thrombolytic Agents

Agent	Streptokinase	Urokinase	APSAC	rt-PA
Fibrin specificity	No	No	No[b]	Yes
Plasma t½, β t½	18 min, 83 min	12–20 min	100 min	4 min, 4–5 min
Allergic sequelae	Yes	No[a]	Yes	No
Patency				
90 min	55%	60%	70%	75%
24 hr	85%	75%	85%	85%
Conventional intravenous dose	1.5 million U/60 min	Bolus 1.5 million U, then 1.5 million U over 90 min	30 U/2–3 min	Bolus 6–10 mg, 50–54 mg over 1st hr. Then 20 mg/hr next 2 hr, total 100 mg/3 hr
Cost[c]	$312.00	$360.00	$1700.00	$2200.00

[a]Not allogenic by strict definition but due to impurities in preparation, shaking, fever, chills etc. may be seen.

[b]Not at clinically used doses.

[c]Our institutional pharmacy cost.

Thus at present it matters less which of the agents are given, but more that one is indeed given and as soon as possible.

The data in Table 39.2 represents a meta-analysis of nine major trials of fibrinolytic therapy for AMI reported by the Fibrinolytic Therapy Trialists' (FTT) Collaborative Group (10). These data are inclusive of all major trials with more than 1000 patients with the exception of the recently completed GUSTO I study (discussed separately below). As clearly shown, for patients presenting within 24 hours of symptom onset and receiving thrombolytic therapy, there was a 9.6% incidence of death during days 0 to 35 as compared with 11.4% deaths among controls. This represents an 18% proportional reduction in 35-day mortality that is highly significant and corresponds to saving 18 lives per 1000 patients treated.

Closer inspection of the information obtained from large, pooled series allows for the evaluation of smaller specific subgroups that may derive particular benefit (and undue risk) from the administration of thrombolytic drugs. As seen in Table 39.2, it is clear that patients with ST-segment elevation on presentation achieve a significant reduction in mortality ($P < .00001$), the magnitude of which is dependent on the area involved (anterior versus inferior, or both). Patients with bundle branch block also received benefit from therapy ($P < .01$). Information on patients with normal ECGs and with suspected infarction is less definitive because of the smaller number of patients in these groups. This group is generally believed to be at low risk and thus not likely to achieve significant benefit from thrombolytic therapy in further analysis, even if larger numbers become available. Present consensus denotes that patients with ST-segment depression appear to be at increased risk from thrombolytic therapy (17), particularly with a higher rate of subsequent myocardial infarction. Therefore in patients presenting with ST-segment depression but without signs of posterior wall myocardial infarction, thrombolytic therapy does not seem to be indicated.

Time to Therapy

In general, maximum benefit from fibrinolytic therapy is obtained with the earliest administration. Rationale for early thrombolysis is predicated on animal work of Reimer and Jennings (18, 19). These investigators in the canine model of coronary thrombosis showed that the degree of myocardial necrosis was proportionally reduced with a shorter time to reperfusion; that is, when flow was restored within 20 minutes, little or no myocardial necrosis resulted (Fig. 39.1). While the com-

Table 39.2.
Mortality Differences During Day 0–35 Subdivided by Presentation Features

Presentation Features[a]	Total Patients (Fibrinolytic & Control)	Deaths During Days 0–35		Proportional Reduction in Odds	Absolute Benefits Per 1000
		Fibrinolytic	Control		
Entry ECG					
BBB	2032	18.7%	23.6%	25% SD 9	49 SD 18**
ST elev, anterior	13230	13.2%	16.9%	25% SD 4	37 SD 6*****
ST elev, inferior	13041	7.5%	8.4%	11% SD 6	8
Other ST elev/ n/k	6050	10.7%	13.4%	23% SD 7	
ST depression	3563	15%	13.8%	−13% SD 10	
Other abnormality	7936	5.2%	5.8%	9% SD 9	
Normal ECG	2029	3.1%	2.5%	−26% SD 30	
Hours from onset					
0–3	19291	8.6%	11.1%	24% SD 4	25 SD 4*****
4–6	17071	9.5%	11.5%	19% SD 5	20 SD 5****
7–12	12702	11.0%	12.6%	15% SD 6	17 SD 6***5
13–14	9537	10.1%	10.6%	5% SD 7	SD 6
Age (years)					
<55	13638	3.7%	4.7%	23% SD 8	10 SD 3***
55–65	16100	7.4%	9.3%	22% SD 5	20 SD 4****
65–74	13155	14.3%	16.5%	16% SD 4	17 SD 6***
75[a]	4988	24.2%	26.1%	8% SD 6	5 SD 6
Sex					
Male	36768	8.5%	10.2%	19% SD 3	18 SD 3*****
Female	11113	14.9%	16.8%	13% SD 5	19 SD 7**
Systolic BP (mm Hg)					
<100	2095	30.0%	35.1%	21% SD 8	51 SD 20*
100–174	42595	9.1%	10.9%	18% SD 3	18 SD
175[a]	3191	7.0%	7.9%	13% SD 13	3*****
					10 SD 9
Heart Rate					
<80	20101	7.4%	8.7%	16% SD 5	13 SD 4****
80-99	9018	9.8%	11.5%	17% SD 6	17 SD 6**
100[a]	4759	17.5%	21.1%	21% SD 7	36 SD 11
Prior MI[b]					
Yes	8721	13.3%	624 (14.5%)	9% SD 6	11 SD 7
No	36959	9.2%	2080 (11.2%)	20% SD 3	21 SD 3*****
Diabetes					
Yes	3436	14.3%	309 (17.9%)	23% SD 8	36 SD 13**
No	29184	9.0%	1514 (10.4%)	14% SD 4	14 SD 3****
ALL PATIENTS	362303	9.6%	3349 (11.4%)	18% SD 2	18 SD 3*****

*, **, ***, ****, ***** correspond to P <.05, <.01, <.005, <.001, <.00001.

[a]ASSET and LATE are excluded from all subdivisions except hours from onset; GISSI-1 from heart rate and diabetes; AIMS from diabetes; and USIM from heart rate and diabetes.

[b]Patients with prior MI excluding GISSI-1 (which generated the hypothesis of less benefit in this subgroup): 425 (12.2%) deaths among 3478 fibrinolytic-allocated patients vs. 466 (13.7%) among 3413 controls; 12% SD 7 proportional reduction; 14 SD 8 lives saved per 1000 (P = .07).

(Adapted from Fibrinolytic Therapy Trialists' (FTT) Collaborative Group. Lancet 1994;343:311–322.)

plexities of the human clinical setting cannot be directly compared with animal models, there is ample clinical evidence to support this concept. A review of 18 early thrombolytic studies by Spann and Sherry (20, 21) showed that global and regional infarct ejection fractions were improved when streptokinase was given within 3 to 4 hours after the onset of symptoms. More recently, there have been several large, controlled trials that have supported this concept (2, 5). First noted in GISSI-1 (2), patients randomized to the active treatment arm (streptokinase 1.5 million units over 60 minutes) within 1 hour of symptom onset had a striking 49% reduction in mortality versus 23% for those randomized within 3 hours. As noted in Figure 39.2, the composite results of both GISSI and ISIS-2 show a substantial time-dependence, most pronounced within the first hour of symptom onset. A reduction in the odds of dying by almost 50% was realized when treatment was started within 1 hour. In the recently completed GUSTO I trial (16) comparing all streptokinase arms to accelerated rt-PA, mortality at 0 to 2 hours from onset of pain was 5.4% and 4.3%, respectively, compared with 9.3% and 8.9%, respectively, for patients presenting 4 to 6 hours into pain. A recent large meta-analysis of large fibrinolytic trials

(10) found that diminution of benefit with delay of therapy was present but perhaps more gradual with a risk reduction of 29% at hours 0 to 1, and 23% at 2 to 3 hours.

Building on the above concepts, several studies (22, 23) have been performed to evaluate the efficacy and feasibility of prehospital thrombolytic therapy in an effort to capture the benefits of very early thrombolysis. Positive results from well-designed and implemented pilot studies (24) gave way to larger randomized trials both in the United States and Europe.

In the Myocardial Infarction Triage and Intervention trial (MITI) (25), patients were treated with rt-PA either in the field or in hospital. Patients randomized to field-initiated therapy were given a 20-mg bolus of rt-PA by the paramedics followed in-hospital by an additional 60 mg of drug (10 mg as a second bolus) over the next 1 hour and then the remaining 20 mg over the second hour. Patients randomized to in-hospital treatment received rt-PA in conventional doses (100 mg). The important findings are depicted in Table 39.3. The effects of treatment assignment were not significantly different, but both groups received thrombolysis in an expedient manner. The mean difference to drug administration from onset of symptoms was 35 minutes in favor of the field-initiated group. However, the average time to treatment for both groups taken together was a short 90 minutes.

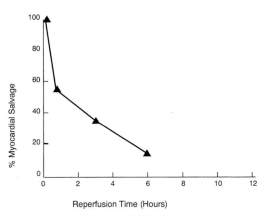

Figure 39.1. Graph shows myocardial salvage (calculated with respect to extent of infarction after 24 hours) as a function of the interval preceding reperfusion in canine model. (Adapted with permission from Reimer KA, Lowe JE, Rasmeussen MM, Jennings RB. Circulation 1977; 56:786–794.)

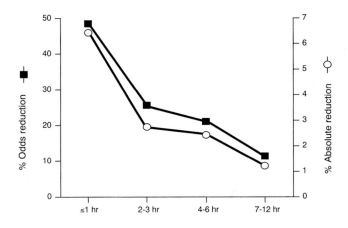

Figure 39.2. Reduction in absolute and relative mortality as a function of time to treatment from symptom onset. Composite results from GISSI-1 and ISIS-2 studies. (Adapted with permission from Anderson JL, Gomez MA, Karagounis LA. Am J Cardiol (Continuing Education Series) 1993;5–12.)

Table 39.3.
Summary of the Key Features of the MITI and EMIP Studies

MITI Study

Comparison	t-PA in-field vs in-hospital
N	360
End points	30-day EF, infarct size (TI-SPECT)
Time to therapy from symptom's onset	
Prehospital group	92 ± 58 min (median 77 min)
In-hospital group	120 ± 49 min (median 110 min)
Difference	33 ± 18 min
Results	1. No significant difference in EF by strategy. No ↓ in composite clinical endpoints
	2. By time to therapy (40 vs 71–180 min)
	↓ Infarct size: 4.9% vs 11.2% of LV, $P < .0001$
	↑ EF: 53% vs 49%, $P < .03$
	↓ Mortality: 1% vs 10%, $P < .03$
	↓ in composite clinical endpoints

EMIP Study

Comparisons	APSAC infield vs inhospital
N	5,454
End points	30-day mortality
Time to therapy from symptoms	
Infield group	Approximately 2 h
Inhospital group	Approximately 3 h
Difference	56 min (median)
Results	1) 17% decrease in 30-day cardiac dath, $P = 0.04$
	2) 13% decrease in 30-day total mortality, $P = 0.1$

MITI, Myocardial Infarction Triage and Intervention; *t-PA*, tissue-type plasminogen activator; *LV*, left ventricle; *EMIP*, European Myocardial Infarction Project; *APSAC*, anisoylated plasminogen-streptokinase activator complex. (Data adapted from MITI and EMIP.)

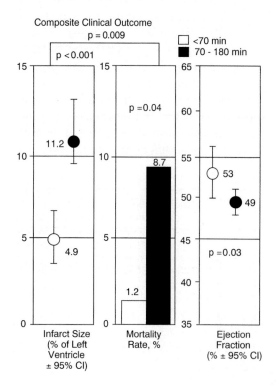

It was rather striking in this study that regardless of where the thrombolytic agent was given (hospital or prehospital), when done so within 70 minutes (versus 71 to 180 minutes) of symptom onset, ejection fraction was improved significantly (53% versus 49%, $P < .03$), infarct size by thallium imaging was attenuated (4.9% versus 11.2% of LV, $P < .001$), and mortality was dramatically lessened (1% versus 10%, $P < .03$) (Fig. 39.3).

The European Myocardial Infarction Project (EMIP) (26) randomized 5454 patients to prehospital versus hospital thrombolytic therapy with APSAC. The results are also shown in Table 39.3. Designed as a mortality trial, it was somewhat underpowered as

Figure 39.3. Composite clinical outcome of patients in the MITI trial. (Adapted with permission from Weaver WD, Cerquerio M, Hallstrom AP, Litwin PE, Martin JS, Kudenchuck PJ, Eisenberg M. JAMA 1993;270:1211–1216.)

Table 39.4.
Left Ventricular Function Following Intravenous Thrombolytic Therapy

Study (Ref.)	Patients[a]	Lytic/Time to RX	Time	Method	TX Group %	Control %	P Value
SK Trials							
ISAM (3)	1,741 (848)	SK	3–4 wks	Contrast	All 56.8	All 53.9	<.005
		<3 hr			57	53.6	<.05
		3–6 hr			56.6	54.4	NS
White (36)	219 (155)	SK/<4 hr	3 wks	Contrast	59	53	<.005
Western (145) Washington	368 (170)	SK/mean 3.5 hr	6–8 wks	RNA	50.8	46.6	<.02
rt-PA Trials							
Nat'l Heart Australia	144 (103)	rt-PA/<3 hr	1 wk	Contrast	57.7	51.1	.04
Guerci (146)	85 (85)	rt-PA/<4 hr	10 d	RNA	53.2	46.4	<.02
O'Rourke (147)	145 (126)	rt-PA/<2.5 hr	3 wk	Contrast	61	54	<.006
ECSG-4 (148)	721 (577)	rt-PA/<6 hr	10–22 d	Contrast	50.7	48.5	<.05
TPAT (149)	115 (115)	rt-PA/<6 hr	9 d	RNA	53.6	47.8	.017
rt-PA vs SK							
TIMI-1 (129)	290 (145)	SK/<7 hr rt-PA/<7 hr	Predischarge	Contrast	49.1 49.9	None	NS
PAIMS (150)	116 (116)	SK/<3 hr rt-PA/<3 hr	Hospital discharge	Echo	51 56	None	.05
White (151)	270 (240)	SK/<3 hr rt-PA/<3 hr	3 wk	Contrast	58 58	None	NS
rt-PA vs UK							
GAUS (152)	157 (101)	UK/<6 hr rt-PA/<6 hr	10–28 d	Contrast	52 53	None	NS
rt-PA vs APSAC							
Bassand (153)	169	APSAC/<5 hr rt-PA/<5 hr	3–7 d	Contrast	50 52	None	NS
TEAM-3 (144)	325 (277)	APSAC/<4 hr rt-PA/<4 hr	7 d (pre-discharge)	RNA	51.3 54.1	None	
	325 (215)	APSAC rt-PA	1 mo (38 d)		50.2 54.8		

[a]Total number of patients randomized is listed. Number in parentheses represents the number undergoing evaluation of LVEF when available.

(Adapted from Cairns JA, Fuster V, Kennedy JW. Chest 1992;102(Suppl):482S with permission.)

enrollment was incomplete primarily because of funding problems. Nonetheless, the numbers were sufficient to show a 17% reduction ($P = .04$) in cardiac mortality at 30 days in patients given APSAC in the prehospital setting. In this trial, patients were treated later than in MITI (3 hours for the in-hospital group, 2 hours for the prehospital group), but field-initiated therapy resulted in saving an additional hour. These data and those of smaller studies illustrate the importance of early thrombolytic administration for maximal chance at infarct artery reperfusion and subsequent myocardial salvage. This so-called time-dependent open-artery concept (27) is predicated on establishing early reperfusion (≤6 hours) and presupposes that benefit is proportional to the rapidity of recanalization and caused by improved myocardial salvage. Left ventricular function is modestly improved (28) (Table 39.4).

Support for the use of thrombolytic therapy given late (6 to 24 hours) has also been accruing. This time-dependent component of restoring infarct artery patency produces survival benefit as well. The two large-scale placebo-controlled trials specifically designed to look at this were LATE (9) and EMERAS (8). The Late Assessment of Thrombolytic Efficacy (LATE) trial randomized a total of 5709 patients with greater than 6 hours of chest pain and either ST-segment elevation (55%) or

Table 39.5.
LATE Trial

Time to Treatment (hr)	Alteplase	Placebo	P Value	% Reduction
6–12	8.7%	11.9%	.033	27.0
12–24	8.7%	9.2%	.542	5.0
6–24	8.8%	10.3%	.079	14.6

Clinical Events In-Hospital		
Event	Alteplase (%)	Placebo (%)
Reinfarction	2.9	3.7
VF	2.0	2.6
Other ventricular arrhythmia	4.9	4.7
Pacemaker	1.3	1.8
Shock	2.7	3.7[a]
HF requiring treatment	30.2	32.9[a]
Angina treatment	45.3	50.7[a]

[a]Statistically significant difference at $P = .05$.

(Data adapted from the LATE Steering Committee. The Lancet 1993; 342:759–66.)

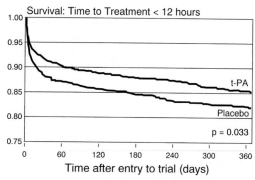

Figure 39.4. Mortality by time to randomization from onset of symptoms. (Adapted with permission from the LATE investigators' presentation at the XIV congress of the European Society of Cardiology. Barcelona, Spain, August 1992.)

other abnormal ECG findings (45%) to alteplase (n = 2836) or placebo (n = 2873). Both groups were balanced with respect to baseline and clinical characteristics. In accordance with the trial design, approximately one-third of patients fell into each of three 6-hour time windows: 6 to 12 hours, 12 to 18 hours, and 18 to 24 hours. Approximately 70% of patients received IV heparin following the infusion of rt-PA. The major results are depicted in Table 39.5. Overall, treatment with rt-PA within 6 to 12 hours of symptom onset resulted in a 25.6% reduction in mortality at 35 days (95% CI 8 to 46%, $P = .023$). As shown in Figure 39.4, overall survival curves seem to favor treatment within 12 hours and extend out to 1 year. Interestingly, however, patients treated in this trial after 12 hours but within 3 hours of hospital admission (presumably because they immediately satisfied entrance criteria) experienced a 22% reduction in mortality. These findings are commensurate with those of ISIS-2 (5), which found a 19% reduction in mortality in the comparable patient group. Thus it can be concluded from this study that treatment with rt-PA within 12 hours of symptom onset in patients with no contraindications is always

beneficial and that patients presenting after 12 hours with clear indications for thrombolytic therapy may benefit substantially.

Data from the South American Estudio Miocardio Estreptoquinasa Republic Americas Sul (EMERAS) study (8, 29), utilizing streptokinase in conventional doses, showed that for patients presenting between 7 and 12 hours the trend toward a lower, 5-week vascular mortality was seen in the thrombolytic versus placebo group (12.6% versus 14.6%, respectively, $P = \text{NS}$).

Numerous hypotheses for the benefit of late thrombolysis have been proposed. Substantial myocardial salvage is not responsible for improved survival since ejection fraction, when measured, is not improved. Acting as a source of collateral blood flow, a patent infarct-related artery may be an important reservoir of additional vascularity in patients with severe multivessel disease. Patency of this vessel may decrease ischemia in the secondary infarct zone and provide a conduit for subsequent coronary revascularization (30). Facilitated access of inflammatory cells to the infarct area may result in less fibrosis and increased scar thickness (33). Left ventricular remodeling following Q-wave myocardial infarction (usually large) may produce successive cavity enlargement and alteration in contractile function (31, 32). Reperfusion of the infarct segment may alter this process in one or more ways. Clinical studies have demonstrated that patients allocated to late (>4 hours from symptom onset) thrombolytic therapy for AMI have lower end-systolic and end-diastolic volumes, and improved regional left ventricular function (34–38) compared with those receiving no thrombolytic treatment.

A reduction in lethal arrhythmias following AMI may play a role in improved survival. Several studies have shown that the propensities for spontaneous and laboratory induction of these events, as well as a decrease in the number of late potentials recorded on signal-average ECG, are reduced after successful thrombolytic administration (39–42). Furthermore, shock-free survival in patients with ICDs appears to be prolonged when the infarct-related artery is patent (43). The mechanism(s) of this benefit is largely unknown. However, improved homogeneity of myocardial substrate (44), reduced left ventricular aneurysm formation, and improved hemodynamics may all play a role (45).

Left Ventricular Function

The impact of thrombolytic therapy on left ventricular function has been evaluated in numerous studies with each of the currently available agents. Table 39.4 details the major trials and the salient findings of each with respect to left ventricular function. As noted, studies on this issue have been extensive, and the currently available data indicate that modest improvement in LVEF can probably be expected after the administration of thrombolytic agents for AMI when these drugs are given within 3 (and perhaps 4) hours of symptom onset (3, 28, 46). No agent given in conventional doses appeared to be superior in improving posttreatment ejection fraction. However, the use of front-loaded rt-PA regimens have yielded more significant gains in

postthrombolytic left ventricular function. In the recently completed GUSTO-1 study (16) patients randomized to the accelerated rt-PA arm had improved TIMI-3 patency, a 66% increase compared with streptokinase (54% versus 30% for accelerated rt-PA versus streptokinase, respectively), and improved left ventricular function even 90 minutes after therapy. By hospital discharge, there was improvement in regional wall motion, ejection fraction, and end-cavity size in patients receiving accelerated rt-PA compared with the other strategies (47).

PRIMARY AND SECONDARY THROMBOSIS: THE ROLE OF ANTITHROMBOTIC AND ANTIPLATELET THERAPIES

The benefits of thrombolytic therapy are clearly defined. However, the overall effectiveness of these drugs remains limited by persistent thrombotic occlusion (48–50) and rethrombosis (49, 51) of the infarct-related artery after timely thrombolysis. These adverse sequelae are important limitations to fibrinolytic efficacy.

Pathogenesis

Reocclusion of the infarct vessel is caused by the complex topography and composition of the atherosclerotic plaque interacting with blood components. Intraarterial thrombosis (and rethrombosis) is a function of vessel wall injury and incomplete thrombolysis. The injury, however, is not uniform with deep injury caused by plaque rupture (52, 53) and superficial vessel wall injury consisting primarily of focal endothelial denudation with loss of endothelium-derived antithrombotic factors (prostacyclin and endothelium-derived relaxing factor). Deep injury generates more thrombin than does superficial injury (54, 55) and is much more likely to result in occlusive coronary arterial thrombosis (56–58).

Clinical Consequences

An exact determination of the incidence of postreperfusion thrombosis and reocclusion is difficult because of methodologic differences in the many studies that have assessed this problem. In general, the highest incidence of reocclusion is seen with drugs that have the shortest half-life and the most fibrin specificity. Thus rt-PA is associated with a higher reocclusion rate than streptokinase, APSAC, or urokinase. In one large, pooled series (28) the angiographic reocclusion rate for rt-PA (given with IV heparin) was 13.5% compared with 8% for streptokinase, urokinase, or APSAC ($P = .002$). This difference may be caused by the extensive systemic fibrin degradation seen with the non–fibrin-specific agents (59).

When it occurs, reocclusion tends to be symptomatic in the majority of patents (60, 61) and is associated with a worsened clinical outcome. Ohman and colleagues (61) reported that reinfarction accounted for 22% of in-hospital deaths. Compared with patients with patent, infarct-related arteries, those with reocclusion (9.2% in this study) had a higher in-hospital mortality (12.8% versus 4.0%) and complication (pulmonary edema, sustained hypotension, respiratory failure, etc.) rate (61). Transient reocclusion, manifested by recurrent ischemic symptoms, has also been linked to worsened outcome following thrombolytic therapy. Califf et al. (62), in an analysis of over 1000 patients in the TAMI trials, found that recurrent ischemia occurred in 18.3% of patients and was associated with a higher mortality and heart failure rate, as well as increased hospital costs, than for patients remaining asymptomatic. To date, there has been little progress in identifying those patients at risk of reinfarction.

Prevention and Treatment

Based on the above discussion, it is clear that attention to ongoing thrombosis and platelet activation is of paramount importance in the setting of thrombolytic therapy. However, neither heparin nor conventional antiplatelet agents in currently utilized doses are completely effective in preventing this occur-

rence (54). There is a large, ongoing investigation into the development of newer and more potent antithrombotic and antiplatelet agents, although at present heparin and aspirin still remain the currently accepted standards (63).

Antithrombotic Therapy

The rationale for the use of anticoagulants along with thrombolytic agents is derived from the belief that the maintenance of coronary artery patency in the infarct-related vessel is the major mechanism by which benefit is obtained and that these agents contribute to that end. The nature of reperfusion is such that dissolution and recurrent thrombosis are cyclic phenomena that often precede sustained arterial patency (64), and antithrombotic agents are thought to contribute, at least in part, to lasting vessel patency. Heparin has been used since 1916 and, although imperfect, currently remains the recommended antithrombotic agent (63). Heparin is a mucopolysaccharide that binds to circulating antithrombin III, requiring this important cofactor for its action but nonetheless providing stronger antithrombin activity. However, the specifics regarding routine use, optimal dose, and timing still have not received uniform consensus.

Various clinical studies as noted in Table 39.6 have been designed to investigate some of these issues. Taken individually, these studies are too small to derive information on mortality; however, a pooled data analysis, including these and other studies, seems to suggest that early mortality is reduced when intravenous heparin is used with rt-PA.

There have been no controlled trials to date evaluating the efficacy of intravenous heparin versus subcutaneous heparin when conventional doses of rt-PA are used. ISIS-3 (7) randomized patients to streptokinase, APSAC, or rt-PA therapy. All patients received aspirin therapy immediately and were randomized to high-dose subcutaneous heparin or no heparin in a factorial design starting 4 hours after

Table 39.6.
Role of Heparin as Adjunctive Therapy to Thrombolytic Agents

Study (Ref.)	Regime	N	Time to Angiogram After Lytic Therapy	Patency (90 Minute)	Reocclusion	Recurrent Ischemia	In-hospital Bleeding	Mortality
Topol (54)	rt-PA with heparin 10,000 U bolus, then IV	134	90 min	79	11	22	13	5
	rt-PA alone			79	5	23	18	9
HART (6)	Heparin continuous IV with rt-PA	205	18 hr	82[a]	12	8	4	1.9
	rt-PA with ASA			85	5	2	5	4.0
Bleich (5)	rt-PA and continuous IV heparin	83	48 hr	71[b]	Not reported	8	12	Not reported
	rt-PA alone			44		9	2	
NHF (1)	Continuous IV heparin after 24 hr	202	7 d	80	Not reported	10	Not reported	Not reported
	ASA and dipyridamole after 24 hr			80		3.8		
SCATI (55)	Continuous subcutaneous heparin ± streptokinse	711		Not reported	Not reported	17	4.4	6[b]
	± streptokinase alone					19	0.6	10

[a]$P < .05$.

[b]$P < .06$.

(Adapted from Popma JJ, Topol EJ. Ann Intern Med. 1991;115:34 with permission.)

completing infusion of the thrombolytic agent. Thirty-five-day vascular mortality was not significantly different for the heparin versus the nonheparin groups (10.0% versus 10.2%, P = NS). However, this did not adequately test the full lytic potential of rt-PA because the delay in heparin therapy may have favored the occurrence of early reocclusion (65).

The value of heparin administration with streptokinase has been quite extensively tested. In the Belgium Optimization Study of Infarct Reperfusion Investigated by ST Monitoring (OSIRIS) (66), 64 patients were randomized to intravenous bolus and continuous infusion of heparin and 1.5 million units of streptokinase and 64 patients to placebo prior to streptokinase therapy for AMI. All patients received aspirin after thrombolytic therapy. Early patency rates assessed via continuous 12-lead electrocardiography at 60 and 90 minutes were higher in the heparin-treated group than in the placebo group (60 minutes:

heparin group 65%, placebo group 52%; 90 minutes: heparin 77%, placebo 60%; P <.05). However, patency at 24 hours, incidence of reinfarction, and clinical outcome were not different.

The utility of subcutaneous heparin with intravenous streptokinase has now been evaluated by trial design in three very large megatrials. ISIS-3 has been discussed. In GISSI-2 (15) patients were randomized to rt-PA or streptokinase followed 12 hours later by subcutaneous heparin 12,500 units subcutaneously every 12 hours until hospital discharge. The composite outcome of vascular death or severe left ventricular damage was not different between the heparin (22.7%) and nonheparin (22.9%) groups. The International tPA/SK Mortality Trial (67) as well showed no difference between the heparin (8.5%) and nonheparin (8.5%) groups. The results of these studies have been more or less validated recently by GUSTO trial (16) (see below). Thus it can be assumed that intravenous heparin confers no benefit over subcutaneous heparin when used with streptokinase in standard doses.

With the exception of ISIS-3, to date there has been relatively little study of antithrombotic adjuvants to APSAC. Routine use of heparin following APSAC therapy was evaluated in the Duke University Clinical Cardiology Studies (DUCCS-1) trial (68, 69). The published results of this randomized trial showed that there were no significant differences in the rates of reinfarction or congestive heart failure and that recurrent ischemia was similar among the intravenous heparin and nonheparin-treated patients. Notably, however, the incidence of total stroke (3% versus 0.8%), hemorrhagic stroke (1.6% versus 0%), and overall mortality (9% versus 7%) was higher in the heparin versus nonheparin groups, respectively. Thus preliminary evidence suggests that omission of intravenous heparin therapy with APSAC does not appear to compromise patient outcome.

Newer Antithrombin Agents

Efforts to improve on the antithrombin activity of heparin and enhance infarct-related artery patency have led to the investigation of newer, more powerful antithrombin agents. Hirudin, a naturally occurring component of leech saliva, now synthesized through recombinant DNA technology, prevents thrombin-induced platelet activation, conversion of fibrinogen to fibrin, and activation of factors V, VIII, and XIII by specific inhibition of thrombin (70, 71). Because of its smaller molecular profile and binding characteristics, hirudin can penetrate into the interstices of the fibrin-bound thrombin complex and thus prevent the growth of thrombus more effectively than the larger heparin molecule (72). In this regard, hirudin has been shown to be more effective at preventing activation of the coagulation cascade during thrombolysis (73).

Recombinant hirudin has been evaluated in several clinical trials. In the TIMI-5 trial

(74) 260 patients were randomized to r-hirudin or heparin in the setting of an acute myocardial infarction. Ninety-minute angiograms in the two groups revealed TIMI-grade 3 flow in 66% of the hirudin-treated patients and in 56% of the heparin-treated patients. Furthermore, reocclusion was reduced in the hirudin group to 2% versus 7% for heparin-treated patients. Although the potential for improved patency has been demonstrated, the risk of excess bleeding remains a concern with more potent thrombin inhibition. This problem has been more clearly defined in several large-scale trials of hirudin use in acute coronary syndromes. GUSTO IIa (73a) randomized 2564 patients with ischemic chest pain and ECG abnormalities in a double-blind fashion to thrombolytic therapy when appropriate and/or adjunctive treatment with adjusted-dose heparin (5000 U bolus and 1000 to 1300 U/hr) over 72 to 120 hours or hirudin (0.6-mg/kg bolus and 0.2-mg/kg/hr infusion). Thrombolytic candidates were eligible to receive either accelerated rt-PA or streptokinase as in the GUSTO I protocol. The heparin group was titrated to maintain an aPTT of 60 to 90 seconds; the hirudin dose was fixed. Although recruitment of 12,000 patients was planned, the trial was stopped early because of excess hemorrhagic strokes in both groups. While overall incidence of hemorrhagic strokes was increased, it was not statistically different between the two antithrombin groups. In the heparin group there were 17 strokes in 1273 treated patients (1.3%; 95% CI, 0.7 to 2.0%) and in the hirudin group nine of 1291 patients treated (0.7%; 95% CI, 0.2 to 1.2%), $P = .11$. When 1264 patients receiving thrombolytic therapy were analyzed separately, all but three of the 26 intracerebral hemorrhages occurred in this group (1.8%) versus 1168 patients not receiving thrombolytic agents (0.3%), a finding that was highly statistically significant ($P < .001$).

Although the incidence of intracerebral

bleeding was not statistically different between the antithrombin groups, patients receiving hirudin tended to have a higher stroke rate in both the nonthrombolytic (0.5% for hirudin versus 0% for heparin; CI, 0 to 1.1% $P = .8$) and the thrombolytic groups (2.2% for hirudin; CI, 0.1 to 3.3% versus heparin; 1.5% CI, 0.5 to 2.5%, $P = .34$).

When the incidence of intracranial hemorrhage was indexed for aggressiveness of anticoagulation as evidenced by the aPTT, patients with hemorrhagic stroke had an aPTT at 12 hours of 110 ± 46 versus 87 ± 36 ($P = .031$) in those without intracranial hemorrhage. This finding was of particular importance since the dose of heparin was 20% higher overall in this study than in GUSTO I. When further compared to GUSTO I (13), an older population with more females and higher systolic blood pressure at enrollment (albeit still within the normal range) was noted in this trial.

Remarkably concordant data have been derived from two similarly randomized trials. In TIMI 9A (73b), patients with evidence of acute myocardial infarction eligible for thrombolytic therapy (accelerated rt-PA or streptokinase) were randomized to conjunctive therapy with intravenous heparin or hirudin in a dosing algorithm similar to GUSTO IIa. Further mirroring GUSTO IIa, enrollment was prematurely halted after randomizing 757 patients because of higher than expected rates of hemorrhage in both treatment arms. Intracranial hemorrhage occurred in six of 345 (1.7%) of hirudin-treated patients and seven (1.9%) of 368 heparin-treated patients ($P = NS$). In both groups the development of major hemorrhage was the principal reason for discontinuation of the study drug. However, hirudin was stopped more frequently for this reason than heparin (16.2% versus 10.9%. $P = .04$). In patients receiving rt-PA, hirudin was discontinued more frequently because of hemorrhage (27.2%) than those randomized to heparin

(17.9%, $P = .008$). As in GUSTO IIa, patients with a higher median aPTT at 12 hours (100s versus 85s) had more major hemorrhages ($P = .001$).

Finally, data from European centers comparing adjunctive heparin and hirudin therapy in patients with acute myocardial infarction treated with accelerated rt-PA conform to the results of the American studies detailed above. In the prospective randomized, double-blind multicenter Hirudin for Improvement of Thrombolysis (HIT) phase III trial (73c), hirudin (from an alternative manufacturer) was compared with heparin in patients receiving accelerated rt-PA for acute myocardial infarction. Once again, enrollment was terminated early (302 patients out of a planned 7000) because of predominance of major bleeding events in the active treatment groups. Both heparin and hirudin were given in a blinded fashion using doses different from that of GUSTO and TIMI 9A. Heparin was administered as a bolus of 70 IU/kg followed by 15 IU/kg/hr to start with dose adjustment based on aPTT. Hirudin was given as a 0.4 mg/kg bolus followed by continuous infusion of 0.15 mg/kg/hr. Dose adjustment was determined by aPTT at regular intervals. Although hirudin was administered in doses lower than that of GUSTO IIIa and TIMI 9A, a predominance of hemorrhagic stroke was still noted in the hirudin group (2.78%) versus heparin (0.0%). Analysis of stroke indexed for aPTT confirmed once again that patients with intracerebral hemorrhage had a higher aPTT value than those without major hemorrhage (106 versus 76 seconds).

Thus, although the use of antithrombotic therapy (principally heparin) has been previously shown to be effective both as a primary treatment in unstable coronary syndromes and conjunctively with thrombolytic agents in acute myocardial infarctions, preliminary evidence supporting additional efficacy using more potent agents such as hirudin is still lacking. Although the studies above were large randomized trials, they shared similar designs and thus may have similar flaws. As has been proposed by workers in the field (74c), more careful analysis of the data is needed prior to abandoning the concept that more complete antithrombin activity is beneficial in unstable coronary syndromes. This concept has previously been found to be sound, and as such a more thorough analysis of patient characteristics (including previous TIAs, ASA and NSAID drug use, etc.) needs to be performed. Furthermore, although more accurate measures of thrombin activity are available (FPA, fragment 1.2, and TATs), they are rarely used clinically, supplanted by the more ubiquitous yet less accurate aPTT and ACT measurements. Since it is reasonable to assume that overaggressive anticoagulation is injurious, perhaps more accurate monitoring is required to reap the benefits of a more potent antithrombin regimen. Thus a reasonable strategy, and one employed by the trialists, is to reduce the dose of the antithrombin agents and continue the trial. Data from GUSTO II and TIMI 9 are forthcoming.

Hirulog, the synthetic peptide analog of hirudin, is another potent antithrombin agent currently under investigation. Lidón et al. (75) evaluated hirulog as the sole anticoagulant (antianginal agents and aspirin were also used) in patients with unstable angina. In this study three dose ranges were chosen, producing elevations in the aPTT of 62 ± 12, 74 ± 5, and 96 ± 10 seconds. Of the 30 patients enrolled, only four developed recurrent ischemic symptoms (two in each of the lower-dose groups). There were no deaths, recurrent myocardial infarctions, or bleeding complications. In a similar trial comparing hirulog with heparin as adjunctive therapy to streptokinase in acute MI, Lidón and colleagues (76) found an angiographic patency rate of 80% for hirulog versus 33% for heparin. Recently, Sharma and coworkers (77) utilized a hirulog (0.2 mg/kg/hr) infusion to treat patients with unstable angina. Only a historical heparin control arm was used for comparison. End-

points were death, myocardial infarction, intractable angina, or intracoronary thrombus. The incidence of combined endpoints for the hirulog group was 19.3% as compared with 45.9% for the historical heparin controls ($P < .01$). Although weakened by the lack of a prospective control group, the findings are more or less consistent with the previously noted heparin-controlled trials. Several additional antithrombotic agents (argatroban and MCI-9038) are in the initial stages of study. Each have been shown to possess potent antithrombotic properties, although clinical experience with them is still lacking. The interested reader is referred to additional references for a more thorough discussion (78–81).

Antiplatelet Therapy

The salutary effects of antiplatelet therapy, in particular aspirin, were unequivocally demonstrated in the ISIS-2 study (5). The overall effect of aspirin was a marked reduction in vascular mortality from 11.8 to 9.4% ($P < .00001$) that persisted through 15 months of follow-up. This benefit was noted across a variety of subgroups according to age, site of infarct, and time to treatment. Importantly, this advantageous effect was achieved with only a small (0.7%) increase in minor bleeding over thrombolytic therapy alone and with a 0.5% decrease in overall stroke rate. Furthermore, the cost of this agent is minimal, making it an effective important therapy in AMI (95).

The role of platelets in the dynamic process of thrombosis and fibrinolysis has been and continues to be the topic of considerable study. The effects of thrombolysis on platelet function are quite complex. In addition to the platelet-activating properties of thrombolytic agents themselves, other local substances in the active clot may play a profound role. Adenosine diphosphate (ADP), collagen, and epinephrine at the site of plaque rupture contribute substantially to the procoagulant milieu (82). Furthermore, platelets contain plasminogen activator inhibitor-1 granules (PAI-1) that may attenuate the action of fibrinolytic agents (83). Platelets also contribute to the cross-linking of fibrin by supplying factor XIII (84, 85). This may at least partially explain the recalcitrance of fibrin mixed with platelets in the deeply fissured plaque to the effects of fibrinolytic agents. Once stimulated, platelet aggregation results in release of vasoactive substances such as thromboxane A_2 that produce attendant vasoconstriction and together with thrombus further compromise the vascular lumen.

Ingestion of aspirin results in immediate and irreversible acetylation of the platelet cyclooxygenase enzyme system. This results in an inability of the platelet to synthesize thromboxane A_2 and other related prostaglandins, impairing their function.

Despite the use of aspirin (and heparin) in patients receiving successful thrombolytic therapy, recurrent ischemia primarily caused by rethrombosis occurs within 1 week in 11 to 21% of patients (86). Platelet aggregation appears to play a pivotal role in this process (87). In this setting recurrent platelet activity, despite the presence of aspirin, may be mediated through stimulation of the glycoprotein IIb/IIIa receptors located in the platelet membrane. This receptor mediates the binding of platelets to sites containing various macromolecular glycoproteins along the vessel wall, including collagen, fibrinogen, fibronectin, and von Willebrand factor (86). The passage of platelets through an area of fixed residual obstruction may result in activation of these receptors and thus platelet function (88, 89). This may occur through a number of cyclooxygenase-independent pathways resulting from the shear forces generated with this motion (89).

Efforts to more thoroughly incapacitate platelet activity have resulted in a search for additional agents capable of targeting areas of platelet function alternate to that affected by aspirin. Among these are compounds that prevent normal function of the glycoprotein

platelet receptors. Two such compounds are the murine monoclonal antibodies 7E3-F{ab′}$_2$ {7E3} and 10E5-F{ab′}$_2$. These agents have been shown to significantly shorten time to reperfusion after thrombotic coronary occlusion (90) and to prevent platelet thrombus formation after vascular injury (91).

Recently, profound inhibition of platelet aggregation after thrombolysis through the use of aspirin plus monoclonal antibody 7E3 Fab was found to be well tolerated and associated with fewer postthrombolysis ischemic events (92). Moreover, infarct-related artery patency in the 7E3 group was 92% versus 56% for the control group. Although not specifically powered for clinical endpoint assessment, the findings remain noteworthy and deserving of larger study.

Compounds that share the same amino acid sequence homology as the glycoprotein IIb/IIIa receptor have been found in nature (snake venom) and synthesized in the laboratory. One of the most promising is integrelin, a highly specific heptapeptide competitive antagonist of the glycoprotein IIb/IIIa complex. This substance is a potent inhibitor of platelet aggregation in animals (93) and humans (94). These two agents and a litany of mechanistically similar ones comprise a new and potentially very useful addition to the antiplatelet armamentarium now dominated by aspirin. These new therapies may be additive to aspirin or supplant its use in acute ischemic syndromes.

ACCELERATED RT-PA AND MODE OF HEPARIN ADMINISTRATION: THE GUSTO-1 TRIAL

Designed to continue the search for improved reperfusion strategies and provide insight into many of the current controversies surrounding thrombolysis in AMI, the Global Utilization of Streptokinase and Tissue Plasminogen Activator for Occluded Coronary Arteries (GUSTO) I trial (16) was designed and carried out. Conceived as a mortality trial, this study effectively randomized

Figure 39.5. GUSTO I randomization strategy.

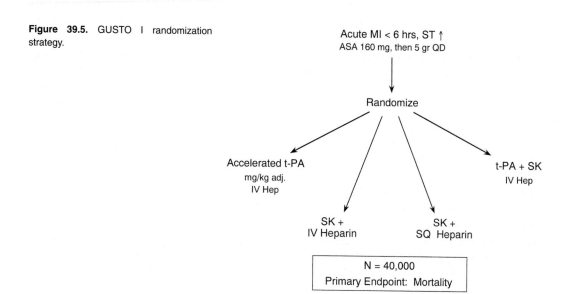

Table 39.7.
Major Clinical Outcomes of the GUSTO Trial

	Streptokinase and Subcutaneous Heparin (N = 9796)	Streptokinase and Intravenous Heparin (N = 10,377)	Accelerated t-PA and Intravenous Heparin (N = 10,344)	Both Thrombolytic Agents and Intravenous Heparin (N = 10,328)	P Value, Accelerated t-PA vs Both Streptokinase Groups
Outcome					
24-hr mortality	2.8	2.9	2.3	2.8	.005
30-day mortality	7.2	7.4	6.3	7.0	.001
Nonfatal stroke	7.9	8.2	7.2	7.9	.006
Nonfatal hemorrhagic stroke	7.4	7.6	6.6	7.4	.004
Nonfatal disabling stroke	7.7	7.9	6.9	7.6	.006

41,021 patients with ≤6 hours of chest pain and ECG evidence of myocardial injury or bundle branch block to one of four treatment arms (Fig. 39.5). To test the efficacy of accelerated rt-PA regimens (96–98) that have been suggested to be more efficacious in smaller studies, 100 mg was given over 90 minutes with a 15-mg bolus. To test the suggestion that postreperfusion reclusion is less with combination therapy (99–101), streptokinase 1 million units and rt-PA 10 mg/kg over 60 minutes were given. These two strategies were compared with conventional streptokinase therapy tested in GISSI-2 (15) and ISIS-3 (7) (1.5 million units IV over 30 to 60 minutes) followed 4 hours later by subcutaneous heparin (12,500 units every 12 hours). Finally, to provide insight into the controversy of intravenous versus subcutaneous heparin, the latter was given (5000 units bolus with infusion 1000 to 1200 units/hour titrated to an aPTT of 65 to 85 seconds) with conventional streptokinase in a fourth arm. Intravenous heparin was similarly administered in the accelerated and combined strategies. Antiplatelet therapy, consisting of aspirin 160 to 325 mg on presentation and then daily, was used. Intravenous followed by oral atenolol therapy was recommended in all patients without contraindications. All other treatment medications were left to the discretion of the physicians.

The major results are shown in Table 39.7. At 30 days there was no significant difference in mortality between streptokinase groups. There was a significant reduction in mortality with accelerated rt-PA when compared with other regimens with an estimated 10 lives saved per 1000 patients treated (risk reduction 14%, 95% CI = 5.9 to 21.3; $P = .001$). This regimen was also significantly better in terms of mortality when compared separately with each of the streptokinase arms. There was no significant difference between the combination regimen and the streptokinase groups. However, the combination arm fared less well than the accelerated rt-PA group

(7.0% versus 6.3% mortality, risk reduction 10% with 95% CI, 0.8 to 19.2; $P = .04$). Thirty-day survival curves for each of the arms is shown in Figure 39.6.

Associated with the improved overall survival in the accelerated rt-PA arm was an excess of two hemorrhagic strokes per 1000 patients treated (absolute excess, 0.2%) for rt-PA as compared with the streptokinase regimens. The combination of thrombolytics carried an excess of four hemorrhagic strokes per 1000 compared with the streptokinase regimens. The net clinical benefit for the accelerated regimen calculated to be the prevention of death or disabling stroke in nine patients per 1000 treated. This reduction was consistent across all prespecified subgroups (Fig. 39.7), although, as expected, most pronounced for patients with anterior infarcts and age less than 75 years.

The improved survival was felt to be the result of obtaining early achievement and maintenance of infarct-related artery patency. An angiographic substudy of 2400 patients (600 in each treatment arm) is consistent with this (47).

The cost differential between rt-PA and streptokinase has been the major subject of controversy with this study. Recombinant tissue plasminogen activator costs $2200 to $2400 per dose. However, an analysis performed with the GUSTO study calculates a cost of approximately $22,000 per year of life saved owing to the average of 10 additional quality-adjusted life years in each of the survivors. This finding compares favorably with $60,000 per year of life saved for dialysis or between $150,000 to 200,000 for some chronic antihypertensive or hypolipidemic therapies.

Thus, for patients presenting to the hospital within 6 hours of chest pain and no contraindication to thrombolysis, management should include chewable aspirin (169 to 325 mg) and the use of a thrombolytic agent. The specifics of which agent is used are less important than the fact that one be used.

Mortality (%)
10
9
8
7
6
5
4
3
2
1
0
0 2 4 6 8 10 12 14 16 18 20 22 24 26 28 30
Days from Randomization
SK (IV)
SK (SubQ)
t-PA + SK
t-PA

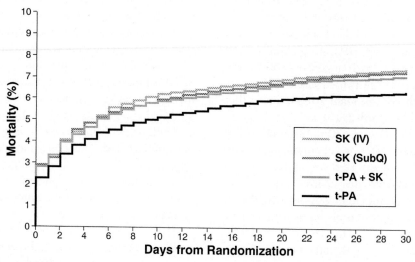

Figure 39.6. GUSTO I 30-day mortality curves. (Adapted with permission from the GUSTO investigators. N Engl J Med 1993;329:673–682.)

Mortality Rates
% of Pts.
SK
t-PA
Odds Ratio & 95% C.I.
Age
< 75 yrs 88% 5.5% 4.4%
≥ 75 yrs 12% 20.6% 19.3%
Infarct Location
Anterior 39% 10.5% 8.6%
Other 61% 5.3% 4.7%
Time to Thrombolytic Therapy
0 to 2 hrs 27% 5.4% 4.3%
> 2 to 4 51% 6.7% 5.5%
> 4 to 6 19% 9.3% 8.9%
> 6 4% 8.3% 10.4%
(2.13)
0.5
1.0
1.5
t-PA better
SK better

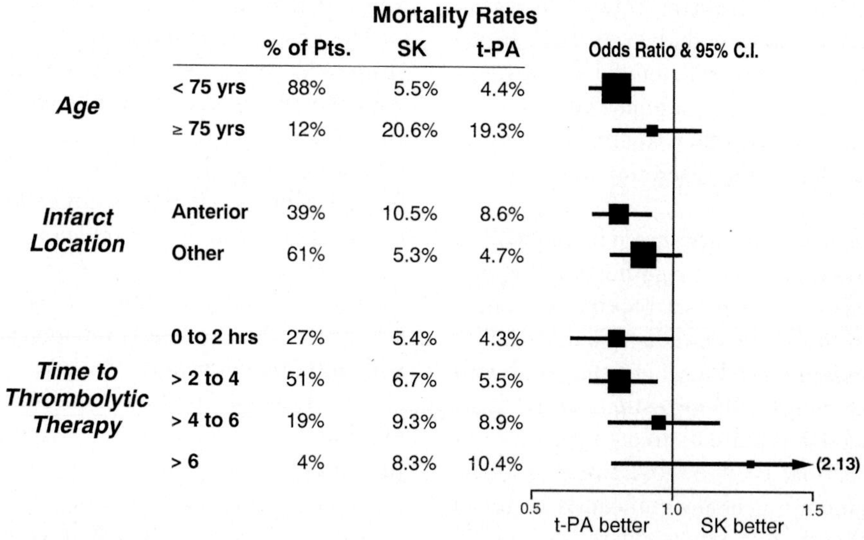

Figure 39.7. GUSTO I prespecified subgroup mortality rates. (Adapted with permission from the GUSTO investigators. N Engl J Med 1993;329:673–682.)

Patients with large infarcts and who are perhaps less than 75 years of age may benefit most from accelerated rt-PA and intravenous heparin titrated to maintain an aPTT of 50 to 70 seconds. If streptokinase is used, there appears to be no benefit and perhaps an increased risk of hemorrhage associated with heparin administration.

CORONARY INTERVENTIONS AND THE USE OF NEWER ANTIPLATELET, ANTITHROMBIN, AND THROMBOLYTIC AGENTS

Since the introduction of percutaneous balloon angioplasty (PTCA) by Andreas Gruenzig in 1977 (102), this innovative modality has seen tremendous growth both in application and in technique. Newer designs have led to the development of novel devices such as rotational and directional atherectomy and coronary stenting. Despite the widespread use of these techniques, their long-term success remains plagued by a restenosis rate of at least 30%. In addition, acute vessel closure from thrombosis, although infrequent, remains a major complication (103). Balloon expansion denudes arterial endothelium and exposes subendothelial structures such as collagen and plaque material to blood, resulting in activation of the coagulation system. Platelet and thrombin play a major role in this process and thus have been the target of pharmacologic agents in efforts to reduce or eliminate this phenomenon.

Conventional Antiplatelet and Antithrombotic Therapy

First-line antiplatelet therapy at present consists primarily of aspirin. This agent, although imperfect, has been shown to reduce acute thrombosis in patients undergoing coronary intervention (104). Ticlopidine, an alternative antiplatelet agent that modifies platelet membrane reactivity, has also been found to decrease acute vessel closure during coronary intervention (104). However, because of its expense and side-effect profile, it is presently indicated for use in patients unable to tolerate aspirin.

New Antithrombotic Agents

The mainstay of anticoagulation and, as such, antithrombotic therapy during coronary intervention and in general is heparin. Given as an intravenous bolus and constant infusion as needed, it is generally used throughout the procedure and discontinued thereafter unless the angiographic results reveal a dissection, filling defect, or "suboptimal" result (105). Because both heparin and aspirin have lessened but not eliminated the risk of abrupt vessel closure secondary to thrombosis (70, 106, 107) and because restenosis has remained unaltered, the use of novel antiplatelet and antithrombotic agents has been actively investigated.

The new agent hirudin and its synthetic analog hirulog are potent antithrombin agents currently undergoing extensive investigation. They act on both free and fibrin-bound thrombin, and this affinity allows for clot penetration. In animal models of balloon injury, hirudin has been shown to be associated with less clot formation (108) and restenosis (109).

In humans both hirudin and hirulog have undergone preliminary investigations. In a dose-ranging trial Topol et al. (109) have shown that high doses of hirulog effectively reduced abrupt vessel closure in patients undergoing coronary angioplasty. When given in a continuous infusion of 1.8 or 2.2 mg/kg/hour after a bolus of 0.45 mg/kg and 0.55 mg/kg, respectively, abrupt vessel closure within 24 hours of the procedure was 3.9% and without significant bleeding sequela. Recombinant hirudin has recently been compared with heparin in patients with stable angina undergoing coronary angioplasty (110). In this trial 113 patients were randomized to hirudin (20 mg bolus, constant infusion 0.16 mg/kg/hour) or heparin in the standard fashion. Of the 39 patients randomized to heparin, four (10.3%) experienced myocardial infarction or underwent emergent surgical revascularization compared with one of 74 patients (1.4%) in the hirudin group. When ST segments were analyzed postprocedurally, ischemic episodes were observed in four patients (11%) in the heparin group and three patients (4%) in the hirudin group.

The salutary effect of hirudin on restenosis following coronary intervention appears to be less substantial. Preliminary data from Europe regarding the use of hirudin compared with heparin on restenosis rates following coronary intervention are available from the HELVETICA trial. Three groups of patients were randomized to IV heparin, IV hirudin, or IV and SQ hirudin in conjunction with their coronary intervention. Preliminary analysis of data revealed no statistically significant difference in complications at 4 days and restenosis rates at 6 months. Restenosis rates and cardiac events averaged about 35% in all three groups at the 6-month follow-up.

New Antiplatelet Agents (Glycoprotein IIb/IIIa Antagonists)

The chimeric 7E3 antibody Fab (c7E3) fragment binds selectively to platelet glycoprotein IIb/IIIa integrin and consists of a genetically reconstructed murine monoclonal IgG molecule. In the recently completed EPIC study (111), in addition to heparin and aspirin, patients given 7E3 as a bolus of 0.25 mg/kg followed by continuous infusion of 10 µg/minute for 12 hours had a 23% overall reduction in major ischemic events (death, MI, urgent revascularization). Furthermore, at 6-month follow-up, there was a 26% reduction in the need for target-vessel revascularization, indicating a reduction in clinical restenosis. When subgroups were evaluated, this reduction in target-vessel revascularization was most significant in patients with angina pectoris but not in acute coronary syndromes.

The salutary benefits of c7E3 appear to be related to a decrease in platelet-mediated thrombosis by more potent platelet inhibition (112), a key component of the unstable coro-

nary syndromes that affected the majority of patients in EPIC. Although used exclusively for acute coronary syndromes in EPIC, Ellis et al. have also confirmed the safety and efficacy of c7E3 in patients with stable angina undergoing elective coronary angioplasty (113).

Thrombolytics and Coronary Intervention

The ability to selectively effect dissolution of coronary thrombus in conjunction with nonsurgical coronary revascularization is an attractive concept. As such, intraarterial thrombolytic therapy in conjunction with coronary intervention, although controversial, may be quite beneficial. Several nonrandomized studies of patients with unstable angina undergoing coronary angioplasty have shown resolution of large intracoronary thrombus with intravenous t-PA, intracoronary streptokinase (114), or intracoronary urokinse (UK) (115).

In a restrospective comparison of high-risk patients undergoing coronary angioplasty, 80 treated with intracoronary UK and 167 without, Pavlides et al. (116) found that patients with intraluminal thrombus appeared to have less ischemic complications (3% versus 18%). However, those with intimal dissection receiving the thrombolytic experienced more ischemic sequelae than those who did not (20.8% versus 9%, respectively).

The Thrombolysis and Angioplasty in Unstable Angina (TAUSA) pilot study (117) suggested that low-dose UK reduced angiographic evidence of thrombus following PTCA. However, the larger, recently completed TAUSA study (117) that enrolled 469 patients in a double-blind, placebo-controlled fashion showed no benefit. In phase I trials 257 patients received a total of 250,000 units of UK (150,000 units before and 100,000 units after PTCA) or placebo. Phase II utilized 500,000 units (250,000 before and 250,000 after PTCA) or placebo in 212 patients; angiograms were performed 15 minutes after the coronary intervention. Results showed that while filling defects were significantly decreased overall with UK, closure and early ischemic events were increased, particularly in phase II (6.7% versus 0% for acute closure and 6.7% versus 1.9% for ischemic episodes in UK and placebo-treated patients, respectively). When patients with unstable angina and myocardial infarction were analyzed separately, filling defects were found to be reduced in the infarct group with UK (10%) versus placebo (20%) at $P = .06$, but acute closure and early events were higher in the unstable angina group (UK 9% vs. placebo 0%, $P <.01$). Furthermore, emergent coronary bypass was higher in the UK unstable angina group as compared with placebo (6% versus 0%, respectively). Thus, based on these recent data, it appears that thrombolytic agents should be avoided in these patients.

Patients with chronic total occlusions present a special revascularization problem. Kahn and Hartzler (118) reported these lesions to be 36% of the total failures. Recently, several preliminary studies have employed the use of intracoronary UK to improve these results. Zidar et al. (119) randomized patients with chronic total occlusions (>3 months) in whom the lesion could not initially be crossed to three groups: group A—0.8 million units, group B—1.6 million units, or group C—3.2 million units of intracoronary UK for 8 hours. PTCA was again attempted after the infusion was complete. In a total of 39 patients given the UK dose, PTCA was successful in 54% (A = 47%, B = 61%, C = 57%; P = NS) of the patients. Bleeding was highest in group C. Only one patient sustained a myocardial infarction, and there were no urgent revascularizations.

The use of UK infusion in conjunction with coronary intervention has been studied in the Recanalization of Chronically Occluded Bypass Grafts with Prolonged Urokinase Infusion Site Trial (ROBUST). In this trial 100 patients received prolonged intracoronary infusions of UK (100,000 to 300,000 units for 3.8 to 54.3 hours) followed by adjunctive balloon angioplasty as required. Preliminary data on 85 patients (120) revealed a recanalization rate of 71% for UK alone and 94% with adjunctive PTCA. There were myocardial infarctions in 5%, an overall stroke rate of 3%, and a 3% death rate. Bleeding requiring transfusion occurred in 16% of patients. Long-term follow-up has yet to be reported. While not innocuous, this may represent an alternative treatment modality in this subset of patients with vein graft disease.

ADVERSE EFFECTS OF THROMBOLYSIS

Complications associated with the use of thrombolytic therapy are principally those of allergic reactions and hemorrhage. The former are encountered with the use of streptokinase and APSAC and are caused by the foreign proteinaceous nature of these compounds. Hemorrhagic complications are clearly increased in patients receiving thrombolytic therapy (121, 122). Although any bleeding complication is generally associated with an increased morbidity, intracranial hemorrhage represents the most devastating and feared complication. Information from a large number of trials provides a forum from which to draw some firm conclusions.

Pooled data from nine large mortality trials (110) show that the overall stroke rate is increased (rt-PA, streptokinase, and APSAC data pooled) and is approximately 1.1% in the thrombolytic group versus 0.7% in control patients (3.7 SD, 0.8 excess strokes per 1000 patients treated, $P <.00001$). All of this excess appeared within the first 24 hours of treatment. Likewise, data from the recently completed GUSTO trial (16) show similar results. Hemorrhagic stroke rate ranged from a low 0.049% in the streptokinase and subcutaneous heparin arm to 0.94% in the combination therapy (rt-PA-streptokinase) and IV heparin arm.

Weighing the risk:benefit ratio when administering thrombolytic therapy is a critical point. Of particular importance is understanding that the fear of cerebral hemorrhage in patients with advanced age (generally ≥75 years) is not a satisfactory reason for withholding thrombolytic therapy when no other contraindications exist. Data from extensive studies reveal that the excess of deaths on days 0 to 1 increase with advancing age but so too did the reduction in deaths from days 2 to 35. This clustering of early deaths has been termed the "early hazard," the cause of which remains incompletely elucidated. Both GISSI-2 (15) and ISIS-3 (7) have shown in a comparative fashion that rt-PA is associated with more bleeding sequelae than streptokinase and that this increases with advancing age. This has also been confirmed in the GUSTO trial where in patients age 75 years or less, hemorrhagic stroke occurred in 0.42% of the streptokinase group and 0.52% of the t-PA (accelerated protocol) group. When compared with patients age 75 years or greater, these values were 1.23% and 2.08%, respectively. Overall, however, the accelerated regimen was associated with an improved clinical outcome score (16). These compelling data solidify the argument that thrombolytic therapy should be given to all patients when the clinical scenario is appropriate without regard for age (123).

CONTRAINDICATIONS

These are based primarily on clinical experience and subject to change as new data are accrued. The only absolute contraindication is active bleeding in a noncompressible site. Patients at risk for intracranial hemorrhage represent the highest risk. Relative contraindications include:

1. Gastrointestinal or genitourinary bleeding within 6 months
2. Major surgery within previous 2 to 4 weeks
3. Prolonged CPR >10 minutes with chest trauma within previous 2 to 4 weeks
4. Intracranial anatomic defect (aneurysm, neoplasm, previous surgery); proliferative diabetic retinopathy
5. Severe, uncontrolled hypertension (systolic BP >200 mm Hg, diastolic BP >120 mm Hg)
6. Pregnancy
7. Cancer
8. Proven bleeding diathesis

In the presence of absolute or relative contraindications, revascularization of the infarct-related artery should be considered and, if possible (given the appropriate setting), attempted utilizing primary angioplasty as this has been shown to produce a survival advantage as well (124).

CURRENT LIMITATIONS AND FUTURE DIRECTIONS

The Illusion of Reperfusion

Reperfusion therapy has undeniably had a major impact on lowering morbidity and mortality associated with AMI. The application of primary PTCA and improvement in administration of thrombolytic, antiplatelet, and perhaps antithrombotic agents have seemingly contributed to a 30% reduction in mortality in large controlled trials (3–6, 13, 125, 126). However, this may leave one with a false sense of security in that they were derived from controlled clinical trials and may not be directly applicable to widespread practice. Furthermore, despite compelling data for the use of thrombolytic therapy in acute MI, it is estimated that only 15 to 30% of patients who are eligible receive the drug in the United States (127–130). Figure 39.8 depicts the

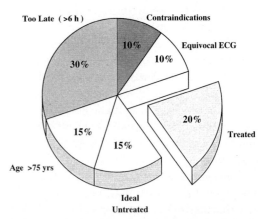

Figure 39.8. The frequency of use of thrombolysis in acute myocardial infarction (AMI) and reasons for exclusions are shown. Note that only 20% of patients with AMI were treated and an additional 15% of eligible patients did not get treated. (Adapted with permission from Muller DW, Topol EJ. Ann Intern Med 1990;113:949–960.)

causes for exclusion in one recent study that addresses this issue. In this particular study only 20% of patients received thrombolytic therapy. An additional 15% were regarded as ideal candidates, but nonetheless were not offered the benefit of chemical reperfusion therapy. These patients have been shown to have a high early and late mortality (131). Sufficient discussion has been given in support of the use of thrombolytic therapy for AMI in all appropriate patients (regardless of age) with ST-segment elevation or bundle branch block presenting within 12 hours of symptom onset.

However, despite the prompt administration of thrombolytic therapy in appropriate individuals, at least 20% of patients will still fail to achieve sustained reperfusion. These patients have a markedly increased morbidity and mortality (132), even after attempts at salvage reperfusion with mechanical devices (133, 134). Current evidence supports several mechanisms for this finding.

Thrombus that is rich in platelets and heavily cross-linked fibrin molecules, as a result of aging, is in general more resistant to the lysis by a thrombolytic agent. More effective lytic strategies are required to impact on these clots. In addition to novel dosing regimens for rt-PA that have been shown to improve patency and decrease mortality (16, 97), newer agents have been under investigation. Molecules such as single-chain urokinase-type plasminogen activator (SCUPA) (135–137) and mutants of rt-PA such as those derived from the saliva of vampire bats (138) have a longer half-life and more potent fibrin lysing capacity, which in experimental models have been shown to be superior to rt-PA and may enhance primary thrombolysis. These await further clinical testing.

Intermittent patency and subsequent reocclusion, as previously described, remain vexing problems. Much of the work in this area is directed toward optimizing the use of currently available antiplatelet and antithrombotic drugs (aspirin and heparin primarily),

while experimentation with more potent agents such as hirudin (55, 71, 73, 75, 139–141) and others (79, 81, 141) are carried out.

Incomplete coronary patency continues to hamper timely thrombolysis. Angiographic outcome postthrombolysis has classically been graded by the Thrombolysis in Acute Myocardial Infarction (TIMI) study group (142). The presence of grades 0 to 1 (no flow-minimal penetration of contrast past thrombus, respectively) was considered as suboptimal or an occluded vessel. Grade 2 (delayed flow past obstruction) and grade 3 (brisk flow) were considered a patent vessel. Presence of the latter two flow patterns after thrombolytic administration has previously been considered evidence of patency. However, numerous recent reports have now challenged that these two flows are equivalent (143–145). Considerable data exist to support the theory that TIMI grade 3 flow alone should be the goal of reperfusion interventions. Pooled data from four German thrombolytic trials (146) found that in-hospital mortality was 7.1% and 6.6% among patients with early TIMI grades 0 to 1 and TIMI grade 2 flow, respectively ($P = $ NS). Patients with TIMI grade 3 flow had an in-hospital mortality rate of 2.7%, which was statistically better ($P <.001$).

At present it remains to be determined whether TIMI grade 2 flow is a cause or marker of worsened outcome after thrombolysis (147). Extensive damage to the distal capillary bed of an infarct vessel caused by cellular and interstitial edema and necrosis may preclude maintenance of brisk reflow following reperfusion therapy. This has been termed the "no-reflow phenomenon." Two groups of investigators have correlated TIMI grade 2 flow to increased reocclusion following reperfusion therapy (148, 149). Ito et al., using contrast echocardiography, described 39 patients with acute anterior wall myocardial infarction in whom reperfusion was obtained using thrombolysis and direct coronary angioplasty (PTCA). Contrast echo demonstrated absence of myocardial reflow despite a patent

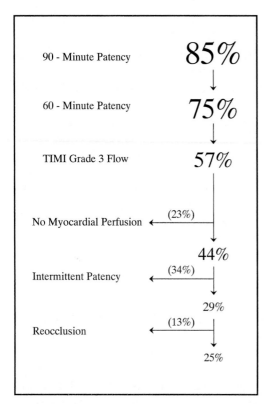

Figure 39.9. Regression of patency after thrombolysis. (Adapted with permission from Lincoff AM, Topol EJ. Circulation 1993;87:1792–1805.)

coronary artery in 23% of the patients; this was thought to be caused by microcirculatory damage. TIMI grade flow was not categorized and indexed for myocardial salvage, but collateral flow was. Graded 0 to 3, collateral flow had no statistically significant effect on improvement of contrast enhancement in the predetermined area of risk.

Based on these and similar arguments, Lincoff and Topol (147) have calculated that optimal reperfusion occurs in 25% or less of patients treated for AMI (Fig. 39.9). Thus, despite the significant advances made in reperfusion therapy for AMI, it is obvious that continued work is needed to further the question for optimal reperfusion. An understanding of the current limitations, coupled with the development and implementation of newer pharmacologic and nonpharmacologic therapeutic strategies, holds the key to the

advancement from the "illusion" to the reality of optimal reperfusion.

REFERENCES

1. Rossi P, Bolognese L. Comparison of intravenous urokinase plus heparin versus heparin alone in acute myocardial infarction. Urochinasi per via Sistemica nell'Infarto Miocardico (USIM) Collaborative Group. Am J Cardiol 1991;68:585–592.
2. Gruppo Italiano por lo Studio della Streptochinasi nell'Infarcto Miacardio (GISSI). Effectiveness of intravenous thrombolytic treatment in acute myocardial infarction. Gruppo Italiano per lo Studio della Streptochinasi nell'Infarto Miocardico (GISSI). Lancet 1986;1:397–402.
3. The ISAM study group. A prospective trial of intravenous streptokinase in acute myocardial infarction (I.S.A.M.). Mortality, morbidity, and infarct size at 21 days. The I.S.A.M. Study Group. N Engl J Med 1986; 314:1465–1471.
4. AIMS Trial study group. Effect of intravenous APSAC on mortality after acute myocardial infarction: preliminary report of a placebo-controlled clinical trial. AIMS Trial Study Group. Lancet 1988;1:545–549.
5. ISIS-2. ISIS-2 (Second International Study of Infarct Survival) collaborative group. ISIS-2 (The Second International Study of Infarct Survival). Randomised trial of intravenous streptokinase, oral aspirin, both, or neither among 17,187 cases of suspected acute myocardial infarction. Lancet 1988;2:349–360.
6. Wilcox RG, von der Lippe G, Olsson CG, Jensen G, Skene AM, Hampton JR. Trial of tissue plasminogen activator for mortality reduction in acute myocardial infarction. Anglo-Scandinavian Study of Early Thrombolysis (ASSET). Lancet 1988;2:525–530.
7. ISIS-3 (Third International Study of Infarct Survival) collaborative group. ISIS-3 (TiSoIS. ISIS-3): a randomised comparison of streptokinase vs tissue plasminogen activator vs anistreplase and of aspirin plus heparin vs aspirin alone among 41,299 cases of suspected acute myocardial infarction. Lancet 1992;339:753–770.
8. Paolasso E. EMERAS Trial: results and discussion. Presented at the 40th annual scientific session of the American College of Cardiology. Atlanta, March 1991.
9. The LATE investigators. The Late Assessment of Thrombolytic Efficacy (LATE) trial. Presented at the XIV congress of the European Society of Cardiology. Barcelona, Spain, August 1992.
10. Fibrinolytic Therapy Trialists' (FTT) collaborative group. Indications for fibrinolytic therapy in suspected acute myocardial infarction: collaborative overview of results on mortality and major morbidity from the randomized trial of more than 1000 patients. Lancet 1994;343(8893):311–322.
11. Neuhaus KL. Thrombolysis in acute myocardial infarction: results of the German-Activator-Urokinase Study. Eur Heart J 1987;8:49.
12. Topol EJ. Advances in thrombolytic therapy for acute myocardial infarction. J Clin Pharmacol 1987;27:735–745.
13. AIMS Trial study group. Long-term effects of intravenous

anistreplase in acute myocardial infarction: final report of the AIMS study. AIMS Trial Study Group. Lancet 1990; 335:427–431.

14. GISSI investigators. Long-term effects of intravenous thrombolysis in acute myocardial infarction: final report of the GISSI study. Gruppo Italiano per lo Studio della Streptochi-nasi nell'Infarto Miocardico (GISSI). Lancet 1987; 2:871–874.

15. Gruppo Italiano por lo Studio della Supravvivenza nell'Infarcto Miacardio. GISSI-2: a factorial randomised trial of alteplase versus streptokinase and heparin versus no heparin among 12,490 patients with acute myocardial infarction. Gruppo Italiano per lo Studio della Sopravvivenza nell'Infarto Miocardico. Lancet 1990;336:65–71.

16. The GUSTO investigators. The international randomized trial comparing four thrombolytic strategies for acute myocardial infarction. N Engl J Med 1993;329:673–682.

17. The TIMI IIIB investigators. TIMI IIIB trial of thrombolysis in unstable angina and non q-wave myocardial infarction. Presented at the 65th scientific session of the American Heart Association. New Orleans, November 1992.

18. Reimer KA, Lowe JE, Rasmeussen MM, Jennings RB. The wave front of ischemic cell death. Myocardial infarct size vs duration of coronary occlusion in dogs. Circulation 1977;56:786–794.

19. Reimer KA, Jennings RB. The "wavefront phenomenon" of ischemic cell death. II. Transmural progression of necrosis within the frame-work of ischemic bed size and collateral flow. Lab Invest 1979;40:633–644.

20. Spann JF, Sherry S, Carabello BA, Mann RH, McCann WD, Gault JH, Gentzler RD et al. High-dose, brief intravenous streptokinase early in acute myocardial infarction. Am Heart J 1982;33:422–466.

21. Spann JF, Sherry S, Carabello BA, Denenberg BS, Mann RH, McCann WD, Gault JH et al. Coronary thrombolysis by intravenous streptokinase in acute myocardial infarction: acute and follow-up studies. Am J Cardiol 1984; 53:655–661.

22. GREAT group. Feasibility, safety, and efficacy of domiciliary thrombolysis by general practitioners: Grampian region early anistreplase trial. Br Med J 1992;305:548–553.

23. Koren G, Weiss AT, Hasin Y, Appelbaum D, Welber S, Rozenman Y, Lotan C et al. Prevention of myocardial damage in acute myocardial ischemia by early treatment with intravenous streptokinase. N Engl J Med 1985; 313:1384–1389.

24. Karagounis L, Ipsen SK, Jessop MR, Gilmore KM, Valenti DA, Clawson JJ, Teichman S et al. Impact on field-transmitted electrocardiography on time to in-hospital thrombolytic therapy in acute myocardial infarction. Am J Cardiol 1990;66:786–791.

25. Weaver WD, Cerqueria M, Hallstrom AP, Litwin PE, Martin JS, Kudenchuck PJ, Eisenberg M. Prehospital-initiated vs hospital-initiated thrombolytic therapy. The Myocardial Infarction Triage and Intervention Trial. JAMA 1993; 270:1211–1216.

26. Boissel JP. The European Myocardial Infarct Project (EMIP). Short-term mortality and nonfatal outcomes. Presented at the 41st annual scientific session of the American College of Cardiology. Dallas, April 1992.

27. Tiefenbrunn AJ, Sobel BE. Timing of coronary recanalization. Paradigms, paradoxes, and pertinence. Circulation 1992;85:2311–2315.

28. Granger CB, Califf RM, Topol EJ. Thrombolytic therapy for acute myocardial infarction. A review. Drugs 1992; 44:293–325.

29. Diaz R. EMERAS trial: study design. Presented at the 40th annual scientific session of the American College of Cardiology. Atlanta, March 1991.

30. Bates ER. Is survival in acute myocardial infarction related to thrombolytic efficacy or the open-artery hypothesis? A controversy to be investigated with GUSTO. Chest 1992;101(Suppl):140S–150S.

31. Pfeffer M, Braunwald E. Ventricular remodeling after myocardial infarction. Circulation 1990;81:1161–1172.

32. White HD, Norris RM, Brown MA, Brandt P, Whitlock R, Wild CJ. Left ventricular end-systolic volume as a major determinant of survival after recovery from acute myocardial infarction. Circulation 1987;76:44–51.

33. Hale SL, Kloner RA. Left ventricular topographic alterations in completely healed rat infarct caused by early and late coronary reperfusion. Am Heart J 1988;116:1508–1513.

34. Topol EJ, Califf RM, Vandormael M, Grines CL, George BS, Sanz ML, Wall T et al. A randomized trial of late reperfusion therapy for acute myocardial infarction. Thrombolysis and Angioplasty in Myocardial Infarction-6 Study Group. Circulation 1992;85:2090–2099.

35. White HD, Norris RM, Brown MA, Takayama M, Maslowski A, Bass NM, Ormiston JA et al. Effect of intravenous streptokinase on left ventricular function and early survival after acute myocardial infarction. N Engl J Med 1987; 317:850–855.

36. Serruys PW, Simoons ML, Suryapranata H, Vermeer F, Wijns W, van den Brand M, Bar F et al. Preservation of global and regional left ventricular function after early thrombolysis in acute myocardial infarction. J Am Coll Cardiol 1986;7:729–742.

37. Bonaduce D, Petretta M, Villari B, Breglio R, Conforti G, Montemurro MV, Lanzillo T et al. Effects of late administration of tissue-type plasminogen activator on left ventricular remodeling and function after myocardial infarction. J Am Coll Cardiol 1990;16:1561–1568.

38. Siu SC, Nidorf SM, Galambos GS, Weyman AE, Picard MH. The effect of late patency of the infarct-related coronary artery on left ventricular morphology and regional function after thrombolysis. Am Heart J 1992; 124:265–272.

39. Kersschot IE, Brugada P, Ramental M, Zehender M, Walldecker B, Stevenson WG, Geibel A et al. Effects of early reperfusion in acute myocardial infarction on arrhythmias induced by programmed electrical stimulation: a prospective, randomized study. Am J Cardiol 1986;7:1234–1242.

40. Sager PT, Perlmutter RA, Rosenfeld LE, McPherson CA, Wackers FJ, Batsford WP. Electrophysiologic effects of

thrombolytic therapy in patients with a transmural anterior myocardial infarction complicated by left ventricular aneurysm formation. J Am Coll Cardiol 1988;12:19–24.

41. Gang ES, Lew AS, Hong M, Wang FZ, Siebert CA, Peter T. Decreased incidence of ventricular late potentials after successful thrombolytic therapy for acute myocardial infarction. N Engl J Med 1989;321:712–716.

42. Ragosta M, Sabia PJ, Kaul S, DiMarco JP, Sarembock IJ, Powers E. Effects of late (1 to 30 days) reperfusion after acute myocardial infarction on the signal-averaged electrocardiogram. Am J Cardiol 1993;71:19–23.

43. Horvitz L, Pietrolungo JF, Suri S, Castle L, Trohman R, Maloney JD. An open infarct-related artery is associated with a lower risk of lethal ventricular arrhythmias in patients with left ventricular aneurysms. Circulation 1992; 86:I315.

44. van der Wall E, van Dijkman P, de Roos A, Doornbos J, van der Laarse A, Manger CV, van Voorthuisen A, Matheijssen NA, Bruschke AV. Diagnostic significance of gadolinium-DTPA (diethylenetriamine penta-acetic acid) enhanced magnetic resonance imaging in thrombolytic treatment for acute myocardial infarction: its potential in assessing reperfusion. Br Heart J 1990;63:12–17.

45. Calkins H, Maughan WL, Weisman HF, Sugiura S, Sagawa K, Levine JH. Effects of acute volume load on refracteriness and arrythmia development in isolated, chronically infarcted dog hearts. Circulation 1989; 79:687–697.

46. Cairns JA, Fuster V, Kennedy JW. Coronary thrombolysis. Chest 1992;102:482–504.

47. The GUSTO angiographic investigators. The comparative effects of tissue plasminogen activator, streptokinase, or both on coronary artery patency, ventricular function, and survival after acute myocardial infarction. N Engl J Med 1993;329:1615–1622.

48. Chesebro JH, Fuster V. Antithrombotic therapy for acute myocardial infarction: mechanisms and prevention of deep venous, left ventricular, and coronary artery thromboembolism. Circulation 1986;III:1–10.

49. Topol EJ, Califf RM, George BS, Kereiakes DJ, Abbottsmith CW, Candela RJ, Lee KL et al. A randomized trial of immediate versus delayed elective angioplasty after intravenous tissue plasminogen activator in acute myocardial infarction. N Engl J Med 1987;317:581–588.

50. National Heart Foundation of Australia Coronary Thrombolysis Group. Coronary thrombolysis and myocardial salvage by tissue plasminogen activator given up to 4 hours after onset of myocardial infarction. National Heart Foundation of Australia Coronary Thrombolysis Group (published erratum appears in Lancet 1988;2(8609):519) Lancet 1988;1:203–208.

51. Ellis SG, Topol EJ, George BS, Kereiaskes DJ, Debowey D, Sigmon KN, Pickel A et al. Recurrent ischemia without warning. Analysis of risk factors for in-hospital ischemic events following successful thrombolysis with intravenous tissue plasminogen activator. Circulation 1989; 80:1159–1165.

52. Mayne R. Collagenous proteins of blood vessels. Arteriosclerosis 1986;6:585–593 (review).

53. Parsons TJ, Haycraft DL, Hoak JC, Sage H. Interaction of platelets and purified collagens in a laminar flow model. Thromb Res 1986;43:435–443.

54. Fuster V, Badimon J. Chesebro J. The pathogenesis of coronary artery disease and acute coronary syndromes. N Engl J Med 1992;326:310–318.

55. Chesebro JH, Webster MW, Zoldhelyi P, Roche PC, Badimon L, Badimon JJ. Antithrombotic therapy and progression of coronary artery disease. Antiplatelet versus antithrombins. Circulation 1992;86(Suppl III):III-100–III-101.

56. Falk E. Plaque rupture with severe pre-existing stenosis precipitating coronary thrombosis. Characterization of coronary atherosclerotic plaques underlying fatal occlusive thrombi. Br Heart J 1983;50:127–134.

57. Davies MJ, Thomas AC. Plaque fissuring: the cause of acute myocardial infarction, sudden ischemic death, and crescendo angina. Br Heart J 1985;53:363–373.

58. Davies SW, Marchant B, Lyons JP, Timmis AD, Rothman MT, Layton CA, Balcon R. Coronary lesion morphology in acute myocardial infarction: demonstration of early remodeling after streptokinase treatment. J Am Coll Cardiol 1990;16:1079–1086.

59. Popma JJ, Califf RM, Ellis SG, George BS, Kereiakes DJ, Samaha JK, Worley SJ et al. Mechanism of benefit of combination thrombolytic therapy for acute myocardial infarction: a quantitative angiographic and hematologic study. J Am Coll Cardiol 1992;20:1305–1312.

60. Dalen JE, Gore JM, Braunwald E, Borer J, Goldberg RJ, Passamani ER, Forman S et al. Six- and twelve-month follow-up of the phase I Thrombolysis in Myocardial Infarction (TIMI) trial. Am J Cardiol 1988;62:179–185.

61. Ohman EM, Califf RM, Topol EJ, Candela R, Abbottsmith C, Ellis S, Sigmon KN et al. Consequences of reocclusion after successful reperfusion therapy in acute myocardial infarction. Circulation 1990;82:781–791.

62. Califf RM, Topol EJ, Ohman EM. Isolated recurrent ischemia after thrombolytic therapy is a frequent, important, and expensive adverse clinical outcome. J Am Coll Cardiol 1992;19:301A (abstract).

63. Gunnar RM, Bourdillon PD, Dixon DW, Fuster V, Karp RB, Kennerdy JW, Klocke FJ et al. Guidelines for the early management of patients with acute myocardial infarcton. A report of the American College of Cardiology/American Heart Association task force on assessment of diagnostic and therapeutic cardiovascular procedures (subcommittee to develop guidelines for the management of patients with acute myocardial infarction). J Am Coll Cardiol 1990;16:249–292.

64. Gold HK, Leinbach RC, Garabedian HD, Yasuda T, Johns JA, Grossbard EB, Palacios I et al. Acute coronary reocclusion after thrombolysis with recombinant human tissue-type plasminogen activator: prevention by a maintenance infusion. Circulation 1986;73:347–352.

65. Webster MI, Chesbro JH, Fuster V. Antithrombotic therapy in acute myocardial infarction: enhancement of thrombolysis, reduction of reocclusion, and prevention of thromboembolism. In: Gersh B, Rahimtoola S, eds. Acute myocardial infarction. New York: Elsvier, 1991.

66. Col J, Decoster O, Hanique G, Deligne B, Boland J,

Pirenne B, Cheron P et al. Infusion of heparin conjunct to streptokinase accelerated reperfusion of acute myocardial infarction. Results of a double-blind randomized study. Circulation 1992;86:I259 (abstract).

67. The International Study Group. In-hospital mortality and clinical course of 20,891 patients with suspected acute myocardial infarction randomised between alteplase and streptokinase with or without heparin. Lancet 1990; 336:71–75.

68. O'Connor CM, Meese R, Navetta F, Smith JE, MacKrell JP, Conn EH, Hartman KW et al. A randomized trial of heparin with anistreplase (APSAC) in myocardial infarction. Circulation 1991;84(Suppl II):II-571.

69. O'Connor CM, Roderick M, Carney R, Smith J, Conn E, Burks J, Hartman C, for the Duke University Clinical Cardiology study group (DUCCS). A randomized trial of intravenous heparin in conjunction with anistreplase (anisoylated plasminogen streptokinase activator complex) in acute myocardial infarction. J Am Coll Cardiol 1994;23:11–18.

70. Heras M, Chesebro JH, Penny WJ, Bailey KR, Badimon L, Fuster V. Effects of thrombin inhibition on the development of acute platelet-thrombus deposition during angioplasty in pigs. Heparin versus recombinant hirudin, a specific thrombin inhibitor. Circulation 1989;79:657–665.

71. Kelly AB, Hanson SR, Marzec U, Harker LA. Recombinant hirudin (r-H) interruption of platelet-dependant thrombus formation. Circulation 1988;80(Suppl II):II-311 (abstract).

72. Hanson SR, Harker LA. Interruption of acute platelet-dependant thrombosis by the synthetic antithrombin D-phenylalanyl-L-propyl-L-argyl chloromethyl ketone. Proc Natl Acad Sci USA 1988;85:3184–3188.

73. Mirshahi M, Soria J, Faivre R, Lu H, Courtney M, Roitswch C, Tripier D et al. Evaluation of the inhibition by heparin and hirudin of coagulation activation during rt-PA–induced thrombolysis. Blood 1989;74:1025–1030.

73a. The GUSTO IIAa Investigators. Randomized trial of heparin versus recombinant hirudin for acute coronary syndromes. Circulation 1994;90:1631–1637.

73b. Antman EM for the TIMI 9A Investigators. Hirudin in acute myocardial infarction. Circulation 1994;90:1624–1630.

73c. Neuhaus KL, Von Essen R, Tebbe U, Jessel A, Heinrichs H, Maürer W, Döring W et al. Safety observations from the pilot phase of the randomized r-hirudin for improvement of thrombolysis (HIT III) study. Circulation 1994;90:1638–1642.

73d. Sobel BE. Intracranial bleeding, fibrinolysis, and anticoagulation. Causal connections and clinical implications. Circulation 1994;90:2147–2151.

74. Cannon CP, McCabe CH, Henery TD, Rodgers WJ, Schweiger M, Gibson RS, Anderson L et al. Hirudin reduces reocclusion compared to heparin following thrombolysis in acute myocardial infarction. Results of the TIMI-5 trial. J Am Coll Cardiol 1993;2(Suppl A):A-136 (abstract).

75. Lidon R-M, Adelman B, Maraganore J, Theroux P. Hirulog, a direct thrombin inhibitor, for the management of unstable angina. Circulation 1992;86(Suppl I):I-386.

76. Lidon RM, Theroux P, Bonan R et al. Hirulog as adjunctive therapy to streptokinase in acute myocardial infarction. J Am Coll Cardiol 1993;21(Suppl A):419A (abstract).

77. Sharma G, Lapsley DE, Vita J, Sharma S, Coccio E, Adelman B, Loscalzo J. Usefulness and tolerability of hirulog, a direct thrombin-inhibitor, in unstable angina pectoris. Am J Med 1993;72:1357–1360.

78. Kerins DM, Roy L, FitzGerald GA, Fitzgerald DJ. Platelet and vascular function during coronary thrombolysis with tissue-type plasminogen activator. Circulation 1989; 80:1718–1725.

79. Jang I-K, Gold HK, Leinbach RC. Acceleration of reperfusion by combination of rt-PA and a selective thrombin inhibitor, argatroban. Circulation 1989;80:II-217 (abstract).

80. Tamao Y, Yamamoto T, Kikumoto R, Hara H, Itoh Z, Hirata T, Mineo K et al. Effects of a selective thrombin inhibitor MCI-9038 on fibrinolysis in vitro and in vivo. Thromb Haemost 1986;56:28–34.

81. Klement P, Boem A, Hirsh J, Maraganore J, Wilson G, Weitz J. The effects of thrombin inhibitors on tissue plasminogen activator–induced thrombolysis in the rat model. Thromb Haemost 1992;68:64–68.

82. Coller BS. Platelets and thrombolytic therapy. N Engl J Med 1990;332:33–40.

83. Kruithof EK, Tran-Thang C, Bachmann F. Studies on the release of plasminogen activator inhibitor from human platelets. Thromb Haemost 1986;55:201–205.

84. Greenberg JP, Packham MA, Guccione MA, Rand ML, Reimers HJ, Mustard JF. Survival of rabbit platelets treated in vitro with chymotrypsin, plasmin, trypsin, or neurominidase. Blood 1976;53:916–927.

85. Harrington RA, Ohman EM. Early reocclusion after thrombolytic therapy. Cardio 1993;4:26–35.

86. Popma JJ, Topol EJ. Adjuncts to thrombolysis for myocardial reperfusion. Ann Intern Med 1991;115:34–44.

87. Golino P, Ashton JH, Glas-Greenwalk P, McNatt J, Buja LM, Willerson JT. Mediation of reocclusion by thromboxane A$_2$ and serotonin after thrombolysis with tissue-type plasminogen activator in canine preparation of coronary thrombosis. Circulation 1988;77:678–684.

88. O'Brien JR. Shear-induced platelet aggregation. Lancet 1990;1:711–713.

89. Fitzgerald DJ, Catella F, Roy L, FitzGerald GA. Marked platelet activation in vivo after intravenous streptokinase in patients with acute myocardial infarction. Circulation 1988;77:142–150.

90. Gold HK, Coller BS, Yasuda T, Saito T, Fallon JT, Guerrero JL, Lienbach RC et al. Rapid and sustained coronary artery recanalization with combined bolus injection of recombinant tissue-type plasminogen activator and monoclonal antiplatelet GPIIb/IIIa antibody in a canine preparation. Circulation 1988;77:670–677.

91. Coller BS, Folts JD, Smith SR, Scudder LE, Jordan R. Abolition of in vivo platelet thrombus formation in primates with monoclonal antibodies to GPIIb/IIIa receptor. Correlation with bleeding time, platelet aggregation, and blockade of the GPIIB/IIIa receptors. Circulation 1989; 80:1766–1774.

92. Kleinman NS, Ohman EM, Califf RM, George BS,

Kerieikes D, Aguirre FV, Weisman H et al. Profound inhibition of platelet aggregation with monoclonal antibody 7E3 Fab after thrombolytic therapy. Results of the Thrombolysis and Angioplasty in Myocardial Infarction (TAMI) 8 pilot study. J Am Coll Cardiol 1993;22:381–389.

93. Song A, Scarborough RM, Phillips DR, Adelman B, Strony J. Integrelin enhances fibrinolysis and prevents arterial occlusion following thrombolysis in canine anodal current model with high-grade stenosis. Circulation 1992;86(Suppl I):8-410 (abstract).

94. Charo IF, Scarborough RM, du Mee CP, Wolf D, Phillips DR, Swift RL. Pharmacodynamics of the GPIIb/IIIa antagonist integrelin: phase I clinical studies in normal healthy volunteers. Circulation 1992;86(Suppl):I-260 (abstract).

95. Ohman EM, Califf RM: Acute myocardial infarction. Thrombolytic therapy: overview of the clinical trials. In Gersh BJ, Rahimtoola SH, eds. New York: Elsevier, 1991.

96. Carney RJ, Murphy GA, Brandt TR, Daley PJ, Pickering E, White HJ, McDonough TJ et al. Randomized angiographic trial of recombinant tissue-type plasminogen activator (alteplase) in myocardial infarction. RAAMI study investigators. J Am Coll Cardiol 1992;20:17–23.

97. Neuhaus KL, von ER, Tebbe U, Vogt A, Roth M, Riess M, Niederer W et al. Improved thrombolysis in acute myocardial infarction with front-loaded administration of alteplase: results of the rt-PA-APSAC patency study (TAPS). J Am Coll Cardiol 1992;19:885–891.

98. Neuhaus KL, Feuerer W, Jeep TS, Niederer W, Vogt A, Tebbe U. Improved thrombolysis with a modified dose regimen of recombinant tissue-type plasminogen activator. J Am Coll Cardiol 1989;14:1566-1569.

99. Califf RM, Topol EJ, Stack RS, Ellis SG, George BS, Kereiakes DJ, Samaha JK et al. Evaluation of combination thrombolytic therapy and timing of cardiac catheterization in acute myocardial infarction. Results of thrombolysis and angioplasty in myocardial infarction—phase 5 randomized trial. TAMI Study Group. Circulation 1991; 83:1543–1556.

100. Grines CL, Nissen SE, Booth DC, Gurley JC, Chelliah N, Wolf R, Blankenship J et al. A prospective, randomized trial comparing combination half-dose tissue-type plasminogen activator and streptokinase with full-dose tissue-type plasminogen activator. Kentucky Acute Myocardial Infarction Trial (KAMIT) group. Circulation 1991; 84:540–549.

101. Topol EJ, Califf RM, George BS, Kereiakes DJ, Rothbaum D, Candela RJ, Abbotsmith CW et al. Coronary arterial thrombolysis with combined infusion of recombinant tissue-type plasminogen activator and urokinase in patients with acute myocardial infarction (TAMI-2). Circulation 1988;77:1100–1107.

102. Gruenzig AR, Turina MI, Schneider JA. Experimental percutaneous dilitation of coronary artery stenosis. Circulation 1976;54:81.

103. Harker LA. Role of platelets and thrombosis in the mechanisms of acute occlusions and restenosis after angioplasty. Am J Cardiol 1987;60:20B–28B.

104. Schwartz L, Bourassa MG, Lesperence J, Aldridge HE, Kazim F, Salvatori VA, Henderson M et al. Aspirin and dipyridamole in the prevention of restenosis after percutaneous transluminal coronary angioplasty. N Engl J Med 1988;318:1714–1719.

105. Ellis SG, Roubin GS, Wilentz J, Douglas JS, King SB. Effect of 18-24 hours heparin administration for prevention of restenosis after uncomplicated coronary angioplasty. Am Heart J 1989;117:777–782.

106. Heras M, Chesebro JH, Webster M, Mruk JS, Grill DE, Penny WJ, Bowie EJ et al. Hirudin, heparin, and placebo during deep arterial injury in the pig. Circulation 1990;82:1476–1484.

107. Chesebro JH, Fuster V. Dynamic thrombosis and thrombolysis: role of antithrombins. Circulation 1991;83:1815–1817.

108. Heras M, Chesebro JH, Penny WJ, Bailey KR, Lam JY, Holmes DR, Reeder GS et al. Importance of adequate heparin dosage in arterial angioplasty in a porcine model. Circulation 1988;78:654–660.

109. Topol EJ, Bonan R, Jewitt D, Sigwart U, Kakkar VV, Rothman M, de Bono D, Ferguson J et al. Use of a direct antithrombin, hirulog, in place of heparin during coronary angioplasty. Circulation 1993;87:1622–1629.

109a. Serruys P et al. for the HELVETICAL trial investigators. Presented at the European Society of Cardiology, Berlin, September 1994.

110. van den Bos AA, Deckers JW, Heyndrickx GR, Laarman G-J, Suryapranata H, Zijlstra F, Close P et al. Safety and efficacy of recombinant hirudin (CGP 39 393) versus heparin in patients with stable angina undergoing coronary angioplasty. Circulation 1993;88:2058–2066.

111. Topol EJ, Califf RM, Weisman HS, Ellis SG, Tcheng JE, Worley S, Ivanhoe R et al. Reduction of clinical restenosis following coronary intervention with early administration of platelet IIb/IIIa integrin blocking antibody. Lancet 1994;343:881–886.

112. Anderson KM, Tannenbaum MA, Sanz ML, Wang AL, Weisman HF. Clinical events following initially successful PTCA are platelet mediated. Results from the EPIC trial. Circulation 1993;88(Suppl):I-506.

113. Ellis SG, Tcheng JT, Navetta FL et al. Safety and antiplatelet effect of murine monoclonal antibody 7E3 Fab directed against platelet glycoprotein IIb/IIIa in patients undergoing elective coronary angioplasty. Cor Art Dis 1993;4:167–175.

114. Grill HP, Brinker JA. Nonacute thrombolytic therapy: an adjunct to coronary angioplasty in patients with large intravascular thrombi. Am Heart J 1989;118:662–667.

115. Kiesz RS, Hennecken JF, Bailey SR. Bolus administration of intracoronary urokinase during PTCA in the presence of intraluminal thrombus. Circulation 1991; 84:II-346 (abstract).

116. Pavlides GS, Schreiber TL, Gangaharan V, Puchrowiz S, O'Neill WW. Safety and efficacy of urokinase during elective coronary angioplasty. Am Heart J 1991;127:731–736.

117. Ambrose JA, Torree SR, Sharma SK, Israel DH, Monsen CE, Weiss M, Untereker W et al. Adjunctive thrombolytic therapy for angioplasty in ischemic rest angina: results of a double-blind randomized pilot study. J Am Coll Cardiol 1992;20:1197–1204.

118. Kahn JK, Hartzler GO. Frequency and causes of failure with contemporary balloon coronary angioplasty and implications for new technologies. Am J Cardiol 1990;66:858–860.

119. Zidar F. Schreiber T, Jones D, Puchrowicz-Ochocki S, Ajluni S, Hollongsworth V, Timmis GC et al. A prospective trial of prolonged urokinase infusion for chronic total occlusion in native coronary arteries. Circulation 1993; 88:I-505 (abstract).

120. Hartman J, McKeever LS, Enger EL, O'Neill WW. Recanalization of chronically occluded bypass grafts with prolonged urokinase infusion site trial. Circulation 1993; 88:I-504 (abstract).

121. Yusuf S, Collins R, Peto R, Furberg C, Stampfer MJ, Goldhaber SZ, Hennekens CH. Intravenous and intracoronary fibrinolytic therapy in acute myocardial infarction: overview of results on mortality, reinfarction, and side effects from 33 randomized controlled trials. Eur Heart J 1985;6:556–583.

122. Fennerty AG, Levine MN, Hirsh J. Hemorrhagic complications of thrombolytic therapy in the treatment of myocardial infarction and venous thromboembolism. Chest 1989;95:885–975.

123. Topol EJ, Califf RM. Thrombolytic therapy for elderly patients. N Engl J Med 1992;327:45–47.

124. Grines CL, Browne KF, Vandormael M, Stone G, O'Keefe J, Overile P, Puchrowicz-Ochocki S et al. Primary angioplasty in Myocardial Infarction (PAMI) trial. Circulation 1992;86:I-641.

125. O'Neill WW, Weintraub R, Grines CL, Meany TB, Brodie BR, Friedman HZ, Ramos RG et al. A prospective, placebo-controlled, randomized trial of intraveous streptokinase and angioplasty versus lone angioplasty therapy of acute myocardial infarction. Circulation 1992;86:1710–1717.

126. Grines CL, Browne KF, Marco J, Rothbaum D, Stone GW, O'Keefe J, Overlie P et al. A comparison of immediate angioplasty with thrombolytic therapy for acute myocardial infarction. The Primary Angioplasty in Myocardial Infarction study group. N Engl J Med 1993;328:673–679.

127. Doorey AJ, Michelson EL, Weber FJ, Dreifus LS. Thrombolytic therapy of acute myocardial infarction: emerging challenges to implementation. J Am Coll Cardiol 1987; 10:1357–1360.

128. Murray N, Lyons J, Layton C, Balcon R. What proportion of patients with myocardial infarction are suitable for thrombolysis? Br Heart J 1987;57:144–147.

129. Jagger JD, Murray RG, Davies MK, Littler WA et al. Eligibility for thrombolytic therapy in acute myocardial infarction. Lancet 1987;1:34–35.

130. Cragg DR, Friedman HZ, Bonema JK, Jaiyesimi IA, Ramos RG, Timmis GC, O'Neill WW et al. Outcome of patients with acute myocardial infarction who are ineligible for thrombolytic agents. Ann Intern Med 1991; 115:173–177.

131. Muller DW, Topol EJ, Califf RM, Sigmon KN, Gorman L, George BS, Kereiakes DJ et al. Relationship between antecedent angina pectoris and short-term prognosis after thrombolytic therapy for acute myocardial infarction. Thrombolysis and Angioplasty in Myocardial Infarction (TAMI) study group. Am Heart J 1990;119:224–231.

132. Califf RM, Topol EJ, George BS, Boswick JM, Lee KL, Stump D, Dillon J et al. Characteristics and outcome of patients in whom reperfusion with intravenous tissue-type plasminogen activator fails: results of the Thrombolysis and Angioplasty in Myocardial Infarction (TAMI) I trial. Circulation 1988;77:1090–1099.

133. Ellis SG, Van de Werf F, Ribeiro dSE, Topol EJ. Present status of rescue coronary angioplasty: current polarization of opinion and randomized trials. J Am Coll Cardiol 1992;19:681–686 (editorial).

134. Ellis SG, Debowey D, Bates ER, Topol EJ. Treatment of recurrent ischemia after thrombolysis and successful reperfusion for acute myocardial infarction. Effects on in-hospital mortality and left ventricular dysfunction. J Am Coll Cardiol 1991;17:752–757.

135. Collen D, Stassen JM, Demarsin E, Kieckens L, Lijnen HR, Nelles L. Pharmacokinetics and thrombolytic properties of chimaeric plasminogen activators consisting of the NH_2-terminal region of human tissue-type plasminogen activator and the COOH-terminal region of human single-chain urokinase-type plasminogen activator. J Vasc Med Biol 1989;1:234–240.

136. Collen D. Designing thrombolytic agents: focus on safety and efficacy. Am J Cardiol 1992;69:71A–81A.

137. Nelles L, Lijnen HR, Collen D, Holmes WE. Characterization of recombinant human single-chain urokinase-type plasminogen activator mutants produced by site-specific mutagenesis of lysine 158. J Biol Chem 1987; 262:5682–5689.

138. Gardell SJ, Ramjit DR, Stabilito JJ, Tsuneo F, Lynch JJ, Cuca GC, Deepak F et al. Effective thrombolysis without marked plasminogenemia following bolus administration of a vampire bat salivary plasminogen activator in rabbits. Circulation 1991;84:244–253.

139. Eisenberg PR. Role of new anticoagulants as adjunctive therapy during thrombolysis. Am J Cardiol 1991; 67:19A–24A.

140. Verstraete M. Advances in thrombolytic therapy. Cardiovasc Drugs Ther 1992;6:111–124.

141. Heras M, Chesebro JH, Penny WJ, Bailey L, Badimon L, Fuster V. Effects of thrombin inhibition on the development of acute platelet-thrombus deposition during angioplasty in pigs: heparin versus recombinant hirudin, a specific thrombin inhibitor. Circulation 1989;79:657–665.

142. Chesebro JH, Knatterud G, Roberts R, Borer J, Cohen LS, Dalen J, et al. Thrombolysis in Myocardial Infarction (TIMI) trial, phase I: a comparison between intravenous tissue plasminogen activator and intravenous streptokinse. Clinical findings through hospital discharge. Circulation 1987;76:142–154.

143. Lincoff AM, Ellis SG, Galeana A, Lee K. Rosenschen U. Is a coronary artery with TIMI grade 2 flow "patent"? Outcome in the Thrombolysis and Angioplasty in Myocardial Infarction trial. Circulation 1992;86(Suppl):I-268 (abstract).

144. Anderson JL, Karagounis LA, Becker LC, Sorensen SG, Menlove RL. TIMI perfusion grade 3 but not grade 2

results in improved outcome after thrombolysis for myocardial infarction. Ventriculographic, enzymatic, and electrocardiographic evidence from the TEAM-3 study. Circulation 1993;87:1829–1839.

145. Karagounis L, Sorensen SG, Menlove RL, Moreno F, Anderson JL. Does thrombolysis in myocardial infarction (TIMI) perfusion grade 2 represent a mostly patent artery or a mostly occluded artery? Enzymatic and electrocardiographic evidence from the TEAM-2 study. Second multicenter thrombolysis trial of eminase in acute myocardial infarction. J Am Coll Cardiol 1992;19:1–10.

146. Vogt A, von ER, Tebbe U, Feuerer W, Appel KF, Neuhaus KL. Impact of early perfusion status of the infarct-related artery on short-term mortality after thrombolysis for acute myocardial infarction: retrospective analysis of four German multicenter studies. J Am Coll Cardiol 1993; 21:1391–1395.

147. Lincoff AM, Topol EJ. Illusion of reperfusion. Does anyone achieve optimal reperfusion during acute myocardial infarction? Circulation 1993;87:1792–1805.

148. Grines CL, Topol EJ, Bates ER, Juni JE, Walton JJ, O'Neill WW. Infarct vessel status after intravenous tissue plasminogen activator and acute coronary angioplasty: prediction of clinical outcome, Am Heart J 1988;115:1–7.

149. Wall T, Mark DB, Califf RM, Collins G, Burgess R, Skelton TN, Hinohara T et al. Prediction of early recurrent myocardial ischemia and coronary reocclusion after successful thrombolysis. An angiographic study. Am J Cardiol 1989;63:423–428.

150. Anderson JL, Becker LC, Sherman SG, Labros KA, Browne KF, Shah PK, Morris DC et al. Anistreplase versus alteplase in acute myocardial infarction: comparative effects on left ventricular function, morbidity, and 1-day coronary artery patency. J Am Coll Cardiol 1992; 20:753–766.

151. Kennedy JW, Martin GV, Davis KB, Maynard C, Stadius M, Sheehan FH, Ritchie JL. The Western Washington intravenous streptokinase in acute myocardial infarction randomized trial. Circulation 1988;77:345–352.

152. Guerci AD, Gerstenblith G, Brinker JA, Chandra NC, Gottlieb SO, Bahr RD, Weiss JL et al. A randomized trial of intravenous tissue plasminogen activator for acute myocardial infarction with subsequent randomization to elective coronary angioplasty. N Engl J Med 1987; 317:1613–1618.

153. O'Rourke M, Baron D, Keogh A, Kelly R, Nelson G, Barnes C, Raftos J et al. Limitation of myocardial infarction by early infusion of recombinant tissue-type plasminogen activator. Circulation 1988;77:1311–1315.

154. Van de Werf F, Arnold AER. Intravenous tissue plasminogen activator and size of infarct, left ventricular function, and survival in acute myocardial infarction (ECSG-4). Br Med J 1988;287:1374–1379.

155. Armstrong PW, Baigrie RS, Daly PA, Haq A, Gent M, Roberts RS, Freeman MR et al. Tissue plasminogen activator: Toronto (TPAT) placebo-controlled randomized trial in acute myocardial infarction. J Am Coll Cardiol 1989; 13:1469–1476.

156. Magnani B. Plasminogen Activator Italian Multicenter Study (PAIMS): comparison of intravenous recombinant single-chain human tissue-type plasminogen activator (rt-PA) with intravenous streptokinase in acute myocardial infarction. J Am Coll Cardiol 1989;13:19–26.

157. White HD, Rivers JT, Maslowski AH, Ormiston JA, Takayama M, Hart HH, Sharpe DN et al. Effect of intravenous streptokinase as compared with that of tissue plasminogen activator on left ventricular function after first myocardial infarction. N Engl J Med 1989;320:817–821.

158. Neuhaus KL, Tebbe U, Gottwik M, Weber MA, Feuerer W, Niederer W, Haerer W et al. Intravenous recombinant tissue plasminogen activator (rt-PA) and urokinase in acute myocardial infarction: results of the German Activator Urokinase Study (GAUS). J Am Coll Cardiol 1988; 12:581–587.

159. Bassand JP, Cassagnes J, Machecourt J, Lusson JR, Anguenot T, Wolf JE, Maublant J et al. Comparative effects of APSAC and rt-PA on infarct size and left ventricular function in acute myocardial infarction. A multicenter randomized study. Circulation 1991;84:1107–1117.

160. Topol EJ, George BS, Kereiakes DJ, Stump DC, Candela RJ, Abbottsmith CW, Aronson L et al. for the TAMI-3 group. A randomized controlled trial of intravenous tissue plasminogen activator and early intravenous heparin in acute myocardial infarction. Circulation 1989; 79:281–286.

161. Hsia J, Hamilton WP, Kleinman N, Roberts R, Chaitman BR, Ross AM. A comparison between heparin and low-dose aspirin as adjunctive therapy with tissue plasminogen activator for acute myocardial infarction. Heparin-Aspirin Reperfusion Trial (HART) investigators. N Engl J Med 1990;323:1433–1437.

162. Bleich SD, Nichols TC, Schumacher RR, Cooke DH, Tate DA, Teichman SL. Effect of heparin on coronary arterial patency after thrombolysis with tissue plasminogen activator in acute myocardial infarction. Am J Cardiol 1990;66;1412–1417.

163. The SCATI (Studio sulla Calciparina nell'Angina e nella Trombosi Ventricolare nell'Infarto) group. Randomised controlled trial of subcutaneous calcium-heparin in acute myocardial infarction. Lancet 1989; 2:182–186.

164. Verstraete M, Bernard R, Bory M, Brower RW, Collen D, Bono D, Erbel R, et al. Randomised trial of intravenous recombinant tissue-type plasminogen activator versus intravenous streptokinase in acute myocardial infarction. Report from the European Cooperative Study Group for Recombinant Tissue-Type Plasminogen Activator. Lancet 1985;1:842–847.

165. Verstraete M, Bleifeld W, Brower RW, Charbonnier B, Collen D, de Bono D, Dunning AJ et al. Double-blind randomised trial of intravenous tissue-type plasminogen activator versus placebo in acute myocardial infarction. Lancet 1985;2:965–969.

166. Topol EJ, Morris DC, Smalling RW, Schumacher RR, Taylor CR, Nishikawa A, Liberman HA et al. A multicenter, randomized, placebo-controlled trial of a new form of intravenous recombinant tissue-type plasminogen activator (activase) in acute myocardial infarction. J Am Coll Cardiol 1987;9:1205–1213.

167. Smalling RW, Schumacher R, Morris D, Harder K, Fuentes F, Valentine RP, Battey LJ et al. Improved infarct-related arterial patency after high dose, weight-adjusted, rapid infusion of tissue-type plasminogen activator in myocardial infarction: results of a multicenter randomized trial of two dosage regimens. J Am Coll Cardiol 1990;15:915–921.

168. Wall TC, Califf RM, George BS, Ellis SG, Samaha JK, Kereiakes DJ, Worley SJ et al. Accelerated plasminogen activator dose regimens for coronary thrombolysis. The TAMI-7 study group. J Am Coll Cardiol 1992;19:482–489.

169. Gemmill JD, Hogg KJ, MacIntyre PD, Booth N, Rae AP, Dunn FG, Hillis WS. A pilot study of the efficacy and safety of bolus administration of alteplase in acute myocardial infarction. Br Heart J 1991;66:134–138.

170. Purvis JA, Trouton TG, Roberts MJ, McKeown P, Mulholland MG, Dalzell GW, Wilson CM et al. Effectiveness of double-bolus alteplase in the treatment of acute myocardial infarction. Am J Cardiol 1991;68:1570–1574.

171. Anderson JL, Gomez MA, Karagounis LA. Very early thrombolysis for acute myocardial infarction. Challenges of thrombolytic therapy. II. Time to treatment. Am J Cardiol (Continuing Education Series) 1993;5–12.

172. Muller DW, Topol EJ. Selection of patients with acute myocardial infarction for thrombolytic therapy. Ann Intern Med 1990;113:949–960.

40. Local Drug Delivery

A. Prospects for Local Drug Delivery

KEITH A. ROBINSON and SPENCER B. KING III

The restenosis rate of 30 to 45% following balloon coronary angioplasty and new interventional procedures remains a major concern (1). Also, while evidence suggests that prosthetic stenting may reduce the lesion recurrence rate in certain patient subgroups (2), the rigorous anticoagulant therapy that may be needed to prevent acute thrombosis raises the specter of hemorrhagic complications (3). These iatrogenic phenomena, restenosis and thrombosis, have been the focus of intense research in the realms of cellular and molecular biology, pharmacology, and bioengineering for a number of years.

While certain systemic drug therapies have been shown effective against arterial injury–induced intimal thickening or smooth muscle cell (SMC) proliferation in some animal models, they have failed in other models, or require doses unattainable in the clinical setting because of side effects. Therefore strategies for the localized delivery of potential antirestenotic, as well as antithrombotic, compounds are under investigation. It is hoped that such systems might eventually provide a means to effectively treat the angioplasty site with pharmaceutical agents at high concentration yet a low total dose. In this way the dilemma inherent in any systemically administered therapy might be avoided; that is, how to achieve an efficacious drug level where it is needed, without producing toxic sequelae.

Experimental approaches for such localized vascular therapy are numerous, but can be grouped into four main categories: (a) use of modified balloon catheters that transfer substances into the arterial wall via balloon perforations, or by means of hydrophilic polymer coatings; (b) delivery of substances at the luminal surface by infusion or at the adventitial surface by polymer implantation or external coating of the artery; (c) luminal implantation of biodegradable or biocompatible polymers, which could incorporate active compounds, as stent material or stent coverings; and (d) cell-mediated delivery such as infusion of endothelial cells (EC) or implantation of EC-seeded stents, or injection of platelets containing substances incorporated by electropermeation. Some of these strategies have little potential practical value for the interventional cardiologist, since they necessitate surgical entry to the arterial site, and will only be considered briefly here as specific studies relate to the pathobiology of the arterial injury response and the concepts of local delivery. Also, many other approaches for targeted drug delivery to specific cells and tissues exist such as linkage to immunoglobulins, but description of these myriad techniques is beyond the scope of this writing. We will instead concentrate primarily on devices and strategies that have laid a foundation for practical application to the problems of iatrogenic restenosis and thrombosis after percutaneous angioplasty of the coronary arteries.

Implicit in many of the current approaches to local delivery is at least the intention, if not the means, to ensure long-term sustained release of the administered compound. Experimental attempts to inhibit intimal thick-ening after arterial injury in animal models by a single perfusion of the arterial wall with substances in simple aqueous solution have largely been negative, although recent stud-ies suggest a positive effect of the cyclic octapeptide angiopeptin (4, 5). Prolonged release from biodegradable polymers (either as stent material, stent covering, or micropar-ticles for wall perfusion) should be feasible by varying the composition of the material to control the degradation rate; however, such material evokes an intense inflammatory response in the coronary arteries of pigs, a species that is considered a reasonable approximation of human coronary arterial injury (6). Therefore it may be of considerable interest to explore the possibility of conjugat-ing active substances such as synthetic pep-tides, oligonucleotides, or DNA constructs to a dense, inert microparticle that could on delivery become entrapped in the tissue at the angioplasty site and remain indefinitely with-out adverse effect while slowly leaching its conjugate to surrounding cells. Accordingly, some of our recent experiments using col-loidal gold, a microparticulate marker sus-pension with potential utility as a delivery vehicle, will be described.

MODIFIED BALLOON CATHETERS

The double-balloon catheter, by which a desired segment of artery can be temporarily isolated from its surroundings and exposed to solutions or suspensions through an acces-sory injection port, was one of the first in what has become a crowded field of complementary gadgets (Fig. 40A.1*A*). This device was used to transfer genetically modified endothelial cells, as well as retrovirus- and liposome-packaged DNA, to balloon-injured iliac arter-ies in microswine (7, 8). These studies not only demonstrated that simple but prolonged exposure (at least 30 min) of the de-endothe-lialized arterial surface could result in effec-tive fluid transfer, but introduced gene ther-apy technology to interventional cardiology.

Unfortunately, successful application of this catheter in the clinical setting may re-quire conditions infrequently encountered in diseased human coronary arteries—a rela-tively long segment without branch arteries—to avoid loss of the infusate. Other technical improvements such as flow-through capacity enabling prolonged inflation may make this device feasible when side-branch runoff is not a problem.

The porous balloon catheter represents the simplest and most straightforward approach to localized delivery and has been shown in a number of studies to enable transfer of mark-ers and labeled pharmaceutical compounds. Four rows of seven laser-drilled 25-μm-sized holes in a PTCA balloon create fluid streams that are intended to saturate the tunica intima and media, and that can penetrate the exter-nal membrane to the adventitia and perivas-cular space with higher driving pressures (Fig. 40A.1*B*).

The arterial wall transfer of aqueous solu-tions using the porous balloon catheter was studied by Wolinsky and Thung (9). They demonstrated that low–molecular weight markers, as well as fluoresceinated heparin and proteins (ferritin, horseradish peroxi-dase), could be deposited in vivo in dog arter-ies and retained for several days. The results were encouraging in terms of the efficacy of fluid uptake and apparent retention, but men-tion was made of the potential for tissue dam-age from high-pressure fluid streaming, including medial dissection and edema.

One of our own experiments examined the histopathologic and dye-penetrating effects of various driving pressures and infusate vol-umes in pig coronary arteries (10). It was ob-served that adequate penetration (to the perivascular space) of 2 ml of methylene blue occurred at only 2 atm. Up to 5 ml vol-ume of 0.9% NaCl solution delivered at this pressure was safe; 10 ml, however, resulted in myocardial hematoma, ventricular fibril-lation, and death in two animals tested. At 2 atm pressure using 3 ml saline, there was lit-

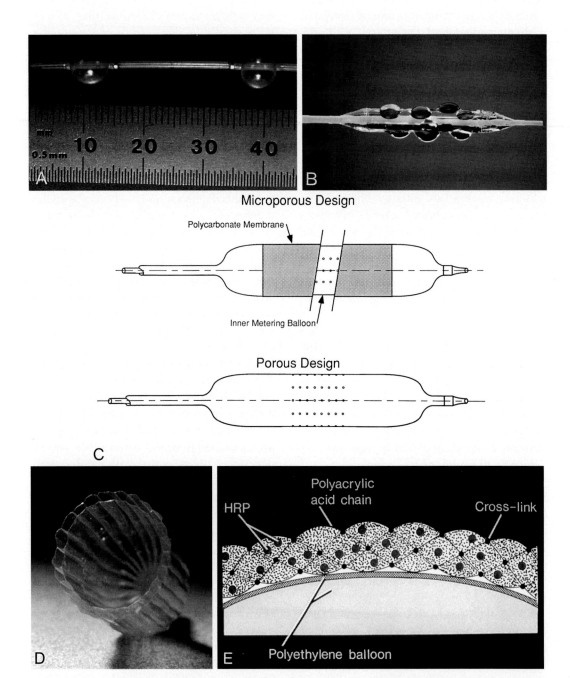

Figure 40A.1. Photographs and diagrams of modified balloon catheters for local drug delivery. **A.** Double-balloon catheter. (Courtesy of Christine Enger, USCI Division, CR Bard, Inc.) **B.** Porous balloon catheter. (Courtesy of Christine Enger, USCI Division, CR Bard, Inc.) **C.** Schematic diagram of microporous infusion catheter compared with porous balloon catheter. (Courtesy of Dr. Charles Lambert, University of S. Alabama, and Steve Rowland, Ph.D., Cordis Inc.) **D.** Channeled balloon catheter seen in cross section. (Courtesy of James Barry, Ph.D., Boston Scientific, Inc.) **E.** Schematic diagram of portion of hydrogel-coated balloon catheter in cross section with horseradish peroxidase marker in hydrogel matrix. (Courtesy of James Barry, Ph.D., Boston Scientific, Inc.)

tle medial damage; at 5 and 10 atm, there was increasing damage, including disorganization of medial SMC, disruption of medial layers, and dissection. Thus safe and efficacious use of the standard porous balloon for 3-mm coronary arteries may take place using infusate volumes of up to 3 ml and low pressures. However, in this study there was no effect of high-dose heparin administration through the porous balloon, at sites of acute overstretch arterial injury in the swine coronaries, on subsequent neointimal thickening. Presumably, if active heparin was indeed transferred to the arterial sites, it was not retained or its efficacy against SMC growth and matrix synthesis was limited.

The effect of porous balloon perfusion of injured pig carotid arteries with the antineoplastic agent methotrexate was analyzed by Muller and coworkers (11). Tritiated methotrexate was injected at the site of angioplasty; scintillation counting revealed significant acute uptake and measurable persistence of activity at 1 week. However, at 2 weeks the beta activity was at background level, and at 4 weeks no effect of porous ballooning with methotrexate on intimal thickening compared with controls receiving saline injection was observed.

A number of possibilities for the failure of this and other attempts to inhibit the restenosis-like response in animal models, using known antiproliferative agents and the porous balloon catheter, have been suggested (11). Two points regarding local delivery strategies are relevant to such a discussion: (a) the presence of fluorescence, radioactivity, or other labels linked to active compounds does not necessarily indicate the presence of biologic activity; (b) the acute deposition and long-term retention patterns of a substance may have considerable effect on its ability to alter cellular functions associated with restenosis, including not only the mitosis of SMCs, but their motile and synthetic capacities, as well as contributory phenomena such as thrombosis and inflammation. If the activity is altered, or if the compound is not where it should be (e.g., within the tunica media, medial and medial/adventitial dissection planes; associated with cells rather than extracellular matrix components), then the functional consequence may be adversely affected.

One way to assess effective transfer from a functional perspective is to perform gene transfer. The porous balloon was used for demonstration of arterial gene transfer by Flugelman and colleagues, who used retroviral carriers to perfuse rabbit aortas with cDNA constructs encoding for either bacterial β-galactosidase or the human LDL receptor, with sequences inserted for neomycin phosphotransferase (12). Analysis of tissues by X-Gal staining, LDL receptor immunohistochemistry, and polymerase chain reaction amplification and Southern blotting of extracted DNA for the phosphotransferase gene yielded sobering results, consistent with an estimated transduction of only one in 10^5 cells of the aortic wall. It is difficult to reconcile these findings with those of Nabel et al. (8), who achieved transmural expression of β-galactosidase up to 5 months after transfection using the double-balloon catheter. It may be that duration of exposure of the arterial tissue to the infused substance is crucial for cellular uptake and functional response.

This concept of duration of exposure received circumstantial support from the work of Chapman and associates, who used a modified version of the porous balloon catheter that allowed blood flow through the catheter body and thus prolonged infusion of a luciferase expression vector into the wall of canine coronary arteries (13). There was some suggestion of increased luciferase activity at 3 to 5 days in arteries transfected by 10 min compared to 1.5 min perfusion, but statistical correlation was not given. Also, the calculated amount of the phosphorescent protein in the entire arterial segment, while statistically different from nontransfected controls, was dismally low (mean = 4.3 pg). Furthermore, 25 ml of infusate was required to achieve even this level of expression, a volume that may induce arrythmogenic complications in the clinical setting.

Another investigative method involves application of microparticle technology, which in theory may enhance both acute deposition and long-term retention of biologically active substances. Wilensky and colleagues injected large (5 μm) polystyrene microspheres into atherosclerotic rabbit iliac arteries, using the porous balloon catheter, to study the feasibility of such a drug delivery system (14). They reported particle retention in the neointima, media, and adventitia for 2 weeks, and suggested that arterial wall injection of biodegradable microparticles containing active

compounds might be the next logical step toward a novel antirestenotic therapeutic strategy. Unfortunately, the delivery of biologically active substances in such a matrix (polylactide, polyglycolide) may introduce other problems, especially leukocytosis as observed when such materials are implanted as vascular grafts or in tandem with metallic stents. Other vehicles may avoid such complications.

One such potential vehicle is colloidal gold. Gold particles have been used as carriers of foreign genes for transfection of plant and animal cells in vitro and in vivo (15, 16) ("microprojectile bombardment," "gene gun," or "biolistic technology"). Not only nucleic

Figure 40A.2. Scanning electron microscopy of luminal surface of pig coronary artery fixed 15 minutes after porous balloon injection of colloidal gold microparticle suspension. **A.** Conventional secondary electron image. **B.** Backscatter electron (BSE) image of same microscopic field. Gold is demonstrated by BSE *(arrows)* in craterlike depression created by fluid stream from porous balloon catheter.

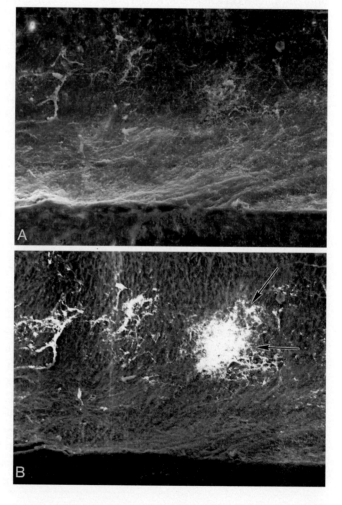

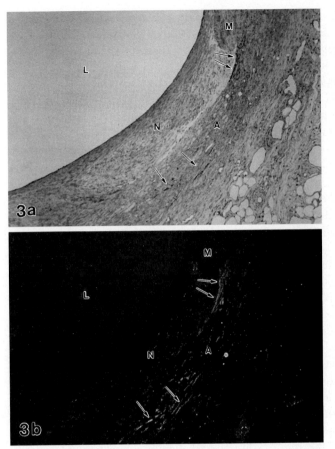

Figure 40A.3. Light microscopy of pig coronary artery perfused in vivo with colloidal gold suspension from porous balloon after balloon overstretch injury harvested at 2 weeks. **A.** Gold deposits are seen persisting in adventitia and around dissected ends of tunica media *(arrows)*. *M,* Media; *L,* lumen; *N,* Neointima; *A,* adventitia. **B.** Same microscopic field photographed under polarized illumination.

acids but a wide range of other compounds, including dextran, polyethylene glycol, and proteins, adhere to colloidal gold through electrostatic adsorption; the latter property provides the basis for its widespread use as an immunolabel for electron microscopy, and by silver enhancement for light microscopy and immunoblotting. We have performed preliminary experiments using colloidal gold as a perfusate suspension in the porous balloon catheter to determine the safety, feasibility, and deposition pattern of such a microparticle delivery strategy, as well as survey its potential for active substance transfer (17). In normal pig coronary arteries at 4 atm of pressure, there is periluminal distribution of the gold suspension with focal heavy deposits associated with craterlike depressions, presumably from fluid jet effects (Fig. 40A.2). Addition-

ally, there is penetration of the arterial wall leaving large perivascular colloidal gold deposits in the adipose tissue. Arteries perfused with the gold suspension after overstretch balloon injury showed gold staining, associated primarily with the medial defect, which persisted at 2 weeks following treatment (Fig. 40A.3).

The amount of arterial injury we observed in specimens acutely perfused with colloidal gold was mild and similar to damage seen in arteries perfused with saline solution at similar pressure and volume (i.e., endothelial desquamation, mild medial disorganization, and edema). Nevertheless, the suspension penetrated to the perivascular tissue in the absence of hematoma or apparent medial dissection, although we cannot rule out the latter. The extravascular deposition we observed may not be an undesirable effect; perivascular application of heparin or antisense oligonucleotides conjugated to biopolymers for sustained release has been effective against balloon injury–induced neointimal formation in rat and rabbit carotid arteries (see below). Quantitation, long-term retention, and drug conjugation characteristics of colloidal gold suspension delivered with the porous balloon are currently under investigation.

The microporous infusion catheter has some similarities to the porous balloon, but eliminates fluid streaming by a double-walled design (Fig. 40A.1C). Large (20 to 25 μm) laser-drilled pores are present in an inner balloon, identical to the porous balloon, which dispense fluid to the inter-balloon space. The outer balloon consists of a polycarbonate membrane with holes 0.8 μm in size, at a density of $3 \times 10^7/cm^2$, which allow fluid to escape to the exterior (18). Potential injurious effects of local therapy are therefore minimized, while the luminal surface of the treated site is saturated with fluid that seeps rather than streams from the interior.

Lambert and associates studied the flow characteristics, as well as dye penetration into agar test blocks, and the histopathologic effects on arteries using the microporous infusion catheter (18). Compared with the porous balloon, which created linear tracts of dye penetration into the agar blocks and at high pressure caused significant tissue damage (including medial disorganization and jet-related crater formation), the microporous infusion catheter showed low-velocity circumferential flow, circumferential dye penetration into agar without dissection tracts, and negligible arterial trauma, consisting of endothelial denudation, subendothelial edema, and fracture of internal elastic lamina related to balloon oversizing.

Experiments performed in our laboratory demonstrated that both tritiated heparin (CN Thomas, manuscript submitted) and colloidal gold microparticles (KA Robinson, manuscript submitted) are successfully transferred to porcine coronary arteries in vivo using the microporous infusion catheter. About 1% of the radioactivity associated with a given quantity of tritiated heparin in solution was detected 3 minutes after infusion into normal, uninjured vessels. Activity persisted at this level in arteries removed up to 60 minutes after infusion. In the second study, a 2-ml volume of colloidal gold microparticles was infused at sites of acute balloon overstretch injury. In this instance microscopic analysis revealed a periluminal distribution of particles, which were associated with damaged endothelial cells, the luminal aspect of exposed elastica interna, and within platelet-fibrin microthrombi.

Another design that can minimize jet effects and related arterial trauma is the *channeled balloon catheter*. This apparatus uncouples balloon inflation from local fluid delivery by a double-walled construction in which the inner high-pressure angioplasty balloon is surrounded by multiple channels, with pores at the outer balloon surface, fed by a separate inflation port (Fig. 40A.1D). These "intramural channels" thus permit local infusion of markers or drugs during vessel dilation. The uptake of markers was studied by Hong et al. who demonstrated medial penetration of horseradish peroxidase and a significant uptake of ^{125}I-insulin in rabbit iliac arteries without evidence of medial dissection from jet effects (19). Experiments performed by our group (CN Thomas, manuscript submitted) indicate that channeled balloon infusion of heparin into preclotted Dacron grafts in a porcine ex vivo arteriovenous shunt model significantly reduces subsequent deposition of ^{111}In-labeled platelets.

The *hydrogel-coated balloon catheter* is a device that obviates concerns over fluid jet-related tissue damage, since substance transfer is achieved by contact of the balloon coating with the arterial intima. To load the catheter, the inflated hydrogel-coated balloon is dipped into an aqueous solution of marker or active compound and allowed to dry. The balloon is then deflated, advanced to the site intended for treatment, and reinflated to transfer the marker or active substance (Fig. 40A.1, *E* and *F*). Fram and colleagues demonstrated successful uptake of horseradish peroxidase into porcine arteries in vitro and in vivo; penetration was deeper with higher pressure and longer duration of inflation (20). Nunes and Scott from our laboratory showed that local delivery of either heparin or the thrombin inhibitor D-Phe-Pro-Arg-chloromethyl ketone to preclotted vascular grafts in the porcine ex vivo shunt model was achieved using the coated balloon (21, 22). A potential problem, however, is the rapid loss of the coating once the prepared catheter is reexposed to an aqueous environment; >90% loss occurs within seconds (23; CN Thomas, unpublished data). A protective peel-back sheath has been developed that may retard this process. Recently, Riessen et al. demonstrated successful transfer of the luciferase expression vector from the hydrogel balloon into rabbit iliac arteries, via a carotid artery approach, using this protective sheath (24). Mitchel and coworkers showed decreased platelet deposition in animal models of arterial injury and lysed coronary thrombus in 15 patients with the device (25).

A different device has been developed but used by the same group to enhance coronary thrombolysis (26). The *"Dispatch" catheter* (not shown) uses a spiral balloon ribbing to approximate a membrane to the artery wall, creating a space into which drug is infused. Since the arterial lumen is left largely open, prolonged residence time is feasible.

Finally, an *iontophoretic balloon* has been produced that uses an electrical current gradient to drive charged molecules in solution into the tissues. This device was found by Fernandez-Ortiz and associates to efficiently load pig carotid arteries with labeled r-hirudin, but 80% loss was measured at 3 hours (27).

ADVENTITIAL DELIVERY AND INFUSION AT THE LUMINAL SURFACE

At least three systems have been developed and shown to achieve biologic effects. Edelman et al. used heparin (both anticoagulant and nonanticoagulant fragments) conjugated to *ethylene-vinyl acetate copolymer* to produce slab-shaped matrices that were implanted adjacent to the common carotid artery in rats after balloon endothelial denudation (28). By further coating the matrix pellet with unconjugated copolymer, allowing matrix degradation through a single needle hole, a near zero-order drug release kinetic was achieved. The percent luminal occlusion of the carotid arteries by neointima formation was significantly reduced compared with arteries in which blank slabs were implanted periadventitially, or when active slabs were placed in the dorsal subcutaneous space. These experiments, while using a system requiring surgical implantation and therefore possessing little immediate applicability for the interventionalist, earmarked the potential efficacy of localized delivery against restenosis.

Biologically active substances can also be mixed with polymer gels and applied as coatings to the adventital aspect of arteries. Okada et al. applied a *heparin-polyvinyl alcohol gel* to the outer surface of balloon de-endothelialized rat carotid arteries, and surrounded it with a Silastic covering to prevent release to other tissues (29). A significant reduction in cross-sectional area of the intima and preservation of the luminal area was observed without change in systemic coagulation parameters.

Antisense c-*myb* oligonucleotides were mixed with a *pluronic copolymer*, which is liquid at 4°C but gels at higher temperature, and applied to the adventitia of injured rat carotid arteries by Simons and colleagues (30). No c-*myb* mRNA could be detected by Northern blot analysis in arteries treated with the antisense oligonucleotide, whereas significant expression was observed when the gel was mixed with a c-*myb* sense oligonucleotide. A reduction in intimal area and intima: media ratio at 2 weeks after injury was achieved with application of the antisense/pluronic mixture, but no effect was seen with mismatch or sense c-*myb* oligonucleotide, or with pluronic gel alone. Interestingly, longitudinal sections of arteries from antisense-treated rats showed that the inhibitory effect on intimal thickening was restricted to the area of local gel application; proximal areas of the carotid that were balloon injured but outside the area of localized delivery showed substantial neointima formation. Again, this technology has no immediate practicality for the angioplasty practitioner, but does demonstrate that localized delivery can be effective against a restenosis-like process. Also, the study showed that inhibition of proto-oncogene expression is a possible therapeutic strategy for the intimal SMC proliferative response to arterial injury.

Hanson and Ku developed a delivery strategy for *high-concentration drug release at the luminal fluid "boundary layer"* (31). A plastic cuff surrounding porous synthetic vascular graft material allows continuous infusion and high-concentration delivery at the distal luminal surface. Using this approach, they demonstrated that the efficiency of local delivery against platelet-dependent thrombus formation on thrombogenic Dacron graft segments just downstream was 720-fold greater than systemic delivery for the thrombin inhibitor D-Pro-Phe-Arg-chloromethyl ketone. Similar studies showed 100-fold dose reduction requirement for local delivery of Arg-Gly-Asp peptide inhibitor of glycoprotein IIb/IIIa, and 23-fold reduction for local hirudin (SR Hanson, personal communication). Thus localized delivery can potentially inhibit thrombosis at sites of vascular intervention while avoiding the bleeding complications associated with systemic anticoagulation or antiplatelet therapy.

LUMINAL IMPLANTATION OF POLYMERS

Conjugation of active compounds to absorbable or biocompatible matrix material, followed by implantation within the arterial lumen by means of catheter or stent delivery, is an antirestenotic and/or antithrombotic local delivery strategy with considerable appeal. Theoretically, this approach would provide sustained release of biologic activity during polymer degradation or tissue interaction while also preventing elastic recoil by mechanical support of a dilated stenosis. Unfortunately, results of initial studies in animals have been mixed, and the future applicability of this technology to interventional cardiology seems uncertain. While polymer-based local drug delivery has been established as an imminently probable clinical modality for such applications as tumor neurosurgery, it has only a fledgling role in cardiology.

Chapman and colleagues implanted *biodegradable stents* composed of filaments of the bioabsorbable suture material poly(L-lactide), which were braided to form an open tubular mesh, into the iliac arteries of dogs (32). There was minimal inflammatory consequence, although similar lack of reaction to metallic stents has also been seen in the dog, and the stent was completely absorbed by 18 months. These results are encouraging and suggest that potential exists for drug release from such a matrix in the form of stent material.

In contrast to the study by Chapman, Murphy et al. found an intense inflammatory foreign body response, with luminally obliterating tissue reaction on implantation of a woven mesh *biocompatible stent* composed of polyethylene terephthalate into swine coronary arteries (33). Most of these reactions were accompanied by formation of ventricular aneurysms. Thus, while mechanically feasible, this choice of biomaterials was deemed unsuitable for further study. However, van Beusekom implanted a similar device of the same material composition into porcine peripheral arteries and found only a mild foreign body reaction (34). It is unknown whether the disparity between these studies is related to anatomic location or methodologic differences.

Both biodegradable (polyglycolide/poly-lactide, polycaprolactone, polyhydroxybu-tyrate valerate) and "biostable" (silicone, polyurethane, polyethylene terephthalate) polymers implanted as longitudinal strips cast over portions of metallic stents (*polymer-coated stents*) evoked severe inflammatory and fibrotic reactions in pig coronaries in studies by Lincoff et al. (35, 36). Only at the sites of polymer covering were histiocytes, granulomas, and medial necrosis observed; modest SMC proliferative response was seen adjacent to areas of stent metal without poly-mer. These experiments seem to indicate that other polymer compounds must be sought for possible clinical use. Exogenous fibrin cover-ing is one possibility (37), but the potential for drug incorporation and release from such a matrix into arterial tissues at angioplasty sites remains to be established.

Polymeric endoluminal paving and sealing is an alternative approach that is under devel-opment and testing. This technique employs thermally activated, structural-phase transi-tions in the polymer material to expand tubu-lar stents into the arterial luminal configura-tion. In addition to bench top and *in vitro* studies, *in vivo* implantations in various ani-mal models were performed by Slepian (38). While the potential for this technology as a drug delivery strategy is recognized, to date no such studies have been reported.

CELL-MEDIATED DELIVERY

A final and intriguing possibility for local delivery involves the use of cells as carriers. In its most basic form this approach would entail introduction of unmodified cells (prob-ably endothelium) whose constitutive molec-ular array (acting as "drugs") would influence thrombosis and/or restenosis. Alternatively, the cells could act as carriers by transfection *in vitro* with cDNA constructs whose products would exert the desired effect by up-regula-tion of endogenous production or by cytoplas-mic uptake using such procedures as elec-tropermeation. Cells, either isolated from the patient's own tissues or obtained from some

other source, could be introduced to the angioplasty site by modified catheters or grown onto stents.

As mentioned above (see "Modified Bal-loon Catheters"), Nabel and colleagues used the double-balloon catheter to introduce autologous, *genetically modified endothelial cells* to the desquamated luminal surfaces of pig iliac arteries (7). In this case the endothe-lium was isolated from excised veins and transfected *in vitro* with an expression vector for bacterial β-galactosidase. After "seeding" the balloon-injured sites, the foreign protein was detected in the treated tissue by histo-chemical staining up to several months after-ward. Dichek et al. transfected vascular endothelial cells and cultured them onto fibronectin-coated, stainless-steel, slotted-tube stents, then demonstrated cell retention and foreign gene expression after balloon catheter expansion of the stents in vitro (39).

We have grown a human microvascular endothelial cell line onto tantalum wire coil stents (40). Cells immortalized with the SV 40 T antigen grew to confluence on bare stents in 3 to 5 days and stained positively by immuno-fluorescence for HLA-A, B, and C (Fig. 40A.4); after balloon expansion in vitro,

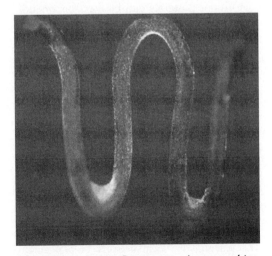

Figure 40A.4. Immunofluorescence microscopy of tan-talum coil stent seeded in vitro with human dermal mi-crovascular endothelial cells for 7 days. Punctate staining indicates presence of the HLA-A, B, and C positive en-dothelial cells.

Figure 40A.5. Scanning electron microscopy of tantalum coil stent that was expanded by balloon catheter in vitro after confluent coverage by human microvascular endothelium and then cultured for an additional 2 days. Recovery of endothelium after substantial balloon-induced cell loss is near complete.

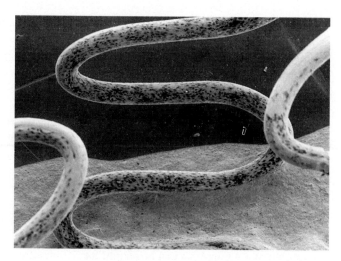

about 30% of cells remained and confluent recovery was achieved in another 3 days (Fig. 40A.5). Seeded stents were frozen and stored for 4 days and, after thawing, cells were morphologically intact and functional, migrating onto culture plates. The cells were also identified by structural characteristics 4 hours after seeded-stent deployment into pig coronary arteries. Further studies are under way to determine effects of endothelial coverage on thrombogenicity and to explore the potential for insertion of genes with desirable functional products.

Cells or platelets can be *electropermeabilized* in vitro to introduce nucleic acids or other molecules, then reinjected to deliver those molecules to the desired locations. Crawford described experiments in which rat platelets were loaded with a stable synthetic prostacyclin analog and then infused at the time of aortic balloon injury (41). This procedure significantly inhibited ^{3}H-thymidine uptake at 3 days into the aortic intima and media, compared with ballooning only. This approach seems promising and warrants further study.

SUMMARY

The potential for local delivery of biologically active compounds is well established. Achieving a high local concentration that is active for an adequate period while avoiding systemic toxicity is reminiscent of Gruentzig's original philosophy of angioplasty. Why subject the whole patient to invasive trauma if a small device targeted to the offending lesion can be effective? It has now been demonstrated that surgically applied, local, adventitial delivery using reservoir devices can inhibit the extent of neointimal development. Local inhibition of thrombosis, a pressing need in this age of stents, has been accomplished in the laboratory without systemic effect. The challenge of how to achieve these effects with practical noninvasive systems is a major but not insurmountable engineering problem. It is encouraging that so many laboratories have taken on the challenge.

REFERENCES

1. Serruys PW, Luitjen HE, Beatt KJ et al. Incidence of restenosis after successful coronary angioplasty: a time-related phenomenon. Circulation 1988;77:361–371.
2. Savage M, Fischman D, Leon M et al. Restenosis risk of single Palmaz-Schatz stents in native coronary arteries: report from the core angiographic laboratory. J Am Coll Cardiol 1992:19:277A (abstract).
3. Serruys PW, Strauss BH, Beatt KJ et al. Angiographic follow-up after placement of a self-expanding coronary artery stent. N Engl J Med 1991;324:13–17.
4. Hong MK, Bhatti T, Matthews BJ et al. The effect of porous infusion balloon-delivered angiopeptin on myointimal hyperplasia after balloon injury in the rabbit. Circulation 1993;88:638–648.
5. Santoian EC, Gravanis MB, Tarazona N et al. Local infusion of angiopeptin into the angioplasty site inhibits neointimal development after overstretch balloon injury in a swine model of restenosis. J Am Coll Cardiol 1993;21:179A (abstract).
6. Karas SP, Gravanis MB, Santoian EC, Robinson KA, Anderberg KA, King SB. Comparison of coronary intimal

proliferation following balloon injury and stenting in swine: an animal model of restenosis. J Am Coll Cardiol 1992;20:467–474.

7. Nabel EG, Plautz G, Boyce FM, Stanley JC, Nabel GJ. Recombinant gene expression in vivo within endothelial cells of the arterial wall. Science 1989;244:1342–1344.

8. Nabel EG, Plautz G, Nabel GJ. Site-specific expression in vivo by direct gene transfer into the arterial wall. Science 1990;249:1285–1288.

9. Wolinsky H, Thung SN. Use of a perforated balloon catheter to deliver concentrated heparin into the wall of the normal canine artery. J Am Coll Cardiol 1990;15:475–481.

10. Santoian EC, Gravanis MB, Schneider JE et al. Use of the porous balloon in porcine coronary arteries: rationale for low pressure and volume delivery. Cathet Cardiovasc Diagn 1993;30:348–354.

11. Muller DWM, Topol EJ, Abrams GD, Gallagher KP, Ellis SG. Intramural methotrexate therapy for the prevention of neointimal thickening after balloon angioplasty. J Am Coll Cardiol 1992;20:460–466.

12. Flugelman MY, Jaklitsch MT, Newman KD, Casscells W, Bratthauer GL, Dichek DA. Low level in vivo gene transfer into the arterial wall through a perforated balloon catheter. Circulation 1992;85:1110–1117.

13. Chapman GD, Lim CS, Gammon RS et al. Gene transfer into coronary arteries of intact animals with a percutaneous balloon catheter. Circ Res 1992;71:27–33.

14. Wilensky RL, March KL, Hathaway DR. Direct intraarterial injection of microparticles via a catheter: a potential drug delivery strategy following angioplasty. Am Heart J 1991;4:1136–1140.

15. Klein TM, Wolf ED, Wu R, Sanford JC. High-velocity microprojectiles for delivering nucleic acids into living cells. Nature 1987;327:70–73.

16. Williams RS, Johnston SA, Riedy M, DeVit MJ, McElligott SG, Sanford JC. Introduction of foreign genes into tissues of living mice by DNA-coated microprojectiles. Proc Natl Acad Sci USA 1991;88:2726–2730.

17. Robinson KA, Sigman SR, Schneider JE et al. Mechanism of fluid transfer from a porous balloon: scanning electron and light microscope study using colloidal gold marker. J Am Coll Cardiol 1993;21:118A (abstract).

18. Lambert CR, Leone JE, Rowland SM. Local drug delivery catheters: functional comparison of porous and microporous designs. Coronary Artery Dis 1993;4:469–475.

19. Hong MK, Farb A, Unger EF, Wang JC, Jasinski LJ, Mehlman MD. A new PTCA balloon catheter with intramural channels for local delivery of drugs at low pressure. Circulation 1992;86:I-380 (abstract).

20. Fram DB, Aretz TA, Mitchel JF et al. Localized intramural delivery of a marker agent during balloon angioplasty: a new technique using hydrogel-coated balloons and active diffusion. Circulation 1992;86:I-380 (abstract).

21. Nunes GL, King SB, Hanson SR, Sahatjian RA, Scott NA. Hydrogel-coated PTCA balloon catheter delivery of an antithrombin inhibits platelet-dependent thrombosis. Circulation 1992;86:I-380 (abstract).

22. Nunes GL, Hanson SR, King SB, Sahatjian RA, Barry JJ, Scott NA. Local heparin delivery with a hydrogel-coated PTCA balloon catheter inhibits platelet-dependent thrombosis. J Am Coll Cardiol 1992;21:117A (abstract).

23. Fram DB, Aretz TA, Mitchel JF, Azrin MA, Gillam LD, McKay RG. Localized intramural delivery of heparin during balloon angioplasty: a new technique using heparin-coated balloons and active diffusion. J Am Coll Cardiol 1992;21:118A (abstract).

24. Riessen R, Blessing E, Takeshita S, Karsch KR, Isner JM. Percutaneous arterial gene transfer using pure DNA applied to a hydrogel-coated angioplasty balloon. Eur Heart J 1993;14:78 (abstract).

25. Mitchel JF, Azrin MA, Fram DB, Hong MK, Wong SC, Barry JJ, Bow LM et al. Inhibition of platelet deposition and lysis of intracoronary thrombus during balloon angioplasty using urokinase-coated hydrogel balloons. Circulation 1994; 90:1979–1988.

26. Mitchel JF, Fram DB, Palme DF, Foster R, Hirst JA, Azrin MA, Bow LM et al. Enhanced intracoronary thrombolysis with urokinase using a novel, local drug delivery system: in vitro, in vivo, and clinical studies. Circulation 1995; 91:785–793.

27. Fernandez-Ortiz A, Meyer BJ, Mailhac A, Falk E, Badimon L, Fallon JT, Fuster V et al. A new approach for local intravascular drug delivery: iontophonetic balloon. Circulation 1994;89:1518–1522.

28. Edelman ER, Adams DH, Karnovsky MJ. Effect of controlled adventitial heparin delivery on smooth muscle cell proliferation following endothelial injury. Proc Natl Acad Sci USA 1990;87:2773–3777.

29. Okada T, Bark DH, Mayberg MR. Localized release of perivascular heparin inhibits intimal proliferation after endothelial injury without systemic anticoagulation. Neurosurgery 1989;25:892–898.

30. Simons M, Edelman ER, DeKeyser J-L, Langer R, Rosenberg RD. Antisense c-myb oligonucleotides inhibit intimal arterial smooth muscle cell accumulation in vivo. Nature 1992;359:67–70.

31. Hanson SR, Ku DN. Efficiency of boundary layer drug delivery for antithrombotic therapy. Thromb Haemostas 1993;69:1240 (abstract).

32. Chapman GD, Gammons RS, Bauman RP et al. A bioabsorbable stent: initial experimental results. Circulation 1990;82:72 (abstract).

33. Murphy JG, Schwartz RS, Edwards WD, Camrud AR, Vlietstra RE, Holmes DR. Percutaneous polymeric stents in porcine coronary arteries: initial experience with polyethylene terephthalate stents. Circulation 1992;86:1596–1604.

34. Van Beusekon HMM, van der Giessen WJ, van Ingen Schenau D, Slager CJ. Synthetic polymers as an alternative to metal in stents? in vivo and mechanical behavior of polyethylene terephthalate. Circulation 1992;86:I-731 (abstract).

35. Lincoff A, Schwartz RS, van der Giessen W et al. Biodegradable polymers can evoke a unique inflammatory response when implanted in the coronary artery. Circulation 1992;86:I-801 (abstract).

36. Lincoff A, van der Giessen W, Schwartz RS et al. Biodegradable and biostable polymers may both cause vigor-

ous inflammatory responses when implanted in the porcine coronary artery. J Am Coll Cardiol 1993;21:179A (abstract).

37. Holmes DR, Edwards WD, Camrud AR, Jorgensen MA, Schwartz RS. Differential arterial response to stents in a porcine coronary model: exogenous fibrin vs. polyurethane vs. polyethylene terephthalate. J Am Coll Cardiol 1993; 21:179A (abstract).

38. Slepian MJ. Polymeric endoluminal paving and sealing: therapeutics at the crossroads of biomechanics and pharmacology. In: Topol EJ, ed. Textbook of interventional cardiology. Philadelphia: WB Saunders, 1990.

39. Dichek DA, Neville RF, Zwiebel JA, Freeman SM, Leon MB, Anderson WF. Seeding of intravascular stents with genetically engineered cells. Circulation 1989;80:1347–1350.

40. Scott NA, Candal FJ, Robinson KA, Ades EW. Seeding of intracoronary stents with human endothelial cells. (abstract). Circulation 1993;88(4):I-150.

41. Crawford N. Electropermeabilized platelets as drug delivery vehicles: possible strategy for prevention of post angioplasty recollusion and restenosis. Proc Restenosis Summit 1993;5:284–294.

B. Local Drug Delivery: Devices and Prospects for Gene Therapy

REIMER RIESSEN and JEFFREY M. ISNER

Vascular injury associated with percutaneous revascularization can initiate a complex cascade of biologic events such as thrombosis, vascular smooth muscle cell migration and proliferation, and production of extracellular matrix. Data from experimental and clinical studies have suggested that smooth muscle cell proliferation is a key event in this process that ultimately leads to restenosis in up to 50% of all patients within the first 6 months after the intervention. The systemic administration of antithrombotic and antiproliferative agents in clinical studies, however, has thus far failed to achieve a significant reduction in the incidence of restenosis. One explanation for the failure of such trials is that submaximal doses of standard pharmacologic agents have been employed because of concern that serious side effects might result from systemic administration of the required doses. The concept of local, intravascular, site-spe-

cific delivery of pharmacologic and/or biologic therapies has evolved as a solution to this potential limitation. This concept presumes that higher concentrations of a therapeutic agent may be achieved directly at the angioplasty site, thus obviating toxicities associated with systemic levels of the therapeutic agent. The inhibition of smooth muscle cell proliferation has been the primary target for local intravascular drug delivery so far. This delivery approach, however, might also prove useful in a variety of other cardiovascular diseases. This includes, for example, the local delivery of antithrombotic agents to vascular segments that are prone to thrombosis and the local deposition of angiogenic factors in or around an ischemic area to promote angiogenesis and neovascularization.

The approaches for local, intravascular, site-specific delivery currently under investigation may be considered according to three strategies: (a) direct deposition of therapeutic agents or genes into the vessel wall via an intravascular delivery system, (b) systemic administration of inactive agents followed by local activation, and (c) systemic administration of agents that have a specific affinity to proliferating smooth muscle cells at the angioplasty site. This discussion will focus principally on intravascular devices designed for direct local delivery into the vessel wall; the last two options will be considered in brief.

DIRECT DEPOSITION OF THERAPEUTIC AGENTS INTO THE VESSEL WALL

Local therapy of restenosis using direct drug delivery should ideally consist of a single-dose application at the time of angioplasty so that further catheterizations for local applications are not necessary. For the therapy of restenosis this is a special challenge because symptoms of restenosis in patients often occur months after the initial angioplasty, indicating that smooth muscle proliferation and/or extracellular matrix production are ongoing for a prolonged time. It cannot be ruled out that drugs targeted to an early step in the sequence of biologic events leading to smooth muscle proliferation could be effective in reducing restenosis, even with a relatively short residence time. It is more likely, however, that drug release over a prolonged time is necessary to achieve an effect on restenosis. The duration of the antiproliferative effect depends both on the pharmacologic properties of the agent and the amount of agent deposited in the arterial wall. The latter depends principally on how the agent is delivered to the artery. Most catheter devices developed for local delivery have been designed to accomplish infusion of aqueous solutions into the vessel wall. Alternatively, polymers designed as microparticles or stents have been modified to provide timed release of the therapeutic agents.

Devices for Intravascular Drug Delivery

DOUBLE-BALLOON CATHETER

The first device used for the localized delivery of drugs or genes was the double-balloon catheter (1, 2). By inflating the two balloons, a sealed compartment is created in which the solubilized therapeutic agent can be instilled after blood has been evacuated from the compartment (Fig. 40B.1A). The injected mixture reaches the arterial wall by diffusion or as a result of applied hydrostatic pressure. It has been recently shown that infusion pressures of about 150 mm Hg (0.2 atm) both are sufficient for the uptake of DNA-plasmids into the arterial wall and are nontraumatic; pressures upward of 500 mm Hg typically create additional injury (3). The double-balloon catheter may be particularly well suited for applications in which the endothelium is the delivery target. In this case the goal of maintaining the endothelium intact is paramount. Clearly, one of the potential advantages not shared by alternative delivery devices is that the double-balloon catheter provides a design option for evacuation, as well as instillation, of the compartment isolated between two inflated balloons. This might be facilitated by a separate infusion and ventilation port that allows introduction and evacuation of solution by flushing the compartment. This is particularly relevant in the case of viral vectors, recombinant fusion toxins, or any other therapeutic agent with features that make systemic circulation of the agent less desirable.

The clinical use of the double-balloon catheter, however, is limited by certain practical problems. Leakage of the solution through side branches, originating at approximately 2 to 4 mm intervals in the case of epicardial coronary arteries, can result in markedly reduced uptake of the therapeutic agent at the target site. Relatively long incubation times of 15 to 30 minutes, thought necessary to permit satisfactory diffusion to occur, require a perfusion thru-port to maintain distal blood flow when such devices are employed in the coronary circulation. Finally, the inflation pressure required to accomplish a satisfactory seal by the two balloons of the delivery compartment can lead to additional vessel injury proximal and distal to the target site; use of latex, in lieu of conventional polyethylene, as the balloon material may assist in solving this particular problem.

POROUS BALLOON CATHETER

The porous balloon (Fig. 40B.1B) was first used for intravascular drug delivery by Wolinsky and Thung (4) and has recently been used for intravascular gene therapy by several investigators (5, 6). Drug or DNA solutions can be injected into the balloon under pressure and are infused into the arterial wall through small balloon perforations that measure 25 μm in diameter. Both the efficacy of and complications inherent to this catheter type are influenced by the infusion pressure. A minimum pressure is necessary to fully inflate the balloon and position it against the arterial wall, so that downstream distribution of the drug does not occur. The depth of penetration of the delivered therapeutic agent is increased with higher pressures. In the case of the Wolinsky balloon, an infusion pressure of 5 atm (3800 mm Hg) was required to

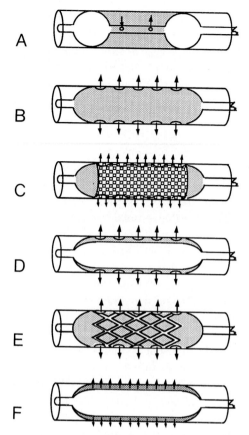

Figure 40B.1. Schematic drawing of several catheter systems used for intravascular drug delivery. **A.** Double-balloon catheter. This catheter is used to infuse drug solution into an arterial compartment isolated by two balloons. **B.** Porous balloon catheter. Agents are injected into the vascular wall through small perforations in the single-lumen balloon catheter. **C.** Microporous balloon. A porous balloon is covered by a permeable polycarbonate membrane (pore size 0.8 μm) to reduce jet-induced injury. **D.** Channel balloon. Drugs are infused through small perforated channels that are located on the surface of an angioplasty balloon. Pressures for balloon inflation and drug infusion can be separated. **E.** Stent-in-a-balloon. A different system for the low-pressure infusion of drugs, using an expandable stent within the balloon to position the balloon against the arterial wall. **F.** Hydrogel catheter. A hydrophilic polymer coating acts as a drug-absorbing sponge. Agents are transferred to the arterial wall during balloon inflation.

achieve transmural deposition of a marker substance during a 1-minute infusion (4). It is important to emphasize, however, that the actual pressure at the balloon-tissue interface is not equivalent to the pressure in the infla-

tion device. The inner resistance of the catheter, which depends on the number and size of the pores, as well as length and diameter of the catheter, results in a considerable pressure drop-off along the catheter. The initial experiments by Wolinsky and Thung (4) demonstrated that an infusion pressure of 3800 mm Hg (5 atm) employed for the "high resistance" porous balloon catheter is equivalent to 500 mm Hg (0.7 atm) for the "low resistance" double balloon. A 1500–mm Hg (2 atm) pressure applied to the porous balloon corresponds only to 0 to 50 mm Hg applied to the double balloon. High infusion pressures (5 to 10 atm), however, increase the likelihood of additional tissue trauma caused by high-velocity fluid jets (7, 8). These jets are particularly problematic when obstructed pores suddenly regain patency, resulting in the explosive release of fluid. In addition to acute complications such as vessel perforation and/or dissection, jet-induced trauma may potentially act to increase the proliferative response (9) or create a nidus for thrombus formation. A recent experimental study investigating the vascular damage caused by porous balloons in a rabbit iliac angioplasty model, however, did not show greater intimal hyperplasia in arteries treated with a porous balloon before angioplasty compared with angioplasty alone (9a). A postmortem study in human atherosclerotic arteries (10) suggested that substances infused via a Wolinsky catheter may enter the arterial tissue preferentially via crevices and dissection planes. Whether these crevices and dissections were caused by a preceding angioplasty versus infusion of the marker substance, however, remains uncertain.

Several modifications of the single porous balloon have been designed to reduce the tissue injury caused by fluid jets. The *microporous balloon* (7) consists of an inner porous balloon with an array of 25-μm holes (Fig. 40B.1C). The inner balloon is surrounded by a small space and covered by a polycarbonate membrane with 0.8-μm pores. The resistance of this catheter to balloon inflation remains high; as a result the high pressure necessary to overcome this resistance leads to leaking of the infusate from the target site. Other prototype catheters have been created with sophisticated designs intended to separate balloon inflation from drug or gene infusion. The *channel balloon* (11) consists of a standard angioplasty balloon that is covered by a layer of perforated tubes that can be perfused independently using a separate pressure via a supplementary thru-port (Fig. 40B.1*D*). This design would theoretically permit balloon angioplasty and local delivery to be accomplished with the same device. Another variation is the *balloon-over-stent* (12) in which a stent within the balloon is used to juxtaposition the balloon against the arterial wall before the drug solution is delivered (Fig. 40B.1*E*). Preliminary experiments have successfully documented that marker substances can be delivered to the arterial wall with all these devices. The optimal delivery protocol for each of these devices has yet to be determined. In addition to infusion and inflation pressures, optimal infusion volume represents another important variable. There is evidence that infusion of smaller volumes of a highly concentrated solution is less traumatic and might be more efficient than the infusion of larger volumes with a low concentration (13); such a concept, however, is likely to depend on the particular agent to be infused. As noted above, the high resistance of some devices may also reduce maximal flow, making it impossible to infuse several milliliters of solution within only a few minutes. Large delivery volumes may cause a portion of the solution to spill into the circulation or into surrounding tissue such as myocardium. Leakage of agents such as fusion toxins or viruses into the circulation increases the risk of systemic side effects. Penetration of drug solutions with unphysiologic pH and ion concentrations into the myocardium could change the local milieu and thereby create an arrhythmogenic focus.

In summary, for all types of porous balloon catheters, the persistent challenge is to combine efficient drug delivery with low tissue damage so that the beneficial effects of the drug outweigh the potentially negative effects of the delivery procedure.

DISPATCH CATHETER

The dispatch catheter represents a new design of an nondilation drug delivery device (13a). It consists of an over-the-wire catheter with a helical inflation coil mounted on its distal tip. The inner part of the helical coil is connected to a urethane sheath that expands after inflation of the catheter's coils, creating an inner lumen that allows for distal blood flow. The outer compartment, delimited by the coil and the sheath, can be filled with therapeutic agents through a separate infusion port. Complete expansion of the inner sheath providing distal perfusion, however, may not be achieved in undilated coronary stenosis or in an undersized artery. Prolonged inflation of the catheter may also lead to ischemia caused by side-branch occlusion by the catheter's coils.

HYDROGEL CATHETER

The hydrogel catheter (Fig. 40B.1*F*) consists of a normal angioplasty balloon coated with a hydrophilic polyacrylic acid polymer that can act as a drug-absorbing sponge (14). The hydrogel coating, which has a thickness of only 5 to 20 μm when dry, swells by a factor of 3 when exposed to an aqueous solution that may include drugs or other molecular agents such as DNA. After drying of the gel, the catheter is coated with a thin layer of therapeutic agent; the latter is subsequently "pressed" into the arterial wall during balloon inflation. In contrast to most of the other catheter devices, the hydrogel catheter permits site-specific intravascular drug delivery to be performed directly during angioplasty with a standard balloon. This delivery system also creates no additional tissue damage. The main disadvantage of this system is that drugs are rapidly washed off the balloon after exposure to the bloodstream. The balloon therefore has to be protected by a sheath as the catheter is advanced toward the target vessel; for the same reason, the time between sheath removal and balloon inflation must be minimized. The hydrogel system may be less well suited for applications in which large amounts of a particular agent are to be deposited in the vessel wall.

STENTS

The treatment of atherosclerotic lesions with metallic stents has the advantage of greater initial gain, less recoil, and a lower risk of dissection, but is frequently complicated by thrombotic occlusions and/or intimal proliferation. The stent may also prove useful as a carrier for sustained local drug delivery of antithrombotic and/or antiproliferative agents. Several approaches are possible to achieve continuous drug release from a stent. First, stents can be seeded with genetically manipulated endothelial cells to produce agents such as tissue plasminogen activator (tPA) (15). Second, stents can be coated directly with drugs or with drug-eluting biodegradable polymers. Third, stents can be manufactured completely of drug-eluting biodegradable polymers (16). The last two options seem most feasible from a practical point of view. Several biodegradable polymers such as polylactide, polyglycolide, polyorthoster, polycaprolactone, and polyethylene oxide/polybutylene terephthalate have been investigated for this purpose (16). Experience with these materials may favor stents made of polylactide, since this material cannot only be used to release drugs, but also causes only a very mild tissue reaction (17); this is in contrast to the other materials, which have been shown to evoke an extensive foreign-body reaction, characterized by fibromuscular proliferation, giant cell formation, and infiltration with macrophages and eosinophils (18). As an alternative drug carrier, fibrin has been used to coat metallic stents and has been reported

to reduce the incidence of stent occlusion without causing a significant foreign-body reaction (19). One concern regarding totally biodegradable stents is that inhomogeneous dissolution of the polymer might predispose to distal embolization. Another question concerns the efficiency of drug delivery from a non-biodegradable stent as long as the stent wires are exposed to the bloodstream.

Potential Therapeutic Agents for Local Drug Delivery

CONVENTIONAL DRUGS

Because of its known antithrombotic and antiproliferative properties, heparin was one of the first drugs used for local drug delivery. After infusion with a porous balloon, heparin is present in the media for up to 48 hours (4). A hydrogel-coated balloon has also been shown to be efficient for delivery of heparin into the vascular wall in vitro (20). For percutaneous applications, the hydrogel balloon has to be protected by a sheath to delay the washout of heparin, which otherwise occurs within 1 minute (21). Local delivery of heparin or a synthetic antithrombin with a hydrogel balloon was found to inhibit platelet-dependent thrombosis in a dacron graft shunt model (22, 22a). Thrombosis and platelet deposition after angioplasty was also shown to be reduced after local delivery of r-hirudin by a double-balloon perfusion catheter in a porcine model (22b). Both hydrogel and dispatch catheters have been used safely and successfully in clinical studies for local delivery of urokinase in patients with evidence of intracoronary thrombus (13a, 22c). A study in atherosclerotic rabbits, however, failed to show any effect on restenosis following local delivery of heparin via a porous balloon (23). Heparin coating of stents also failed to reduce intimal proliferation in several experimental studies (24, 25). The only agent shown thus far to have a mild beneficial effect on experimental intimal hyperplasia when delivered intraluminally is angiopeptin (26, 27); this effect, may be mediated through the stimulation of endothelial regrowth. Local delivery of antiproliferative agents such as thiol protease inhibitors (28), colchicine (29), doxorubicin (9), or methotrexate via a porous balloon (30) or a stent (24) had no significant effect on the development of intimal hyperplasia; one possible explanation for the failure of these experimental studies may be that the residence time of these agents was insufficient to exert a favorable effect. Both by convection and diffusion, molecules can be cleared rapidly from the arterial wall. More than 90% of deposited colchicine, for example, is cleared within a few hours following intramural injection (29). One approach to minimize drug washout is the use of nondiffusible, drug-eluting microparticles. Similar to biodegradable stents, these microparticles can be manufactured from a variety of synthetic polymers (e.g., polylactide) or natural substances such as proteins or polysaccharides. Variables such as the total dose of drug or gene, as well as the kinetics of release, can be manipulated. Again, biocompatibility of the material is a major issue to be resolved because of the concern of potentially detrimental effects related to a foreign-body reaction against the polymer. Microparticles can be injected efficiently into the arterial wall via a porous balloon (31) or a balloon over a stent (12) and are retained in the arterial wall, as well as in the periadventitial tissue, for at least 2 weeks. While biodegradable microparticles releasing colchicine have been shown to inhibit smooth muscle cell proliferation in vitro (32), the efficacy of this approach in vivo could not be demonstrated (32a). Another drug that may be tested with this delivery system in the near future is dexamethasone, shown previously to inhibit neointimal proliferation in the balloon-injured, rat carotid artery model when delivered locally from a silicone polymer implanted in the adventitia (33). It is possible, of course, to consider "combination chemotherapy," that is, delivery of several agents that act in combination to retard vessel narrowing via multiple mechanisms; agents that block protein synthesis, extracellular matrix production, and thrombus formation could thus be applied in combination.

GENE THERAPY

In parallel with local delivery of pharmacologic agents, much attention over the past years has focused on the concept of local, site-specific gene therapy (2) for the treatment of vascular disease such as restenosis and thrombosis and has gained much attention recently. Dramatic progress in the field of molecular biology has provided the tools required to transiently express recombinant DNA in the cells of the vascular wall in vivo. The resulting gene products can be selected in a rational fashion to modulate biologic processes in the vascular wall such as cell proliferation or matrix production by autocrine means. Recent reports by Nabel et al. have demonstrated that intravascular gene transfer with plasmids encoding for the histocompatibility gene HLA-B7 (34) or the growth factors PDGF-B (3) and basic-FGF (35) can result in a marked inflammatory or proliferative response, respectively, localized to the treated region. Applied to the problem of restenosis, any strategy involving gene therapy must begin with consideration of a very fundamental distinction: whether the protein products resulting from successful gene expression will be retained intracellularly or whether they will be secreted. Overexpression of nonsecreted growth inhibiting genes, for which certain tumor suppressor genes are potential candidates (36), would be limited only to those cells that were successfully transfected. Another approach is to transfect arteries with the herpes simplex virus thymidine kinase gene, which renders vascular cells sensitive to the cytotoxic effects of the nucleoside analog ganciclovir (36a, 36b). Assuming that there is not a clonal population of cells that is principally responsible for generating the restenotic lesion, transfection of a very high percentage of cells would likely be required. In contrast, a lower transfection efficiency might be sufficient for secreted gene products that can exert an effect on surrounding cells. Whether secreted gene products can be identified that have a clear antiproliferative effect remains to be shown. Potential candidates include genes for nitric oxide synthetase, somatostatin, and interferon-γ. Local intravascular gene therapy, of course, may also prove useful for over-expression of protein products designed to prevent thrombosis or for secretion of angiogenic growth factors intended to facilitate regional revascularization of ischemic myocardium, brain, and/or limbs.

In addition to the gene, a catheter-based intravascular gene delivery system includes several other components that may have an important impact on the transfection efficiency. First, the gene must be delivered in an appropriate *gene carrier*. Expression of marker genes can be achieved with pure plasmid DNA (6, 37) or a mixture of plasmid DNA with cationic liposomes (2, 6, 38). The latter has been previously shown to increase transfection efficiency in cell culture, although the use of liposomes in vivo continues to be compromised by a low transfection efficiency. The precise mechanism by which liposomes facilitate cellular uptake of DNA and subsequent translocation from cytoplasm to nucleus remains enigmatic. Retroviral vectors have been used effectively for gene transfer (39) and represent a potential alternative to lipofection. In the case of vascular gene transfer, use of retroviral vectors must accommodate the requirement that the target cells be proliferating (40). A variety of strategies to address this issue are currently under investigation, including use of growth factors such as vascular endothelial growth factor to stimulate endothelial cell DNA synthesis and thereby facilitate transfection (R. Mulligan, personal communication). More recently, experience with replication-defective adenoviruses in nonvascular gene transfer has been applied to the cardiovascular system. The receptor-mediated uptake of these viruses results in highly efficient gene transfer to the endothelium (41), myocardium (42), and vascular smooth muscle cells (41a, 43). Several modifications of viral gene transfer have been described in which inactivated viruses are employed in lieu of replication defective viruses. Inactivated viral particles can be used to enhance uptake of plasmid DNA, either in conjunction with liposomes (44, 45) or polylysine linkers (46).

Second, the expression of the gene has to be driven by a *promoter*. The highest levels of expression reported in vascular smooth muscle cells to date have been achieved using promiscuous viral promoters such as the cytomegalovirus, Rous Sarcoma virus, or Simian virus 40 promoter. These promoters are not tissue specific. To restrict gene expression to certain cell types at the transfection site, especially when very efficient gene carriers such as adenoviruses are used, tissue-specific endogenous promoters—for example, an actin promoter if the target cells are smooth muscle cells—are an option that may refine gene transfer. This strategy is based on the concept that regulation of a given gene in a particular cell or a certain tissue is accomplished by interactions of DNA-binding proteins and/or other transcription factors specific to certain tissues or cells.

Third, gene and carrier have to be delivered to the vessel wall by a *gene delivery device*. The first device used for intravascular gene delivery of marker genes such as β-galactosidase and luciferase was the double-balloon catheter (2, 38). Advantages and limitations of this catheter type have been discussed earlier. In our hands, transfections performed with luciferase plasmids, mixed with liposomes, and applied via a double-balloon system in a rabbit model resulted in low levels and frequency of gene expression (38). In contrast, arterial gene transfer with pure luciferase DNA via a hydrogel balloon was successful in all animals, and mean luciferase expression was about 100 times higher than in the previous experiments using the double-balloon system (37). Others have used porous balloons to perform gene transfer with retroviruses or plasmid DNA (5, 6). These devices have also been evaluated for adenoviral gene transfer (41a, 43).

Another approach to intravascular gene therapy is to remove the cells targeted for gene transfer from an individual and transfer the recombinant gene into those cells in vitro. The successfully transfected cells can be selected and reimplanted at a specific recipient site in vivo. Both endothelial cells and smooth muscle cells have been reimplanted at a site of previous denudation using a double-balloon catheter (47, 48). Alternatively, stents can be seeded with genetically engineered endothelial cells prior to transvascular introduction (15).

ANTISENSE OLIGONUCLEOTIDES

Antisense oligonucleotides constitute a molecular strategy distinct from gene therapy. These are short segments of synthetic DNA that are usually chemically modified to resist enzymatic degradation by intra- or extracellular nucleases. After cellular uptake, antisense oligonucleotides can bind in a relatively specific manner to a complementary mRNA; the action of RNase H on the resulting DNA/RNA hybrid renders this segment of mRNA unavailable for translation. The advantage of antisense oligonucleotides is that they can be specifically targeted against mRNAs for proteins that are essential for cell proliferation. Certain of these proteins are strategically located near the final common pathway into which multiple, partially redundant, signal-transduction pathways (including growths factors and their receptors) converge. Antisense oligonucleotides targeted against a variety of mRNAs, including proliferating cell nuclear antigen (PCNA) (49), nonmuscle myosin (50), and the protooncogenes c-myb (50) and c-myc (51), have been shown to partially inhibit smooth muscle cell proliferation in vitro. This effect can last in culture for several days after exposure for only 2 hours; the effect, however, is typically reversible. In several studies antisense oligonucleotides administered in vivo were shown to reduce neointimal formation after denudation in rat carotid arteries. For example, c-myb or c-myc antisense oligonucleotides were applied to the adventitia in combination with a pluronic gel (52, 52a); in another study, antisense oligonucleotides to the cyclin cdc2 were mixed with inactivated viral particles, liposomes, and a nuclear protein, and were subsequently injected into the lumen of a ligated rat carotid artery (53). Percutaneous delivery of c-myc antisense oligonucleotides via a porous balloon has successfully been used to reduce neointima formation in porcine coronary arteries (53a). Clinical studies testing this approach are planned.

SYSTEMIC ADMINISTRATION OF INACTIVE AGENTS FOLLOWED BY LOCALIZED ACTIVATION

Photodynamic therapy (PDT) constitutes a form of local therapy in which the activity of light-excitable photosensitizers is exploited to produce injury of targeted cells. Photosensitizers are relatively nontoxic substances unless they are activated by the appropriate wavelength of light. Hematoporphyrin derivatives, activated by red light with a wavelength of 635 nm, have been used for the treatment of neoplastic disorders. These substances accumulate in proliferating tissues such as tumors and have also been shown to be present in higher concentrations in atherosclerotic plaque than in normal artery after systemic administration (54). Cultured smooth muscle cells from atherosclerotic plaques show also a higher sensitivity to hematoporphyrins than smooth muscle cells from normal arteries (55). Catheter-based light delivery systems are now available for intravascular PDT (56). PDT involving administration of a hematoporphyrin derivative, followed by flash-lamp irradiation delivered via a quartz fiber catheter with a diffusing tip was shown to inhibit neointima foundation in a rabbit model (57). This effect, achieved when the treatment was delayed for 1 week after balloon injury, was associated with extensive medial smooth muscle cell necrosis. It remains to be shown whether this latter effect predisposes to vascular complications such as aneurysmal dilation or perforation, but clinical experience with laser balloon angioplasty (58) suggests this is unlikely to be a frequent concern. The clinical use of hematoporphyrins in the past has been limited by a cutaneous photosensitivity that can last for several weeks. To reduce the systemic phototoxicity, lower doses of novel hematoporphyrin derivatives have been administered locally via a porous balloon (59). Likewise, chloroaluminium-sulfonated phtalocyanin, which has an absorption peak of light at 695 nm, inhibited neointima formation in rats after balloon injury and also produced necrosis of the media (60). Psoralen represents an alternative photosensitizer currently under investigation as an agent to be administered in conjunction with ultraviolet irradiation (PUVA). This photosensitizer, used routinely for the treatment of dermatologic disorders, has limited systemic toxicity. A single exposure to PUVA was shown to result in complete stasis of cell proliferation over a 28-day period without cell necrosis (61). Finally, preliminary studies have suggested that very low doses of ultraviolet radiation generated from a diode laser and delivered locally to an isolated segment of rat carotid artery in vivo can inhibit smooth muscle cell proliferation and cause medial necrosis even when used alone, with no photoactive agent (Fig. 40B.2).

The effect observed in these applications of PDT on smooth muscle cells in the media may be desirable. It is conceivable that a population of smooth muscle cells at risk to proliferate and migrate from the media to an intimal location might be eliminated. Moreover,

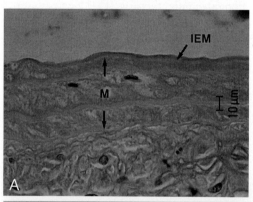

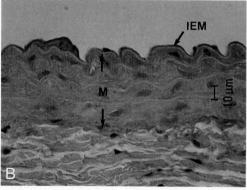

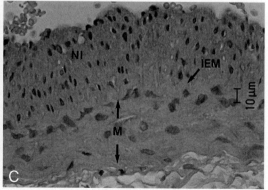

Figure 40B.2. **A.** Section of a rat carotid artery 3 weeks after balloon denudation followed by radiation with low doses of ultraviolet light generated from a diode laser in the absence of any photosensitizers. The presence of only very few cell nuclei in the media *(M)* indicates smooth muscle cell necrosis. The artery does not show any neointimal proliferation. *IEM,* Internal elastic membrane. **B.** Normal uninjured artery. **C.** Untreated rat carotid artery 3 weeks after balloon injury demonstrating a thick neointima *(NI).*

clinical applications of PDT would invariably target arteries with a larger volume of plaque interposed between the lumen and media. Clinical experience with the Spears laser-balloon catheter (58) suggests that aneurysm formation following medial injury is rare. A second issue, for which there are limited data (62) but considerable concern, is the possibility that proteins released from necrotic cells might represent potent mitogens capable of initiating a secondary wave of cell proliferation.

SYSTEMIC ADMINISTRATION OF AGENTS WITH A SPECIFIC AFFINITY TO PROLIFERATING SMOOTH MUSCLE CELLS

Proliferating smooth muscle cells, in comparison with quiescent cells, often express higher numbers of cell surface receptors for a variety of growth factors. Differential expression of growth factor receptors may provide the opportunity to use cytotoxic agents that specifically target proliferating smooth muscle cells. Targeted delivery of cytotoxins to specific cell surface receptors may be accomplished with recombinant fusion proteins. These chimeric agents combine a potent toxin with peptide ligands to cell surface receptors. After receptor binding and internalization of the protein, action of the toxin results in cell death. For the receptor-targeting component, several growth factors have been used, including transforming growth factor α (63), epidermal growth factor (EGF) (64), basic fibroblast growth factor (bFGF) (65, 66), and interleukin-2 (67). Toxins that have been used to complete the hybrid include a modified Pseudomonas exotoxin (63, 65), diphtheria toxin (64), and saporin (66), a toxin directed at ribosomal RNA. In cell culture these fusion toxins preferentially kill rapidly proliferating smooth muscle cells, as compared with quiescent cells (63, 66). A recombinant cytotoxin specific for the EGF receptor also was shown to prevent smooth muscle cell outgrowth from human atherosclerotic plaque in culture (64). We (68) and

others (66) have used the balloon-injured rat carotid artery model to study the effects of recombinant fusion proteins on neointima formation in vivo. Systemic intravenous delivery of a fusion protein was shown by Casscells et al. (66) and more recently by Pickering et al. (68) to inhibit intimal proliferation, but was also associated with systemic toxicity, manifested principally as weight loss. Such systemic toxicity is not altogether unanticipated because of the fact that growth factor receptors are not exclusively expressed by proliferating smooth muscle cells but are also present on cells from other organs such as the liver and gut. Previous nonvascular use of these fusion toxins suggests that the doses employed in the rat would be unlikely to exhibit similar toxicity in humans. Nevertheless, even in the case of a systemically administered agent designed to be activated locally, there may well be a role for local delivery. Preliminary experience in our laboratory has demonstrated that local administration of the fusion protein to a segment of balloon-injured rat carotid artery resulted in markedly reduced neointimal formation with markedly reduced systemic side effects. Thus, while this treatment strategy was originally designed as targeted systemic therapy, its future clinical use might well be local delivery via an intravascular delivery system. Several questions, however, must first be resolved. These include foremost the optimal time at which to apply the toxin; application immediately postangioplasty might be most practical, but uncertainty regarding the time interval between balloon injury and the onset of increased expression of receptors in proliferating cells remains a concern. Second, the long-term consequences of intimal and/or medial cell necrosis, as discussed above in conjunction with photodynamic therapy, are unclear. Presumably, an agent such as a fusion toxin, which aborts protein production, would generate a lesser amount of mitogens available for release on cell death; what has not been fully excluded is the potential effect of preexisting stored mitogens generated prior to toxin administration.

SUMMARY

Local drug delivery represents a potentially valuable adjunct to the treatment of restenosis and other vascular diseases. Several prototype devices have been developed and tested in vivo. Further modifications are expected to achieve more efficient delivery without concomitant tissue damage. Additional studies will be required (a) to demonstrate the logical but as yet unproved concept that the efficacy and safety of pharmacologic substances conventionally administered systemically are superior when these substances are delivered locally, and (b) to clarify the efficacy and safety of alternative, locally targeted strategies such as gene therapy, antisense oligonucleotides, photodynamic therapy, and recombinant fusion proteins.

ACKNOWLEDGMENTS

The contributions of Guy Leclerc, J. Geoffrey Pickering, Satoshi Takeshita, Christopher Pastore, Marianne Kearney, and Jaclynn Jekanowski to work discussed in this manuscript is gratefully acknowledged.

REFERENCES

1. Jorgensen B, Tonnesen KH, Bülow J et al. Femoral artery recanalisation with percutaneous angioplasty and segmentally enclosed plasminogen activator. Lancet 1989; 1:1106–1108.

2. Nabel EG, Plautz G, Nabel GJ. Site-specific gene expression in vivo by direct gene transfer into the arterial wall. Science 1990;249:1285–1288.

3. Nabel EG, Yang Z, Liptay S et al. Recombinant platelet-derived growth factor B gene expression in porcine arteries induces intimal hyperplasia in vivo. J Clin Invest 1993; 91:1822–1829.

4. Wolinsky H, Thung SN. Use of a perforated balloon catheter to deliver concentrated heparin into the wall of the normal canine artery. J Am Coll Cardiol 1990;15:475–481.

5. Flugelman MY, Jaklitsch MT, Newman KD, Casscells W, Bratthauer GL, Dichek DA. Low-level in vivo gene transfer into the arterial wall through a perforated balloon catheter. Circulation 1992;85:1110–1117.

6. Chapman GD, Lim CS, Gammon RS et al. Gene transfer into coronary arteries of intact animals with a percutaneous balloon catheter. Circ Res 1992;71:27–33.

7. Lambert C, Leone JE, Rowland SM. Local drug delivery catheters: functional comparison of porous and microporous designs. Coronary Artery Dis 1993;4:469–475.

8. Santoian EC, Gravanis MB, Schneider JE, Tarazona N, Cipolla GD, Robinson KA, King SBI. Use of the porous balloon in porcine coronary arteries: rationale for low pressure and volume delivery. Cathet Cardiovasc Diagn 1993; 30:348–354.

9. Franklin SM, Kalan JM, Currier JW et al. Effects of local delivery of doxorubicin or saline on restenosis following angioplasty in atherosclerotic rabbits. Circulation 1992; 86:I-52 (abstract).

9a. Plante S, Dupuis G, Mongeau CJ, Durand P. Porous balloon catheters for local delivery: assessment of vascular damage in a rabbit iliac angioplasty model. J Am Coll Cardiol 1994;24:820–824.

10. Wolinsky H, Lin C-S. Use of the perforated balloon catheter to infuse marker substances into diseased coronary artery walls after experimental postmortem angioplasty. J Am Coll Cardiol 1991;17:174B–178B.

11. Hong MK, Farb A, Unger EF, Wang JC, Jasinski LJ, Mehlman MD. A new PTCA balloon catheter with intramural channels for local delivery of drugs at low pressure. Circulation 1992;86:I-380 (abstract).

12. Wilensky RL, March KL, Gradus-Pizlo I, Schauwecker DS, Hathaway DR. Enhanced localization and retention of microparticles following intramural delivery into atherosclerotic arteries using a new delivery device. J Am Coll Cardiol 1993;21:185A (abstract).

13. French BA, Mazur W, Finnigan JP et al. Gene transfer into intact porcine coronary arteries via infusion balloon catheter: influences of delivery volume and pressure. Circulation 1992;86:I-799 (abstract).

13a. Mitchel JF, Fram DB, Palme DF, Foster R, Hirst JA, Azrin MA, Bow LM et al. Enhanced intracoronary thrombolysis with urokinase using a novel, local drug delivery system. Circulation 1995;91:785–793.

14. Fram DB, Aretz T, Azrin MA, Mitchel JF, Samady H, Gillam LD, Sahatjian R et al. Localized intramural drug delivery during balloon angioplasty using hydrogel-coated balloons and pressure-augmented diffusion. J Am Coll Cardiol 1994;23:1570–1577.

15. Dichek DA, Neville RF, Zwiebel JA, Freeman SM, Leon MB, Anderson WF. Seeding of intravascular stents with genetically engineered endothelial cells. Circulation 1989; 80:1347–1353.

16. Murphy JG, Schwartz RS, Huber KC, Holmes DR. Polymeric stents: modern alchemy or the future? J Invasive Cardiol 1991;3:144–148.

17. Zidar JP, Gammon RS, Chapman GD et al. Short and long-term vascular tissue response to the Duke bioabsorbable stent. J Am Coll Cardiol 1993;21:439A (abstract).

18. Murphy JG, Schwartz RS, Edwards WD, Camrud AR, Vliestra RE, Holmes DR. Percutaneous polymeric stents in porcine coronary arteries. Initial experience with polyethylene terephthalate stents. Circulation 1992;86:1596–1604.

19. Holmes DR, Camrud AR, Jorgenson MA, Edwards WD, Schwartz RS. Polymeric stenting in the porcine coronary artery model: differential outcome of exogenous fibrin sleeves versus polyurethane-coated stents. J Am Coll Cardiol 1994;24:525–531.

20. Azrin MA, Mitchel JF, Fram DB, Pedersen CA, Cartun RW, Barry JJ, Bow LM et al. Decreased platelet deposition and smooth muscle cell proliferation after intramural heparin

delivery with hydrogel-coated balloons. Circulation 1994; 90:433–441.

21. Sheriff MU, Khetpal V, Spears JR. Method of application of local high-dose heparin during balloon angioplasty. J Am Coll Cardiol 1993;21:188A (abstract).

22. Nunes GL, Hanson SR, King SB, Sahatjian RA, Barry JJ, Scott NA. Local heparin delivery with a hydrogel-coated PTCA balloon catheter inhibits platelet-dependent thrombosis. J Am Coll Cardiol 1993;21:117A (abstract).

22a. Nunes GL, Hanson SR, King SBI, Sahatjian RA, Scott NA. Local delivery of a synthetic antithrombin with a hydrogel-coated angioplasty balloon catheter inhibits platelet-dependent thrombosis. J Am Coll Cardiol 1994;23:1578–1583.

22b. Meyer BJ, Fernandez-Ortiz A, Mailhac A, Falk E, Badimon L, Don Michael A, Chesebro JH et al. Local delivery of r-hirudin by a double-balloon perfusion catheter prevents mural thrombosis and minimizes platelet deposition after angioplasty. Circulation 1994;90:2474–2480.

22c. Mitchel JF, Azrin MA, Fram MA, Hong MK, Wong SC, Barry JJ, Bow LM et al. Inhibition of platelet deposition and lysis of intracoronary thrombus using urokinase-coated hydrogel balloons. Circulation 1994;90:1979–1988.

23. Gimple LW, Gertz SD, Haber HL et al. Effect of chronic subcutaneous or intramural administration of heparin on femoral artery restenosis after balloon angioplasty in hypercholesterolemic rabbits. A quantitative and histopathological study. Circulation 1992;86:1536–1546.

24. Cox DA, Anderson PG, Roubin GS, Chou C, Agrawal SK, Cavender JB. Effect of local delivery of heparin and methotrexate on neointimal proliferation in stented porcine coronary arteries. Coronary Artery Dis 1992;3:237–248.

25. Zidar JP, Jackman JD, Gammon RS et al. Serial assessment of heparin coating on vascular responses to a new tantalum stent. Circulation 1992;86:I-185 (abstract).

26. Hong MK, Bhatti T, Matthews BJ, Stark KS, Cathapermal SS, Foegh ML, Ramwell PW et al. The effect of porous infusion balloon-delivered angiopeptin on myointimal hyperplasia after balloon injury in the rabbit. Circulation 1993;88:638–648.

27. Santoian EC, Gravanis MB, Tarazona N et al. Local infusion of angiopeptin into the angioplasty site inhibits neointimal development after overstretch balloon injury in a swine model of restenosis. J Am Coll Cardiol 1993;21:179A (abstract).

28. Wilensky RL, March KL, Hathaway DR. Restenosis in an atherosclerotic rabbit model is reduced by a thiol protease inhibitor. J Am Coll Cardiol 1991;17:268A (abstract).

29. Wilensky RL, Gradus-Pizlo I, March KL, Sandusky GE, Hathaway DR. Efficacy of local intramural injection of colchicine in reducing restenosis following angioplasty in the atherosclerotic rabbit model. Circulation 1992;86:I-52 (abstract).

30. Muller DWM, Topol EJ, Abrams GD, Gallagher KP, Ellis SG. Intramural methotrexate therapy for the prevention of neointimal thickening after balloon angioplasty. J Am Coll Cardiol 1992;20:460–466.

31. Wilensky RL, March KL, Hathaway DR. Direct intraarterial wall injection of microparticles via a catheter: a potential drug delivery strategy following angioplasty. Am Heart J 1991;122:1136–1140.

32. March KL, Mohanraj S, Ho PPK, Wilensky RL, Hathaway DR. Biodegradable microspheres containing a colchicine analogue inhibit DNA synthesis in vascular smooth muscle cells. Circulation 1994;89:1929–1933.

32a. Gradus-Pizlo I, Wilensky RL, March KL, Michaels M, Hathaway DR: Local delivery of biodegradable microparticles containing colchicine or colchicine analog does not block restenosis in atherosclerotic rabbit femoral arteries. Circulation 1993;88:I-311 (abstract).

33. Villa AE, Guzman LA, Chen W, Golomb G, Levy RJ, Topol EJ. Local delivery of dexamethasone for prevention of neointimal proliferation in a rat model of balloon angioplasty. J Clin Invest 1994;93:1243–1249.

34. Nabel EG, Plautz G, Nabel GJ. Transduction of a foreign histocompatibility gene into the arterial wall induces vasculitis. Proc Natl Acad Sci USA 1992;89:5157–5161.

35. Nabel EG, Yang ZY, Plautz G et al. Recombinant fibroblast growth factor-1 promotes intimal hyperplasia and angiogenesis in arteries in vivo. Nature 1993;362:844–846.

36. Chang MW, Barr E, Seltzer J, Jiang YQ, Nabel GJ, Nabel EG, Parmacek MS et al. Cytostatic gene therapy for vascular proliferative disorders with a constitutively active form of the retinoblastoma gene product. Science 1995; 267:518–522.

36a. Ohno T, Gordon D, San H, Pompili VJ, Imperiale MJ, Nabel GJ, Nabel EG. Gene therapy for vascular smooth muscle cell proliferation after arterial injury. Science 1994;265:781–784.

36b. Guzman RJ, Hirschowitz EA, Brody SL, Crystal RG, Epstein SE, Finkel T. In vivo suppression of injury-induced vascular smooth muscle cell accumulation using adenovirus-mediated transfer of the herpes simplex virus thymidine kinase gene. Proc Natl Acad Sci USA 1994; 91:10732–10736.

37. Riessen R, Rahimizadeh H, Blessing E, Takeshita S, Barry JJ, Isner JM. Arterial gene transfer using pure DNA applied directly to a hydrogel-coated angioplasty balloon. Hum Gene Ther 1993;4:749–758.

38. Leclerc G, Gal D, Takeshita S, Nikol S, Weir L, Isner JM. Percutaneous arterial gene transfer in a rabbit model. Efficiency in normal and balloon-dilated atherosclerotic arteries. J Clin Invest 1992;90:936–944.

39. Mulligan RC. The basic science of gene therapy. Science 1993;260:926–932.

40. Miller DG, Adam MA, Miller AD. Gene transfer by retrovirus vectors occurs only in cells that are actively replicating at the time of infection. Mol Cell Biol 1990;10:4239–4242.

41. Lemarchand P, Jones M, Yamada I, Crystal RG. In vivo gene transfer and expression in normal uninjured blood vessels using replication-deficient recombinant adenovirus vectors. Circ Res 1993;72:1132–1138.

41a. Steg PG, Feldman LJ, Scoazec JY, Tahlil O, Barry JJ, Bouchlefar S, Ragot T et al. Arterial gene transfer to rabbit endothelial and smooth muscle cells using percutaneous delivery of an adenoviral vector. Circulation 1994;90:1648–1656.

42. Stratford-Perricaudet LD, Makeh I, Perricaudet M, Briand P. Widespread long-term gene transfer to mouse skeletal muscles and heart. J Clin Invest 1992;90:626–630.

43. Willard JE, Landau C, Glamann DB, Burns D, Jessen ME, Pirwitz MJ, Gerard RD et al. Genetic modification of the vessel wall. Comparison of surgical and catheter-based techniques for delivery of recombinant adenovirus. Circulation 1994;89:2190–2197.

44. Kaneda Y, Iwai K, Uchida T. Increased expression of DNA cointroduced with nuclear protein in adult rat liver. Science 1989;243:375–378.

45. Morishita R, Gibbons GH, Kaneda Y, Ogihara T, Dzau VJ. Novel in vitro gene transfer method for study of local modulators in vascular smooth muscle cells. Hypertension 1993;21:894–899.

46. Cotten M, Wagner E, Zatloukal K, Phillips S, Curiel DT, Birnstiel ML. High-efficiency receptor-mediated delivery of small and large (48 kilobase) gene constructs using the endosome-disruption activity of defective or chemically inactivated adenovirus particles. Proc Natl Acad Sci USA 1992;89:6094–6098.

47. Nabel EG, Plautz G, Boyce FM, Stanley JC, Nabel GJ. Recombinant gene expression in vivo within endothelial cells of the arterial wall. Science 1989;244:1342–1344.

48. Plautz G, Nabel EG, Nabel GJ. Introduction of vascular smooth muscle cells expressing recombinant genes in vivo. Circulation 1991;83:578–583.

49. Speir E, Epstein SE. Inhibition of smooth muscle cell proliferation by an antisense oligodeoxynucleotide targeting the messenger RNA encoding proliferating cell nuclear antigen. Circulation 1992;86:538–547.

50. Simons M, Rosenberg RD. Antisense nonmuscle myosin heavy chain and c-myb oligonucleotides suppress smooth muscle cell proliferation in vitro. Circ Res 1992; 70:835–843.

51. Biro S, Fu YM, Yu ZX, Epstein SE. Inhibitory effects of antisense oligodeoxynucleotides targeting c-myc mRNA on smooth muscle cell proliferation and migration. Proc Natl Acad Sci USA 1993;90:654–658.

52. Simons M, Edelman ER, DeKeyser JL, Langer R, Rosenberg RD. Antisense c-myb oligonucleotides inhibit intimal arterial smooth muscle cell accumulation in vivo. Nature 1992;359:67–70.

52a. Edelman ER, Simons M, Sirois MG, Rosenberg RD. C-myc in vasculoproliferative disease. Circ Res 1995; 76:176–182.

53. Morishita R, Gibbons GH, Ellison KE, Nakajima M, Zhang L, Kaneda Y, Ogihara T et al. Single intraluminal delivery of antisense cdc2 kinase and proliferating-cell nuclear antigen oligonucleotides results in chronic inhibition of neointimal hyperplasia. Proc Natl Acad Sci USA 1993; 90:8474–8478.

53a. Shi Y, Fard A, Galeo A, Hutchinson HG, Vermani P, Dodge GR, Hall DJ et al. Transcatheter delivery of c-myc antisense oligomers reduces neointimal formation in a porcine model of coronary artery balloon injury. Circulation 1994; 90:944–951.

54. Spears JR, Serur J, Shropshire D, Paulin S. Fluorescence

55. Dartsch PC, Ischinger T, Betz E. Responses of cultured smooth muscle cells from human nonatherosclerotic arteries and primary stenosing lesions after photoradiation: implications for photodynamic therapy of vascular stenoses. J Am Coll Cardiol 1990;15:1545–1550.

56. Tang G, Hyman S, Schneider JH, Gianotta SL. Application of photodynamic therapy to the treatment of atherosclerotic plaques. Neurosurgery 1993;32:438–443.

57. Asahara T, Usui M, Amemiya T et al. Pathological effects of balloon Xe-Hg flash lamp irradiation as photodynamic therapy for the prevention of restenosis. J Am Coll Cardiol 1993;21:185A (abstract).

58. Reiss GJ, Pomerantz RM, Jenkins RD et al. Laser balloon angioplasty: clinical, angiographic and histologic results. J Am Coll Cardiol 1991;18:193–202.

59. Gonschior P, Erdemci A, Gerheuser F et al. Selective hematoporphyrin derivative (HMD) application in arterial vessels using a porous balloon catheter results in equivalent levels as compared to high-dose systemic administration. Z Kardiol 1991;80:738–745.

60. Ortu P, LaMuraglia GM, Roberts G, Flotte TJ, Hasan T. Photodynamic therapy of arteries. A novel approach for the treatment of experimental intimal hyperplasia. Circulation 1992;85:1189–1196.

61. March KL, Patton BL, Wilensky RL, Hathaway DR. 8-methoxypsoralen and longwave ultraviolet irradiation are a novel antiproliferative combination for vascular smooth muscle. Circulation 1993;87:184–191.

62. Gajdusek CM, Schwartz SM. Comparison of intracellular and extracellular mitogenic activity. J Cell Physiol 1984; 121:316–322.

63. Epstein SE, Siegall CB, Biro S, Fu YM, FitzGerald D, Pastan I. Cytotoxic effects of a recombinant chimeric toxin on rapidly proliferating vascular smooth muscle cells. Circulation 1991;84:778–787.

64. Pickering JG, Bacha P, Weir L, Jekanowski J, Nichols JC, Isner JM. Prevention of smooth muscle cell outgrowth from human atherosclerotic plaque by a recombinant cytotoxin specific for the epidermal growth factor receptor. J Clin Invest 1993;91:724–729.

65. Biro S, Siegall CB, Fu YM, Speir E, Pastan I, Epstein SE. In vitro effects of a recombinant toxin targeted to the fibroblast growth factor receptor on rat vascular smooth muscle and endothelial cells. Circ Res 1992;71:640–645.

66. Casscells W, Lappi DA, Olwin BB et al. Elimination of smooth muscle cells in experimental restenosis: targeting of fibroblast growth factor receptors. Proc Natl Acad Sci USA 1992;89:7159–7163.

67. Miller DD, Paige SB, Tio FO et al. Lymphocyte/monocyte interleukin-2 receptor targeted fusion toxin therapy with DAB486-IL2 prevents proliferative post-angioplasty restenosis. Circulation 1991;84:II-70 (abstract).

68. Pickering JG, Gal D, Bacha P et al. Inhibition of injury-induced intimal thickening in the rat carotid artery by a recombinant cytotoxin specific for the epidermal growth factor receptor. J Am Coll Cardiol 1993;21:178A (abstract).

SECTION V

SUMMARY AND FUTURE DIRECTIONS

41. Summary

DAVID R. HOLMES JR.

The field of interventional cardiology continues to expand. From the initial, highly selected lesions treated by Gruentzig, the technique has evolved and is now used to treat a wide variety of complex lesion subtypes, including calcified lesions, long diffuse disease, vein graft segments, chronic total occlusions, ostial lesions, and highly angulated and bifurcation lesions. From the initial, very limited, rather bulky nonsteerable devices, the equipment available has also evolved and changed dramatically with multiple iterations of competing balloon technology and an ever-increasing number of new "widgets." Interventional cardiologists have become increasingly experienced in assessing complex lesions and deciding on the "optimal" approach. There is more often art than science involved in this process—more often anecdote than well-selected broad observations. Although the field of interventional cardiology is moving toward the concept of device-specific/lesion-specific technology, it is not yet there. One only has to attend one of the multiple invasive cardiology meetings to realize that there are often several approaches to any specific lesion or clinical situation. Sometimes what is used is what is available; at other times, all options are available and an attempt is made to select the one that "fits best," although the definition of "best fit" changes from course to course and year to year. Not all new approaches are effective either on the whole or in the specific patient—sometimes this lack of effectiveness is the result of technical failure, for example, failure to be able to deliver a large bulky device to a distant arterial segment. Sometimes it is the result of factors about which little is known, for example, the interaction in a specific lesion between barotrauma of an inflatable device and the compliance of the segment treated. What is important is to continue the process of determining which approaches work.

It has been the purpose of this book to explore the potential approaches to problematic patient and lesion issues in the arena of interventional cardiology. Such a problem-solving approach facilitates procedures, but does not necessarily guarantee their success. It has been evident that there are a variety of approaches to solving these common problems. Interventional cardiologists will have found that many of these approaches have common bases, although some at least are radically different.

At the end of the day we will all use what has worked in the past. As knowledge accumulates and approaches are tested, we will be able to continue to try to identify specific lesion subsets and select the optimal approach in our own setting for the specific patient at hand.

It is the hope for the future to change Galen's remark from "All who drink of this remedy recover in a short time, except those whom it does not help, who all die. Therefore it is obvious that it only fails in incurable cases," to "All who drink of this remedy recover in a short time, except those whom it does not help in whom we try something else which then works."

Index

Page numbers followed by t and f indicate tables and figures, respectively.